D0336398

Diseases of the Kidney

Diseases of the Kidney

SECOND EDITION

Editors

Maurice B. Strauss, M.D.
Professor of Medicine and Associate Dean,
Tufts University School of Medicine, Boston

Louis G. Welt, M.D.
Alumni Distinguished Professor and Chairman,
Department of Medicine, University of North Carolina
School of Medicine, Chapel Hill

By 59 Authors

Volume II

Little, Brown and Company
Boston

Second Edition

Second Printing

Library of Congress catalog card No. 70-146340

ISBN 0-316-81911

Published in Great Britain
by Churchill/Livingstone, Edinburgh and London

Printed in the United States of America

Slipcase and binding design
by Vincent Ceci

Contents

Volume I

Volume II

Diseases of the Kidney

19

Nephrosclerosis

Solomon Papper and Carlos A. Vaamonde

In its literal sense the term *nephrosclerosis* (hardening of the kidney) might be used with varying exactness to describe the kidneys in several disease states of diverse origin. In its traditional application the term refers to the pathologic processes associated with the following disorders involving the renal vasculature: arteriosclerosis, arteriolar (benign) nephrosclerosis, and the accelerated (malignant) phase of hypertensive disease.

Arteriosclerosis (Atherosclerosis)

Atherosclerosis of the major renal arteries or their main branches is also referred to as arterial nephrosclerosis or senile nephrosclerosis. The latter term seems inappropriate in view of the fact that atherosclerosis is certainly not limited to the aged. For the most part, renal atherosclerosis occurs in association with similar lesions in other vessels throughout the body and is a part of the generalized process of atherosclerosis.

PATHOLOGY

The appearance of the kidney varies considerably, depending largely upon the site and number of narrowed or occluded vessels and the presence or absence of other renal lesions, especially pyelonephritis and arteriolar sclerosis. The latter is commonly found in association with disease of the major arteries, although the causes of these two types of vascular lesions may be quite different.

In the absence of narrowing of the main renal artery or of a significant degree of associated arteriolar sclerosis, the kidneys are generally normal in size. If only a few of the major arterial branches are involved, the kidneys may appear normal except for the presence of scars due to areas of ischemic atrophy. With increasing vascular involvement, the surface of the kidney may appear irregular because of large, depressed, scarred areas separated by smooth portions. If there is also a significant degree of arteriolar nephrosclerosis, the kidney demonstrates the fine granularity associated with that lesion in addition to the coarser irregularity produced by the atherosclerotic lesions. If the main renal artery itself is narrowed significantly, the entire kidney may be decreased uniformly in size and appear pale.

Microscopic examination reveals the same characteristic intimal proliferation of atherosclerosis that is seen in vessels elsewhere in the body. The intima may be disrupted and exhibit plaque formation with narrowing, and even thrombus formation with complete occlusion. The parenchyma distal to the occluded vessel is a wedge-shaped fibrotic area with sclerosis of glomeruli and fibrous replacement of tubules. Further details of the renal pathology may be found elsewhere [1, 11, 45, 65, 141].

CLINICAL FEATURES

It is difficult to determine the precise clinical significance of this variety of renal arteriosclerosis. In a certain number of patients with occlusion of a main renal artery hypertension develops, a situation apparently analogous to the experimental variety of renal hypertension described by Goldblatt [51]. On the other hand, arteriosclerotic stenosis of the main renal artery is often found in normotensive subjects [42, 68]. Aside from instances of renovascular hypertension, however, it is generally believed that renal arteriosclerosis is of little clinical importance and is usually not associated with any abnormality other than minimal proteinuria in some patients [45].

AGING AND RENAL FUNCTION

Shock and his associates [111, 150] have made an extensive study of renal function in relation to aging in persons without clinical evidence of cardiovascular disease. They found that glomerular filtration rate (GFR) and renal plasma flow (RPF) at age 90 were approximately 50 per cent of the normal values at age 20, with the major changes commencing after age 40. (Lewis and Alving [92] have made similar observations with the more commonly employed clinical tests; the mean blood urea nitrogen (BUN) at ages 30 to 40 was 12.9 mg. per 100 ml. and was 21.2 mg. per 100 ml. after age 70.) Shock and his associates also observed that tubular function decreased with age; the tubular maximum for glucose (Tm_G) and concentrating ability were both reduced. More recently, decreased renal function with age has been confirmed. However, the response of the aged kidney to suboptimal doses of vasopressin is not appreciably altered [94]. Shock's group found evidence of normal acid-base equilibrium when patients were resting [150], but they noted that after acidosis was induced with ammonium chloride, recovery was decidedly slower in the aged than in the young individual. Whether or not any of the observed decrease in renal function associated with aging is a result of atrophy secondary to atherosclerosis as distinguished from an intrinsic involutional process is difficult to assess in view of the very high correlation between aging and atherosclerosis.

In summary, it seems that, aside from certain instances of renovascular hypertension, atherosclerosis of the major renal arteries does not lead to serious or symptomatic renal functional alterations. Although present evidence is not entirely adequate, the possibility exists that if the vascular lesions are severe and plentiful, they may contribute to the described decrease in renal function associated with aging, and may make the kidney less able to withstand sudden alterations in acid-base equilibrium or abrupt changes in renal blood flow due to any cause.

Arteriolar (Benign) Nephrosclerosis

Arteriolar nephrosclerosis, also called benign nephrosclerosis, is so intimately associated with essential hypertension that a description of the anatomic features of arteriolar nephrosclerosis is followed by a brief consideration of essential hypertension in general and its relation to this renal lesion.

PATHOLOGY

The pathology of arteriolar nephrosclerosis has been extensively studied [1, 11, 25, 26, 45, 65, 70, 80, 113, 142, 144, 159, 160, 162]. The kidneys may be of normal or slightly reduced weight. In general they are not as small as those observed in the advanced stages of glomerulonephritis or pyelonephritis; however, severe contraction may occur. Indeed, in the end stages of arteriolar nephrosclerosis it may be difficult, if not impossible, in some instances to distinguish, grossly or histologically, this lesion from "primary" renal disease. While characteristically the surface of the kidney has a fine generalized granular appearance frequently likened to that of scotch grain leather, the surface may appear normal if the microscopic lesions are not extensive. This granular appearance is due to the fine areas of atrophy separating normal or hypertrophic areas of the kidney. In addition to fine granularity, there may be the larger and more prominent scars of the associated lesions of atherosclerosis or pyelonephritis.

The histologic appearance of the kidney in arteriolar nephrosclerosis also shows considerable variation in intensity and extent. Although all renal structures may be involved, the arteriolar lesion attracts the most attention. In its earliest diagnosable stage the characteristic abnormality consists of a thickened afferent arteriole, with hyalinization of the arteriolar wall which apparently begins subendothelially (Fig. 19-1). Subsequently, hyalinization involves the media as well, with ultimate narrowing of the lumen. The hyaline lesion may be distributed in patchy fashion along the entire length of the afferent arteriole, but it is especially noted at its proximal end [65]. The efferent arteriole has little if any hyaline change unless there is associated diabetes mellitus [159].

Pathologists continue to show great interest in the possible mechanisms accounting for the development of the hyaline lesion [13, 34, 65, 105, 106, 155]. The hyaline material itself has been considered by some to represent degenerated smooth muscle. Others proposed overproduction of collagen as the explanation. One of the major views has been that the hyaline is a result of degenerated basement membranes. The demonstration of fibrin and other plasma proteins within the hyaline deposit strongly indicates some hematogenous derivation.

Although the stages of evolution of the lesion are not clear, the hypothesis, albeit not proved, of Sommers et al. [159, 162] is of interest. These investigators reported meticulous and extensive observations on kidney tissue collected by biopsy during sympathectomy for hypertension. They view the renal arteriolar lesion as evolving through four stages. There may be significant variation in the distribution and severity of the vascular lesions observed in any one kidney, resulting in a microscopic appearance lacking in uniformity. The first stage is spasm, which they infer from increased concentric overlapping of the smooth muscle cells in the walls of morphologically normal afferent arterioles; they carefully point out the hazards of defining spasm of vessels in fixed tissues. The second stage is thickening of the vessel wall due to edema of the smooth muscle cells; at this stage larger arterioles appear somewhat dilated. The third stage is hypertrophy of the smooth muscle cells. The fourth stage is characterized by hyaline degeneration of the vessel wall.

Besides arteriolar lesions, Sommers et al. [159, 162] have observed unexplained dilatation of renal venules and collecting cortical veins. Of some note is the further observation that the kidney biopsy specimen from patients with benign hypertension may demonstrate fibrinoid necrosis of the afferent arterioles, a lesion sometimes thought to be diagnostic of the malignant phase of the disease [145].

In addition to the vascular lesions of arteriolar nephrosclerosis there are abnormalities of glomeruli, tubules, and interstitial areas that are generally believed to be secondary to the ischemia which results from arteriolar insufficiency.

Many glomeruli are normal, while others show ischemic changes of two types: (1) shrinkage and hypocellularity of the glomerular tuft resulting ultimately in a small eosinophilic area, and (2) the appearance of a

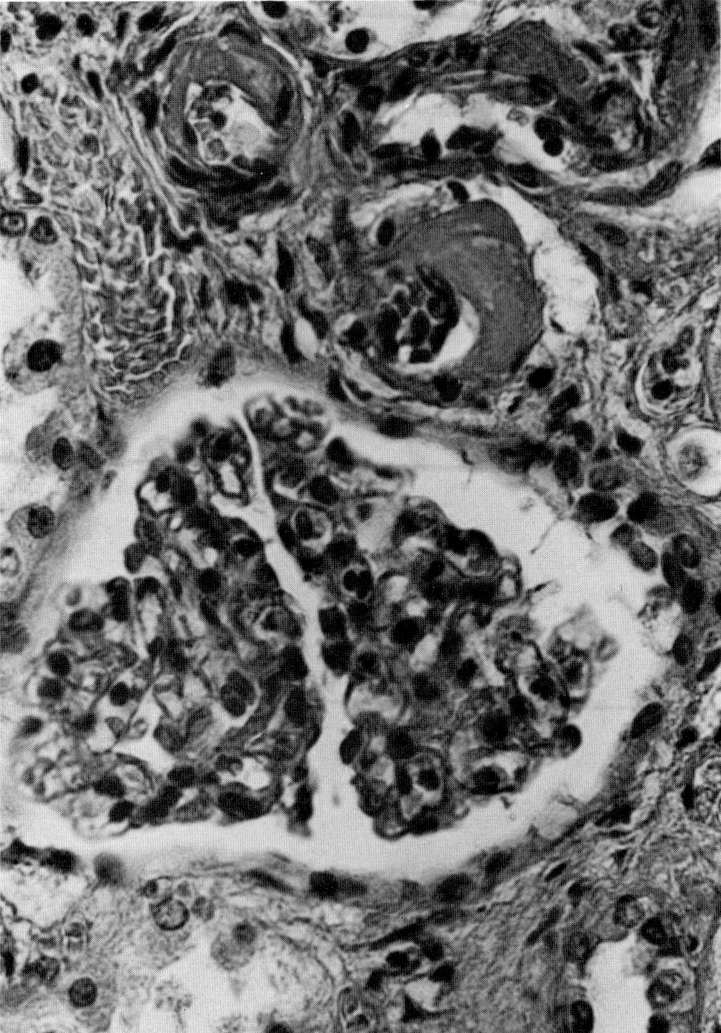

Figure 19-1. Benign arteriolar nephrosclerosis showing arterioles with prominent hyaline thickening in their walls. The glomerulus is not remarkable. Hematoxylin and eosin. ×128.

collagen-like material internal to Bowman's capsule beginning near the hilus and spreading ultimately throughout the glomerulus. Some glomeruli are completely sclerosed.

The earliest evidences of ischemia are probably the cloudy swelling and dilatation of the proximal convoluted tubules, as well as the presence of lymphocytic aggregates in the stroma. Ultimately many tubules become atrophic or may be lost entirely in some areas.

Since the arteriolar lesions develop at an irregular rate and may be focal in distribution, the renal parenchyma may be normal in appearance in certain areas but show complete hyalinization of glomeruli and severe tubular atrophy in others. As the vascular lesions become more widespread and more intense, there are increasing areas of ischemic atrophy and interstitial fibrosis and fewer areas of normal renal tissue.

PATHOGENESIS

For many years investigators have sought to determine the precise relationship between essential hypertension and arteriolar nephrosclerosis. The important question is which comes first, the high blood pressure or the renal lesion.

The possibility that hypertension may be secondary to renal disease was apparently first suggested by Bright [19, 20], who made this prediction without measurement of blood pressure. Subsequently, this relationship has been clearly noted in the common occurrence of hypertension in association with a variety of "primary" renal diseases [45]. Hypertension secondary to unilateral renal artery occlusion (renovascular hypertension) added considerably to the interest in the possibility that a similar mechanism is active in essential hypertension, although surely the argument by analogy alone is hazardous.

The thesis that the blood pressure elevation may be responsible for the renal lesion finds its support in the following observations:

1. Similar arteriolar lesions are found in other organs of the body as well as the kidney, suggesting that the vascular disease is a generalized phenomenon and not a specific renal lesion, although it is more prominent in the kidneys [38, 44].

2. Renal arteriolar sclerosis is observed in a variety of other diseases associated with hypertension, including "primary" renal disease (pyelonephritis, glomerulonephritis, and polycystic disease) and pheochromocytoma [45].

3. While the overwhelming majority of patients with essential hypertension have renal arteriolar sclerosis, Bell and Clawson [12] observed little or none in 10 per cent of their cases. Bell [11] reported that 17.5 per cent of patients with essential hypertension without renal failure had normal renal arterioles and prearterioles. Similarly, Sommers and his associates [162], studying kidney specimens obtained by renal biopsy at sympathectomy, found a small number (less than 2 per cent) of patients with persistent hypertension who did not have a significant degree of renal arteriolar sclerosis.

4. The lesion of renal arteriolar sclerosis may occur in the absence of hypertension. Thus Bell [11] has noted that renal arteriolar sclerosis occurs in 16.5 per cent of people over age 50 who do not have hypertension. Smith [155] found a comparable degree of hyaline arteriosclerosis in kidneys from normotensive subjects and from those with early hypertension. In normotensive subjects, the frequency increased with age, while in hypertensive patients the frequency and severity of the lesion increased with chronicity. Fisher et al. [46], in electron microscopic studies, found ultrastructural foci of hyalinization in normal arterioles.

5. Patients with hypertension elsewhere, as in the lesser circuit, similarly develop vascular disease of the pulmonary bed [114].

6. Patients early in the course of essential hypertension may have normal total renal blood flow and no functional evidence of ischemia [6, 27].

7. There are data to indicate that there may be an inverse relationship between renal function and the height of the blood pressure, although this relationship is not precise [115–117].

On the other hand, there is evidence that is consistent with the view that the hypertension is secondary to renal arteriolar sclerosis. In some instances the substantiating data are the same as those summarized above, differently interpreted:

1. It may be emphasized that arteriolar sclerosis in patients with hypertension is far more common in the kidney than elsewhere [45]. If arteriolar sclerosis is to be regarded as a generalized lesion secondary to hypertension, its unusual predilection for the kidney must be accounted for.

2. The fact that the same vascular lesion is encountered in other renal disease may indicate that a variety of conditions may result in arteriolar nephrosclerosis.

3. The observation that arteriolar nephrosclerosis of significant degree is not found in

a certain number of renal-biopsy [159, 162] and postmortem [11, 12] specimens does not preclude the possible role of arteriolar insufficiency and ischemia. In fact, Sommers et al. [159, 162] believed that all but one of the kidneys without evidence of arteriolar sclerosis in their series showed spasm which might have accounted for the findings consistent with ischemia.

4. The fact that mild renal arteriolar sclerosis occurs in some people over the age of 50 in the absence of hypertension may be interpreted to indicate that the lesion in these instances was not sufficiently severe or lasting to have produced hypertension.

5. Goldblatt [52] implies that there is no proof that the pulmonary arterial sclerosis associated with pulmonary hypertension is a direct result of the elevated blood pressure per se. Rather, the vascular lesion may be due to some other concomitant of the disease state which results in pulmonary hypertension.

6. Work by Baldwin and his associates [6] and Chasis and Baldwin [27] revealed a striking disparity in certain measures of renal function in the two kidneys of patients with hypertensive disease. One interpretation of this finding is that the disparity may be due to differences in the degree of renal ischemia in the two kidneys, a situation that is consistent with a primary role for the kidney in essential hypertension. Thus normal total renal blood flow in the presence of hypertension cannot necessarily be assumed to be evidence that there is no underlying renal functional disturbance. This aspect is more thoroughly considered by Chasis and Baldwin [27], who, after pointing out that the anatomic approach cannot clearly discriminate between primary and secondary vascular changes, emphasize that the observed functional alterations early in essential hypertension "favor a primary renal mechanism." This is discussed more fully below.

7. The reported general inverse relationship between renal function and the height of the blood pressure may indicate that the two variables have a common cause without bearing a causal relationship to each other. If one accepts the possibility that abnormalities in renal function may go undetected early in hypertension, or that abnormalities may be expressed as a disparity in the contribution to renal function made by each kidney, then a causal relationship may exist in the direction of abnormal renal function producing hypertension.

One may consider the available data and interpret the relationship of hypertension to renal arteriolar sclerosis in a more complex fashion than acceptance of a simple primary role for one and secondary role for the other. One view may be that hypertension due to any cause can result in renal arteriolar sclerosis and that the latter, if severe enough or of long enough duration (or both), may serve to aggravate or sustain the elevation of blood pressure. Another approach is that high blood pressure and renal arteriolar sclerosis are independent processes that may serve to intensify each other. Thus, on the one hand, the hypertensive process may damage the vessel wall, with resultant acceleration of renal arteriolar sclerosis; on the other hand, the renal vascular process may produce certain changes in the kidney, perhaps associated with ischemia, which serve to promote, aggravate, or sustain the elevated blood pressure. Conceptual formulations such as these allow a reconciliation of many of the confusing observations already discussed, although reconciliation per se does not constitute evidence or proof of the correctness of such interpretations. These approaches also give greater importance to the observations that hypertension may persist even after a known cause (e.g., pheochromocytoma, coarctation of the aorta, Cushing's syndrome) has been corrected. Among explanations offered for this phenomenon has been the possibility that the prolonged elevation of blood pressure results in renal arteriolar sclerosis which in turn is responsible for the continued elevation of blood pressure.

While the issue of the precise relationship

between arteriolar nephrosclerosis and essential hypertension remains undecided, it is probably reasonable to state that the majority of present investigators favor a primacy of hypertension in the production of the renal arteriolar lesion. It is now commonly held that hyaline arteriosclerosis is associated with aging in the normal subject and that hypertension accelerates the development of the lesion. This does not exclude the possibility that subsequent development of arteriolar nephrosclerosis in and of itself may play a role in sustaining or even aggravating the elevated blood pressure. That some relationship exists between arteriolar nephrosclerosis and hypertension seems clear from the fact that the kidneys of most patients with hypertension who are studied have some stage of the renal vascular lesion, and from the suggestive evidence that in a general way the elevation of blood pressure correlates with the degree of renal arteriolar involvement. However, one may see hypertension without apparent arteriolar sclerosis and vice versa, indicating that the relationship is not likely to be simple and direct. Reasonable argument has been made also for the primacy of renal arteriolar sclerosis, but final proof is not yet available.

In the course of the continuing controversy over the exact relationship between arteriolar nephrosclerosis and essential hypertension, certain other concepts relating the role of renal circulatory factors to the development of essential hypertension have evolved. Thus, Evans [40], in performing rather extensive and meticulous studies on the major arteries of the kidney, has advanced the thesis that the basic disturbance in essential hypertension is a congenital hypoplasia of the muscle in the media of the renal artery. He has further hypothesized that this hypoplasia is accompanied by a proliferation of the intima which narrows the lumen, producing renal ischemia, which in turn results in hypertension. Others [36], however, believe that the arterial abnormalities described by Evans are more likely to be the result, rather than the cause, of high blood pressure.

Another approach to renal circulatory factors in hypertension was taken by Ljungqvist [98], who combined histologic and stereomicroangiographic studies of the kidneys of 15 patients with benign nephrosclerosis. He found cortical ischemia which he attributed to degenerated arterioglomerular units in the cortex. These anatomic studies also suggested that the decreased cortical flow may have been accompanied by increased medullary perfusion. Recently, Hollenberg and associates [67a] have shown arteriographic abnormalities in the distal interlobar and arcuate arteries of patients with essential hypertension. The degree of the vascular lesions correlated with renal hemodynamic abnormalities, age of the patients, and with the duration, severity, and presence of complications of hypertension.

In addition to the specific question of which comes first, renal arteriolar sclerosis or essential hypertension, at least brief consideration must be given to several renal mechanisms (perhaps related to arteriolar disease) that have been proposed as having some causal role in the development of hypertension.

A variety of experimental observations point to the possibility that the kidney may elaborate a substance or substances that ultimately produce an elevation of blood pressure. In this regard the renin-angiotensin-aldosterone system has received considerable attention. A variety of observations indicate that the juxtaglomerular (JG) cells found in the wall of the afferent arteriole near the glomerulus are the source of renin, and that the latter is produced in response to altered renal perfusion [173, 174]. Although reduced renal arterial pressure will result in increased granules in the juxtaglomerular cells, it is not clear that pressure changes per se, as distinguished from other circulatory changes, are required to stimulate renin secretion. Renin reacts with a plasma globulin (hypertensinogen) to produce angiotensin, a substance with vasoconstrictor properties [17, 51, 122, 166]. In addition, angiotensin stimulates the adrenal cortical secretion of aldosterone. It is very difficult to interpret the role of the renin-angiotensin-aldosterone system in the genesis of human essential hypertension [123, 167]. Genest et al. [49, 50] have shown that the average blood angiotensin level is above normal in essential hypertension; however, 50 per cent of these hypertensive persons have no detectable angiotensin in the blood. These authors interpret their findings to indicate that maintenance of hypertension is not caused by elevated angiotensin levels. Such observations do not preclude an initiating role of angiotensin. Laragh [86] has found normal or low serum levels of aldosterone and renin in patients with essential hypertension. On theoretical grounds Laragh [86] postulates that there might be a small increase in angiotensin early in essential hypertension which is no longer present because of adjustments related to feedback mechanisms and altered vascular reactivity. In addition, others have found elevated renin secretion rates in patients with essential hypertension who have moderately severe small renal artery disease and reduced renal blood flow, while patients with uncomplicated essential hypertension had low renin secretion rates [67a, 67b]. Relatively little help is obtained from anatomic observations indicating that patients with essential hypertension may have enlargement of the juxtaglomerular cells [161, 162] because so many variables, in particular those related to sodium metabolism, influence these findings. Therefore, for the present one must conclude that the role of the juxtaglomerular apparatus and the renin-angiotensin-aldosterone system in the development of essential hypertension is not known.

Other pressor substances originating in the kidney have also been implicated from time to time without proof. Excellent studies by Shorr and his group [151, 152] have suggested a possible role for a substance called vasoexcitor material (VEM), which originates in the kidney and is capable of increasing vascular constrictor responsiveness to epinephrine. These investigators have demonstrated a relative excess of this material in the blood of animals with hypertension due to renal artery occlusion, as well as in the blood of patients with essential hypertension. There is no firm or conclusive evidence, however, that any of these substances plays any role in the pathogenesis of essential hypertension in man [16, 17, 168].

The kidney has been related to the development of hypertension in experiments in which hypertension develops following bilateral nephrectomy [58, 85]. On the basis of these studies, it has been postulated that the kidney either produces an antihypertensive agent or inactivates a hypertensive substance. Thus, under circumstances in which hypertension exists, there may be a deficiency of renal depressor activity rather than an excess of a pressor material of renal origin. The prostaglandins, a group of unsaturated cyclic fatty acids found in the renal medulla, have been demonstrated to have antihypertensive properties [90]. Whether the prostaglandins have any relevance to essential hypertension is entirely unknown.

While the precise relationship of pyelonephritis to the development of essential hypertension is not known, it is clear that an appreciable number (12 to 25 per cent) of patients with hypertension have histologic evidence of pyelonephritis [83, 159, 162, 183]. Furthermore, it is known that hypertension may result from unilateral or bilateral pyelonephritis [83]. Finally, a damaged kidney (perhaps one with arteriolar nephrosclerosis) may be more susceptible to bacterial invasion [143]. Shapiro [149] surmises from experiments in rats that pyelonephritis per se does not result in hypertension. Rather, he suggests that pyelonephritis makes the individual more prone to hypertensive disease, aggravates existing hypertension, and indicates that the hypertensive kidney is predisposed to develop pyelonephritis. More extensive epidemiologic studies are required to define further the relationship between pyelonephritis, arteriolar nephrosclerosis, and essential hypertension [77].

CLINICAL COURSE

Because of the close relationship of arteriolar nephrosclerosis to essential hypertension, certain broad clinical aspects of essential hypertension, with particular reference to the kidney, are briefly considered. Several comprehensive articles and books provide a more thorough exposition of essential hypertension [2, 53, 69, 121, 138, 139, 154].

Any study of the natural history of essential hypertension is made extremely difficult by virtue of the following factors: In the first place, there is no assurance that all hypertensive disease otherwise unexplained is due to one process, and therefore all cases of it may justifiably be studied as a group. Second, there is considerable discussion concerning the definition of high blood pressure itself; long-term observation of patients with intermittent hypertension makes it clear that there is considerable variation in the development of vascular "complications" [9, 28, 39, 53, 57, 69, 89, 91, 125, 130, 131, 138, 154]. This diversity may reflect great variation in the course of a single disease process in different individuals, or it may be due to a fundamental lack of homogeneity in the original group of patients studied. Finally, there are relatively few detailed long-term follow-up studies of untreated patients with elevated blood pressure [181, 182].

The studies of Perera [130] are of particular value and emphasize that most patients are less than 50 years old when their blood pressure becomes elevated. They may be expected to live approximately 20 years from the onset of increased blood pressure. In general, 15 of these years, although interspersed with vague symptoms of nervousness, headache, dizziness, and palpitation in some patients, are characterized by an absence of vascular "complications" involving the heart, brain, or kidneys. Thereafter, for the five years prior to death, there is evidence of a variable degree of organ involvement. A very small proportion of patients (variously estimated at from 1 to 8 per cent), either at the beginning of their course or at some time during it, enter the accelerated phase of the disease (discussed below) which, if untreated, is generally fatal in one to two years [53, 82, 112, 133, 146]. This is the overall view of the course of the disease, but the enormous individual variation from patient to patient cannot be overemphasized. Some have high blood pressure for months, with a rapid and extensive organ deterioration, while others have hypertension for more than 20 years without serious or clinically significant complications [10, 18, 102].

Although most patients with essential hypertension have anatomic lesions of the kidney and a large number — probably most patients with established hypertension — have demonstrable renal functional abnormalities, only a relatively small proportion of patients with essential hypertension have serious renal functional impairment or die directly as a result of renal insufficiency. The statistics on this point vary somewhat, depending upon definition, case selection, and follow-up period, but the proportion is seldom given as greater than 10 per cent [53, 69, 130, 154]. Only a small number of these patients (1 per cent of all patients with essential hypertension) are thought to die of chronic progressive renal disease clinically similar in its course to "primary" renal disease, such as pyelonephritis or glomerulonephritis [53]. Most patients with essential hypertension who die in uremia do so as the result of an acute accelerated course of renal failure included in the syndrome known as malignant hypertension. Perera [130] estimates that in addition to those deaths *due* to the complications of renal failure, in a further 10 per cent of deaths among patients with essential hypertension, renal insufficiency is a contributory factor.

The development of sustained azotemia is probably the most meaningful prognostic sign in essential hypertension according to Hagans and Brust [60]. In their last patients, death occurred within three months of the deterioration of renal function to the point of sustained azotemia. Whether or not their data agree precisely with the observations of others, they certainly support the view that sustained renal failure in essential hypertension is an ominous sign.

RENAL FUNCTION

Urinalysis in the absence of renal failure may give normal results, or there may be a slight degree of proteinuria with a few hyaline and granular casts [45, 69]. In general, significantly increased numbers of white blood cells and red blood cells are not noted in the urine under these circumstances.

Many observations and reports in the literature [6] indicate that "early" in the course of essential hypertension the results of detailed renal function tests may be within normal limits. However, some evidence indicates that overall function may be normal in the presence of abnormal variations in the discrete functions of the two kidneys. This latter observation is debated.

The initial detailed work on the subject was reported in 1941 by Goldring and Chasis and their associates [53, 55], who have continued their interest and excellent research in this area over the ensuing years. Their data, confirmed by those of other investigators, indicate that the earliest impairment in overall renal function is a decrease in the tubular maximum for para-aminohippurate (Tm_{PAH}), probably a measure of functional tubular tissue. This is almost always associated with a reduction in renal plasma flow (RPF), although the glomerular filtration rate (GFR) may remain normal in the early stages. Thus, the filtration fraction (FF) — that is, that proportion of the renal plasma flow which is filtered by the glomeruli per unit time (GFR/RPF) — is generally increased. In addition to the elevated FF and increased ratio of GFR to Tm_{PAH}, there is characteristically a relative reduction of renal blood flow to functional tubular mass (RPF/Tm_{PAH}) in essential hypertension. These observations were interpreted to indicate an increase in efferent arteriolar resistance, the formation of "impotent" tubules, and renal ischemia of the residual functioning renal tissue.

More recently Lowenstein et al. [96], employing dye-dilution technics, studied the distribution of intrarenal blood flow in 12 patients with essential hypertension and in eight normotensive subjects. The results suggest that blood flow is reduced uniformly throughout the renal vascular bed, although the technic employed may not permit this conclusion with complete certainty. Indeed, more recent studies of intrarenal hemodynamics with the ^{133}Xe washout technic suggest a decrease in cortical renal blood flow out of proportion to the reduction in other parts of the kidney [67a]. No matter how the observed functional changes are interpreted, however, it is clear that the altered function is not entirely due to altered structure.

Thus, the kidney in a patient with the characteristic alterations of arteriolar nephrosclerosis and essential hypertension is capable of acute change in function under certain experimental circumstances. The administration of pyrogen to most patients with hypertension results in an increase in RPF and hyperemia (increased RPF/Tm_{PAH}) very similar to the effects in a normotensive individual [53, 55, 56]. Similarly, the administration of epinephrine results in a reduction in renal blood flow without apparent alteration of the intrarenal distribution of blood in normotensive and hypertensive subjects [96].

As indicated above, in their earlier reports Goldring and Chasis [53] stated the possibility that hypertensive patients may be suffering from renal ischemia due to functional efferent arteriolar constriction (despite the anatomic lesions in the afferent arteriole) secondary to some humoral factor. At present, whether or

trol group. Other similar observations are recorded in the proceedings of an international symposium on antihypertensive therapy [59].

Magee et al. [100], participants in the Veterans Administration Cooperative Study of Antihypertensive Agents, have approached the problem directly. Patients with essential hypertension had detailed assessment of renal function annually for three to five years, during which time some received placebos while others received antihypertensive drugs. In this period of study, inulin and para-aminohippurate clearances were no different in the patients without change in blood pressure, as compared with those in patients whose blood pressure decreased. Similar results were obtained by Reubi [141] in a group of 56 patients with grade 1 or 2 ocular fundi followed one to five years with and without treatment. In a series of patients with diastolic blood pressure under 130 mm. Hg, Moyer et al. [116, 117] found no difference in renal function after mean follow-up periods of approximately 28 months, between the 14 treated and 8 untreated patients. Although detailed studies of renal function were not reported in the Veterans Administration Cooperative Study of Antihypertive Agents, it is noteworthy that 6 of 264 placebo-treated hypertensive patients had evidence of renal damage while none of 259 drug-treated patients did [181, 182].

In some instances, support for the beneficial effects of antihypertensive treatment in the prevention or amelioration of benign nephrosclerosis is sought from data indicating that reduction in blood pressure in the malignant phase inhibits the rapidly lethal deterioration of renal function that characterizes this syndrome. Such observations are not necessarily relevant to the situation prevailing in the benign phase. The mechanisms producing the two renal lesions and the impaired renal function may be quite different in the two phases.

Having enumerated some of the possible advantages of blood pressure reduction in patients with arteriolar nephrosclerosis, one must mention a possible disadvantage of prescribing medication that reduces blood pressure. There is reason to believe that a reduction in blood pressure in a patient who already has impairment in renal function may result in further deterioration of renal function [35, 59, 69, 147]; however, such an adverse effect is not invariable or inevitable [147].

In the relatively few patients in whom serious renal insufficiency develops in the course of arteriolar nephrosclerosis in the benign phase of the disease, the treatment is that of chronic renal failure in general as described in earlier chapters. It should be added, however, that if lowering of the blood pressure is undertaken, it must be done with considerable caution. In the presence of congestive heart failure, the decreased pressure may well result in improvement in the circulatory status, which in turn may result in improvement in renal function. However, in the absence of congestive heart failure, reduction of blood pressure in the patient with renal failure due to arteriolar nephrosclerosis bears the hazard of causing further deterioration in renal function.

In summary, there is relatively little incontrovertible evidence that reduction in blood pressure either prevents the development of arteriolar nephrosclerosis or arrests its rate of progression once it is present. There is a body of evidence (considered above), however, which is consistent with the possibility that elevated blood pressure itself may be a factor in the production of arteriolar nephrosclerosis. Treatment of hypertension must be considered in relation not only to the associated nephrosclerosis but also to other features of the disease, especially cardiovascular and cerebrovascular involvement. A strong case has been presented for the view that a reduction in blood pressure may minimize, or indeed obviate, some of the cardiac and cerebrovascular problems associated with hypertension [69, 115, 181, 182]. The data in this regard may be more impressive than those on the relation of blood pressure to the renal lesion. Two brief summaries of somewhat divergent interpretations of the data by outstanding authorities in the field are of interest in this regard [54, 127]. Perhaps the majority of workers in the field regard the presently available evidence as favoring lowering the blood pressure in patients with unequivocal evidence of persistent hypertension. Some would also treat patients with intermittent hypertension.

Malignant Nephrosclerosis

Arteriolar nephrosclerosis has been described as it generally occurs: a process characterized by a gradual and often imperceptible decrease in renal function, the lesion only infrequently being severe enough to cause the clinical picture of renal failure. In fact, slow progressive renal failure due to arteriolar nephrosclerosis probably accounts for death in uremia in not more than 1 per cent of the hypertensive population. In contradistinction to this condition is malignant nephrosclerosis, a process characterized by rapid deterioration of renal function.

The term *malignant nephrosclerosis* is sometimes used interchangeably with malignant hypertension, but this is probably not entirely proper. Although both terms may be subject to criticism, they are in common usage and therefore require further consideration. There is confusion concerning the definition of malignant hypertension, although virtually all definitions are basically clinical in nature. Thus, some workers have considered papilledema in a patient with high blood pressure as the sole criterion for the diagnosis, while others have defined the term on the basis of the level of the diastolic blood pressure alone. Most students of this disease consider malignant hypertension to be a much broader term than malignant nephrosclerosis, the former describing a clinical situation characterized by an acute and, if untreated, almost invariably fatal form of hypertensive disease. In general, this rapid deterioration is associated with papilledema, progressive renal failure, and cardiac and central nervous system manifestations. As a rule, but not invariably, this clinical syndrome has as one of its important anatomic counterparts a histologic lesion called malignant nephrosclerosis. Some patients, however, have a rapidly progressive course of the disease characterized by papilledema or cerebrovascular deterioration (or both) without uremia and without the histologic features of malignant nephrosclerosis. On the other hand, a certain number of patients (5 per cent, Kincaid-Smith et al. [82]; 16 per cent, Goldring and Chasis [53]) have a similarly fulminating clinical course with uremia and malignant nephrosclerosis but without papilledema.

The term *malignant hypertension* in this chapter refers to a clinical syndrome generally featured by papilledema and the development of uremia, although a similarly rapid clinical deterioration may occur with only one present; the term *malignant nephrosclerosis* is used to indicate a specific histologic lesion that is seen in most patients with the clinical course we have defined as malignant hypertension. Patients with a similar clinical picture but without uremia usually do not have the same histologic lesion. A term that has been proposed to describe cases in which renal failure is prominent — the accelerated renal phase of hypertensive disease — is perhaps preferable to either malignant hypertension or malignant nephrosclerosis.

INCIDENCE

The incidence of malignant nephrosclerosis in the course of benign arteriolar nephrosclerosis is not clearly established. Obviously an accurate estimate would be difficult to derive in view of the problems of definition and case selection. Nonetheless, there are a few appraisals that suggest an order of magnitude. Perera's data [130] and those of Goldring and Chasis [53] indicate that malignant nephrosclerosis develops in 6 and 8 per cent, respectively, of patients with essential hypertension. Kincaid-Smith et al. [82] thought that figures of this magnitude were due to selection of cases demanding specialized care; their data, which are related to certain assumptions regarding the general incidence of hypertension, give a figure close to 1 per cent. Bechgaard [10] similarly stated that the malignant course develops in 1 per cent of patients with the benign phase.

Although arteriolar nephrosclerosis is the most common background for the development of malignant nephrosclerosis, a clinical and histologic picture apparently identical with that of malignant nephrosclerosis may be superimposed upon a variety of diseases associated with hypertension — for example, glomerulonephritis, pyelonephritis, renovascular disease, and polycystic renal disease. Interestingly, malignant nephrosclerosis and malignant hypertension may develop de novo — that is, without prior hypertension [45, 133, 137]. Although McMichael [107] has properly pointed out how difficult it is to be certain that a patient with malignant nephrosclerosis has had no prior hypertension, we believe that there is reasonable evidence that such a condition exists. In the very interesting study of Kincaid-Smith et al. [82] of patients with the clinical syndrome of malignant hypertension, histologic material was available for precise diagnosis in 124 cases. Approximately 40 per cent of these patients had arteriolar nephrosclerosis as the underlying lesion, approximately 21 per cent had chronic pyelonephritis, and 15 per cent had chronic glomerulonephritis; in the rest, polyarteritis nodosa, unilateral renal artery obstruction, postpartum malignant hypertension, radiation nephritis, congenital renal disease, hydronephrosis, Cushing's syndrome, nephrocalcinosis, scleroderma, and tuberculous pyelonephritis were the underlying lesions. Similar findings had previously been described in 51 cases reported by Heptinstall [63].

PATHOLOGY

It is apparent from the foregoing discussion that in addition to the diagnostic renal features of malignant nephrosclerosis, pathologic examination will usually reveal evidence of underlying renal disease, such as arteriolar nephrosclerosis, pyelonephritis, or glomerulonephritis. Thus, the size of the kidney and whether it has the granularity of arteriolar nephrosclerosis or the large scars of pyelonephritis or other renal lesions will be determined primarily by the underlying renal disease rather than by the process of malignant nephrosclerosis.

In those instances in which malignant nephrosclerosis has apparently developed de novo, the kidneys are normal in size. In any case, in addition to some congestive mottling which may be present on gross inspection, the diagnostic feature is the presence of small petechiae, especially in the cortex, which are due to arteriolar rupture. In some instances of malignant nephrosclerosis, petechiae are not seen on gross inspection; and there is no indication whatever that the characteristic microscopic lesions of malignant nephrosclerosis will be found.

The histologic appearance of the kidney in malignant nephrosclerosis, which has been extensively reviewed by numerous writers [1, 11, 45, 65, 80, 138, 142, 160, 161], presents three major changes: (1) proliferative endarteritis, (2) necrotizing arteriolitis, and (3) necrotizing glomerulitis. While many outstanding investigators [65] regard necrotizing arteriolitis as the hallmark of malignant nephrosclerosis, Kincaid-Smith et al. [82] and Robbins [142] are of the opinion that the proliferative endarteritis is the most specific lesion. In any case both lesions are most striking and commonly seen in malignant nephrosclerosis.

Proliferative endarteritis occurs in the afferent arterioles and small interlobular arteries and produces an appearance sometimes referred to as "onion peel" or "onion skin" (Fig. 19-2). It is generally believed that this pro-

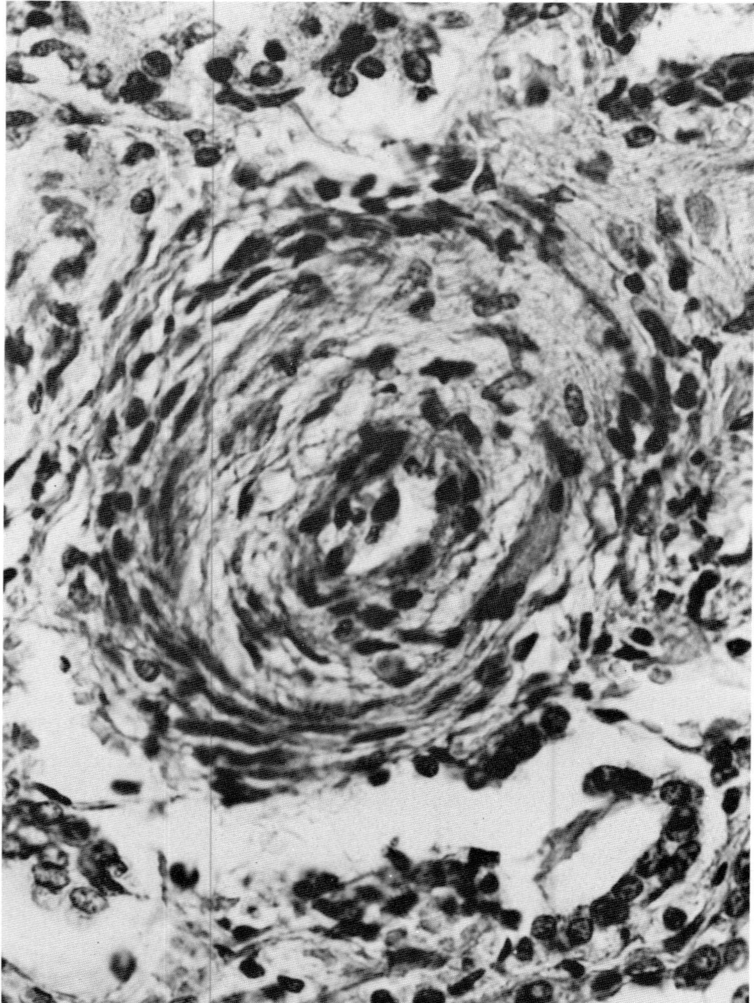

Figure 19-2. Malignant arteriolar nephrosclerosis showing prominent endothelial proliferation (onion skinning) of small artery. Hematoxylin and eosin. ×128.

liferation is one of fibroblasts derived from subendothelial connective tissue. This thickening can apparently develop with great rapidity and produce narrowing of the lumina of the vessels which in turn results in parenchymal change distal to the narrowed vessels. Ljungqvist [98], employing microangiographic technics, has demonstrated extensive narrowing and obliteration of the vascular lumen by this process. This obliterative lesion is probably primarily responsible for the severe renal ischemia. The degree of ischemic changes, including tubular atrophy, varies with the underlying disease and the duration of the malignant phase.

Necrotizing arteriolitis is found in the afferent arterioles and is characterized by deposition of fibrinoid material and polymorphonuclear cells in the arteriolar wall (Fig. 19-3). Often thromboses are present in the lumina of the vessels; these vessels are often ruptured, producing small hemorrhages into the tubular structures or the stroma of the kidney. These are the hemorrhagic lesions often seen on gross

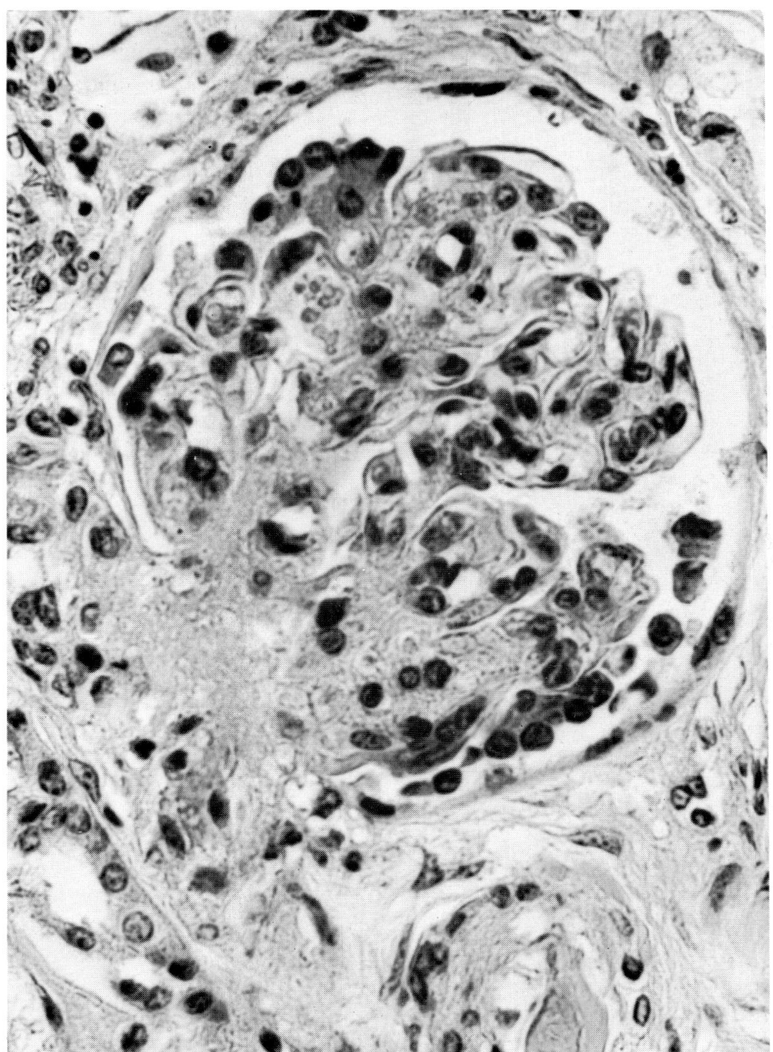

Figure 19-3. Malignant arteriolar nephrosclerosis with necrotizing arteriolitis and focal necrotizing glomerulitis. Hematoxylin and eosin. ×128.

inspection as petechiae. Saltz et al. [145] have observed the same lesion in biopsy specimens from patients undergoing sympathectomy for a disease process which had none of the clinical evidences of malignant hypertension and no other pathologic features of malignant nephrosclerosis, suggesting that the lesion may not be pathognomonic of malignant nephrosclerosis.

The third lesion noted in malignant nephrosclerosis is glomerulitis with necrosis (Fig. 19-3). This was originally thought to represent an inflammatory process similar perhaps to glomerulonephritis. Glomerular necrosis, however, bears a strong relationship to the necrotizing arteriolitis of the afferent arterioles — in fact, the glomeruli involved are usually immediately distal to afferent arterioles demonstrating necrotizing arteriolitis. These glomeruli are characterized by precipitation of fibrinoid material within the tuft with some infiltration of polymorphonuclear leukocytes.

Generally, that portion of the glomerulus adjacent to the afferent arterioles is most involved; and in some sections, it is quite clear that the observed necrosis is a direct extension of a similar process in the arteriole (Fig. 19-3). These glomerular changes may progress to cellular proliferation, giving an appearance similar to the chronic lesions of glomerulonephritis. However, in the latter condition the lesions are widespread, whereas the glomerular lesions seen in association with malignant nephrosclerosis are irregular in their distribution and rarely involve more than one-third of all the glomeruli.

In addition to the three lesions characteristic of malignant nephrosclerosis (i.e., proliferative endarteritis, necrotizing arteriolitis, and glomerular necrosis), in most instances the features diagnostic of benign arteriolar nephrosclerosis will be found. In other cases, as indicated above, there will be definite evidence of chronic glomerulonephritis, pyelonephritis, and other varieties of renal disease which also predispose to the development of malignant nephrosclerosis pathologically and an accelerated clinical course.

In the course of malignant nephrosclerosis, arteriolar necrosis and proliferative endarteritis may occur in other organs, such as the gastrointestinal tract, the liver, and the pancreas, although it is apparent that the vascular lesion is rarely widespread in organs other than the kidney. On occasion, however, the arteriolar lesion has resulted in ischemia in organs, producing areas of infarction.

PATHOGENESIS

The pathogenesis of these lesions is not conclusively established, although many students of this condition [45, 65, 138, 139] are of the opinion that the high level of blood pressure in itself is responsible for the characteristic abnormalities observed in malignant nephrosclerosis. There is indeed an impressive body of evidence, both clinical and experimental, to support this contention. In the first place, a variety of renal disorders having diverse causes but all sharing elevated blood pressure as a prominent feature of the clinical picture may be associated with the changes we have characterized as malignant nephrosclerosis. Second, the patients in whom this condition develops generally have extremely high levels of diastolic blood pressure. In Heptinstall's series, vascular necrosis correlated with the level of blood pressure [64]. Severe hypertension produced by marked renal artery constriction results in arteriolar necrosis and intimal thickening in many blood vessels of the body, sparing the kidney, the organ protected from the high blood pressure by virtue of the presence of the constricting clamp. Similarly, Wilson and Byrom [184, 185] produced hypertension in rats by partial constriction of a renal artery. This was followed by arteriolar necrosis, glomerulitis, and intimal proliferation in the contralateral kidney but not in the clamped one — findings again consistent with the role of high blood pressure itself in the development of these lesions. Necrotizing lesions in the pulmonary arterial tree have also been observed in instances of pulmonary hypertension of diverse cause [165]. Finally, the work of Pickering et al. [140] demonstrates that lowering the blood pressure experimentally may result in subsidence of the necrotic lesion of the arterioles, while McCormack et al. [103] have made similar observations in man with malignant nephrosclerosis.

Although these data supporting an important role for hypertension itself in the development of malignant nephrosclerosis are quite impressive, other observations suggest that elevation of blood pressure in and of itself may not account completely for the pathogenesis of malignant nephrosclerosis. First, Kincaid-Smith et al. [82] compared blood pressure in a carefully matched series of patients suffering from malignant nephrosclerosis with that in a series of patients demonstrating the features of benign nephrosclerosis, and were unable to find any striking difference in the two groups.

Second, Perera [129] has presented six patients in whom retinopathy and papilledema developed at a time when their blood pressures were actually normal. Similarly, papilledema has been observed to regress while blood pressure remained elevated. Third, Bali and Goldblatt [7] observed that following the clamping of a renal artery, arteriolitis in the dog occurred only in the presence of renal failure. This suggested the possible causative importance of a toxic factor. Muirhead et al. [118, 119] noted necrotizing arteriolitis in dogs that had undergone bilateral nephrectomy and did not have hypertension.

Exploration of the possibility that some factor associated with the development of uremia has a role in the development of arteriolitis is a difficult problem. Fleming [47] produced acute arteriolitis in rabbits that developed uremia following renal artery clamping and contralateral nephrectomy. Despite comparable blood pressure elevation, those animals not developing uremia did not demonstrate any acute lesions of the arteries similar to those of malignant nephrosclerosis. (On the other hand, Fasciolo and Cramer [43] found arteriolar lesions occurring in the presence of a normal blood urea concentration in experimentally induced hypertension.)

Clinical evidence presented by Perera and his associates [133, 135, 136] is relevant to this problem. That an additional mechanism other than the rapidly increased blood pressure may be involved received some support from their careful studies, in which the data suggest that patients with accelerated hypertension have clinical characteristics that differ from those of patients with essential or benign nephrosclerosis, and to some extent set them apart from such persons. First, it has been documented that malignant hypertension has developed in patients known to have been normotensive within a month of the onset of the clinical manifestations of the accelerated phase. Second, the preponderance of male patients in Perera's series represents a distinct reversal of the statistical incidence in patients with benign arteriolar nephrosclerosis. Kincaid-Smith et al. [82], who noted the same sex distribution differences in their series, attributed them to a difference in the course of the disease in patients over 50 years of age. They interpreted the divergence simply as confirmation of the fact that the disease is more benign in women of this age group. In Perera's series as well as in Kincaid-Smith's series, the age distribution curves of patients with malignant nephrosclerosis and of those with essential hypertension are quite dissimilar. Perera's data also indicated that women with malignant hypertension had significantly different body build than women with benign essential hypertension. In addition, blood group A was rare in Negro women with malignant nephrosclerosis. Unexplained weight loss and an elevated erythrocyte sedimentation rate in their patients with malignant hypertension are interesting general findings reported by Kincaid-Smith et al. and Perera which are not noted in patients with benign nephrosclerosis. Finally, patients with malignant hypertension seem to benefit from sympathectomy whether or not the blood pressure has been reduced following surgery [133]. It is clearly pointed out by Perera that this kind of information does not necessarily prove that factors other than blood pressure elevation play a role in the development of malignant hypertension. However, these data require explanation, which at present cannot be found simply in an acute elevation of blood pressure. It may be that the changes of malignant nephrosclerosis result from other factors that are most readily operative in the presence of hypertension although not a direct result of it.

There is evidence indicating increased production of renin, angiotensin, and aldosterone in malignant nephrosclerosis, presumably due to the many areas of renal ischemia secondary to the vascular lesions [49, 50, 67b, 86, 88, 123]. The precise relationship of this increased activity of the renin-angiotensin-aldosterone system to the initiation or maintenance of malignant hypertension is not clear.

CLINICAL FEATURES

A number of reports describe the clinical manifestations of malignant hypertension very completely [45, 53, 69, 79, 82, 112, 121, 133, 138, 139, 146, 154]. Therefore, only major characteristics are considered here.

While malignant nephrosclerosis does not present a uniform clinical picture, there are certain characteristics that allow fairly accurate diagnosis. According to Kincaid-Smith et al. [82] the peak incidence of this syndrome for men is found between the ages of 50 and 54, and for women between the ages of 45 and 54. Perera [133] found the ages at peak incidence to be 44 for men and 36 for women, figures comparable to those reported in the series of Schottstaedt and Sokolow [146], who noted the average age at onset to be 44 years in men and 41 years in women. Whether the higher age in the study of Kincaid-Smith et al. [82] can be accounted for by case selection or by an earlier onset of the accelerated renal phase of hypertension in the United States than in Great Britain is not clear. As we have indicated, the incidence of the accelerated phase is higher in men than in women; and in the study of Kincaid-Smith et al., this is particularly true after the age of 50.

One of the most characteristic symptoms, although not an invariable one, is the abrupt onset of severe headache or a fairly sudden increase in its intensity. It is not at all unusual for headache to be the first and the most distressing symptom of malignant hypertension. Although the headache is often described as constant, occipital and most severe in the morning, it may actually be diffuse or localized to any part of the head, occur at any time of the day or night, and be intermittent or constant. The intensity of the headache does not necessarily parallel the development of papilledema or the elevation of spinal fluid pressure, both of which are common findings in this syndrome. On occasion, especially when the headache is occipital, it may be associated with general feelings of stiffness of the neck; nuchal rigidity has been described under such circumstances [45].

Blurring of vision is a very common symptom in malignant nephrosclerosis, and sometimes visual symptoms precede any others. Often they are associated with papilledema and may be attributable to it, but it is important to recognize that sometimes no such correlation exists. Similarly anorexia, nausea, vomiting, and even abdominal pain may be associated with uremia, but they may also be present and unexplained in the absence of profound renal failure.

A very interesting symptom of malignant nephrosclerosis is weight loss, observed and emphasized in the studies of Kincaid-Smith et al. [82] and Perera [133]. The cause of weight loss is not clear from these studies; Perera states specifically that it is not related to anorexia, and both groups of authors state that it is not correlated with other evidences of uremia. Indeed, weight loss may antedate any other clinical manifestation of the accelerated phase of hypertensive disease.

From this brief account of some of the major symptoms, it can readily be seen that a patient who presents with sudden onset of violent headache, blurring of vision, and vomiting might well be suspected of having a brain tumor. If in addition the patient has any of the major evidences commonly associated with vascular disease of the brain, such as seizures, pareses, confusion or coma, papilledema, and a high spinal fluid protein concentration, the suspicion of brain tumor may be strengthened considerably.

Physical examination reveals high blood pressure and perhaps a large heart. The results of neurologic examination vary over a broad range from normal findings to a host of neurologic abnormalities associated with cerebral vascular disease. There may in addition be evidence of debility, especially if severe renal failure is present. In most instances, but not all, bilateral papilledema and severe hypertensive retinopathy are observed. The swollen disc is generally also hyperemic in appearance. The papilledema may precede or follow the development of the characteristic retinal changes of cotton-wool exudates and hemorrhages, both linear and flame-shaped. Although it is frequently assumed that the papilledema is a reflection of an increased cerebrospinal fluid pressure, Kincaid-Smith et al. [82] and Schottstaedt and Sokolow [146] cast some doubt upon this relationship, in that papilledema in several of their cases was present while cerebrospinal fluid pressure was normal.

The characteristic urinary finding is the rather abrupt development of marked albuminuria, or a striking increase in proteinuria in a patient previously known to have small amounts of albumin in the urine. In addition, the urine frequently contains red blood cells. While Fishberg [45] stated that gross hematuria is not a common manifestation of malignant hypertension, Goldring and Chasis [53] place the incidence at approximately 20 per cent and Schottstaedt and Sokolow [146] at 26 per cent. In the latter series gross hematuria was an initial symptom in 8 per cent. In our own experience, gross hematuria is common and has been noted as an early complaint in several patients. There may be some hyaline and granular casts and occasional white cells, but pyuria is not a prominent feature except in patients with pyelonephritis. Renal failure may not be present at the onset of the malignant phase, but it generally ensues and often progresses with great rapidity.

We have mentioned the interesting finding, reported by both Kincaid-Smith et al. [82] and Perera [133], of an elevation in the erythrocyte sedimentation rate — a finding that remains unexplained. In the studies reported by Kincaid-Smith and her associates, approximately two-thirds of the patients had an increase in cerebrospinal fluid pressure, and a similar number had an increase in the protein concentration of the spinal fluid.

While there is some variation in the statistics relating to prognosis in malignant nephrosclerosis, it is clear that in untreated patients death is virtually inevitable in a relatively short time. In 1939 Keith et al. [78] reported that 80 per cent of their group of hypertensive patients with papilledema were dead in one year and 90 per cent in two years; only a few lived for three years. Of 104 patients with malignant hypertension reported on by Schottstaedt and Sokolow in 1953 [146], two-thirds died within nine months, and all but three were dead in two and one-half years. These three lived more than five years and may be classified as having had spontaneous remission. Spontaneous remission is unusual but is well documented. In the study of Kincaid-Smith et al. [82] 55 per cent of patients with malignant hypertension were dead in a year, while one patient had a spontaneous remission.

Of the untreated patients described by Kincaid-Smith et al. [82], approximately 50 per cent died of a combination of uremia and congestive heart failure, and an additional 17 per cent died in uremia alone, while 20 per cent had cerebral vascular accidents as a direct cause of death. In the series of Milliez et al. [112] 18 of 27 patients died in uremia, while Heptinstall [63] observed 70 per cent of the patients died in uremia.

TREATMENT

Although the value of lowering the blood pressure in patients with arteriolar benign nephrosclerosis remains a subject of controversy, treatment with measures that reduce the blood pressure seems clearly associated with clinical improvement and a better prognosis in many patients with malignant nephrosclerosis. That this benefit is somehow related to a decrease in blood pressure itself is suggested by the many observations that it can be caused by a diverse group of therapeutic measures apparently having in common the effect of lowering the blood pressure: sympathectomy, pyrogens, rice diet, hypotensive drugs, and nephrectomy in cases due to unilateral renal arterial occlusion [33, 116, 117, 120, 124, 147, 156]. (As indicated earlier, the actual role of lowering blood pressure may be questioned in instances of a favorable response to sympathectomy unaccompanied by a reduction in blood pressure. On the other hand, perhaps the surgery resulted in fewer acute striking increments in blood pressure in these cases.) From the very nature of this syndrome, it is apparent that it would be extremely difficult to secure a meticulously randomized study of treated and untreated subjects that would provide a complete, unequivocal interpretation. Nonetheless, with this limitation in mind, there seem to be enough data to support the opinion that prognosis is favorably affected by treatment, that cardiovascular status may be favorably influenced, that retinopathy may be markedly improved, and that further deterioration of renal function may be prevented. Doubt remains, however, that renal function may be significantly improved by lowering blood pressure.

Much material is available on the treatment of malignant nephrosclerosis [31, 59, 62, 69, 108, 137, 139, 153, 157, 158]. In 1958 Moyer et al. [116, 117] reported the clinical results in a nonrandomized group of 31 patients with malignant hypertension, 13 of whom were treated with hypotensive drugs and 18 of whom remained untreated. Of the treated group, 11 were alive after an average follow-up period of 30 months, while 17 of the 18 untreated patients had died, the average survival time being 14 months. Twelve of the 17 patients died in uremia. Of this group of 31 patients, detailed studies of renal function were available in 21 — 12 treated and 9 untreated. After an average follow-up period of 29 months, two of the 12 treated patients and all of the untreated patients had died, with an average survival time of 12 months. Renal function did not change in the treated group during the average follow-up time of 28 months, as shown by the fact that mean control values of BUN (31 mg. per 100 ml.), GFR (66 ml. per minute), and RPF (513 ml. per minute) remained unchanged. The 9 untreated patients experienced a deterioration of 60 per cent from control values in these same functions in only 10 months. The treated patients also demonstrated significant improvement in their cardiovascular status. In this study, then, there was no improvement in renal function with therapy, but the implication is that treatment prevented rapid deterioration. Similar data are available from other studies [31, 62, 108, 157, 158]. Additional support for the beneficial effects of antihypertensive treatment in malignant nephrosclerosis is found in the studies of McCormack et al. [103], who demonstrated regression of arteriolar necrosis in patients so treated.

There is much in the literature expressing doubt that treatment of the accelerated renal phase of hypertension favorably alters the course of the disease in patients whose renal function has already deteriorated to the point at which a BUN higher than 60 to 65 mg. per 100 ml. is sustained in the absence of dehydration, heart failure, or other reversible cause of uremia. This view has been challenged in the excellent study of Woods and Blythe [186], who treated 20 patients with malignant hypertension and a BUN of 50 mg. per 100 ml. or higher (mean BUN of 79 mg. per 100 ml., with a range of 50 to 148 mg. per 100 ml.). Their conclusions in part are quoted: ". . . of the 11 (55 percent) who lived for one year, 9 (45 percent) are still alive. The follow-up period is approaching four years in 2, between two and three years in 2 and between one and two years in 5. In the surviving patients, the glomerular filtration rate has decreased slightly in 1, remained unchanged in 3, and increased an average of 15 ml. per minute in 5. Reduction of blood pressure in patients with malignant hypertension complicated by renal insufficiency does not necessarily result in deterioration of renal function and may result in improved survival rates." Perry et al. [137] have had a similar experience. In view of these and other observations [117a], it seems clear that previous views must be modified. Patients with malignant nephrosclerosis and an elevated BUN should be treated vigorously with antihypertensive medications along with meticulous attention to the management of renal failure.

The results of therapy of malignant hypertension may be expressed in general terms as follows: Without treatment 85 to 90 per cent of patients are dead within 15 months; with drug treatment this figure is reduced to approximately 10 to 20 per cent mortality. Long-term survival figures in treated patients are now being reported. Thus, Perry et al. [137], who reported a one-year survival rate of 85 per cent, observed a 38 per cent survival in nonazotemic patients after 12 years. The data at Hammersmith Hospital, reported by Dollery [31], is interesting in this regard. The one-year survival rate of patients with a blood *urea* level under 60 mg. per 100 ml. was 73 per cent, while in patients with higher initial blood urea levels the survival rate was 15 per cent. After five years, the survival figures were 33 and 8 per cent, respectively. It is interesting to note, however, that the patients with blood urea concentrations below 60 mg. per 100 ml. had a 21 per cent survival rate after 10 years.

When the organ systems are differently affected by treatment, as often seems to be the case, one cannot help wondering if, as Perera [132] has pointed out so carefully, the mechanisms responsible for the retinopathy are necessarily identical with those responsible for the renal damage and the cardiovascular damage. Perera has emphasized that the fact that treatment of patients in the accelerated renal phase of hypertension may prolong life does not necessarily imply that a reversal of the fundamental pathologic process involved takes place.

Summary

Three major conditions involving the blood vessels are included in the term nephrosclerosis. The first is concerned with atherosclerosis of the large vessels of the kidney. For the most part, except in those instances associated with renovascular hypertension, this lesion is not accompanied by any significant reduction in renal function. Whether or not it is responsible for any of the observed decrease in renal function occurring in the process of aging remains unclear. The possibility also exists that this process may be linked with a decrease in the capacity of the kidney to withstand acute changes in the internal environment of the organism or acute circulatory insufficiency due to any cause.

The most common lesion in nephrosclerosis is arteriolar nephrosclerosis, which is intimately associated with essential hypertension, although the precise nature of this relationship is not clear. For the most part, patients with this disease have a long course without any clinically significant deterioration in renal function. Approximately 1 per cent of them die with renal failure and a kidney similar to that observed in patients with primary renal disease. In a number of these patients, varying from 1 to 8 per cent according to the particular series reported, the accelerated or malignant phase of this disease will develop. Most patients with arteriolar nephrosclerosis die of heart disease, cerebral vascular disease, or intercurrent illness rather than of renal failure. In benign nephrosclerosis the effect of treatment designed to lower the blood pressure on the kidney cannot be conclusively evaluated at this time.

At any time in the course of arteriolar nephrosclerosis or other varieties of renal disease, there may be an abrupt onset of an accelerated renal phase of the disease, often initiated by retinopathy including papilledema. At the same time, or more usually soon thereafter, there may be increased proteinuria, red cells in the urine, rapidly progressive uremia, and death. The clinical course of this malignant phase may be ameliorated by treatment designed to reduce the blood pressure. Renal function is generally not improved significantly by treatment, but progressive deterioration seems to be prevented in many instances. While patients with moderate to marked renal insufficiency have a less favorable prognosis, even in this group, treatment may be beneficial.

Acknowledgments

This work was supported in part by Research Grant 07765 from the National Heart Institute, United States Public Health Service.

Photomicrographs were generously provided by Dr. Stanley Weitzner, Department of Pathology, Albuquerque Veterans Administration Hospital, University of New Mexico School of Medicine, Albuquerque, New Mexico.

References

1. Allen, A. C. *The Kidney: Medical and Surgical Diseases.* New York: Grune & Stratton, 1951.
2. Andrus, E. C. (Editor). *Second National Conference in Cardiovascular Disease.* Vol. 1, Research. Washington, D.C. 1964.
3. Baldwin, D. S., Biggs, A. W., Goldring, W., Hulet, W. H., and Chasis, H. Exaggerated natriuresis in essential hypertension. *Amer. J. Med.* 24:893, 1958.
4. Baldwin, D. S., Gombos, E. A., and Chasis, H. Urinary concentrating mechanism in essential hypertension. *Amer. J. Med.* 38:864, 1965.
5. Baldwin, D. S., Gombos, E. A., and Chasis, H. Changes in sodium and water excretion induced by epinephrine and l-norepinephrine in normotensive and hypertensive subjects. *J. Lab. Clin. Med.* 61:832, 1963.
6. Baldwin, D. S., Hulet, W. H., Biggs, A. W., Gombos, E. A., and Chasis, H. Renal function in the separate kidneys of man: II. Hemodynamics and excretion of solute and water in essential hypertension. *J. Clin. Invest.* 39:395, 1960.
7. Bali, T., and Goldblatt, H. On pathogenesis of vascular lesions of malignant hypertension in rat; role of elevated blood pressure and renal functional failure. *Exp. Med. Surg.* 12:460, 1954.

7a. Bank, N., Aynedjian, H. S., Bansal, U. K., and Goldman, D. M. Effect of acute hypertension on sodium transport by the distal nephron. *Amer. J. Physiol.* 219:275, 1970.

8. Barraclough, M. A., and Jones, N. F. Effect of fluid retention following vasopressin on sodium excretion by hypertensive subjects. *Clin. Sci.* 23:433, 1962.
9. Bechgaard, P. Arterial hypertension; follow-up study of 1000 hypertonics. *Acta Med. Scand.* Suppl. 172:3, 1946.
10. Bechgaard, P. The Natural History of Benign Hypertension. In Bock, K. D., and Cottier, P. T. (Eds.), *Essential Hypertension: An International Symposium.* Berlin: Springer-Verlag, 1960. P. 198.
11. Bell, E. T. *Renal Diseases.* Philadelphia: Lea & Febiger, 1946.
12. Bell, E. T., and Clawson, B. J. Primary (essential) hypertension; study of 420 cases. *Arch. Path.* 5:939, 1928.
13. Biava, C. G., Dyrda, I., Genest, J., and Bencosme, S. A. Renal hyaline arteriosclerosis: An electron microscope study. *Amer. J. Path.* 44:349, 1964.

14. Biron, P., Koiw, E., Nowaczynski, W., Brouillet, J., and Genest, J. The effects of intravenous infusions of valine-5 angiotensin II and other pressor agents on urinary electrolytes and corticosteroids, including aldosterone. *J. Clin. Invest.* 40:338, 1961.
15. Black, D. A. K. Salt and hypertension. *Brit. J. Nutr.* 6:428, 1952.
16. Braun-Menendez, E. Prohypertensive and antihypertensive actions of the kidney. *Ann. Intern. Med.* 49:717, 1958.
17. Braun-Menendez, E., Fasciolo, J. C., Leloir, L. F., Muñoz, J. M., and Taquini, A. C. *Renal Hypertension.* Springfield, Ill.: Thomas, 1946.
18. Breslin, D. J., Gifford, R. W., Jr., and Fairbairn, J. F., II. Essential hypertension: 20 years' follow-up study. *Circulation* 33:87, 1966.
19. Bright, R. *Reports of Medical Cases Selected with a View of Illustrating the Symptoms and Cure of Diseases by a Reference to Morbid Anatomy.* London: Longman, 1827.
20. Bright, R. Tabular view of the morbid appearances in 100 cases connected with albuminous urine with observation. *Guy. Hosp. Rep.* 1:396, 1836.
21. Brodsky, W. A., and Graubarth, H. N. Excretion of water and electrolytes in patients with essential hypertension. *J. Lab. Clin. Med.* 41:43, 1953.
22. Bucht, H., Ek, J., Josephson, B., Thomasson, B., Varnauskas, E., and Werko, L. Rapid infusion and renal function. *Clin. Sci.* 15:617, 1956.
23. Buckalew, V. M., Jr., Puschett, J. B., Kintzel, J. E., and Goldberg, M. Mechanism of exaggerated natriuresis in hypertensive man: Impaired sodium transport in the loop of Henle. *J. Clin. Invest.* 48: 1007, 1969.
24. Cannon, P. J. Effects of five percent dextrose-water infusions in normal and hypertensive man. *Circulation* 37:832, 1968.
25. Castleman, B., and Smithwick, R. H. Relation of vascular disease to hypertensive state based on study of renal biopsies from 100 hypertensive patients. *J.A.M.A.* 121: 1256, 1943.
26. Castleman, B., and Smithwick, R. H. Relation of vascular disease to hypertensive state; adequacy of renal biopsy as determined from study of 500 patients. *New Eng. J. Med.* 239:729, 1948.
27. Chasis, H., and Baldwin, D. S. The kidney in essential hypertension: Victim or culprit. *Circulation* 34:921, 1966.
28. Clark, E. G., Glock, C. Y., and Vought, R. L. Studies in hypertension: I. An epidemiologic approach to the study of the natural history of essential hypertension. *J. Chronic Dis.* 4:231, 1956.
29. Cottier, P. T., Weller, J. M., and Hoobler, S. W. Effect of an intravenous sodium chloride load on renal hemodynamics and electrolyte excretion in essential hypertension. *Circulation* 17:750, 1958.
30. Deleon, A. C., Jr., Dreifus, L. S., and Bellet, S. Urinary osmolar concentration, a means of evaluating early renal function changes in essential hypertension. *Amer. J. Med. Sci.* 239:144, 1960.
31. Dollery, C. T. Treatment of malignant hypertension. *Mod. Treatm.* 3:39, 1966.
32. Dustan, H. P., Poutasse, E. F., Corcoran, A. C., and Page, I. H. Separated renal function in patients with renal arterial disease, pyelonephritis and essential hypertension. *Circulation* 23:34, 1961.
33. Dustan, H. P., Schneckloth, R. E., Corcoran, A. C., and Page, I. H. The effectiveness of long-term treatment of malignant hypertension. *Circulation* 18:644, 1958.
34. Dustin, P., Jr. Arteriolar Hyalinosis. In Richter, G. W., and Epstein, M. A. (Eds.), *International Review of Experimental Pathology.* New York: Academic, 1962. Vol. 1, p. 73.
35. Editorial. Hypotensive drugs and renal function. *Lancet* 1:84, 1957.
36. Editorial. Renal changes in essential hypertension. *Lancet* 1:586, 1960.
37. Ek, J. Influence of heavy hydration on renal function in normal and hypertensive man. *Scand. J. Clin. Lab. Invest.* 7 (Suppl. 19):1, 1955.
38. Evans, G. A contribution to the study of arterio-sclerosis with special reference to its relation to chronic renal disease. *Quart. J. Med.* 14:215, 1921.

39. Evans, W. Hypertonia or uneventful high blood pressure. *Lancet* 2:53, 1957.
40. Evans, W. The aetiology of systemic hypertension. *Brit. Heart J.* 22:17, 1960.
41. Evelyn, K. A., Singh, M. M., Chapman, W. P., Perera, G. A., and Thaler, H. Effect of thoracolumbar sympathectomy on the clinical course of primary (essential) hypertension. *Amer. J. Med.* 28:188, 1960.
42. Eyler, W. R., Clark, M. D., Garman, J. E., Rian, R. L., and Meininger, D. E. Angiography of the renal areas including a comparative study of renal arterial stenosis in patients with and without hypertension. *Radiology* 78:879, 1962.
43. Fasciolo, J. C., and Cramer, F. K. Las lesiones oculares en la hipertension arterial por isquemia renal. *Rev. Soc. Argent. Biol.* 14:393, 1938.
44. Fishberg, A. M. Anatomic findings in essential hypertension. *Arch. Intern. Med.* 35:650, 1925.
45. Fishberg, A. M. *Hypertension and Nephritis* (5th ed.). Philadelphia: Lea & Febiger, 1954.
46. Fisher, E. R., Perez-Stable, E., and Pardo, V. Ultrastructural studies in hypertension: I. Comparison of renal vascular and juxtaglomerular cell alterations in essential and renal hypertension in man. *Lab. Invest.* 15:1409, 1966.
47. Fleming, H. A. Factors involved in production of acute arterial lesions in rabbits with experimental renal hypertension. *J. Path. Bact.* 65:441, 1953.
48. Freis, E. D. Hemodynamics of hypertension. *Physiol. Rev.* 40:27, 1960.
49. Genest, J. Studies on the mechanism of human arterial hypertension. *Dis. Chest* 45:351, 1964.
50. Genest, J., Boucher, R., deChamplain, J., Veyrat, R., Chretien, M., Biron, P., Tremblay, G., Roy, P., and Cartier, P. Studies on the renin-angiotensin system in hypertensive patients. *Canad. Med. Ass. J.* 90:263, 1964.
51. Goldblatt, H. *The Renal Origin of Hypertension.* Springfield, Ill.: Thomas, 1948.
52. Goldblatt, H. Anatomical Considerations of Hypertension. In Bell, E. T. (Ed.), *Hypertension, A Symposium.* Minneapolis: University of Minnesota Press, 1951. P. 18.
53. Goldring, W., and Chasis, H. *Hypertension and Hypertensive Disease.* New York: The Commonwealth Fund, 1944.
54. Goldring, W., and Chasis, H. Antihypertensive drug therapy: An appraisal. *Arch. Intern. Med.* (Chicago) 115:523, 1965.
55. Goldring, W., Chasis, H., Ranges, H. A., and Smith, H. W. Effective renal blood flow in subjects with essential hypertension. *J. Clin. Invest.* 20:637, 1941.
56. Gombos, E. A., Lee, T. H., Solinas, J., and Mitrovic, M. Renal response to pyrogen in normotensive and hypertensive man. *Circulation* 36:555, 1967.
57. Griep, A. H., Barry, G. R., Hall, W. C., and Hoobler, S. W. Prognosis in arterial hypertension: Report on 117 patients under 53 years of age, followed 8 to 10 years. *Amer. J. Med. Sci.* 221:239, 1951.
58. Grollman, A. The Role of the Kidney in the Pathogenesis of Hypertension as Determined by a Study of the Effect of Nephrectomy on the Blood Pressure of Normal and Hypertensive Animals. In *Transactions of the Second Conference on Factors Regulating Blood Pressure.* New York: Josiah Macy, Jr. Foundation, 1948.
59. Gross, F. (Ed.). *Antihypertensive Therapy: Principles and Practice: An International Symposium.* New York: Springer-Verlag, 1966.
60. Hagans, J. A., and Brust, A. A. The natural history of hypertension. *Amer. J. Med.* 28:905, 1960.
61. Hanenson, I. B., Taussky, H. H., Polasky, N., Ransohoff, W., and Miller, B. F. Renal excretion of sodium in arterial hypertension. *Circulation* 20:498, 1959.
62. Harrington, M., Kincaid-Smith, P., and McMichael, J. Results of treatment of malignant hypertension: A 7-year experience in 94 cases. *Brit. Med. J.* 2:969, 1959.
63. Heptinstall, R. H. Malignant hypertension: A study of fifty-one cases. *J. Path. Bact.* 65:423, 1953.
64. Heptinstall, R. H. Renal biopsies in hypertension. *Brit. Heart J.* 16:133, 1954.
65. Heptinstall, R. H. *Pathology of the Kid-*

ney. Boston: Little, Brown, 1966.

66. Hollander, W. Effects of intravenous hydration and Pitressin on renal function in subjects with essential hypertension. *Circulation* 19:691, 1959.
67. Hollander, W., and Judson, W. E. Electrolyte and water excretion in arterial hypertension: I. Studies in non-medically treated subjects with essential hypertension. *J. Clin. Invest.* 36:1460, 1957.
67a. Hollenberg, N. K., Epstein, M., Basch, R. I., and Merrill, J. P. "No man's land" of the renal vasculature. An arteriographic and hemodynamic assessment of the interlobar and arcuate arteries in essential and accelerated hypertension. *Amer. J. Med.* 47:845, 1969.
67b. Hollenberg, N. K., Epstein, M., Basch, R. I., Couch, N. P., Hickler, R. B., and Merrill, J. P. Renin secretion in essential and accelerated hypertension. *Amer. J. Med.* 47:855, 1969.
68. Holley, K. E., Hunt, J. C., Brown, A. L., Kincaid, O. W., and Sheps, S. G. Renal artery stenosis: A clinical-pathologic study in normotensive and hypertensive patients. *Amer. J. Med.* 37:14, 1964.
69. Hoobler, S. W. *Hypertensive Disease: Diagnosis and Treatment.* New York: Hoeber, 1959.
70. Hudson, R. E. B. *Cardiovascular Pathology*. Baltimore: Williams & Wilkins, 1965.
71. Hulet, W. H., Baldwin, D. S., Biggs, A. W., Gombos, E. A., and Chasis, H. Renal function in the separate kidneys in man: I. Hemodynamics and excretion of solute and water in normal subjects. *J. Clin. Invest.* 39:389, 1960.
72. Hulet, W. H., Hagedorn, C. W., Richardson, J. R., Jr., and Hartley, B. J. Hydrogen ion excretion in the separate kidneys of normal and hypertensive man. *Proceedings of the Second International Congress of Nephrology*. New York: Karger, 1964. P. 819.
73. Hulet, W. H., and Richardson, J. R., Jr. Postural natriuresis and renal concentrating capacity in essential hypertension. *Amer. J. Med.* 33:27, 1962.
74. Hulet, W. H., Richardson, J. R., Jr., and Hagedorn, C. W. Renal hemodynamics, tubular excretion, and urine-concentrating capacity in the separate kidneys of subjects with essential hypertension. *J. Lab. Clin. Med.* 62:787, 1963.
75. Hunt, J. C., Maher, F. T., and Greene, L. F. Functional characteristics of the separate kidneys in hypertensive man. *Amer. J. Cardiol.* 17:493, 1966.
76. Josephson, B., Bergström, J., Bucht, H., and Hultman, E. On the influence of body water volume and potassium supply on the aldosterone excretion in arterial hypertension. *Scand. J. Clin. Lab. Invest.* 14:47, 1962.
77. Kass, E. H. Discussion in Stauber, J., Stamler, R., and Pullman, T. N. (Eds.), *The Epidemiology of Hypertension.* New York: Grune & Stratton, 1967. P. 68.
78. Keith, N. M., Wagener, H. P., and Barker, N. W. Some different types of essential hypertension: Their course and prognosis. *Amer. J. Med. Sci.* 197:332, 1939.
79. Keith, N. M., Wagener, H. P., and Kernohan, J. W. Syndrome of malignant hypertension. *Arch. Intern. Med.* 41:141, 1928.
80. Kimmelstiel, P., and Wilson, C. Benign and malignant hypertension and nephrosclerosis: Clinical and pathological study. *Amer. J. Path.* 12:45, 1936.
81. Kimmelstiel, P., and Wilson, C. Inflammatory lesions in glomeruli in pyelonephritis in relation to hypertension and renal insufficiency. *Amer. J. Path.* 12:99, 1936.
82. Kincaid-Smith, P., McMichael, J., and Murphy, E. A. The clinical course and pathology of hypertension with papilloedema (malignant hypertension). *Quart. J. Med.* 27:117, 1958.
83. Kleeman, C. R., Hewitt, W. L., and Guze, L. B. Pyelonephritis. *Medicine* (Balt.) 39: 3, 1960.
84. Koch, K. M., Aynedjian, H. S., and Bank, N. Effect of acute hypertension on sodium reabsorption by the proximal tubule. *J. Clin. Invest.* 47:1696, 1968.
85. Kolff, W. J., and Page, I. H. Blood pressure reducing function of kidney: Reduc-

tion of renoprival hypertension by kidney perfusion. *Amer. J. Physiol.* 178:75, 1954.

86. Laragh, J. H. Renin, angiotensin, aldosterone and hormonal regulation of arterial pressure and salt balance. *Fed. Proc.* 26:39, 1967.
87. Laragh, J. H., Sealey, J. E., and Kirshman, J. S. Natriuretic activity in plasma and urine of salt-loaded man and sheep. *J. Clin. Invest.* 48:49a, 1969.
88. Laragh, J. H., Sealey, J. E., and Sommers, S. C. Patterns of adrenal secretion and urinary excretion of aldosterone and plasma renin activity in normal and hypertensive subjects. *Circ. Res.* 18 and 19 (Suppl. 1): 158, 1966.
89. Leading Articles. Prognosis of hypertension. *Brit. Med. J.* 1:1461, 1959.
90. Lee, J. B. Antihypertensive activity of the kidney: The renomedullary prostaglandins. *New Eng. J. Med.* 277:1073, 1967.
91. Leishman, A. W. D. Observations on prognosis in hypertension. *Brit. Med. J.* 1:1131, 1953.
92. Lewis, W. H., Jr., and Alving, A. S. Changes with age in renal function in adult men; clearance of urea; amount of urea nitrogen in blood; concentrating ability of kidneys. *Amer. J. Physiol.* 123:500, 1938.
93. Lewy, J. E., and Windhager, E. E. Peritubular control of proximal tubular fluid reabsorption in the rat kidney. *Amer. J. Physiol.* 214:943, 1968.
94. Lindeman, R. C., Lee, T. D., Jr., Yiengst, M. J., and Shock, N. W. Influence of age, renal disease, hypertension, diuretics and calcium on the antidiuretic responses to suboptimal infusions of vasopressin. *J. Lab. Clin. Med.* 68:206, 1966.
95. Lowenstein, J., Beranbaum, E. R., Chasis, H., and Baldwin, D. S. Intrarenal pressure and exaggerated natriuresis in essential hypertension. *Clin. Sci.* 38:359, 1970.
96. Lowenstein, J., Steinmetz, P. R., Effros, R. M., Demeester, M., Chasis, H., Baldwin, D. S., and Gomez, D. M. The distribution of intrarenal blood flow in normal and hypertensive man. *Circulation* 35:250, 1967.
97. Lowitz, H. D., Stumpe, K. O., and Ochwadt, B. Natrium- und Wasserresorption in den verschiedenen Abschnitten des Nephrons beim experimentellen renalen Hochdruck der Ratte. *Pflueger. Arch.* 304: 322, 1968.
98. Ljungqvist, A. The intrarenal arterial pattern in essential hypertension. A microangiographic and histological study. *J. Path. Bact.* 84:313, 1962.
99. Madeloff, M. S., Schwartz, F. D., Borges, F. J., Entwisle, G., Revell, S. T. R., Jr., and Young, J. D., Jr. Differential renal clearance patterns in the evaluation of hypertension. *J. Urol.* 87:258, 1962.
100. Magee, J. H., Unger, A. M., and Richardson, D. W. Changes in renal function associated with drug or placebo therapy of human hypertension. *Amer. J. Med.* 36: 795, 1964.
101. Martino, J. A., and Earley, L. E. Demonstration of a role of physical factors as determinants of the natriuretic response to volume expansion. *J. Clin. Invest.* 46:1963, 1967.
102. Mathisen, H. S., Løken, H., Brox, D., and Stokke, H. Prognosis in essential hypertension. *Scand. J. Clin. Lab. Invest.* 17 (Suppl. 84) :257, 1965.
103. McCormack, L. J., Beland, J. E., Schneckloth, R. E., and Corcoran, A. C. Effects of antihypertensive treatment in the evolution of renal lesions in malignant nephrosclerosis. *Amer. J. Path.* 34:1011, 1958.
104. McDonald, S. J., and de Wardener, H. E. The relationship between the renal arterial perfusion pressure and the increase in sodium excretion which occurs during an infusion of saline. *Nephron* 2:1, 1965.
105. McGee, W. G., and Ashworth, C. T. Fine structure of chronic hypertensive arteriopathy in the human kidney. *Amer. J. Path.* 43:273, 1963.
106. McKinney, B. The pathogenesis of hyaline arteriosclerosis. *J. Path. Bact.* 83:449, 1962.
107. McMichael, J. Discussion following Perera [133].
108. McMichael, J., and Murphy, E. A. Methonium treatment of severe and malignant hypertension. *J. Chronic Dis.* 1:527, 1955.

109. Mertz, D. P. The concentrating power of the kidneys in essential hypertension. *German Med. Monthly* 11:125, 1966.
110. Metzger, R. A., Vaamonde, L. S., Vaamonde, C. A., and Papper, S. Renal excretion of sodium during oral water administration in patients with systemic hypertension. *Circulation* 38:955, 1968.
111. Miller, J. H., and Shock, N. W. Age differences in renal tubular response to antidiuretic hormone. *J. Geront.* 8:446, 1953.
112. Milliez, P., Tcherdakoff, P., Samarcq, P., and Rey, L. P. The Natural Course of Malignant Hypertension. In Bock, K. D., and Cottier, P. T. (Eds.), *Essential Hypertension: An International Symposium.* Berlin: Springer, 1960. P. 214.
113. Moritz, A. R., and Oldt, M. R. Arteriolar sclerosis in hypertensive and non-hypertensive individuals. *Amer. J. Path.* 13:679, 1937.
114. Moschcowitz, E. Cause of arteriosclerosis. *Amer. J. Med. Sci.* 178:244, 1929.
115. Moyer, J. H. (Ed.). *Hypertension* (*First Hahnemann Symposium on Hypertensive Disease.*) Philadelphia: Saunders, 1959.
116. Moyer, J. H., Heider, C., Pevey, K., and Ford, R. V. The vascular status of a heterogeneous group of patients with hypertention with particular emphasis on renal function. *Amer. J. Med.* 24:164, 1958.
117. Moyer, J. H., Heider, C., Pevey, K., and Ford, R. V. The effect of treatment of the vascular deterioration associated with hypertension, with particular emphasis on renal function. *Amer. J. Med.* 24:177, 1958.
117a. Mroczek, W. J., Davidov, M., Gavrilovich, L., and Finnerty, F. A., Jr. The value of aggressive therapy in the hypertensive patient with azotemia. *Circulation* 40:893, 1969.
118. Muirhead, E. E., Turner, L. B., and Grollman, A. Hypertensive cardiovascular disease; vascular lesions of dogs maintained for extended periods following bilateral nephrectomy or ureteral ligation. *A.M.A. Arch. Path.* 51:575, 1951.
119. Muirhead, E. E., Turner, L. B., and Grollman, A. Hypertensive cardiovascular disease; nature and pathogenesis of arteriolar sclerosis induced by its tinctorial characteristics. *A.M.A. Arch. Path.* 52:266, 1951.
120. Newborg, B., and Kempner, W. Analysis of 177 cases of hypertensive vascular disease with papilledema: 126 patients treated with rice diet. *Amer. J. Med.* 19:33, 1955.
121. Page, I. H., and Corcoran, A. C. *Arterial Hypertension: Its Diagnosis and Treatment.* Chicago: Year Book, 1945.
122. Page, I. H., and Corcoran, A. C. *Experimental Renal Hypertension.* Springfield, Ill.: Thomas, 1948.
123. Page, I. H., and McCubbin, J. W. *Renal Hypertension.* Chicago: Year Book, 1968.
124. Page, I. H., Taylor, R. D., and Corcoran, A. C. Pyrogens in the Treatment of Malignant Hypertension. In Bell, E. T. (Ed.), *Hypertension: A Symposium.* Minneapolis: University of Minnesota Press, 1951.
125. Palmer, R. S., and Muench, H. Course and prognosis of essential hypertension; follow-up of 453 patients 10 years after original series was closed. *J.A.M.A.* 153:1, 1953.
126. Papper, S., Belsky, J. L., and Bleifer, K. H. The response to the administration of an isotonic sodium chloride-lactate solution in patients with essential hypertension. *J. Clin. Invest.* 39:876, 1960.
127. Pears, M. A., and Pickering, G. W. Antihypertensive drug therapy; another appraisal. *Arch. Intern. Med.* 115:526, 1965.
128. Peart, W. S., and Brown, J. J. Effect of angiotensin (Hypertensin or angiotonin) on urine flow and electrolyte excretion in hypertensive patients. *Lancet* 1:28, 1961.
129. Perera, G. A. Development of hypertensive manifestations after disappearance of hypertension. *Circulation* 10:28, 1954.
130. Perera, G. A. Hypertensive vascular disease; description and natural history. *J. Chronic Dis.* 1:33, 1955.
131. Perera, G. A. Relation of blood pressure lability to prognosis in hypertensive vascular disease. *J. Chronic Dis.* 1:121, 1955.
132. Perera, G. A. Hypertensive vascular disease: Therapeutic principles and objectives. *J. Chronic Dis.* 1:472, 1955.
133. Perera, G. A. The accelerated form of hy-

pertension, a unique entity? *Trans. Ass. Amer. Physicians* 71:62, 1958.

134. Perera, G. A. Antihypertensive drug versus symptomatic treatment in primary hypertension: Effect of survival. *J.A.M.A.* 173:11, 1960.
135. Perera, G. A., and Adler, G. ABO blood groups in the accelerated form of hypertension. *Ann. Intern. Med.* 53:84, 1960.
136. Perera, G. A., and Damon, A. Height, weight and their ratio in the accelerated form of primary hypertension. *A.M.A. Arch. Intern. Med.* 100:263, 1957.
137. Perry, H. M., Jr., Schroeder, H. A., Cantanzaro, F. J., Moore-Jones, D., and Carmel, G. H. Studies on the control of hypertension: VIII. Mortality, morbidity and remissions during twelve years of intensive therapy. *Circulation* 33:958, 1966.
138. Pickering, G. W. *High Blood Pressure* (2nd ed.). New York: Grune & Stratton, 1968.
139. Pickering, G. W. Hyperpiesis: High blood pressure without evident cause; essential hypertension. *Brit. Med. J.* 2:959, 1021, 1965.
140. Pickering, G. W., Wright, A. D., and Heptinstall, R. H. Reversibility of malignant hypertension. *Lancet* 2:952, 1952.
141. Reubi, F. C. The Late Effects of Hypotensive Drug Therapy on Renal Functions of Patients with Essential Hypertension. In Bock, K. D., and Cottier, P. T. (Eds.), *Essential Hypertension: An International Symposium*. Berlin: Springer-Verlag, 1960. P. 317.
142. Robbins, S. L. *Textbook of Pathology*. Philadelphia: Saunders, 1957.
143. Rocha, H., Guze, L. B., Freedman, L. R., and Beeson, P. B. Experimental pyelonephritis: III. The influence of localized injury in different parts of the kidney on susceptibility to bacillary infection. *Yale J. Biol. Med.* 30:341, 1958.
144. Salomon, M. I., Narasimhan, P., Bruno, M. S., and Ober, W. B. Renal lesions in essential hypertension. *Angiology* 13:216, 1962.
145. Saltz, M., Sommers, S. C., and Smithwick, R. H. Clinico-pathologic correlations of renal biopsies from essential hypertensive patients. *Circulation* 16:207, 1957.
146. Schottstaedt, M. F., and Sokolow, M. Natural history and course of malignant hypertension with papilledema (malignant hypertension). *Amer. Heart J.* 45:331, 1953.
147. Schroeder, H. A. Hypertensive vascular disease: Therapy with modern drugs and its limits. *J. Chronic Dis.* 1:497, 1955.
148. Selkurt, E. E., Womack, I., and Dailey, W. N. Mechanism of natriuresis and diuresis during elevated renal arterial pressure. *Amer. J. Physiol.* 209:95, 1965.
149. Shapiro, A. P. Experimental pyelonephritis and hypertension: Implications for the clinical problem. *Ann. Intern. Med.* 59:37, 1963.
150. Shock, N. W. The Role of the Kidney in Electrolyte and Water Regulation in the Aged. In *Ciba Foundation Colloquia on Ageing. Vol. IV. Water and Electrolyte Metabolism in Relation to Age and Sex.* Boston: Little, Brown, 1958. P. 229.
151. Shorr, E. Participation of hepatorenal vasotropic factors in experimental renal hypertension. *Amer. J. Med.* 4:120, 1948.
152. Shorr, E., and Zweifach, B. W. Hepatorenal vasotropic factors in blood during chronic essential hypertension in man. *Trans. Ass. Amer. Physicians* 61:350, 1948.
153. Simpson, F. O., and Smirk, F. H. The treatment of malignant hypertension. *Amer. J. Cardiol.* 9:868, 1962.
154. Smirk, F. H. *High Arterial Pressure.* Springfield, Ill.: Thomas, 1957.
155. Smith, J. P. Hyaline arteriosclerosis in the kidney. *J. Path. Bact.* 69:147, 1955.
156. Smithwick, R. H. Hypertensive vascular disease; results of and indications for splanchnicectomy. *J. Chronic Dis.* 1:477, 1955.
157. Sokolow, M., and Perloff, D. Five year survival of consecutive patients with malignant hypertension treated with antihypertensive agents. *Amer. J. Cardiol.* 6:858, 1960.
158. Sokolow, M., and Perloff, D. The choice of drugs and the management of essential

hypertension. *Progr. Cardiovasc. Dis.* 8:253, 1965.

159. Sommers, S. C. Pathology of the Kidney and Adrenal Gland in Relationship to Hypertension. In Moyer, J. (Ed.), *Hypertension. (First Hahnemann Symposium on Hypertensive Disease.)* Philadelphia: Saunders, 1959.

160. Sommers, S. C. Pathology of Essential Hypertension. In Moyer, J. (Ed.), *Cyclopedia Medica.* Philadelphia: Davis, 1964. Vol. 4, p. 9.

161. Sommers, S. C. Hypertension and kidney disease. *Progr. Cardiovasc. Dis.* 8:210, 1965.

162. Sommers, S. C., Relman, A. S., and Smithwick, R. H. Histologic studies of kidney biopsy specimens from patients with hypertension. *Amer. J. Path.* 34:685, 1958.

163. Sporn, I. N., Lancestremere, R. G., Vaamonde, C. A., and Papper, S. Acute renal conservation of sodium in hypertension. *Arch. Intern. Med.* (Chicago) 111: 439, 1963.

164. Steinmetz, P. R., Eisinger, R. P., Gombos, E. A., Chasis, H., and Baldwin, D. S. Excretion of free water and solute during maximal water diuresis in normal and hypertensive subjects. *J. Lab. Clin. Med.* 64: 238, 1964.

165. Symmers, W. St. C. Necrotizing pulmonary arteriopathy associated with pulmonary hypertension. *J. Clin. Path.* 5:36, 1952.

166. Symposium. *Ciba Foundation on Hypertension. Humoral and Neurogenic Factors.* Boston: Little, Brown, 1954.

167. Symposium. Angiotensin, sodium and hypertension. *Canad. Med. Ass. J.* 90:153, 1964.

168. Symposium. Proceedings of conference on basic mechanisms of arterial hypertension. University of Michigan. *Circulation* 17:641, 1958.

169. Talbott, J. H., Castleman, B., Smithwick, R. H., Melville, R. S., and Pecora, L. J. Renal biopsy studies correlated with renal clearance observations in hypertensive patients treated by radical sympathectomy. *J. Clin. Invest.* 22:387, 1943.

170. Taquini, A. C., Plesch, S. A., Capris, T. A., and Badano, B. N. Some observations on water and electrolyte metabolism in essential hypertension. *Acta Cardiol.* (Brux.) 11:109, 1956.

171. Thompson, J. E., Silva, T. F., Kinsey, D., and Smithwick, R. H. Effect of acute salt loads on urinary sodium output of normotensive and hypertensive patients before and after surgery. *Circulation* 10:912, 1954.

172. Thurau, K., and Deetjen, P. Die Diurese bei arteriellen Drucksteigetungen. *Pflueger. Arch. Ges. Physiol.* 274:567, 1962.

173. Tobian, L. Physiology of the juxtaglomerular cells. *Ann. Intern. Med.* 52:395, 1960.

174. Tobian, L. Interrelationship of electrolytes, juxtaglomerular cells and hypertension. *Physiol. Rev.* 40:280, 1960.

175. Tobian, L., Coffee, K., Ferreira, D., and Meuli, J. The effect of renal perfusion pressure on the net transport of sodium out of distal tubular urine as studied with the stop-flow technique. *J. Clin. Invest.* 43:118, 1964.

176. Toor, M., Dulfano, M., and Yahini, J. The Effect of Increased Intra-pulmonary, Intracardiac and Intra-arterial Blood Pressure on Renal Sodium Excretion. In Moyer, J. (Ed.), *Hypertension. (First Hahnemann Symposium on Hypertensive Disease.)* Philadelphia: Saunders, 1959. P. 31.

177. Ulrych, M., Hofman, J., and Hejl, Z. Cardiac and renal hyperresponsiveness to acute plasma volume expansion in hypertension. *Amer. Heart J.* 68:193, 1964.

178. Vaamonde, C. A., Sporn, I. N., Lancestremere, R. G., Belsky, J. L., and Papper, S. Augmented natriuretic response to acute sodium infusion after blood pressure elevation with metaraminol in normotensive subjects. *J. Clin. Invest.* 43:496, 1964.

179. Vaamonde, C. A., Vaamonde, L. S., Morosi, H. J., and Papper, S. Augmented natriuretic response to acute sodium infusion in normotensive patients with chronic pulmonary disease. *J. Clin. Invest.* 44:1106, 1965.

180. Vagnucci, A. I., and Wesson, L. G., Jr.

Diurnal cycle of renal hemodynamics and excretion of chloride and potassium in hypertensive subjects. *J. Clin. Invest.* 43:522, 1964.

181. Veterans Administration Cooperative Study Group on Antihypertensive Agents. Effects of treatment on morbidity in hypertension: I. Results in patients with diastolic blood pressures averaging 115 through 129 mm. Hg. *J.A.M.A.* 202:1028, 1967.

182. Veterans Administration Cooperative Study Group on Antihypertensive Agents. Effects of treatment on morbidity in hypertension: II. Results in patients with diastolic blood pressure averaging 90 through 114 mm. Hg. *J.A.M.A.* 213:1143, 1970.

183. Weiss, S., and Parker, F., Jr. Pyelonephritis: Its relation to vascular lesions and to arterial hypertension. *Medicine* (Balt.) 18: 221, 1939.

184. Wilson, C., and Byrom, F. B. Renal changes in malignant hypertension, experimental evidence. *Lancet* 1:136, 1939.

185. Wilson, C., and Byrom, F. B. The vicious circle in chronic Bright's disease. Experimental evidence from the hypertensive rat. *Quart. J. Med.* 34:65, 1941.

186. Woods, J. W., and Blythe, W. B. Management of malignant hypertension complicated by renal insufficiency. *New Eng. J. Med.* 277:57, 1967.

20

Hypertension Due to Renal Vascular Disease, Renal Infarction, Renal Cortical Necrosis

James W. Woods and T. Franklin Williams

Hypertension Due to Renal Vascular Disease

From the time of Bright, there has been sustained interest in the relation between renal disease, including renal vascular disease, and generalized cardiovascular disease with hypertension. The still unresolved question of the role of the kidney in the pathogenesis of essential hypertension is discussed in Chapter 19. The present section deals with the experimental and clinical features of partial obstruction to the renal circulation and the associated hypertension.

By the latter part of the nineteenth century the lines of experimental study of this problem, which have proved most fruitful in recent years, had already been undertaken. Cohnheim is said to have attempted, without success, to produce a rise in systemic arterial pressure by constriction of the renal arteries [1]. Tigerstedt and Bergman [392], in 1898, showed that injection of extracts of kidneys produced hypertension. However, other observers were unable to confirm this work [1].

The problem of obtaining reproducible experimental results in this field persisted until 1934, although it may be noted in retrospect that Janeway [193] in 1906 described one dog which had hypertension for 105 days after constriction of a renal artery, and Cash [66] in 1924 noted that production of almost total nephrectomy, or production of renal infarcts, induced hypertension in some dogs.

In 1934 the publication by Goldblatt and his colleagues [141] of a dependable method for producing sustained hypertension in dogs by partial constriction of one or both renal arteries gave an immense impetus to the study of this relationship. By 1946 a "thorough summary of the work performed to date" contained over 1200 references [50], almost all dated after 1934. In succeeding years continuing efforts have been made to answer the same fundamental questions about the mechanism of participation of the kidney in systemic hypertension and the diagnosis of curable renal causes of hypertension in patients. Probably the most significant recent advances have been the identification and synthesis of angiotensin, improvement in methods for assay of renin, the elucidation of the interrelationships of angiotensin and aldosterone, and their clinical applications in the alleviation of hypertension.

This field has continued to be one of unusual controversy, with numerous examples of experimental results which appear at first to be contradictory. Upon further examination these contradictions can usually be attributed to differences in methodology or differences between species of animals studied (or both).

EXPERIMENTAL PRODUCTION OF RENAL ARTERIAL HYPERTENSION

Partial obstruction of the arterial supply to one or both kidneys, as by application of the nonirritating silver clamp of Goldblatt [141], results in hypertension which begins in 24 to 72 hours and reaches its maximal level in about one week. Other methods [72, 95] are equally effective, although the hypertension may be slower in developing. The effect has been demonstrated in many mammalian species; most experimental work has been done in the dog, rat, cat, and rabbit [37, 50, 72, 139–141, 301, 320, 421]. The magnitude of the effect is roughly proportional to the amount of constriction of the renal arteries: Moderate constriction leads to hypertension without evidence of deterioration of renal function; severe constriction results in more severe hypertension and the rapid development of generalized arteriolar necrosis and renal insufficiency — a picture closely resembling human malignant hypertension. Once the blood pressure has reached a stable high level or has begun to fall, further constriction usually leads to a further rise in pressure.

Bilateral arterial constriction, or unilateral constriction combined with removal of the opposite kidney, produces longer-lasting effects than simple unilateral constriction. Unilateral constriction alone has rarely produced permanent hypertension in the dog, but it will do so approximately two-thirds of the time in the rat [140, 413, 414]. Removal of the constriction (or removal of the constricted kidney with the other kidney intact, provided, in certain species, that the hypertension has not been present longer than six to eight weeks) results in a return to normal systemic pressure, usually within a few hours [37, 117, 139, 319, 335].

Certain other methods for production of hypertension probably share the same mechanism as renal arterial constriction. These include constriction of the whole kidney by wrapping with cellophane or silk [298], and production of partial infarction of the kidney either by almost total occlusion of the main renal artery or by occlusion of one or more branches. As noted in the section on *Renal Infarction* (see below), the associated hypertension is not invariably present, and may or may not persist indefinitely. The survival of some abnormal renal tissue surrounding the infarct appears to be necessary for the occurrence of hypertension — that is, total infarction of the kidney is rarely associated with sustained hypertension [37, 112, 133].

Other technics that may produce hypertension by the same or a different mechanism, such as ligation of the ureters, pyelonephritis, or irradiation, will not be included in this discussion.

PATHOLOGY OF EXPERIMENTAL RENAL ARTERIAL HYPERTENSION

Pathologic changes in the kidney beyond an arterial constriction have been found to be variable. There may be no recognizable abnormalities; or some atrophic but apparently viable tubules, or areas of definite infarction surrounded by areas of atrophic but viable tubular cells, may be present. In general, the severity of pathologic findings in the affected kidney parallels the degree of constriction and also the severity of the hypertension, but definite and sustained hypertension has been described in animals in which no abnormality in the constricted kidney could be recognized other than increased collateral circulation in the renal capsule [50, 72, 140, 413, 414].

Elsewhere in the body, the extent of vascular disease is well correlated with the degree of systemic hypertension [415]. Wilson and Byrom [413, 414] used this experimental approach (unilateral renal arterial constriction in the rat) to obtain evidence for their view, now widely accepted, that the hypertension itself leads to all degrees of vascular damage, including that associated with malignant hypertension. They found vascular lesions (cellular intimal proliferation and intimal and medial necrosis) in the interlobular arteries and afferent arterioles of the kidney *exposed* to the hypertension, and also in the arterioles of the pancreas, intestine, mesentery, stomach, and heart. There were no vascular lesions in the kidney, which was *protected* from the hypertension by the arterial constriction. Further corroboration comes from the demonstration, by Masson et al. [262], in rats with partial renal infarction, that as long as hypertension is prevented by administration of hydralazine, no vascular lesions develop, but with discontinuance of hydralazine and appearance of hypertension vascular lesions develop within 7 to 14 days. Allison et al. [3] have shown that arteriolar necroses underwent resolution and healing in rabbits when the clip was removed from the renal artery and the blood pressure fell.

PATHOGENESIS OF RENAL ARTERIAL HYPERTENSION

The mechanism whereby renal arterial constriction leads to a change in the kidney, which then leads to increased systemic pressure, remains unclear. It has been proposed that a decrease in renal blood flow (RBF) — i.e., ischemia — is a constant event [374], and there is no question that severe renal arterial constriction results in a definite decrease in RBF [30, 231]. However, it was shown by Corcoran and Page [79] and Warthin and Thomas [406] that mild to moderate arterial constriction in dogs could result in sustained systemic hypertension with only a transient decrease in RBF, followed by a return to control values. A rapid increase in collateral circulation to these kidneys is a constant feature [140], and either this or thinning of the vessel wall beneath the clamp, allowing more blood to pass, may account for the return of normal blood flow. Furthermore, autoregulation of RBF occurs, as has been known for some time. There is also evidence that decrease in oxygen supply is not the stimulus that leads to hypertension: Making animals anoxic by breathing gas mixtures poor in oxygen [187], or perfusion of the kidney with venous blood [93], does not lead to hypertension. The relationship of ischemic tubular atrophy to renovascular hypertension is uncertain since it may be absent both in the kidneys of dogs with experimental renal hypertension and in some human kidneys, the removal of which has resulted in cure of the hypertension. Thus there is no unequivocal evidence that renal ischemia is an essential element in pathogenesis. However, the negative evidence does not entirely discount it.

Another possible mechanism is the effect on some renal processes of a lowered perfusion pressure beyond the constriction. Levy et al. [231] found that the systolic pressure beyond the constriction in dogs was at control levels even though it was below the femoral systolic pressure, which had risen above control values as a result of the constriction. Mason et al. [261] in further similar studies found that, after an initial fall, the distal pressure tended to rise with time toward control levels.

Bounous and Shumacker [44], utilizing surgical constriction of one renal artery (without removal of the opposite kidney) in dogs, were able to produce moderate sustained hypertension in 65 of 90 animals. They found the mean blood pressure distal to the stenosis to be within the normal range in almost all cases despite the elevation of pressure proximally. As is discussed later (see page 784), cure of human renovascular hypertension is not always associated with the presence of a large pressure gradient across the stenosis. However, in normal dogs, Skinner et al. [365] found renin in increased amounts in renal venous blood when mean perfusion pressure was reduced as little as 5 to 10 mm. Hg from resting levels of around 100 mm. Hg. Thus, if the renin-angiotensin system is involved in the pathogenesis of renovascular hypertension, very small hemodynamic changes may be sufficient to activate mechanisms which result in systemic hypertension. There is no strong evidence to support the concept that decreased pulse pressure beyond a renal artery constriction is responsible for the accompanying hypertension [216, 300].

MEDIATION OF RENAL ARTERIAL HYPERTENSION

It was shown early in studies by Blalock and Levy [37] and by Collins [72] that denervated kidneys with renal arterial constriction produced the same degree of hypertension as normally innervated kidneys. Denervation included transplantation of the kidneys to a different site. Early studies also showed that constriction of other arterial areas, such as the splenic or femoral arteries [140, 141], did not result in hypertension. As already mentioned, except in chronic preparations in rats, the removal of the constricted kidney, with the opposite kidney intact, leads to a rapid return to normal pressure. Thus a constriction of the blood supply to the kidney produces hypertension which is contingent upon the continued presence of that organ in the circulation, is probably unique for the kidney, and is not mediated through the nerve supply of the kidney. Three logical alternative explanations exist: (1) The kidney has increased its secretion of some vasopressor substance or precursor into the bloodstream; (2) a renal mechanism for removing some vasopressor substance (or substances) from the systemic circulation has been impaired; or (3) the production of some vasodepressor substance by the kidney has been diminished.

Renal Secretion of a Vasopressor Substance: The Renin-Angiotensin System. In 1898 Tigerstedt and Bergman [392] reported careful observations on the intravenous injection of saline extracts of rabbit kidneys into normal rabbits, following which a distinct rise in blood pressure occurred in 80 to 100 seconds. They then demonstrated that extracts of boiled kidney, or boiled extract of normal kidney, would produce no effect, that the hypertensive substance in the extract was not soluble in alcohol, that it could stand temperatures as high as 54 to 56°C., and that it was not dialyzable — thus it had the properties of a protein. They gave this substance the name renin. They showed that it resided mainly in the renal cortex (i.e., very little was extractable from renal medullary tissue), that it was effective in nephrectomized as well as in normal animals, and that section of the vagus nerves, or section at the base of the brain, or removal of the spinal cord made no difference in the hypertensive response to the injection. They noted that there was a rise in diastolic pressure with no change in heart rate and concluded that the effect was on peripheral vessels, not on the heart. Further knowledge of the preparation and properties of renin has recently been reviewed [302, 310]. Refinements in methods of extraction continue to be made [363]; however, chemically pure renin is yet to be obtained.

The evidence that renin is secreted by the juxtaglomerular apparatus of the kidney is convincing and is as follows: (1) The abundance of secretory granules in the cytoplasm of the juxtaglomerular cells closely parallels the amount of extractable renin in a kidney under various physiologic conditions [394]; (2) the abundance of granules parallels the secretion of renin; (3) microdissection studies have shown that the bulk of extractable renin is located at the vascular poles of the glomeruli (where the juxtaglomerular apparati are located) [33, 78]; (4) fluorescein-labeled renin antibodies localize only in the cytoplasm of the juxtaglomerular cells, where the secretory granules are located [166], and do not stain the macula densa. It appears reasonable to conclude from the last evidence that the macula densa does not contain renin [77].

In 1939 Page [299] and Braun-Menendez and his colleagues [49] discovered that renin had the properties of an enzyme, splitting a plasma substrate into a smaller molecule now known as angiotensin. Then, in 1956, came the determination of the amino acid sequence of angiotensin [106, 309, 364], followed the next year by the synthesis of angiotensin [54, 346]. It is now known that renin splits a plasma substrate, an alpha-2 globulin, forming a decapeptide, angiotensin I, which has virtually no pressor activity. Angiotensin I in the presence of an enzyme found largely in the pulmonary capillary bed [290a, 293a] is converted to an octapeptide, angiotensin II, an extremely potent vasopressor substance. In subsequent discussion, the word angiotensin will refer to angiotensin II. The chemistry of angiotensin and its analogues has been reviewed in detail [301, 310].

An interrelationship between renin and the suprarenal glands was suspected from animal studies by Deane and Masson [88] and Gross [152]. The former had shown that injection of renin in rats resulted in an increase in the size of the zona glomerulosa, the region of the adrenal cortex which is the source of aldosterone. The latter showed that the amount of renin present in the kidney, and probably in the circulation, of the rat was markedly diminished by administration of desoxycorticosterone. In 1960 Genest et al. [134] and Laragh et al. [224] demonstrated that angiotensin stimulated the adrenal glands in man to produce aldosterone, by far the most potent mineralocorticoid known. Davis and his colleagues [65, 86, 87], in an impressive series of experiments, have demonstrated the essential role of the kidney in the secretion of aldosterone. Removal of the kidney prevented the rise of aldosterone secretion normally produced by bleeding the animals. Nephrectomy in dogs with chronic thoracic caval constriction and high levels of aldosterone secretion resulted in a fall in the rate of secretion. The injection of an extract of the kidney, or renin, or angiotensin produced a rise in aldosterone secretion in hypophysectomized, nephrectomized animals, whereas injection of liver extracts did not. From these and subsequent data, it now appears reasonably certain that angiotensin is the principal aldosterone-stimulating hormone, although the potassium ion and adrenocorticotropin have a weaker stimulating effect. Many of the complex functions and characteristics of the renin-angiotensin-aldosterone system have been reviewed in recent years [152a, 301, 310, 326a].

Despite remarkable advances in our understanding of this system in the past decade, the critically important problem of the nature of control of renin secretion has not yet been resolved. Vander [400] has reviewed and analyzed the various theories proposed. Of these, the theory that the juxtaglomerular apparatus serves as a renal baroreceptor sensitive to changes in mean arterial pressure, and the theory that the sodium load to the macula densa is detected and that there exists a reciprocal relationship between sodium load and renin release, are being considered most seriously. There is also evidence that the sympathetic nervous system can alter renin release and synthesis. In addition, Michelakis et al. [271] have demonstrated in vitro stimulation of renin production in dog renal-cell suspensions by epinephrine, norepinephrine, and adenosine-3′, 5′-monophosphate. They suggest that agents that are known to influence renin production in the intact animal may exert their effects, at least in part, through direct chemical actions on the renal cells and that adenosine-3′, 5′-monophosphate may play a role as an intracellular mediator of the renin-stimulating action of catecholamines. It seems likely that the juxtaglomerular apparatus may be a site for integration of several diverse inputs.

Despite establishment of the fact that renin is released in increased amounts from the experimentally constricted or ischemic kidney during the first week or two, the extent of its participation in the sustained hypertension produced by renal arterial constriction continues to be a controversial subject. Many investigators have found increased renin or angiotensin activity in the renal venous blood or systemic blood of laboratory animals soon after the induction of hypertension by arterial constriction or similar technics. However, more often than not, no increased renin or angiotensin has been found in the chronic, benign, sustained stage of hypertension [246]. The same is true for aldosterone secretion. Both renin and aldosterone are usually increased in malignant hypertension in both dogs and man. The failure to establish a pathogenetic relationship between renin-angiotensin and chronic experimental renovascular hypertension may be due to inadequate methods of measurement, now improving, or to various other possibilities:

1. Renovascular hypertension may not be etiologically related to renin-angiotensin. The studies of MacDonald et al. [247a] in rabbits immunized against angiotensin II which nonetheless developed hypertension provides strong evidence for this possibility.
2. Renal hypertension may at first be due to a humoral cause, but later, in the chronic phase, it may become predominantly neurogenic in nature [329].
3. The chronic phase of renal hypertension may be due to small amounts of angiotensin that, with time, act on the sympathetic nervous system to enhance the cardiovascular effects of its normal activity [246].
4. Angiotensin released when renal perfusion is threatened may stimulate increased aldosterone secretion which causes renal sodium and water retention which, in turn, markedly increases pressor sensitivity to angiotensin [223].

Whether one of these hypotheses or yet another will eventually prove correct remains for the future. Deeper exploration, as in many biological problems, has led to greater complexity. Improved methods for renin assay and for measurement of plasma aldosterone [53], recent development of a radioimmunoassay for angiotensin [46, 68, 153], and the interest of many competent investigators promise clarification of unsolved problems.

Relation of Renal Vascular Hypertension to Renoprival Hypertension and to the Function of a Remaining Normal Kidney. The occurrence of hypertension in bilaterally nephrectomized dogs was first described by Harrison et al. [164]. Grollman et al. [151] made similar but more extensive observations over a period of weeks, utilizing intermittent peritoneal irrigation. The fact that hypertension may develop after bilateral nephrectomy is now accepted, but the pathogenesis of the hypertension is debated. One view, held by Grollman and colleagues, ascribes its occurrence to the loss of a humoral antihypertensive principle of renal origin which is necessary for the maintenance of normal blood pressure. The other view rejects the idea of a hormonal deficiency and attributes the hypertension to changes in water and electrolyte stores resulting from loss of excretory function. Studies in animals have not resolved the argument. In previously normotensive men, bilateral nephrectomy does not result in hypertension, provided body hydration is rigidly controlled by fluid and salt restriction. An increase in blood pressure always follows expansion of blood volume and extracellular fluid volume. Hypertension is often improved by bilateral nephrectomy and usually remits completely after successful kidney grafting [268, 269].

The interrelationships of the two kidneys in experimental renovascular hypertension are of interest. Removal of the opposite normal kidney in an animal with unilateral renal arterial constriction usually leads to a worsening of the hypertension [139, 141]. The transplantation of a normal kidney into the neck of a dog with renal arterial constriction and hypertension often results in a decrease in blood pressure [217]. Thus the normal kidney restrains, but does not completely prevent or reverse, hypertension due to renal arterial constriction. Blaquier et al. [38, 142] similarly observed a fall in blood pressure upon transplanting normal kidneys into rats with hypertension due to figure-of-eight ligatures on their one remaining kidney. They also found that transplantation of such kidneys into nephrectomized rats with hypertension induced by infusion of hog renin did not lower the blood pressure; thus under the conditions of their experiments the transplanted kidneys do not appear to work by inactivating renin.

Tobian et al. [395] have carried this approach even further, and have found that when a connection between the transplanted normal kidney and the animal with Goldblatt hypertension is made with a short length of polyethylene tubing, such that the added kidney is perfused at a high pressure, the blood pressure of such animals changes 90 per cent toward normal in two and one-half hours; when the perfusion is kept at a low pressure through a longer connecting tubing, the blood pressure falls only 35 per cent toward normal. Thus the antihypertensive action of the normal kidney is apparently stimulated by elevated pressure, not by the composition of the blood perfusing it.

Furthermore, this renal vasodepressor effect is due to some nonexcretory function of the kidney. Transplantation of the ureter of the normal kidney into the inferior vena cava does not alter any of the results already described [117, 151, 335].

Removal of the arterial constriction almost invariably reverses the hypertension, even in chronic renal hypertensive animals, and even when the opposite kidney has been removed [117–119]. Thus, the constricted kidney is also potentially capable of counteracting the hypertensive mechanism, but is restrained from doing so by the arterial constriction. Denervation makes no difference in any of these reversals.

All of the foregoing evidence has led to the speculation that the constricted kidney secretes some substance, which may be renin, that suppresses the normal kidney's antihypertensive function. The normal kidney may be so much more sensitive to small amounts of renin than other tissues that the amount of renin required to suppress its antihypertensive function may be too small to be detected by current methods [119, 393].

There is current interest in vasodepressor renomedullary prostaglandins [178], vasodepressor renomedullary lipid [284], and a phospholipid found in kidney and plasma which inhibits renin [350, 368]. The last compound also reduces the blood pressure of rats with acute and chronic renal hypertension, but it has no effect on the blood pressure of normotensive rats. The exact role of these factors in renal hypertension remains to be determined.

ROLE OF RENAL ARTERIAL CONSTRICTION IN HUMAN HYPERTENSION

Even before Goldblatt's demonstration that unilateral arterial constriction could produce significant systemic hypertension, an association between unilateral renal disease and hypertension had been noted in clinicopathologic material. Ask-Upmark [16], in 1929, had reported five cases of girls who at postmortem examination had malignant nephrosclerosis and unilateral renal abnormalities, consisting of difference in the size of the kidneys, deformity with duplication of the renal pelvis and vessels, and poor development of the renal pelvis. However, just as in experimental work, also in clinical investigation, it was Goldblatt's 1934 publication which stimulated a great interest in unilateral renal lesions as a cause of hypertension.

The first report of this diagnosis in life, and of cure of the hypertension by unilateral nephrectomy, was that of Butler [58] in 1937, of two instances of unilateral pyelonephritis in children. The first report of a stenotic lesion of a renal artery causing hypertension and cured by nephrectomy was that of Leadbetter and Burkland [226] in 1938. In their patient, a 5½-year-old child, who had had hypertension since the age of 3, the hypertension was cured by removal of a small kidney supplied by a partially occluded renal artery which, in retrospect, may have shown the changes of fibromuscular dysplasia [424]. The glomeruli and tubules of the excised kidney were said to be normal in appearance. The youngest reported case is that of a male infant with malignant hypertension and congestive heart failure who was cured by nephrectomy on the eighth day of life [76]. Numerous types of lesions have since been shown to result in renovascular hypertension. The following list summarizes the lesions reported; references give illustrative cases or reviews.

LESIONS PRODUCING RENOVASCULAR HYPERTENSION*

A. Intrinsic renal vascular lesions
   1. Atherosclerosis (see pages 777–778)
   2. Fibromuscular dysplasia (see pages 777–778)
   3. Renal artery aneurysm [209]
   4. Thrombosis or embolism [185, 209, 245, 352]
   5. Renal arteriovenous fistula [209]
   6. Miscellaneous arteritides
      a. Takayashu's disease [17, 399]
      b. Thromboangiitis [255]
      c. Syphilitic arteritis [325]
      d. Periarteritis nodosa [230]
   7. Renal vein thrombosis [147]
B. Extrinsic lesions
   1. Atherosclerotic or dissecting aneurysm of the aorta [158]
   2. Trauma [221]
   3. Ganglioneuroma or lymphosarcoma in renal pedicle [39, 80, 155]
   4. Extrinsic fibrous or musculotendinous bands [82]
   5. Other intraabdominal tumors or cysts [110, 218]
   6. Coarctation of the abdominal aorta [90]

* Pyelonephritis and other renal inflammatory diseases not considered here.

Prevalence of Renovascular Hypertension. The prevalence of renovascular hypertension is unknown and will not likely be determined from the study of unselected hypertensive populations until simple definitive tests become available. Earlier large surveys [47, 372] may have underestimated the frequency of this condition since they were based on autopsy and surgical material and were carried out before the widespread use of renal arteriography. Smith [372] concluded that less than 2 per cent of all patients with diastolic hypertension are candidates for therapeutic renal surgery, but unilateral renal disease in the majority of his cases was due to pyelonephritis, unilateral renal atrophy, or hydronephrosis. Abdominal aortography frequently reveals stenosis of one or both renal arteries in hypertensive patients, especially beyond the age of 40, but this method does not discriminate between the functionally significant and the functionally insignificant lesions. It has been amply demonstrated that such lesions are not uncommon in normotensive subjects as well [100, 108, 181, 386].

Of 525 selected hypertensive patients studied by Perloff et al. [316], 195 had major arterial lesions; 122 were operated on and of these 76 had a subsequent fall in blood pressure, 45 (8.6 per cent) to normal levels. Of 220 selected but consecutive patients entering a study carried out by Foster et al. [122], 208 underwent an extensive battery of tests, and 44 (21 per cent) were judged to have functionally significant stenosis. The judgment in each case was based on a composite interpretation of the arteriogram, split renal function study, measurement of pressure gradient at operation, and response to operative treatment.

Recent epidemiologic studies in the United States [145, 308] are in agreement that high blood pressure is exceedingly common (approximately 15 per cent of adults with levels of 160/95 mm. Hg or greater). If the hypertension in 3 per cent of these persons has a renovascular cause, the number of potentially curable cases is large. It is probable that this cause exceeds the sum of all other known surgically correctible causes of hypertension, including primary aldosteronism [113, 204, 227].

Clinical and Pathologic Features. On the basis of accumulating experience with larger groups of patients, most workers now agree that on the whole, there is little in the history and physical examination, aside from an upper-abdominal bruit, to distinguish those hypertensive patients with renal artery stenosis from those without it [20, 21, 122, 188, 212, 265, 280, 302, 311, 416]. Males or females affected predominate in a given experience depending largely on whether the obstruction (or obstructions) is due to fibromuscular dysplasia or to atherosclerosis in the majority of cases; fibromuscular dysplasia most often affects females in the third or fourth decade, while atherosclerosis more often affects males in the fifth to seventh decades. Atherosclerotic obstruction of the renal artery appears to be less frequent in the Negro male than in the white male [122, 423] just as is the prevalence of coronary heart disease different between the two groups [247]. A family history of hypertension is as frequent in those with renovascular hypertension as in those with essential hypertension. The onset of renovascular hypertension is insidious, may be mild or severe [416], and is rarely accompanied by a history of flank pain, hematuria, or trauma. The mean duration of hypertension at the time of diagnosis is about 5 years. While abrupt onset, especially of the malignant phase, or sudden acceleration of the disease should arouse the suspicion of the clinician, this is not seen in most patients. The presence of an upper-abdominal bruit, especially if continuous throughout systole and diastole, correlates best with the presence of partial renal artery obstruction, and its frequency in such cases probably depends on the care and skill used in the search for it.

Hunt et al. [188] strongly suspect renovascular hypertension when severe retinal arteriolar narrowing and focal constrictions without any, or only slight, chronic hypertensive sclerosis are found on examination of the optic fundus in patients with hypertension of one year's duration or longer and in whom parenchymal renal disease and pheochromocytoma have been excluded. Hypokalemia appears to correlate with the severity of the hypertensive process rather than with the presence of a renovascular etiology [265].

While many pathologic processes (see above) may produce renovascular hypertension, obstruction of the renal arteries or their branches by atherosclerosis or fibromuscular dysplasia are by far the most common. Atherosclerosis usually involves a relatively short segment of the proximal portion of the main renal artery and is eccentric in location [245, 280] (Fig. 20-1). It occasionally involves a main branch supplying one pole or an accessory artery. Fibromuscular dysplasia is an interesting vascular disease or collection of diseases being found with increasing frequency [163, 244, 265, 305]. Women are affected more often

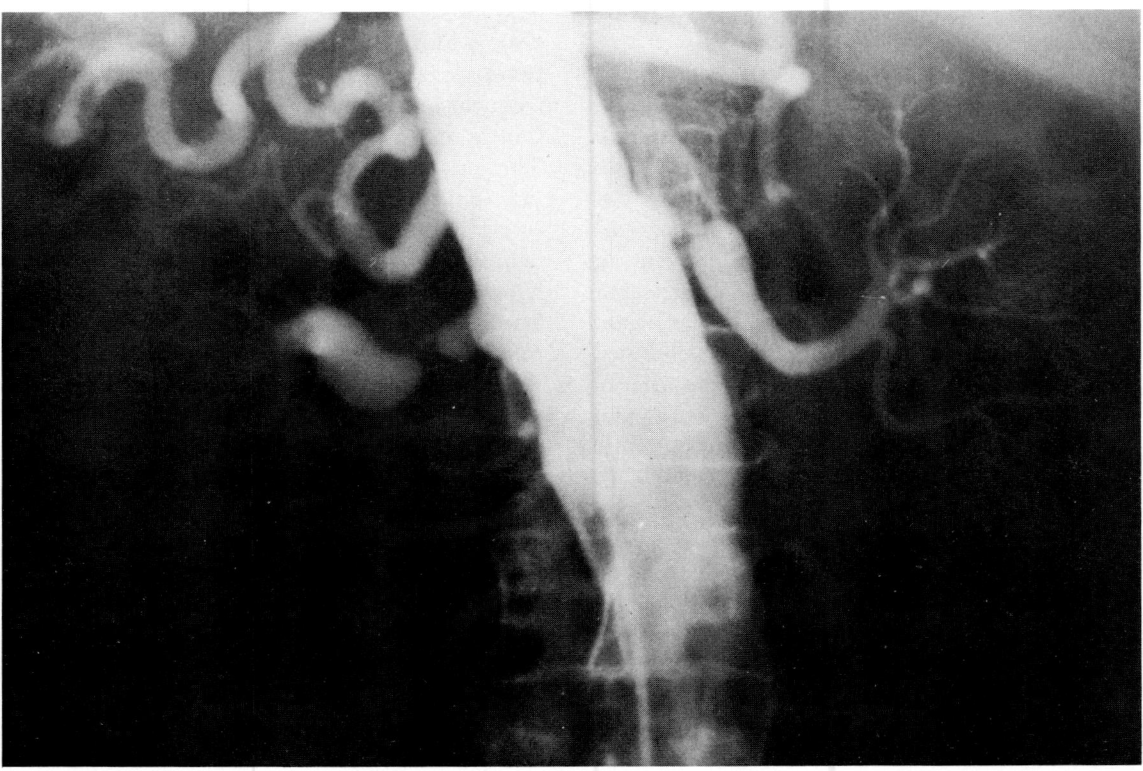

Figure 20-1. Atherosclerotic lesions in the proximal portions of both renal arteries producing severe stenosis and poststenotic dilatation.

than men (3:1) at an average age of 38 years. The lesion may be focal, multifocal ("string of beads"), or tubular, unilateral or bilateral, and characteristically involves the distal two-thirds of the artery (Fig. 20-2). Its occurrence in extrarenal arteries has been reported recently [163, 305, 327]. Palubinskas et al. [305] found that of the group of 70 patients with fibromuscular dysplasia of the renal arteries seen by them, 5 have one or more intracranial aneurysms, even though fewer than 15 per cent of the group have had cerebral angiography. There is a report [161] of two sisters in whom hypertension developed at ages 20 and 23; both sisters had fibromuscular dysplasia of the renal arteries (confirmed at autopsy), and both died of subarachnoid hemorrhage. Another report describes fibromuscular dysplasia (radiographic diagnosis only) occurring in each of three hypertensive sisters [157]. The etiology is entirely unknown.

The pathologic changes in human kidneys to which the arterial supply has been constricted or obstructed have shown the great degree of variability already described for experimental renal artery constriction (see page 770), including cases in which there were no significant renal lesions [245]. Ischemic tubular atrophy has been found to be better correlated with renovascular hypertension than any other pathologic finding [74, 210, 229]. The vessels of the two kidneys show differences, but these are not as clear-cut — i.e., normal "protected" vessels distal to the stenosis —

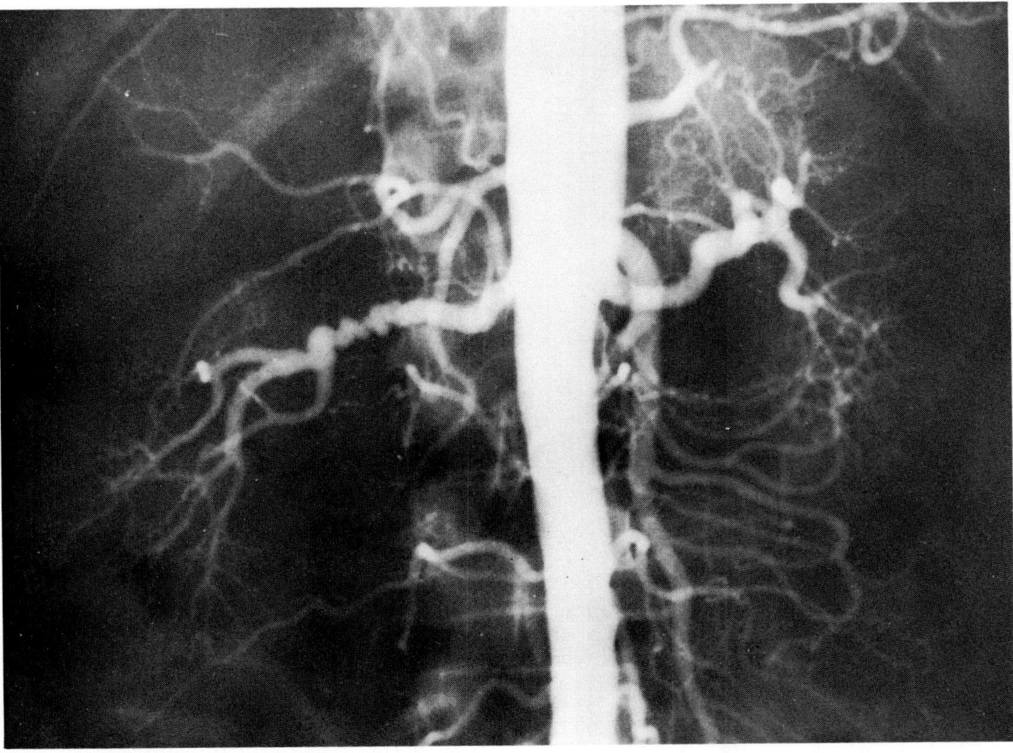

Figure 20-2. Fibromuscular dysplasia involving the distal two-thirds of both renal arteries.

as those reported in animals [210]. While the degree of nephrosclerosis may bear some correlation to the success of surgery [21], the evidence is strong that its presence even in moderately severe degree does not preclude an excellent result [21, 122, 342, 384]. The presence of characteristic histologic changes in the juxtaglomerular apparatus in human renovascular hypertension is controversial [265]. This is not surprising since the changes (predominantly hyperplasia rather than granulation as in animals) are unevenly distributed throughout the renal cortex [306]. Therefore, a biopsy from only part of the depth of the cortex, such as is often obtained in a percutaneous or open renal biopsy, may not indicate the overall change.

Diagnosis of Occlusive Renal Vascular Disease Associated with Hypertension. Except for the presence of an upper-abdominal bruit, no other aspect of the history or physical examination has consistent predictive value in differentiating essential from renovascular hypertension. Thus, there is an obvious need for a practical screening test. An ideal one has not been found, but rapid-sequence intravenous pyelography best approaches it. It is the single most readily available procedure of proved value. The isotope renogram has adherents, and at least one group [122] proposes that renal arteriography be done in any patient with diastolic hypertension in whom operative correction would be recommended if a significant lesion were found.

Advantages, disadvantages, results, and complications of proposed procedures must be

Table 20-1. Examples of Results with Three Diagnostic Tests

Author and Classification	Excretory Urogram No.	Excretory Urogram %	Renogram No.	Renogram %	Differential Excretion Test No.	Differential Excretion Test %
Prior summary [412]						
False positive	—		—		7/63	11
False negative	—		—		14/42	13
Baker et al. [21][a]						
False positive	6/20	30	3/15	20	1/17	6
False negative	1/14	7	1/10	10	2/12	17
Wilson et al. [416]						
False positive	11/127	8	—			
False negative	36/128	28	—		27/56[b]	48
Foster et al. [122]						
False positive	25/163	15	50/162	30	8/133	6
False negative	12/44	27	14/44	32	6/40[c]	15
Hunt et al. [188, 189]						
False positive	—		—		0/36	0
False negative	25/99	26	25/85	29	7/74	9

[a] Aortography revealed bilateral stenosis in 12 patients; surgery directed against the most affected side.
[b] 9 false-positive results in 29 patients with unilateral disease.
[c] 3 of 6 with false-negative results had bilateral disease.

considered. Examples of results with intravenous urography, renography, and differential excretion tests from several centers are shown in Table 20-1. Rapid-sequence films were utilized for urography, except in the series of Wilson et al. [416]. The Howard differential excretion test was used in all series except that of Foster et al. [122], who used the Stamey modification. False-positive and false-negative results of tests are judged solely on the basis of surgical results in the several series summarized before 1962 and in that of Baker et al. [21]; the judgment is based on a composite interpretation of all studies and on the response to surgery, when carried out, in the remainder. More prospective studies of large numbers of patients, all studied by means of multiple tests and followed for several years after surgery, are needed. The report of Foster and colleagues [122] stands out in this regard.

RAPID-SEQUENCE INTRAVENOUS PYELOGRAPHY. Howard et al. [182] first suggested the usefulness of the pyelogram in renovascular hypertension, and Maxwell et al. [264] demonstrated the value of early films. Its advantages include availability, relative safety, simplicity, and cheapness. The usual technic includes catharsis on the preceding afternoon or evening, overnight dehydration, rapid injection of dye, and exposure of films at 1, 2, 3, 4, 5, 10, and 15 minutes. At 15 minutes, oblique views and a spot film of the bladder are also desirable. In addition, a postvoiding film may provide an important clue with respect to lower urinary tract obstruction.

Occlusive disease of the renal arteries reduces renal plasma flow (RPF). The reduction in RPF decreases the volume of glomerular filtrate, which, in turn, leads to the excretion of urine with characteristics such that the ratio of water excreted to that filtered is diminished. This leads to increased concentrations of filtered, nonreabsorbed substances such as contrast media or creatinine. A decreased glomerular filtration rate (GFR) may result in delayed appearance of dye in the pelviocalyceal system. With severe grades of stenosis, atrophy of the kidney occurs. The majority of renovascular lesions are unilateral, but even with bilateral involvement both kidneys are not usually affected to an equal degree. It is on these pathophysiologic changes that most of the diagnostic tests are based and from these changes that the following criteria of a positive pyelogram have evolved:

1. Difference in kidney length, especially if this is progressive with time (1.5 cm. or greater difference usually considered significant)
2. Delayed appearance of contrast medium or hypoconcentration on one side in early films
3. Unilateral increased density of contrast medium in late films
4. Ureteral notching by collateral vessels [156]
5. Defects in renal silhouette in the nephrogenic phase suggestive of segmental infarction or atrophy

The presence of one or more of these criteria on a given side enhances the possibility that a major arterial lesion will be found. Manipulation of the pyelographic appearance by water loading or the production of an osmotic diuresis after the early films, by increasing the urine flow more in the unaffected kidney, may occasionally show relative hyperconcentration in the ischemic kidney, but probably does not justify the added labor involved.

Analysis of results in the recent, larger series reveals that a positive pyelogram was present in 72 [122, 188, 416] to 90 per cent [116, 213, 264] of proved cases (10 to 28 per cent false negative) and in 8 to 15 per cent of patients shown to have essential hypertension (false-positive results) [122, 416].

RENOGRAPHY WITH ^{131}I-LABELED HIPPURAN. This test, introduced by Taplan et al. [388], is based on external detection of the level of radioactivity in the kidney as the test agent is transported from blood to urine through the renal parenchyma. Disease entities interfering with renal blood flow, tubular function, or the urine evacuation system produce a change in the tracing. Renograms from unilaterally diseased kidneys may show either a general depression in all segments of the tracing or a marked prolongation of the excretory phase. The radioisotope renogram has the advantages of rapidity of performance and lack of hazard or trauma to the patient. The major limitations lie in lack of availability to most clinicians, in aiming of the collimated tubes collecting counts from the kidneys, and lack of specificity as regards renal artery stenosis. It may be superseded by the scintillation camera of Anger [8], which permits constant visual monitoring of the passage of the test agent through the parenchyma and pelvis of the kidney concomitant with the inscription of the renogram curve [55].

Although, with equipment in current use, the renogram is a reasonably sensitive method of detecting disparity of function between the two kidneys and has been judged useful in screening hypertensive patients for renal artery stenosis by some workers [21, 56, 418], nevertheless, most have been discouraged by the technical problems, and the high frequency of false-positive and false-negative tests [122, 135, 265, 311].

A renal scintiscan using chlormerodrin (Neohydrin) labeled with ^{203}Hg, in which the test agent accumulates in viable renal tubular cells, reveals tumors, cysts, and infarcts as negative patterns, but has not proved useful as a screening test for renovascular hypertension.

RENAL ANGIOGRAPHY. Renal angiography [209] is required for proof in all patients suspected of having renovascular hypertension and for delineation of the site and extent of the lesion when surgery is contemplated. In addition, it has the potentiality of detecting two curable lesions that may not be detected by any other procedure with the possible exception of renal vein renin determinations [272, 417]: (1) bilateral arterial constriction, in instances in which this is more or less equal on the two sides [102, 322], and (2) narrowing or occlusion of one branch of a renal artery, in which instances the function of the kidney may not be altered enough to be detectable [272]. Aortography is not infallible, however. At times technical difficulties make interpretation uncertain or impossible.

Percutaneous transfemoral catheterization of the aorta or renal arteries is the technic of choice in most patients today (see Chapter 4). Retrograde abdominal aortography by insertion of a catheter into the exposed femoral artery was introduced by Farinas in 1941. Pierce devised a percutaneous method of catheter insertion in 1951, and this was subsequently modified by Seldinger in 1953. This method can be used in all patients except those with evidence of advanced aortoiliac atheromatous disease and those in whom transfemoral catheterization is unsuccessful owing either to the presence of atheromatous disease or to extreme torsion of the iliac arteries. In such patients, some alternate technic must be employed if pursuit of the examination is deemed worthwhile. After aortorenal angiography has been performed, if better visualization of specific areas is required, selective injection of the individual renal arteries may be carried out as part of the same procedure. In addition to providing the ultimate in detailed visualization of the renal vessels, selective renal angiography avoids the superimposition of other visceral arteries often unavoidably opacified by aortorenal angiography and allows for oblique views that may better delineate the degree and length of the stenosis. Lesions that appear on the postero-anterior projection to be amenable only to nephrectomy can sometimes be shown to be suitable for reconstruction in selective oblique arteriograms.

In 22 patients with atherosclerotic renal artery stenosis and a pressure gradient of greater than 25 mm. Hg, Bookstein [42] found one or more arteriographic features indicating hemodynamic significance in 21 of 23 lesions. Klatte et al. [213], in 36 patients with unilateral renal artery stenosis, found an excellent correlation between the degree of stenosis as judged from renal angiograms and surgical cure in patients with atherosclerotic lesions and no correlation in patients with fibromuscular dysplasia.

Renal angiography, by the Seldinger technic and in experienced hands, is accompanied by complications infrequently, though they may on rare occasions be extremely serious or even fatal. Complications due to the contrast medium include allergic reactions and renal and neurologic damage. Based on experience with intravenous urography, 8.6 deaths per million urograms, or about one death in 120,000 injections can be expected [313]. Renal damage has been the most frequently reported serious complication of abdominal aortography [242, 274], but it can be avoided with careful technic and the proper choice and dosage of contrast medium [209]. Spinal cord damage is a very rare but important complication of abdominal aortography. Since 90 per cent of the cases of neurologic damage reported by Killen and Foster [208] were due to the older and more toxic medium, Urokon, it is expected that neurologic damage will be considerably less with newer media.

Local complications at the site of arterial catheterization include hematoma, hemorrhage, arterial thrombosis, embolization from dislodgement of atheromatous plaques, subintimal contrast-medium dissection of the artery, arteriovenous fistulas, formation of a false aneurysm, perforation of the vessel wall by the guide wire, and infection.

DIFFERENTIAL RENAL EXCRETION. The diagnostic use of separate measurements of renal excretion has grown out of the experimental observations of Blake et al. [36] and Mueller et al. [283a] that unilateral renal arterial constriction (or a controlled decrease in renal perfusion pressure [349]) results in a marked decrease in the rate of excretion of water and sodium on the constricted side. Selkurt [349] and many others [391a] have demonstrated the importance of changes in peripheral resistance or, autoregulation, in the distal vascular bed of the kidney. Selkurt's data showed that RPF, GFR, urinary flow, and sodium excretion did not change until the obstruction in the main renal artery produced a gradient of at least 40 mm. Hg distal to the stenosis. Mann et al. [256] had shown earlier that the lumen of an artery may be reduced 50 per cent without any change in blood flow, and that it can be reduced as much as 90 per cent before a 50 per cent reduction in blood flow occurs. Differential renal function studies may thus detect those lesions on angiography that have exceeded both a critical reduction (50 per cent) in cross-sectional area and the capacity of the renal vascular bed to maintain RPF.

In 1954 Howard et al. [182] utilized these observations in the establishment of a diagnostic test for renovascular hypertension. In their original and subsequent reports [74, 183, 184] they found that curable cases of hypertension due to unilateral renal disease almost invariably show the affected kidney to have a 50 per cent or greater reduction in urine volume, a 50 per cent increase in urine creatinine concentration, and a 15 per cent decrease in urinary sodium concentration as compared with the unaffected kidney.

A number of methods have subsequently been used in an attempt to improve the performance or interpretation of split renal function tests. Rapoport [328] suggested that the fraction of the filtered sodium which is excreted might be more discrepant between the two kidneys, and thus be a more sensitive indicator of unilateral renal disease than the criteria of Howard. Furthermore, by expressing this difference between the kidneys as a ratio (a "tubular-rejection-fraction ratio"), one does not need quantitative measurements of urine flow: The ratio can be calculated simply from the concentration of sodium and creatinine or inulin in the urine from the two sides (accepting the known error in the assumption that creatinine is filtered and neither secreted nor reabsorbed). Rapoport found the value for this ratio in 37 patients with essential hypertension or other forms of renal disease without evidence of renal arterial obstruction to be in the range of 0.62 to 1.62. In 7 patients with unilateral renal arterial obstruction he found ratios outside these limits, and found similar positive results upon calculating other reported data.

Stamey et al. [375, 377], recalling that experimental unilateral renal arterial constriction is followed by a relatively increased reabsorption of water by the affected kidney, independent of antidiuretic hormone activity [30], pointed out that the urine from such a kidney should contain a smaller volume and a higher concentration of inulin, para-aminohippurate (PAH), or creatinine than that from the unaffected side. These measurements can be made in the presence of a constant infusion of vasopressin plus urea in saline, an arrangement that produces an osmotic diuresis with constant, maximal antidiuretic activity and simplifies the collection of urine samples.

Birchall et al. [34] have advocated comparison of the urinary sodium-creatinine ratios in the two kidneys as the most sensitive determination of the differential excretion test. This differs from the Rapoport method only in the final method of expressing results.

A comparison of results obtained with differential renal excretion tests over the past decade by several groups of workers is shown in Table 20-1. It is apparent that the ability of the test to predict a favorable surgical outcome has varied in different hands, and that it has erred more toward false-negative results than false-positive results. It is generally agreed that the test is fallible in the presence of bilateral renal artery lesions and branch lesions. In a comparison of modifications of the differential excretion test in 101 hypertensive patients with either essential hypertension or unilateral renal artery stenosis [341] there were no clear differences between the accuracy of the Howard, Rapoport, or Stamey tests. There were few positive tests in the group with essential hypertension. Those with renovascular hypertension usually had positive tests.

While a positive differential excretion test indicates a functionally significant lesion, cure of the patient's hypertension depends on other factors as well. Surgical competence obviously varies, and skill in revascularization technics has improved markedly when recent results are compared with those of even five years ago. In addition, the function of the contralateral kidney is especially important when removal of the ischemic kidney is necessary. It has been found by at least three groups [341, 376, 403] that surgical cure is less likely when RPF to the "unaffected" kidney is less than 200 ml. per minute. This appears to be a more valid means of assessing the unaffected kidney than by morphologic changes in specimens obtained by renal biopsy, although exceptions occur with both. Thus it is important to incorporate measurements of RPF into the differential excretion test.

It must be noted that ureteral catheterization is technically unsuccessful 10 to 20 per cent of the time even in the most experienced hands [75], and carries some risk for the patient in terms of morbidity [83].

PRESSURE GRADIENTS. Determination of the pressure gradient in the renal artery at the time of operation has been used in an attempt to select those patients who are likely to obtain relief of hypertension. Stewart et al. [380] found that good results were obtained in 89 per cent of their patients with mean pressure gradients greater than 40 mm. Hg. Baker et al. [21] found that all patients in their cured group had gradients of 60 mm. Hg or greater. Most workers have not had such decisive results (see Chapter 4).

In recent studies in dogs, two groups [241, 390] have demonstrated that the pressure gradient is not constant but depends on pressure proximal to the stenosis and, more importantly, on vasomotor tone distal to the stenosis. They concluded that multiple hemodynamic events present during an operative procedure may alter renovascular resistance, and that these changes tend to negate the value of the pressure gradient in a stenotic renal artery as a criterion for operative repair. If a large gradient is found, there is a good correlation with a curable lesion; but the absence of a large gradient is an unreliable observation on which to base operative decisions. It also has the obvious limitation of being of possible help only after the patient has undergone laparotomy.

RENAL VEIN RENIN. Despite the attractiveness of the hypothesis that the renin-angiotensin system is etiologically related to human renovascular hypertension and that measurement of renin or angiotensin might be helpful diagnostically, many conflicting reports have appeared [286, 312]. The methods have been fraught with difficulty and only recently have reasonably sensitive and specific bioassay technics evolved. Several variables that may affect plasma renin levels [174, 190, 400], including exercise, posture, sodium balance, blood volume, drugs, and the accelerated phase of hypertension, have not always been taken into account. In addition, Gordon et al. [144] have shown that there is a diurnal rhythm in plasma renin activity in man. Finally, it now appears that the plasma renin activity in the peripheral veins is at approximately the same level as that in the renal vein of the unaffected kidney in patients with renovascular hypertension [417]. It is therefore not surprising that a direct correlation between peripheral vein renin activity and the presence or absence of renovascular hypertension has not been found in many studies.

On the other hand, a comparison or ratio between the renin activity of the two renal veins might yield information that is diagnostically or predictively important, and several recent studies support this possibility. Helmer and

Table 20-2. Renal Vein Renin Activity in the Diagnosis of Renovascular Hypertension

Author and Classification	Result No.	Result %	Ratio Between the Two Veins	Renin Assay Method	Type of Hypertension
Michelakis et al. [272]					
False positive	1/13	7.7	>1.4	Boucher	Essential
False negative	1/18	5.5	<1.5	Boucher	Renovascular
Winer et al. [417]					
False positive	1/10	10	>1.4	Helmer	Essential
False negative	0/9[a]	0	<1.5	Helmer	Renovascular
Fitz [114]					
False positive	3/14	21	>1.4[b]	Pickens	Essential
False negative	1/9	11	<1.5[b]	Pickens	Renovascular

[a] Includes 2 patients with branch lesions.
[b] Author's criteria were ratio > 2 and renin from diseased kidney > normal (4.1 nanograms per milliliter).

Judson [175] were the first to report success in predicting the outcome of surgery by measuring renin in renal venous blood. Successful results have subsequently been reported by several other groups [202, 254, 270, 272, 282, 417]. Rather than renin, one of these groups has measured angiotensin [282] and another assays undefined pressor activity [254]. Results from three laboratories [114, 272, 417] where sufficient details are given for comparison and results of surgery are known, are shown in Table 20-2. It appears that a ratio of renal vein renin activity between the affected and nonaffected kidneys of 1.5 or greater has predictive value which is at least as good as, and perhaps better than, other tests in use. Each of these workers used a different assay method.

Peart [312] has raised the important question of whether such measurements of renin *concentration* may be only a slightly elaborate way of determining renal plasma flow since if renin production from a kidney remained the same while renal flow were halved, the concentration in the renal vein would be doubled. Woods and Michelakis [422] have examined this question in a group of patients in whom bilateral renal vein plasma renin activity, effective renal plasma flow, and the results of surgery were known. The data indicated that increased renin activity reflected increased renin secretion by the kidney with arterial stenosis in the majority of the patients. Since the quantitative evaluation of renin release requires measurement of total renin secretory rates, the data required are renal venous–arterial renin differences and total renal plasma flow. Renal plasma flow in these circumstances could be determined by an indicator-dilution technic. The latter technic has been successfully used for the measurement of renal blood flow [71, 211].

Differences in renin between affected and nonaffected kidneys can be exaggerated by such maneuvers as lowering of mean blood pressure by drugs [202], by drugs independent of a fall in blood pressure [190], and by upright posture. A prediction that the modest disparity of renal vein renin ratios of the recumbent patient with unilateral renal artery stenosis would show maximal disparity after changing from recumbent to upright posture and minimal disparity after changing from upright to recumbent posture has been confirmed in a study by Michelakis et al. [273] and is shown in Figure 20-3. The near equality of renin concentration from the two renal veins after resumption of recumbency is thought

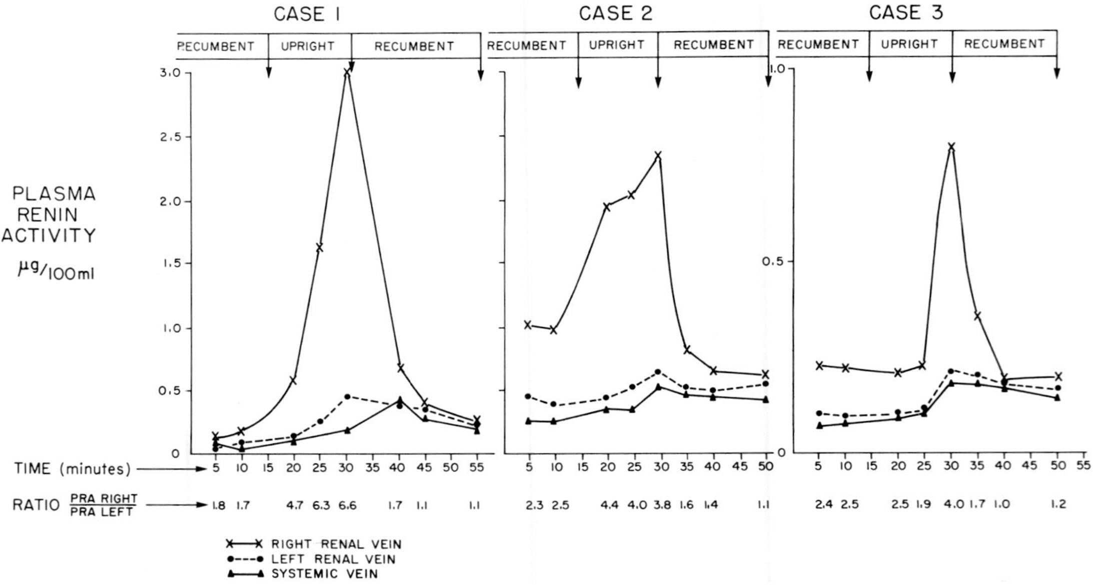

Figure 20-3. Plasma renin activity (PRA) from the two renal veins and antecubital veins of three patients with right-renal-artery stenosis. Samples were obtained simultaneously at five-minute intervals after nine hours of recumbency, during 15 minutes of erect posture, and after resumption of the supine posture. Peripheral PRA mirrors PRA from the unaffected kidney; the ratio between renal veins increases with erect posture; and, immediately after return to recumbency, the ratio approaches unity.

to be due to recirculation of renin through the unaffected kidney since the half-life of renin is in the order of 20 minutes. Peripheral vein renin activity was similar to that of the unaffected kidney. It is thus apparent that a rigid protocol should be followed in the collection of renal vein samples.

Catheterization of the renal veins in our hands results in fewer technical problems and a lower morbidity than does catheterization of the two ureters. This procedure like the others previously described, except for intravenous urography, is largely limited to medical centers at the present time.

ANGIOTENSIN INFUSION TEST. This test was proposed by Kaplan and Silah [204] as an indirect estimation of the amount of circulating angiotensin. It is based on the assumption that patients with increased endogenous levels of angiotensin will require a greater amount of exogenous angiotensin to obtain a given pressor response. Their results enabled complete separation of patients with functionally significant renovascular hypertension from those with benign hypertension. It did not allow identification of renovascular hypertension in those with accelerated or malignant hypertension. Several others who have evaluated the test have found that while those with renovascular hypertension *as a group* are resistant to infused synthetic angiotensin II and those with benign essential hypertension *as a group* are sensitive to the pressor effect of this agent, there is overlap between the groups, and the test is not highly reliable in the individual patient [51, 115, 291, 361]. Fitz et al. [115] found no correlation between results of the test and plasma renin levels in nine patients, and Nicotero et al. [291] found a depressed response nonspecific since it also occurred with phenyllysine vasopressin.

In summary, the most reasonable approach to the diagnosis at present is to offer rapid-sequence pyelography to all patients with significant diastolic hypertension (e.g., a diastolic pressure greater than 95 mm. Hg). In those with positive studies, and who would be acceptable operative risks if a surgical lesion is found, aortography should follow. If a matching anatomic lesion is present, bilateral renal vein renin determination or differential renal function studies, or both, should be done. If the patient has an upper-abdominal bruit, malignant hypertension (because of its gravity), onset in childhood or sudden onset especially beyond age 50 [316], or acceleration of the disease, aortography should be carried out despite a normal intravenous pyelogram. As aortography is not infallible, in exceptional cases the examination of differential renal excretion and renal vein renin levels may be considered despite a normal arteriogram.

It is apparent that tests in current use have greater precision in indicating a functionally significant lesion than in predicting the outcome of surgery when several variables are involved. Also, it is not necessarily true that the excretory and endocrine functions of the kidney can be correlated. As has been discussed earlier, large gradients in pressure across stenotic lesions of the renal artery are required to affect excretory functions, whereas small gradients may induce renin production [365].

Management of Renovascular Hypertension. Surgical correction of the renal vascular lesion or segmental or total nephrectomy, in certain patients, offers the possibility of a marked improvement in their condition. In Table 20-3 are given surgical results in twelve series reported since 1962 in which comparisons are possible. Of 1045 operated patients, an average 47 per cent were cured and 76 per cent cured or improved; the average mortality during the immediate postoperative period was 6 per cent.

Despite these beneficial effects on the hypertension, a note of caution is in order regarding the ultimate prognosis for patients with atherosclerotic renovascular disease. In a study of 109 such patients, Wollenweber et al. [420] concluded that improved prognosis for life but not for symptomatic cardiovascular episodes results from good blood pressure control by either surgical or medical means. When advanced atherosclerotic disease is present in the renal artery (or arteries), the frequency of associated atherosclerotic vascular disease is high, and the disease is apt to progress. Owen [296] has reported a similar experience. Consequently, surgical repair should be undertaken only when the hypertension is severe or, apart from hypertension, in order to restore renal function. Data bearing on the natural history of fibromuscular dysplasia are also needed.

The preceding section discusses the current status of methods for diagnosing renal arterial disease with hypertension and for attempting to predict which patients would benefit from surgery. The converse question must also be considered: What are the circumstances under which surgery of this type would be contraindicated even though evidence for a "curable" lesion had been found?

Page et al. [303] have suggested that surgery may be ill-advised if any of the following conditions is present:

1. The patient has extensive cerebral or coronary atherosclerosis.
2. Renal function is severely impaired.
3. An aortic aneurysm is present in the thorax as well as in the abdomen.
4. The patient is elderly.
5. Renal function has not deteriorated and the hypertension is mild, in a middle-aged person.
6. The surgeon's experience is inadequate.

These have been sound general guides. Some modification based on subsequent expe-

Table 20-3. Results of Surgery from Several Centers

	Author	No. of Patients	% Cured	% Cured or Improved[a]	% Operative Mortality	% Nephrectomy/ % Angioplasty	Criteria of Cure: Blood Pressure (mm. Hg.) Duration
1962	Stewart et al. [380]	43	40	82	4	51/49	"Normotensive" 2–24 mo.
1962	Baker et al. [21]	23	39	65	8	21/79	Diastolic ≤ 90 > 1 yr.
1963	Dustan et al. [101]	76	62	78	10	41/59	Normal[b] > 1 yr.
1964	Kaufman & Maxwell [206]	67	37	82	4	40/60	≤ 140/90 ≥ 1 yr.
1964	Owen [296]	63	43	69	9	37/63	Diastolic ≤ 90 > 1 yr.
1965	Hejnal et al. [173]	43	68	80	2	20/80	"Normal" > 6 mo.
1966	Fenton et al. [111]	15	53	67	0	87/13	Diastolic ≤ 90 > 1 yr.
1966	Morris et al. [280]	432	41	81	7	0/100	≤ 140/90 > 1 yr.
1966	Foster et al. [122]	35	46	77	6	46/54	≤ 140/90 > 3–40 mo.
1967	Hunt et al. [188]	100	55	84	0	47/53	Diastolic ≤ 90 > 1 yr.
1967	Baird et al. [20]	26	38	79	8	0/100	Normal[b] blood pressure[b] > 1 yr.
1967	Perloff et al. [316]	122	37	65	8	45[c]/55	≤ 150/90 > 1 yr.
	Total	1045					
	Average		47	76	6		

[a] Criteria of improved category variable — usually, easily controlled on mild drugs.
[b] Age adjusted.
[c] 22 per cent listed here had segmental renal resection for fibromuscular dysplasia.

rience may be made. Reconstructive surgery is not necessarily contraindicated in the presence of renal insufficiency if this is due to renal artery stenosis although the operation should obviously be approached cautiously. Baird et al. [20] have operated upon 10 such patients. Although the only two postoperative deaths in their series occurred in this group, they state that neither was directly attributable to inadequate renal function. Of the eight surviving patients, the BUN decreased postoperatively in five and was unchanged in three. Hypertension was cured or significantly improved in five and unchanged in three. Morris et al. [279] have described eight azotemic patients with extreme bilateral renal artery stenosis or marked unilateral renal artery narrowing with absence of the contralateral kidney who survived operation. Improvement in renal function followed operation in each patient, and hypertension was corrected or significantly reduced in all. The follow-up period was from 8 to 36 months in four.

Since branch-artery lesions in patients with fibromuscular dysplasia frequently necessitate nephrectomy, a trial of medical therapy should probably be undertaken first [188]. The same approach appears to be wise in children under 8 to 10 years of age because of the technical difficulty with reconstructive surgery involving very small vessels. Nephrectomy should not be done in children with fibromuscular dysplasia, unless drug therapy proves impossible, because of the possibility of later involvement of the contralateral renal artery [123]. Antihypertensive drug therapy has been found to be effective in many patients with renovascular hypertension who were not candidates for surgical repair [101, 360].

The surgical approach to renovascular hy-

enough to be easily palpated, and quite tender [267].

There is usually a leukocytosis. Albuminuria is the most common urinary finding, and microscopic hematuria has occurred in most reported cases in which symptoms have been present; however, this has often been described as only three to four red cells per high-power field. Gross hematuria has been noted only rarely [22, 143]. In several cases hemoglobinuria has been found [84, 185, 232, 373].

There is likely to be a temporary rise in serum and urinary lactic dehydrogenase and alkaline phosphatase, and serum glutamic oxalacetic transaminase. The possible diagnostic usefulness of these changes is discussed under *Diagnosis and Management.*

When the infarction involves a large part of one kidney, the excretory function of the whole organ disappears at least temporarily [28, 255]. Rarely, a large perirenal hematoma may develop, with the appearance of a mass, displacement of the kidney and ureter, and obliteration of the psoas shadow [7, 295].

Hypertension is a common development. Typically the blood pressure begins to rise four to eight days after the infarction [2, 11, 28, 45, 112, 143, 182, 232, 255, 258, 326, 340, 352, 382, 426]. It may remain elevated for two to three weeks and then subside coincident with the disappearance of other signs and symptoms, or it may be sustained. Discussion of the relation between renal infarction and hypertension is included in the first part of this chapter.

By three weeks, in instances of massive infarction, distinct diminution in the size of the kidney can be detected on x-ray examination [11, 143]. When only partial infarction has occurred, return of function has been seen by intravenous pyelogram or retrograde studies within one to two months [26, 28].

Thus, an episode of renal infarction typically pursues a self-limited course; it may not even be recognized while it is in process. Eventually there may be no evidence of residual effects, or there may be persistent hypertension with or without a detectable change in size or function of the injured kidney.

PATHOLOGY

Human kidneys, when examined within a few days after renal infarction has occurred, have been slightly to moderately enlarged, with tense capsules, and mottled discoloration over the surface of the infarcted area. Such an area almost invariably involves cortex and medulla to an equal degree, in striking contrast to the entity of renal cortical necrosis (see below). A thin rim of subcapsular tissue [201], and small portions of the medulla closest to the renal pelvis, may remain more or less normal, presumably due to the blood supply to these areas from capsular, ureteral, and pelvic vessels not involved in the major vessel obstruction.

The infarcted area itself typically consists of a central portion of necrotic tissue, in which, as time passes, there is loss of all cellular details. At the edge of the necrotic area, an area of infiltration with neutrophils is seen in the early days of the infarction. Surrounding this is an area of hyperemia and hemorrhage, the hemorrhage extending irregularly into the viable tissue adjacent to the infarcted area [2, 45, 84, 185, 201, 232, 408].

With the passage of time, the infarcted area shrinks and becomes replaced by scar tissue. There may be some revascularization of the area. Renal tissue at the edge of the infarcted area may show histologic evidence of recovery.

PATHOGENESIS: EXPERIMENTAL RENAL INFARCTION

The sequence of changes in the kidney following obstruction to the renal circulation has been of continuing interest to experimental pathologists. Cohnheim [71a], after studying experimental occlusion of the arterial supply to kidneys and other organs, concluded that the hyperemia which develops following such occlusion was due to reflux flow of blood through the veins. This view was refuted by Litten [236] and Welch [407], who showed that hemorrhage developed in the area of a kidney peripheral to the occlusion of an artery quite early, and at a time when the pressure in the veins was zero. Litten concluded that the hyperemia and hemorrhage came from the collateral circulation to the edges of the infarcting area, rather than from venous reflux. His findings have been repeatedly confirmed [205, 333, 354].

A number of careful descriptions exist of the day-to-day development of the changes following experimental occlusion by various technics [27, 120, 162, 205, 252, 253, 353, 354, 407]. Karsner and Austin [205] in particular stressed the appearance of hyperemia throughout the occluded area within two hours of occlusion. Beginning about four hours after occlusion, loss of hemoglobin from the red cells in the central area in which infarction is developing began to occur; by 48 hours loss of the color of the red cells in this area was almost complete. At 48 hours experimental infarcts have the same general appearance as human renal infarcts of the same duration.

At two days after arterial occlusion in rabbits, Sheehan and Davis [354] noted the appearance of occlusive thrombi in the small arteries at the point at which they crossed the edge of the necrotic tissue. They described much fibrin in the thrombi, which implied a constant bathing of this area with fresh blood from the living end of the vessels. Calcification may begin to appear in the dead tubules at the edges of the necrotic area within two or three days after arterial occlusion [103, 235, 354].

The development of collateral circulation around and to some extent into an infarcted area has been the subject of considerable study. Results suggest that there is both perfusion through existing peritubular anastomoses [239] and growth of new vessels [27, 253].

Very little attention has been given to the sequence of functional changes produced by partial renal infarction. As already referred to in the description of the clinical picture, a moderately large infarct is accompanied by disappearance of all excretory function, followed in the next few weeks by return of urine formation and the excretion of iodopyracet (Diodrast) or similar substances in sufficient quantity to give a satisfactory intravenous pyelogram. The temporary functional impairment may be the result of increased intrarenal pressure, but this has not been established. Marshall and Kolls [259], in 1919, reported one experiment in dogs in which they ligated the renal arterial branch supplying the posterior one-third of one kidney. The urine flow and excretions of creatinine, chloride, urea, and phenol red on the affected side all declined immediately to one-half those of the control kidney, a result equivalent to simple removal of a portion of the nephrons.

DIAGNOSIS AND MANAGEMENT OF RENAL INFARCTION

As already noted, an episode of renal infarction may pass entirely unnoticed by a patient or his physician. Even when present, the pain associated with renal infarction has often been poorly localized and has been mistaken for pain due to appendicitis and gallbladder disease. Evidence of a source of emboli may help guide the physician's thinking to the kidney.

When renal infarction is suspected, performance of intravenous pyelography is indicated provided overall renal function appears to be adequate for satisfactory visualization (see Chapter 3). Within the first two weeks after larger renal infarctions, pyelograms will be likely to show absence of or marked diminution in excretion of radiopaque dye on the involved side. Radiorenograms may also indicate nonfunction. However, areas of renal infarction large enough to produce sustained hypertension have been associated in some cases with normal or minimally abnormal pyelograms [258]. In such instances, renal scintiscanograms may be useful in identifying segmental areas of infarction [170, 220, 366, 419].

Because on intravenous pyelography the appearance of impaired excretion could also be due to obstruction of the ureter, retrograde study with ureteral catheterization of the involved side is indicated as the next step. In renal infarction without other renal abnormalities, this procedure will reveal a normal-appearing, nondilated pelvis and collecting system. Little or no urine will be found on that side, and intravenously injected dye (phenol red or indigo carmine) will appear very late if at all from the ureteral catheter.

With renal vein thrombosis, there may be wide separation of the calyces, presumably by renal edema, resembling polycystic kidneys [97, 427]. On retrograde study extravasation of dye into necrotic renal parenchyma may occur, producing a "smudged" appearance [97, 427].

The combination of history, signs and symptoms, virtual absence of excretory function on the involved side, and a normal collecting system, is strong evidence for renal infarction [28, 172, 255]. If renal arterial occlusion (as opposed to renal vein thrombosis) seems likely, and if an attempt to relieve the occlusion is to be considered, then arteriography should be performed [194, 220].

With the recent advent of procedures for measuring, in blood and urine, enzymes emanating from injured or necrotic tissue, increases in enzyme activities have been observed in a number of patients with renal infarction, and may help in differential diagnosis [6, 70, 97, 125, 130, 238, 358]. Typically, *serum* concentration of lactic dehydrogenase (LDH) and glutamic oxalacetic transaminase (GOT) rise on the first to second day after the onset of flank pain. The GOT usually returns to normal earlier (e.g., by the fourth day), whereas the LDH remains elevated for 14 or more days. The serum alkaline phosphatase begins to rise later, about the fifth day, and remains elevated longer, up to 28 days [97, 125, 130, 238]. *Urinary* LDH is elevated by the fourth day and returns to normal over the next four days; urinary alkaline phosphatase rises by the second day — sooner than the serum concentration — and returns to normal by the ninth day [130, 238]. These findings have been confirmed in experimental studies in animals [32, 125, 402], except that serum alkaline phosphatase rose within 24 hours in dogs [179].

Amador et al. [6] have discussed urinary alkaline phosphatase and LDH activities in the differential diagnosis of renal disease, and they report that, in addition to necrosis of renal parenchyma, urinary elevation of both enzymes is found in acute glomerulonephritis, lupus erythematosus involvement of the kidney, diabetic glomerulosclerosis, renal and prostatic carcinoma, and adrenocortical adenomas and carcinomas. It is possible that, through use of both serum and urinary measurements and inclusion of GOT, the differentiating value of enzyme activities will be greater. This may also be enhanced by separation of LDH into its isozymes: In one case of renal infarction studied in this way, only the $alpha_1$ and $alpha_2$ serum isozymes were increased, as in myocardial infarction and hemolytic anemia, and the isozyme pattern was different from those in a number of other diseases [70].

In instances of infarction due to arterial occlusion, radiologic evidence of diminution in renal size, observable as early as two weeks after infarction [143], is corroborative evidence for this diagnosis. Calcium deposits may be seen radiologically [98]. The extent of return of function may be evaluated by repeated intravenous pyelography at intervals of a month or more.

With increasing awareness of renal infarction and availability of arteriography for locating occlusions, surgery for relief of arterial obstruction is being reported, often with recovery of renal function [52, 98, 240, 315, 370]. Most reported cases were operated on within two to four days of onset of symptoms, but one patient had recovery of renal function with surgery 39 days after obstruction probably occurred [315]. Thus, although early diagnosis and intervention is highly desirable, an attempt at restoring arterial supply even at a later time is probably justifiable — for example, in cases in which the sole kidney carrying on the major or only renal function suffers arterial occlusion. The presence of even small amounts of arterial blood flow, such as through a partially obstructed vessel [26] or through collateral vessels [52, 315, 370], may be sufficient to sustain viable renal tissue. Support of these clinical data exists in the demonstration by Morris et al. [281] that a renal arterial pressure of 12 to 38 mm. Hg will protect the dog kidney against the extensive functional and histologic damage produced by total arterial obstruction for two to two and one-half hours.

In renal vein thrombosis with infarction, there is some evidence that early surgical removal of the involved kidney is associated with better survival rate [330, 362]. Attention should be given to the identification of the underlying process that led to the renal infarction and to the prevention of further episodes insofar as possible.

The only reasonable indications for surgical removal of all or part of a kidney with infarction due to arterial occlusion are the development of infection in the damaged tissues or the appearance of significant hypertension. By "significant hypertension" is meant either an initial hypertension so severe that it is life-threatening in itself and is not readily controlled by safe antihypertensive measures, or the persistence of hypertension beyond the first two to three months after the infarction has occurred [182, 362]. The indications, contraindications, and details of surgery for hypertension of renal origin are discussed earlier in this chapter.

Renal Cortical Necrosis

The term *renal cortical necrosis* is a pathologic, descriptive name for a rare, usually fatal disorder characterized by death of all types of tissues throughout much of the cortex of both kidneys, with sparing of the medullary portions. Both pathologically and in the related clinical features this disorder presents striking findings that distinguish it from simple renal infarction due to occlusion of a major vessel and from acute tubular necrosis. The diagnosis may be suspected clinically but can be established only from the typical pathologic findings in tissue obtained by renal biopsy or on postmortem examination. The pathogenetic sequence of events has been debated throughout the more than 70 years since the distinctive picture was first recognized, and unanswered questions continue to stimulate study of the pathology and attempts to reproduce the entity in laboratory animals.

Most of the original literature dealing with the clinical and pathologic features is in the form of case reports. In addition, good reviews have appeared from time to time [15, 96, 99, 160, 234, 348, 357].

CLINICAL FEATURES

Since the first descriptions in 1883, approximately 300 cases of renal cortical necrosis have been reported in the medical literature. More specific indication of its rarity is the fact that Ash [15], in 1933, found only two cases in the files of the Army Medical Museum. Other more recent series of patients with acute renal failure [225, 387] or of general autopsies [428] agree. An unusual concentration of cases — 13 in a period of only 17 months — was noted at the Cincinnati General Hospital by Wells et al. [409]. No explanation was found.

Cases of renal cortical necrosis have been reported at all ages. More than 30 cases are recorded in infancy and childhood, including onset in the antepartum period [63, 89, 107, 317, 339, 369, 405, 428]. Published data [351, 357] allow the crude estimation that renal cortical necrosis will develop in one in every 100 to 200 patients with premature separation of the placenta with concealed hemorrhage. Among women with premature separation of the placenta, the frequency of renal cortical necrosis appears to be higher over the age of

30 [96]; the frequency of the disease in this group is not related to parity, but is related to the weeks of gestation in that its occurrence is much higher between the twenty-third and thirty-first weeks than when placental separation occurs later in pregnancy [44, 94, 96, 233, 357, 369, 405]. No explanation for this last observation has been offered. If the cases associated with premature placental separation are excluded, then the incidence of reported cases is higher among men than women [96].

Even though the relationship between underlying disease and the events that result in renal cortical necrosis is not yet clear, it is still true that in almost all cases some other pathologic process or physiologic stress (e.g., pregnancy) has been present at the time renal cortical necrosis appeared. Conditions associated with the onset of renal cortical necrosis are:

1. Pregnancy, often but not always with preeclampsia or eclampsia with:
   a. Premature separation and concealed hemorrhage [15, 69, 96, 248, 292, 347, 357, 405, 409, 410]
   b. Septic abortion [18, 176, 234, 251, 331]
   c. Other infections [94, 128, 405]
   d. Nonseptic abortion [405]
   e. Placenta praevia
   f. External puerperal hemorrhage and shock [248, 307]
   g. Postpartum hemorrhage [48, 57]
   h. Rupture of dissecting aneurysm [233] [233]
   i. Possible sulfonamide reaction [405]
   j. Thrombosis of renal veins [338, 396]
   k. Preexisting renal disease [149, 225]
   l. Diabetes (postpartum onset of renal cortical necrosis) [44]
   m. No abnormality other than eclampsia, probably [81, 186, 345]
2. Cases in infancy and childhood, associated with:
   a. Vomiting, diarrhea, usually fever [63, 89, 99, 107, 369, 409, 428]
   b. Infections: pharyngitis, tonsillitis, scarlatina, tuberculosis, peritonitis, staphylococcal septicemia, pneumonia [9, 63, 91, 107, 199, 404, 428]
   c. Transfusion reaction [405]
   d. Shock following traumatic delivery [428]
   e. Antepartum hemorrhage in the mother [339]
   f. Phosphorus poisoning [317]
3. Cases in adults not associated with pregnancy, associated with:
   a. Infection: tonsillitis, pneumonia, diphtheria, tuberculosis, peritonitis [9, 96, 99, 357, 381, 409]
   b. Vomiting and/or diarrhea [15, 99]
   c. Shock [96, 314, 409]
   d. Myocardial failure [404]
   e. Possible overdosage of epinephrine for a Stokes-Adams attack [154]
   f. Diethylene glycol poisoning [131]
   g. Cadminum poisoning [31]
   h. Alcoholism, ingestion of almond extract, injection of camphor (all in one patient) [96]
   i. Shock and ruptured liver [127]
   j. Second- and third-degree burns
   k. Snake-bite [294]
   l. Following resection of abdominal aneurysm
   m. Probable intravascular coagulation [383]
   n. Hemolytic anemia associated with thrombotic thrombocytopenia [129]
   o. No other disease or abnormality [15, 146, 409]

Premature separation of the placenta has been present in approximately half of all reported cases. Among infants, the most frequent associated problem is diarrhea or vomiting or both, usually accompanied by dehydration. Infections of various types constitute the second most common associated illness in children and adults. Most of the remaining cases have been associated with shock from some other cause or with the ingestion of a toxic substance such as phosphorus or diethylene glycol.

Among the obstetrical cases preexisting toxemia of pregnancy has been very common [23, 248, 292] but is not invariably present [425]. A number of cases give documentation for the absence of toxemia or of any abnormal urinary findings up to the time of the catastrophic event which ushered in the renal cortical necrosis [128, 348, 357, 359, 396].

The actual onset of anuria may occur with or without any clinical or historical evidence of shock or hypotension. In most of the patients with premature separation a shock-like state has been described [357]. Even though the blood pressure has often fallen only to normal levels, such levels may be hypotensive for many of these patients who were previously hypertensive as a part of their toxemia. In other patients shock and hypotension have occurred for periods up to several hours [232, 248, 251, 405, 409]. In infants who had diarrhea and vomiting it seems likely that dehydration and resultant contraction in circulating blood volume was a factor in precipitating the renal cortical necrosis. In most cases associated with infections, there has been no evidence to suggest a contracted circulating blood volume or a redistribution of blood volume. Thus the presence of shock or hypotension is a less constant finding in patients with renal cortical necrosis than in those with acute tubular necrosis [176, 387, 405, 425].

The body temperature is usually normal throughout most of the course of the anuria. However, MacGillivray [249] pointed out that in all eight patients with renal cortical necrosis observed by him a slight to moderate rise in temperature occurred on the second to third day after onset of anuria. This may be a useful differentiating point between renal cortical necrosis and acute tubular necrosis, for in the latter such a transient rise in temperature is said to occur only rarely [249].

These patients are repeatedly described as feeling well and mentally clear. Abnormal physical findings are minimal; there may be some tenderness in the costovertebral angle [91, 137, 409], but even this is often not present. A tendency for these patients to show more retinal edema and spasm of arterioles than other uremic pregnant patients has been claimed [263]. Very commonly a leukocytosis (up to 25,000 per cubic millimeter), predominantly neutrophils, is found in the first few days after the onset of anuria.

The rate of urine formation in most patients with renal cortical necrosis is very low and, particularly in the first few days, is often zero [409]. This point perhaps is of some value in attempting to distinguish these patients from those with acute tubular necrosis where total anuria is rare. Beginning at about the fourth or fifth day in the patients with renal cortical necrosis, there has frequently been an increase in the urine volume, up to 300 to 500 milliliters per day but rarely more than this.

Urinalysis, when urine is available, has invariably shown marked albuminuria and usually either gross or microscopic hematuria; the latter finding is more common in renal cortical necrosis than in acute tubular necrosis [409]. White cells are present in the urine in varying degrees; granular or hyaline casts have been mentioned only rarely. The pH, specific gravity, and chemical constituents of the urine have received little attention. In one case in which recovery occurred, the specific gravity, four days after onset, was reported as 1.020; the albumin content of the urine was not mentioned [146].

The clinical course of these patients is that of the development of the uremic syndrome, with nausea and vomiting, sometimes diarrhea which may become bloody, and ultimately convulsions and death. The duration of survival of patients in whom the daily urine has remained very small has been similar to that of patients with acute tubular necrosis [5, 136].

The blood pressure, if normal initially, has remained normal or only slightly elevated in most patients throughout the course of their anuria or oliguria, until death. However, hypertension [57, 136, 225, 409], or exacerbation of previous hypertension [69], has developed in a few patients late in the course. Effersøe et al. [105] have speculated that the decortication may prevent hypertension.

Calcification within the necrotic renal parenchyma is identifiable pathologically as early as the fifth day of anuria, and radiologically by the twenty-fourth day after onset [411]. In patients surviving longer than that, radiologic evidence of renal calcification is usually [4, 15, 91, 104, 105, 243, 276, 294], but not always [69, 192], present. At times it outlines the borders of necrotic tissue and gives a double or "tramline" appearance [237, 401].

The occurrence of focal areas of necrosis in other organs is commented upon below in the section on *Pathology*; in general, the correlation of clinical signs and symptoms with these lesions is poor. Patients with intestinal lesions have often had diarrhea, but whether this intestinal involvement is due to the same process that caused the renal cortical necrosis or is secondary to the uremia is not clear. MacGillivray [248] found that the blood urea levels in four patients with renal cortical necrosis and simultaneous necrosis of the anterior pituitary were lower than one might expect in typical anuric patients; this is consistent with the known effects of hypophysectomy on catabolism.

Ultimate survival of patients with renal cortical necrosis proved by biopsy has been reported in at least 17 cases [4, 43, 67, 69, 81, 92, 104, 105, 146, 150, 192, 225, 294, 383, 401, 411]. The histologic findings indicated that focal or patchy necrosis was present. Most cases have occurred since 1955, in association with prolongation of life by the use of extracorporeal hemodialysis until renal function returned. The longest period of severe oliguria (less than 50 ml. of urine per day), with survival, was 21 days [146].

PATHOLOGY

Gross Pathology of the Kidneys. The gross anatomic changes in a case of fully developed renal cortical necrosis are so characteristic that the description by Juhel-Rénoy [200] in 1886, one of the first reports of this entity in the medical literature,* may be presented as typical. His patient was a 16-year-old girl in whom anuria developed on approximately the ninth day after a sore throat and scarlatina; she died six days later. At autopsy:

> Each [kidney] is subjected to exact weight; each weighed 290 grams; they are thus very notably increased in size. Their consistency to palpation gives the impression of an almost woody hardness. The exterior surface is a violet red; it appears bulging in places. The capsule is detached very easily, without carrying along any of the renal parenchyma . . . The aspect of the two substances (cortex and medulla) is as different as possible. The cortical substance, *light yellowish in appearance,* in certain areas golden yellow, reminding one of laudable pus, forms a veritable band, a sort of shell which surrounds the limits of the medullary substance . . . In many places one notes variable degrees of extravasation of blood . . . The pyramids, in contrast, are dark purple, and in some places the color is frankly dark black. [Translated from the French.]

An excellent early picture of the gross appearance is reproduced as Figure 20-4. The gross features enumerated by Juhel-Rénoy may be discussed in more detail in the light of subsequent experience.

The size of the kidneys has been found to be increased in all patients for two to three weeks after the onset of anuria. Among those who have survived longer, kidney size has gradually diminished as documented radiologically [276] and pathologically. In two patients who

* The earliest recorded case appears to be one included by Frielander [126] in an article on nephritis in scarlatina, in 1883. The first reported case associated with the puerperium was that of Bradford and Lawrence [48] in 1898. It is somewhat puzzling that this entity, which has such a characteristic gross appearance, was not recognized by earlier pathologists.

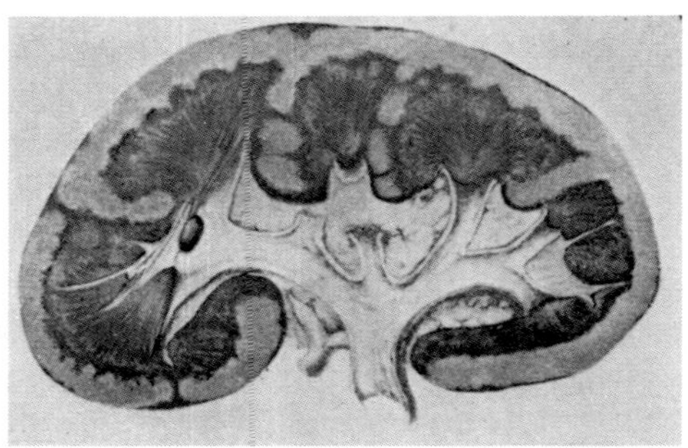

Figure 20-4. An early illustration of the kidney in renal cortical necrosis. The patient was a 36-year-old woman, previously healthy, whose seventh pregnancy terminated with a stillbirth with considerable loss of blood. She was anuric from the time of delivery until death, seven days later. (Reproduced, by permission, from Bradford and Lawrence [48].)

survived 79 and 116 days, renal size diminished to approximately 40 per cent of normal [5, 276]. The *capsule* usually is not thickened and strips easily from the kidney. Almost invariably 1 to 2 mm. of cortical tissue underlying the capsule has remained viable, even in instances of otherwise total renal cortical necrosis [2, 357, 381]. The *medulla* usually appears congested with blood but is otherwise normal; very rarely the boundary of the medulla has shown some necrosis [96, 347, 348, 369].

The variability in the extent of the cortical necrosis has come to be recognized as this condition has been studied more carefully. Sheehan and Moore [357], in patients with renal cortical necrosis following premature separation of the placenta, described typical lesions that ranged in size from small foci of cortical necrosis, not larger than 1 mm. in diameter, to gross necrosis of virtually the entire cortex, including the columns of Bertin. Cases described by others also show this variable degree of involvement. The few patients who have survived, in whom the diagnosis has been made by biopsy, have probably had incomplete, patchy necrosis. It is likely that other patients have had such minimal degrees of cortical necrosis that the presence of renal disease was not recognized or was considered to be acute tubular necrosis with recovery.

On gross examination, the renal vessels have shown abnormalities only occasionally. Thrombosis is never present in the main renal artery or its interlobar branches, and inconstantly in the arcuate branches or the interlobular arteries [214]. In only two case reports has generalized thrombosis of the renal veins in association with renal cortical necrosis been described [338, 396]. In occasional patients there has been gross or microscopic evidence of arteriosclerosis in the larger renal arteries [48, 137, 196, 225, 292].

The cortical necrosis has almost always involved both kidneys in approximately the same degree. Furthermore, in cases in which the necrosis is focal or patchy, the different individual lesions appear to be the same age both grossly and microscopically. One exceptional case has been reported as unilateral renal cortical necrosis — a patient whose opposite kidney was "protected" by narrowing of the main renal artery [12]. However, the data in the case protocol might also be consistent with malignant nephrosclerosis or embolic damage in the affected kidney.

Microscopic Pathology of the Kidneys. The microscopic findings show a characteristic sequence of events with passage of time after the initiation of renal cortical necrosis. Elucidation of this sequence in patients, principally through the work of Sheehan and Moore [357], has contributed importantly to the understanding of the pathogenesis of this disorder. (For a summary of these changes, the reader is referred to the first edition of this text [page 530], or to the original work.) The microscopic changes are discussed in relation to pathogenesis, below.

The full extent of the microscopic changes is reached by 36 to 72 hours after onset, the changes then persisting with little further alteration for two to three weeks. This is the stage usually seen in biopsy or postmortem material [96, 171, 233, 348, 357]. In areas of complete necrosis, the characteristic feature is the death of cells of all types without significant distortion or disappearance of the basic structural details [214, 220]. In the *glomeruli*, the capillary loops are distended with dehemoglobinized red cells, and all cells show pyknosis or loss of nuclei. *Tubular cells* show all types of "coagulation necrosis," with pyknosis or loss of nuclei and a stripping away of the cells from the basement membrane [214]. The afferent arterioles are lined with a thrombus composed, probably, of fibrin and platelets (containing very few red cells). The thrombus often occludes the lumen of the afferent arteriole and extends into some of the glomerular capillaries; usually it extends back into the intralobular arteries, more or less to the edge of the area of complete necrosis. In older lesions (7 to 14 days or more), organizing thrombus is frequently found in intralobular and arcuate arteries just outside the area of complete necrosis [177, 332, 357, 381]. The afferent arterioles and intralobular arteries in the necrotic area may show varying degrees of loss of intima, disintegration of the media, and diapedesis of red cells into the media. These vessels are almost always dilated. The veins in the necrotic area usually appear empty.

In the center of areas of complete necrosis there is evidence of a slight increase in interstitial fluid but no cellular infiltration. As one proceeds toward the periphery of a necrotic area, one finds a distinct zone of infiltration by polymorphonuclear leukocytes, a band 100 to 200 micra wide and occurring 200 to 400 micra inside the edges of the necrotic area [195, 348, 357]. This infiltration is well developed by the third or fourth day; the leukocytes disintegrate beginning about the sixth day, but a "smudgy" staining by their nuclear debris persists for some days [357].

The edge of the necrotic area characteristically shows a very abrupt change to normal renal tissue [2, 15]; many illustrations in the literature show one-half of the contents of a single glomerulus necrotic, the other half normal. Some degeneration of tubular cells may extend outside the zone of complete necrosis.

Few examples of the kidneys in renal cortical necrosis with survival beyond two to three weeks are available [5, 91, 136, 199, 276, 357]. Gradual shrinkage of the necrotic tissue and replacement by scar tissue appears to occur. There is some revascularization of necrotic vascular channels, including necrotic glomeruli. Deposition of calcium is a frequent occurrence, in necrotic tubules and necrotic glomeruli, beginning as early as five and one-half days and becoming more marked with the passage of time [5, 91, 132, 136, 225, 276, 405]. Typically it occurs in necrotic tissue immediately adjacent to surviving tissue [318]. The remaining areas of surviving nephrons show regeneration and hypertrophy of glomeruli and tubules [91, 357].

Pathologic Changes in Other Organs. The most important observation is the *infrequency* of pathologic changes in other organs. In a number of well-studied cases, including obstetrical cases, no lesions have been found in other organs [15, 48, 136, 214, 233, 428]. However, there are instances among obstetric patients with renal cortical necrosis in which necrosis has also been found in the anterior pituitary gland [186, 199, 248, 331, 359, 409], other parts of the brain [186, 196, 251, 331, 359, 369], liver [63, 137, 186, 195, 248, 338, 359, 428], pancreas [251], gastrointestinal tract [63, 194], spleen [94, 132], and adrenal glands [176, 251, 359]. These changes in other organs may or may not have the same pathogenesis as the renal cortical necrosis.

PATHOGENESIS

Hypotheses Based on Sequential Changes. From their sequential observations Sheehan and Moore [357] proposed the following explanation for the sequence of changes found in renal cortical necrosis.

First, an initial ischemic period lasting probably four to six hours is required to produce the death of tubular and glomerular cells which is seen in the earliest specimens. This ischemia may have its origin no more proximal in the vascular system than the glomerulus itself. There is then a *return of flow of blood* through these areas; the development of necrotic changes seen at 8 to 12 hours after onset requires exposure of the previously ischemic tissues to the circulation, and the fibrin thrombi in the glomeruli also bespeak some passage of blood through them.

Second, at approximately 12 hours another period of ischemia begins. Sheehan and Moore attribute this to "operative spasm" of the intralobular arteries, of six to eight hours' duration or longer, inasmuch as it is followed by death of the peripheral portion of the intralobular arteries and the afferent arterioles. This period of ischemia is then followed by a brief *second period of return of flow,* as indicated by the dilatation of the glomeruli and arterioles which occurs at 17 to 24 hours, the crowding of glomerular capillaries with red cells, and the appearance of thrombi in the dying arteries and arterioles. This is the last flow of blood into the necrotic tissue, as indicated by the fact that only 12 to 14 hours later (36 to 48 hours after onset) the red cells in the glomeruli lose their hemoglobin, thus establishing the presence of stasis and ischemia for the preceding 12 to 24 hours [353]. The very slow rate of autolysis that occurs thereafter in the central necrotic areas is also evidence for failure of any further circulation in these areas.

In summary, the basic abnormal process, in the view of Sheehan and Moore, is ischemia, probably due to vasospasm in the small renal vessels and not due primarily to thrombosis or to toxic damage to these vessels. Only in the final stage, after probably two periods of ischemia, is leakage of plasma out of and thrombosis within dying vessels implicated as a contributing cause to the failure of continued blood flow. It is proposed that the second period of vasospasm in the intralobular arteries is a "reflex" backward propagation of vasospasm set off by the first period of spasm and ischemia in the glomerular capillaries or afferent arterioles.

The hypothesis that ischemia as a result of vasospasm within the smaller vessels of the kidneys is the basic pathogenetic mechanism has also been proposed by a number of earlier authors [15, 96, 126, 197, 198, 348]. Three other major theories about the pathogenetic sequence have been advanced: In the first place, it has been proposed that a toxic agent damages the glomerular capillary epithelium allowing extravasation of plasma and a conglutination of red cells within the glomerulus, which is then followed by stasis and thrombosis [99, 171, 194, 369]. Secondly, the primary change may be thrombosis within the afferent arterioles and intralobular arteries [24]. Specifically, in patients with premature separation and concealed hemorrhage, it has been proposed that the release of thromboplastin into the bloodstream from the placenta causes increased clotting, with the appearance of thrombi in these vessels of the kidney and other organs [250, 344]. Thirdly, it has been proposed that toxic substances, such as bacterial toxins, cause necrosis of the afferent arterioles and intralobular arteries, with resultant vasodilatation, stasis, and thrombosis [251, 289, 338, 367, 405]. McKay et al. [251] offer this sequence as an explanation for the changes found in patients with massive infection such as septic abortions, in which death may occur very rapidly (within less than 24 hours) with areas of necrosis in many organs in addition to the kidneys.

It is possible that the ultimate picture of renal cortical necrosis is arrived at through more than one sequence of changes [160, 171]. However, at least in the group of patients with premature separation of the placenta, the early findings described by Sheehan and Moore tend to eliminate all three of the above explanations. In other cases examined pathologically relatively soon after onset, thrombosis has also been minimal [15]. Furthermore, the almost invariable sparing of the subcapsular nephrons is consistent with this area's being protected from ischemic damage by its proximity to circulation in the capsule, whereas there would be no reason to expect that circulating toxins would avoid this tissue. Similarly, the occasional sparing of juxtamedullary nephrons would be surprising for a direct toxic mechanism, but can be correlated with the fact that the intralobular arteries usually remain patent for the first 0.5 to 1.0 mm. beyond their origin from the arcuate arteries, which allows preservation of circulation to the first branches of the intralobular arteries into the juxtamedullary glomeruli [357].

Any theory about the event or events precipitating renal cortical necrosis must account for the following observations which seem to be clearly established in the many case reports:

1. The precipitating process in the majority of instances affects the renal cortex without producing recognizable damage in any other organ. As Klotz [214] stated in 1908, "what is most striking is that a very definite part of a functioning organ should be completely affected by a process of infarction." In the minority of cases in which focal necrosis or thrombosis in other organs has been found, there have been no features to set them apart from the cases without such involvement.

2. There need be no underlying disease of renal parenchyma or renal vessels, although arteriosclerosis in the renal arteries, occasionally present, may in some way predispose to the development of renal cortical necrosis.

3. A general failure of the systemic circulation, as evidenced by a serious fall in blood pressure or clinical signs of shock, is not a necessary element in initiating renal cortical necrosis (see pages 794–797) [176, 357, 405, 425].

4. No known external toxin or type of infection is a necessary part of the development of renal cortical necrosis, as demonstrated by the large number of cases associated with pregnancy, in most of which there was no evidence for infection. On the other hand, certain specific external agents can apparently initiate the process.

The above points, composed largely of factors which are *not* necessary for the initiation of renal cortical necrosis, narrow the site to the kidneys themselves. The evidence reviewed in the preceding section appears to support most strongly the view that the initiating event produces ischemia due to vasospasm of the smaller arteries and afferent arterioles. The initiating factor could conceivably be either the action of some circulating substance that directly stimulates vasospasm of the small renal vessels, or the action of a neurogenic mechanism that affects the renal vessels alone or out of proportion to neurogenic effects in any other areas. A circulating vasospastic substance in a relatively small number of cases could be an extrinsic substance, but in most instances it would have to be something elaborated by the person himself—either a normal substance such as epinephrine or oxytocin, elaborated in abnormal amounts; or an abnormal substance such as an "eclamptic" toxin; or a normal substance acting upon renal vessels which were unusually hypersensitive to it, such as may occur in pregnancy. The experimental studies reviewed below throw some light on these possibilities.

Experimental Production of Lesions Resembling Renal Cortical Necrosis. A pathologic picture resembling human renal cortical necrosis has been produced experimentally by several technics.

OBSTRUCTION OF MAJOR RENAL VESSELS, AND SUSTAINED HYPOTENSION. Sheehan and Davis have made a systematic study of the pathologic effects of constriction of the major renal vessels of rabbits [353–355]. Their findings relevant to renal cortical necrosis indicated, first, that permanent ischemia leads to a much more rapid sequence of changes in the necrotic tissue than is seen in human renal cortical necrosis; and second, that the *medulla* is more sensitive to temporary general ischemia than the cortex. These results supported the view [357] that in human renal cortical necrosis periods of vasospasm are followed by temporary reflow of blood, and that the origin of the ischemia must be localized in cortical intralobular arteries or more peripherally.

By clamping the renal pedicle for two and one-half to six hours and then removing the clamp, Sheehan and Davis [355], by frequent sequential observation, found evidence of a return of pulsation and blood flow for 30 to 60 minutes which then faded away, to be followed by generalized necrosis. This sequence begins to resemble that postulated by Sheehan and Moore in human renal cortical necrosis. However, Sheehan and Davis were unable to establish the cause of the failure to sustain the renal circulation after this brief period of return flow. Sequential studies using radiographic technics to look for evidence of spasm developing during this early period would be informative. Daniel et al. [85] have observed by angiography rather marked patchy vasoconstriction of the peripheral cortical vessels in the kidneys of rabbits, 24 and 48 hours after clamping the pedicle for two hours. They did not make earlier observations. Other studies in rats [215a] and dogs [41, 385] tend to corroborate the findings of Sheehan and Davis in rabbits.

NEUROGENIC VASOSPASM AND ISCHEMIA. The possible role of neurogenic stimuli to the small arteries of the kidney in producing cortical vasospasm and ischemia has been the subject of repeated but inconclusive investigation. Milles et al. [275], in 1932, demonstrated radiographically that a denervated rabbit kidney responded to chilling of the animal with less vasoconstriction of the peripheral renal arteries than did the opposite control kidney. Trueta et al. [398] presented evidence in rabbits that various neurogenic stimuli would cause marked blanching of the renal cortex with preservation of or increase in radiographic material in the juxtamedullary and medullary vessels. This and other similar lines of evidence were used to support the hypothesis of a juxtamedullary shunting of blood under nervous control. Subsequent functional and radiographic studies have given variable results which in general have tended to support neither the concept of a juxtamedullary shunt nor the role of nervous stimuli in bringing on renal cortical necrosis. The functional evidence was reviewed by Smith [371] and Bergstrand [29]. Neither Oliver et al. [293] nor Schlegel and Moses [343], in experimental studies of the renal circulation in rabbits by the fluorescent-dye technic, were able to find evidence for a medullary shunt.

Massive electrical stimulation of the nerves to the kidney will produce a temporary cessation of blood flow through the kidney, but after about a half hour there is a patchy return of blood flow which ultimately reaches normal levels [40]. The medulla may appear congested at a time when there is actually no flow through cortex or medulla [41]. Clamping one renal artery of a dog, or insertion of a catheter into one renal vein, will also produce temporary anuria and a fall in renal plasma flow and creatinine clearance in the opposite kidney, with return to normal within three hours.

Thus, in all these studies it has not been possible to show a sustained vasospastic and ischemic effect by neurogenic pathways. The possibly necessary role of the sympathetic nervous system in endotoxin-induced renal cortical necrosis is discussed below.

EFFECTS OF BACTERIAL TOXINS AND SIMILAR SUBSTANCES. The intravenous [138, 290, 334, 403a] or renal arterial [369] injection of staphylococcal toxin in rabbits produces renal damage which when fully developed grossly resembles the later changes seen in human renal cortical necrosis. However, the early changes are quite different from those observed by Sheehan and Moore [357] in their early cases of human renal cortical necrosis.

Glynn [138] made sequential observations after injecting staphylococcal toxin and found beginning dilatation of glomerular capillaries and afferent arterioles, and changes in the mitochondria of convoluted tubules, within five minutes after injection. Necrosis began as early as five hours and was extensive by 24 hours. The early lesions followed a segmental distribution, suggesting that the site of damage was in the intralobular arteries or beyond them, and that certain areas were more sensitive to the injected toxin than others. Furthermore, there is evidence of contraction of vessels and necrosis before thrombosis is visible in arteries or glomeruli — that is, evidence more consistent with a primary vasospastic process [266, 288]. The cases reviewed by McKay et al. [251] and Powell [323] may be examples of human renal cortical necrosis of similar origin. There are distinct species differences in degree of renal damage produced by this toxin [403a].

Injections of either washed meningococcus bacteria [35] or toxin derived from meningococcus or *Serratia marcescens* [390b, 391] or filtrates of cultures of *Salmonella typhosa, S. paratyphosa,* meningococcus, and *E. coli* [10], or purified *E. coli* endotoxin [25], given to rabbits either in frequent repeated or continuous intravenous injections or in two injections 24 hours apart, produce a picture that grossly resembles human renal cortical necrosis. There is usually hemorrhage in many other organs as well. This has been referred to as the "generalized Shwartzman phenomenon." The earliest change, seen within a few hours, is obstruction of glomeruli with eosinophilic-staining material which also stains with periodic acid–Schiff's reagent [390a]. The renal cortex, within 24 hours, shows thrombotic and necrotic changes of the intralobular arteries and afferent arterioles, packing of the glomeruli with red cells, and necrosis of glomeruli and tubules. *There is also frequently some necrosis in the medulla.* The renal cortical lesion will develop in pregnant [10] or cortisone-treated [390a, 391] rabbits after a single intravenous injection of bacterial toxin.

Most recent evidence, including infusion of thrombin and fibrin under various conditions, suggests that this type of experimental renal cortical necrosis is due to obstruction of glomeruli and small arteries by fibrin or fibrin-like material, leading to thrombosis. This in turn is due to endotoxin-induced defects in fibrinolysis or reticuloendothelial removal of fibrin, or both [73, 228, 336]. Defective fibrinolysis may be potentiated in pregnancy [257]. An intact sympathetic nervous system is necessary for the endotoxin-initiated effects [285, 304]. Endotoxin may produce its effects through an action on circulating antibodies [229].

This apparently conditioned type of response in the rabbit renal cortex to certain, generally gram-negative, bacterial toxins is more suggestive of the timing and pathology of human renal cortical necrosis than is the reaction to staphylococcal toxin. However, the glomerular lesion and the medullary necrosis suggest that this technic does not produce as specifically localized changes as the human disease. Furthermore, Apitz [10] was unable to produce similar effects in rats or mice and only to a minor degree in guinea pigs.

Other infectious agents or related substances which have produced renal cortical necrosis are the hog cholera virus, when injected in massive amounts into hogs [337], and horse serum or bovine gamma globulin containing killed, dried, group A beta-hemolytic streptococci, injected into rabbits [278]. The former agent produced thrombosis and necrosis of the arcuate arteries as well as smaller vessels. The latter substances produced areas of medullary necrosis. Generalized hemorrhagic lesions in other organs were present. These experimental models therefore also differ in several ways from the human picture.

THE EFFECTS OF NORMALLY OCCURRING HORMONES. Among normally occurring circulating substances, the experimental injection of epinephrine, vasopressin, oxytocin, or serotonin, each in abnormally large amounts, can produce the picture of renal cortical necrosis. Penner and Bernheim [314], by repeated daily injections of epinephrine intraperitoneally into dogs, induced renal lesions varying from simple increase in protein content of Bowman's space to necrosis of glomeruli and tubules. They attributed the damage to spasm in individual afferent arterioles, inasmuch as nephrons supplied by certain afferent arterioles were necrotic and those supplied by other afferent arterioles from the same intralobular artery were viable. One case report, that of a 54-year-old woman with complete heart block who received large amounts of epinephrine and ephedrine and developed renal cortical necrosis, suggests that this mechanism may be reproduced in humans [154]. However, that patient also had a period of asystole of at least 10 minutes and probably some further periods of shock. The "shock-like" appearance of most patients with premature placental separation and concealed hemorrhage, in the presence of maintained blood pressure, suggests the possibility of secretion of large amounts of epinephrine or norepinephrine.

Vasopressin injected into rats in very large doses (5 to 40 units daily) produced visible ischemia of the cortex and, within 24 hours, areas of necrosis of the renal cortex with sparing of the cells immediately subcapsular and sparing of the pyramids [60]. Smaller doses given repeatedly produced only tubular degeneration. In further similar studies, Byrom [61] and Byrom and Pratt [62] found that both oxytocin and vasopressin would produce renal cortical necrosis in ovariectomized rats treated with estrogen and progesterone. In these "sensitized" rats approximately 0.5 unit of oxytocin or 5.0 units of vasopressin were the threshold doses for the production of cortical necrosis. Both doses are very large in comparison to any physiologic amount of these hormones in the rat. However, it is highly interesting that rats "sensitized" with the hormones that might be circulating near term in pregnancy are susceptible to developing renal cortical necrosis when oxytocin, a hormone associated with labor, is injected, whereas the rat is not susceptible to injected oxytocin under other conditions. These authors point out that there is no evidence in human beings for an increased vascular sensitivity to oxytocin at the time of the increased uterine sensitivity (at term). The possibility of oxytocin poisoning has been raised in at least one case [176], a woman with a septic abortion who had received large amounts of Pituitrin for delivery of the placenta. She also went into severe shock. Postmortem examination five days later showed renal cortical necrosis and necrosis of both adrenal glands. Another possibility is that the shock and renal cortical necrosis were related to bacterial toxins from the septic abortion. Hypophysectomy will prevent oxytocin-induced renal cortical necrosis in estrogen-treated rats [219].

Page and Glendening [297] gave a five- to seven-hour infusion of serotonin and produced renal cortical damage with some areas of infarction and damage to arterioles. They reasoned that in human beings premature separation of the placenta releases thromboplastic proteins into the circulation resulting in clotting of blood. It is known that platelets upon being involved in thrombosis release serotonin into the circulation; this could be a source of serotonin which could produce renal cortical necrosis. Until there is more direct evidence for this hypothesis, it must be considered speculative.

OTHER TOXIC SUBSTANCES. The fatal human cases of diethylene glycol poisoning which resulted from the use of this vehicle for an early preparation of sulfanilamide showed renal cortical necrosis [131]. Studies in animals (rabbit, rat, and dog) showed that diethylene glycol alone would produce these lesions [131, 289]; there is more necrosis of small arteries of the renal cortex than is seen in most human cases. De Navasquez [289] emphasized the intensity of necrotic changes in the small arteries of the renal cortex. Reyna [332] produced similar lesions in rabbits by the injection of lithium carmine over several days; adrenal cortical necrosis also occurred. The sequential development of these lesions has not been studied.

An entirely different possible pathogenetic mechanism is suggested by the result of experimental choline or methionine deficiency in young rats or pregnant rats, in which varying degrees of hemorrhagic necrosis of the kidneys is a prominent feature [148, 277]. Hartroft [167], however, in discussing this experimental model, has emphasized that choline deficiency causes primarily tubular degeneration, and only inconstantly glomerular and vascular changes. He thinks that the latter changes are secondary to tubular swelling and obstruction of capillaries.

These various experimental studies demonstrate that severe damage to renal cortical tissue can be produced by a number of different technics that cause only inconstant damage to other tissues. This suggests, as does the analysis of evidence in the human cases of renal cortical necrosis, that the small vessels of the renal cortex are unusually sensitive to a variety of noxious agents and events. Whether these affect the kidney through a single common pathway, such as neurogenic vasospasm or vasospasm due to action of circulating substances directly on arteries and arterioles, is not yet clear. It may be that in certain circumstances the two possibilities just listed operate, while in other circumstances there is primary deposition of fibrin clots, and actual toxic damage to arteriolar and capillary walls.*

The fact that this disorder appears only rarely among those patients who have one of the apparently predisposing diseases (premature separation of the placenta, infections, etc.) suggests that there is something special about the individual in whom renal cortical necrosis develops. Duff and More [96] proposed that these persons may have an unusual degree of hypersensitivity of their renal cortical vessels to noxious stimuli.

As a part of future efforts to understand the pathogenesis of this disorder, it seems important to obtain more sequential information about its development, such as may now be done with serial percutaneous renal biopsies, and to attempt to design experimental models, particularly in pregnant mammals, which mimic more closely the conditions under which the human disease develops.

PREVENTION AND TREATMENT

Inasmuch as renal cortical necrosis, of whatever extent, results in permanent loss of the involved portions of the kidneys, with death the usual outcome among cases recognized to date, any feasible measures to prevent its occurrence would have obvious value. Unfortunately, as already described, there are thus far only minor clues available to help in predicting situations in which this disorder might be likely to occur. Therefore, the physician usually becomes aware of its presence when obvious anuria is noted, some time after any conceivable preventable steps might be taken. Furthermore, until the pathogenesis is better understood, only very tentative recommendations about prophylactic steps can be made.

Several types of experimental evidence give some hope that preventive measures may ultimately be found. The first is the finding of Sheehan and Davis [356], in rabbits, that deep anesthesia prevents the generalized renal necrosis caused by constriction of the renal pedicle for two to three hours. It is not clear just how the anesthesia exerted a protective action. Several lines of further inquiry seem indicated: the effect of the anesthesia on metabolic processes within the kidney tissues; its effect

* There is recent experimental evidence that swelling of perivascular cells in the brain following brief anoxia, probably due to the lack of availability of metabolic energy for the cellular sodium pump, leads to obstruction of the vascular lumen and failure of return of blood flow [69a]. It has been suggested that this sequence may operate in other instances of tissue necrosis, including renal [213].

upon the body temperature and any possible relations between hypothermia and protection of the kidney against ischemia; and the effect of anesthesia on neurogenic stimuli to the ischemic kidney.

Second, several studies show that denervation of the kidney, or the use of a ganglionic blocking agent or alpha-adrenergic blocking agents, will prevent vasoconstriction or cortical or tubular damage in certain experimental situations [275, 285, 304, 324]. If more reproducible evidence can be obtained for the role of neurogenic vasoconstriction in the onset of renal cortical necrosis, then various measures, pharmacologic and surgical, directed at blocking the nervous pathways, can be studied.

Third, Hatcher et al. [168] have reported that the production of a mannitol diuresis results in much better survival of dogs in which renal shutdown is produced by a 60- to 75-minute infusion of epinephrine. Finally, Thomas and Good [391] demonstrated that the renal cortical necrosis produced by two intravenous injections of bacterial toxins (or one injection in a cortisone-treated rabbit) could be prevented by administering nitrogen mustard three days before the injections of the toxin. This protective action of nitrogen mustard is probably related to its production of marked granulocytopenia [379, 391]. When granulocytes are present there is thought to be a reaction between them and the injected toxin, with release of substances toxic to the kidneys. Other more reliable ways of preventing this reaction may be found.

Until further knowledge is acquired, the only sound preventive recommendations appear to be to watch carefully and repeatedly for, and to take steps to reverse immediately, any signs of dehydration (particularly in infants) or hypotension or shock (particularly in the presence of pregnancy).

The management of patients with anuria or oliguria due to renal cortical necrosis is the same as that of any patient with acute renal failure of any type (see Chapters 10 and 17). The importance of differentiating renal failure from obstruction of the urinary tract warrants reemphasis. Although certain clinical features may suggest the presence of renal cortical necrosis rather than acute tubular necrosis, these entities cannot be distinguished with certainty except by renal biopsy. Even when a diagnosis of renal cortical necrosis has been established by this technic, one can never be certain in advance about the extent of the necrosis and about the degree of reversibility which may occur with time. Therefore, the object of management is the same as in acute tubular necrosis — namely, to sustain the patient by all appropriate measures, including dialysis where indicated, to allow time for recovery of all possible function. Again, it should be noted that a growing, albeit still small, number of patients with this condition have survived after having been sustained by repeated hemodialyses for as long as a month [4] (see page 797) — thus, no arbitrary time limit for the use of dialysis. Chronic dialysis or homotransplantation of kidneys will probably be the only ultimate solution to this usually fatal disease.

References

1. Allbutt, C. *Diseases of the Arteries Including Angina Pectoris.* London: Macmillan, 1915. Vol. 1, chap. 5, p. 309.
2. Allen, A. C. *The Kidney — Medical and Surgical Diseases.* New York: Grune & Stratton, 1951.
3. Allison, P. R., Bleehan, N., Brown, W., Pickering, G. W., Robb-Smith, A. H. T., and Russell, R. P. The production and resolution of hypertensive vascular disease in the rabbit. *Clin. Sci.* 33:39, 1967.
4. Alwall, N. Die aktive Therapie der Nier-

eninsuffizienz. *Deutsch. Med. Wschr.* 83: 1008, 1958.

5. Alwall, N., Erlanson, P., Tomberg, A., Moëll, H., and Fajers, C. M. Two cases of gross renal cortical necrosis in pregnancy with severe oliguria and anuria for 116 and 79 days respectively. *Acta Med. Scand.* 161: 93, 1958.
6. Amador, E., Dorfman, L. E., and Wacker, W. E. C. Urinary alkaline phosphatase and LDH activities in the differential diagnosis of renal disease. *Ann. Intern. Med.* 62:30, 1965.
7. Amar, A. D., and Gray, C. P. Perirenal hematoma following renal infarction. *J. Urol.* 89:652, 1963.
8. Anger, H. O. Scintillation camera. *Rev. Sci. Instrum.* 29:28, 1958.
9. Apert, M. E., and Bach, E. Insuffisance rénale aigue chez un tuberculeux. Necrobiose frappant exclusivement toute l'éntendue de la substance corticale des deux reins. *Bull. Soc. Med. Hop. Paris* 52:471, 1928.
10. Apitz, K. A study of the generalized Shwartzman phenomenon. *J. Immun.* 29: 255, 1935.
11. Arnold, M. W., Goodwin, W. E., and Colston, J. A. C. Renal infarction and its relation to hypertension. *Urol. Survey* 1: 191, 1951.
12. Aronson, S., and Sampson, M. C. Unilateral renal cortical necrosis and unilateral benign and malignant nephrosclerosis. *A.M.A. Arch. Path.* 51:30, 1951.
13. Aschner, P. W. The clinical importance of aseptic infarction of the kidney. *Amer. J. Med. Sci.* 164:386, 1922.
14. Aschner, P. W. Thrombosis and thrombophlebitis of the renal vein. *J. Urol.* 17: 309, 1927.
15. Ash, J. E. Bilateral cortical necrosis of the kidneys (angioneurotic anuria). *Amer. J. Med. Sci.* 185:71, 1933.
16. Ask-Upmark, E. Über juvenile maligne Nephrosklerose und ihr Verhältnis zu Störungen in der Nierentwicklung. *Acta Path. Microbiol. Scand.* 6:383, 1929.
17. Ask-Upmark, E. On the pathogenesis of the hypertension in Takayashu's syndrome. *Acta Med. Scand.* 169:467, 1961.
18. Atherton, H. E. Bilateral cortical necrosis of the kidneys in pregnancy: Preliminary case report. *Memphis Med. J.* 21:56, 1946.
19. Avery, M. E., Oppenheimer, E. H., and Gordon, H. H. Renal-vein thrombosis in newborn infants of diabetic mothers. *New Eng. J. Med.* 256:1134, 1957.
20. Baird, R. J., Wilson, D. R., Sider, R. C., and Rapoport, A. Renal artery surgery in patients with presumptive renovascular hypertension. *Canad. Med. Ass. J.* 96:1299, 1967.
21. Baker, G. P., Jr., Page, L. B., and Leadbetter, G. W., Jr. Hypertension and renovascular disease. *New Eng. J. Med.* 267: 1325, 1962.
22. Barney, J. D., and Mintz, E. R. Infarcts of the kidney. *J.A.M.A.* 100:1, 1933.
23. Bartholomew, R. A., Colvin, E. D., Grimes, W. H., and Fish, J. S. Facts pertinent to a rational concept of abruptio placentae. *Amer. J. Obstet. Gynec.* 57:69, 1949.
24. Bell, E. T. *Renal Diseases.* Philadelphia: Lea & Febiger, 1950. P. 258.
25. Beller, F. K., and Graeff, H. Deposition of glomerular fibrin in the rabbit after infusion with endotoxin. *Nature* (London) 215:295, 1967.
26. Bellman, S., and Oden, B. An unusual case of renal embolism. *Acta Chir. Scand.* 120:276, 1960.
27. Belt, A. E., and Joelson, J. J. The effect of ligation of branches of the renal artery. *Arch. Surg.* 10:117, 1925.
28. Ben-Asher, S. Hypertension caused by renal infarction. *Ann. Intern. Med.* 23:432, 1945.
29. Bergstrand, A. Studies on the Oxford shunt. *Acta Chir. Scand.* Suppl. 166, 1952.
30. Berliner, R. W., and Davidson, D. G. Production of hypertonic urine in the absence of pituitary antidiuretic hormone. *J. Clin. Invest.* 36:1416, 1957.
31. Beton, D. C., Andrews, G. S., Davies, H. J., Howells, L., and Smith, G. F. Acute cadmium poisoning. Five cases with one death from renal necrosis. *Brit. J. Industr. Med.* 23:292, 1966.

32. Bett, M. M., Skeggs, J. D., Johnston, G., and Hershey, F. B. Lactic dehydrogenase activity of dog plasma and urine following renal injury. *Surg. Forum* 9:65, 1958.
33. Bing, J., and Kazimierczak, J. Renin content of different parts of the periglomerular circumference. *Acta Path. Microbiol. Scand.* 50:1, 1960.
34. Birchall, R., Batson, H. M., Jr., and Brannan, W. Contribution of differential renal studies to the diagnosis of renal arterial hypertension. *Amer. J. Med.* 32:164, 1962.
35. Black-Shaffer, B., Hiebert, T. G., and Kerby, G. P. Experimental study of purpuric meningococcemia in relation to the Shwartzman phenomenon. *Arch. Path.* 43:28, 1947.
36. Blake, W. D., Wégria, R., Ward, H. P., and Frank, C. W. Effect of renal arterial constriction on excretion of sodium and water. *Amer. J. Physiol.* 163:422, 1950.
37. Blalock, A., and Levy, S. E. Studies on the etiology of renal hypertension. *Ann. Surg.* 106:826, 1937.
38. Blaquier, P., Gomez, A. H., and Hoobler, S. W. Role of the intact kidney in experimental hypertension. *Fed. Proc.* 17:16, 1958.
39. Blatt, E., and Page, I. H. Hypertension and constriction of the renal arteries in man: Report of a case. *Ann. Intern. Med.* 12:1690, 1939.
40. Block, M. A., Wakim, K. G., and Mann, F. C. Circulation through kidney during stimulation of the renal nerves. *Amer. J. Physiol.* 169:659, 1952.
41. Block, M. A., Wakim, K. G., Mann, F. C., and Bennett, W. A. Renal lesions and function following prolonged experimental hypotension. *Surgery* 32:551, 1952.
42. Bookstein, J. J. Appraisal of arteriography in estimating the hemodynamic significance of renal artery stenoses. *Invest. Radiol.* 1:281, 1966.
43. Boucot, N. G., Guild, W. R., and Merrill, J. P. Bilateral renocortical necrosis with recovery. *New Eng. J. Med.* 257:416, 1957.
44. Bounous, G., and Shumacker, H. B., Jr. Experimental unilateral renal artery stenosis. *Surg. Gynec. Obstet.* 114:415, 1962.
44a. Bourne, W. A. Nephrectomy in hypertension due to renal artery infarction with superinfection of streptococcal endocarditis by fungus. *Brit. Med. J.* 2:271, 1954.
45. Boyd, C. H., and Lewis, L. G. Nephrectomy for arterial hypertension. *J. Urol.* 39:627, 1938.
46. Boyd, G. W., Landon, J., and Peart, W. S. Radioimmunoassay for determining plasma levels of angiotensin II in man. *Lancet* 2:1002, 1967.
47. Braasch, W. F. Renal disease as a factor in hypertension. *Amer. J. Surg.* 56:209, 1942.
48. Bradford, J. R., and Lawrence, T. W. P. Endarteritis of the renal arteries, causing necrosis of the entire cortex of both kidneys. *J. Path. Bact.* 5:195, 1898.
49. Braun-Menendez, E., Fasciolo, J. C., Leloir, L. F., and Muñoz, J. M. La substancia hipertensora de la sangre del riñon isquemiado. *Rev. Soc. Argent. Biol.* 15:420, 1939.
50. Braun-Menendez, E., Fasciolo, J. C., Leloir, L. F., Muñoz, J. M., and Taquini, A. C. *Renal Hypertension.* Translated by L. Dexter. Springfield, Ill.: Thomas, 1946.
51. Breckenridge, A. Angiotensin-infusion test. *Lancet* 2:209, 1965.
52. Brest, A. N., Bower, R., and Heider, C. Renal functional recovery following anuria secondary to renal artery embolism. *J.A.M.A.* 187:540, 1964.
53. Brodie, A. H., Shimizu, N., Tait, S. A. S., and Tait, J. F. A method for the measurement of aldosterone in peripheral plasma using ^{3}H-acetic anhydride. *J. Clin. Endocr.* 27:997, 1967.
54. Bumpus, F. M., Schwarz, H., and Page, I. H. Synthesis and pharmacology of the octapeptide angiotensin. *Science* 125:886, 1957.
55. Burke, G., Halko, A., and Coe, F. L. Dynamic clinical studies with radioisotopes and the scintillation camera: I. Sodium iodohippurate ^{131}I renogram. *J.A.M.A.* 197:85, 1966.
56. Burrows, B. A., and Farmelant, M. H. The use of radioactive isotopes in the diagnosis of hypertension. *Progr. Cardiovasc. Dis.* 8:159, 1965.
57. Burt, R. L., and Kearns, P. R. Bilateral

cortical necrosis of the kidneys. A case report with laboratory and necropsy findings. *Obstet. Gynec.* 2:484, 1953.

58. Butler, A. M. Chronic pyelonephritis and arterial hypertension. *J. Clin. Invest.* 16: 889, 1937.
59. Buttarazzi, P. J., Devine, P. C., Devine, C. J., Jr., and Poutasse, E. F. The indications, complications, and results of partial nephrectomy. *J. Urol.* 99:376, 1968.
60. Byrom, F. B. Morbid effects of vasopressin in the organs and vessels of rats. *J. Path. Bact.* 45:1, 1937.
61. Byrom, F. B. The effects of estrogenic and other sex hormones on the response of the rat to vasopressin. *Lancet* 1:129, 1938.
62. Byrom, F. B., and Pratt, O. E. Oxytocin and renal cortical necrosis. *Lancet* 1:753, 1959.
63. Campbell, A. C. P., and Henderson, J. L. Symmetrical cortical necrosis of the kidneys in infancy and childhood. *Arch. Dis. Child.* 24:269, 1949.
64. Campbell, M. F., and Matthews, W. F. Renal thrombosis in infancy: Report of two cases in male infants urologically examined and cured by nephrectomy at thirteen and thirty-three days of age. *J. Pediat.* 20:604, 1942.
65. Carpenter, C. C. J., Davis, J. O., and Ayers, C. R. Relation of renin, angiotensin II, and experimental renal hypertension to aldosterone secretion. *J. Clin. Invest.* 40: 2026, 1961.
66. Cash, J. R. A preliminary study of the blood pressure following reduction of renal substance with a note on simultaneous changes in blood-chemistry and blood-volume. *Bull. Johns Hopkins Hosp.* 35:168, 1924.
67. Caton, W., and Sheldon, W. Referred to by Ober, W. E., Reid, D. E., Romney, S. L., and Merrill, J. P. Renal lesions and acute renal failure in pregnancy. *Amer. J. Med.* 21:781, 1956.
68. Catt, K. J., Cain, M. C., and Fohlan, J. P. Measurement of angiotensin II in blood. *Lancet* 2:1005, 1967.
69. Chervony, A. M., Biava, C. G., Schwartz, M. A., and West, M. Bilateral renal cortical necrosis, malignant hypertension, probable pituitary insufficiency, with survival. *Amer. J. Med.* 39:147, 1965.

69a. Chiang, J., Kowada, M., Ames, A., II, Wright, R. L., and Majno, G. Cerebral ischemia: III. Vascular changes. *Amer. J. Path.* 52:455, 1968.

70. Cohen, L., Djordjerich, J., and Ormiste, V. Serum lactic dehydrogenase isozyme patterns in cardiovascular and other diseases, with particular reference to acute myocardial infarction. *J. Lab. Clin. Med.* 64:355, 1964.
71. Cohn, J., and Gombos, E. A. Unilateral renal hemodynamics studied by dilution technique in man. *Amer. J. Cardiol.* 16: 820, 1965.

71a. Cohnheim, J. *Untersuchungen Über die Embolischen Processe.* Berlin: August Hirschwald, 1872.

72. Collins, D. A. Hypertension from constriction of the arteries of denervated kidneys. *Amer. J. Physiol.* 116:616, 1936.
73. Collins, R. D., Robbins, B. H., and Mayes, C. E. Studies on the pathogenesis of the generalized Shwartzman reaction: Production of glomerular thrombosis and renal cortical necrosis by intraaortic thrombin infusion in normal and leukopenic rabbits. *Johns Hopkins Med. J.* 122:375, 1968.
74. Connor, T. B., Berthrong, M., Thomas, W. C., Jr., and Howard, J. E. Hypertension due to unilateral renal disease — with a report on a functional test helpful in diagnosis. *Bull. Johns Hopkins Hosp.* 100: 241, 1957.
75. Connor, T. B., Thomas, W. C., Jr., Haddock, L., and Howard, J. E. Unilateral renal disease as a cause of hypertension: Its detection by ureteral catheterization studies. *Ann. Intern. Med.* 52:544, 1960.
76. Cook, G. T., Marshall, V. F., and Todd, J. E. Malignant renovascular hypertension in a newborn. *J. Urol.* 96:863, 1966.
77. Cook, W. F. The detection of renin in juxtaglomerular cells. *J. Physiol.* (London) 194:73P, 1968.
78. Cook, W. F., and Pickering, G. W. The location of renin within the kidney. *J. Physiol.* (London) 143:78, 1958.

79. Corcoran, A. C., and Page, I. H. Renal blood flow in experimental renal hypertension. *Amer. J. Physiol.* 135:361, 1941–42.

80. Cornell, S. H., and Kirkendall, W. M. Neurofibromatosis of the renal artery: An unusual cause of hypertension. *Radiology* 88:24, 1967.

81. Crook, A. Communication on necrosis of the cortex of the kidney after labour. *Proc. Roy. Soc. Med.* (Section of *Obstet. Gynec.*) 20:1249, 1926–27.

82. D'Abreu, F., and Strickland, B. Developmental renal-artery stenosis. *Lancet* 2:517, 1962.

83. Dahl, D. S., O'Connor, V. J., Jr., Walker, C. D., and Simon, N. M. The morbidity of differential renal function studies. *J.A.M.A.* 202:857, 1967.

84. Danhiez, P. Les grands infarctus rénaux. *J. Urol. Med. Chir.* 23:481, 1927.

85. Daniel, P. M., Prichard, M. M. L., and Ward-McQuaid, J. N. The renal circulation after temporary occlusion of the renal artery. *Brit. J. Urol.* 26:118, 1954.

86. Davis, J. O. Importance of the Renin-Angiotensin System in the Control of Aldosterone Secretion. In Williams, P. C. (Ed.), *Hormones and the Kidney.* New York: Academic, 1963. P. 325.

87. Davis, J. O., Carpenter, C. C. J., Ayers, C. R., Holman, J. E., and Bahn, R. C. Evidence for secretion of an aldosterone-stimulating hormone by the kidney. *J. Clin. Invest.* 40:684, 1961.

88. Deane, H. W., and Masson, G. M. C. Adrenal cortical changes in rats with various types of experimental hypertension. *J. Clin. Endocr.* 11:193, 1951.

89. DeAngelis, C., and Sochan, O. Bilateral cortical necrosis of the kidneys in a twenty-seven day old infant. *Amer. Practit.* 10:429, 1959.

90. De Bakey, M. E., Garrett, H. E., Howell, J. F., and Morris, G. C., Jr. Coarctation of the abdominal aorta with renal artery stenosis: Surgical considerations. *Ann. Surg.* 165:830, 1967.

91. DeGraeff, J., and DeBaan, P. Bilateral renal cortical necrosis: Recovery of urinary output after an anuric period of 31 days. *Acta Med. Scand.* 163:341, 1959.

92. Derot, M., Prunier, P., Roudier, R., and Prunier, Mme. Deux cas de nécrose corticale du rein. *Bull. Soc. Med. Hop. Paris* 76:812, 1960.

93. Divry, A. The mechanism of the hypertensive action of the kidney. *Arch. Int. Physiol.* 59:211, 1951.

94. Dolman, C. L. A., and Herd, J. A. Acute pancreatitis in pregnancy complicated by renal cortical necrosis and cerebral mucormycosis. *Canad. Med. Ass. J.* 81:562, 1951.

95. Drury, D. R. The production by a new method of renal insufficiency and hypertension in the rabbit. *J. Exp. Med.* 68:693, 1938.

96. Duff, G. L., and More, R. H. Bilateral cortical necrosis of the kidneys. *Amer. J. Med. Sci.* 201:429, 1941.

97. Duggan, M. L. Acute renal infarction. *J. Urol.* 90:669, 1963.

98. Duncan, D. A., and Dexter, R. N. Anuria secondary to bilateral renal-artery aneurysm. *New Eng. J. Med.* 266:971, 1962.

99. Dunn, J. S., and Montgomery, G. L. Acute necrotizing glomerulonephritis. *J. Path. Bact.* 52:1, 1941.

100. Dustan, H. P., Humphries, A. W., de Wolfe, V. G., and Page, I. H. Normal arterial pressure in patients with renal arterial stenosis. *J.A.M.A.* 187:1028, 1964.

101. Dustan, H. P., Page, I. H., Poutasse, E. F., and Wilson, L. An evaluation of treatment of hypertension associated with occlusive renal arterial disease. *Circulation* 27:1018, 1963.

102. Dustan, H. P., Poutasse, E. F., Corcoran, A. C., and Page, I. H. Separated renal functions in patients with renal arterial disease, pyelonephritis, and essential hypertension. *Circulation* 23:34, 1961.

103. Edwards, E. Acute renal calcification: An experimental and clinicopathologic study. *J. Urol.* 80:161, 1958.

104. Effersøe, P., Gormsen, H., Iversen, P., and Raaschou, F. Nyre biopsi-og Dialyseproblemer. *Ugeskr. Laeg.* 116:1715, 1954.

105. Effersøe, P., Raaschou, F., and Thomsen,

A. C. Bilateral renal cortical necrosis. A patient followed up over eight years. *Amer. J. Med.* 33:455, 1962.

106. Elliott, D. F., and Peart, W. S. The amino acid sequence in a hypertensin. *Biochem. J.* 65:246, 1957.

107. Eskeland, G., and Skogrand, A. Bilateral cortical necrosis of the kidneys in infancy. *Acta Paediat.* (Uppsala) 48:277, 1959.

108. Eyler, W. R., Clark, M. D., Garman, J. E., Rian, R. L., and Meininger, D. E. Angiography of the renal areas including a comparative study of renal artery stenosis in patients with and without hypertension. *Radiology* 78:879, 1962.

109. Falci, E. Sur la nécrose du rein. *J. Urol. Med. Chir.* 18:449, 1924.

110. Farrell, J. I., and Young, R. H. Hypertension caused by unilateral renal compression. *J.A.M.A.* 118:711, 1942.

111. Fenton, S. S. A., Lyttle, J. A., and Pantridge, J. F. Diagnosis and results of surgery in renovascular hypertension. *Lancet* 2:117, 1966.

112. Fishberg, A. M. Hypertension due to renal embolism. *J.A.M.A.* 119:551, 1942.

113. Fishman, L. M., Küchel, O., Liddle, G. W., Michelakis, A. M., Gordon, R. D., and Chick, W. T. Incidence of primary aldosteronism in uncomplicated "essential hypertension": A prospective study using elevated aldosterone secretion and suppressed plasma renin activity as diagnostic criteria. *J.A.M.A.* 205:497, 1968.

114. Fitz, A. Renal venous renin determinations in the diagnosis of surgically correctable hypertension. *Circulation* 36:942, 1967.

115. Fitz, A. E., Valenca, M., and Kirkendall, W. M. Angiotensin infusion test in normals and hypertensive subjects. *Clin. Res.* 13:206, 1965.

116. Fleming, R. J., Ellis, K., Meltzer, J. I., and Laragh, J. H. Hypertension and unilateral renal disease: The usefulness of modified intravenous urography. *Circulation* 32:682, 1965.

117. Floyer, M. A. The Role of the Kidney in the Mechanism of Experimental Hypertension. In Wolstenholme, G. E. W., and Cameron, M. P. (Eds.), *Ciba Foundation Symposium on Hypertension.* Boston: Little, Brown, 1954. P. 155.

118. Floyer, M. A. Further studies on the mechanism of experimental hypertension in the rat. *Clin. Sci.* 14:163, 1955.

119. Floyer, M. A. Role of the kidney in experimental hypertension. *Brit. Med. Bull.* 13:29, 1957.

120. Foà, P. Ueber Niereninfarkte. *Beitr. Path. Anat.* 5:275, 1889.

121. Folsom, A. I., and Alexander, J. C. Total infarction of right kidney: Fibrotic atrophy of left kidney. *Urol. Cutan. Rev.* 38:197, 1934.

122. Foster, J. H., Oates, J. A., Rhamy, R. K., Klatte, E. C., Pettinger, W. A., Burko, H. C., Younger, R. K., and Scott, H. W., Jr. Detection and treatment of patients with renovascular hypertension. *Surgery* 60:240, 1966.

123. Foster, J. H., Pettinger, W. A., Oates, J. A., Rhamy, R. K., Klatte, E. C., Burko, H. C., Bolasny, B. L., Gordon, R., Puyau, F. A., and Younger, R. K. Malignant hypertension secondary to renal artery stenosis in children. *Ann. Surg.* 164:700, 1966.

124. Freeman, N. E., Leeds, F. H., Elliott, W. G., and Roland, S. I. Thromboendarterectomy for hypertension due to renal artery occlusion. *J.A.M.A.* 156:1077, 1954.

125. Frahm, C. T., and Folse, R. Serum oxaloacetic transaminase levels following renal infarction. Report of a case and experimental observations following ligation of the renal arteries. *J.A.M.A.* 180:209, 1962.

126. Friedlander, C. Ueber Nephritis Scarlatinosa. *Fortschr. Med.* 1:81, 1883.

127. Furtwaengler, A. Diffuse Rindennekrose beider Nieren nach Leberruptur. *Krankheits Forshung.* 4:349, 1927.

128. Gaspar, I. A. Bilateral cortical necrosis of the kidneys. *Amer. J. Clin. Path.* 8:281, 1938.

129. Gasser, C., Gautier, E., Steck, A., Siebenmann, R. E., and Oechslin, R. Hämolytisch-urämishe Syndrome: Bilaterale Nierenrindennekrosen bei akuten erwobenen hämolytischen Anämien. *Schweiz. Med. Wschr.* 85:905, 1955.

130. Gault, M. H., and Steiner, G. Serum and urinary enzyme activity after renal infarction. *Canad. Med. Ass. J.* 93:1101, 1965.

131. Geiling, E. M. K., and Cannon, P. R. Pathologic effects of elixir of sulfanilamide (diethylene glycol) poisoning: A clinical and experimental correlation: final report. *J.A.M.A.* 111:919, 1938.

132. Geipel, P. Nierenrindennekrose und Fleckmilz bei Eklampsie. *Arch. Gynaek.* 124:231, 1925.

133. Gellman, D. D. Reversible hypertension and unilateral renal artery disease. *Quart. J. Med.* 27:103, 1958.

134. Genest, J., Nowaczynski, W., Koiw, E., Sandor, T., and Biron, P. Adrenocortical Function in Essential Hypertension. In Bock, K. D., and Cotter, P. T. (Eds.), *Essential Hypertension: An International Symposium.* Berlin: Springer-Verlag, 1960. P. 126.

135. Gifford, R. W., Jr., and Poutasse, E. F. Renal vascular hypertension: Diagnosis and treatment. *Progr. Cardiovasc. Dis.* 8: 141, 1965.

136. Gjørup, S., Killmann, S. A., and Thaysen, J. N. Bilateral cortical necrosis. A case followed during 51 days by means of hemodialytic treatment. *Acta Med. Scand.* 158:47, 1957.

137. Glynn, E. E., and Briggs, H. Symmetrical cortical necrosis of the kidney in pregnancy. *J. Path. Bact.* 19:321, 1914–15.

138. Glynn, J. H. The pathogenesis of cortical necrosis of the kidneys in rabbits following the injection of staphylococcus toxin. *Amer. J. Path.* 13:593, 1937.

139. Goldblatt, H. Studies on experimental hypertension: V. The pathogenesis of experimental hypertension due to renal ischemia. *Ann. Intern. Med.* 11:69, 1937–38.

140. Goldblatt, H. *The Renal Origin of Hypertension.* Springfield, Ill.: Thomas, 1948.

141. Goldblatt, H., Lynch, J., Hanzal, R. F., and Summerville, W. W. Studies in experimental hypertension: I. The production of persistent elevation of systolic blood pressure by means of renal ischemia. *J. Exp. Med.* 59:347, 1934.

142. Gomez, A. H., Hoobler, S. W., and Blaquier, P. Effect of addition and removal of a kidney transplant in renal and adrenocortical hypertensive rats. *Circ. Res.* 8:464, 1960.

143. Goodyer, W. E., and Beard, D. E. Diagnosis and management of renal-artery thrombosis: Report of a case. *New Eng. J. Med.* 237:355, 1947.

144. Gordon, R. D., Wolfe, L. D., Island, D. P., and Liddle, G. W. A diurnal rhythm in plasma renin activity in man. *J. Clin. Invest.* 45:1587, 1966.

145. Gordon, T., and Devine, B. *Hypertension and Hypertensive Heart Disease in Adults. United States. 1960–1962.* Vital and Health Statistics, Data from the National Health Survey. National Center for Health Statistics, Series 11, No. 13. U.S. Dept. of Health, Education and Welfare, U.S. Govt. Printing Office, Washington, D.C. 1966.

146. Gormsen, H., Iversen, P., and Raaschou, F. Kidney biopsy in acute anuria with a case of acute bilateral cortical necrosis. *Amer. J. Med.* 19:209, 1955.

147. Gregg, J. A., Shirger, A., and Harrison, E. G., Jr. Thrombosis of the renal veins associated with hypertension: Report of a case. *Proc. Mayo Clin.* 36:550, 1961.

148. Griffith, W. H., and Wade, N. J. Some effects of low choline diets. *Proc. Soc. Exp. Biol. Med.* 41:188, 1939.

149. Griffith, W. S. A., and Herringham, W. P. A case of necrosis of the entire renal cortex of both kidneys, together with thrombosis of all the cortical arteries, occurring in the puerperal state. *J. Path. Bact.* 11:237, 1906–07.

150. Groen, J., and Lindeboom, G. A. Solutio placentae gevolgd door anurie. *Nederl. T. Geneesk.* 84:688, 1940; quoted by Effersøe et al. [105].

151. Grollman, A., Muirhead, E. E., and Vanatta, J. Role of the kidney in pathogenesis of hypertension as determined by a study of the effects of bilateral nephrectomy and other experimental procedures on the blood pressure of the dog. *Amer. J. Physiol.* 157: 21, 1949.

152. Gross, F. Adrenocortical Function and

Renal Pressor Mechanisms in Experimental Hypertension. In Bock, K. D., and Cotter, P. T. (Eds.), *Essential Hypertension: An International Symposium*. Berlin: Springer-Verlag, 1960. P. 92.

152a. Gross, F., Bruner, H., and Ziegler, M. Renin-angiotensin system, aldosterone, and sodium balance. *Recent Progr. Hormone Res.* 21:119, 1965.

153. Haber, E., Page, L. B., and Jacoby, G. A. Synthesis of antigenic branch-chain copolymers of angiotensin and poly-l-lysine. *Biochemistry* (Wash.) 4:693, 1965.

154. Haft, D. E., and Prior, J. T. Bilateral cortical necrosis of the kidneys following treatment of an unusual case of heart block. *Ann. Intern. Med.* 34:1483, 1951.

155. Halpern, M., and Currarino, G. Vascular lesions causing hypertension in neurofibromatosis. *New Eng. J. Med.* 273:248, 1965.

156. Halpern, M., and Evans, J. A. Coarctation of the renal artery with "notching" of the ureter. *Amer. J. Roentgen.* 88:159, 1962.

157. Halpern, M. M., Sanford, H. S., and Viamonte, M., Jr. Renal-artery abnormalities in three hypertensive sisters: Probable familial fibromuscular hyperplasia. *J.A.M.A.* 194:512, 1965.

158. Halprin, H. Dissecting aneurysm of the entire aorta with partial bilateral renal artery occlusion: Report of a case. *U.S. Naval Med. Bull.* 41:1098, 1943.

159. Hamburger, J., Richet, G., Crosnier, J., Funck-Brentano, J. L., Antoine, B., Ducrot, H., Mery, J. P., and de Montera, H. *Nephrology,* Trans. by A. Walsh. Philadelphia: Saunders, 1968. Vol. II, p. 1206.

160. *Ibid.* P. 1217.

161. Hansen, J., Holten, C., and Thorborg, J. V. Hypertension in two sisters caused by so-called fibromuscular hyperplasia of the renal arteries. *Acta Med. Scand.* 178:461, 1965.

162. Harrington, S. W. The effect on the kidney of various surgical procedures on the blood supply, capsule, and on the ureters. *Arch. Surg.* 2:547, 1921.

163. Harrison, E. G., Jr., Hunt, J. C., and Bernatz, P. E. Morphology of fibromuscular dysplasia of the renal artery in renovascular hypertension. *Amer. J. Med.* 43:97, 1967.

164. Harrison, T. R., Mason, M. F., Resnik, H., and Rainey, J. Changes in blood pressure in relation to experimental renal insufficiency. *Trans. Ass. Amer. Physicians* 51: 280, 1936.

165. Hartmann, H. R., Newcomb, A. W., Barnes, A., and Lowman, R. M. Renal infarction following selective renal arteriography. *Radiology* 86:52, 1966.

166. Hartroft, P. M., Sutherland, L. E., and Hartroft, W. S. Juxtaglomerular cells as the source of renin: Further studies with the fluorescent antibody technique and the effect of passive transfer of antirenin. *Canad. Med. Ass. J.* 90:163, 1964.

167. Hartroft, W. S. Discussion of paper by Griffith, W. G. The renal lesions in choline deficiency. *Amer. J. Clin. Nutr.* 6:263, 1958.

168. Hatcher, C. R., Jr., Gagnon, J. A., and Clarke, R. W. The effects of hydration in epinephrine-induced renal shutdown in dogs. *Surg. Forum* 9:106, 1958.

169. Hawthorne, E. W., Perry, S. L. C., and Pogue, W. G. Development of experimental renal hypertension in the dog following reduction of renal artery pulse pressure without reducing mean pressure. *Amer. J. Physiol.* 174:393, 1953.

170. Haynie, T. P., Stewart, B. H., Nofal, M. M., Carr, E. A., Jr., and Bierwaltes, W. H. Renal scintiscans in the diagnosis of renal vascular disease. *J. Nucl. Med.* 2:272, 1961.

171. Heggie, J. F. Discussion on the pathological features of cortical necrosis of the kidney and allied conditions associated with pregnancy. *Proc. Roy. Soc. Med.* 42:380, 1949.

172. Heitzman, E. R., and Perchik, L. Radiographic features of renal infarction. *Radiology* 76:39, 1961.

173. Hejnal, J., Hejhal, L., Firt, P., and Michal, V. Surgical management of vasorenal hypertension. *J. Cardiovasc. Surg.* (Torino) 6:400, 1965.

174. Helmer, O. M. Renin activity in blood from patients with hypertension. *Canad. Med. Ass. J.* 90:221, 1964.

175. Helmer, O. M., and Judson, W. E. The Presence of Vasoconstrictor and Vasopressor Activity in Renal Vein Plasma of Patients with Arterial Hypertension. In *Hypertension,* New York: Amer. Heart Ass., 1960. Vol. 8, p. 38.

176. Hertig, A. T., and Mallory, T. B. Case records of the Massachusetts General Hospital, #32121. *New Eng. J. Med.* 234:416, 1946.

177. Herzog, G. Über Hyaline Thrombose der Kleinen Nierengefässe und einen Fall von Thrombose der Nierenvene. *Beitr. Path. Anat.* 56:175, 1913.

178. Hickler, R. B., Lauler, D. P., Saravis, C. A., Vagnucci, A. I., Steiner, G., and Thorn, G. W. Vasodepressor lipid from the renal medulla. *Canad. Med. Ass. J.* 90:280, 1964.

179. Highman, B., Thompson, E. C., Roche, J., and Altland, P. D. Serum alkaline phosphatase in dogs with experimental splenic and renal infarction and with endocarditis. *Proc. Soc. Exp. Biol. Med.* 75:109, 1957.

180. Hirschberg, H. A., and Soll, S. N. Renal infarction of traumatic origin. *J.A.M.A.* 119:1088, 1942.

181. Holley, K. E., Hunt, J. C., Brown, A. L., Jr., Kincaid, O. W., and Sheps, S. G. Renal artery stenosis: A clinical-pathologic study in normotensive and hypertensive patients. *Amer. J. Med.* 37:14, 1964.

182. Howard, J. E., Berthrong, M., Gould, D. M., and Yendt, E. R. Hypertension resulting from unilateral renal vascular disease and its relief by nephrectomy. *Bull. Johns Hopkins Hosp.* 94:51, 1954.

183. Howard, J. E., and Connor, T. B. Hypertension produced by unilateral renal disease. *Arch. Intern. Med.* (Chicago) 109:8, 1962.

184. Howard, J. E., and Connor, T. B. Use of differential renal function studies in the diagnosis of renovascular hypertension. *Amer. J. Surg.* 107:58, 1964.

185. Hoxie, H. J., and Coggin, C. B. Renal infarction: Statistical study of two hundred and five cases and detailed report of an unusual case. *Arch. Intern. Med.* 65:587, 1940.

186. Hügin, W. Über Nierenrinden — und hypophysenvorderlappennekrose bei Gravidität. *Gynaecologia* (Basel) 121:269, 1946.

187. Huidobro, F., and Braun-Menendez, E. The secretion of renin by the intact kidney. *Amer. J. Physiol.* 137:47, 1942.

188. Hunt, J. C., Bernatz, P. E., and Harrison, E. G., Jr. Factors determining diagnosis and choice of treatment of renovascular hypertension. *Circ. Res.* 21:II-211, 1967.

189. Hunt, J. C., Maher, F. T., Greene, L. F., and Sheps, S. G. Functional characteristics of the separate kidneys in hypertensive man. *Amer. J. Cardiol.* 17:493, 1966.

190. Huvos, A., Yagi, S., Mannick, J. A., and Hollander, W. Stimulation of renin secretion by hydralazine: II. Studies in renovascular hypertension. *Circulation* 32:II-118, 1965.

191. Iumgano, M. Necrosi bilaterale del rene per embolia dell'arteria renale. *Rinascensza Med.* (Napoli) 4:372, 1927.

192. Irvine, R. O. H. The twin-coil artificial kidney in the treatment of acute oliguric renal failure, with case reports of renal cortical necrosis, fatal hemolysis following bee stings and Weil's disease treated with the artificial kidney. *New Zeal. Med. J.* 61:184, 1962.

193. Janeway, T. C. Note on the blood pressure changes following reduction of the renal arterial circulation. *Proc. Soc. Exp. Biol. Med.* 6:109, 1908-09.

194. Janower, M. L., and Weber, A. L. Radiologic evaluation of acute renal infarction. *Amer. J. Roentgen.* 95:309, 1965.

195. Jardine, R., and Kennedy, A. M. Three cases of symmetrical necrosis of the cortex of the kidneys associated with puerperal eclampsia and suppression of urine. *Lancet* 1:1291, 1913.

196. Jardine, R., and Kennedy, A. M. Suppression of urine in pregnancy and the puerperium — its relation to symmetrical necrosis of the renal cortex. *Lancet* 2:116, 1920.

197. Jardine, R., and Teacher, J. H. Two cases of necrosis of the cortex of the kidneys associated with puerperal eclampsia and suppression of the urine. *J. Path. Bact.* 14:141, 1909.

198. Jardine, R., and Teacher, J. H. Two cases of symmetrical necrosis of the cortex of the kidneys associated with puerperal eclampsia and suppression of urine. *J. Path. Bact.* 15:137, 1910–11.
199. Joekes, A. M., and Bull, G. M. Accidental hemorrhage with bilateral cortical necrosis of the kidneys, treated by artificial kidney. *Proc. Roy. Soc. Med.* 41:678, 1948.
200. Juhel-Rénoy, E. De l'anurie précoce scarlatineuse. *Arch. Gen. Med.* VII serie, Tome 17: 385, 1886.
201. Kaiser, T. F., and Ross, R. R. Total infarction of the kidneys from bilateral arterial emboli. *J. Urol.* 66:500, 1951.
202. Kaneko, Y., Ikeda, T., Takeda, T., and Ueda, H. Renin release during acute reduction of arterial pressure in normotensive subjects and patients with renovascular hypertension. *J. Clin. Invest.* 46:705, 1967.
203. Kaplan, N. M. The steroid content of adrenal adenomas and measurements of aldosterone production in patients with essential hypertension and primary aldosteronism. *J. Clin. Invest.* 46:728, 1967.
204. Kaplan, N. M., and Silah, J. G. The angiotensin-infusion test: A new approach to the differential diagnosis of renovascular hypertension. *New Eng. J. Med.* 271:536, 1964.
205. Karsner, H. T., and Austin, J. H. Studies in infarction: Experimental bland infarction of the kidney and spleen. *J.A.M.A.* 57:951, 1911.
206. Kaufman, J. J., and Maxwell, M. H. Surgery for renovascular hypertension: Analysis of 67 cases. *J.A.M.A.* 190:709, 1964.
207. Kaufman, J. J., and Moloney, P. J. Results of synthetic grafts in the treatment of renal artery stenosis. *J. Urol.* 98:140, 1967.
208. Killen, D. A., and Foster, J. H. Spinal cord injury as a complication of aortography. *Ann. Surg.* 152:211, 1960.
209. Kincaid, O. W. (Ed.). *Renal Angiography.* Chicago: Year Book, 1966.
210. Kincaid-Smith, P. The Diagnostic Value of Renal Biopsy in Renovascular and Other Forms of Renal Hypertension. In Gross, F. (Ed.), *Antihypertensive Therapy.* Berlin: Springer-Verlag, 1966.
211. Kioschos, J. M., Kirkendall, W. M., Valenca, M. R., and Fitz, A. E. Unilateral renal hemodynamics and characteristics of dye-dilution curves in patients with essential hypertension and renal disease. *Circulation* 35:229, 1967.
212. Kirkendall, W. M., Fitz, A. E., and Lawrence, M. S. Renal hypertension. *New Eng. J. Med.* 276:479, 1967.
213. Klatte, E. C., Babb, O. W., Burko, H. C., Foster, J. H., Rhamy, R. K., and Oates, J. R. The radiographic pre- and postoperative assessment of patients with renovascular disease. *Radiology* (in press).
214. Klotz, O. Infarction of renal cortex in pregnancy. *Amer. J. Obstet.* 58:619, 1908.
215. Kobernick, S. D., Moore, J. R., and Wiglesworth, F. W. Thrombosis of the renal veins with massive hemorrhagic infarction of the kidneys in childhood. *Amer. J. Path.* 27:435, 1951.
215a. Koletsky, S., and Gustafson, G. E. The effects of temporary cessation of renal blood flow in rats. *J. Clin. Invest.* 26:1072, 1947.
216. Kolff, W. J. Discussion. In Hoobler, S. W. (Ed.), *Proceedings of the Conference on Basic Mechanisms of Arterial Hypertension. Circulation* 17:677, 1958.
217. Kolff, W. J. Reduction of Experimental Renal Hypertension by Kidney Perfusion. In Hoobler, S. W. (Ed.), *Proceedings of the Conference on Basic Mechanisms of Arterial Hypertension. Circulation* 17:702, 1958.
218. Koons, K. M., and Ruch, M. K. Hypertension in a 7-year-old girl with Wilms's tumor relieved by nephrectomy. *J.A.M.A.* 115:1097, 1940.
219. Kovács, K., Dávid, M. A., and László, F. A. Effect of hypophysectomy on the development of renal cortical necrosis induced by posterior pituitary extract in oestrone pretreated rats. *Brit. J. Exp. Path.* 45:415, 1964.
220. Lang, E. K. Arteriographic diagnosis of renal infarctions. *Radiology* 88:1110, 1967.
221. Lange, K., Nagamatsu, G., and Altman, A. Nonpenetrating abdominal trauma as a cause of renal vascular hypertension. *J.A.M.A.* 198:673, 1966.
222. Langley, G. J., and Platt, R. Hypertension

and unilateral kidney disease. *Quart. J. Med.*, n.s. 16:143, 1947.

223. Laragh, J. H. Aldosterone and Angiotensin in Hypertensive Vascular Disease. In Manger, W. M. (Ed.), *Hormones and Hypertension*. Springfield, Ill.: Thomas, 1966. P. 121.

224. Laragh, J. H., Angers, M., Kelly, W. G., and Lieberman, S. S. Hypertensive agents and pressor substances: The effect of epinephrine, norepinephrine angiotensin II, and others on the secretory rate of aldosterone in man. *J.A.M.A.* 174:234, 1960.

225. Lauler, D. P., and Schreiner, G. E. Bilateral renal cortical necrosis. *Amer. J. Med.* 24:519, 1958.

226. Leadbetter, W. F., and Burkland, C. F. Hypertension in unilateral renal disease. *J. Urol.* 39:611, 1938.

226a. Leaf, A. Regulation of intracellular fluid volume and disease. (Editorial.) *Amer. J. Med.* 49:291, 1970.

227. Ledingham, J. G. G., Bull, M. B., and Laragh, J. H. The meaning of aldosteronism in hypertensive disease. *Circ. Res.* 21:II-177, 1967.

228. Lee, L. Reticuloendothelial clearance of circulating fibrin in the pathogenesis of the generalized Shwartzman reaction. *J. Exp. Med.* 115:1065, 1962.

229. Lee, L. Antigen-antibody reaction in the pathogenesis of bilateral renal cortical necrosis. *J. Exp. Med.* 117:365, 1963.

229a. LeFebvre, R., and Genest, J. Study of renal ischemic tubular atrophy in 79 patients with arterial hypertension. *Canad. Med. Ass. J.* 82:1249, 1960.

230. Leiter, L. Unusual hypertensive renal disease. 1. Occlusion of renal arteries (Goldblatt hypertension). 2. Anomalies of urinary tract. *J.A.M.A.* 111:507, 1938.

231. Levy, S. E., Light, R. A., and Blalock, A. The blood flow and oxygen consumption of the kidney in experimental renal hypertension. *Amer. J. Physiol.* 122:38, 1938.

232. Libman, E., and Fishberg, A. M. Unilateral hemoglobinuria: Its occurrence in infarction of the kidney. *Ann. Intern. Med.* 11:1344, 1937–38.

233. Lindeboom, G. A., and Bouwer, W. F. Dissecting aneurysm (and renal cortical necrosis) associated with arachnodactyly (Marfan's disease). *Cardiologia* (Basel) 15:12, 1949–50.

234. Lindqvist, B., Erlamson, P., and Brun, A. A case of renal cortical necrosis probably caused by a human equivalent of the Shwartzman reaction. *Acta Med. Scand.* 173:561, 1963.

235. Litten, M. Ueber pathologische Verkalkungen und Kalkmetastasen in den Nieren. *Virchow. Arch.* [Path. Anat.] 83:508, 1881.

236. Litten, M. Der hamorrhagische Niereninfarct. (Embolischer Infarct oder embolischer Necrose). *Klin. Handbuch der Harn und Sexualortane.* Herausgegeben von W. Zuelzer. 1. Abtheil. 284, 1894.

237. Lloyd-Thomas, H. G., Balme, R. H., and Key, J. J. Tram-line calcification in renal cortical necrosis. *Brit. Med. J.* 1:909, 1962.

238. London, I. L., Hoffsten, P., Perkoff, G. T., and Pennington, T. G. Renal infarction: Elevation of serum and urinary lactic dehydrogenase (LDH). *Arch. Intern. Med.* (Chicago) 12:87, 1968.

239. Loomis, D., and Jett-Jackson, C. E. Plastic studies in abnormal renal architecture: VI. An investigation of the circulation in infarcts of the kidney. *Arch. Path.* 33:735, 1942.

240. Loomis, L., Ocker, J. M., Jr., and Hodges, C. V. Dynamic treatment of renal artery embolism: A case report and review of the literature. *J. Urol.* 96:131, 1966.

241. Lupu, A. N., Kaufman, J. J., and Maxwell, M. H. Renal artery constriction: Physiological determinants of pressure gradients. *Ann. Surg.* 167:246, 1968.

242. McAfee, J. G. A survey of complications of abdominal aortography. *Radiology* 68:825, 1957.

243. McAlister, W. H., and Nedelman, S. H. The roentgen manifestations of bilateral renal cortical necrosis. *Amer. J. Roentgen.* 86:129, 1961.

244. McCormack, L. J., Noto, T. J., Jr., Meaney, T. F., Poutasse, E. F., and Dustan, H. P. Subadventitial fibroplasia of the renal artery, a disease of young women. *Amer. Heart J.* 73:602, 1967.

245. McCormack, L. J., Poutasse, E. F., Meaney, T. F., Noto, T. J., Jr., and Dustan, H. P. A pathologic-arteriographic correlation of renal arterial disease. *Amer. Heart J.* 72: 188, 1966.

246. McCubbin, J. W., and Page, I. H. A Unifying View of Renal Hypertension. In Manger, W. M. (Ed.), *Hormones and Hypertension*. Springfield, Ill.: Thomas, 1966. P. 104.

247. McDonough, J. R., Hames, C. G., Stulb, S. C., and Garrison, G. E. Coronary heart disease among Negroes and whites in Evans County, Georgia. *J. Chronic Dis.* 18:443, 1965.

247a. MacDonald, G. J., Louis, W. J., Renzini, V., Boyd, G. W., and Peart, W. S. Renal-clip hypertension in rabbits immunized against angiotensin II. *Circ. Res.* 27:197, 1970.

248. MacGillivray, I. Combined renal and anterior pituitary necrosis. *J. Obstet. Gynaec. Brit. Emp.* 57:924, 1950.

249. MacGillivray, I. Bilateral renal cortical necrosis in obstetric patients. *J. Obstet. Gynaec. Brit. Emp.* 58:92, 1951.

250. McKay, D. G., Merrill, S. J., Weiner, A. E., Hertig, A. T., and Reid, D. E. The pathologic anatomy of eclampsia, bilateral renal cortical necrosis, pituitary necrosis, and other acute fatal complications of pregnancy and its possible relationship to the generalized Shwartzman phenomenon. *Amer. J. Obstet. Gynec.* 66:507, 1953.

251. McKay, D. G., Jewett, J. F., and Reid, D. E. Endotoxin shock and the generalized Shwartzman reaction in pregnancy. *Amer. J. Obstet. Gynec.* 78:546, 1959.

252. MacNider, W. deB. The pathological changes which develop in the kidney, as a result of occlusion, by ligature, of one branch of the renal artery. *J. Med. Res.* 22: 91, 1910.

253. MacNider, W. deB. The pathological changes which develop in the kidney as a result of occlusion by ligature of one branch of the renal artery. Part II. *J. Med. Res.* 24:425, 1911.

254. McPaul, J. J., Jr., McIntosh, D. A., Williams, L. F., Gritti, E. J., and Grollman, A. Correlation of the pressor activity of the renal venous effluent with excretory function and other tests in focal, parenchymal, and vascular renal disease. *Circulation* 33:781, 1966.

255. Malisoff, S., and Macht, M. B. Thromboangiitic occlusion of the renal artery with resultant hypertension. *J. Urol.* 65:371, 1951.

256. Mann, F. C., Herrick, J. F., Essex, H. E., and Baldes, E. J. The effect on the blood flow of decreasing the lumen of a blood vessel. *Surgery* 4:249, 1938.

257. Margaretten, W., Zucker, W. O., and McKay, D. G. Production of the generalized Shwartzman reaction in pregnant rats by intravenous infusion of thrombin. *Lab. Invest.* 13:552, 1964.

258. Margolin, E. G., Merrill, J. P., and Harrison, J. H. Diagnosis of hypertension due to occlusion of the renal artery. *New Eng. J. Med.* 256:581, 1957.

259. Marshall, E. K., Jr., and Kolls, A. D. Studies on the nervous control of the kidney in relation to diuresis and urinary secretion: IV. Unilateral ligation of one branch of one renal artery and unilateral splanchnotomy. *Amer. J. Physiol.* 49:335, 1919.

260. Marshall, S., and Whapham, E. Case of bilateral renal infarction in a newly born infant. *Lancet* 2:428, 1936.

261. Mason, M. F., Robinson, C. S., and Blalock, A. Studies on the renal arterial blood pressure and the metabolism of kidney tissue in experimental hypertension. *J. Exp. Med.* 72:289, 1940.

262. Masson, G. M. C., McCormack, L. J., Dustan, H. P., and Corcoran, A. C. Hypertensive vascular disease as a consequence of increased arterial pressure. *Amer. J. Path.* 34:817, 1958.

263. Mateer, F. M., Borecky, D. C., Balash, W. R., Bonessi, J. V., and Danowski, T. S. Uremia in pregnancy. *Amer. J. Obstet. Gynec.* 86:249, 1963.

264. Maxwell, M. H., Gonick, H. C., Wiita, R., and Kaufman, J. J. Use of the rapid-sequence intravenous pyelogram in the diagnosis of renovascular hypertension. *New Eng. J. Med.* 270:213, 1964.

265. Maxwell, M. H., Lupu, A. N., and Franklin, S. S. Clinical and physiological factors determining diagnosis and choice of treatment of renovascular hypertension. *Circ. Res.* 21:II-201, 1967.

266. Meili, A. Experimentolle Erzeugung von symmetrischen Nierenrindennekrosen bei Ratten mit Staphylokokken-toxin. *Z. Ges. Exp. Med.* 136:405, 1963.

267. Melick, W. F., and Vitt, A. E. Thrombosis of the renal vein. *J. Urol.* 51:587, 1944.

268. Merrill, J. P., Giordano, C., and Heetderks, D. R. The role of the kidney in human hypertension: I. Failure of hypertension to develop in the renoprival subject. *Amer. J. Med.* 31:931, 1961.

269. Merrill, J. P., and Schupak, E. Mechanisms of hypertension in renoprival man. *Canad. Med. Ass. J.* 90:328, 1964.

270. Meyer, P., Milliez, P., Alexandre, J. M., and Devaux, C. Renal-vein renin in renovascular hypertension. *Lancet* 1:1429, 1966.

271. Michelakis, A. M., Caudle, J., and Liddle, G. W. Stimulation and inhibition of renin production in vitro. *Clin. Res.* 16:75, 1968.

272. Michelakis, A. M., Foster, J. H., Liddle, G. W., Rhamy, R. K., Küchel, O., and Gordon, R. D. Measurement of renin in both renal veins: Its use in diagnosis of renovascular hypertension. *Arch. Intern. Med.* (Chicago) 120:444, 1967.

273. Michelakis, A. M., Woods, J. W., Liddle, G. W., and Klatte, E. C. A predictable error in the use of renal vein renin determinations in the diagnostic evaluation of renovascular hypertension. *Arch. Intern. Med.* (Chicago) 123:359, 1969.

274. Miller, G. M., Wylie, E. J., and Hinman, F., Jr. Renal complications from aortography. *Surgery* 35:885, 1954.

275. Milles, G., Müller, E. F., and Petersen, W. F. Renal denervation: The effect of snake venom and chilling in the renal circulation. *Arch. Path.* 13:233, 1932.

276. Moëll, H. Gross bilateral renal cortical necrosis during long periods of oliguria-anuria: Roentgenologic observations in two cases. *Acta Radiol.* (Stockholm) 48:355, 1957.

277. Moore, H. C. The renal lesions associated with intra-uterine hemorrhage and foetal death in pregnant rats given progesterone and an experimental diet. *J. Path. Bact.* 84:137, 1962.

278. More, R. H., and Kobernick, S. D. Arteritis, carditis, glomerulonephritis and bilateral renal cortical necrosis induced in rabbits. *A.M.A. Arch. Path.* 51:361, 1951.

279. Morris, G. C., Jr., De Bakey, M. E., and Cooley, D. A. Surgical treatment of renal failure of renovascular origin. *J.A.M.A.* 182:609, 1962.

280. Morris, G. C., Jr., De Bakey, M. E., Crawford, E. S., Cooley, D. A., and Zanger, L. C. C. Late results of surgical treatment for renovascular hypertension. *Surg. Gynec. Obstet.* 122:1255, 1966.

281. Morris, G. C., Jr., Heider, C. F., and Moyer, J. H. The protective effect of subfiltration arterial pressure on the kidney. *Surg. Forum* 6:623, 1956.

282. Morris, R. E., Jr., Ransom, P. A., and Howard, J. E. Studies on the relationship of angiotensin to hypertension of renal origin. *J. Clin. Invest.* 41:1386, 1962.

283. Morrow, I., and Amplatz, K. Embolic occlusion of the renal artery during aortography. *Radiology* 86:57, 1966.

283a. Mueller, C. B., Surtshin, A., Carlin, M. R., and White, H. L. Glomerular and tubular influences on sodium and water excretion. *Amer. J. Physiol.* 165:411, 1951.

284. Muirhead, E. E., Leach, B. E., Daniels, E. D., and Hinman, J. W. Lapine renomedullary lipid in murine hypertension. *Arch. Path.* (Chicago) 85:72, 1968.

285. Müller-Berghaus, G., and McKay, D. G. Prevention of the generalized Shwartzman reaction in pregnant rats by α-adrenergic blocking agents. *Lab. Invest.* 17:276, 1967.

286. Mulrow, P. J. Renal pressor substances in the diagnosis of hypertension. (Editorial.) *Ann. Intern. Med.* 61:977, 1964.

287. Munger, H. V. Renal thrombosis. *J. Urol.* 71:144, 1954.

288. Nakai, H., and Margaretten, W. Effect of staphylococcal toxin on the rabbit kidney. *Arch. Path.* (Chicago) 76:38, 1963.

289. de Navasquez, S. The histology and

pathogenesis of bilateral cortical necrosis of the kidney in pregnancy. *J. Path. Bact.* 41: 385, 1935.

290. de Navasquez, S. Experimental symmetrical cortical necrosis of the kidneys produced by staphylococcus toxin: A study of the morbid anatomy and associated circulatory and biochemical changes. *J. Path. Bact.* 46:47, 1938.

290a. Ng, K. K. F., and Vane, J. R. Conversion of angiotensin I to angiotensin II. *Nature* (London) 216:762, 1967.

291. Nicotero, J. A., Moutsos, S. E., Perez-Stable, E., Turrian, H. E., and Shapiro, A. P. Diagnostic and physiologic implications of the angiotensin infusion test. *New Eng. J. Med.* 274:1464, 1966.

292. Ober, W. E., Reid, D. E., Romney, S. L., and Merrill, J. P. Renal lesions and acute renal failure in pregnancy. *Amer. J. Med.* 21:781, 1956.

293. Oliver, J., MacDowell, M., and Tracy, A. The pathogenesis of acute renal failure associated with traumatic and toxic injury: Renal ischemia, nephrotoxic damage and the ischemic episode. *J. Clin. Invest.* 30: 1307, 1951.

293a. Oparil, S., Sanders. C. A., and Haber, E. In-vivo and in-vitro conversion of augiotension to angiotension II in dog blood. *Circ. Res.* 26:591, 1970.

294. Oram, S., Ross, G., Pell, L., and Winteler, J. Renal cortical calcification after snakebite. *Brit. Med. J.* 1:1647, 1963.

295. Ouimet-Oliva, D., Charron, J., and Bélanger, R. Renal infarct with perirenal hematoma. *Amer. J. Roentgen.* 98:70, 1966.

296. Owen, K. The surgery of renal artery stenosis. *Brit. J. Urol.* 36:7, 1964; and personal communication.

297. Page, E. W., and Glendening, M. B. Production of renal cortical necrosis with serotonin (5-hydroxy tryptamine). *Obstet. Gynec.* 5:781, 1955.

298. Page, I. H. The production of persistent arterial hypertension by cellophane perinephritis. *J.A.M.A.* 113:2046, 1939.

299. Page, I. H. On the nature of the pressor action of renin. *J. Exp. Med.* 70:521, 1939.

300. Page, I. H. Initiation and maintenance of renal hypertension. *Amer. J. Surg.* 107: 26, 1964.

301. Page, I. H., and Corcoran, A. C. *Experimental Renal Hypertension.* Springfield, Ill.: Thomas, 1948.

302. Page, I. H., and McCubbin, J. W. (Eds.) *Renal Hypertension.* Chicago: Year Book, 1968.

303. Page, I. H., Dustan, H. P., and Poutasse, E. F. Mechanisms, diagnosis and treatment of hypertension of renal vascular origin. *Ann. Intern. Med.* 51:196, 1959.

304. Palermo, C., Ming, S. C., Frank, E., and Fine, J. The role of the sympathetic nervous system in the generalized Shwartzman reaction. *J. Exp. Med.* 115:609, 1962.

305. Palubinskas, A. J., Perloff, D., and Newton, T. H. Fibromuscular hyperplasia: An arterial dysplasia of increasing clinical importance. *Amer. J. Roentgen.* 98:907, 1966.

306. Parker, R. A. Distribution of the changes in the juxtaglomerular apparatus in human renal artery stenosis. *Nephron* 4:315, 1967.

307. Parker, R. T., McIntosh, H. D., Johnson, H. W., and Donnelly, J. F. The development and management of acute renal failure in the obstetric patient. *Southern Med. J.* 52:251, 1959.

308. Paul, O., and Ostfeld, A. M. Epidemiology of hypertension. *Progr. Cardiovasc. Dis.* 8:106, 1965–66.

309. Peart, W. S. The isolation of a hypertensin. *Biochem. J.* 62:520, 1956.

310. Peart, W. S. The renin-angiotensin system. *Pharmacol. Rev.* 17:143, 1965.

311. Peart, W. S. Diagnosis of Renal Artery Stenosis. In Gross, F. (Ed.), *Antihypertensive Therapy.* Berlin: Springer-Verlag, 1966.

312. Peart, W. S. Pressor Assays in the Evaluation of Renal Hypertension. *Proceedings of the Third International Congress of Nephrology,* Washington, 1966. Vol. 3, p. 140. Basel/New York: Karger, 1967.

313. Pendergrass, H. P., Tondreau, R. L., Pendergrass, E. P., Ritchie, D. J., Hildreth, E. A., and Askovitz, S. I. Reactions associated with intravenous urography: Historical and statistical review. *Radiology* 71:1, 1958.

314. Penner, A., and Bernheim, A. I. Acute ischemic necrosis of the kidney: A clinicopathologic and experimental study. *Arch. Path.* 30:465, 1940.

315. Perkins, R. P., Jacobson, D. S., Feder, F. P., Lipchick, E. O., and Fine, P. H. Return of renal function after late embolectomy. *New Eng. J. Med.* 276:1194, 1967.

316. Perloff, D., Sokolow, M., Wylie, E. J., and Palubinskas, A. J. Renal vascular hypertension, further experiences. *Amer. Heart J.* 74:614, 1967.

317. Perry, J. W. Phosphorus poisoning with cortical necrosis of the kidney: A report of two fatal cases. *Aust. Ann. Med.* 2:94, 1953.

318. Phillips, M. J. Bilateral renal cortical necrosis associated with calcification: Report of a case and a review of aetiology. *J. Clin. Path.* 15:31, 1962.

319. Pickering, G. W. The role of the kidney in acute and chronic hypertension following renal artery constriction in the rabbit. *Clin. Sci.* 5:229, 1944–45.

320. Pickering, G. W., and Prinzmetal, M. Experimental hypertension of renal origin in the rabbit. *Clin. Sci.* 3:357, 1937–38.

321. Poutasse, E. F. Occlusion of a renal artery as a cause of hypertension. *Circulation* 13: 37, 1956.

322. Poutasse, E. F., Humphries, A. W., McCormack, L. J., and Corcoran, A. C. Bilateral stenosis of renal arteries and hypertension. *J.A.M.A.* 161:419, 1956.

323. Powell, D. E. B. Non-suppurative lesions in staphylococcal septicemia. *J. Path. Bact.* 82:141, 1961.

324. Powers, S. R., Nesbitt, R. E. L., Jr., Boba, A., and Stein, A. Mechanism and prevention of distal tubular necrosis in dogs following experimental placental abruption. *Surg. Gynec. Obstet.* 107:469, 1958.

325. Price, R. K., and Skelton, R. Hypertension due to syphilitic occlusion of the main renal arteries. *Brit. Heart J.* 10:29, 1948.

326. Prinzmetal, M., Hiatt, N., and Trogerman, L. M. Hypertension in a patient with bilateral renal infarction. *J.A.M.A.* 118:44, 1942.

326a. Proceedings of the International Symposium on Angiotensin, Sodium and Hypertension. *Canad. Med. Ass. J.* 90:153, 1964.

327. Rainer, W. G., Cramer, G. G., Newby, J. P., and Clarke, J. P. Fibromuscular hyperplasia of the carotid artery causing positional cerebral ischemia. *Ann. Surg.* 167:444, 1968.

328. Rapoport, A. Modification of the "Howard test" for the detection of renal-artery obstruction. *New Eng. J. Med.* 263:1159, 1960.

329. Reed, R. K., Sapirstein, L. A., Southard, F. D., Jr., and Ogden, E. The effects of Nembutal and yohimbine on chronic renal hypertension in the rat. *Amer. J. Physiol.* 141:707, 1944.

330. Regan, F. C., and Crabtree, E. G. Renal infarction: A clinical and possible surgical entity. *J. Urol.* 59:981, 1948.

331. Reid, D. E., and Davis, J. C. Case records of the Massachusetts General Hospital. *New Eng. J. Med.* 258:1215, 1958.

332. Reyna, F. G. Über die toxische Wirkung der intravenösen Lithium-Karmininjektionen und ihre Beziehung zu der Totalnekrose der Nieren und Nebennierenrinde. *Beitr. Path. Anat.* 97:261, 1936.

333. Ribbert. Beitrage zart Kenntnis der Nierinfarckte. *Virchow. Arch.* [Path. Anat.] 155:201, 1899.

334. Rigdon, R. H., Joyner, A. L., and Ricketts, E. T. A study of the action of a filterable staphylococcal toxin on the kidneys of normal rabbits. *Amer. J. Path.* 10:425, 1934.

335. Rodbard, S., and Katz, L. N. The role of renal metabolism in hypertension and uremia. *J. Exp. Med.* 73:357, 1941.

336. Rodriguez-Erdmann, F. Pathogenesis of bilateral renal cortical necrosis. Its production by means of exogenous fibrin. *Arch. Path.* (Chicago) 79:615, 1965.

337. Röhrer, H. Pathologisch-anatomische und histologische Studien bei akuter Schweinepest, inbesondere an Leber und Niere. Mit einem Anhaug über totale Nierenrindennekrosen. *Virchow. Arch.* [Path. Anat.] 284:201, 1932.

338. Rolleston, H. D. Symmetrical necrosis of the cortex of the kidneys — associated with suppression of the urine in women shortly after delivery. *Lancet* 2:1173, 1913.

339. Sanerkin, N. G., and Evans, D. M. D. Bilateral renal cortical necrosis in infants, associated with maternal antepartum haemorrhage. *J. Path. Bact.* 90:269, 1965.
340. Saphir, O., and Ballinger, J. Hypertension (Goldblatt) and unilateral malignant nephrosclerosis. *Arch. Intern. Med.* 66:541, 1940.
341. Schacht, R. A., Conway, J., and Stewart, B. H. Split renal function studies in hypertension. *Arch. Intern. Med.* (Chicago) 119:588, 1967.
342. Schacht, R. A., Zweifler, A. J., and Conway, J. Renal artery stenosis. *New Eng. J. Med.* 271:55, 1964.
343. Schlegel, J. U., and Moses, J. B. A method for visualization of kidney blood vessels applied to studies of the crush syndrome. *Proc. Soc. Exp. Biol. Med.* 74:832, 1950.
344. Schneider, C. L. Thromboplastin Complications of Late Pregnancy. In Hammond, J., Browne, F. J., and Wolstenholme, G. E. W. (Eds.), *Ciba Foundation Symposium. Toxaemias of Pregnancy—Human and Veterinary.* Philadelphia: Blakiston, 1950. P. 163.
345. Shüppel, A. Ein Fall von doppelseitiger totaler Nierenrindennekrose bei Eklampsia, nebst Kurzen Abriss über den derzeitigen Stand der Eklampsiefrage. *Arch. Gynaek.* 103:243, 1914.
346. Schwyzer, R., Iselin, B., Kappeler, H., Riniker, B., Rittel, W., and Zuber, H. Synthese hockswirksamer Oktapeptide mit der vermutlichen Amino-säurese quenz des noch unbekannten Hypertensin II aus Rinderserum (Val_5-Hypertensin II und Val_5-Hypertension II–Asp-B-amid) *Helv. Chim. Acta* 41:1287, 1958.
347. Scriver, W. deM. A case of anuria due to diffuse infarctions of the renal cortex. *Canad. Med. Ass. J.*, n.s. 19:701, 1928.
348. Scriver, W. deM., and Oertel, H. Necrotic sequestration of the kidneys in pregnancy (symmetrical cortical necrosis): A clinical and anatomic-pathogenetic study. *J. Path. Bact.* 33:1071, 1930.
349. Selkurt, E. E. Effect of pulse pressure and mean arterial pressure modification on renal hemodynamics and electrolyte and water excretion. *Circulation* 4:541, 1951.
350. Sen, S., Smeby, R. R., and Bumpus, F. M. Isolation of a phospholipid renin inhibitor from kidney. *Biochemistry* (Wash.) 6:1572, 1967.
351. Sexton, L. I., Hertig, A. T., Reid, D. E., Kellogg, F. S., and Patterson, W. S. Premature separation of the normally implanted placenta: A clinicopathologic study of 476 cases. *Amer. J. Obstet. Gynec.* 59:13, 1950.
352. Shea, J. D., Schwartz, J. W., and Kobilak, R. E. Thrombosis of the left renal artery with hypertension: Case report. *J. Urol.* 59:302, 1948.
353. Sheehan, H. L., and Davis, J. C. Complete permanent renal ischaemia. *J. Path. Bact.* 76:569, 1958.
354. Sheehan, H. L., and Davis, J. C. Patchy permanent renal ischaemia. *J. Path. Bact.* 77:33, 1959.
355. Sheehan, H. L., and Davis, J. C. Renal ischaemia with failed reflow. *J. Path. Bact.* 78:105, 1959.
356. Sheehan, H. L., and Davis, J. C. The protective effect of anesthesia in experimental renal ischaemia. *J. Path. Bact.* 79:337, 1960.
357. Sheehan, H. L., and Moore, H. C. *Renal Cortical Necrosis and the Kidney of Concealed Accidental Hemorrhage.* Springfield, Ill.: Thomas, 1953.
358. Sheinin, J., and Cohen, L. Serum enzymes and diagnosis of acute myocardial infarction. *Postgrad. Med.* 36:594, 1964.
359. Sheldon, W. H., and Hertig, A. T. Bilateral cortical necrosis of the kidney. A report of two cases. *Arch. Path.* 34:866, 1942.
360. Sheps, S. G., Osmundson, P. J., Hunt, J. C., Schirger, A., and Fairbairn, J. F., II. Hypertension and renal artery stenosis: Serial observations on 54 patients treated medically. *Clin. Pharmacol. Ther.* 6:700, 1965.
361. Simmons, J. L., Payne, R. B., Ajzen, H., and Woods, J. W. The angiotensin infusion test. *J. Urol.* 96:115, 1966.
362. Sivack, G. C., and Lich, R., Jr. Renal infarction. *Southern Med. J.* 51:329, 1958.
363. Skeggs, L. T., Lentz, K. E., Kahn, J. R., and

Hochstrasser, H. Studies on the preparation and properties of renin. *Circ. Res.* 21:II-91, 1967.

364. Skeggs, L. T., Lentz, K. E., Kahn, J. R., Shumway, N. P., and Woods, K. R. Amino acid sequence of hypertensin II. *J. Exp. Med.* 104:193, 1956.
365. Skinner, S. L., McCubbin, J. W., and Page, I. H. Control of renin secretion. *Circ. Res.* 15:64, 1964.
366. Sklaroff, D. M., Berk, N., and Kravitz, C. The renal scintogram in urologic work-up. *J.A.M.A.* 178:418, 1961.
367. Skjörten, F. Bilateral renal cortical necrosis and the generalized Shwartzman reaction. *Acta Path. Microbiol. Scand.* 61:394, 1964.
368. Smeby, R. R., Sen, S., and Bumpus, F. M. A naturally occurring renin inhibitor. *Circ. Res.* 21:II-129, 1967.
369. Smith, A., and Muirhead, E. E. Bilateral cortical necrosis of kidneys: Report of two cases and consideration of pathogenesis. *Texas J. Med.* 47:88, 1951.
370. Smith, H. T., Shapiro, F. L., and Messner, R. P. Anuria secondary to renovascular disease. *J.A.M.A.* 204:928, 1968.
371. Smith, H. W. *The Kidney. Structure and Function in Health and Disease.* New York: Oxford University Press, 1951.
372. Smith, H. W. Unilateral nephrectomy in hypertensive disease. *J. Urol.* 76:685, 1956.
373. Smith, L. H., Jr., and Morgan, W. S. Case records of the Massachusetts General Hospital. *New Eng. J. Med.* 258:237, 1958.
374. Stamey, T. A. Functional characteristics of renovascular hypertension with emphasis on the relationship of renal blood flow to hypertension. *Circ. Res.* 11:209, 1962.
375. Stamey, T. A. *Renovascular Hypertension.* Baltimore: Williams & Wilkins, 1963.
376. Stamey, T. A. Renovascular hypertension — 1965. (Editorial.) *Amer. J. Med.* 38:829, 1965.
377. Stamey, T. A., Nudelman, I. J., Good, P. H., Schwentker, F. N., and Hendricks, F. Functional characteristics of renovascular hypertension. *Medicine* (Balt.) 40:347, 1961.
378. Stegeman, W. Renal vessel thrombosis (Do we sometimes cause this?). *Urol. Cutan. Rev.* 52:710, 1948.
379. Stetson, C. A., and Good, R. A. Studies on the mechanism of the Shwartzman phenomenon: Evidence for the participation of polymorphonuclear leucocytes in the phenomenon. *J. Exp. Med.* 93:49, 1951.
380. Stewart, B. H., DeWeese, M. S., Conway, J., and Correa, R. J., Jr. Renal hypertension. *Arch. Surg.* (Chicago) 85:617, 1962.
381. Stoekinius, W. Über fast vollständige doppelseitige Nierenrindennekrose bei Diphtherie. *Beitr. Path. Anat.* 69:373, 1921.
382. Strandness, D. E., Smith, J. H., and Pate, V. A. Acute hypertension and renal infarction. *U.S. Armed Forces Med. J.* 11: 584, 1960.
383. Straub, P. W., von Felton, A., and Frick, P. G. Recurrent intravascular coagulation with renal cortical necrosis and recovery. *Ann. Intern. Med.* 64:643, 1966.
384. Strickler, W. L. Surgical cure of malignant hypertension with intrarenal arteriosclerosis. *J.A.M.A.* 194:233, 1965.
385. Stueber, P. J., Koletsky, S., and Persky, L. The effect of intermittent clamping of the renal pedicle. *Surg. Forum* 10:887, 1959.
386. Sutton, D., Brunton, F. J., and Starer, F. Renal artery stenosis. *Clin. Radiol.* 12:80, 1961.
387. Swan, R. C., and Merrill, J. P. The clinical course of acute renal failure. *Medicine* (Balt.) 32:215, 1953.
388. Taplan, G. V., Meredith, O. M., Jr., Kade, H., and Winter, C. C. The radioisotope renogram: An external test for individual kidney function and upper urinary tract patency. *J. Lab. Clin. Med.* 48:886, 1956.
389. Teplick, J. G., and Yarrow, M. W. Arterial infarction of the kidney. *Ann. Intern. Med.* 42:1041, 1955.
390. Thomas, C. S., Jr., Brockman, S. K., and Foster, J. H. Variability of the pressure gradient in renal artery stenosis. *Surg. Gynec. Obstet.* 126:339, 1968.

390a. Thomas, L. The Generalized Shwartzman Reaction in Rabbits Infected with Group A Hemolytic Streptococci. In Thomas, L. (Ed.), *Rheumatic Fever.* (A symposium held at the University of Minnesota on November 29, 30, and December 1, 1951, under the sponsorship of the Minnesota Heart Association.) Minneapolis: University of Minnesota Press, 1952.

390b. Thomas, L., and Good, R. A. Bilateral cortical necrosis of the kidneys in cortisone-treated rabbits following ingestion of bacterial toxin. *Proc. Soc. Exp. Biol. Med.* 76:604, 1951.

391. Thomas, L., and Good, R. A. The effect of cortisone on the Shwartzman reaction: The production of lesions resembling the dermal and generalized Shwartzman reactions by a single injection of bacterial toxin in cortisone-treated rabbits. *J. Exp. Med.* 95:409, 1952.

391a. Thurau, K. Renal hemodynamics. *Amer. J. Med.* 36:698, 1964.

392. Tigerstedt, R., and Bergman, P. G. Niere und Kreislauf. *Skand. Arch. Physiol.* 8:223, 1898.

393. Tobian, L. Interrelationships of electrolytes, juxtaglomerular cells and hypertension. *Physiol. Rev.* 40:280, 1960.

394. Tobian, L., Janecek, J., and Tomboulian, A. Correlation between granulation of juxtaglomerular cells and extractable renin in rats with experimental hypertension. *Proc. Soc. Exp. Biol. Med.* 100:94, 1959.

395. Tobian, L., Winn, B., and Janecek, J. The influence of arterial pressure on the antihypertensive action of a normal kidney, a biological servomechanism. *J. Clin. Invest.* 40:1085, 1961.

396. Torrens, J. A. Massive infarction of the renal cortex. *Lancet* 1:99, 1911.

397. Traube, L. *Über den Zusammenhang von Herz — und Nieren — Krankheiten.* Berlin: Verlag von August Hisschwald, 1856. P. 77.

398. Trueta, J., Barclay, A. E., Daniel, P. M., Franklin, K. J., and Pritchard, M. M. L. *Studies of the Renal Circulation.* Springfield, Ill.: Thomas, 1947.

399. Ueda, H. Renovascular hypertension as a manifestation of aortitis syndrome. (Editorial.) *Jap. Heart J.* 8:209, 1967.

400. Vander, A. J. Control of renin release. *Physiol. Rev.* 47:359, 1967.

401. Vernon-Parry, J., and Williams, R. T. Renal cortical necrosis with survival. *Brit. Med. J.* 2:903, 1963.

402. Verrilli, R. A., Vick, N. F., and Uhlman, R. C. Studies of alkaline phosphatase in various pathological conditions of the kidney: II. Renal vascular and ureteral obstruction. *J. Urol.* 86:525, 1961.

403. Vertes, V., Genuth, S., Leb, D. E., and Galvin, J. B. Unilateral renal plasma flow in the assessment of correctable renovascular hypertension. *New Eng. J. Med.* 273:855, 1965.

403a. VonGlahn, W. C., Jr., and Weld, J. T. The effect of *Staphylococcus aureus* toxin in the kidney. *J. Exp. Med.* 61:1, 1935.

404. VonZalka, E. Über symmetrische Rindennekrose der Niere. *Virchow. Arch.* [Path. Anat.] 290:57, 1933.

405. Wahle, G. H., Jr., and Muirhead, E. E. Bilateral renal cortical necrosis in a child associated with an incompatible blood transfusion. *Texas J. Med.* 49:770, 1953.

406. Warthin, T. A., and Thomas, C. B. Studies in experimental hypertension: I. Phenol red excretion and renal blood flow in hypertension of renal origin. *Bull. Johns Hopkins Hosp.* 72:203, 1943.

407. Welch, W. H. Hemorrhagic infarction. *Trans. Ass. Amer. Physicians* 2:121, 1887.

408. Welch, W. H. Embolism. In Albutt, T. C., and Rolleston, H. D. (Eds.), *A System of Medicine.* London: Macmillan, 1909. Vol. 4, p. 803.

409. Wells, J. D., Margolin, E. G., and Gall, E. A. Renal cortical necrosis: Clinical and pathologic features in twenty-one cases. *Amer. J. Med.* 29:257, 1960.

410. Westman, A. Two cases of necrosis of the renal cortex in toxicosis of pregnancy. *Acta Obstet. Gynaec. Scand.* 7:235, 1928.

411. Whelan, J. G., Jr., Ling, J. T., and Davis, L. A. Antemortem roentgen manifestations of bilateral renal cortical necrosis. *Radiology* 89:682, 1967.

412. Williams, T. F. Renal Cortical Necrosis, Renal Infarction, and Hypertension due to Renal Vascular Disease. In Strauss, M. B., and Welt, L. G. (Eds.), *Diseases of the Kidney.* Boston: Little, Brown, 1963. P. 557.

413. Wilson, C., and Byrom, F. B. Renal

changes in malignant hypertension. *Lancet* 1:136, 1939.

414. Wilson, C., and Byrom, F. B. The vicious circle in chronic Bright's disease: Experimental evidence from the hypertensive rat. *Quart. J. Med.* 10:65, 1941.
415. Wilson, C., and Pickering, G. W. Acute arterial lesions in rabbits with experimental renal hypertension. *Clin. Sci.* 3:343, 1937–38.
416. Wilson, L., Dustan, H. P., Page, I. H., and Poutasse, E. F. Diagnosis of renal arterial lesions. *Arch. Intern. Med.* (Chicago) 112: 270, 1963.
417. Winer, B. M., Lubbe, W. F., Simon, M., and Williams, J. A. Renin in the diagnosis of renovascular hypertension. *J.A.M.A.* 202:121, 1967.
418. Winter, C. C. Renograms and other radioisotope tests in the diagnosis of renal hypertension. *Amer. J. Surg.* 107:43, 1964.
419. Wisoff, C. P., and Chambers, D. F. Subtotal renal infarctions. *Amer. J. Roentgen.* 98:63, 1966.
420. Wollenweber, J., Sheps, S. G., and Davis, G. D. Clinical course of atherosclerotic renovascular disease. *Amer. J. Cardiol.* 21: 60, 1968.
421. Wood, J. E., Jr., and Cash, J. R. Experimental hypertension-observations on sustained elevation of systolic and diastolic blood pressure in dogs. *J. Clin. Invest.* 15: 543, 1936.
422. Woods, J. W., and Michelakis, A. M. Renal vein renin in renovascular hypertension. *Arch. Intern. Med.* (Chicago) 122:392, 1968.
423. Woods, J. W., and Williams, T. F. Unpublished observations.
424. Wylie, E. J., and Wellington, J. S. Hypertension caused by fibromuscular hyperplasia of the renal arteries. *Amer. J. Surg.* 100:183, 1960.
425. Young, J. Discussion of the pathological features of cortical necrosis of the kidney and allied conditions associated with pregnancy. *Proc. Roy. Soc. Med.* (Section of *Obstet. Gynaec.*). 42:375, 1949.
426. Yulie, C. L. Obstructive lesions of the main renal artery in relation to hypertension. *Amer. J. Med. Sci.* 207:394, 1944.
427. Zheutlin, N., Hughes, D., and O'Loughlin, B. J. Radiographic findings in renal vein thrombosis. *Radiology* 73:884, 1959.
428. Zuelzer, W. W., Charles, S., Kurnetz, R., Newton, W. A., and Fallon, R. Circulatory diseases of the kidneys in infancy and childhood. *Amer. J. Dis. Child.* 81:1, 1951.

21

Renal Involvement in Myeloma, Amyloidosis, Systemic Lupus Erythematosus, and Other Disorders of Connective Tissue

W. Gordon Walker, A. McGehee Harvey, and John H. Yardley

The features common to all the disorders considered in this chapter include an abnormality of one or more of the plasma proteins and progressive renal disease that usually terminates fatally and often dominates the clinical picture. In most instances, the derangement of plasma proteins involves some fraction of the immunoglobulins. In some of the disorders the existence of antigen-antibody complexes within the kidney has been established by one or more technics [96]. Although the exact mechanism of renal injury remains incompletely understood, it seems likely that these abnormal accumulations of plasma proteins within the kidney are important in the pathogenesis of the progressive renal disease [44, 65].

Myelomatosis

Since 1848, when Sir Henry Bence Jones described a unique protein in the urine of a patient with multiple myeloma [13], the relation between the abnormal proteins recognized in myeloma and the renal disease has been the object of much study [12, 19, 26, 150]. The availability of more precise methods of studying these abnormal proteins has increased understanding of their role in the clinical manifestations of these diseases. The clinical features of renal disease may result from the development of one or more of three aberrations in protein metabolism: (1) production of large amounts of an abnormal serum protein, M protein or myeloma globulin [137, 138, 153]; (2) urinary excretion of Bence Jones protein; and (3) development of a form of amyloidosis resembling primary amyloidosis. The hypercalcemia frequently seen in myelomatosis may also result in severe renal disease.

PROTEIN ABNORMALITIES

The presence of some type of protein abnormality can be demonstrated in approximately 90 per cent of patients with mutiple myeloma if the refined technics presently available are used routinely. In all but two cases in a series of 80, abnormal proteins were found in either the serum or urine [33, 135]. Serum abnormalities were found on immunoelectrophoretic analysis in 85 per cent of the patients of another series [10, 92, 126, 127]. On paper electrophoresis, the myeloma protein appears as a heavily staining homogenous discrete spot, the electrophoretic mobility varying in different cases but remaining constant in any single case [136, 137]. In the series of 112 patients studied by Carbone and associates [24] 60 per cent had IgG myeloma protein, whereas 20 per cent had synthesized only Bence Jones protein. More recently Fahey and associates have reported a number of cases of plasma cell myeloma with D-myeloma protein (IgD). They estimate that it occurs in less than 1 per cent of patients with myeloma [52].

The source of these abnormal serum proteins is the abnormal plasma cell (myeloma cell) seen in multiple myeloma. Evidence is now fairly conclusive that in general a single "line" or clone of plasma cells is responsible for the production of the single specific globulin [123]. There are, however, several well-documented instances of a single cell type producing two distinct types of protein [37, 151].

CLINICAL FEATURES

Myelomatosis rarely develops earlier than the fourth decade. Onset and early course are usually insidious, accompanied by progressive weakness, loss of appetite and weight, and gastrointestinal symptoms such as nausea and vomiting. Severe bone pain due to expansion of myelomatous tissue in the bone marrow is a hallmark of the disease. Nervous system manifestations may develop as a result of spinal cord compression or nerve root compression by a plasmacytoma, cellular infiltration of perineural structures, vascular occlusions in local areas of the nervous system, vertebral collapse producing cord or nerve root compression, and in addition amyloid deposits, particularly in the peripheral nervous system, may produce neuropathies. The polyneuropathy of obscure origin associated with other malignant tumors has also been described in patients with myeloma. In the later stages, renal involvement and complicating infections play an important role [51, 107, 156].

RENAL DISEASE

Proteinuria occurs in well over half the cases of myeloma, and progressive renal insufficiency with death in uremia is a common occurrence. In most cases, Bence Jones protein can be demonstrated in the urine, although occasionally proteinuria is seen in the absence of demonstrable Bence Jones proteins. The pathologic finding of extensive cast formation with plugging of the tubules and atrophy of the tubular epithelium has been responsible for the view that this is the principal mechanism of renal failure [161]. However, multiple factors including decreased renal blood flow, increased viscosity of the blood, hypercalcemia with nephrocalcinosis, precipitation of protein with plugging of the tubular lumen, and probably accumulation of abnormal proteins within the tubular epithelial cells all play a significant role in the progressive renal impairment. The relative importance of each factor varies with the individual case [97].

Functional studies, including the measurement of glomerular filtration rate (GFR), renal plasma flow (RPF), and tubular excretory maximum of para-aminohippurate (Tm_{PAH}), in two series of patients with myelomatosis showed a fairly close parallelism between changes in RPF and GFR, except in advanced renal impairment when a disproportionate depression of glomerular filtration function (low filtration fraction) was observed [7, 69]. A similar disparity between glomerular and tubular function was observed by comparing GFR and Tm_{PAH}. Furthermore, no correlation was noted between functional impairment and the presence or absence of Bence Jones proteinuria. Three patients in one series showed functional impairment without proteinuria. This disproportionate glomerular involvement would not be expected on the basis of simple obstruction of the tubules by occluding casts.

Roussak and Oleesky [146] reported marked polyuria of sudden onset in association with myelomatosis. Persistent hyposthenuria and polyuria were noted, with urine output varying between 3.5 and 5 liters per day. Water deprivation, hypertonic saline infusion, and vasopressin administration failed to significantly increase the specific gravity of the urine. The patient was hypercalcemic throughout the study, and Bence Jones protein was constantly present. Microdissection studies at postmortem examination showed "massive precipitation of structureless protein-like material — most marked in the collecting ducts," atrophied epithelium of the collecting ducts, and in places denudation of the tubular epithelium without evident regeneration. Histologic changes in the collecting duct and hypercalcemia may both have contributed to this hyposthenuria. It has been demonstrated that correction of hypercalcemia in multiple myeloma may be associated with marked improvement in the concentrating function of the kidney (Fig. 21-1).

Patients with myelomatosis and the aggregate of renal tubular abnormalities referred to as Fanconi's syndrome have been reported [50, 155, 174]. Generalized aminoaciduria, low plasma amino acid levels, renal glycosuria, mild renal acidosis, hypokalemia, hypophosphatemia, elevated alkaline phosphatase activity, hypouricemia, and normal urea clearance were the major findings in these reports. Bence Jones protein was usually present although one patient had proteinuria without demonstrable Bence Jones protein. The demonstration of rod-shaped inclusion bodies resembling crystals in the tubular epithelial cells of one patient and similar cells in the plasma cells of the bone marrow has led to the suggestion that this clinical picture may be the result of specific tubular damage produced by intracellular accumulation of the Bence Jones protein [155]. In support of this view, it is interesting that Wilson and his co-workers [174] have reported several patients with renal tubular acidosis associated with quantitative abnormalities in IgA, IgG, and IgM immunoglobulins although they could not demonstrate immunoglobulin deposition in material obtained at renal biopsy in one patient. Three patients with multiple myeloma and adult Fanconi syndrome have now been studied, however, with demonstration of inclusion bodies within the renal tubular cells. Levi and his co-workers have demonstrated the presence of Bence Jones proteins of lambda and kappa type within the tubular cells in areas of tubular atrophy in myeloma kidneys [102]. It thus seems reasonable that the intracellular accumulation of gamma-globulin fragments may indeed interfere with some of the transport functions of the renal tubular cells.

Despite the several different types of renal impairment that may develop in patients with

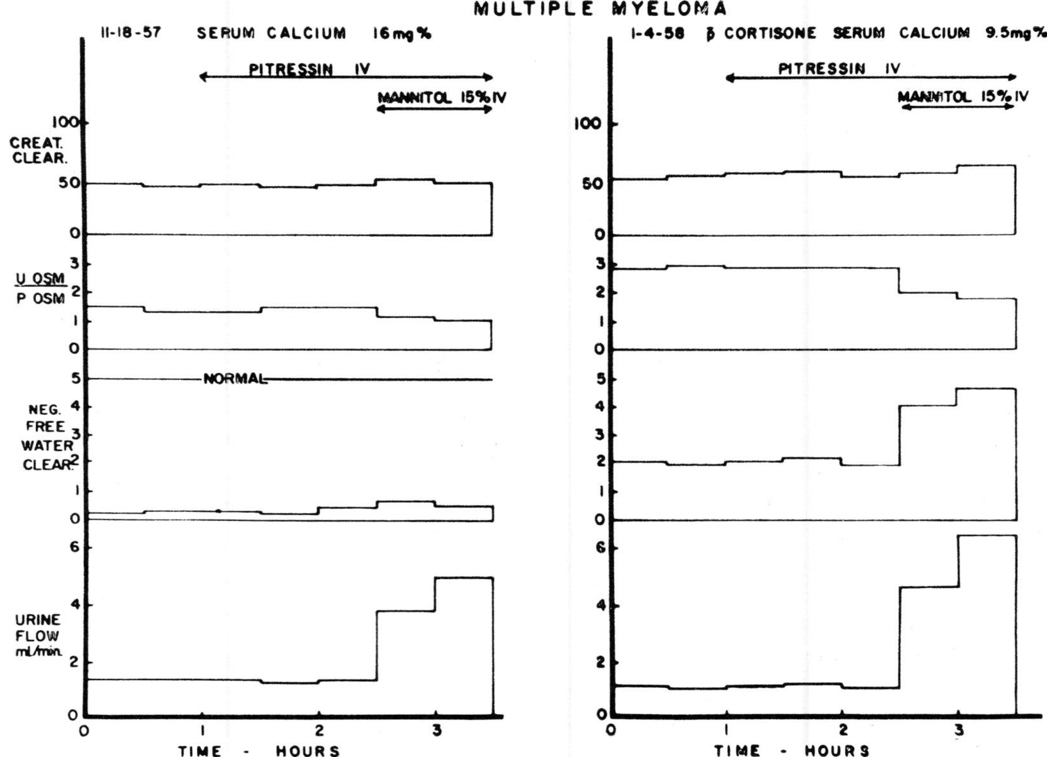

Figure 21-1. Renal concentrating ability in patient with multiple myeloma and hypercalcemia. The studies were performed during infusion of 50 milliunits of Pitressin per kilogram per hour. During the last hour, urine flow was augmented by administration of hypertonic mannitol. Negative free water clearance ($T^{C}_{H_2O}$) was markedly impaired when first measured during hypercalcemia, but was virtually normal two weeks later when serum calcium had returned to normal during cortisone administration.

myelomatosis, it is not possible to establish a unique relationship between a specific alteration of renal function and any one of the several factors that have been implicated in the renal impairment.

On histologic examination of myeloma kidneys, numerous casts are seen that do not differ from those seen in other forms of renal disease, but the proteinaceous deposits taking the form of eosinophilic, frequently lamellated casts are unique to myelomatosis although they are not constantly seen. These casts have a hard, glassy appearance and are frequently associated with varying degrees of giant cell reaction (Fig. 21-2A) [43, 94, 177]. The giant cells, which often appear to be engulfing the casts, are frequently in continuity with the tubular epithelium and basement membrane (Fig. 21-2B). They may represent a syncytial mass of tubular epithelium rather than giant cells derived from histiocytes. Such cast formation is associated with tubular dilatation, atrophy, occasional apparent rupture, and interstitial fibrosis. The obstruction and atrophy with tubular damage and acute inflammatory change is occasionally most striking in the collecting system (Fig. 21-3). When extensive, these changes may provide an adequate explanation for the clinically evident renal insufficiency, but as pointed out by Levi and his co-workers [102],

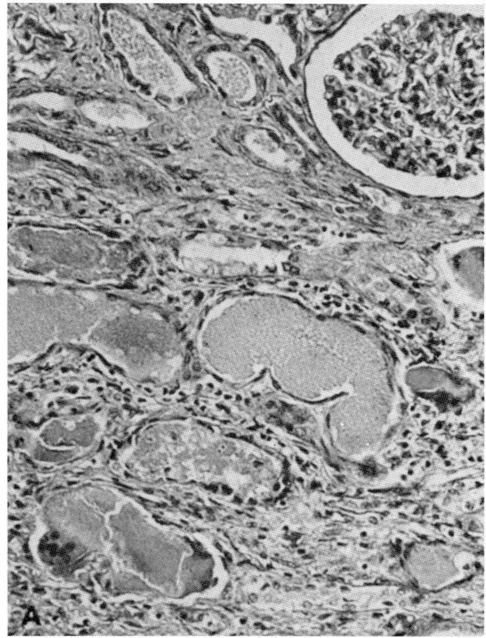

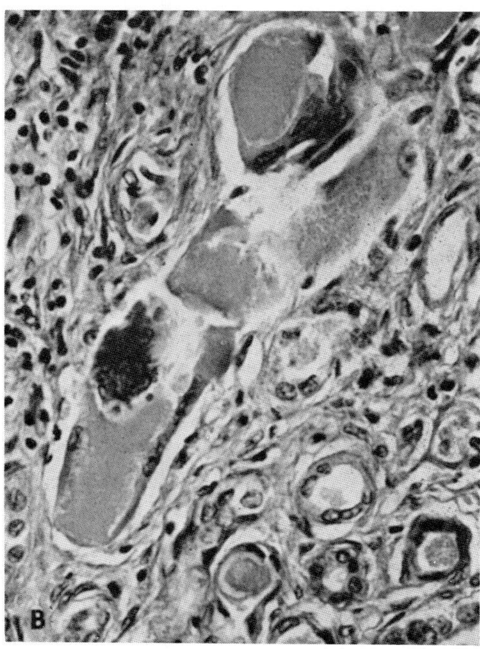

Figure 21-2. Myeloma kidney disease. A. Large dilated tubules filled with amorphous casts. Giant cells are present; atrophy of tubules and chronic inflammation are also seen. Glomeruli are normal. Hematoxylin and eosin. ×200. B. Giant cells showing probable origin from epithelium. Hematoxylin and eosin. ×400.

tubular atrophy more often correlates better with renal insufficiency than does the presence or extent of casts. Their finding of intraepithelial proteins as well as the previously mentioned crystalline inclusions in tubular cells suggests that the abnormal proteins may exert a direct effect upon the functional integrity of the nephron.

Recent immunofluorescent studies of the casts found in multiple myeloma indicate that the casts contain albumin, IgG, as well as kappa and lambda light chains, and in many instances fibrinogen [177]. This confirms earlier work that indicated that the casts were composed of a complex mixture of proteins [43].

Although it is evident that the pathologic picture associated with renal impairment is variable, there is general agreement that the infiltrates of plasma cells occasionally seen within the kidney are usually not associated with any clinically recognizable disturbance in renal function.

The tubular epithelium and its basement membrane frequently show extensive calcium deposition with secondary destruction. The associated damage, particularly in the convoluted tubules, may be extensive (Fig. 21-4). One of the renal effects in experimental hypercalcemia is a reduction in the medullary sodium concentration. This abnormality, plus the extensive calcium deposition in the region of the tubular basement membrane, reduces the efficiency of water movement in the distal convolutions and collecting ducts, resulting in urine concentration varying from isotonicity to hypotonicity. The observations of Roussak and Oleesky [146] suggest that, in addition, the deposition of proteinaceous material and resulting injury to the epithelium may also

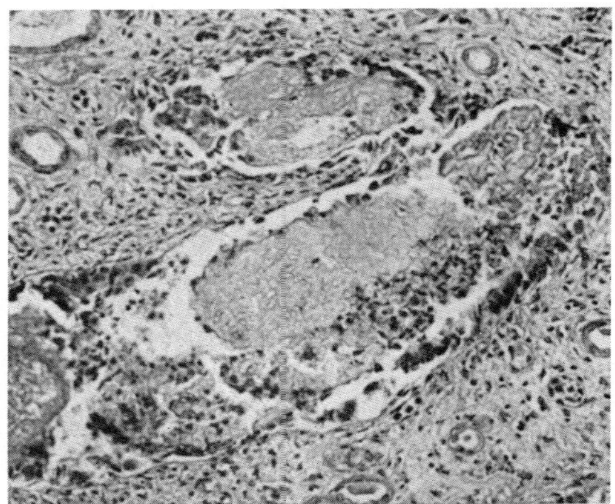

Figure 21-3. Myeloma kidney disease. Casts in collecting ducts showing acute inflammation and fragmentation. Hematoxylin and eosin. ×150.

play a role in the disturbance observed in the renal-concentrating mechanism.

MYELOMATOSIS AND AMYLOID DEPOSITS

Amyloid deposits are found in about 10 per cent of autopsy cases of multiple myeloma. The generalized deposition of amyloid seen in this disease usually falls into the distribution pattern of primary amyloidosis (see below). The mesenchymal tissues and blood vessels are characteristically involved. Deposition within glomeruli is considerably less than that seen in secondary amyloidosis. While it is generally thought that the amyloid deposits must in some way be related to the abnormal protein produced in myelomatosis, and several authors have pointed out that membranous thickening of glomerular capillaries may be prominent in some patients with multiple myeloma, immunofluorescent studies have failed to demonstrate the deposition of light chains of Bence Jones protein within the glomerulus [102]. The relation between these two disorders is considered further in the section on *Amyloidosis* below.

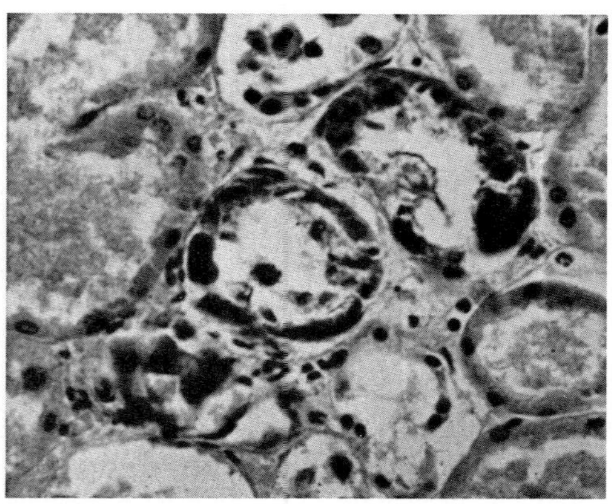

Figure 21-4. Myeloma renal disease. Calcification of epithelium and basement membrane in convoluted tubules. Hematoxylin and eosin. ×300.

DIAGNOSIS

Although clinical renal disease is rarely the presenting manifestation of multiple myeloma, Bence Jones proteinuria may be seen very early in the disease and its recognition is so simple and of such importance that a screening test for its detection should occupy an important place among simple laboratory procedures of value in diagnosis. However, false-negative and false-positive tests may be encountered unless special precautions are taken. For routine screening, a salting-out method has been found to be of considerable value [49] and the reversible heat precipitation described by Putnam and Udin [137] is also of great value for rapid screening. It is clear, however, from recent studies of large numbers of patients with multiple myeloma that neither of these tests can be relied upon to identify all cases of Bence Jones proteinuria and if clinical circumstances make the diagnosis of myeloma likely some type of screening electrophoretic procedure on the serum or urine is indicated [24, 87, 102].

Several reports noting the hazards of intravenous pyelography have appeared. Oliguria has been reported to follow this procedure, particularly in patients with preexisting evidence of renal disease [121, 129]. For this reason, it has been recommended that pyelography be avoided whenever the diagnosis of renal involvement with myeloma is entertained; or if employed, the patient should be well hydrated.

TREATMENT

The variable course of the disease makes objective evaluation of therapeutic agents difficult. Urethane, stilbamidine, alkylating agents, folic acid antimetabolites, steroids, ACTH, and 6-mercaptopurine have all been used with questionable benefit [148]. There is no good evidence that any of these agents are of value in reversing the renal lesions associated with myeloma or in changing the clinical course once renal failure has appeared. There is some evidence that L-phenylalanine mustard therapy may have a beneficial effect in those patients synthesizing kappa-type Bence Jones protein and that treatment of this group may result in longer survival than in those with lambda-type Bence Jones protein [24].

Although it is doubtful that any of the chemotherapeutic agents will successfully reverse renal damage, a recent report emphasizes that occasionally the combination of widespread myelomatosis and acute renal failure is not a hopeless situation, the combination of hemodialysis and phenylalanine mustard being adequate to produce marked clinical improvement [19]. This merits particular emphasis in view of the relative frequency with which acute renal failure follows dehydration and such procedures as intravenous pyelography in patients with severe multiple myeloma [129].

Hypercalcemia, with its attendant renal effects, merits specific mention. Hypercalcemia may be the most striking manifestation of myelomatosis on occasion, with serum calcium values exceeding 15 to 20 mg. per 100 ml. The marked nephrotoxicity of such calcium levels, as well as the damage to other tissues, makes early recognition and treatment of this aspect of the disease imperative. Most cases respond to steroid administration by dramatic reduction in serum calcium levels. Even more dramatic reduction in serum calcium can be effected by the production of an osmotic diuresis with a large divalent anion such as sulfate [18, 27, 90]. The accompanying increase in calcium excretion can be potentiated by such diuretics as furosemide and ethacrynic acid; the benzothiadiazides have an opposite effect [172]. The effects of such treatment are transient, and the serum calcium begins to rise again shortly after the infusion has been discontinued. The hazards of such therapy have been emphasized [18, 79], and it should be employed with caution. The use of phosphate should be avoided [18]. The principal usefulness of such therapy probably lies in its use as an adjunctive measure combined with steroid administration in the acute hypercalcemic crisis occasionally seen in patients with myeloma and other malignant tumors. The early renal manifestations associated with hypercalcemia are usually easily reversed with this treatment (Fig. 21-1), but there is no evidence that it has any effect on the advanced stages of renal insufficiency associated with nephrocalcinosis.

Amyloidosis

Amyloidosis is the term used to signify the group of diseases characterized by the accumulation of an extracellular, eosinophilic, hyaline substance distributed irregularly and in varying degrees through virtually all organs of the body. During the period of more than a century since it was first described by Rokitansky and Virchow, much of the effort devoted to the study of amyloidosis has been directed toward obtaining a suitable classification of this group of disorders [22, 31, 170]. Amyloidosis may occur as a late development in a number of chronic diseases, including suppurative diseases such as osteomyelitis as well as tuberculosis, leprosy, and rheumatoid arthritis, or occasionally may be found in previously healthy individuals without coexistent or antecedent illness. The latter form has been termed *primary amyloidosis* to distinguish it from the secondary variety which complicates the long course of the illnesses listed above. Amyloid also occurs in perhaps 5 to 10 per cent of patients with myelomatosis and has also been described in association with medullary thyroid carcinoma and with islet cell tumors of the pancreas [31]. In addition, three distinct hereditary forms have been recognized [4, 16, 147, 158]. Thus, using these clinical features, it is possible to classify amyloidosis as primary, secondary, hereditary, or amyloidosis associated with neoplastic disease [1, 4–6, 10]. An alternate classification based upon the anatomic features of the amyloid deposits has been proposed [80] and challenged [31].

Heller, Missmahl, and their associates[80] have proposed a classification of amyloid based upon the site of earliest deposition of the amyloid material, indicating that amyloid may appear first either along reticulin fibers and hence be termed perireticular amyloid or, alternately, along collagen fibers and be termed pericollagen. The former type appears within the intima of blood vessels and spreads toward the media, while the latter or pericollagen type appears first within the adventitial layer of blood vessels. Included in the perireticular amyloid classification are some of the hereditary amyloidoses (familial Mediterranean fever and the syndrome of deafness and urticaria, with amyloid deposits) as well as the amyloid associated with chronic inflammation. The pericollagen included the familial amyloidosis with neurologic involvement, amyloidosis seen in myeloma, and classic primary amyloidosis. They used polarization microscopy to facilitate identification of the early lesions and considered that classification was improved thereby [80]. Other workers have questioned whether this pathologic classification does provide a sharp distinction between the various clinical types of amyloidosis [31].

Osserman's [126] observations that patients with primary amyloidosis almost all had some abnormal paraprotein analogous to that seen in myeloma led to the belief, supported by some experimental studies, that amyloidosis was in some way the result of deposition of such abnormal globulins in the tissues [33, 126, 167]. More recent studies have failed to confirm this notion, however [10, 31].

Electron microscopy of amyloid-laden tissues has demonstrated a fibrillar structure to the amyloid [31]. Studies by Cohen and Calkins [32] on isolated preparations of these fibrils failed to demonstrate any specific association or reaction with tagged anti-gamma-globulin antibodies. These fibrils represent a fibrous protein composed of laterally aggregated filaments demonstrating longitudinal periodicity or beading distinct from collagen, and possibly containing a small amount of carbohydrate. The amyloid fibril is distinct from gamma globulin and does not appear to contain any of this globulin in isolated preparations [32]. Regardless of the source of material studied, whether from amyloid experimentally induced in animals or from any of the several distinct clinical forms of amyloidosis, the chemical and ultrastructural features of the material are the same. Both experimental and electron microscopic observations suggest that this particular substance arises from the reticuloendothelial cell. Despite the remarkable clinical association between the presence of amyloidosis and abnormalities of the immunoglobulins or the presence of significant quantities of Bence Jones protein, the significance of this association remains obscure. It has been suggested that this is a reflection of an abnormality which arises in some precursor stem cell that gives rise to both abnormal reticuloendothelial elements and plasma cells so that the presence of these two abnormal cell types gives rise to the production of both amyloid and abnormal immunoglobulins [10, 31].

The frequency of amyloidosis, as judged solely by histologic evidence at postmortem examination, varies between 0.4 and 0.5 per cent. In a series of 4000 autopsies from the Massachusetts General Hospital, the diagnosis was made 21 times. The majority of these cases occurred in patients with rheumatoid arthritis and multiple myeloma [21]. In 20,000 consecutive autopies at the Johns Hopkins Hospital, amyloidosis was noted in 79 cases. In 46, the lesion was associated with chronic inflammatory disease such as tuberculosis, bronchiectasis, pyelonephritis, or some other chronic suppurative process. Five cases were associated with multiple myeloma. In the remaining 28 cases, there was no association with any other major disease process. Renal involvement was demonstrated in 16 of the 79 cases, being noted much more frequently in the cases associated with inflammatory disease.

CLINICAL MANIFESTATIONS OF RENAL AMYLOIDOSIS

Proteinuria is the most common manifestation of renal involvement in amyloidosis, and it may be present for many years as the sole renal abnormality. In this circumstance, the patient's major symptoms are associated with amyloid deposition in other organs, proteinuria representing only an incidental finding. When clinically manifest renal disease occurs, it usually presents either as renal insufficiency with progressive uremia or as the nephrotic syndrome. Renal vein thrombosis and a clinical picture resembling that of diabetes insipidus have also been reported [8, 25, 46, 77].

Severe renal insufficiency leading to death from uremia results from extensive replacement of renal tissue by amyloid accumulations. In a series of 100 cases proved at autopsy, only 10 per cent showed significant azotemia (blood urea nitrogen greater than 35 mg. per 100 ml.), and in only four instances did the blood urea nitrogen exceed 100 mg. per 100 ml. [11, 46]. Heptinstall and Joekes [83] report similar findings in a smaller group of cases diagnosed by renal biopsy. Thus, uremia as the presenting manifestation of renal amyloidosis is relatively uncommon.

It is generally stated that hypertension is an infrequent consequence of diffuse renal amyloidosis. In Heptinstall's series, however, 5 of 11 patients had significant elevation of the arterial blood pressure [83]. In our experience, the majority of patients have been normotensive when first seen, and blood pressure usually has fallen as the disease progressed. Bell [11], however, noted hypertension in nearly half of those cases in which severe amyloid deposition and azotemia were present.

The nephrotic syndrome is commonly the presenting manifestation of renal amyloidosis and exhibits the characteristic features of edema, hypoproteinemia, and hypercholesterolemia. Urinary protein loss may range from 4 to 20 gm. or more per day, and urinary sedimentary changes may include microscopic hematuria, granular casts, and some fatty casts. The frequency of the nephrotic syndrome has varied in different series. Calkins and Cohen [21] reported an incidence of 50 per cent in secondary amyloidosis, while Heptinstall and Joekes [83] found significant edema associated with hypoproteinemia in only 2 of 11 cases diagnosed by biopsy. Bell [11] noted that approximately one-third of his cases had significant edema with hypoproteinemia. In the extensive review by Rukavina et al. [147], a correlation was noted between the presence and severity of the nephrotic syndrome and the severity of the renal involvement as judged histologically. In our experience, the diagnosis has been made from biopsy material in seven patients; six of these exhibited the nephrotic syndrome and all but one were instances of primary amyloidosis.

In a study of nine cases of thrombosis of the renal vein, Harrison et al. [77] found four to be associated with renal amyloidosis. It was not possible to ascertain the chronologic sequence of events, but it appeared likely that amyloidosis preceded the thrombosis. In three of these cases, the clinical picture was that of rapidly progressive uremia. In the fourth case, sudden onset of the nephrotic syndrome with preservation of other aspects of renal function was noted. These observations have been confirmed by Barclay and his associates [8], who reported nine similar cases.

Carone and Epstein [25] reported on a patient with marked polyuria as a feature of amyloidosis associated with chronic osteomyelitis. The daily urinary output of this patient ranged from 3 to 6 liters. Proteinuria was persistently present, but the total amount of protein excreted was small. The patient was normotensive, exhibited a slight reduction in phenolsulfonphtalein (PSP) excretion, and had a normal blood nonprotein nitrogen. Urinary hypotonicity persisted despite hypertonic saline infusion and intravenous administration of vasopressin. At autopsy, amyloid deposition was demonstrated in the medulla of the kidney; heavy deposits surrounded the collecting ducts and involved many of the vasa recta. It was concluded that these deposits restricted the movement of water out of the collecting ducts to such a degree that the urine remained persistently hypotonic. Polyuria had been previously noted [46] but was attributed to the osmotic diuresis associated with renal insufficiency. Polyuria was sufficiently severe to be mentioned as a symptom in only one of the 79 cases seen at the Johns Hopkins Hospital.

More information about the clinical course of amyloidosis has been obtained through the study of patients with familial Mediterranean fever than perhaps in any other situation in which amyloidosis may be encountered [80, 81, 158]. Sohar and his associates [158], in their review of more than 800 cases of familial Mediterranean fever, obtained a detailed picture both of the importance of amyloidosis in this condition and of the natural history of renal involvement by amyloid deposition. Amyloidosis in this condition is genetically determined and appears to account basically for all deaths seen in familial Mediterranean fever. In virtually every case death is the result of renal involvement. The frequency of amyloidosis in the group which they studied was about 28 per cent, but it was noteworthy that follow-up study of these cases revealed that the rate of development of new cases of amyloidosis was approximately equal to the rate at which cases of familial Mediterranean fever were diagnosed and added to the group.

The clinical course of the amyloid nephropathy of familial Mediterranean fever is divided into four stages of variable duration: the preclinical stage, proteinuria, nephrosis, and finally uremia. The preclinical state is not well studied but has been clearly documented in several cases in which biopsies, performed for one reason or another, have revealed amyloidosis in vessels of the kidney or elsewhere in the complete absence of symptoms. How long such a state can exist is unknown, but in one instance in Sohar's series it was present for six years. The authors were able to observe the appearance of proteinuria in 30 cases among the patients whom they followed. A look at the subsequent history of these patients reveals that 19 remain in the stage of proteinuria for periods ranging between 2 and 10 years; in the remaining 11, the proteinuria was followed after a variable period of time by the appearance of the nephrotic syndrome. The duration between onset of proteinuria and onset of the nephrotic syndrome ranged between two and nine years, the majority of cases falling between three and five years. The duration of the nephrotic syndrome averaged between one and two years and was followed in virtually every instance by the appearance of progressive uremia. This usually was present for an additional year to year and a half. Thus, although proteinuria may be present for a decade or more, the appearance of the nephrotic syndrome usually heralds the beginning of the terminal phase of the illness, and in general, patients live about three years after the nephrotic syndrome first appears.

In the uremic stage, the kidneys may indeed become small. Interestingly enough, hypertension accompanies progressive renal insufficiency of the uremic phase in nearly one-half the total cases.

HISTOPATHOLOGY OF RENAL AMYLOIDOSIS

The most marked accumulations of amyloid occur in the glomeruli, although deposition of amyloid may be seen in the peritubular basement membranes, interstitium, and blood vessels. The earliest glomerular changes detectable by light microscopy are hyaline widening of the intercapillary or mesangial regions accompanied by some thickening of the capillary basement membranes (Figs. 21-5, 21-6). As the disease progresses, deposition of amyloid occurs in both locations until in the late stages large nodular masses and greatly thickened capillary basement membranes are evident. Significant reduction in the number and size of the capillary lumina is a late manifestation.

By electron microscopy [31, 32, 119] the amyloid material is seen to be a fibrillar substance lying against the basement membrane, usually between the endothelium and the basement membrane of the glomerulus. Eventually, this material develops along either side, lifting off the epithelial or endothelial cytoplasm (Figs. 21-6, 21-7). The true basement membrane tends to remain as a definite line of greater density even when it passes through large masses of amyloid, although at times it may become indistinct (Fig. 21-7). It is clear from both light and electron microscopy that the mesangium is the site of much, if not most, of the amyloid deposition (Fig. 21-6). The larger deposits almost completely obliterate the mesangial cytoplasm.

In the glomeruli showing amyloid deposits, there is replacement of individual epithelial foot processes by a continuous cytoplasmic sheet. Such a change is also noted in other conditions associated with significant proteinuria and is generally believed to be a secondary or nonspecific phenomenon [134].

Atrophic tubules are commonly seen in instances of advanced glomerular amyloidosis. However, significant amounts of amyloid are often found in the basement membrane surrounding the tubules. The tubules may be dilated and filled with eosinophilic casts, resembling the alterations characteristically found in chronic pyelonephritis [83]. Fibrosis, lymphocytic infiltration, and additional amyloid deposition may be noted in the interstitial tissue in advanced cases. In several of our patients histologic study has revealed

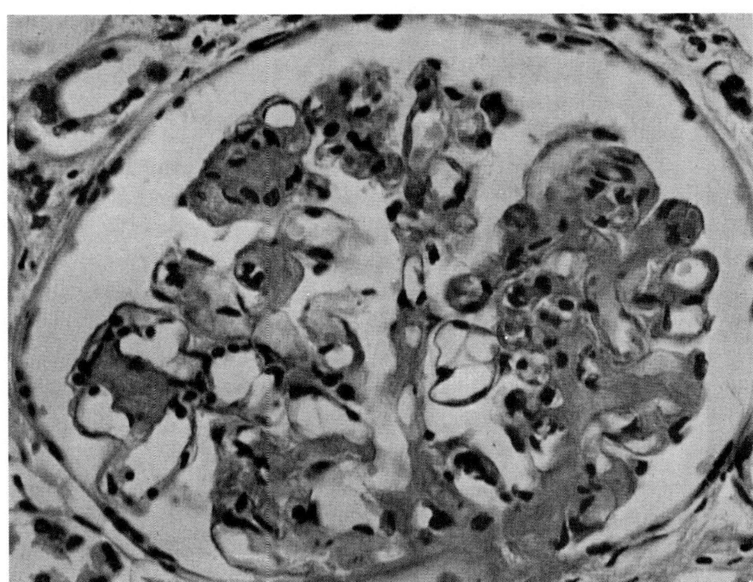

Figure 21-5. Amyloidosis. Early glomerular amyloid deposition. Hematoxylin and eosin. ×500, before 25% reduction.

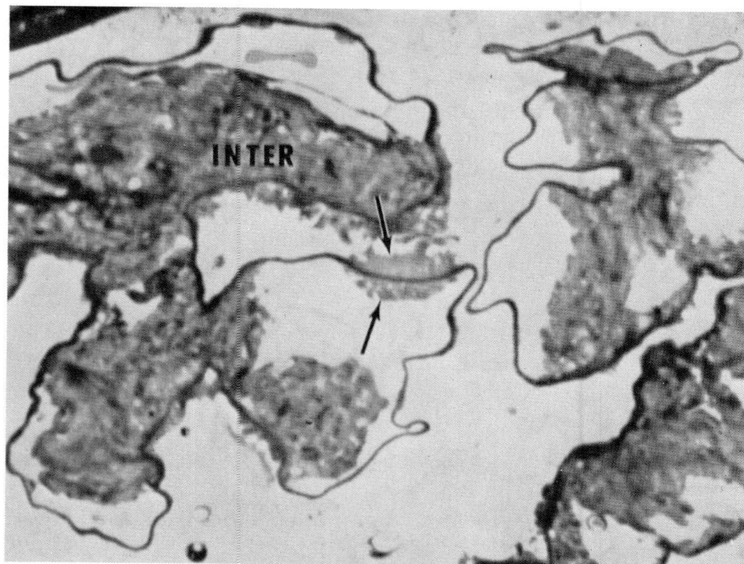

Figure 21-6. Amyloidosis. Osmic-fixed, methacrylate-embedded section of a glomerulus cut 1 micron thick. Deposition in intercapillary areas (INTER) is most marked. Amyloid is also present (*arrows*) on both sides of the darkly stained capillary basement membrane. Methenamine-silver stain. ×2000, before 25% reduction.

amyloid deposited around the thin limb of the loops of Henle and the nearby capillary loops (Fig. 21-8). The occurrence of vascular amyloidosis in the kidney is variable in both primary and secondary types of deposits, but no significant arterial obstruction develops even with extreme deposition. Thus far, light and electron microscopy have failed to demonstrate any distinct structural differences between amyloid observed in human material and that in experimentally induced material nor have any consistent structural differences been identified between the several clinically recognized types of human amyloidosis [31, 142].

The histologic features of amyloidosis are ordinarily quite apparent in material stained with hematoxylin and eosin, but the definitive differentiation of amyloid from other hyaline and proteinaceous substances requires special staining technics. This is especially true in needle-biopsy material where only a few glo-

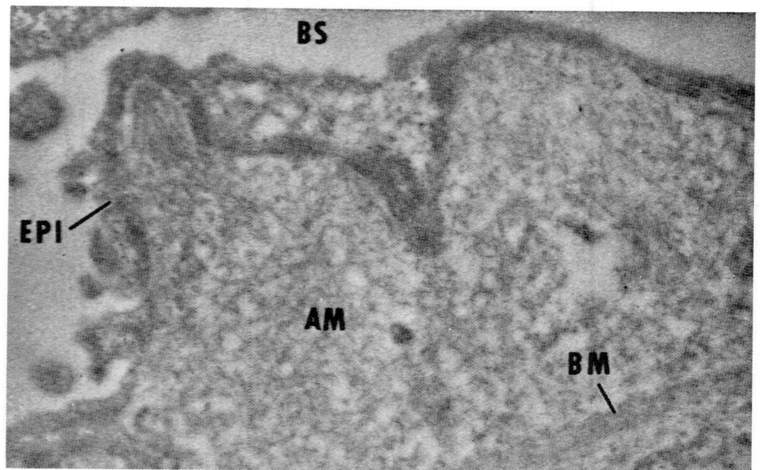

Figure 21-7. Amyloidosis. Electron micrograph of a capillary loop showing fibrillar-appearing amyloid (AM) on both sides of a still recognizable true basement membrane (BM). The epithelium (EPI) no longer shows the usual foot processes adjacent to Bowman's space (BS). ×36,000, before 25% reduction.

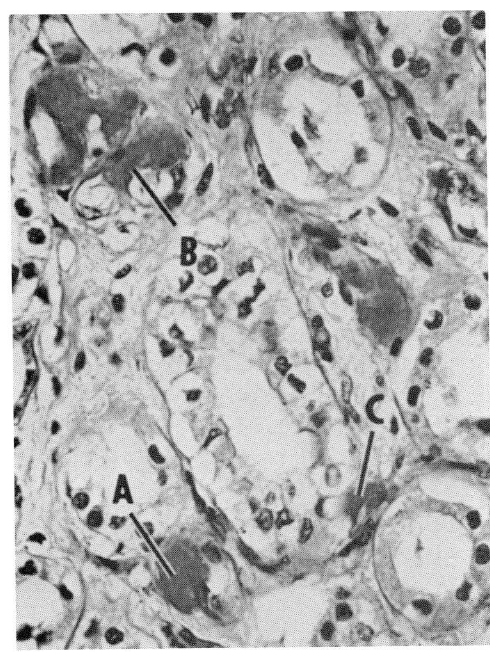

Figure 21-8. Amyloidosis. Medullary amyloid deposits involving the thin limbs (A), capillaries (B), and basement membranes of the collecting ducts (C). Hematoxylin and eosin. ×400.

meruli may be available for study and a reliable diagnosis is difficult. The staining characteristics of amyloid may vary greatly from case to case, and none of the metachromatic stains are specific for the detection of amyloid. Cohen [31] has recently reviewed the staining properties of amyloid. Although the deposition of fibrillar amyloid deposits as demonstrated by electron microscopy is the most specific, the combination of Congo-red staining and demonstration of birefringence by polarization microscopy appears to be the most useful technic for demonstrating amyloid by light microscopy. The use of fluorescent dyes offers no unique advantages [31, 167, 168].

DIAGNOSIS

The occurrence of proteinuria in association with chronic suppurative disease or other inflammatory diseases such as rheumatoid arthritis should always raise the suspicion of renal amyloidosis. In addition, the diagnosis should always be entertained in any adult presenting with the nephrotic syndrome. Proteinuria accompanied by mild to marked renal failure and abnormal blood pressure should create suspicion also, especially if associated with normal or large renal shadows on x-ray examination. The various hereditary forms of amyloidosis such as the syndrome of deafness, urticaria, and amyloidosis, familial Mediterranean fever, and the familial form described by Andrade are sufficiently distinctive that the disease can be suspected on clinical grounds [1, 4, 5].

The diagnosis can be established with certainty only by histologic examination. The value of liver and renal biopsy as well as rectal biopsy have been well demonstrated. However, untoward results characterized by life-endangering and occasionally fatal hemorrhage have been recorded following liver biopsy in three patients [21]. Consequently, it has been recommended by some authors that liver biopsy not be undertaken if amyloidosis is suspected. Alternatively, renal biopsy appears to be a safe procedure in the presence of amyloidosis. Heptinstall found renal amyloidosis in over 10 per cent in a series of nearly 100 consecutive renal biopsies. In our experience, this diagnosis has been encountered somewhat less commonly, being made seven times in approximately 300 renal biopsies.

Routine blood and urine examinations reveal no specific abnormalities. Commonly there is an elevation of the erythrocyte sedimentation rate. Anemia usually parallels the degree of renal insufficiency. Proteinuria is the most common and most reliable index of renal involvement. Hematuria is infrequently seen, occurring in less than 5 per cent of cases. Hyaline and granular casts are relatively common, particularly in patients exhibiting marked proteinuria. Serum protein electrophoresis may reveal an abnormal spike (monoclonal gammopathy), but as has been adequately demonstrated recently, this is not seen in all cases so that absence of such a finding does not exclude the disease [10, 108].

TREATMENT

No specific treatment for amyloidosis exists. Antimetabolites known to depress the rate of formation of gamma globulins have been ineffective when used in those cases of amyloidosis associated with abnormal globulin production. Steroids have been of little or no value.

The general supportive measures of importance in treatment of the nephrotic syndrome have been discussed elsewhere in this book (Chapter 16) as have the principles of management of renal insufficiency when it appears.

Systemic Lupus Erythematosus

Systemic lupus erythematosus (SLE) is a connective tissue disorder with varied clinical manifestations, occurring predominantly in women in the reproductive period of life [47, 78, 91]. The course of this disease is frequently chronic, being associated with exacerbations and remissions over many years. Even when acute and severe manifestations occur, they may be followed by dramatic, spontaneous improvement. One or more of a large family of serum protein abnormalities may be present, including the factor responsible for the formation of the LE cell [86].

GENERAL CLINICAL FEATURES

The clinical pattern of this syndrome is variable. The joints and the dermis are most frequently involved, but changes in the pleura, pericardium, and lymph nodes are often seen, and renal involvement is one of the leading causes of death. In addition to the signs due to specific organ lesions, constitutional alterations such as fever, fatigability, and weight loss are common. There is no single characteristic pattern as the disease evolves. Often it presents as a puzzling combination of clinical events involving multiple systems and showing little continuity. Nearly all patients exhibit one or more hematologic abnormalities during the course of the disease, and in some a blood disorder such as hemolytic anemia or thrombocytopenic purpura is the presenting or dominant feature. Leukopenia is commonly found, and 80 per cent of the patients have a mild or moderate normocytic, normochromic anemia due to retarded erythropoiesis. A false-positive serologic test for syphilis may precede the initial clinical manifestations by many years [115]. The serum gamma globulin concentration is frequently elevated, while serum albumin may be reduced. In the active phase, serum complement activity may be reduced. Plasma fibrinogen levels are increased. Less common evidences of plasma protein dysfunction are autoagglutination of red cells, a circulating anticoagulant, a positive Coombs test, and the presence of cryoglobulins [78].

In addition to the hematologic evidences of an autoimmune disorder (hemolytic anemia, thrombotic thrombocytopenic purpura), abnormal reactions of gamma globulins have been identified [34, 152]. Serum from patients suffering with SLE contains gamma globulins that react with constituents of cell nuclei. One of these, an antinucleoprotein factor, is responsible for the production of the LE-cell phenomenon, the most commonly used diagnostic test for SLE. The reactions that these substances exhibit characterize them as antibodies, and the use of standard immunologic technics has identified antibodies to single-stranded and double-stranded deoxyribonucleic acid (DNA), to nucleoproteins, to the nonhistone proteins of the nucleus, and to the Sm antigen [95]. In addition, antibodies to various cytoplasmic constituents including antiribosomal antibodies have been identified [42, 96].

The significance of these antibodies in the pathogenesis of SLE remains incompletely understood. They do not appear to play a primary etiologic role since they exert no cytotoxic effect upon transplacental transfer or when given to laboratory animals. LE cells are rarely found in vivo (see Fig. 21-15), and the artificial conditions required for their production suggest that the antibody responsible for their production is effective only against damaged cells [36, 96]. In addition, virtually all the clinical manifestations of the disease may exist in the absence of all these factors. More recent evidence has assigned a role for at least some of these antibodies in the pathogenesis and progression of the renal lesions in SLE. Both DNA antigen and DNA antibody have been identified as circulating constituents of the serum and as components of the renal lesions in SLE.

PATHOLOGIC CHANGES

The chief pathologic alterations in SLE may be considered in three general categories: fibrinoid alterations, lesions involving cellular necrosis and nuclear alterations, and the granulomatous reaction.

Fibrinoid Alterations. The lesion termed fibrinoid alteration (also called fibrinoid degeneration, fibrinoid necrosis, or simply fibrinoid by various authors) refers to the presence of a homogeneous, markedly eosinophilic material histologically resembling fibrin. This material is part of a nonspecific reaction seen under a variety of conditions, but its common occurrence in the connective tissue diseases is well recognized [88, 131]. As an isolated finding, fibrinoid alteration is principally seen in the ground substance in lupus erythematosus. Immunologic studies in SLE and other connective tissue disorders have demonstrated that the fibrinoid material contains gamma globulin [68].

Cellular Necrosis and Nuclear Alterations. Gross [74] believed that the hematoxylin bodies of SLE, which he first noted in endocardial lesions in autopsy material, represented pyknotic nuclei. It is now almost universally agreed that they are the best if not the only histologic finding specific for SLE. Studies have demonstrated clearly that the phagocytized inclusion body of the LE cells is identical with the hematoxylin bodies. Small masses of this material, approximately the size of individual nuclei, may coalesce to form large extracellular aggregates scattered throughout the tissues [70, 71].

Various tissues — including vessel walls, connective tissue in different organs, and lymph nodes — may show foci of fresh necrosis. These lesions are most common in autopsy material from patients exhibiting a fulminant and rapidly fatal course clinically. Such necrotic sites commonly contain hematoxylin bodies. Indeed, the predominant occurrence of these structures at injury sites in acute SLE has been offered as evidence that the integrity of the cell must be interrupted before the nucleus can react with the serum factor. This concept gains support from the observation that in vitro demonstration of the LE-cell phenomenon is enhanced by a variety of procedures that subject the cells to trauma and mechanical injury [36].

Granulomatous Reaction. Teilum [164] described epithelioid cell granulomas and nodular areas of necrosis in the serous membranes, lungs, and lymph nodes in two fatal cases of SLE. This is an unusual reaction in which foci of necrosis, fibrinoid alteration, and sometimes hematoxylin bodies may be surrounded by an accumulation of epithelioid cells. Giant cells, which may enclose masses of fibrinoid material, are frequently present.

RENAL INVOLVEMENT

Lupus nephritis is probably the most serious of the many manifestations of SLE. Despite the effectiveness of the corticosteroids in suppressing most of the other manifestations of the disease, renal disease remains the leading cause of death in this disorder. Renal involvement appears to be more common in the younger patients. In the 90 patients reported by Soffer et al. [157], 62 per cent of the 56 patients with renal disease were under the age of 30 years, while 65 per cent of the 34 patients without renal involvement were past the age of 30. Morbidity and mortality from renal involvement were also nearly twice as great in the younger patients [157]. Patients who exhibit renal involvement are much more likely to do so early in the course of their illness [145, 157], although we have seen fulminant renal disease develop in one woman more than 15 years after the onset of the SLE.

Clinical manifestations of renal lupus include hypertension, edema, and on occasion oliguria or anuria with rapidly progressing uremia. Hypertension in SLE is seen almost exclusively in patients with renal involvement, but it is not a constant feature of lupus nephritis. The clinical spectrum of renal involvement ranges from proteinuria and hematuria without any accompanying symptoms to a picture of severe glomerulonephritis with uremia or the nephrotic syndrome, or both.

Hypertension is rarely seen early in the course of the disease. In general, it roughly parallels the degree of renal involvement and is usually severe when lupus nephritis has damaged the kidney severely. Even when therapy has been successful in arresting the activity of the disease in these cases with advanced renal damage, hypertension persists and is often sufficiently severe to represent an additional threat of further renal damage.

In about 20 per cent of patients with lupus nephritis the nephrotic syndrome develops at some stage during the illness, with the typical findings of heavy proteinuria, hypoalbuminemia, hypercholesteremia, and doubly refractile fat bodies in the urine [157]. The earlier finding of Muehrcke and his associates [120] that the presence of a low serum cholesterol value in patients with the nephrotic syndrome and lupus nephritis heralded a particularly poor prognosis has not been borne out in subsequent studies [145, 157]. Although as a group lupus patients with nephrosis fare poorly and have a higher mortality rate than the total group of patients with lupus nephritis, subsequent studies have failed to identify any association between cholesterol levels and mortality rate.

Urinary findings vary from slight proteinuria and a few red and white blood cells on microscopic examination to a "telescoped" urine sediment that contains all the casts and other formed elements seen in the various stages of ordinary glomerulonephritis. In general, the urinary findings correlate well with the histologic findings on renal biopsy [178]. In general, patients with the minimal renal involvement that characterizes lupus glomerulitis (see below) excrete less than 1 gm. of protein in the urine per 24 hours, and the urine sediment contains only moderate numbers of leukocytes and a few red blood cells. RBC casts are rarely seen in this group. Those cases with more advanced and widespread histologic changes exhibit much heavier proteinuria, and the urine sediment includes many RBC casts as well as granular casts, erythrocytes, and leukocytes [98, 104].

HISTOLOGY

The earliest visible change that can be seen by light microscopy in lupus nephritis is the appearance of minute foci of hypercellularity at the periphery of some of the glomerular capillary tufts (Fig. 21-9). The hypercellularity appears attributable to endothelial proliferation associated with localized fibrinoid change, leading to thickening of the basement membrane of the glomerulus. This lesion is termed *local glomerulitis* since only part of a tuft is usually involved. With increase in size of hypercellular areas, glomerular ischemia presumably develops, inflammatory cells appear, and early necrotic changes with karyorrhexis may be noted. Small fibrinous adhesions may be seen bridging Bowman's space. Later, dense fibrous adhesions appear attached to Bowman's capsule (Fig. 21-10). With progress of the disease, these hypercellular areas become more numerous and may eventually fuse to involve entire glomeruli, although the

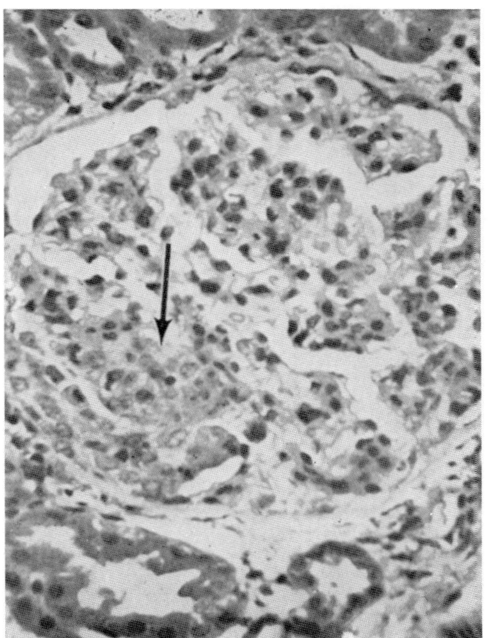

Figure 21-9. Systemic lupus erythematosus. Glomerulus showing local necrosis and hypercellularity (*arrow*) and adjacent adhesion formation. This corresponds to the stage of "local glomerulitis" described by Muehrcke et al. [72]. Hematoxylin and eosin. ×300.

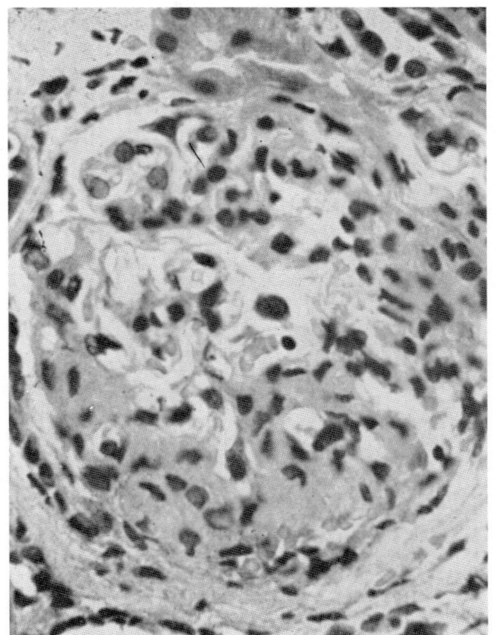

Figure 21-10. Systemic lupus erythematosus. Local fibrosis of a glomerulus. Hematoxylin and eosin. ×500.

disease often remains focal in that some glomeruli are spared. Eosinophilic thickening of the basement membrane is evident. This stage has been called *general glomerulitis* (Fig. 21-11). On the other hand, when fibrinoid thickening of the glomerular membrane is the dominant change, with endothelial proliferation less striking, the lesion is described as *membranous glomerulonephritis.* In contrast to the ordinary type of membranous glomerulonephritis, however, the membrane thickening is not always uniform. Extreme membranous thickening of single capillary loops is designated the wire-loop lesion (Fig. 21-11). Material described as fibrinoid or hyaline in appearance may also fill the capillary lumina to form structures referred to as hyaline thrombi (Fig. 21-12). Occasionally these contain Feulgen-positive basophilic material having the characteristics of a hematoxylin body (Figs. 21-13, 21-14).

Lesions fitting the description of subacute glomerulonephritis are frequently seen, usually in patients who exhibit clinical manifestations of the nephrotic syndrome [59, 120]. In addition to the hypercellular change and membrane thickening, fibroepithelial crescents of Bowman's capsule are present, and there is evidence of degeneration in the renal tubules. Edema and inflammatory cells in the interstitial tissue are frequently seen. In those patients who die of renal insufficiency there is widespread renal damage with lesions of the type referred to as local fibrinous glomerulonephritis or lesions of subacute and chronic glomerulonephritis indistinguishable from glo-

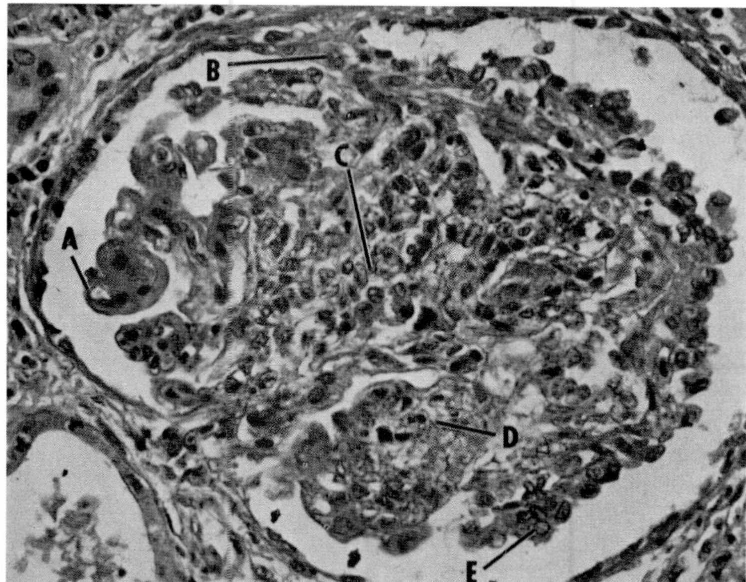

Figure 21-11. Systemic lupus erythematosus. A wire-loop lesion is visible peripherally (A). There are also an adhesion (B), local hypercellularity (C), necrosis (D), and proliferation of epithelial cells (E). Hematoxylin and eosin. ×500, before 25% reduction.

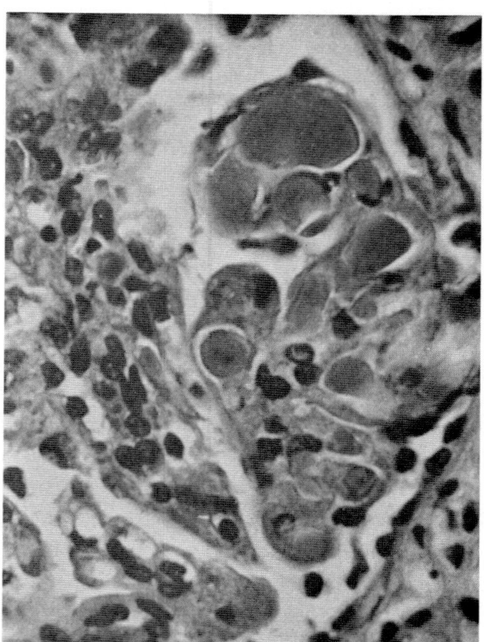

Figure 21-12. Systemic lupus erythematosus. Hyaline thrombi in glomerular capillary lumina. This patient presented with the clinical picture of thrombotic thrombocytopenic purpura, although hyaline thrombi may be found in SLE in the absence of that syndrome. Hematoxylin and eosin. ×500.

merulonephritis due to other causes. The characteristic wire-loop lesions and hematoxylin bodies may be found. The latter may be found either in the glomeruli or in the interstitium. LE cells are a great rarity (Fig. 21-15). Although the lesions described above are the typical findings in lupus nephritis, they are not diagnostic, since all these changes, except for hematoxylin bodies, may be seen in a variety of renal diseases. It is not possible to diagnose SLE from renal biopsy findings in the absence of hematoxylin bodies.

Earlier studies led to the inference that the different pictures described above were really stages in the progression of changes that were encountered in all cases of lupus nephritis [120]. This concept has been questioned as a result of longer follow-up periods of patients with lupus nephritis. More recent studies suggest either that the earlier stage of lupus glomerulitis does not progress to the more destructive later stages, or alternately that it is much more susceptible to arrest and reversal by therapy than the more widespread changes of the membranous glomerulonephritis or proliferative glomerulonephritis of lupus [133, 145].

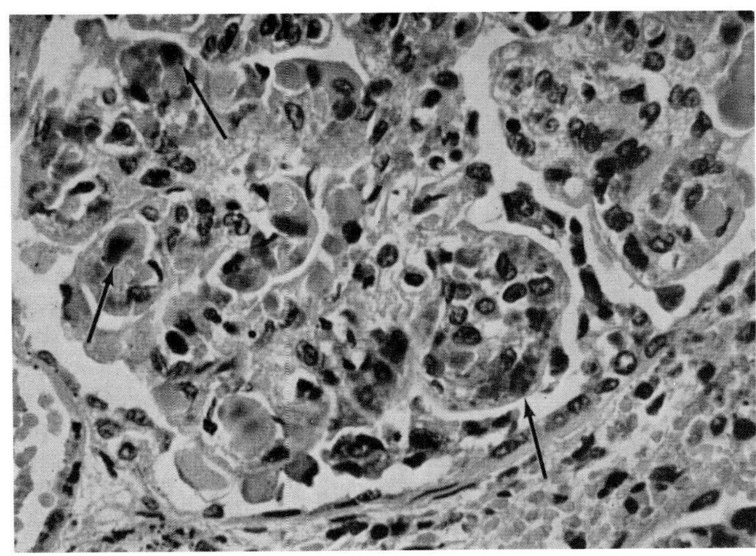

Figure 21-13. Systemic lupus erythematosus. Another glomerulus from the same case as Figure 21-12. Some thrombi contain basophilic, irregular masses (*arrows*). Hematoxylin and eosin. ×600, before 25% reduction.

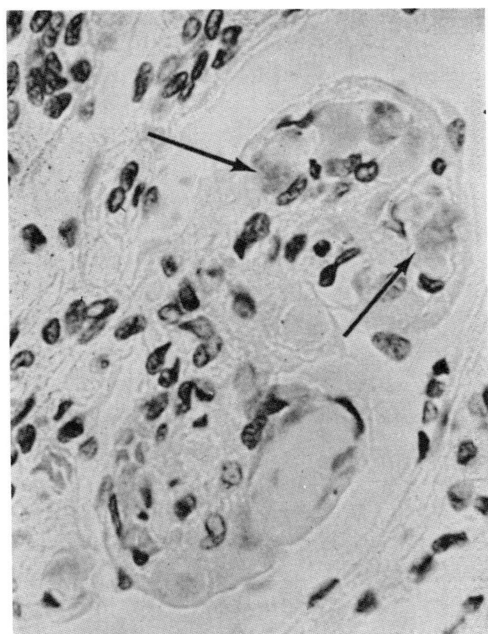

Figure 21-14. Systemic lupus erythematosus. Feulgen staining shows that the basophilic material seen in Figure 21-13 gives a positive reaction for DNA (*arrows*). ×600.

Ultrastructural Changes, Immunofluorescent Studies, and Functional Abnormalities. Electron microscopy and immunofluorescent studies have added substantially to an understanding of the pathogenesis of some of the glomerular changes in lupus nephritis [34, 54, 60, 95]. Among the earlier changes recognized by electron microscopy, generalized thickening of the basement membrane was the most prominent. Subsequent studies recognized the pro-

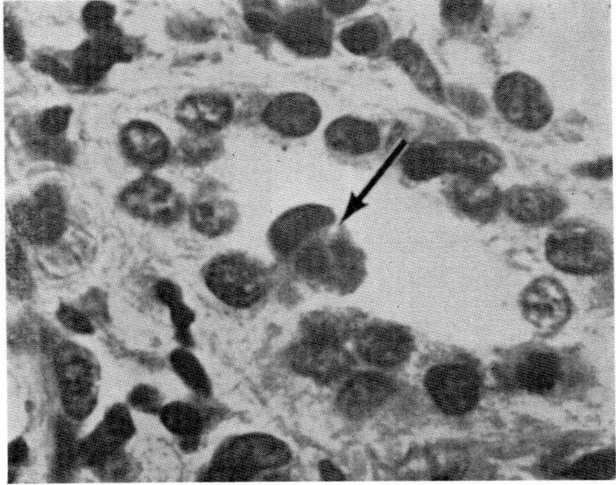

Figure 21-15. Systemic lupus erythematosus. An LE cell (*arrow*) is seen in a tubular lumen. This is a rare finding. Hematoxylin and eosin. ×750.

liferative endothelial changes and variable severe changes in the epithelial cells, with loss of foot processes [54, 134]. Subendothelial electron-dense deposits, noted originally by Farquhar et al. [54], were recognized as a common finding by other workers [35]. This material has been equated with the fibrinoid changes seen by light microscopy and is apparently responsible for producing the wire-loop appearance of capillary loops seen in sections stained with hematoxylin and eosin. These deposits were subsequently identified in subepithelial locations also (see Fig. 21-18) [54]. Even in the absence of such deposits, the basement membrane may reach a thickness that is four to six times normal size (Fig. 21-16). When this change is pronounced, accumulations of basement membrane-like material (mesangial matrix) may be visible in the mesangial area also [159, 160].

Comerford and Cohen [35] reported ultrastructural studies on 13 patients with SLE and variably severe renal involvement. They were able to arrange their findings into three groups that correlated well with clinical severity of renal involvement. Group 1 changes included thickening and nodularity of the basement membrane but no electron-dense deposits. These changes were seen regularly in persons with only minimal urinary findings. At times, this basement membrane thickening may be so uniform (Fig. 21-16) as to go unappreciated unless actual measurements of membrane thickness are made (Fig. 21-17). Group 2 findings included subepithelial or intramembranous electron-dense deposits in addition to variable thickening of the basement membrane. Group 3 represented those cases characterized by marked subendothelial electron-dense deposits situated beneath the endothelium adjacent to the basement membranes. They also reported electron-dense deposits within the endothelial cytoplasm, the latter apparently representing phagocytic activity of the endothelium. These latter two groups were seen in association with more severe renal involvement. Groups 2 and 3 are not mutually exclusive since both subendothelial and subepithelial electron-dense deposits may be seen in the same patient (Fig. 21-18).

The recent demonstration of virus-like intracellular inclusions in glomerular endothelial cytoplasm in almost all (29 of 30) electron photomicrographic material from kidney biopsies obtained from patients with proved systemic lupus erythematosus is an observa-

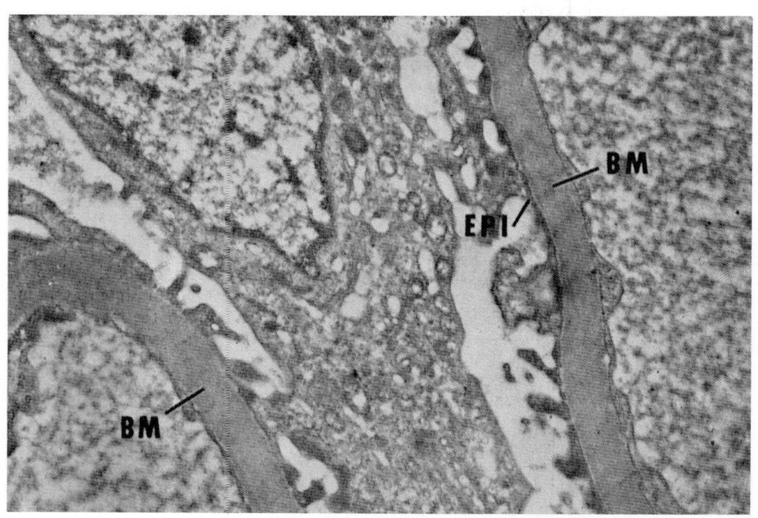

Figure 21-16. Systemic lupus erythematosus. Electron micrograph showing widened basement membranes (BM) without evidence of a denser deposit like that shown in Figure 21-18. The foot processes of an epithelial cell (EPI) show a tendency to fuse. ×12,800, before 25% reduction.

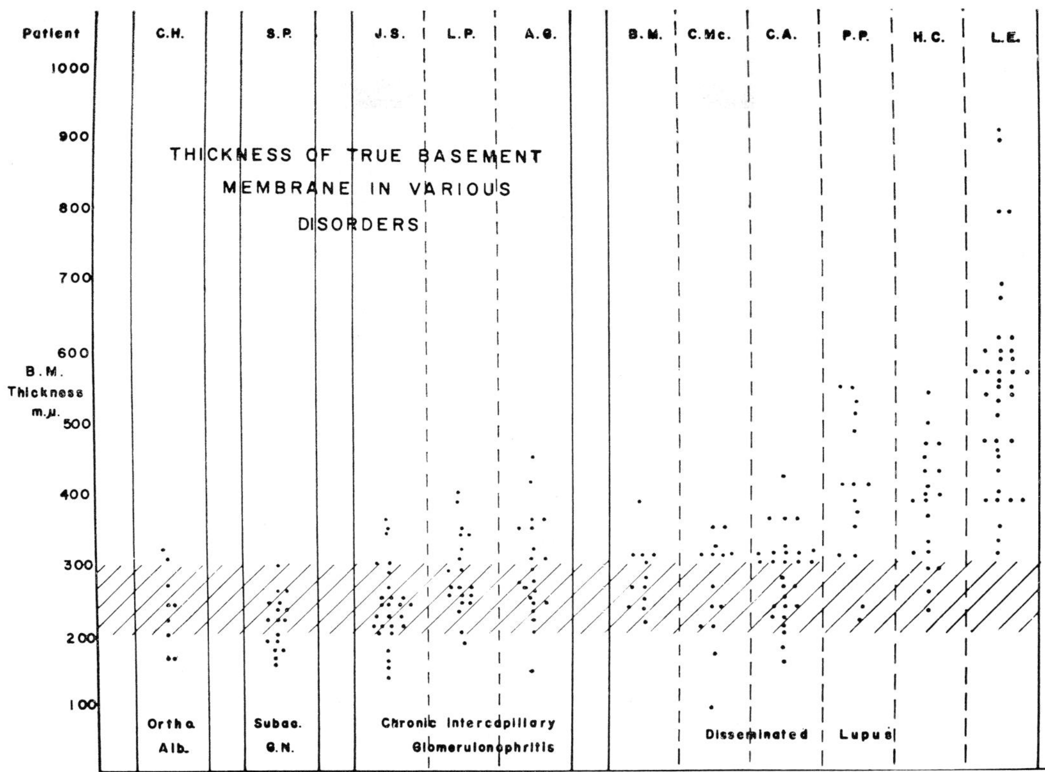

Figure 21-17. Histogram of random measurements made from electron micrographs of glomerular basement membranes. Visible deposits were not included in the measurements. The hatched interval shows the range for normal human glomeruli. Note that there are an increased range and mean thickness for ordinary chronic nephritis, but the basement membrane thickness in some lupus cases exceeds that found in the other diseases. These include orthostatic albuminuria and subacute glomerulonephritis.

tion of great interest [72a]. Careful examination of comparable material from non-lupus renal lesions failed to yield any such structures. The observations reported thus far do not establish that these are indeed virus particles nor do they provide any clues to their possible etiologic significance. Nevertheless, the observation is an important one that merits careful study. Quite apart from pathogenetic or etiologic considerations, the fact that these structures could be identified in virtually all specimens of renal tissue in cases of proved lupus has important diagnostic implications.

Immunofluorescent studies have identified proteinaceous deposits within the glomeruli that apparently correspond with at least some of the electron-dense deposits seen by electron microscopy. The various immunoreactive substances in the serum of patients with SLE have been the subject of intensive study, particularly in respect of their localization within the glomeruli of the kidneys of patients with lupus [95, 96]. Beginning with the demonstration of deposition of gamma globulin and beta$_{1c}$-globubin within the glomerulus by immunofluorescent technics, a series of elegant experiments has strongly supported the view that antigen-

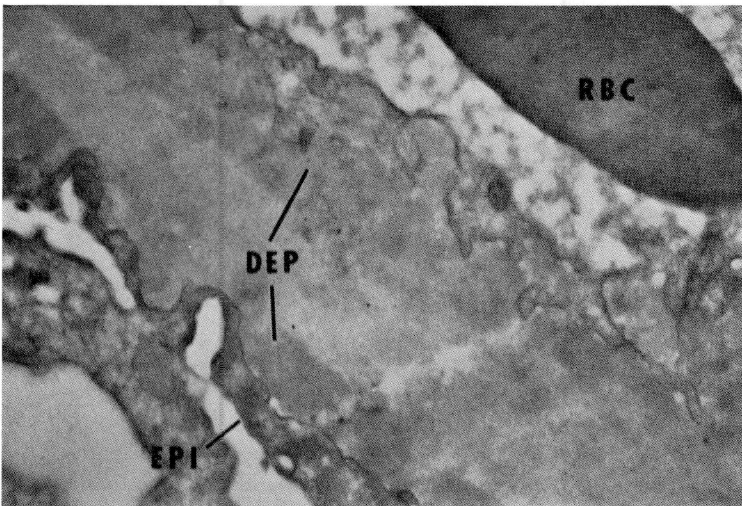

Figure 21-18. Systemic lupus erythematosus. Electron micrograph of a wire loop. A red cell (RBC) indicates the capillary lumen. The epithelial foot processes (EPI) have fused. Irregular, electron-dense deposits (DEP) have markedly thickened the basement membrane region. ×20,000, before 25% reduction.

antibody complexes are deposited within the glomerulus, predominantly along the glomerular basement membrane [96, 111]. Of the several antibodies capable of reacting with various components of the cell that have been identified in the serum of patients with SLE, the one that has been studied most intensively in relation to its possible role in lupus nephritis is the anti-DNA antibody [96]. The use of an acid buffer wash on glomeruli isolated from kidneys of patients dying with lupus erythematosus yields antibodies directed against DNA. Quantities obtained indicated that these antibodies are concentrated in the kidneys [95]. The use of deoxyribonuclease, an enzyme known to release anti-DNA antibody from anti-DNA-DNA complexes, also yields anti-DNA antibody when exposed to isolated glomeruli from patients with lupus. By combining dilution technics and immunofluorescent staining it has been possible to identify DNA antigen within the kidneys of patients with lupus [95, 96]. Thus the combination of these technics has produced strong evidence that antigen-antibody complexes of DNA are deposited within the glomeruli of patients with lupus nephritis. Furthermore, in over two-thirds of patients with lupus nephritis, circulating anti-DNA antibodies are demonstrable, and the titer of these antibodies fluctuates in a pattern that correlates well with clinical evidence of activity of the disease [152]. As pointed out by Koffler and Kunkel [96] in a review of the above studies, it is likely that other antigen-antibody complexes existing in SLE may also be responsible for renal injury, but they have not been studied in such detailed fashion. Until similar studies are performed on other antigen-antibody systems known to appear in patients with SLE, it is not possible to assign a unique role to the anti-DNA-DNA complexes in the production of lupus nephritis.

The experimental evidence that antigen-antibody complexes can produce renal disease that may under certain circumstances progress to chronic glomerulonephritis is quite persuasive. Following Germuth's [64] initial observation that glomerular lesions develop during the immune phase of antigen elimination from the circulation and regress when excess circulating antibody appears, Germuth and McKinnon [65] noted that soluble antigen-antibody complexes could induce anaphylaxis in unsensitized guinea pigs. They suggested that soluble antigen-antibody complexes were responsible for the vascular and renal lesions of hypersensitivity and reported preliminary experiments supporting this suggestion. Dixon and his associates [45] subsequently confirmed this and reported a careful series of experiments showing that it was possible to produce chronic glomerulonephritis by exposing animals to circulating antigen-antibody complexes over long periods.

These studies included immunofluorescent demonstration of antigen-antibody complexes in the renal lesions. Further studies by Germuth and his associates [67] established that soluble complexes were more likely to form during repeated immunizations of animals that were poor antibody producers, a situation establishing favorable conditions of slight antigen excess for production of soluble complexes. By varying the dosage of antigen used, they were able to produce either chronic membranous glomerulonephritis with low doses or obliterative glomerulonephritis with higher doses [67]. It is noteworthy that virtually all these experiments were carried out with bovine serum albumin or similar antigens unrelated to the kidney, a fact that suggests the possibility that a wide variety of immune complexes may produce renal disease under appropriate circumstances [44, 67]. There is remarkable similarity in the histologic appearance of this type of experimental nephritis with that seen in SLE and other forms of human glomerulonephritis both with respect to immunofluorescent and ultrastructural appearance as well as by light microscopy.

The mechanisms ultimately responsible for producing glomerular injury in response to immune-complex deposition remain imperfectly understood. The analogy between the local fibrinoid glomerulitis of SLE and the obliterative glomerulonephritis described by Germuth in experimental immune-complex disease seems clear since both appear to be the result of occlusion of segments of the glomerular tuft by excessive deposition of fibrinoid material. The paradox of extensive and apparently mechanical deposition of dense proteinaceous material and diffuse thickening of the glomerular basement membrane associated with increased loss of protein in the urine is more difficult to reconcile. It has been well established by both ultrastructural and functional studies that the basement membrane is the effective barrier to diffusion and ultrafiltration [53, 55]. Similarly, function studies in pathologic states such as the nephrotic syndrome encountered in lupus nephritis and other nephritides indicate a change in permeability of the basement membrane so that the permeance of larger protein molecules is increased [28, 73, 76, 161, 162]. Ultrastructural studies suggest that all three types of cells within the glomerulus (mesangial, endothelial, and epithelial) are responsible for production and maintenance of the basement membrane [112]. It has also been reported that the glomerulus exhibits a high rate of protein turnover, a major portion of this latter activity apparently occurring within the basement membrane [171], since both electronmicroscopic and immunofluorescent studies indicate that some, and perhaps all, of the cell types of the glomerulus also serve a scavenger function in reclaiming protein deposited within the glomerulus.

It seems possible that the increased burden placed on the metabolic machinery of these cells by the combined load of glomerular basement membrane maintenance and the greatly increased scavenger function imposed by the trapping of these immune complexes could result in relative metabolic insufficiency or a form of "high output" failure of the cells of the glomerulus, leading to inadequate maintenance of the integrity of the glomerular basement membrane. Direct evidence bearing on this possibility is unavailable, but the observations of Comerford and Cohen [35] on the ultrastructural glomerular changes in lupus nephritis have revealed that the presence of electron-dense deposits is associated with greater degrees of proteinuria, a finding consistent with the above view.

TREATMENT

The initial report of Pollak and his associates [132] concerning the influence of steroid therapy on the course of lupus nephritis appeared to show a rather striking difference between high-dosage therapy with prednisone (40 to 60 mg. daily for six months before reduction below 40 mg. per day) in one group of patients and lower steroid dosage in a second group. There was histologic evidence of progression of the renal lesions in subsequent biopsies obtained in the patients receiving the lower-steroid-dosage regimen — that is, all 10 patients in this group died, with an average survival time of about 15 months beyond the initial biopsy. In the group receiving the higher dosage of steroids, of five who were azotemic when treatment began, all but one died within five months and the remaining patient survived 26 months. Of the 11 who were not azotemic when the high-steroid regimen was begun, two died 22 and 41 months after therapy was begun, and the remaining nine were alive with an average duration of treatment of 40 months at the time of reporting [132].

The experience of Rothfield et al. [145] is somewhat different from that reported by Pollak. Of 52 patients in their series 29 had renal disease, and the response to therapy appeared to correlate well with other evidences of activity of their SLE. Similarly, the response of the renal lesion to steroid therapy paralleled the response of systemic evidence of activity to steroid treatment. Four patients who were initially azotemic died of renal insufficiency after treatment had begun. Five patients who were azotemic at the beginning of therapy had survived an average of five years at the time of reporting. Of these, two still had persistent proteinuria as the only evidence of renal involvement, while three had no evidence of renal disease. In their experience the coexistence of azotemia and the nephrotic syndrome was an extremely poor prognostic sign; all three patients in this group died within four months of beginning therapy. The steroid regimen employed by these investigators varied according to the severity of the disease, but the average maintenance dosage was 10 mg. of prednisone per day. The initial dose ranged from 40 to 60 mg. per day, but this was reduced as soon as the patients became asymptomatic. The majority of the patients in this series had focal glomerular lesions, and these authors concluded that the outlook was more favorable in this group than in cases where glomerular lesions were severe and diffuse.

In a subsequent report covering a larger group of patients with longer follow-up period, Pollak et al. [133] reported their experience with 87 patients with SLE that included 40 patients followed for a total of 160 patient years with diagnoses of either normal kidneys, lupus glomerulitis, or membranous lupus glomerulonephritis. Of this group, only two developed mild lupus glomerulonephritis and responded to therapy. Two others developed severe lupus glomerulonephritis and died of chronic renal failure. On the basis of these results they concluded that progression of the milder forms of renal involvement to severe disease was uncommon. Of the patients in the total group who had active lupus glomerulonephritis at the beginning of the study, most died with severe renal failure. It was their impression that high dosages of steroids slowed, and on occasion, halted the progress of the renal involvement in this group.

Zweiman and his associates [178], reporting on 40 patients followed an average of 30 months, noted similar results. Patients with normal kidneys or mild glomerulitis did well. Those with severe clinical and histologic evidence of renal disease did poorly. All deaths from renal disease occurred in this group; four patients died within the first 15 months of therapy. There were no other deaths due to renal disease in the follow-up period. Gary et al. [63] report results consistent with the above series.

None of the studies reviewed briefly above

are without bias of various sorts, and it is often difficult to identify the direction and degree of bias. Several generalizations appear warranted, however. There appears to be a concensus that patients with mild clinical and/or histologic changes do well and show no more than a slight tendency to develop progressive and severe renal disease. Conversely, the prognosis is guarded in patients with major clinical manifestations of renal involvement and histologic evidence of active lupus glomerulonephritis. Although the survival time in this group is short, it appears that high dosages of steroids do possess distinct therapeutic potential and at times may arrest progress of the disease. The problems presented by hypertension in this group merit emphasis. Frequently, even though steroids are successful in arresting progress of the disease, renal damage has already become so extensive that severe hypertension becomes the major clinical problem. Vigorous antihypertensive treatment with careful follow-up observation is mandatory if the clinical progress achieved with steroids is to be maintained.

Between the two extremes of the clinical spectrum of lupus nephritis described above, there is a fairly large group of patients with renal involvement about whom few generalizations can be made with regard to therapy. The best and safest course appears to be careful clinical evaluation and the use of steroids in adequate doses to suppress clinical signs of activity of the disease, including those related to the kidney. There appears to be no inherent therapeutic advantage to continuing high dosages of steroid beyond the period required to suppress activity, and tapering of the drug dosage should be started shortly after the clinical manifestations of the disease have been controlled and should continue to the lowest level consistent with reasonable control of the symptoms of the disease. In cases in which significant renal involvement has been documented, it is doubtful whether steroids should be discontinued until the patient has been completely free of evidence of renal disease for a period of at least nine months to a year. Use of azathioprine and similar antimetabolites appears to offer additional promise in those patients with active severe disease, but for the present this therapy should still be regarded as under evaluation [113, 173].

Polyarteritis (Periarteritis Nodosa)

Polyarteritis is characterized histologically by inflammation and fibrinoid necrosis of medium-sized or small arteries and clinically by a variable multisystem disorder, the manifestations of which depend on the location of the vascular lesions. Among the early clinical findings are fever, tachycardia, loss of weight, and diffuse aching and tenderness of the extremities. Early local symptoms are commonly related to the joints, alimentary tract, kidneys, and peripheral nervous system [143]. Leukocytosis is frequent and eosinophilia is common in patients with pulmonary involvement. Rose and Spencer [144], in their review of the natural history of polyarteritis in 100 histologically proved cases, divided the disease into two major groups, one with and the other without lung involvement. Lung involvement was present in about one-third of the total group. These cases were distinguished by at least three of the following features. (1) a characteristic respiratory illness preceding the onset of systemic polyarteritis; (2) high blood eosinophilia; (3) numerous eosinophils in the acute polyarteritic lesions; (4) pulmonary polyarteritis; (5) granulomatous polyarteritis; (6) giant cells in polyarteritic lesions; and (7) the presence in viscera of necrotizing or granulomatous lesions not demonstrably related to arteries. From their study of previous reports, they concluded that such pulmonary cases have been given a variety of names by other authors, including Wegener's granulomatosis, Loeffler's syndrome, necrotizing granulomatosis and angiitis, diffuse eosinophilic arteritis, and allergic granulomatosis. There was, however, no substantial difference in the clinical patterns of renal disease that distinguished the group without pulmonary involvement from those with pulmonary involvement.

RENAL INVOLVEMENT

Renal involvement is common in polyarteritis, its incidence varying between 75 and 85 per cent. Although other manifestations of the disease may overshadow the symptoms due to renal involvement, back pain, dysuria, nocturia, and hematuria are frequently encountered. Proteinuria and hematuria herald the onset of renal damage and should arouse suspicion of polyarteritis when associated with either weight loss or signs of a multisystem disorder. Occasionally, polyarteritis may present as an illness resembling acute glomerulonephritis without hypertension. In such patients renal manifestations may dominate the picture, completely obscuring the more common clinical manifestations of polyarteritis. Such an onset may be followed by a fulminant course, with rapidly developing uremia leading to death early in the course of the disease. Patients with less severe renal involvement survive longer, but eventually progressive hypertension develops ending in the maligant phase. Clinical manifestations of renal involvement fail as reliable guides for identification or exclusion of renal polyarteritis. Although only 8 to 10 per cent of patients may have complaints (predominantly flank pain and hematuria) referable to the genitourinary system, renal involvement as judged by the presence of azotemia and abnormal urine is present in over 80 per cent [143].

There are two characteristic renal lesions: (1) renal polyarteritis, and (2) a distinctive form of glomerulonephritis first clearly recognized by Davson et al. [41]. The two lesions may be seen separately or together. Renal polyarteritis is associated clinically with proteinuria, small numbers of red blood cells in the urine, and sometimes hyaline and granular casts. Such abnormalities may be present intermittently; hence repeated urine examination is important. Renal polyarteritis (Fig. 21-19) is the most common change found histologically, the majority of lesions occuring in the arterial vessels. The kidneys may be grossly enlarged, often showing a bossing of the surface due to cortical infarcts or areas of ischemic atrophy of varying size and shape. The microscopic lesion in the vessels is similar to that seen in other organs, and most commonly, healed polyarteritic lesions are abundantly evident. Seventy-six per cent of the cases studied by Rose and Spencer [144] showed some healed lesions, and in 48 per cent only healed lesions were seen (Fig. 21-20). The glomerulitis presents a clinical illness that resembles ordinary glo-

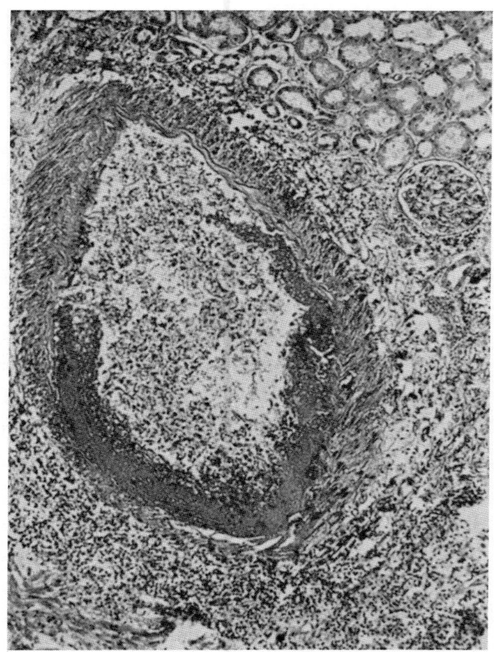

Figure 21-19. Polyarteritis. An acute intrarenal lesion showing fresh arterial wall necrosis, fibrinoid change, and acute inflammation. Hematoxylin and eosin. ×75.

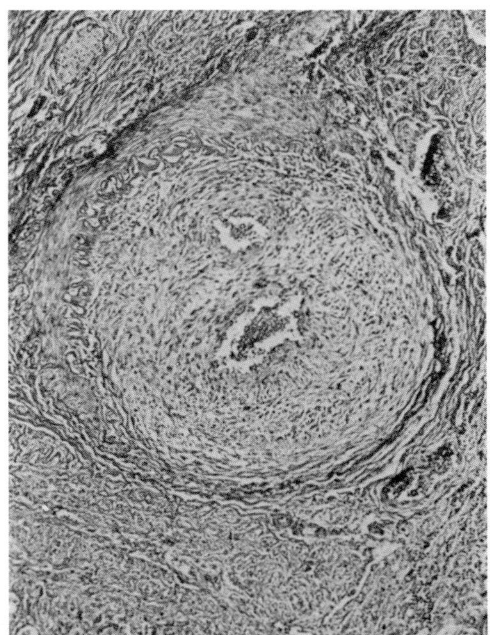

Figure 21-20. Polyarteritis. A healed arterial lesion with almost complete obliteration of the lumen by a recanalized thrombus. There is *segmental* replacement of the wall by fibrosis and loss of the internal elastic membrane. Hematoxylin and eosin. ×75.

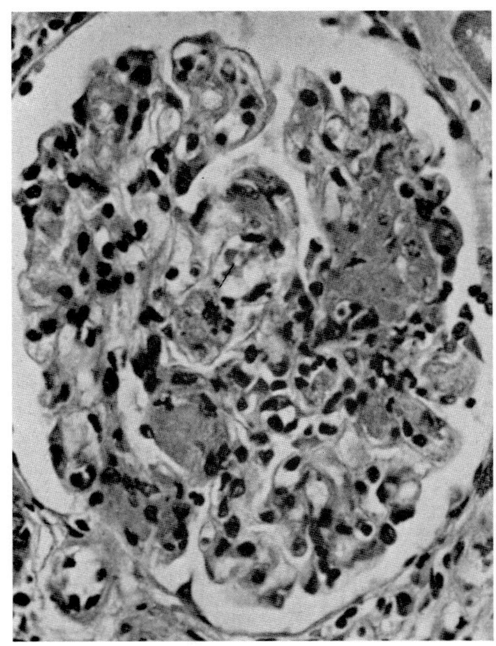

Figure 21-21. Polyarteritis. Local acute necrosis in a glomerulus showing fibrinoid change and capillary thrombi. Hematoxylin and eosin. ×400.

merulonephritis in many respects. The onset is usually acute, and renal failure develops rapidly with the presence of proteinuria, numerous red blood cells, and red blood cell and other types of casts. Edema often appears, but the blood pressure remains normal.

Glomerular lesions not attributable to ischemia resulting from polyarteritis or hypertension may be seen in 30 per cent of autopsy cases. The kidneys may be large, and the capsule usually strips easily, with some paleness of the underlying cortex. Histologically there can be either proliferative or destructive glomerular involvement. In the initial phase of the renal disorder, capillary microthrombi are common. There is frequently fibrinoid change involving a part or all of a tuft (Figs. 21-21, 21-22). The tufts are often adherent to Bowman's capsule, with proliferation and crescent formation (Fig. 21-23). Hemorrhage into the capsular space or tufts may be seen, but the glomerular capillaries usually appear bloodless and may show some polymorphonuclear infiltration. All gradations are seen from the picture of the acute glomerulonephritis to complete hyalinization and fibrosis (Fig. 21-24). The disease may be diffuse or local with sparing of variable numbers of glomeruli. Tubules also may show severe damage with dilatation, atrophy, and intraluminal collections of casts and cellular debris.

If the patient survives the initial phase of glomerulonephritis, progressive hypertension may appear, leading to further deterioration in renal function and death in uremia. This is usually associated with histologic evidence of widespread glomerular and tubular damage. A few specific lesions (Fig. 21-25) may remain,

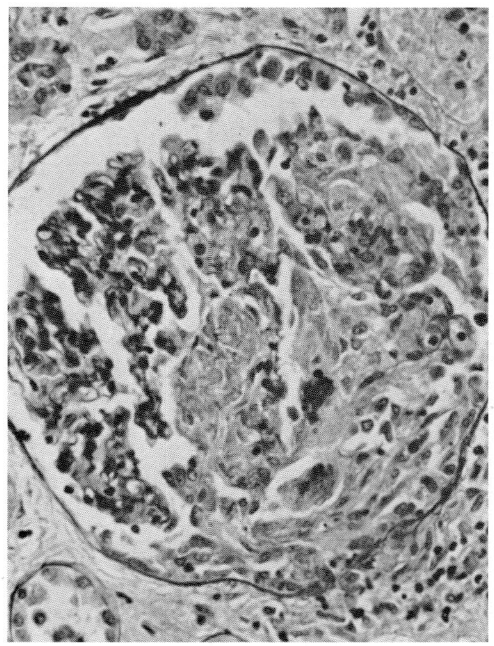

Figure 21-22. Polyarteritis. A slightly older local lesion with some epithelial and possibly endothelial proliferation. PAS. ×300.

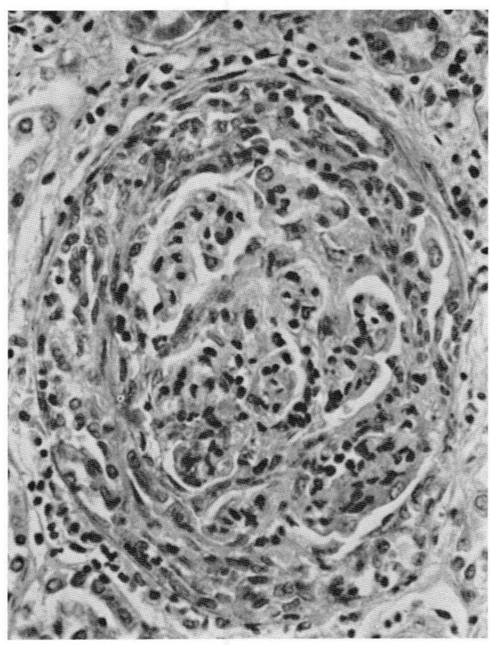

Figure 21-23. Polyarteritis. Glomerulonephritis of the subacute variety with crescent formation. Hematoxylin and eosin. ×300.

but the major change is similar to that seen in ordinary chronic glomerulonephritis.

In contrast to the unimpressive numbers of red cells seen with the pathologic picture of renal polyarteritis alone, the glomerular lesions usually can be recognized clinically by the appearance of macroscopic or heavy microscopic hematuria. The glomerulonephritis of polyarteritis usually occurs more frequently in the older age groups (40 to 70 years of age). Hypertension is not a feature of the early or acute phases of the nephritis of polyarteritis. The frequency of the characteristic glomerulitis in cases with generalized polyarteritis seems far too high to be due to chance alone. Another point emphasized by Krupp [98] is the finding of the telescoped urinary sediment in polyarteritis in which one sees simultaneously all of the elements seen separately in various stages of ordinary glomerulonephritis.

Darmady et al. [40] described an unusual case of polyarteritis in which the renal functional impairment was primarily tubular. This was manifested by loss of large quantities of sodium, chloride, and to a lesser extent potassium in the urine. The urine was persistently hypotonic even during continuous infusion of vasopressin. At postmortem examination, multiple infarcted areas and polyarteritis of the renal arteries were noted. In addition, microdissection of nephrons in noninfarcted areas showed widespread tubular damage and relatively intact glomeruli.

In the group of patients reported by Rose and Spencer [144], necrotizing or granulomatous lesions not demonstrably related to arteries were seen in the kidneys in 10 of the 24 cases of pulmonary involvement (Fig. 21-26). They were sometimes numerous. In the smaller lesions, a focus of necrosis was sur-

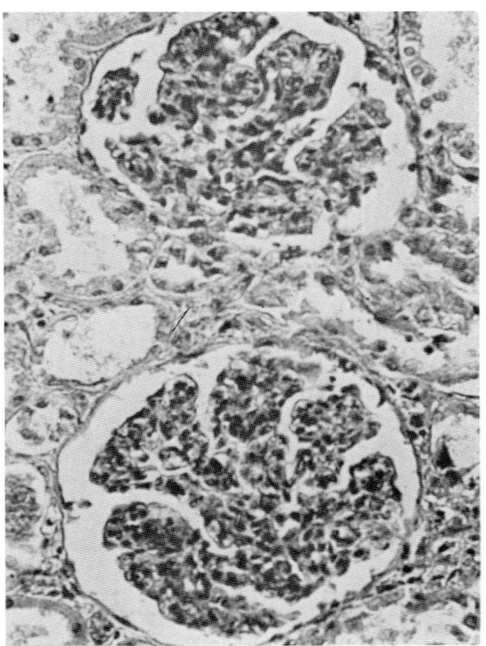

Figure 21-24. Polyarteritis. In this instance the principal renal lesion is acute diffuse proliferative glomerulonephritis. A focal or local character was not evident in this case. Hematoxylin and eosin. ×250.

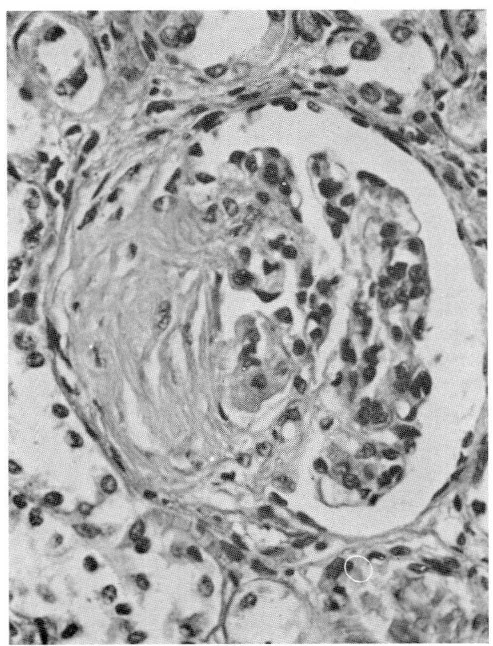

Figure 21-25. Polyarteritis. A fibrosed local glomerular lesion of the type found in more chronic cases. Hematoxylin and eosin. ×400.

rounded by an acute inflammatory reaction in which eosinophils were prominent. In others resembling tubercles, the eosinophils were replaced by chronic inflammatory cells including giant cells. In our experience, however, this type of granulomatous lesion is not confined to polyarteritis with lung involvement. Serial blood pressure measurements were available in only half the cases reported by Rose and Spencer, and of these, 24 remained normotensive throughout the illness. In this group without hypertension, recent arterial and glomerular lesions were commonly encountered, while healed lesions with associated ischemic changes were found in only one case. In 15 patients in whom hypertension developed during the course of the disease, there was evidence of prior renal involvement. At autopsy in 12 of these cases healed renal polyarteritis or

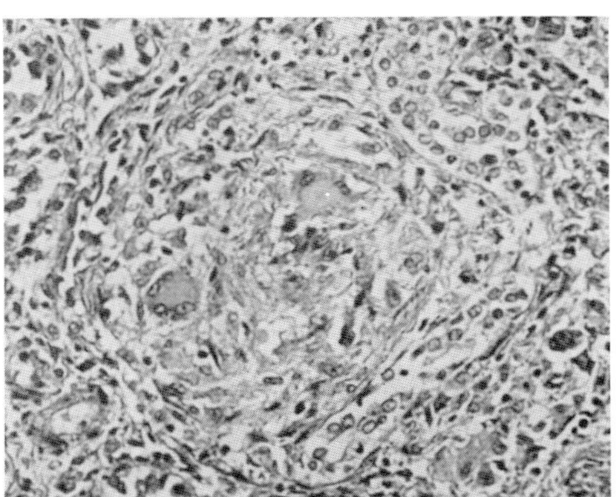

Figure 21-26. Polyarteritis. An epithelioid tubercle (granuloma) in the interstitial tissue. Giant cells are evident. Distinguishing such lesions from those of tuberculosis or sarcoid may be difficult, yet they can indeed be a specific feature of polyarteritis. Hematoxylin and eosin. ×200.

chronic glomerulitis was noted. Rose and Spencer concluded that hypertension was usually a sequel to renal polyarteritis or glomerulitis in these cases and postulated that the blood pressure rose during healing of the active lesions. Frohnert and Sheps [61] also observed that hypertension developed during the course of the illness and after steroid therapy had been started in approximately one-fourth of their cases. These data support the concept that hypertension in polyarteritis is not a precursor of the disease but follows it and appears to be related to the onset of renal ischemia. These findings are at variance with earlier views [93, 163].

EXPERIMENTAL ARTERITIS

Since Gruber [75] first suggested in 1925 that periarteritis nodosa might represent a general hyperergic reaction to either infectious or toxic agents, considerable work has been done on the relationship of hypersensitivity to the pathogenesis of inflammatory vascular lesions. Much of the activity and controversy in this field followed the report of Rich [140], in 1942, of necrotizing vascular lesions in cases of serum sickness and in association with hypersensitivity to sulfonamides. In the following year, Rich and Gregory [141] produced necrotizing arteritis in rabbits by injecting large doses of horse serum intravenously. In both the clinical cases and the laboratory animals, the lesions were morphologically indistinguishable from those seen in polyarteritis. Others who have observed necrotizing vascular lesions at autopsy in patients receiving a potentially allergenic drug have reported differences in the type and distributions of the lesions in these cases when compared with those seen in spontaneous polyarteritis [175, 176].

The term *hypersensitivity angiitis* has been used to designate the drug-induced vascular lesions. In human cases, this angiitis is described as an acute necrotizing inflammation in and around the smallest branches of blood vessels, both arterial and venous. In advanced cases, the process spreads to larger vessels. The initial lesion is said to be fibrinoid necrosis occurring in the intima or subendothelial ground substance. The necrosis rapidly involves the whole vessel wall. There is an intense cellular reaction, frequently containing eosinophils and surrounded by interstitial edema. In the kidney, a necrotizing glomerulitis is often present. Zeek [175] reported that, in contrast to polyarteritis, arteritic lesions are often found in the pulmonary vessels along with small foci or necrotizing pneumonia. This statement is reminiscent of the description of polyarteritis and pulmonary lesions in the study by Rose and Spencer. In Zeek's experience, however, the lesions in a given case were usually of about the same age and no chronic or healed lesions were noted. The clinical manifestations were those of hypersensitivity complicating the symptoms of the infectious disease for which the therapy had been initiated. However, from the point of view of renal disease, renal involvement is about as common in association with this group of drug-induced or hypersensitivity angiitis as in polyarteritis.

Some observers are unconvinced of the distinction between drug-induced cases and spontaneously occurring cases of polyarteritis. Rose questions the evidence incriminating drugs as a causative factor in human polyarteritis. Nevertheless, lesions have been produced in laboratory animals, by the administration of foreign protein, that appear to be histologically similar to polyarteritis in man. It is also clear that polyarteritis often develops in a setting in which no drugs have been administered. Germuth and Pollack [66] demonstrated that deposition of insoluble antigen-antibody complexes in the tissues of animals produced a necrotizing vasculitis in laboratory animals that resembles polyarteritis histologically. This finding suggests that polyarteritis may represent a disturbance produced by the precipitation of insoluble antigen-antibody complexes within the tissues that is comparable to soluble immune-complex disease discussed in the preceding section.

TREATMENT

The use of steroid therapy usually controls the systemic manifestations of polyarteritis, although frequently large doses are necessary to accomplish this [139]. Concomitant with control of the clinical manifestations there is usually suppression of the histologic evidence of inflammation and healing of the necrotic arterial lesions. In some patients, evidence of renal involvement may greatly improve or disappear. The available evidence suggests that the most important factor in prognosis is the extent and stage of the renal lesions before treatment is started. Frohnert and Sheps [61], in a follow-up study of 130 patients, noted that in those patients who received no treatment there was only a 10 per cent survival in five years, whereas over 40 per cent were living at 10 years when treated with intensive steroid therapy. Within the treated group, those patients without evidence of renal disease or hypertension fared better than when either of these complicating features was present. Nevertheless, there was substantial improvement in the survival data among patients who had hypertension as well as those with marked renal disease. In the hypertensive group, over 30 per cent were surviving at the end of five years, and the comparable figure for the group with renal disease was approximately 35 per cent. Thus, steroid therapy is effective as a means of suppressing the acute manifestations of the disease as well as substantially prolonging life.

The occasional dramatic response of the acute glomerulonephritis of polyarteritis to steroid therapy warrants special emphasis. Occasionally, patients exhibit dramatic reversal of severe uremia under steroid therapy when treatment is begun during the early acute phase of the illness. However, when severity of renal disease in acute polyarteritis progresses to the anuric state, the prognosis worsens significantly, and any major improvement in this group of patients is extremely rare if it ever occurs [99].

Primary Systemic Sclerosis (Scleroderma)

Diffuse scleroderma or primary systemic sclerosis is a relatively rare but grave systemic disease characterized by extensive induration of the skin and variable visceral manifestations. It usually presents as a skin disorder, with edema of the skin a prominent early manifestation. Raynaud's phenomenon is also seen early and may, on occasion, precede any structural alteration in the skin. These changes are associated with, or followed by, a progressive induration of the skin which most often involves the face and upper extremities. The skin ultimately becomes board-like and rigidly fixed to the underlying tissues. Such changes around joints lead to marked limitation of motion. Erythema, cyanosis, patchy areas of hyperpigmentation and depigmentation, with loss of hair, as well as marked trophic changes, ulceration, and gangrene may be seen. Visceral changes, including gastrointestinal involvement with motility disturbances as well as cardiovascular and pulmonary involvement, are also seen.

RENAL INVOLVEMENT

Clinical evidences of renal disease are relatively uncommon, although laboratory evidence of damage to the kidneys is obtained in as many as one-fourth of cases. Usually, the only manifestation of renal involvement is proteinuria. This may be present for extended periods without clinical evidence of progressive renal dysfunction. Renal clearance data on such patients indicate that in a majority of patients, there is a significant reduction in renal plasma flow [165]. In an occasional case, the disease appears to accelerate suddenly, with the appearance of severe hypertension and associated oliguria leading rapidly to uremia and death [114].

D'Angelo and his associates [39] tabulated the postmortem findings in 58 cases of scleroderma and compared them to a group of matched controls. Renal lesions that were encountered more frequently than in the control group included fibrinoid necrosis in the afferent arteriole or glomerulus, hyperplasia of interlobular arteries, and thickening of the glomerular basement membrane (i.e., wire-loop lesion). Each of these lesions was observed in approximately one-third of the cases studied, and at least one of these findings was present in nearly 60 per cent of the autopsies on patients with scleroderma. It has been recognized for many years that arterial lesions may occur in patients with primary systemic sclerosis, not only in the skin and subcutaneous tissues but also in other areas, including the intestinal tract and the lung. Renal abnormalities resembling those seen in systemic lupus erythematosus, including wire-loop glomerular lesions, have been reported [17, 56]. In other cases renal vascular lesions having points of similarity to those seen in periarteritis nodosa have been described [23, 130]. Such observations have suggested that there is an overlap in the renal vascular lesion seen in the various connective tissue diseases.

However, a specific type of lesion may in rare instances develop in the renal cortical arteries in patients with primary systemic sclerosis. This type of lesion has been seen in cases of severe parenchymal damage accompanied by oliguria, severe hypertension, and rapidly progressive renal failure leading to death in a few weeks. Some authors have thought that this complication might be associated with the administration of adrenal steroids, but there are reports of cases in which the fulminating renal lesions developed although no steroids had been administered [23, 30, 58]. Whenever sufficient clinical data are available, the extent and severity of these renal lesions appear to correlate with the degree of hypertension and renal failure [56].

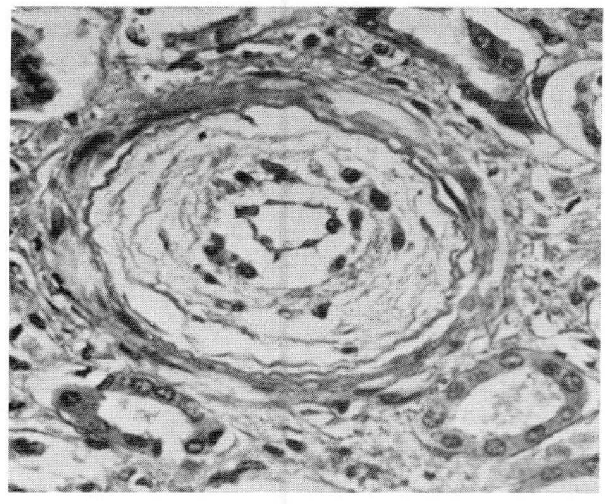

Figure 21-27. Primary systemic sclerosis. Mucinoid change and cellular proliferation in the intima of an interlobular artery. The internal elastic membrane is intact. Hematoxylin and eosin. ×300.

The renal arterial lesions fall into two distinct histologic types which seem to differ in their time of onset. The clinical and pathologic findings have led to the interpretation that the initial lesion is the dilatation of long segments of the proximal portion of the interlobular arteries associated with mucoid thickening and cellular proliferation of the intima (Fig. 21-27). This lesion appears to develop only a few weeks before death and leads to ischemic atrophy of those portions of the renal cortex nourished by the affected arteries. In the reported cases this parenchymal atrophy has been assessed to have been from two to four weeks old [23, 114] when death occurred.

The other prominent change is fibrinoid alteration in the distal portions of the interlobular arteries and afferent arterioles (Fig. 21-28). It is less common than the mucoid and proliferative intimal lesion seen in the larger arterial branches, but may be related to it. The fibrinoid change most commonly is seen within the arterial or arteriolar wall, completely replacing it. On the other hand, it may occur subintimally — that is, between the thickened

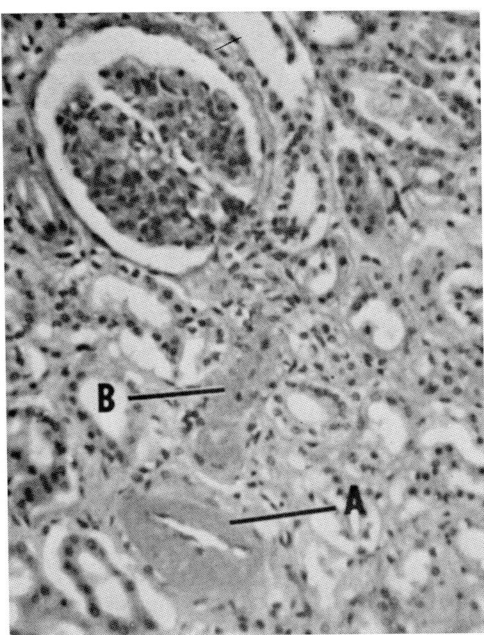

Figure 21-28. Primary systemic sclerosis. Fibrinoid change in interlobular artery (A) and afferent arteriole (B). This patient had no hypertension by history or during the three months he was followed before death occurred. Hematoxylin and eosin. ×200.

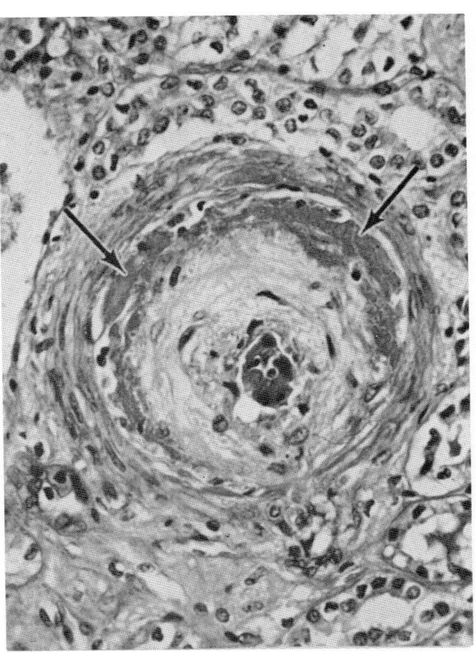

Figure 21-29. Primary systemic sclerosis. Another interlobular artery from the case shown in Figure 21-28. There is fibrinoid material (*arrows*) that by elastic stain was seen to be inside the internal elastic lamella and within the mucoid, proliferating intima. Note stretching and flattening of the media associated with dilatation. Hematoxylin and eosin. ×300.

intima and the internal elastic membrane in a manner resembling a dissection (Fig. 21-29). It is in this form that the fibrinoid alteration suggests a deposited substance and is unique to systemic sclerosis. The more commonly occurring fibrinoid change in the arterial or arteriolar media, on the other hand, is indistinguishable from that seen in malignant hypertension with nephrosclerosis. At such sites there may be associated necrotic cellular debris, the vessel lumina are thrombosed, but acute inflammation is usually absent [30]. This absence of associated inflammation is a characteristic feature of scleroderma and serves to distinguish it from the similar fibrinoid change seen in polyarteritis.

Since the lesions often show no evidence of healing, they are considered to develop usually only a few days before death. Further deterioration of renal function follows the acute ischemic changes that occur mainly in the outer half of the cortex and range from multiple cortical infarcts (Fig. 21-30) to necrosis or damage to the convoluted tubules only. These preterminal changes appear to be an adequate explanation of the oliguria frequently seen in such cases.

In the reported cases the percentage of involved glomeruli has ranged from less than 5 to 60 per cent [56]. The focal cortical infarctions and the lack of glomerular obsolesence are emphasized as an indication of acute renal ischemia. There may be focal glomerular lesions with localized or diffuse thickening of basement membranes. Wire-loop lesions are occasionally seen.

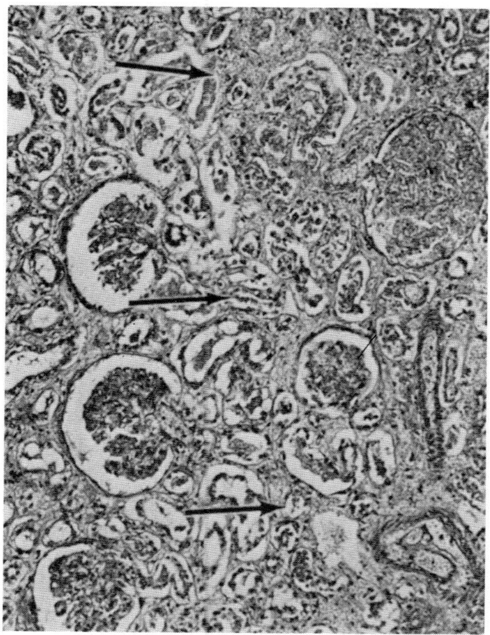

Figure 21-30. Primary systemic sclerosis. Edge of a fresh infarct (*arrows*) produced by arterial lesions of the type shown in Figures 21-27, 21-28, and 21-29. Hematoxylin and eosin. ×100.

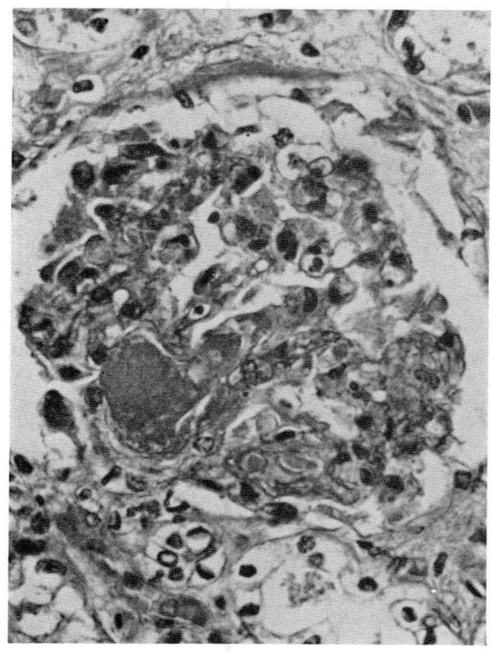

Figure 21-31. Primary systemic sclerosis. A hyaline thrombus is seen at the root of the tuft. Cells in the tuft are undergoing necrosis. Hematoxylin and eosin. ×400.

In severely involved kidneys homogeneous and granular eosinophilic masses may develop in the lumina of glomerular capillaries (Fig. 21-31). Many capillaries appear to be replaced by this fibrinoid material, and at times this is seen in continuity with similarly altered arterioles. Marked degenerative change in tubules characterized by flattening and hyperchromasia of the epithelial cells of convoluted tubules and hyaline-droplet formation may be noted. The interlobular stroma may contain increased amounts of fibrous tissue with varying degrees of lymphocytic and plasma cell infiltration.

It is apparent from correlation of autopsy findings with clinical information available just prior to death that the renal abnormalities in the aggregate occur more than twice as frequently as does hypertension in scleroderma. This finding suggests that, in a significant number of cases, the renal changes either precede or occur in the absence of hypertension.

It has been suggested that these vascular lesions represent a primary manifestation of the sclerodermatous process and are in turn responsible for the development of hypertension and renal failure. It may be pointed out that with the possible exception of the subintimal fibrinoid alteration described above, patients with malignant nephrosclerosis show glomerular, tubular, and vascular lesions morphologically and tinctorially identical with those described in patients with primary systemic sclerosis. The intimal mucoid of the interlobular arteries in both diseases has been characterized as acid mucopolysaccharide of the hyaluronic acid type, and the evidence suggests that this vascular change in the scleroderma kidney may represent the early or acute phase in the development of the vascular hyalinization seen in the chronic phase of nephrosclerosis.

In those scleroderma patients who die without the fulminant renal disease (the more common course of events), the renal arteries often show marked narrowing indistinguishable from ordinary arteriosclerosis. It is possible that the arterial lesion resembling arteriosclerosis is the healed version of the more acute arterial disease.

The relation of renal sclerodermatous involvement to the terminal malignant hypertension that occurs rarely in the disease is not clearly understood. Although the majority of patients exhibiting the unique renal lesions with uremia and oliguria have had severe hypertension during the terminal phase of the illness, such lesions have been described in the absence of hypertension. The patient in the illustrative case shown here (Figs. 21-27 through 21-31) exhibited severe cardiac involvement with congestive heart failure followed by azotemia, oliguria, and death in uremia, but at no time during the terminal three months of the illness was an elevated blood pressure recorded. Thus, the entire sequence of renal involvement occurred in the absence of hypertension. It has been suggested that perhaps the sudden appearance of hypertension is associated with vasospasm of the renal arteries, in view of the frequent occurrence of Raynaud's phenomenon in other vessels in scleroderma. It is of interest that erosion studies following plastic perfusion of kidneys from a patient exhibiting hypertension, oliguria, and uremia, demonstrated marked narrowing of the arcuate arteries and failure to perfuse nearly all the afferent glomerular arterioles [165].

The present treatment of scleroderma is unsatisfactory. Penicillamine and dextran may provide modest benefit for the skin manifestations of the disease but are of no value in treating visceral involvement. Steroids are without benefit and may be harmful in the presence of advanced renal disease inasmuch as they may produce further obliterative changes within the renal vascular bed. Perhaps the most important therapeutic approach is the careful control of hypertension when it appears. Although adequate data are lacking on the effectiveness of such control in prolonging life in systemic sclerosis, the authors have followed a patient with scleroderma presenting with malignant hypertension and mild azotemia who has remained stable for four years on no other treatment than effective control of her blood pressure.

Thrombotic Thrombocytopenic Purpura

Thrombotic thrombocytopenic purpura is a syndrome characterized by thrombocytopenic purpura, hemolytic anemia, and bizarre symptoms and signs of central nervous system involvement. The first case was described by Moschcowitz [117] in 1925 under the title "An Acute Febrile Pleiochromic Anemia with Hyaline Thrombosis of the Terminal Arterioles and Capillaries." Microscopic examination showed what were interpreted as hyaline thrombi thought to represent platelet thrombi in the terminal arterioles and capillaries. The term thrombotic thrombocytopenic purpura was first applied to this condition by Singer and his co-workers [154] in 1947. The characteristic lesions are commonly seen in the renal cortex, and may lead to renal failure with nitrogen retention [9].

The onset of the disease is usually acute, and is associated with malaise, headache, fatigability, and myalgia. Fever is uniformly present, and nausea, vomiting, and abdominal pain are frequently noted. There is pallor, but icterus is usually mild. Enlargement of the liver and spleen, as well as lymphadenopathy, has been observed. The cardiac manifestations include tachycardia, a gallop rhythm, and occasionally a systolic murmur. The onset may be distinguished by psychotic behavior. Other nervous system manifestations include confusion, delirium, and stupor. Focal neurologic signs such as convulsions, cranial nerve palsies, hemiplegia, and aphasia may develop. The hemolytic anemia is associated with abnormally shaped erythrocytes designated helmet cells or schizocytes. The clinical and laboratory manifestations of thrombocytopenia with purpura are similar to those seen in purpura due to other causes. On occasion, dramatic remission may be induced with therapy [85].

The histologic picture consists of occlusions of small arterial vessels and capillaries by an amorphous acidophilic material. It was first thought that these were platelet thrombi, but later it was demonstrated that the material is composed of an immunochemically reactive derivative of fibrinogen or fibrin [38]. Occasionally, it occupies the entire thickness of the vessel wall, and in the region of the lesion the endothelial cells appear larger than normal and are often present in multiple layers. Frequently, the elastic fibers are interrupted at the site of the lesion. Aneurysmal dilatation of vessels may be noted, and in certain instances recanalization may occur. This is of interest in view of the fluctuating clinical manifestations in some cases. Moore and Schoenberg [116] suggest that endothelial damage is the first event in the pathogenesis of the lesion, and that the endothelial cells respond by the elaboration of an abnormal amount of mucopolysaccharide intimately associated with protein. If platelets play any role, it appears to be secondary to this initial tissue change. These lesions are commonly seen in the myocardium, adrenal glands, kidney cortex, pancreas, and gray matter of the brain.

The kidneys are often involved in thrombotic thrombocytopenic purpura. Proteinuria, gross or microscopic hematuria, white blood cells, and casts are frequently seen, and renal insufficiency is common. Histologically,

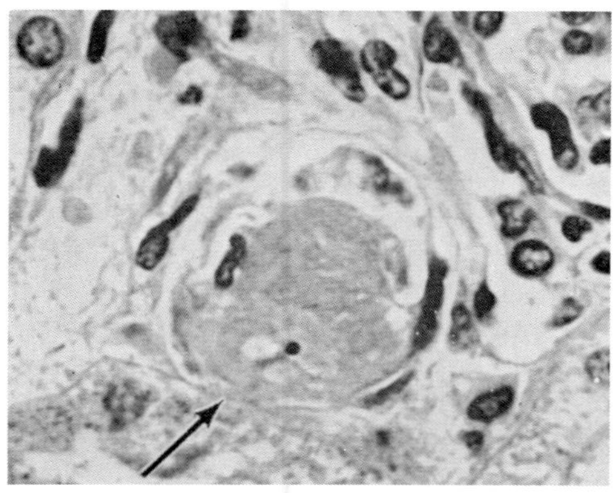

Figure 21-32. Thrombotic thrombocytopenic purpura. Hyaline thrombus in an afferent arteriole. There may be necrosis of the endothelium at one point (*arrow*). Hematoxylin and eosin. ×750.

eosinophilic thrombi in the arterioles and locally within the glomerular capillaries are characteristic (Figs. 21-11, 21-32). The glomerular changes are seen only in those areas adjacent to the capillary lesions, the remainder of the glomerulus being normal in appearance.

Lukes et al. [105] noted renal abnormalities in 47 of 49 cases of thrombotic thrombocytopenic purpura, with severe proteinuria in 30, and azotemia in 37. Amorosi and Ultmann [3] reviewed all the published cases in 1966, representing a total of 274 cases of thrombotic thrombocytopenic purpura. There was evidence of renal involvement in 191 of 217 cases, the principal manifestations being significant proteinuria, hematuria, pyuria, and casts as well as azotemia.

The greater difficulties arising in differential diagnosis are related to the similar appearance of symptomatic hemolytic anemia and thrombocytopenia in systemic lupus erythematosus. Both disorders may lead to anemia as well as to depression of platelets. The angiopathy of thrombotic purpura may sometimes appear along with the vascular changes of lupus or polyarteritis. Features of SLE or polyarteritis have been described in about 10 per cent of the

swelling and proliferation of the endothelium, foot-process changes, vasculization of the epithelial changes, and accumulation of polymorphonuclear leukocytes occur. These changes are also similar to those described in other diseases where immune-complex deposition is thought to play an etiologic role [15, 35, 118].

TREATMENT

The variability in the clinical course of the nephritis associated with Schönlein-Henoch purpura makes interpretation of therapeutic results difficult. In our experience, steroids have occasionally appeared to be of benefit in suppressing activity of the disease and in arresting the rate of progression of renal damage. Intensive immunosuppressive therapy appears to be of benefit, but this must receive more intensive evaluation before it can be recommended as a standard form of therapy [113, 173].

Lung Hemorrhage in Glomerulonephritis

In 1955 Parkin and his associates [128] described seven patients in whom hemoptysis was an early and important symptom heralding the onset of an illness characterized by rapidly progressing renal failure leading to death in uremia. Postmortem examination revealed a proliferative glomerulonephritis. Subsequently, more than 100 cases have been reported [48, 89, 149], several authors noting that the original description appeared to be that by Goodpasture [72], who described a case of severe hemoptysis following influenza in an 18-year-old man. Postmortem examination revealed extensive pulmonary hemorrhage and a proliferative glomerulonephritis. In a number of reports, one or more of the patients had polyarteritis, but this did not necessarily involve the pulmonary vascular bed. Some of the reported cases exhibited hemoptysis only after the uremia had become clinically severe [109]. When these two groups are excluded, the typical picture is characterized by the appearance of severe hemoptysis in patients with normal renal function and occasionally with an initially normal urinalysis [48]. This initial event is followed in a variable but usually short time by rapidly progressive renal failure that usually terminates fatally in a few weeks or months. The hemoptysis tends to be episodic, the attacks of hemoptysis of varying severity being punctuated by intervals of freedom. In one case followed by one of the authors, the bouts of hemoptysis appeared to be associated with more rapid progression of the renal disease.

The renal disease is characterized initially by hematuria that tends to become more severe as the disease progresses. It is usually grossly visible; at times, the packed red cell volume of the urine may exceed 2 or 3 per cent. Red blood cell casts are numerous and usually appear early in the course of the disease. Proteinuria is usually heavy once renal involvement becomes clinically evident; it may exceed 8 to 10 gm. daily and produce some or all the clinical manifestations of the nephrotic syndrome. Hypertension is seldom seen early in the disease, although it may appear as the disease progresses [14].

Histologically, the earliest change seen in the kidney is a local and focal glomerulonephritis that appears relatively benign and is indistinguishable from the changes seen in early nephropathy of Schönlein-Henoch purpura. Indeed, it has been suggested that this is a variant of anaphylactoid purpura, with the lung being involved in the vascular abnormality rather than the vessels of the skin, joints, and digestive tract [149]. Local glomerular necroses are probably more common in the earlier stages of this disorder than in the Schönlein-Henoch nephropathy. As the disease progresses, the histologic picture changes to that of a severe diffuse glomerulonephritis with extensive necroses within the glomeruli, marked crescent formation, and many red blood cells in Bowman's space and in the tubules. The tubules show large areas of atrophy with some interstitial inflammation and some areas of tubular necrosis [14, 48, 84]. These late changes are also not clearly distinguishable from those seen in the most advanced and severe forms of Schönlein-Henoch nephritis.

Electron microscopy reveals changes similar to those encountered in many other diffuse renal diseases, particularly those seen in Schönlein-Henoch purpura. These changes include endothelial swelling and proliferation, increase in mesangial matrix, subendothelial electron-dense deposits of fibrillar material that exhibits a periodicity similar to that of fibrin, as well as granular dense bands or ovoid masses of material deposited within the basement membranes. There may also be marked scalloping of the basement membrane. Abnormal inclusion bodies within some of the cells of the glomerulus, thought possibly to represent virus particles, have also been described [48].

Immunofluorescent studies have identified gamma globulin and β_1 C-globulin deposited in an uninterrupted linear fashion along the basement membrane of the glomerulus. Fibrinogen or fibrin has also been identified by this technic [48]. The gamma globulin thus identified can be eluted off with an acid buffer at a pH known to disassociate antigen-antibody complexes [101]. The predominant class of immunoglobulins obtained by this elution is IgG. Elaborate studies on this eluted material have established that the major portion represents specific antiglomerular basement membrane antibody. In addition to reacting with glomerular basement membrane, this material has also been demonstrated to react with basement membrane from pulmonary tissue [110]. The convincing demonstration that these eluted antibodies can produce severe and rapidly progressive renal disease when given to monkeys provides support for the suggestion that antiglomerular basement membrane antibody may play a cardinal pathogenic role in the evolution of Goodpasture's syndrome by the production of immunologic injury to both glomerular basement membrane and pulmonary basement membrane [44, 101].

There is ample evidence, however, that this antiglomerular basement membrane antibody is not uniquely confined to those patients with lung hemorrhage as an early manifestation of glomerulitis. Similar antibodies have been obtained from patients with subacute and chronic glomerulonephritis. Antibodies obtained from patients with these diseases appear to differ from the antiglomerular basement membrane antibody in those patients with pulmonary hemorrhage only in the quantitative intensity of the reactions observed. In particular, the degree of cross-reactivity with basement membrane from lung is significantly greater with antibody from the latter group than that from other forms of glomerulonephritis [101, 110]. No information is available concerning the mechanism whereby this material is produced.

The term *Goodpasture's syndrome* has been used to identify the group of patients with severe hemoptysis and glomerulonephritis, but perhaps it is well to emphasize that the term may encompass a group of disorders or a spectrum of disease rather than a single entity. In a number of reports beginning with that of Parkin et al. [84, 128], several of the patients have exhibited clear histologic evidence of polyarteritis. Although in a majority of reported cases hemoptysis developed as the initial manifestation of the disorder, antedating the development of renal disease, other patients were apparently uremic when hemoptysis was recognized [109]. Histologically, the changes occurring in this group of patients cannot easily be distinguished from those seen in several other disorders, including polyarteritis and Schönlein-Henoch disease [15]. The antibody to glomerular basement membrane that has been identified in some patients with pulmonary hemorrhage is not uniquely limited to this disorder, since it has been identified in other, apparently unrelated conditions. Although the proposal has been made to limit the term Goodpasture's syndrome only to those patients without polyarteritis who develop hemoptysis prior to the appearance of renal involvement, it is not completely clear that such distinction is warranted [84]. One of the cases described by Goodpasture exhibited arteriolar vascular lesions in the gut [72]. Several reports have included cases with clinical features that are typical of the disorder, but the diagnosis of polyarteritis was established histologically. Among the five patients we have had an opportunity to follow, one patient showed typical lesions of polyarteritis on muscle biopsy, but at postmortem examination only the pulmonary hemorrhagic changes and glomerulonephritis could be identified. Another patient exhibited recurrent episodes of gross hemoptysis and rapidly progressing glomerulonephritis and in addition he had purpuric lesions scattered over the skin that were typical of the lesions seen in Schönlein-Henoch purpura.

TREATMENT

The results of therapy in this group of cases have been disappointing. The majority of cases reported have terminated fatally within a few months of onset. The few cases reported as surviving for an appreciable length of time have all had treatment with large doses of steroids initiated early in the course of the disease [14, 84, 89]. Thus early and vigorous steroid therapy may be indicated in such cases. More recently, a number of these cases have been reported in which pulmonary hemorrhage has ceased after the patient has been placed on chronic hemodialysis and subjected to nephrectomy [29]. A few patients have had renal transplants without recurrence of the pulmonary manifestations [106].

References

1. Abruzzo, J., Amanti, C. M., and Heimer, R. Primary amyloidosis with monoclonal immunoglobulin A proteinuria. *Amer. J. Med.* 45:460, 1968.
2. Allen, A. C. *The Kidney. Medical and Surgical Diseases.* New York: Grune & Stratton, 1951.
3. Amorosi, E. L., and Ultmann, J. E. Thrombotic thrombocytopenic purpura: Report of 16 cases and review of the literature. *Medicine* (Balt.) 45:139, 1966.
4. Anderson, V., Buch, N. H., Jensen, M. K., and Killman, S. A. Deafness, urticaria and amyloidosis. *Amer. J. Med.* 42:449, 1967.
5. Andrade, C. A peculiar form of peripheral neuropathy: Familial generalized amyloidosis with special involvement of the peripheral nerves. *Brain* 75:408, 1952.
6. Apitz, K. Die Paraproteinosum (Über die Storung des Eiweisstoffwechsels bei Plasmacytom). *Virchow. Arch. Path. Anat.* 306:631, 1940.
7. Armstrong, J. B. Study of renal function in patients with multiple myeloma. *Amer. J. Med. Sci.* 219:488, 1950.
8. Barclay, G. P. T., Cameron, H. MacD., and Loughridge, L. A. Amyloid disease of the kidney and renal vein thrombosis. *Quart. J. Med.* 29:137, 1960.
9. Barondess, J. A. Thrombotic thrombocytopenic purpura: Review of the literature and report of three cases. *Amer. J. Med.* 12:294, 1952.
10. Barth, W. F., Willerson, J. T., Waldmann, T. A., and Decker, J. L. Primary amyloidosis. *Amer. J. Med.* 47:259, 1969.
11. Bell, E. T. Amyloid disease of the kidneys. *Amer. J. Path.* 9:185, 1933.
12. Bell, E. T. Renal lesions associated with multiple myeloma. *Amer. J. Path.* 9:393, 1933.
13. Bence Jones, H. On a new substance occurring in the urine of a patient with mollities ossium. *Phil. Trans.* 138:55, 1848.

14. Benoit, F. L., Rulon, D. B., Theil, G. B., Doolan, P. D., and Watten, R. H. Goodpasture's syndrome: A clinicopathologic review. *Amer. J. Med.* 37:424, 1964.
15. Berger, J. IgA glomerular deposits in renal disease. *Transplantation Proc.* 1:933, 1969.
16. Bergman, F., and Warmenius, S. Familial perireticular amyloidosis in a Swedish family. *Amer. J. Med.* 45:601, 1968.
17. Bevans, M. Pathology of scleroderma, with special reference to the changes in the gastrointestinal tract. *Amer. J. Path.* 21:25, 1945.
18. Breuer, R. I., and LeBauer, J. Caution in the use of phosphates in the treatment of severe hypercalcemia. *J. Clin. Endocr.* 27:695, 1967.
19. Bryan, C. W., and Healy, J. K. Acute renal failure in multiple myeloma. *Amer. J. Med.* 44:128, 1968.
20. Bywaters, E. G. L., Isdale, I., and Kempton, J. J. Schoenlein-Henoch purpura: Evidence for a group A beta hemolytic streptococcal etiology. *Quart. J. Med.* 25:161, 1957.
21. Calkins, E., and Cohen, A. S. Diagnosis of amyloidosis. *Bull. Rheum. Dis.* 10:215, 1960.
22. Calkins, E., Cohen, A. S., and Larsen, B. Amyloidosis: Preliminary chemical, clinical and experimental observations. *Ann. N.Y. Acad. Sci.* 86:1033, 1960.
23. Calvert, R. J., and Owen, T. K. True scleroderma kidney. *Lancet* 2:19, 1956.
24. Carbone, P. P., Kellerhouse, L. E., and Gehan, E. Plasmacytic myeloma: A study of the relationship of survival to various clinical manifestations and anomalous protein type in 112 patients. *Amer. J. Med.* 42:937, 1967.
25. Carone, F. A., and Epstein, F. H. Nephrogenic diabetes insipidus caused by amyloid disease. *Amer. J. Med.* 29:539, 1960.
26. Carson, C. P., Ackerman, L. P., and Maltby, J. D. Plasma cell myeloma: Clinical, pathologic and roentgenologic review of 90 cases. *Amer. J. Clin. Path.* 25:849, 1959.
27. Chakmakjian, Z. H., and Bethune, J. E. Sodium sulfate treatment of hypercalcemia. *New Eng. J. Med.* 275:862, 1966.
28. Chinard, F. P., Lauson, H. D., Eder, H. A., Greif, R. L., and Hiller, A. A study of the mechanism of proteinuria in patients with the nephrotic syndrome. *J. Clin. Invest.* 33:621, 1954.
29. Cleveland, R. J., Lee, H. M., Prout, G. R., and Hume, D. M. Preservation of cadaver kidney for renal homotransplantation in man. *Surg. Gynec. Obstet.* 119:991, 1964.
30. Clinicopathologic Conference. Scleroderma with congestive heart failure. *Amer. J. Med.* 14:231, 1953.
31. Cohen, A. S. The constitution and genesis of amyloid. *Int. Rev. Exp. Path.* 4:159, 1965.
32. Cohen, A. S., and Calkins, E. A. Study of the fine structure of the kidney in casein-induced amyloidosis in rabbits. *J. Exp. Med.* 112:479, 1960.
33. Combined Staff Clinic. Multiple myeloma. *Amer. J. Med.* 23:283, 1957.
34. Combined Staff Clinic. Systemic lupus erythematosus. *Amer. J. Med.* 28:416, 1960.
35. Comerford, F. R., and Cohen, A. S. The nephropathy of systemic lupus erythematosus. *Medicine* (Balt.) 46:425, 1967.
36. Conley, C. L. The L.E. cell test. *J. Chronic Dis.* 5:275, 1957.
37. Costea, N., Yakulis, V. L., Libnoch, J. A., Pilzce, C. G., and Heller, P. Two myeloma globulins in one subject and one cell line. *Amer. J. Med.* 42:630, 1967.
38. Craig, J. M., and Gitlin, D. The nature of the hyaline thrombi in thrombotic thrombocytopenic purpura. *Amer. J. Path.* 33:251, 1957.
39. D'Angelo, W. A., Fries, J. F., Masi, A. T., and Shulman, L. E. Pathologic observations in systemic sclerosis (scleroderma). *Amer. J. Med.* 46:428, 1969.
40. Darmady, E. M., Griffiths, W. S., Spencer, H., Mattingly, D., Stranck, F., and de Wardener, H. E. Renal tubular failure associated with polyarteritis nodosa. *Lancet* 1:378, 1955.
41. Davson, J., Ball, J., and Platt, R. Kidney in periarteritis nodosa. *Quart. J. Med.* 17:175, 1948.
42. Deicher, H. R. G., Holman, H. R., and Kunkel, H. G. Anticytoplasmic factors in

the sera of patients with systemic lupus erythematosus and certain other diseases. *Arthritis Rheum.* 3:1, 1960.

43. Dent, C. E., and Rose, G. A. The Bence Jones protein of multiple myelomatosis, its methionine content and its possible significance in relation to the etiology of the disease. *Biochem. J.* 44:610, 1949.
44. Dixon, F. J. The pathogenesis of glomerulonephritis. *Amer. J. Med.* 44:493, 1968.
45. Dixon, F. J., Feldman, J. D., and Vazquez, J. J. Experimental glomerulonephritis. *J. Exp. Med.* 113:899, 1961.
46. Dixon, H. M. Renal amyloidosis in relation to renal insufficiency. *Amer. J. Med. Sci.* 187:401, 1934.
47. Dubois, E. L., and Tuffanelli, D. L. Clinical manifestations of systemic lupus erythematosus. *J.A.M.A.* 190:104, 1964.
48. Duncan, D. A., Drummond, K. N., Michael, A. F., and Vernier, R. L. Pulmonary hemorrhage and glomerulonephritis. *Ann. Intern. Med.* 62:920, 1965.
49. Effersøe, P., and Tidstrom, B. Detection of myeloma protein in urine by a new quick method. *J. Lab. Clin. Med.* 50:134, 1957.
50. Engle, R. L., Jr., and Wallis, L. A. Multiple myeloma and the adult Fanconi syndrome. *Amer. J. Med.* 22:5, 1957.
51. Faden, R. S. Differentiation of plasmocytic response from myelomatous diseases on the basis of bone-marrow findings. *Cancer* 5:128, 1952.
52. Fahey, J. L., Carbone, P. P., Rowe, D. S., and Bachman, R. Plasma cell myeloma with D-myeloma protein (IgD myeloma). *Amer. J. Med.* 45:373. 1968.
53. Farquhar, M. G., and Palade, G. E. Segregation of ferritin in glomerular protein absorption droplets. *J. Biophys. Biochem. Cytol.* 7:297, 1960.
54. Farquhar, M. G., Vernier, R. L., and Good, R. A. An electron microscope study of the glomerulus in nephrosis, glomerulonephritis, and lupus erythematosus. *J. Exp. Med.* 106:649, 1957.
55. Farquhar, M. G., Wissig, S. L., and Palade, G. E. Glomerular permeability: I. Ferritin transfer across the normal glomerular wall. *J. Exp. Med.* 113:47, 1961.
56. Fisher, E. R., and Rodman, G. P. Pathologic observations concerning the kidney in progressive systemic sclerosis. *A.M.A. Arch. Path.* 65:29, 1958.
57. Forbus, W. D., Perlzwig, W. A., Parfentjev, I. A., and Burwell, J. C., Jr. Bence-Jones protein excretion and its effect upon the kidney. *Bull. Johns Hopkins Hosp.* 57: 47, 1935.
58. Fred, H. L., and Ramho, O. N. Acute renal failure due to scleroderma kidney. *A.M.A. Arch. Intern. Med.* 100:813, 1957.
59. Freedman, P. Lupus Nephritis. In Milne, M. D. (Ed.), *Recent Advances in Renal Disease.* (The Proceedings of a conference held in London at the Royal College of Physicians of London.) Philadelphia: J. B. Lippincott, 1960.
60. Freedman, P., Peters, J. H., and Kark, R. M. Localization of gamma globulin in the diseased kidney. *A.M.A. Arch. Intern. Med.* 105:524, 1960.
61. Frohnert, P. P., and Sheps, S. G. Long-term follow-up study of periarteritis nodosa. *Amer. J. Med.* 43:8, 1967.
62. Gairdner, D. The Schönlein-Henoch syndrome (anaphylactoid purpura). *Quart. J. Med.* 17:95, 1948.
63. Gary, N. E., Maher, J. F., and Schreiner, G. E. Lupus nephritis: Renal function after prolonged survival. *New Eng. J. Med.* 276:73, 1967.
64. Germuth, F. G., Jr. A comparative histologic and immunologic study in rabbits of induced hypersensitivity of the serum sickness type. *J. Exp. Med.* 97:257, 1953.
65. Germuth, F. G., Jr., and McKinnon, G. E. Studies on the biologic properties of antigen-antibody complexes: I. Anaphylactic shock induced by soluble antigen-antibody complexes in unsensitized normal guinea pigs. *Bull. Johns Hopkins Hosp.* 101:13, 1957.
66. Germuth, F. G., Jr., and Pollack, A. D. Immune complex disease: III. The granulomatous manifestations. *Johns Hopkins Med. J.* 121:254, 1967.
67. Germuth, F. G., Jr., Senterfit, L. B., and Pollack, A. D. Immune complex disease: I. Experimental acute and chronic glomer-

ulonephritis. *Johns Hopkins Med. J.* 120: 225, 1967.

68. Gitlin, D., Craig, J. M., and Janeway, C. A. Studies on the nature of fibrinoid in the collagen disease. *Amer. J. Path.* 33:55, 1957.
69. Goldman, R., Adams, W. S., and Luchsinger, E. B. Renal function in multiple myeloma. *J. Lab. Clin. Med.* 40:519, 1952.
70. Goodman, G. C., and Deitch, A. D. A cytochemical study of the L.E. bodies of systemic lupus erythematosus: I. Nucleic acids. *J. Exp. Med.* 106:575, 1957.
71. Goodman, G. C., and Deitch, A. D. A cytochemical study of the L.E. bodies of systemic lupus erythematosus: II. Proteins. *J. Exp. Med.* 106:593, 1957.
72. Goodpasture, E. W. The significance of certain pulmonary lesions in relation to the etiology of influenza. *Amer. J. Med. Sci.* 158:863, 1919.
72a. Grausz, H., Earley, L. E., Stephens, B. G., Lee, J. C., and Hopper, J., Jr. Virus-like particles in glomerular endothelium of patients with SLE. *New Eng. J. Med.* 283: 506, 1970.
73. Gregoire, F., Malmendier, C., and Lambert, P. P. The mechanism of proteinuria, and a study of the effects of hormonal therapy in the nephrotic syndrome. *Amer. J. Med.* 25:516, 1958.
74. Gross, L. The Heart in Atypical Verrucous Endocarditis. In Epstein, A. A. et al. (Eds.), *Contributions to the Medical Sciences in Honor of Emanuel Libman.* New York: International Press, 1932. Vol. 2, p. 527.
75. Gruber, G. B. Zur Frage der Periarteritis Nodosa, mit besonderer Berucksichtigung der Gallenblasen-und Nieren-Beteiligung. *Virchow. Arch. [Path. Anat.]* 258:441, 1925.
76. Hardwicke, J., and Squire, J. R. The relationship between plasma albumin concentration and protein excretion in patients with proteinuria. *Clin. Sci.* 14:509, 1955.
77. Harrison, C. V., Milne, M. D., and Steiner, R. E. Renal vein thrombosis. *Quart. J. Med.* 25:285, 1956.
78. Harvey, A. M., Shulman, L. E., Tumulty, P. A., Conley, C. L., and Schoenrich, E. H. Systemic lupus erythematosus; a review of the literature and clinical analysis of 138 cases. *Medicine* (Balt.) 33:291, 1954.
79. Heckman, B. A., and Walsh, J. H. Hypernatremia complicating sodium sulfate therapy for hypercalcemic crisis. *New Eng. J. Med.* 276:1082, 1967.
80. Heller, H., Missmahl, H. P., Sohar, E., and Gafni, J. Amyloidosis: Its differentiation into peri-reticulin and peri-collagen types. *J. Path. Bact.* 89:15, 1964.
81. Heller, H., Sohar, E., Gafni, J., and Heller, J. Amyloidosis in familial Mediterranean fever. *Arch. Intern. Med.* (Chicago) 107: 539, 1961.
82. Heptinstall, R. H. Diseases of the Kidney. In Harrison, C. V. (Ed.), *Recent Advances in Pathology* (7th ed.). Boston: Little, Brown, 1960.
83. Heptinstall, R. H., and Joekes, A. M. Renal amyloid: A report on 11 cases proven by renal biopsy. *Ann. Rheum. Dis.* 19:126, 1960.
84. Heptinstall, R. H., and Salmon, M. V. Pulmonary hemorrhage with extensive glomerular disease of the kidney. *J. Clin. Path.* 12:272, 1959.
85. Hill, J. M., and Loeh, E. Massive hormonal therapy and splenectomy in acute thrombotic · thrombocytopenic purpura. *J.A.M.A.* 173:778, 1960.
86. Holman, H. R., Deicher, H. R. G., and Kunkel, H. G. The L.E. cell and the L.E. serum factors. *Bull. N.Y. Acad. Med.* 35: 409, 1959.
87. Jarnum, I. A new diagnostic test in amyloidosis. *Lancet* 1:1007, 1960.
88. Johnson, G. *Diseases of the Kidney.* London: John W. Parker & Son, 1852. P. 76.
89. Johnson, J. R., and McGovern, V. J. Goodpasture's syndrome and Wegener's granulomatosis. *Aust. Ann. Med.* 11:250, 1962.
90. Kahie, M., Orman, B., Gyorky, F., and Brown, H. Hypercalcemia. Experience with phosphate and sulfate therapy. *J.A.M.A.* 201:721, 1967.
91. Kemperer, P. General Considerations on Collagen Disease. In Asboe-Hansen, G. (Ed.), *Connective Tissue in Health and*

Disease. New York: Philosophical Library, 1957.

92. Klein, H., and Block, M. Bone marrow plasmacytosis: Review of 60 cases. *Blood* 8:1034, 1953.
93. Knowles, H. C., Jr., Zeek, P. M., and Blankenhorn, M. A. Studies on necrotizing angiitis. *A.M.A. Arch. Intern. Med.* 92: 789, 1953.
94. Kobernick, S. D., and Whiteside, J. N. Renal glomeruli in multiple myeloma. *Lab. Invest.* 6:478, 1957.
95. Koffler, D., Agnello, V., Carr, R. I., and Kunkel, H. G. Anti-DNA antibodies and renal lesions in patients with systemic lupus erythematosus. *Transplantation Proc.* 1: 933, 1969.
96. Koffler, D., and Kunkel, H. Mechanism of renal injury in systemic lupus erythematosus. *Amer. J. Med.* 45:165, 1968.
97. Kopp, W. L., Bierne, G. J., and Burns, R. O. Hyperviscosity syndrome in multiple myeloma. *Amer. J. Med.* 43:141, 1967.
98. Krupp, M. A. Urinary sediment in visceral angiitis (periarteritis nodosa, lupus erythematosus, Libman-Sacks disease): Quantitative studies. *Arch. Intern. Med.* 71:54, 1943.
99. Ladefoged, J., Nielson, G., Raaschou, F., and Sorenson, A. Acute anuria due to polyarteritis nodosa. *Amer. J. Med.* 46:827, 1969.
100. Laszlo, M. H., Alvarez, A., and Feldman, F. The association of thrombotic thrombocytopenic purpura and disseminated lupus erythematosus: Report of a case. *Ann. Intern. Med.* 42:1308, 1955.
101. Lerner, R. A., Glassock, R. J., and Dixon, F. J. The role of antiglomerular basement membrane antibody in the pathogenesis of human glomerulonephritis. *J. Exp. Med.* 126:989, 1967.
102. Levi, D. F., Williams, R. C., Jr., and Lindstrom, F. D. Immunofluorescent studies of the myeloma kidney with special reference to light-chain disease. *Amer. J. Med.* 44:922, 1968.
103. Levitt, L. M., and Burbank, B. Glomerulonephritis as a complication of Schönlein-Henoch syndrome. *New Eng. J. Med.* 248: 530, 1953.
104. Lippman, R. N. *Urine and the Urinary Sediment* (2d ed.). Springfield, Ill.: Thomas, 1962.
105. Lukes, R. J., Rath, C. E., Steussy, C. N., and Mailliard, J. Thrombotic thrombocytopenic purpura — clinical and pathological findings in 49 cases. *Blood* 17:366, 1961.
106. Maddick, R. K., Stevens, L. E., Reemstma, K., and Bloomer, H. A. Goodpasture's syndrome: Cessation of pulmonary hemorrhage after bilateral nephrectomy. *Ann. Intern. Med.* 67:1258, 1967.
107. Magnus-Levy, A. Multiple myeloma. *Acta Med. Scand.* 95:217, 1938.
108. Mawas, C., Sors, C., and Bernier, J. J. Amyloidosis with primary agammaglobulinemia, severe diarrhea and familial hypogammaglobulinemia. *Amer. J. Med.* 46: 624, 1969.
109. McCaugher, W. T., and Thomas, J. B. Pulmonary hemorrhage and glomerulonephritis. *Amer. J. Clin. Path.* 38:577, 1962.
110. McPhaul, J. J., Jr., and Dixon, F. J. Characterization of human anti-glomerular basement membrane antibodies eluted from glomerulonephritic kidneys. *J. Clin. Invest.* 219:308, 1970.
111. Mellors, R. C., Ortega, L. G., and Holman, H. R. Role of gamma globulins in pathogenesis of renal lesions in systemic lupus erythematosus and chronic glomerulonephritis, with an observation on the lupus erythematosus cell reaction. *J. Exp. Med.* 106:191, 1957.
112. Menefee, M. G., and Mueller, C. B. Some Morphological Considerations of Transport in the Glomerulus. In Dalton, A. J., and Haguenau, F. (Eds.), *Ultrastructure of the Kidney*. New York: Academic Press, 1967.
113. Michael, A. F., Vernier, R. L., Drummond, K. N., Levitt, J. L., Herdman, R. C., Fish, A. J., and Good, R. A. Immunosuppressive therapy of chronic renal disease. *New Eng. J. Med.* 276:817, 1967.
114. Moore, H. C., and Sheehan, H. L. The kidney in scleroderma. *Lancet* 1:68, 1952.
115. Moore, J. E., Shulman, L. E., and Scott, J. T. The natural history of systemic lupus

erythematosus: An approach to its study through chronic biologic false positive reactors. *J. Chronic Dis.* 5:282, 1957.

116. Moore, R. D., and Schoenberg, M. D. A polysaccharide component in the vascular lesions of thrombotic thrombocytopenic purpura. *Blood* 15:511, 1960.
117. Moschcowitz, E. An acute febrile pleiochromic anemia with hyaline thrombosis of the terminal arterioles and capillaries: An undescribed disease. *Arch. Intern. Med.* 36:89, 1925.
118. Movat, H. Z. Electron Microscopy of Kidney Biopsies from Children and Adolescents. In Metcoff, J. (Ed.), *Proceedings of the Eleventh Annual Conference on the Nephrotic Syndrome.* New York: National Kidney Disease Foundation, 1960. P. 228.
119. Movat, H. Z. The fine structure of the glomerulus in amyloidosis. *Arch. Path.* (Chicago) 69:323, 1960.
120. Muehrcke, R. C., Kark, R. N., Pirani, C. L., and Pollak, V. E. Lupus nephritis; a clinical and pathologic study based on renal biopsies. *Medicine* (Balt.) 36:1, 1957.
121. Myhre, J. R., Brodwall, E. G., and Knudsen, S. B. Acute renal failure following intravenous pyelography in cases of myelomatosis. *Acta Med. Scand.* 158:43, 1957.
122. Norkin, J., Freedman, H. H., and Evans, G. W. Thrombotic thrombocytopenic purpura in siblings. *Amer. J. Med.* 43:294, 1967.
123. Nossal, G. J., and Lederburg, J. Antibody production by single cells. *Nature* (London) 181:1419, 1958.
124. Oliver, J. New directions in renal morphology: A method, its results and its future. *Harvey Lect.* 40:102, 1944–1945.
125. Osler, W. The visceral lesion of purpura and allied conditions. *Brit. Med. J.* 1:517, 1914.
126. Osserman, E. F. Plasma cell myeloma: 2. Clinical aspects. *New Eng. J. Med.* 261: 952, 1959.
127. Osserman, E. F., and Lawlor, B. P. Abnormal serum and urine proteins in 35 cases of multiple myeloma, as studied by filter paper electrophoresis. *Amer. J. Med.* 18:462, 1955.
128. Parkin, T. W., Rusted, I. E., Burchall, N. D., and Edwards, J. E. Hemorrhagic and interstitial pneumonitis with nephritis. *Amer. J. Med.* 18:220, 1955.
129. Perillie, P. B., and Conn, H. O. Acute renal failure after intravenous pyelography in plasma cell myeloma. *J.A.M.A.* 167:2186, 1958.
130. Platt, R., and Davson, J. A clinical and pathological study of renal disease: II. Diseases other than nephritis. *Quart. J. Med.* 19:33, 1950.
131. Pollack, A. D. Some observations on the pathology of systemic lupus erythematosus. *J. Mount Sinai Hosp. N.Y.* 26:224, 1959.
132. Pollak, V. E., Kark, R. M., and Pirani, C. L. Corticosteroid therapy in lupus nephritis: Importance of adequate dosage. *Bull. Rheum. Dis.* 11:249, 1961.
133. Pollak, V. E., Pirani, C. L., and Schwartz, F. D. The natural history of renal manifestations of systemic lupus erythematosus. *J. Lab. Clin. Med.* 63:537, 1964.
134. Post, R. S. The Effects of Glomerular Structure of Proteinuria Induced in Normal Rats, Determined by Electron Microscopy. In Metcoff, J. (Ed.), *Proceedings of the Eleventh Annual Conference on the Nephrotic Syndrome.* New York: National Kidney Disease Foundation, 1960. P. 222.
135. Putnam, F. W. Aberration of protein metabolism and multiple myeloma: Interrelationships of abnormal serum globulins and Bence-Jones proteins. *Physiol. Rev.* 37: 512, 1957.
136. Putnam, F. W. Plasma cell myeloma and macroglobulinemia: 1. Physiochemical, immunochemical and isotopic turnover studies of the abnormal serum and urinary proteins. *New Eng. J. Med.* 261:902, 1959.
137. Putnam, F. W., and Udin, B. Proteins in multiple myeloma: 1. Physical chemical study of serum proteins. *J. Biol. Chem.* 202:727, 1953.
138. Renier, M., and Stern, K. G. Electrophoretic studies on protein distribution in serum of multiple myeloma patients. *Acta Haemat.* (Basel) 9:19, 1953.
139. Report to Medical Research Council by Collagen Disease and Sensitivity Panel.

Treatment of polyarteritis nodosa with cortisone: Results after 3 years. *Brit. Med. J.* 1:1399, 1960.

140. Rich, A. R. Role of hypersensitivity in periarteritis nodosa as indicated by seven cases developing during serum sickness and sulfonamide therapy. *Bull. Johns Hopkins Hosp.* 71:123, 1942.

141. Rich, A. R., and Gregory, J. E. Experimental demonstration that periarteritis nodosa is a manifestation of hypersensitivity. *Bull. Johns Hopkins Hosp.* 72:65, 1943.

142. Richter, G. W. The resorption of amyloid under experimental conditions. *Amer. J. Path.* 30:239, 1953.

143. Rose, G. A. The natural history of polyarteritis. *Brit. Med. J.* 2:1148, 1957.

144. Rose, G. A., and Spencer, H. Polyarteritis nodosa. *Quart. J. Med.* 26:43, 1957.

145. Rothfield, N., McCluskey, R. T., and Baldwin, D. S. Renal disease in systemic lupus erythematosus. *New Eng. J. Med.* 269:537, 1963.

146. Roussak, N. J., and Oleesky, S. Water losing nephritis. *Quart. J. Med.* 23:147, 1954.

147. Rukavina, H. V., Black, W. G., Jackson, C. E., Falls, H. F., Carey, J. H., and Curtis, A. C. Primary systemic amyloidosis. *Medicine* (Balt.) 35:239, 1956.

148. Rundles, R. W., and Coonrad, E. V. Treatment of multiple myeloma. In American Cancer Society, Inc. and National Cancer Institute, U.S. Public Health Service, *Proceedings of the Third National Cancer Conference, Detroit, Michigan, June 4–6, 1956.* Philadelphia: Lippincott, 1957.

149. Rusby, N. L., and Wilson, C. Lung purpura with nephritis. *Quart. J. Med.* 29:501, 1960.

150. Sanchez, L. M., and Domz, C. A. Renal patterns in myeloma. *Ann. Intern. Med.* 52:44, 1960.

151. Sanders, J. H., Fahey, J., Finegold, I., Ein, D., Reisfeld, R., and Berard, C. Multiple anomalous immunoglobulins: Clinical, structural and cellular studies in 3 patients. *Amer. J. Med.* 47:43, 1969.

152. Schur, P. H., and Sandson, J. Immunologic factors and clinical activity in systemic lupus erythematosus. *New Eng. J. Med.* 278:533, 1968.

153. Shapiro, S., Ross, V., and Moore, D. H. Viscous protein obtained in large amount from serum of a patient with multiple myeloma. *J. Clin. Invest.* 22:137, 1943.

154. Singer, K., Bornstein, F. P., and Wile, S. A. Thrombotic thrombocytopenic purpura: Hemorrhagic diathesis with generalized platelet thromboses. *Blood* 2:542, 1947.

155. Sirota, J. H., and Hammerman, D. Renal studies in an adult subject with Fanconi syndrome. *Amer. J. Med.* 16:138, 1954.

156. Snapper, I., Turner, L. B., and Moscovitz, H. L. *Multiple Myeloma.* New York: Grune & Stratton, 1953.

157. Soffer, L. J., Southrew, A. L., Weiner, H. E., and Wolf, R. L. Renal manifestations of systemic lupus erythematosus; a clinical and pathological study of 90 cases. *Ann. Intern. Med.* 54:215, 1961.

158. Sohar, E., Gafni, J., Pras, M., and Heller, H. Familial Mediterranean fever: A survey of 470 cases and review of the literature. *Amer. J. Med.* 43:227, 1967.

159. Spiro, D. The structural basis of proteinuria in man. *Amer. J. Path.* 35:47, 1959.

160. Spiro, D. Electron Microscopic Studies of Renal Biopsies on Patients with Proteinuria. In Metcoff, J. (Ed.), *Proceedings of the Eleventh Annual Conference on the Nephrotic Syndrome.* New York: National Kidney Disease Foundation, 1960. P. 171.

161. Squire, J. R. Functional Pathology. In Milne, M. D. (Ed.), *Recent Advances in Renal Disease.* (Proceedings of a Conference held in London at the Royal College of Physicians of London.) Philadelphia: Lippincott, 1960.

162. Stevens, M. B., and Knowles, B. Significance of urinary gamma globulin in lupus nephritis: Electrophoretic analysis. *New Eng. J. Med.* 267:1159, 1962.

163. Summers, W. M. C., and Gillett, R. Polyarteritis nodosa, associated with malignant hypertension, disseminated platelet thrombosis, "wire-loop" glomeruli, pulmonary silicotuberculosis and sarcoidosis-like lymphadenopathy. *A.M.A. Arch. Path.* 52:489, 1951.

164. Teilum, G. Miliary epitheloid cell granulomas in lupus erythematosus. *Acta Path. Microbiol. Scand.* 22:73, 1945.
165. Urai, L., Munkacsi, I., and Szinay, G. New data on the pathology of "true scleroderma kidney." *Brit. Med. J.* 1:713, 1961.
166. Urizar, R. E., Michael, A. F., Sisson, S. P., and Vernier, R. L. Anaphylactoid purpura: II. Immunofluorescent and electron microscopic studies of the glomerular lesions. *Lab. Invest.* 19:437, 1968.
167. Vasquez, J. J., and Dixon, F. J. Immunohistochemical analysis of amyloid by fluorescence technique. *J. Exp. Med.* 104:727, 1956.
168. Vassar, P. I., and Culling, C. F. A. Fluorescent stains with special reference to amyloid and connective tissue. *A.M.A. Arch. Path.* 68:487, 1959.
169. Vernier, R. L., Worthen, H. G., Peterson, R. D., Colle, E., and Good, R. A. Anaphylactoid purpura: I. Pathology of the skin and kidney and frequency of streptococcal infection. *Pediatrics* 27:181, 1961.
170. von Sallman, L. (Moderator) Primary amyloidosis: Clinical Staff Conference at the National Institutes of Health. *Ann. Intern. Med.* 52:668, 1960.
171. Walker, W. G., and Hulter, H. N. Some observations on the metabolic activity of glomeruli. *Trans. Amer. Clin. Climat. Ass.* 81:174, 1969.
172. Walser, M. Renal Excretion of Alkaline Earths. In Comar, C. L., and Bronner, F. (Eds.), *Mineral Metabolism*. New York: Academic, 1969. Vol. III.
173. White, R. H. R., Cameron, J. S., and Trounce, J. R. Immunosuppressive therapy in steroid resistant proliferative glomerulonephritis accompanied by the nephrotic syndrome. *Brit. Med. J.* 2:283, 1966.
174. Wilson, I. D., Williams, R. C., Jr., and Tobian, L. Renal tubular acidosis: Three cases with immunoglobin abnormalities in the patients and their kindreds. *Amer. J. Med.* 43:356, 1967.
175. Zeek, P. M. Periarteritis nodosa and other forms of necrotizing angiitis. *New Eng. J. Med.* 248:764, 1953.
176. Zeek, P. M., Smith, C. C., and Weeter, J. C. Studies on periarteritis nodosa: III. Differentiation between vascular lesions of periarteritis nodosa and of hypersensitivity. *Amer. J. Path.* 24:889, 1948.
177. Zinneman, H. H., Glenchur, H., and Gleason, D. F. The significance of urine electrophoresis in patients with multiple myeloma. *Arch. Intern. Med.* (Chicago) 106:172, 1960.
178. Zweiman, B., Kornbloom, E. A., Carnog, J., and Hildreth, E. A. The prognosis of lupus nephritis: Role of clinicopathologic correlations. *Ann. Intern. Med.* 69:441, 1968.

22

Diabetic Renal Disease

Jacob Churg and Henry Dolger

It has been recognized for some time that renal disease is an almost invariable though initially insidious concomitant of diabetes. Currently the definition of diabetes mellitus, in addition to insulin insufficiency and its associated metabolic expressions, includes associated or concomitant premature vascular degeneration as an integral part of the clinical picture. These two manifestations develop at different velocities so that at first only the insufficiency of insulin is evident in the juvenile diabetic patients, while adult diabetic patients may exhibit any or all of the concomitants before the onset of any chemical abnormality is expressed clinically (Fig. 22-1).

The interest in renal aspects of diabetes was kindled by the report of Kimmelstiel and Wilson [38] on nodular glomerulosclerosis. Subsequent studies have demonstrated that prolongation of life by means of insulin and antibiotics was often at the cost of renal disease. Dolger [20] found albuminuria and hypertension in 50 per cent of all juvenile diabetic patients with retinopathy — all three findings appearing within an average of 13 years of the onset of diabetes. This duration between the onset of diabetes and the appearance of vascular and renal damage was shortened in the older diabetic patients in whom, of course, the initial picture was often asymptomatic.

Fanconi [21] reported that of 87 juvenile diabetic patients all had nephropathy within 16 years of the onset of the underlying disease. In fact, within 21 years all 87 had died, with uremia as the most frequent cause of death. In some of the more recent investigations, over 50 per cent of all patients (juvenile and mature) who have had diabetes for 10 to 20 years were found to be in renal failure [34, 55]. The renal disease in diabetes may affect any and all structural elements of the kidney from the glomerulus to the interstitial tissue, and give rise to a variety of clinical manifestations often terminating in uremia. Most of the renal lesions occurring in diabetes, such as arteriosclerosis and pyelonephritis, are similar to those of nondiabetic patients but are more frequent and more severe. Some, such as nodular glomerulosclerosis, are virtually diagnostic of diabetes.

For the purposes of description and also of differential diagnosis, we shall discuss separately renal disease manifesting itself as an alteration of blood vessels — arteries, arterioles, and capillaries — and that due to infection and

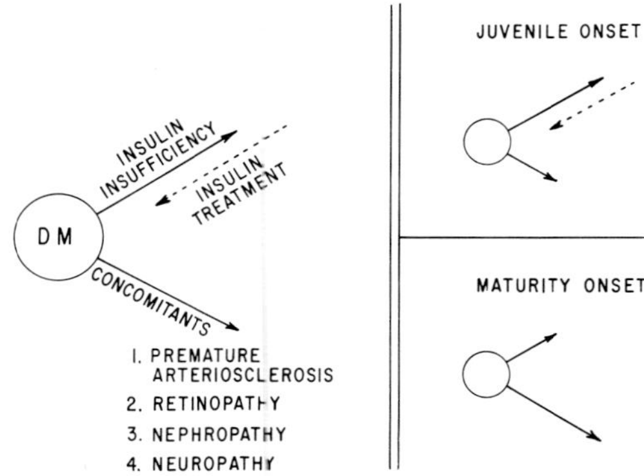

Figure 22-1. Concomitants of diabetes mellitus (DM) — juvenile onset and maturity onset.

inflammation — pyelitis, pyelonephritis, and papillary necrosis. In practice, the vascular and infectious processes often coexist, producing a spectrum of clinical signs and symptoms. Though minor tubular changes, varying from deposition of glycogen and lipid in the cells to basement membrane thickening, are common, they are omitted because their functional and clinical significance is largely unknown.

Vascular Disease

Renal arteriosclerosis and arteriolosclerosis are presented in detail in Chapter 19. The changes discussed here are those with demonstrable relation to diabetes.

The renal vascular tree in diabetic patients is altered in the same manner as that in nondiabetic persons — namely, by thickening of the wall and narrowing of the lumen. The main processes that lead to thickening of the walls are different in each segment of the vascular tree though not necessarily unrelated: In the arteries, it is intimal fibrosis and lipid deposition (atheromatosis); in the arterioles, hyalinization of the intima and the media; and in the glomeruli, widening of the capillary basement membranes and proliferation of the intercapillary tissue (mesangium). It has been noted that in diabetes smaller arteries are frequently affected by proliferative lesions of the endothelium [27].

ARTERIOSCLEROSIS

Sclerosis of the main renal artery and its major branches is more frequent and more severe in diabetic patients than in nondiabetic persons of the same age [6, 42]. This includes atheromatosis characterized by lipid deposition as well as simple intimal fibrosis. Narrowing of the vascular channels may lead to segmental or to more diffuse parenchymal atrophy, but unless this is severe, there are few clinical evidences. Severe narrowing of the main renal artery or its major branches, sufficient to cause renal ischemic hypertension, is often the result of diabetes [62]. One of the more recent illuminating concepts in clinical medicine has been the realization that even preclinical diabetes may be associated with increased severity and frequency of arteriosclerosis [15, 31], at least in the coronary arteries, just as it may produce a host of pathologic alterations in other tissues.

ARTERIOLOSCLEROSIS

As with arteriosclerosis, hyaline arteriolosclerosis is more common and more severe in diabetic than in nondiabetic persons and also occurs at an earlier age. Furthermore, it is more extensive, frequently involving the efferent as well as the afferent arterioles [6].

The nature of arteriolar hyalinization is still under debate. *Hyalin* is defined as an acidophilic, homogeneous or finely granular material consisting of, or containing, globulins, fibrinogen, and other proteins and lipids. Under the electron microscope, hyalin is dense and usually finely granular [9, 24]. It is first detected in the intima between intact cells and elastic fibers; later it invades the media, replacing muscle cells. It has been suggested in the past that hyalin may be derived from the smooth muscle [49] or from elastic fibers [48]. However, most investigators are now inclined to the hypothesis that hyalin is deposited by escape from the blood [24].

In addition to hyaline deposition, the affected arterioles usually show thickening of the basement membranes, including those that surround smooth muscle fibers (sarcolemma) [10]. The relation of arterioles to hypertension is more complex in diabetic than in nondiabetic persons. In the latter, arteriolosclerosis is almost invariably accompanied by hypertension, whereas many persons with diabetes show hyalinization of arterioles but remain normotensive. Bell [6] proposed that in these patients, hyalinization is due to diabetes per se and that hypertension in diabetes follows narrowing of arterioles. This chain of events explains the increased frequency of hypertension in diabetes. However, malignant hypertension and malignant nephrosclerosis are rare [6].

GLOMERULOSCLEROSIS

The term *diabetic glomerulosclerosis* is applied to several more or less distinct and usually coexistent pathologic alterations: nodular glomerulosclerosis, diffuse glomerulosclerosis, thickening of capillary basement membranes and of Bowman's capsule, and the so-called exudative or hyaline lesions. On gross examination the kidneys affected by diabetic glomerulosclerosis tend to be larger than normal not only early in the disease but even in the later stages, with considerable arteriolosclerosis and glomerular alteration leading to renal failure [56]. The surfaces remain smooth for a long time, though eventually they tend to acquire a fine granularity. These changes contrast with those of arteriolosclerosis in the kidneys of nondiabetic persons, which are smaller than normal and distinctly granular. The difference probably lies in the fact that in diabetes neither the arterioles nor the glomeruli become severely compromised until very late in the disease. Furthermore, glomeruli and tubules tend to be larger than normal, partly counteracting the contraction due to scarring [56].

Histology. Nodular glomerulosclerosis was originally described by Kimmelstiel and Wilson [38] under the name of "intercapillary glomerulosclerosis." It is now generally agreed that the nodules arise in the intercapillary tissue or mesangium (for the discussion of mesangium, see Chapter 1). The nodules occupy the centers of individual lobules along the periphery of the glomerulus and away from the hilus (Fig. 22-2). They vary considerably in size and number per glomerulus. Their shape is usually oval or round, and the texture is slightly fibrillar; older lesions tend to be lamellated. In the early stages of the disease, the nodules may be moderately cellular but tend to become acellular with aging. Sometimes a narrow rim of nuclei remains along the periphery of the nodule. The staining reactions are similar to those of the normal mesangium and the basement membrane — that is, red with the periodic acid–Schiff reagent (PAS), indicating the presence of mucopolysaccharides or glycoproteins; blue or green with "connective tissue" (triphenylmethane) dyes, in the same manner as collagen. The nodules are invariably associated with at least some degree of diffuse glomerulosclerosis, and, in fact, transitional forms can often be demonstrated.

Diffuse glomerulosclerosis consists of disseminated thickening of the branching mesangial stalk, from the hilus to the peripheral lobules (Fig. 22-2). The thickened stalk is finely fibrillar and stains in the same manner as the normal mesangium. Lesser degrees of diffuse glomerulosclerosis shade imperceptibly into normal and may be difficult to distinguish from the slight thickening observed in nondiabetic hypertensive patients and in older normotensive individuals.

Electron microscopy demonstrates that the thickening of the mesangium is caused by an increase in the number and bulk of strands of the mesangial matrix (basement membrane branches, basement membrane-like material) [7, 18, 22, 23, 40, 51, 60, 61] (Figs. 22-3, 22-4).

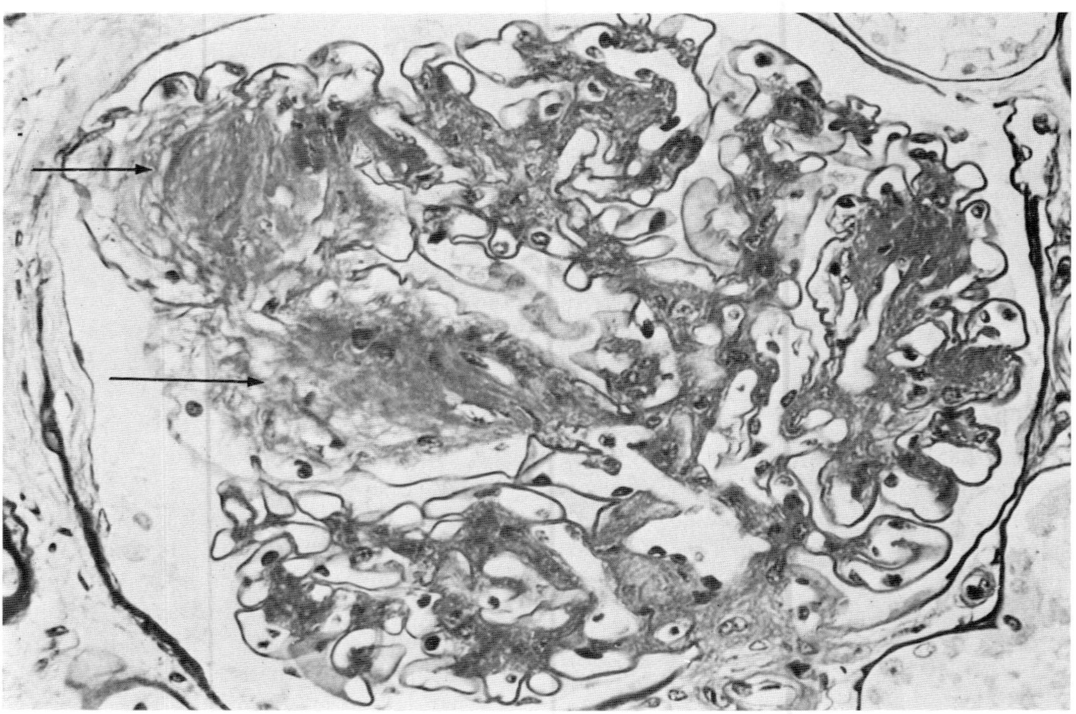

Figure 22-2. Diffuse and nodular diabetic glomerulosclerosis. Nodules are indicated by arrows. ×465, before 9% reduction.

There may be also a slight increase in mesangial cells. The structure of the matrix and its relation to the mesangial cells is at first altered but little. With progression of the lesion there is gradual compression and disappearance of the cells, which are replaced by an increasing amount of matrix. In the lobular centers the matrix becomes compacted into nearly homogeneous or lamellated masses characteristic of nodular glomerulosclerosis (Figs. 22-5, 22-6). Thus, on the electron microscopic level the nodules are merely the most advanced form of the diffuse disease. The lobular centers probably represent the most distensible portions of the mesangial stalk and are the site of predilection not only of the diabetic nodules but also of certain inflammatory processes (lobular glomerulonephritis) and of extraneous deposits (amyloid). In addition to the large amount of matrix, the more advanced diabetic nodules often contain a small amount of collagen and sometimes also deposits of protein and lipid (see section on *Hyaline Lesions*) (Fig. 22-5).

Electron microscopy also reveals something else that can be little appreciated by light microscopy — namely, that the capillary basement membranes are thickened (Figs. 22-3, 22-4). This thickening is usually coincidental with, but not necessarily proportional to, the increase in mesangial matrix. Some authors believe that basement membrane thickening is a late phenomenon [37, 52], but we have observed it quite early in the disease. Thickening may be focal at first, but soon becomes diffuse, and often leads to structures five to ten times the normal width [18], which is impressive even under the light microscope. The thickened basement membrane tends to be layered

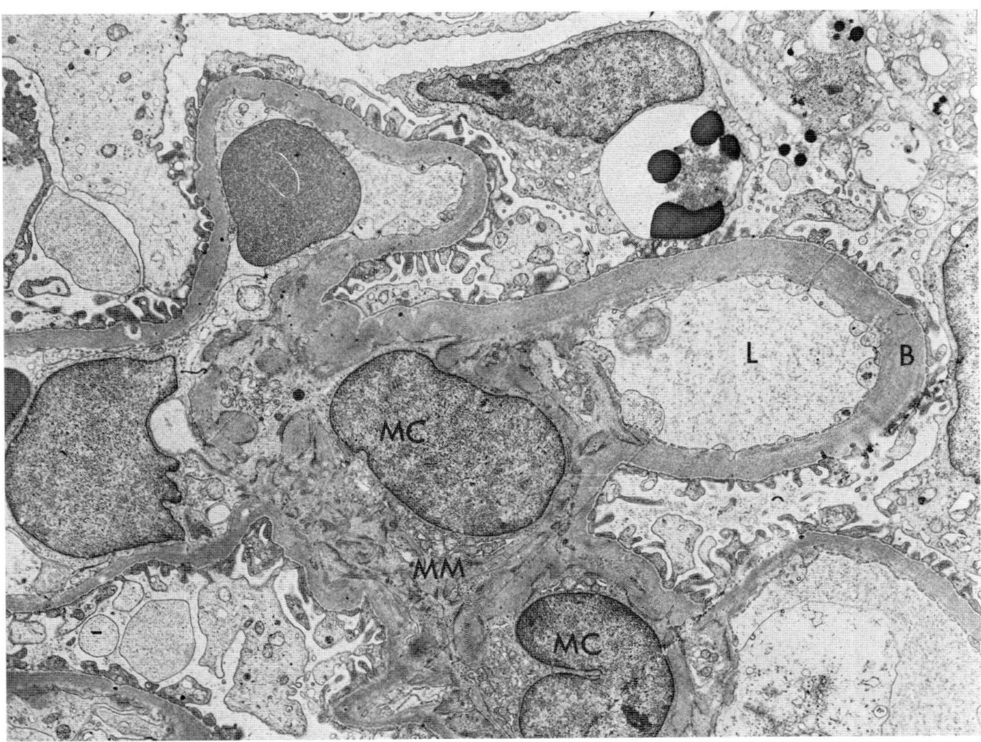

Figure 22-3. Early diffuse diabetic glomerulosclerosis. A single glomerular lobule with a widened mesangial stalk and a wreath of capillaries showing thick basement membranes. MC = mesangial cell; MM = mesangial matrix; L = capillary lumen; B = basement membrane. ×3700. (Reproduced with permission of the *American Journal of Pathology.*)

and nonhomogeneous. Protein and lipid deposits are often encountered in the basement membrane, or between the basement membrane and the epithelial cells or between the basement membrane and the endothelial cells.

Thickening and lamellation of Bowman's capsule is not specific for diabetes since it occurs with any type of glomerular obsolescence. Similarly, thickening of the tubular basement membrane is nonspecific. However, both of these changes occur in diabetes early in the disease and are more severe than in other types of pathologic process. In fact, thickening of basement membranes around rather well-preserved tubules is helpful in the recognition of diabetic nephropathy.

The capillary lumina of the glomeruli affected by sclerosis become gradually compressed but remain patent until very late stages of the disease. Some of the capillaries may undergo aneurysmal dilatation [3]. This is particularly true of capillaries that encircle a nodular lesion.

Hyaline Lesions. Hyaline lesions are known under a variety of names: exudative lesions [29], fibrinoid caps [68], and hyaline caps [76]. They consist of homogeneous or faintly granular eosinophilic material lying in the capillary lumen, in Bowman's space, or attached to Bowman's capsule ("capsular drop"). The material is very similar to that seen in hyalinized arterioles. It is PAS positive,

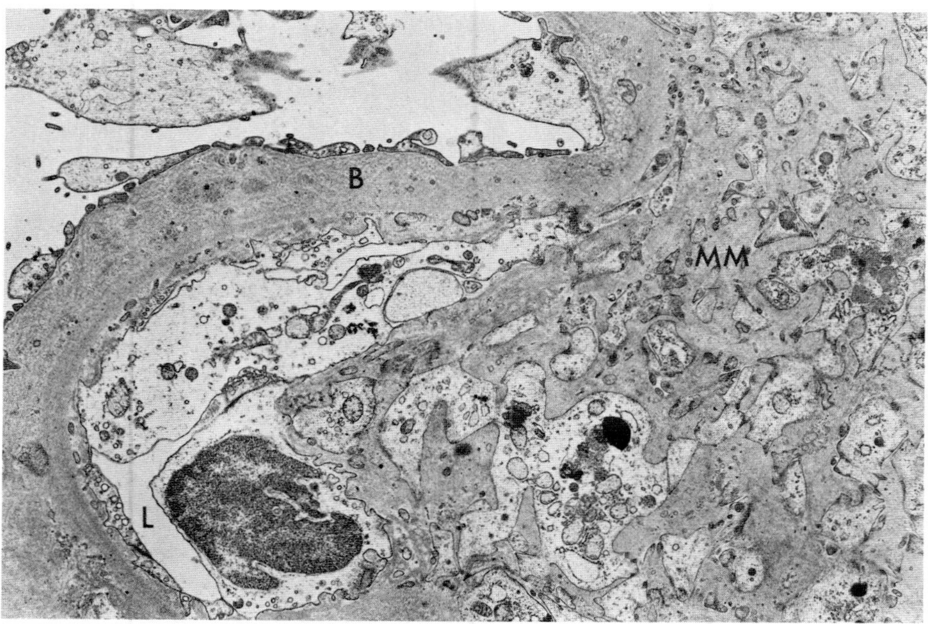

Figure 22-4. Advanced diffuse diabetic glomerulosclerosis. Marked increase in mesangial matrix (MM) and thickening of basement membrane (*B*). L = capillary lumen. ×5500.

though less strongly so than the basement membrane or the mesangial matrix. In contrast to the latter, hyalin always stains red with connective tissue stains and contains a good deal of lipid. Under the electron microscope it appears dense and finely granular, the granules measuring about 35 to 70A [24].

In addition to the locations mentioned above, hyalin may also be present, though usually in small amounts, in the mesangial nodules (Fig. 22-5). Nodules containing appreciable amounts of hyalin tend to assume a red coloration with connective tissue stains or an intermediate color between red and blue. Such nodules also give a positive staining reaction for lipids [56].

The most common hyaline lesions are those that fill the capillary lumen in the manner of thrombi (Fig. 22-7). They attain considerable size and may be confused with mesangial nodules. However, they are distinguished from the latter by their homogeneous appearance and by the fact that they are closely invested by a basement membrane. The intracapillary hyaline thrombus begins actually as a subendothelial deposit which gradually enlarges, pushing the endothelium into the lumen and eventually breaking through the endothelium to fill the lumen.

With the possible exception of the capsular drop, hyaline deposits are not specific for diabetes but occur in a variety of glomerular diseases, particularly in their more advanced stages. In diabetic glomerulosclerosis, however, these deposits are more abundant, stain more eosinophilically, and occur in the earlier stages of the disease.

Pathogenesis. The basic lesion of diabetic glomerulosclerosis may be conceived of as an accumulation of excessive amounts of basement membrane and mesangial matrix in the glomeruli. The excess material is similar in

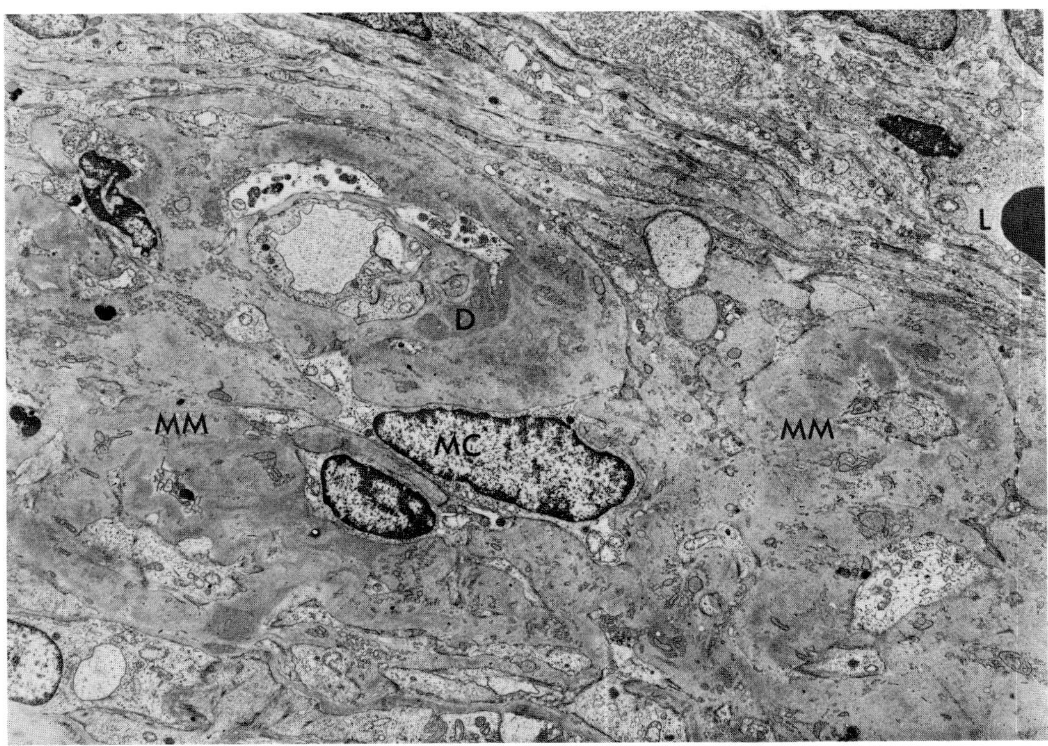

Figure 22-5. Early nodular diabetic glomerulosclerosis. Compression of mesangial cells and beginning compaction of abundant mesangial matrix. Small hyaline deposits (D) are seen in the nodule. MM = mesangial matrix; L = capillary lumen. ×4250.

texture and appearance to its normal counterpart, but it is probably abnormal in function. Superimposed on the sclerosis are the hyaline, or exudative, lesions. Histochemical and chemical studies demonstrate protein, carbohydrate, and lipid in the normal as well as in diabetic glomeruli [77]. Hydrolysis of the protein reveals considerable amounts of hydroxyproline, the characteristic amino acid of collagen [14, 41]. Though typical collagen fibrils are hardly ever seen in normal glomeruli (and are present only in small amounts in diabetic glomeruli), it must be assumed that a modified form of collagen or a related scleroprotein is an important constituent of both basement membrane and mesangial matrix. This is also consistent with the staining reactions with triphenylmethane dyes. Diabetic glomeruli contain a higher proportion of hydroxyproline than normal glomeruli [14].

Carbohydrates constitute only a small portion of the dry weight of the basement membrane (5 to 10 per cent). The main components are glucose and galactose and their hexosamines [67]. The significance of these carbohydrates lies in the compounds they form by themselves or with proteins, such as mucopolysaccharides, mucoproteins, and glycoproteins. These substances have been called "structural carbohydrates" [61]. They probably constitute the "ground substance" in which scleroproteins are embedded, or with which

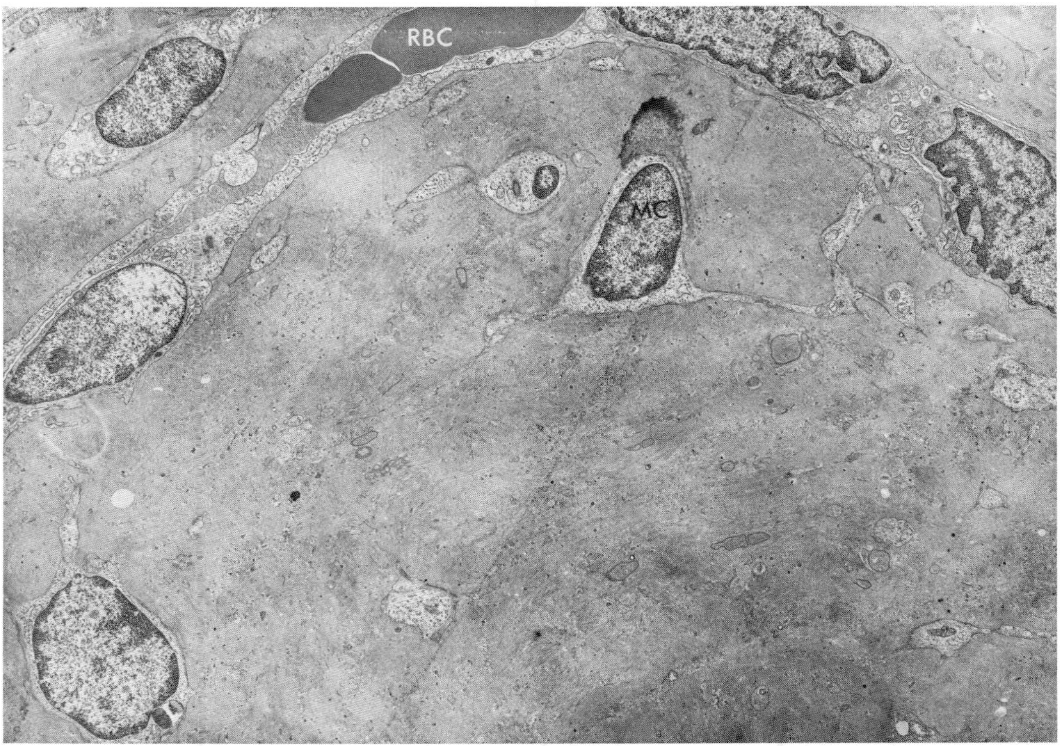

Figure 22-6. Advanced nodular diabetic glomerulosclerosis. Finely fibrillar mesangial matrix fills the mesangium. Only a few remnants of mesangial cells (MC) are seen. A compressed capillary containing red blood cells (RBC) runs in an arc at the top of the illustration. ×4600, before 22% reduction. (Reproduced with permission of the *American Journal of Pathology.*)

they chemically combine to form a compact gel. Structural carbohydrates probably play an important role in maintaining the continuity and integrity of the basement membranes. The proportion of carbohydrates to other substances is about the same in the glomeruli of the patient with diabetic glomerulosclerosis as in those of a normal subject, but the absolute amount is considerably increased. This increase may be due either to overproduction, or as suggested by some, to decreased turnover [41].

Two theories have been proposed to explain the excessive accumulation of structural carbohydrates: (1) a metabolic defect caused by relative or absolute deficiency of insulin resulting in persistent hyperglycemia, or (2) a genetic abnormality parallel to, but independent of, the metabolic defect. There is also a third suggestion — namely, that the lesions are the result of sensitization to the injected or to the autochthonous insulin [13]. This has received but little support and in any event would not easily explain the overproduction of structural carbohydrates. However, there is considerable support for the other two theories.

The most convincing evidence in favor of the metabolic theory is the frequent development of glomerulosclerosis in diabetes secondary to the destruction of the pancreas. In man, such destruction has been caused by acute or chronic pancreatitis, by cancer, or by hemo-

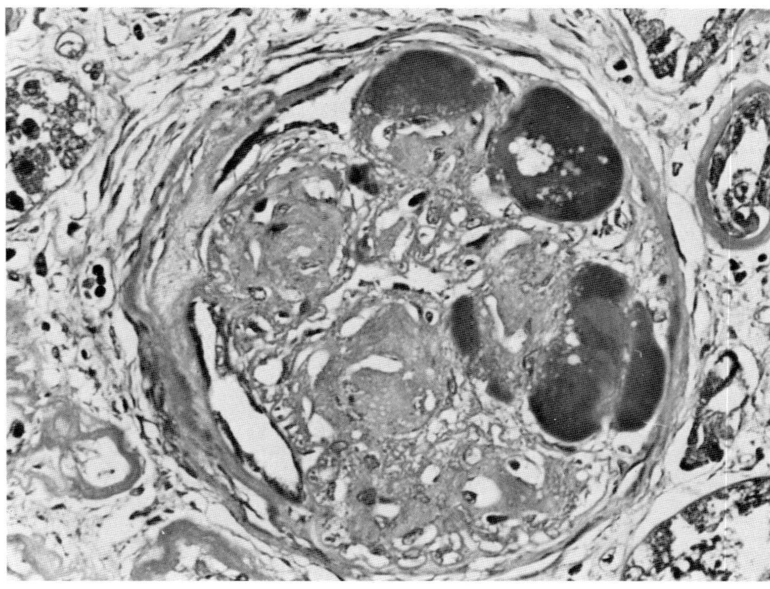

Figure 22-7. Advanced diabetic glomerulosclerosis. Nodules are gray, hyaline (exudative) lesions are black. ×465, before 20% reduction.

chromatosis [32]. The glomerular lesions vary from basement membrane thickening to true nodules [32]. Conversely, amelioration of diabetes in man by successful pituitary ablation apparently leads to reduction in thickness of the abnormal glomerular capillary basement membranes [33].

Animals made diabetic by alloxan [28] or by pancreatectomy [25] develop glomerular lesions similar to diffuse diabetic glomerulosclerosis in man. These consist of focal or diffuse thickening of the capillary basement membrane and an increase in the mesangial matrix, together with some cellular proliferation. Such lesions can be prevented by insulin therapy [30]. Nodules have also been described in animals with long-standing, poorly controlled diabetes [12], though their identity with human nodular disease has not been conclusively proved.

Recent studies have suggested some possible pathways between the abnormal glucose metabolism and glomerulosclerosis. Spiro [66] has studied alloxan-induced diabetes in rats. Because the synthesis of glucosamine is not controlled by insulin, Spiro proposed that deficiency of insulin causes diversion of excessive amounts of glucose into noninsulin-controlled channels, such as formation of structural carbohydrates. Winegrad and Burden [78] demonstrated that in diabetes there is increased utilization of glucose via the glycuronic acid pathway and suggested that this may have a role in the excessive formation of structural carbohydrates.

Against the metabolic theory may be adduced the fact that glomerulosclerosis correlates poorly with the severity of diabetes and with the blood glucose levels. Furthermore, not all persons with pancreatic diabetes develop glomerulosclerosis, and those who do are sometimes suspected of having a genetic predisposition.

In favor of the genetic theory — that is, of a genetic defect independent of glucose metabolism — are cases of glomerulosclerosis occurring in the very early stages of diabetes [20, 38] or even in "prediabetes," as in the clinically nondiabetic children of two diabetic parents [74]. It is possible that such persons do in fact suffer from very mild unrecognized diabetes of long duration, but the very mildness of such disease suggests that glomerulosclerosis is not merely a matter of excess glucose in the blood. Further support for the genetic theory is provided by the study of Siperstein et al. [65] on the muscle capillaries. Some 98 per cent of genetic diabetics and 50 per cent of prediabetics (children of two diabetic parents) showed significant thickening of the capillary basement membranes. However, the occurrence of basement membrane thickening in acquired human and experimental diabetes cannot be completely disregarded. Possibly one can do no better at the moment than entertain both theories and postulate a genetic defect which may or may not be reinforced by a metabolic abnormality as suggested by the eloquent simplicity of the title of an address to the Sixth Congress of the International Diabetes Federation [16a]: " 'What Is Inherited — What Is Added'. Hypothesis for the Pathogenesis of Diabetes Mellitus." (See also [45].)

Though the basement membranes and mesangial matrix in diabetic glomerulosclerosis are chemically similar to the corresponding normal structures, their function is obviously altered. The basement membranes, although thicker, are more permeable to larger molecules such as protein. This increased permeability does not correlate well with its light or electron microscopic appearance and so is probably related to disturbance in molecular arrangement. There is also a suggestion that basement membranes in the diabetic kidney are mechanically weaker as evidenced by the tendency of the capillaries to form aneurysms.

The pathogenesis of the hyaline (exudative) lesions is different from that of the sclerotic lesions. Hyalin, whether in the glomeruli, or in the arterioles, contains a variety of proteins, including glycoproteins, albumin, globulin, fibrinogen, and complement; mucopolysaccharides; and lipids such as triglycerides, fatty acids, phosphatides, and cholesterol [19, 50]. The chemical composition and structure of hyalin suggests that it is a precipitate of substances found in the circulating blood. Secondary degeneration of local elements such as connective tissue or smooth muscle may augment the deposits. Deposition of hyalin in diabetes is probably related to the increased permeability, and perhaps also to the enhanced affinity of the altered tissue for large molecules (proteins and lipoproteins).

Microangiopathy. It is now generally believed that glomerulosclerosis constitutes a part of a much wider process — diabetic microangiopathy — which affects small vessels throughout the body. This subject is discussed in detail in several recent reports [47, 69, 78]. Microangiopathy has been noted in the retina, skin, muscles, and other locations. Its outstanding feature is thickening of the vascular basement membranes [1, 4, 65, 80]. Because of the variability of normal measurements, the extent and frequency of this thickening is still a matter of debate. Its existence is accepted by the majority of investigators but not without some opposition [26, 73]. In addition to the thickened basement membrane, the affected vessels may also show other changes, already noted, in the glomerulus. The retinal capillaries exhibit a striking tendency to the formation of aneurysms which may become filled with hyaline material. Exudates may be present in the retina due, at least in part, to the leakage of protein from the affected capillaries. Although it has been suggested that the term *microangiopathy* be applied only to the capillary lesions [35], most authors use it also in reference to arteriolosclerosis. In fact, the changes in the arterioles are quite similar to those in the capillaries comprising both the basement membrane thickening and the hyaline deposition in the wall.

Microangiopathy is most important clinically in its renal and retinal expressions. The early detection of proteinuria along with the first appearance of retinal microaneurysms on ophthalmoscopic examination invariably indicates the beginning of accelerated vascular damage on a more generalized basis. Although these obvious lesions portend the imminence of other organ involvement (e.g., neuropathy and premature coronary artery disease), the rate of vascular deterioration is unpredictable for each patient. Even in the juvenile subject with long-standing diabetes it is not unusual to find little or relatively static signs of such damage. Unfortunately the degree of "control" of the underlying diabetes offers no correlation with the onset of microangiopathy; this is understandable because obvious lesions of diffuse glomerulosclerosis are already present in a significant number of middle-aged and elderly patients at the time of onset of overt diabetes.

The functional significance of microangiopathy other than in the kidney and in the eye has not been established. A suggestion has recently been made that certain forms of idiopathic edema result from microangiopathy of diabetic type [63]. It is customary to separate microangiopathy from the disease of larger vessels. As previously indicated, the latter is often interpreted as an exaggeration of nondiabetic arteriosclerosis possibly secondary to the high blood lipid levels prevailing in diabetes. In some respects, however, the lesions of the large vessels are analogous to those of the small vessels [17]. Arterial intima contains a good deal of structural carbohydrates in the ground substance of its connective tissue. Presumably these carbohydrates are altered in diabetes either quantitatively or qualitatively, rendering the intima more permeable to lipids and proteins and more likely to become the site of their deposition. It has been reported that atherosclerotic plaques in diabetes contain increased amounts of mucopolysaccharides or carbohydrates as compared with nondiabetic atherosclerosis [11, 57].

One can carry the above reasoning even further and postulate that all connective tissue, vascular or extravascular, is altered in diabetes because of changes in the structural carbohydrates of its ground substance [17]. An example of such connective tissue disease in diabetes may be lipoid necrobiosis. Though usually regarded as a form of ischemic necrosis of skin caused by occlusive arteriolosclerosis, evidence suggests that the accompanying vascular lesions are part of the necrobiosis and not its cause and that the primary disease is in the connective tissue itself [44]. Accumulation of lipid in the affected areas may be analogous to the lipid deposits in atheromas.

Frequency of Glomerulosclerosis in Diabetes. Glomerulosclerosis is extremely frequent in diabetes. Some degree of mesangial and basement membrane thickening can be demonstrated by electron microscopy in nearly 100 per cent of patients [18] and by light microscopy in over 60 per cent [39]. However, nodular lesions are distinctly less common; their prevalence depends to a degree upon the criteria of individual observers. In a large series of nearly 1500 autopsies of diabetic persons, Bell [5] found nodules in 12.8 per cent of males and 19.4 per cent of females; Warren et al. [74] quote a figure of 25 per cent. Nodules are most frequently seen in long-standing diabetes, especially in the juvenile form of long duration, and perhaps more often in mild than in severe diabetes. However, they occasionally occur in early cases or even in asymptomatic chemical diabetes. It is possible, of course, that such patients have had unrecognized mild diabetes for a long time, with periods of improvement and relapse.

Clinical Manifestations. The clinical triad of albuminuria, hypertension, and the nephrotic syndrome which characterizes the patient with advancing diabetic glomerulosclerosis is further complicated by the added factors of secondary anemia, congestive cardiac failure, mounting uremia, and increasing insulin sensitivity. Surprisingly, this formidable combination may be consistent with fairly long survival with the judicious aid of repeated transfusions of packed red blood cells, and digitalization. Correction of the anemia and cardiac failure may enhance limited renal function and may even reduce the nephrotic picture. In the face of uremia, however, extreme dietary sodium restriction, diuretics, and antihypertensive drugs should be avoided. The interesting phenomenon of the decreasing insulin requirements, even to the point of discontinuance, has been explained only partly by the decreased food intake due to anorexia and the presence of metabolic products enhancing the action of insulin. Despite our knowledge of the progressive reduction of renal function in these patients with diabetic kidneys, wise therapeutic efforts can often be fruitful in prolonging life as well as in ameliorating some of the disabling symptoms.

Pyelonephritis

The increased susceptibility of diabetic patients to infections and their frequent exposure to instrumentation are well known. There seems to be little doubt that in the preantibiotic era acute pyelonephritis was a common and severe complication, several times more frequent in persons with than those without diabetes [58]. To what extent this is true today is somewhat uncertain. Asymptomatic bacteriuria is two to three times more frequent in diabetic than in nondiabetic persons [53, 72]. While people with bacteriuria often develop pyelonephritis, the presence of even large numbers of bacteria in the urine does not necessarily prove an infection of the kidneys. It appears that evidence of infection, or at least of inflammation, is much more common at autopsy than in biopsy material. The latter seldom reveals specific histologic changes and seldom gives positive bacteriologic cultures even in the presence of clinical disease [16, 70]. However, this may be true in part because of the focal nature of pyelonephritis and the limited involvement of the kidney in the early stages. The needle biopsy, after all, is a small sample that may easily miss focal lesions. We have observed diabetic patients in whom renal biopsy revealed no inflammation and who at autopsy a year or two later had extensive acute and chronic inflammation of both kidneys with hardly any uninvolved areas. The presumption is that pyelonephritis was present the year before but was focal, and that biopsy missed a lesion. (For the general discussion of pyelonephritis and the diagnostic problems it presents to the clinicians and the pathologists, the reader is referred to Chapter 18.)

The situation is even more complex when dealing with chronic pyelonephritis. This may follow the acute disease or may develop insidiously. The commonly used criteria for histologic diagnosis of chronic pyelonephritis were established by Weiss and Parker [75] in their cases of known infection of the kidneys (see Chapter 18). Taken individually these changes are nonspecific and can be found in many renal diseases. Even the complete assortment of gross and histologic criteria cannot be used as incontestable proof of chronic infection, unless confirmed by bacteriologic cultures of kidney tissue. Such bacteriologic studies often have been disappointing [16]. Nevertheless, it appears that even if bacteria die out, their antigens may remain in the macrophages and in the tubular cells and possibly maintain inflammation. Such antigens can be demonstrated by immunofluorescent technics [71]. Even in the absence of any further stimuli, scarring may develop in the areas of inflammation and eventually interfere with kidney function. Vascular lesions produce areas of tissue degeneration and necrosis that go through an inflammatory stage that may be mistaken for pyelonephritis.

The reported frequency of chronic pyelonephritis in the general autopsy population varies widely, from 2 to 20 per cent [36]. This prevalence figure depends not only upon the type of material but even more so upon the anatomic criteria. Warren et al. [74], in a careful study in the period from 1960 to 1963, found histologic evidence of chronic pyelonephritis in 128 out of 351 (36.5 per cent) autopsies of patients with diabetes. However, polymorphonuclear leukocytes and necrosis were often absent, and it is uncertain whether these cases represent a smoldering infectious process or interstitial inflammation of noninfectious origin. At the moment it does not seem possible to offer even approximately accurate figures for the frequency of pyelonephritis in diabetes. However, in view of the greater susceptibility and greater exposure of diabetic patients to infection, a high index of suspicion and active treatment on the basis of clinical judgment appear to be justified.

NECROSIS OF RENAL PAPILLAE

Necrosis of renal papillae is several times more frequent in diabetic patients than in the general population [59]. The other two common causes are: urinary obstruction and overuse of analgesic drugs, especially phenacetin. Morphologically papillary necrosis has the appearance of an anemic infarct involving the inner part of the medulla and the papilla. Usually several or all papillae are involved, often bilaterally. The necrotic papillae tend to slough off, and the characteristic fragments of necrotic tissue may be found in the urine.

Papillary necrosis is usually associated with and is secondary to severe infection. Conversely, infection may develop secondarily to the presence of necrotic tissue and obstruction of the urinary flow.

Necrosis of the papillae has been produced in animals by several methods: administration of certain chemicals [46], injection of human serum [43, 54], ureteral obstruction without infection [64], and occlusion of the renal vein [8]. The mechanism of necrosis probably varies with each experimental model: chemicals may damage the tissue after becoming concentrated in the medulla; human serum causes platelet thrombi in the vasa recta [54], while ureteral obstruction causes compression of the vessels at the base of the papillae via the raised pressure in the pelvis.

It seems likely that vascular, especially venous, obstruction plays an important role in the pathogenesis of papillary necrosis. Diabetic patients are probably unusually susceptible to papillary necrosis because of their tendency to both vascular disease and renal infection. The latter leads to edema of the tissues and inflammation of venous walls, with compression and thrombosis. Thrombi are often found in various branches adjacent to or leading from the areas of papillary necrosis [75], though at autopsy it may not be easy to ascertain whether thrombosis is the cause or the sequela of necrosis.

Clinical diagnosis of papillary necrosis is often difficult but should be suspected in a variety of situations [59], especially in a diabetic patient who has severe acute urinary infection or an exacerbation of chronic infection, has acidosis complicated by pyelonephritis and uremia, has obstructive uropathy and develops sudden signs of infection, uses large amounts of phenacetin or other analgesics, or acquires uremia of undetermined etiology.

Patients with papillary necrosis are often very toxic. They may have colic and hematuria and, as mentioned earlier, may pass fragments of necrotic papillae. On x-ray examination, characteristic changes of papillary necrosis may be found, and if the patient survives long enough, renal calculi form with radiolucent centers representing sloughed off renal papillae encrusted by mineral deposits.

The prognosis for papillary necrosis is apparently better in nondiabetic than in diabetic patients; few of the latter survive the attack [2, 79]. Nephrectomy has been advocated in the past but is actually contraindicated because of frequent bilateral involvement. In addition to energetic treatment of infection, dialysis may be required to deal with uremia.

Acknowledgment

This study was supported in part by U.S. Public Health Service Research Grant AM 00918 from the National Institute of Arthritis and Metabolic Diseases.

References

1. Aagenaes, O., and Moe, H. Light and electron microscopic study of skin capillaries of diabetics. *Diabetes* 10:253, 1961.
2. Abdulhayoglu, S., and Marble, A. Necrotizing renal papillitis (papillary necrosis) in diabetes mellitus. *Amer. J. Med. Sci.* 248: 623, 1964.
3. Allen, A. C. So-called intercapillary glomerulosclerosis. A lesion associated with diabetes mellitus: Morphogenesis and significance. *Arch. Path.* 32:33, 1941.
4. Banson, B. B., and Lacy, P. E. Diabetic microangiopathy in human toes, with emphasis on the ultrastructural change in dermal capillaries. *Amer. J. Path.* 45:41, 1964.
5. Bell, E. T. *Renal Diseases* (2nd ed.). Philadelphia: Lea & Febiger, 1950.
6. Bell, E. T. A postmortem study of vascular disease in diabetics. *A.M.A. Arch. Path.* 53:444, 1952.
7. Bergstrand, A., and Bucht, H. Electronmicroscopic investigation on the glomerular lesions in diabetes mellitus (diabetic glomerulosclerosis). *Lab. Invest.* 6:293, 1957.
8. Beswick, I. P., and Schatzki, P. F. Experimental renal papillary necrosis. *A.M.A. Arch. Path.* 69:733, 1960.
9. Biava, C. G., Dyrda, T., Genest, J., and Bencosme, S. A. Renal hyaline arteriolosclerosis: An electron microscope study. *Amer. J. Path.* 44:349, 1964.
10. Bloodworth, J. M. B., Jr. Histochemistry and Electronmicroscopy of Diabetic Retinopathy. In Siperstein, M. D., Colwell, A. R., Sr., and Meyer, K. (Eds.), *Small Blood Vessel Involvement in Diabetes Mellitus.* Washington, D.C.: American Institute of Biological Sciences, 1964. P. 81.
11. Bloodworth, J. M. B., Jr. Discussion in Siperstein, M. D., Colwell, A. R., Sr., and Meyer, K. (Eds.), *Small Blood Vessel Involvement in Diabetes Mellitus.* Washington, D.C.: American Institute of Biological Sciences, 1964. P. 232.
12. Bloodworth, J. M. B., Jr. Experimental diabetic glomerulosclerosis: II. The dog. *Arch. Path.* (Chicago) 79:113, 1965.
13. Blumenthal, H. T., Hirata, Y., Owens, C. T., and Berns, A. W. A Histo- and Immunologic Analysis of the Small Vessel Lesion of Diabetes in the Human and in the Rabbit. In Siperstein, M. D., Colwell, A. R., Sr., and Meyer, K. (Eds.), *Small Blood Vessel Involvement in Diabetes Mellitus.* Washington, D.C.: American Institute of Biological Sciences, 1964. P. 279.
14. Bonting, S. L., De Bruin, H., and Pollak, V. E. Quantitative histochemistry of the nephron: VI. Hydroxyproline in the human glomerulus. *J. Clin. Invest.* 40:177, 1961.
15. Braunsteiner, H., DiPauli, R., Sailer, S., and Sandhofer, F. Myokardinfarkt und latent diabetische Stoffwechsellage. *Klin. Wschr.* 43:585, 1965.
16. Brun, C., Raaschon, F., and Eriksen, K. R. Simultaneous Bacteriologic Studies of Renal Biopsies and Urine. In Kass, E. H. (Ed.), *Progress in Pyelonephritis.* Philadelphia: Davis, 1965. P. 461.

16a. Cerasi, E., and Luft, R. "What is inherited — what is added." Hypothesis for the pathogenesis of diabetes mellitus. *Diabetes* 16:615, 1967.

17. Churg, J., and Dachs, S. Diabetic Renal Disease: Arteriosclerosis and Glomerulosclerosis. In Sommers, S. C. (Ed.), *Pathology Annual, 1966.* New York: Appleton-Century-Crofts, 1966.
18. Dachs, S., Churg, J., Mautner, W., and Grishman, E. Diabetic nephropathy. *Amer. J. Path.* 44:155, 1964.
19. Davies, M. J., Woolf, N., and Carstairs, K. C. Immunohistochemical studies in diabetic glomerulosclerosis. *J. Path. Bact.* 92: 441, 1966.
20. Dolger, H. Clinical evaluation of vascular damage in diabetes mellitus. *J.A.M.A.* 134: 1289, 1947.
21. Fanconi, G., Botstejn, A., and Kousmine, C. Nephropathie beim kindlichen diabetes mellitus. *Helv. Paediat. Acta* 3:341, 1948.
22. Farquhar, M. G., Hopper, J., Jr., and Moon, H. D. Diabetic glomerulosclerosis, electron and light microscopic studies. *Amer. J. Path.* 35:721, 1959.
23. Fiaschi, E., Scuro, L. A., and Naccarato, R.

Intorno alle prime alterazioni morfologiche del rene nel diabete giovanil recente. *Minerva Nefrol.* 10:95, 1963.

24. Fisher, E. R., Perez-Stable, E., and Pardo, V. Ultrastructural studies in hypertension: I. Comparison of renal vascular and juxtaglomerular cell alterations in essential and renal hypertension in man. *Lab. Invest.* 15: 1409, 1966.
25. Foglia, V. G., Mancini, R. E., and Cardeza, A. F. Glomerular lesions in diabetic rat. *A.M.A. Arch. Path.* 50:75, 1950.
26. Friederici, H. H. R., Tucker, W. R., and Schwartz, T. B. Observations on small blood vessels in skin in normal and diabetic patients. *Diabetes* 15:233, 1967.
27. Goldenberg, S., Alex, M., Joshi, R. A., and Blumenthal, H. T. Nonatheromatous peripheral vascular disease of the lower extremity in diabetes mellitus. *Diabetes* 8:261, 1959.
28. Greenberg, S. R. Glomerular changes in chronic alloxan diabetes. *Arch. Path.* (Chicago) 73:263, 1962.
29. Hall, G. F. M. The significance of atheroma of the renal arteries in Kimmelstiel-Wilson's syndrome. *J. Path. Bact.* 64:103, 1952.
30. Hansen, R. O., Lundbaek, K., Olsen, T. S., and Orskov, H. Kidney lesions in rats with severe long term alloxan diabetes: III. Glomerular ultrastructure. *Lab. Invest.* 17:675, 1967.
31. Herman, M. V., and Gorlin, R. Premature coronary artery disease and preclinical diabetic state. (Editorial.) *Amer. J. Med.* 38: 481, 1965.
32. Ireland, J. T., Patnaik, B. K., and Duncan, L. J. P. Glomerular ultrastructure in secondary diabetes and in normal subjects. *Diabetes* 16:628, 1967.
33. Ireland, J. T., Patnaik, B. K., and Duncan, L. J. P. Effect of pituitary ablation on the renal arteriolar and glomerular lesions in diabetes. *Diabetes* 16:636, 1967.
34. Kasanen, A., and Forsstrom, J. Njurkomplikationer vid diabetes. *Nord. Med.* 72: 1264, 1964.
35. Kimmelstiel, P. Diabetic Nephropathy. In Becker, E. L. (Ed.), *Structural Basis of Renal Disease.* New York: Harper & Row, 1968.
36. Kimmelstiel, P., Kim, O. J., Beres, J. A., and Wellman, K. Chronic pyelonephritis. *Amer. J. Med.* 30:589, 1961.
37. Kimmelstiel, P., Osawa, G., and Beres, J. Glomerular basement membrane in diabetes. *Amer. J. Clin. Path.* 45:21, 1966.
38. Kimmelstiel, P., and Wilson, C. Intercapillary lesions in the glomeruli of the kidney. *Amer. J. Path.* 12:83, 1936.
39. Laipply, T. C., Eitzen, O., and Dutra, F. R. Intercapillary glomerulosclerosis. *Arch. Intern. Med.* 74:354, 1944.
40. Lannigan, R., Blainey, J. D., and Brewer, D. B. Electron microscopy of the diffuse glomerular lesion in diabetes mellitus with special reference to early changes. *J. Path. Bact.* 88:255, 1964.
41. Lazarow, A., and Speidel, E. The Chemical Composition of the Glomeruli. Basement Membrane and Its Relationship to the Production of Diabetic Complications. In Siperstein, M. D., Colwell, A. R., Sr., and Meyer, K. (Eds.), *Small Blood Vessel Involvement in Diabetes Mellitus.* Washington, D.C.: American Institute of Biological Sciences, 1964. P. 127.
42. LeCompte, P. M. Vascular lesions in diabetes mellitus. *J. Chronic Dis.* 2:178, 1955.
43. Lee, J. C., French, S. W., Wizzird, J. P., and Hopper, J., Jr. Early morphologic changes in serum-induced renal papillary necrosis in the rat: III. Light and electron microscopic studies. *Lab. Invest.* 17:458, 1967.
44. Lever, W. F. *Histopathology of the Skin* (4th ed.). Philadelphia: Lippincott, 1967.
45. Luft, R. What is inherited in diabetes mellitus and what precipitates the disease? *Nord. Med.* 78:929, 1967.
46. Mandel, E. E., and Popper, H. Experimental medullary necrosis of the kidney. *A.M.A. Arch. Path.* 52:1, 1951.
47. Marble, A. Angiopathy in diabetes: An unsolved problem. *Diabetes* 16:825, 1967.
48. McGee, W. G., and Ashworth, C. T. Fine structure of chronic hypertensive arteriopathy in the human kidney. *Amer. J. Path.* 43:273, 1963.
49. Montgomery, P. O., and Muirhead, E. E.

A characterization of hyaline arteriolar sclerosis by histochemical procedures. *Amer. J. Path.* 30:521, 1954.

50. Muirhead, E. E., Montgomery, P. O'B., and Booth, F. The glomerular lesions of diabetes mellitus: Cellular hyaline and acellular hyaline lesions of "intercapillary glomerulosclerosis" as depicted by histochemical studies. *A.M.A. Arch. Intern. Med.* 98:146, 1955.
51. Ormos, J., and Solbach, H. G. Beitrag zur Morphologie de Niere bei Diabetes Mellitus. *Frankfurt. Z. Path.* 72:379, 1963.
52. Osawa, G., Kimmelstiel, P., and Seiling, V. Thickness of glomerular basement membranes. *Amer. J. Clin. Path.* 45:7, 1966.
53. Oseasohn, R., Liebow, I. M., and Newill, V. R. Incidence of bacteriuria and urinary tract infection in a group of diabetic women. *Amer. J. Med. Sci.* 247:661, 1964.
54. Patrick, R. L., Kroc, D. J., and Klavins, J. V. Renal papillary necrosis induced by heterologous serum. *Arch. Path.* (Chicago) 78: 108, 1964.
55. Ramel, C. The kidney in diabetes. *Schweiz. Med. Wschr.* 95:416, 1965.
56. Randerath, E. Intercapillary glomerulosclerosis. *Virchow Arch. Path. Anat.* 323: 483, 1953.
57. Randerath, E., and Dietzel, F. B. Vergleichende histochemische Untersuchungen der Arteriosklerose bei Diabetes Mellitus und ohne Diabetes Mellitus. *Deutsch. Arch. Klin. Med.* 205:523, 1959.
58. Robbins, S. L., and Tucker, A. W. Cause of death in diabetes: Report of 307 autopsied cases. *New Eng. J. Med.* 231:865, 1944.
59. Rutner, A. B., and Smith, D. R. Renal papillary necrosis. *J. Urol.* 85:462, 1961.
60. Sabour, M. S., MacDonald, M. K., and Robson, J. S. An electron microscopic study of the human kidney in young patients with normal renal function. *Diabetes* 11:291, 1962.
61. Samarcq, P., Morand, J. C., Lubetski, J., and Agerad, E. Diabetic kidney: Optical and electron microscopic studies. Anatomicochemical correlation. *Path. Biol.* (Paris) 12:659, 1964.
62. Shapiro, A. P., Perez-Stable, E., and Moutsos, S. E. Coexistence of renal arterial hypertension and diabetes mellitus. *J.A.M.A.* 192: 813, 1965.
63. Shaw, R. A., Kryston, L. J., Fleishmajer, R., Kashatus, W. C., Segal, B. L., Gambeseia, J. M., and Mills, L. C. The rationale for treatment of idiopathic edema. *Amer. J. Cardiol.* 21:115, 1968.
64. Sheehan, H. L., and Davis, J. C. Experimental hydronephrosis. *A.M.A. Arch. Path.* 68:185, 1959.
65. Siperstein, M. D., Unger, R. H., and Madison, L. L. Studies of muscle capillary basement membranes in normal subjects, diabetic, and pre-diabetic patients. *J. Clin. Invest.* 47:1973, 1968.
66. Spiro, R. G. Glycoproteins and diabetes. *Diabetes* 12:223, 1963.
67. Spiro, R. G. Studies on the renal glomerular basement membrane: Preparation and chemical composition. *J. Biol. Chem.* 242: 1915, 1967.
68. Spuhler, O., and Zollinger, H. U. Die diabetische Glomerulosclerose. *Deutsch. Arch. Klin. Med.* 190:321, 1943.
69. Story, H. C. Disease of small blood vessels in diabetes mellitus. *Amer. J. Med. Sci.* 252: 357, 1966.
70. Thomsen, A. C. The Significance of Renal Biopsy for the Diagnosis of Pyelonephritis in Diabetic Patients. In Wolstenholme, G. E. W., and Cameron, M. P. (Eds.), *Renal Biopsy.* Boston: Little, Brown, 1961. P. 281.
71. Tuttle, E. P. In discussion of Definition of Chronic Pyelonephritis. In Kass, E. H. (Ed.), *Progress in Pyelonephritis.* Philadelphia: Davis, 1965. P. 381.
72. Vejlsgaard, R. Bacteriuria in Patients with Diabetes Mellitus. In Kass, E. H. (Ed.), *Progress in Pyelonephritis.* Philadelphia: Davis, 1965. P. 478.
73. Vracks, R., and Strandness, D. E., Jr. Basal lamina of abdominal skeletal muscle capillaries in diabetics and nondiabetics. *Circulation* 35:690, 1967.
74. Warren, S., LeCompte, P. M., and Legg, M. A. (Eds.). *The Pathology of Diabetes Mellitus* (4th ed.). Philadelphia: Lea & Febiger, 1966. P. 227.

75. Weiss, S., and Parker, F. Pyelonephritis: Its relation to vascular lesions and to arterial hypertension. *Medicine* (Balt.) 18:211, 1939.
76. Wernley, M. La glomerulosclerose diabetique. *Rev. Med. Suisse Rom.* 64:615, 1944.
77. Windrum, G. M., Kent, P. W., and Eastoe, J. E. The constitution of human renal reticulin. *Brit. J. Exp. Path.* 36:49, 1955.
78. Winegrad, A. I., and Burden, C. L. L-xylulose metabolism in diabetes mellitus. *New Eng. J. Med.* 274:298, 1966.
79. Wright, J., Morin, L. J., and Dunn, L. J. Renal papillary necrosis: Eight-year survival in a diabetic. *Diabetes* 16:664, 1967.
80. Yamashita, T., and Becker, B. The basement membrane in the human diabetic eye. *Diabetes* 10:167, 1961.

23

Urate Nephropathy

Frank H. Tyler

Renal disease in association with abnormalities of uric acid metabolism has become an important current subject. It has long been recognized that uric acid stones are common in patients with gout, but recognition of the importance of renal disease as a cause of death in gouty patients is of more recent origin. More exciting has been the development of therapeutic agents with which these processes can be considerably modified. Improved understanding of the renal handling of urate has provided the opportunity to develop technics for protection of the kidney from damage by excess loads of uric acid.

Urate Metabolism

In the human being uric acid is the end product of purine metabolism. It presents a problem because of its sparing solubility. There is a remarkable divergence of purine metabolism among the various animal species. A physiologic advantage accrues to certain reptiles and birds as the result of their ability to convert the majority of their nitrogenous wastes to uric acid for excretion. Urate is concentrated in the cloaca and excreted in semisolid form in the absence of large volumes of water. At the other extreme, most mammalian species excrete little or no uric acid because it is converted by uricase to alantoin which is quite soluble and easily metabolized. Among the primates, however, uricase has been lost along the evolutionary pathway, with the result that a considerable excretory load of uric acid is present. Ingested purines and those derived from nucleic acid metabolism must be excreted as uric acid. Dietary purines usually form only a small fraction of the total urate load but may become important with unusual diets.

Urate is excreted mainly by two routes. One fraction, which varies with the plasma level of urate and other factors, is excreted into the gastrointestinal tract where it is converted into alantoin, alantoic acid, ammonia, and carbon dioxide by the bacterial flora of the gastrointestinal tract. A second fraction (60 to 85 per cent of the total) is excreted by the kidneys.

Renal excretion of uric acid has been the subject of extensive study by many investigators. A large measure of uncertainty about interpretation of data from animals cannot be resolved because of the many evolutionary changes which urate metabolism has undergone. Therefore the bulk of the useful work has been done in man despite his limitations as an experimental animal.

Uric acid, which has a pKa of about 5.75, is present in plasma mostly as the biurate ion (monosodium urate). Nearly all urate exists in freely filtrable form and appears in the glomerular filtrate at about the same concentration as in plasma water. (A small fraction, less than 5 per cent, appears to be bound to beta globulin in normal man, with lesser amounts in gout.) Only a fraction, approximately 8 per cent, of the filtered load appears in the urine. For many years it was assumed that urinary urate consisted of that part of the filtered load not reabsorbed by the tubules. However, the paradoxical effect of salicylate on urate excretion suggested that the process might be more complex. At low concentrations salicylate decreases urate excretion, while at high concentrations it is uricosuric. Many other substances, including the diuretic thiazides, lactate and beta-hydroxybutyric acid, angiotensin, and norepinephrine, share this phenomenon of decreasing urate excretion. Studies with pyrazinimide, which can nearly completely prevent tubular urate secretion but does not block reabsorption, have demonstrated that at least 98 per cent of the filtered urate is reabsorbed under ordinary circumstances [18]. It seems probable that virtually all of the filtered urate is reabsorbed in the proximal tubule. Secretion then accounts for most of the uric acid that is excreted. The ability of salicylate and other substances to block each process at different plasma levels accounts for the observed paradoxical effects.

Within very wide limits the capacity of the tubule to reabsorb the filtered load of urate is not exceeded. Indeed, no Tm for the process has been demonstrated even at plasma levels above 15 mg. per 100 ml. However, as the plasma level of urate rises, the proportion secreted rises so that the plasma level does not rise in proportion to the urate load. These physiologic complexities and the many modifications by pathophysiologic and pharmacologic variables have made the regulation of serum urate and the magnitude of urate excretion a confusing and controversial subject.

Urate nephropathy occurs in patients with gouty arthritis and in a number of other circumstances. Some of the causes of urate nephropathy are:

- Familial gout
- Hyperuricemia of unknown origin without gout
- Hyperuricosuria
  - Myeloproliferative disorders
    - Polycythemia rubra vera
    - Secondary polycythemia
    - Myeloid metaplasia
    - Chronic myelocytic leukemia
  - Lymphoma
  - Multiple myeloma
  - Lesch-Nyhan syndrome
- Hyperuricemia of renal origin
  - Glycogen storage disease
  - Fasting
  - Uremia
- Henneman-Wallach syndrome

It is convenient to divide consideration of the effects of uric acid on the kidney into uric acid nephrolithiasis and the intrarenal effects of urate deposition. In addition, patients with gout or hyperuricemia, or both, acquire other kinds of nephritis and vascular disease which are not clearly related to the abnormal urate metabolism. The causes of renal disease in gout are uric acid stone, tophaceous deposits in the kidney, interstitial nephritis, and vascular disease of the kidney.

Urinary urate stones consist almost entirely of uric acid which is less soluble than sodium biurate and is the form which predominates at usual urinary pH (i.e., less than 5.75). Tophaceous deposits in the kidney, as well as in other tissues, are made up of needle-like crystals of sodium biurate — the form in which it is present at plasma pH of 7.4.

In the following discussions the term *gout* refers to that particularly torturing kind of arthritis which apparently results from microcrystalline sodium biurate within the synovial membrane. Most gouty subjects who suffer from this disorder do so as the result of a process which leads to hyperuricemia because of excess urate production or impaired urate excretion (or both). It is assumed that most of these are instances in which an inborn genetic factor, perhaps on occasion influenced by factors in the environment, results in the urate excess and its deposition in tissue. This disorder has usually been called primary gout. It should be recognized that the use of this term does not necessarily imply that all of these disorders are caused by the same mechanism. The term should not serve to obscure the fact that these processes are still not understood. The designation secondary gout is used for cases in which the mechanism of hyperuricemia is understood. Secondary gout may result from overproduction of uric acid, as in the patient with a myeloproliferative disorder, or from impaired urate excretion, as in type 1 glycogenosis in which the chronic hyperlacticemia impairs urate excretion [5]. Similarly, primary and secondary hyperuricemia will be used in the same way when referring to those subjects who have elevated plasma urate levels but who have not experienced gouty arthritis. We shall also be concerned with a group of patients who, despite normal serum urate values, tend to form uric acid stones.

Uric Acid Nephrolithiasis

FREQUENCY

The association of gouty arthritis and uric acid nephrolithiasis has been well recognized through the ages. Stones in the urinary tract are an uncommon event in the general population of most countries. In the United States the estimate has been made that the frequency of nephrolithiasis is 1 per 1000 persons and that only approximately 10 per cent of these stones are composed of uric acid. On the other hand, at least 10 per cent of the patients with primary gout experience difficulties with urinary tract stones in the course of their disease. In some series this proportion reaches values as high as 22 per cent [22]. Thus the prevalence of uric acid stones appears to be at least a thousand times greater in patients with primary gout than in the general population. On the other hand, stones, gravel, and sand in the urinary tract are even more common among those patients with secondary gout. In the recent report by Yü and Gutman [22] 42 per cent of their patients with secondary gout had experienced these difficulties.

Most patients with primary gout excrete about the same amount of uric acid as is found in the urine of normal subjects; a few patients show clearly excessive excretion. The distribution is not bimodal. In the series of Yü and Gutman [22] one-half the persons who excreted more than 1100 mg. of urate per day had experienced urolithiasis. However, even among the patients with normal urate excretion the frequency of urolithiasis was also considerably increased. In secondary gout the frequency of uric acid stone was more clearly related to excess urate excretion.

MECHANISM OF URIC ACID LITHIASIS

Why do patients with primary gout but normal uric acid excretion have increased frequency of stones? Sodium biurate is much more soluble than uric acid. Thus as urinary pH drops below the pKa (5.75), the urine becomes progressively supersaturated with uric acid even at normal rates of uric acid excretion. The risk of uric acid precipitation is obvious. Indeed, the curious fact is not that urolithiasis occurs in primary and secondary gout, but that uric acid stones do not develop in all human beings, for we all frequently excrete urine with pH below 5.5. There appear to be two mechanisms that protect most normal subjects from the development of uric acid lithiasis. The first has to do with the peculiar solubility characteristics of uric acid. This compound is particularly apt to form supersaturated solutions; indeed, it is frequently extremely difficult, even in the presence of extreme hypersaturation, to induce initial crystallization of the compound without seeding. Most normal morning urines are considerably supersaturated with uric acid, but stone formation is uncommon. Secondly, with food and fluid ingestion the urine usually becomes relatively dilute and tends to become alkaline (the so-called postprandial alkaline tide). The solubility is not exceeded in many daytime urines. This clearly reduces the opportunity for uric acid stone formation. In primary gout, on the other hand, urinary pH in early morning specimens tends to be even lower than in normal subjects and to fail to show the daytime rise. Thus, it is not unreasonable that the combination of persistently acid urines and to a lesser degree increased urate excretion are responsible for the increased frequency of uric acid lithiasis in patients with primary gout.

The reason for the very acid urines in patients with primary gout is not entirely clear. Yü and Gutman [22] have presented evidence that at a given urinary pH, subjects with primary gout excrete less ammonia and relatively more titratable acid than normal subjects. This phenomenon appears to be characteristic of both the gouty subjects with stone and those without stone, but is more striking in the former. Ammonia is formed in the kidney from glutamine, and the suggestion has been made that the defect relates to an error in glutamine metabolism. Because glutamine is also a precursor of uric acid in the liver, it also has been proposed that the glutamine nitrogen is diverted to urate formation and therefore unavailable to the kidneys for ammonia formation. However, it is clear that with acid loading the patient with primary gout can strikingly increase his ammonia formation just as can the normal subject. Regardless of the underlying mechanism, it is clear that the secretion of a persistently acid urine is a major contributor to the frequency of uric acid stone in the patient with primary gout.

Urolithiasis also occurs in patients with hyperuricemia but not gouty arthritis. Population studies have failed to show a clear-cut group of hyperuricemic subjects. The range of serum urate levels in nongouty subjects is clearly unimodal. Thus a definition of primary hyperuricemia must be arbitrary. Nonetheless, when looked at from the other point of view, it is clear that the majority of subjects who experience uric acid lithiasis do have high serum urate values and presumably belong to the same population in whom gout develops.

There is clear evidence that primary gout and primary hyperuricemia are not caused by a single pathophysiologic process. The description by Lesch and Nyhan [11] of a syndrome of hyperuricemia and self-mutilation initiated a series of investigations by Seegmiller and Frazier [17] of the enzymes concerned with purine synthesis and degradation. It is clear that the Lesch-Nyhan syndrome results from a lack of a specific enzyme which feeds hypoxanthine back into nucleotide formation. In its absence, greatly excess amounts of uric acid are formed. Partial deficit in this enzyme appears to account for hyperuricemia and hyperuricosuria in some adults. How many similar anomalies exist is unclear at the present. Whether the major proportion of the remaining patients with gout and uric acid lithiasis have similar defects is unknown.

Special mention should be made of one group of patients in whom uric acid stones develop in the absence of either hyperuricemia or excess urate excretion. They represent the extreme end of a spectrum which begins with patients who have secondary gout with extremely high urate production and excretion rates but normal regulation of urinary acid excretion.

TREATMENT

It may be a truism, but the first point of any discussion of the management of uric acid stone is that its prevention is the best treatment. Once stone has formed, the complications of obstruction, back pressure on the kidneys, and the development of a bacterial infection secondary to the obstruction may present insoluble problems. In addition, once stone has formed there is a marked tendency for recurrence. This may be related to the presence of submacroscopic particles which persist or to the structural damage resulting from the mechanical and infectious insult.

Preventive Therapy. From the prior discussion of the mechanism which leads to stone formation it is obvious that the objective must be to reduce the concentration of uric acid (as contrasted to urate) in the urine. This can be accomplished in three fashions: (1) reducing the load of urate which must be excreted; (2) increasing the volume of the urinary flow, thus decreasing the concentration; and (3) increasing the pH of the urine. All decrease the uric acid concentration and thereby avoid the persistent supersaturation.

Until recent years most of our efforts had to be restricted to the latter two maneuvers, and both proved to be extraordinarily difficult and relatively unsatisfactory. Most patients find it difficult to increase their fluid intake sufficiently to modify their total urinary output consistently. The process is an effective one if it can be accomplished but requires continuous monitoring of urinary volume and a program of fluid ingestion which the patient must look on as medicine. Superficially simple as the process may seem, it is truly impractical except in unusually compulsive individuals or those who have been conditioned by the intense pain of nephrolithiasis. The problem is entirely comparable to that of inducing an obese patient to follow a diet of limited caloric content; the outcome is equally unsuccessful.

Alkalinization of the urine on a long-time basis is also very difficult. Large amounts of base must be administered. The dose required obviously depends on many factors, the most important of which is the acid load ingested in the diet. Although it is possible to provide an alkaline ash diet, this restricts most meats and many other palatable foods; most patients also find the diet rather objectionable. It seems better, therefore, to make only modest restrictions in protein intake and to compensate for the sulfate and phosphate which derive from these sources by the administration of added base. The exact salt to be used in providing the excess base is a matter of convenience and acceptability to the patient. In point of fact, it is frequently impossible to provide sufficient base in any other form than sodium or potassium bicarbonate because of the large doses required. In patients who tolerate a sodium load well, 10 to 30 gm. of sodium bicarbonate taken as powdered baking soda rather than as tablets may be the simplest technic. The use of citrate-containing solutions such as Shohl's may occasionally be more acceptable to the patient. In achieving alkalinization there is no substitute for frequent checking of urinary pH, as can be done conveniently with nitrazine paper at the time of voiding. In establishing the initial regimen the check should be made at least four times a day, and urines of pH 7 or above should be achieved with regularity.

Drug Therapy. The addition of a carbonic anhydrase inhibitor such as acetazolamide is very useful in two circumstances: (1) in the initial achievement of alkalinization when the problem is urgent, and (2) in the prevention of relapse to an acid pH overnight. In addition, it may have a minor effect in helping to compensate for the tendency to sodium retention induced by the high sodium load administered. One must remember, however, that urinary alkalinization is achieved at the expense of a loss of total base from the body and that, unless this deficit is repaired, the problem of urinary acidity will recur in even more severe fashion once the effect of the carbonic anhydrase inhibition has worn off.

There was concern when the effective uricosuric agent, probenecid, was introduced to clinical management of gouty arthritis and tophaceous disease that a marked increase in nephrolithiasis might result because of the rapid excretion of the excessive body pool of urate. The problem has been a relatively minor one, however, although in an occasional patient previously unrecognized nephrolithiasis does become evident following the initiation of probenecid therapy. Prophylaxis against the problem can be achieved by large urinary outputs and alkalinization as described above. When uricosuric agents are provided in a regular fashion, the continuing increment in urate excretion is relatively small, and in the chronic management of patients with probenecid and other uricosuric agents, it appears that uric acid lithiasis is no more common than it is in untreated patients with gout.

The simplest and therefore most effective means of management of the problem of uric acid stones is by the administration of allopurinol. This compound is an analogue of hypoxanthine. It competes effectively with both xanthine and hypoxanthine for the xanthine oxidase and prevents their conversion to uric acid. Both hyperuricemia and hyperuricosuria are controlled, with obvious benefit to the patient in whom these phenomena are producing problems. As would be expected, an excess of hypoxanthine and xanthine results and must be excreted. Xanthine itself is extremely insoluble, even more so than uric acid. Initially there was concern that xanthine stones might result from the use of allopurinol in the management of hyperuricemia and hyperuricosuria, but extensive experience has not resulted in the development of this problem. The reasons appear to be twofold: (1) In the doses administered clinically allopurinol is only partially effective in producing blockade of xanthine oxidase activity; and (2) some patients appear to produce a total of hypoxanthine, xanthine, and uric acid equivalent to their prior urate production, but in others a considerable deficit is observed. The latter are the very patients in whom the xanthine might present the most serious problem — that is, those patients with markedly increased total urate production. The reason for this effect is somewhat uncertain at the present time, but the reasonable suggestion has been made that the accumulation of hypoxanthine results in reincorporation of it and its precursors into the nucleotide pool. Total purine formation is thus inhibited by a feedback mechanism.

Allopurinol has proved to be a remarkably effective medication. Toxicity from the compound is uncommon and rather benign in character. A few patients experience minor gastrointestinal disturbances which are usually relieved by reducing the dosage. A scaly erythematous dermatitis, which is frequently self-limited or which disappears on reduction of the dosage, occurs in some patients. Serious drug reactions have been remarkably uncommon, and it is uncertain that they are actually produced by the drug itself. On the other hand, it should be remembered that this compound has come into general usage only within the last years, and it is still possible that occasional severe reactions to the drug will not become apparent until it has been used over a longer period of time and in a much larger group of patients. Nonetheless in patients with urate nephropathy it is frequently the best therapy available. In appropriate circumstances it can be combined with the other modalities of therapy which have been described.

Other Kidney Disease in Patients With Gouty Arthritis

TOPHACEOUS RENAL DISEASE

Tophaceous deposits in the kidney, as well as in the cartilaginous structures, occur in patients with gouty arthritis. These may result in extensive destruction of kidney substance and occasionally in renal insufficiency. Talbott

[19] made a classic study of the kidney in gouty patients some years ago. In 191 postmortem examinations of patients with gouty arthritis he found histologic evidence of kidney damage in all but three. Nearly half (90 out of 191) the total number showed well-developed urate deposits, and an additional 38 showed minimal but definite urate deposition. Thus, two-thirds of the total group had intrarenal deposition of identifiable tophaceous material.

The sodium biurate is usually deposited in the interstitial tissues of the medullary pyramid and produces a histologic picture, with fibrosis and lymphocyte infiltration, entirely similar to that of chronic bacterial infection in the obstructed kidney. Although this process has usually been referred to as pyelonephritis, it is not known in how many instances actual bacterial infection has contributed to the lesion. It may well be that in many instances a similar chronic inflammatory and scarring process is initiated by the urate deposit per se rather than by complicating bacterial infection. On the other hand, in a few instances massive acute purulent pyelonephritis develops in the absence of obstruction by stone.

An even larger number of the kidneys showed moderate to marked vascular changes. In about a quarter of the total number of patients the damage to the kidney was of such severity that it led to progressive renal insufficiency. Early death in gouty patients is most frequently the result of uremia. In a considerably greater number proteinuria, pyuria, or hematuria was present, usually in association with hypertension.

The correlation between the severity of clinical gouty arthritis and the degree of renal involvement was evident but of only moderate degree. Some of the patients with mild gout had severe tophaceous renal disease with scarring and vascular changes leading to renal insufficiency, while a few of the patients with severe gout had only minimal changes in the kidney. In a small proportion of the patients the evidence of renal disease had antedated the development of gouty arthritis.

It is clear that urate nephropathy may develop in the absence of gouty arthritis, just as uric acid lithiasis may occur in such circumstances. The frequency of intrarenal urate deposits in patients with blood dyscrasias leading to hyperuricemia and hyperuricosuria makes it clear that the process is most likely to develop in patients with a large excess urate load. On the other hand, the phenomenon occurs occasionally in hyperuricemic patients who excrete only the usual amounts of urate.

HYPERURICEMIA AND RENAL DISEASE

Two additional questions need to be discussed concerning the relationship between hyperuricemia and renal disease. The first is concerned with the effect of therapy on the renal complications and the second is concerned with the relation of the patient with asymptomatic hyperuricemia to this problem.

The documentation by Talbott and Terplan [20] of the frequent occurrence of renal disease in patients with gout led to considerable enthusiasm for the treatment of gouty hyperuricemia in an attempt to prevent progression of the renal damage with its obvious threat to the survival of the patient. Deposition of sodium biurate crystals in the pyramids of the kidney can be prevented by controlling the hyperuricemia and by alkaline diuresis. Documentation of the effectiveness of these procedures is difficult, however, and at present one must proceed in large part on the analogy with their effectiveness on tophaceous deposits about joints and on renal stones. On the other hand, the hypothesis is so self-evident that it seems wise to accept it. The frequency of significant renal involvement among patients with tophaceous gout adds another strong incentive to proceed with vigorous therapy. Whether or not patients who have vascular nephritis are benefited by this therapy is less obvious, but there is no reason to believe the vascular nephritis is made worse by such management and they, too, may be in some fashion related to the urate excess and ameliorated by appropriate management [4a].

The problem in the patient with asymptomatic primary hyperuricemia is more difficult. Many physicians have concluded that the argument outlined above is equally valid in patients with hyperuricemia alone and, therefore, have recommended vigorous therapy of the hyperuricemia in such subjects. Hyperuricemia is very much more common than gouty arthritis, and although it clearly antedates the arthritis in some patients with typical gout, the conclusion that patients with hyperuricemia alone belong to the same group as those who will develop gouty arthritis is not justified a priori.

Until recently few data were available on which one could make a judgment concerning this important and most difficult problem. Recent studies have been carried out in several different population groups [6]. In at least two of these the population has been followed particularly to look for the development of vascular disease and other cardiovascular complications. Several pieces of interesting information have developed from these studies. In the first place, patients who developed gout frequently were hyperuricemic at the initial examination. However, as the study has progressed the rate at which these asymptomatic hyperuricemic patients are acquiring gouty arthritis has fallen off, thus suggesting that the hyperuricemia has different significance in different subjects. It appears from these data that a majority of asymptomatic hyperuricemic subjects belong to the group that will not develop gout; therefore, one cannot use the evidence that patients with gouty arthritis have renal damage from urate deposit as a justification for treatment of primary hyperuricemia.

Another reason suggested for the treatment of hyperuricemia was the presumption that cardiovascular disease, particularly coronary occlusion, was more common among subjects with gouty arthritis [1], as well as the belief that something about the hyperuricemia led to the development of the vascular disease. This clinical impression has not been clearly borne out by the studies to date [6]. Here again there seems no fully documented justification for the treatment of hyperuricemia per se.

The population group with hyperuricemia cannot be considered as a unit. It has become clear, as stressed elsewhere, that hyperuricemia is induced by many different processes. It seems probable that, even among those patients in whom present technics do not allow clear differentiation of the mechanism of the hyperuricemia, there are several subgroups. As technics for identification of such subgroups improve, it may well be that one will be able to identify patients in whom therapy of the hyperuricemia is desirable. For the moment, however, it seems unjustified, except in those instances in which it is clear that the hyperuricemia reflects a remarkably large production of uric acid. In such subjects uric acid lithiasis is a real threat to the survival of the patient, and allopurinol and alkaline diuresis seem justified.

URATE NEPHROPATHY AND MYELOPROLIFERATIVE DISORDERS

Urate nephropathy occurs in a number of other disorders. Two of these are leukemia and other myeloproliferative diseases, and hyperuricemia resulting from impaired excretion of uric acid (see page 899).

The occurrence of gouty arthritis and urate nephropathy in patients with chronic myeloproliferative disorders has long been recognized. The pathogenic process in these disorders appears to be simply excess urate production from the metabolism of the nucleoprotein provided by the accelerated turnover of myeloid cells. A similar process also develops occasionally in disorders that are concerned with accelerated lymphocyte turnover such as lymphosarcoma. The higher prevalence of urate nephropathy in myeloid disorders may reflect their chronicity as compared with the shorter course of the more malignant processes.

Management in these chronic processes is not different from that which one would provide for patients with familial gouty arthritis with overproduction of uric acid. Allopurinol alone may suffice to control both hyperuricemia and hyperuricosuria [3]. If not, alkaline diuresis should be added.

Acute Urate Nephropathy. A specific variety of urate nephropathy that has become prominent in recent years is a by-product of the development of effective means for the management of certain lymphomas and other tumors. Acute episodes of excess urate production occasionally occur in the course of the leukemias and lymphomas. With the advent of nitrogen mustard and other effective agents for the treatment of these cancers the frequency of these crises has been remarkably increased, acute urate nephropathy being one of the serious complicating problems in therapy [10]. Again, the mechanism appears to be simply the very rapid release of large amounts of nucleoprotein which are metabolized to uric acid. These enormous urate loads frequently exceed the capacity of the kidney to maintain their excretion, and extreme degrees of hyperuricemia not infrequently develop.

Pathologic manifestations in the kidney are somewhat different and consist of the deposition in the collecting tubules and interstitium of the pyramid of multiple minute biurate crystals, sometimes associated with passage of sand or amorphous sediment in the urine. This frequently leads to acute renal shutdown. External obstruction by sand or stone in the pelvis and ureters occasionally occurs, but most frequently the oliguria is associated with the intrarenal process, which unless it can be promptly relieved, results in irreversible damage. If anuria occurs, these patients do very poorly although they sometimes run the course observed in patients with acute tubular necrosis with diuresis occurring in the second or third week. If the extreme hyperuricemia is recognized before serious urinary manifestations begin, alkaline diuresis may prevent the progression to more serious manifestations. In this crisis it is obvious that the administration of carbonic anhydrase inhibitors and intravenous bicarbonate, as well as the provision of a large fluid intake, may be essential and urgent. Simultaneous administration of allopurinol in relatively large dosage is desirable. A considerable experience now has not demonstrated the development of xanthine stones as had been predicted by some observers.

A better means of management is the attempt to prevent the development of the crisis. All patients with disorders of this type should have at least a serum uric acid determination. Even high-normal or slightly elevated values may reflect marked urate overproduction. It must be remembered that rather marked uricosuria may develop in the absence of striking hyperuricemia in these patients with normal renal urate excretion. Measurement of urinary uric acid may be essential.

As long as these values are normal, no special precautions are necessary unless an effective therapeutic agent is to be given. When such agents are administered, one should not only keep a careful watch for the development of hyperuricemia but also take reasonable precautions in terms of assuring a urine volume of at least 1500 ml. and administrating allopurinol before the administration of the antitumor agent. A number of groups have now published studies of such a regimen and have demonstrated its effectiveness [1, 14].

HYPERURICEMIA DUE TO IMPAIRED URIC ACID EXCRETION

Hyperuricemia also develops in patients who have specifically impaired excretion of uric acid. This is found most characteristically in patients who have an excess of lactate or ketone bodies in the circulation. This is a relatively common cause for the transient elevation of serum uric acid values in many circumstances, including the hyperlacticemia of anoxic shock, eclampsia in the pregnant patient, during fasting, and that which results simply from prolonged vigorous muscular exercise.

When the hyperlacticemia is recurrent or chronic, a considerable number of the patients will develop uric acid stones. An example is the patient with glycogen storage disease of type 1 (von Gierke's disease or glucose 6-phosphatase deficiency) [5]. Among the abnormalities which these patients experience is a marked increase in serum lactate resulting from accelerated anaerobic glycolysis. They also frequently experience ketosis, which contributes to the urate retention, and appear to have a modest increase in urate production, presumably because of the acceleration of incorporation of amino acid precursors into the purine synthetic process. Hyperuricemia, however, results primarily from impaired urate excretion. One might anticipate that the increased gastrointestinal disposition of urate would lead to chronic reduction in urinary urate excretion and protection of the patient from urinary stones, but the fact is that uric acid stones are remarkably common in adolescent and adult patients with von Gierke's disease. It is less clear whether or not intrarenal deposition of biurate occurs, but it may well.

The occurrence of urinary stone probably relates to two processes. In the first place, the magnitude of hyperlacticemia and ketosis varies in these subjects depending on the availability of glucose from external sources, and thus although urate excretion is continually inhibited, the magnitude of the inhibition varies from time to time, with relative or absolute hyperuricosuria occurring at intervals. Secondly, the patient continually experiences a metabolic acidosis because of the lactate-pyruvate excess which is accentuated when ketosis is also present. The kidney therefore excretes a remarkably acid urine in an attempt to compensate for the continuous organic acid acidosis. This acid medium in the urine greatly favors uric acid precipitation and undoubtedly is a major contributor to the frequency of uric acid lithiasis in patients with glycogen storage disease.

Management is not different from that used in the patient with gouty arthritis, although there seems no purpose in the administration of uricosuric agents to such subjects if allopurinol controls the hyperuricemia.

References

1. Barlow, K. A. Hyperlipidemia in primary gout. *Metabolism* 17:289, 1968.
2. Barzel, U. S., Sperling, O., Frank, M., De Vries, A. Renal ammonium excretion and urinary pH in idiopathic uric acid lithiasis. *J. Urol.* 92:1, 1964.
3. Deconti, R. C., and Calabresi, P. Use of allopurinol for prevention and control of hyperuricemia in patients with neoplastic disease. *New Eng. J. Med.* 274:481, 1966.
4. Drenick, E. J. Hyperuricemia, acute gout, renal insufficiency and urate nephrolithiasis due to starvation. *Arthritis Rheum.* 8: 988, 1965.

4a. Editorial. Hyperuricaemia, hypertension, and vascular disease. *Lancet* 1:87, 1967.

5. Fine, R. N., Strauss, J., and Donnell, G. N. Hyperuricemia in glycogen-storage disease type 1. *Amer. J. Dis. Child.* 112:572, 1966.
6. Hall, A. P., Barry, P. E., and Dawber, T. R. Epidemiology of gout and hyperuricemia: A long-term population study. *Amer. J. Med.* 42:27, 1967.
7. Henneman, P. H., Wallach, S., and Dempsey, E. F. The metabolic defect responsible for uric acid stone formation. *J. Clin. Invest.* 41:537, 1962.
8. Holland, P., and Holland, N. Y. Preven-

tion and management of acute hyperuricemia in childhood leukemia. *J. Pediat.* 72: 358, 1968.

9. Krakoff, I. H. Use of allopurinol in preventing hyperuricemia in leukemia and lymphoma. *Cancer* 19:1489, 1966.
10. Krakoff, I. H., and Murphy, M. L. Hyperuricemia in neoplastic disease in children: Prevention with allopurinol, a xanthine oxidase inhibitor. *Pediatrics* 41:52, 1968.
11. Lesch, M., and Nyhan, W. L. A familial disorder of uric acid metabolism and central nervous system function. *Amer. J. Med.* 36: 561, 1964.
12. Lonsdale, K., and Mason, P. Uric acid, uric acid dihydrate, and urates in urinary calculi, ancient and modern. *Science* 152: 1511, 1966.
13. Morriss, R. H., and Beeler, M. F. X-ray diffraction analysis of 464 urinary calculi. *Amer. J. Clin. Path.* 48:413, 1967.
14. Muggia, F. M., Ball, T. J., and Ultmann, J. E. Allopurinol in the treatment of neoplastic disease complicated by hyperuricemia. *Arch. Intern. Med.* (Chicago) 120:12, 1967.
15. Rapoport, A., Crassweller, P. O., and Husdan, H. The renal excretion of hydrogen ion in uric acid stone formers. *Metabolism* 16:176, 1967.
16. Rieselbach, R. E., Bentzel, C. J., Cotlove, E., Frei, E., III, and Freireich, E. J. Uric acid excretion and renal function in the acute hyperuricemia in leukemia: Pathogenesis and therapy of uric acid nephropathy. *Amer. J. Med.* 37:872, 1964.
17. Seegmiller, J. E., and Frazier, P. D. Biochemical considerations of the renal damage of gout. *Ann. Rheum. Dis.* 25:668, 1966.
18. Steele, T. H., and Rieselbach, R. E. The renal mechanism for urate homeostasis in normal man (the contribution of residual nephrons within the chronically diseased kidney to urate homeostasis in man). *Amer. J. Med.* 43:868, 1967.
19. Talbott, J. H. *Gout* (2nd ed.). New York: Grune & Stratton, 1964.
20. Talbott, J. H., and Terplan, K. L. The kidney in gout. *Medicine* (Balt.) 39:405, 1960.
21. Watts, R. W. E., Watkins, P. J., Matthias, J. Q., and Gibbs, D. A. Allopurinol and acute uric acid nephropathy. *Brit. Med. J.* 1:205, 1966.
22. Yü, T., and Gutman, A. B. Uric acid nephrolithiasis in gout (predisposing factors). *Ann. Intern. Med.* 67:1133, 1967.

24

Calcium Nephropathy

Franklin H. Epstein

Impairment of the function of the kidneys, ranging from minimal derangement of concentrating capacity to progressive renal failure, may complicate a variety of diseases characterized by hypercalcemia or hypercalciuria or both. In order to understand the pathogenesis and physiology of the nephropathy of hypercalcemia, it is helpful to appreciate some experimental facts concerning the relationship between calcium and the kidney.

Renal Handling of Calcium

One of the factors controlling renal excretion of calcium is the quantity of calcium filtered by the glomeruli. If the concentration of calcium in serum and glomerular filtrate falls, thereby decreasing the amount of calcium filtered per minute, urinary calcium decreases and calcium reabsorption approaches 100 per cent. If serum proteins are normal, urinary calcium is generally negligible when serum calcium is below 7.5 mg. per 100 ml. [4]. Acute reductions in glomerular filtration rate also reduce calcium excretion [19, 118, 166]. Chronic depression of the glomerular filtration rate tends to decrease calcium clearance [83], and may result in normal or low values for urinary calcium despite an increase in the concentration of filtrable calcium in serum. Once renal insufficiency has supervened, calcium excretion may be less than 200 mg. per day even when the serum calcium is elevated in, for example, the milk-alkali syndrome, or in hyperparathyroidism.

RELATIONSHIPS BETWEEN THE EXCRETION OF CALCIUM AND SODIUM

Approximately 9 or 10 gm. of calcium is filtered by the glomeruli of a healthy adult in the course of a day. Ninety-eight per cent of this is normally reabsorbed by the renal tubules. An important fact about the renal tubular handling of calcium is that it is remarkably similar to that of sodium. For example, Walser [161] observed that in diuretic dogs the clearance of free calcium ion equaled the clearance of sodium. When the proximal tubule of the rat is perfused with solutions containing calcium in varying concentrations, there is a striking similarity between Ca^{++} and Na^{+} in terms of outward transport, influx into the lumen of the proximal convolution, and the concentration ratio between tubular fluid and plasma at equilibrium [62]. The bulk of calcium reabsorption, like that of sodium, takes place in the proximal tubule [41, 99]. The concentration of calcium in proximal tubular fluid is equal to that of an ultrafiltrate of plasma, implying that under normal circumstances in the proximal tubule calcium is absorbed with water in the proportion that exists in the glomerular filtrate. An active transport mechanism can be inferred from the fact that during mannitol diuresis, the concentration of Ca^{++} in the proximal tubule can fall to as low as 21 per cent of the plasma concentration. In the distal tubule, even under nondiuretic conditions, calcium concentration is reduced to 60 per cent of the ionized calcium of plasma. Like sodium, the concentration of calcium increases in renal tissue along a gradient from cortex to medulla [157]. This is presumably a consequence of active reabsorption of calcium in high concentration by the ascending limb of Henle's loop, and trapping of calcium in medullary tissue by countercurrent flow in medullary capillaries.

It might be predicted from these considerations that urinary calcium would be influenced by the quantity of sodium ingested in the diet and excreted by the kidneys. In fact, changing from a diet containing 25 mEq. of sodium to one containing 350 mEq. of sodium daily, can change calcium excretion from 180 mg. to as much as 580 mg. per day [91]. Clearly, the sodium content of diet and urine must be controlled — or at least recorded — if the clinical significance of urinary calcium is to be properly appreciated.

The obvious analogies between renal behavior toward Ca^{++} and Na^{+} suggest that these ions share a common pathway of active transport. There is no direct evidence for this, however, and the way in which Ca^{++} is transported by kidney cells and across cell membranes is unknown. Schatzmann [143] has shown that human erythrocyte ghosts extrude Ca^{++} in a reaction linked to hydrolysis of adenosine triphosphate. This important finding suggests that the plasma membranes of other cells, including renal cells, share the ability to transport Ca^{++} actively.

The link between sodium and calcium excretion appears to be forged most strongly at the level of the proximal tubule. It is therefore most apparent when the excretion of sodium is altered in response to changes in the volume of extracellular fluids. For example, rapid infusion of isotonic saline increases the excretion of both sodium and calcium, as a result of diminished reabsorption of fluid in the proximal tubule [103]. The dual effects of mineralocorticoids upon sodium and calcium excretion provide another illustration of this principle. Acute administration of deoxycorticosterone causes a fall in urinary sodium, owing primarily to an action on sodium reabsorption in the distal tubule. The excretion of calcium is unchanged by this maneuver, resulting in a dissociation between urinary calcium and sodium [101, 120]. When deoxycorticosterone injections are continued and sodium is permitted in the diet, sodium is retained and extracellular fluid volume expands. Absorption of glomerular filtrate in the proximal tubule is then inhibited, and sodium excretion rises to control levels, the resultant of diminished proximal and enhanced distal absorption. The excretion of calcium, on the other hand, becomes greatly elevated above baseline levels, since decreased proximal absorption of calcium is not counterbalanced by a stimulus to distal reabsorption [119]. This effect of the chronic administration of deoxycorticosterone to increase calcium excretion is abolished by a salt-free diet [152]. It is therefore related to volume expansion rather than to a direct action of the hormone on tubular handling of calcium.

The influence of the volume of body fluids on calcium excretion is illustrated in another way by the action of diuretics. Calcium excretion is enhanced initially during the acute phase of action of almost all diuretics. When diuretics are given chronically, however, the urinary output of calcium falls to very low levels, even though sodium excretion continues so as to equal sodium intake [105, 129]. The fall in calcium excretion can be prevented by giving enough salt to prevent sodium depletion and contraction of the extracellular fluid [151]. Though there is some tendency for glomerular filtration rate to fall when mild salt depletion is produced by diuretics, this is not necessarily responsible for the decrease in calciuria, since urinary calcium may decline remarkably without a measurable change in creatinine clearance [129]. There is indirect evidence that reabsorption in the proximal tubule is greatly enhanced under these circumstances [43]. The decrease in calcium excretion produced by chronic thiazide administration is presumably mediated through a secondary stimulation of proximal tubular reabsorption of both sodium and calcium, on behalf of a depleted extracellular fluid.

PARATHYROID HORMONE

Just as aldosterone influences tubular absorption of sodium without greatly affecting that of calcium, so parathyroid hormone alters renal tubular reabsorption of calcium without changing the excretion of sodium. Renal excretion of calcium is abruptly reduced when parathyroid hormone is infused intravenously or into the renal artery, a result of increased tubular reabsorption of calcium [89, 166]. Stop-flow experiments indicate that the accelerated reabsorption takes place in the distal tubule [166]; parathyroid extracts do not alter the flux of calcium across the proximal tubule of the rat [62]. This effect of parathyroid hormone should be distinguished from its well-known action to increase the renal excretion of phosphate by retarding its absorption from glomerular filtrate. It seems likely that fine adjustments in the level of renal reabsorption of calcium and its excretion by the kidneys are normally accomplished through the mediation of the parathyroid glands.

OTHER INFLUENCES ON CALCIUM EXCRETION

In subjects eating normally, calcium excretion, like that of sodium and potassium, exhibits a *diurnal variation,* being greater during the day than at night [77]. Like the univalent ions, it is unaffected by water diuresis [77, 171]. The excretion of calcium is altered in a special way by *food*. Calcium excretion is increased by glucose [134] (whether given orally or intravenously) and by protein [55, 95]. It is therefore increased by an ordinary meal, and the normal daytime increase in urinary calcium is reversed by fasting [77]. These changes occur without concomitant changes in glomerular filtration rate or creatinine clearance. The use of the calcium-creatinine concentration ratio in random specimens of urine as a guide to the excretion of calcium over 24 hours may therefore be subject to considerable error. The calciuric effect of carbohydrate is said to be exaggerated in certain patients with renal stones, suggesting a role in the genesis of renal calculi [102].

When *dietary calcium* is reduced, renal conservation of calcium is variable and sluggish [113]. Calcium continues to be excreted in urine and feces for many days to weeks after normal persons are placed on a low-calcium diet. In patients whose intake of calcium has been excessive and whose calcium stores are presumably larger than normal, urinary losses of calcium may continue for several months after calcium intake is interrupted [82]. It may be erroneous, therefore, to interpret the continued excretion of calcium in the urine under these circumstances as a primary renal defect [86]. If the skeleton is sufficiently depleted, on the other hand, the kidneys are apparently capable of retaining calcium avidly. Thus, Liu et al. [111] found urines practically free of calcium in their patient with osteomalacia, despite a normal serum calcium and an adequate intake (1000 mg.).

Increases in the intake of *inorganic phosphate* diminish the urinary output of calcium although in man absorption of calcium from the intestinal tract is unchanged [55, 114]. The mechanism therefore presumably involves the deposition of calcium and phosphorus in bone. Infusions of phosphate have been shown to decrease serum calcium slightly while greatly augmenting the secretion of parathyroid hormone [146]. The fall in urinary calcium produced by phosphate in normal persons is probably secondary both to a slight fall in filtered calcium and to accelerated reabsorption of calcium in the distal tubule stimulated by parathyroid hormone. Because of its powerful action in encouraging calcium deposition in bone (and perhaps sometimes in soft tissues), inorganic phosphate is an effective way to treat hypercalcemia, regardless of etiology [68].

Metabolic acidosis is regularly attended by hypercalciuria, whether or not the parathyroids are present [100]. Respiratory acidosis, on the other hand, does not increase urinary calcium [104, 167]. In addition to decreasing calcium reabsorption by renal tubules, metabolic acidosis appears to impair intestinal transport of calcium and to increase the amount of calcium appearing in the feces [72]. It is not yet certain whether this is due to a primary action of acidosis on the transporting cells or a secondary effect on kidney and intestine of the mobilization of calcium from bone.

An excess of *cortisone* has long been known to increase calcium excretion via the feces and the urine as well as producing osteoporosis. The action of cortisone thus appears to be antagonistic to vitamin D at two levels (bone and intestine) and to parathyroid hormone at two sites (intestine and kidney). The increases in fecal and urinary calcium produced by adrenal steroids do not, however, depend on the presence of the parathyroid hormone or on changes in parathyroid secretion, since they are easily demonstrated in hypoparathyroid subjects [160]. The antagonism between vitamin D and glucocorticoids is readily observed in several clinical situations. There is a dramatic increase in the calciferol requirements of hypoparathyroid patients when adrenal steroids are prescribed for a coincidental disorder [127]. Conversely, prednisone is an effective treatment for vitamin D intoxication [168]. Finally, the response of hypercalciuria to cortisone in Boeck's sarcoid is most conveniently explained by the hypersensitivity of patients with sarcoid to vitamin D [6].

Thyrocalcitonin is said to increase renal excretion of calcium and phosphorus in normal as well as hyperparathyroid humans [10]. *Thyroid hormone* increases the turnover of calcium by the skeleton [96] and may cause excessive excretion of calcium in the urine, the feces, or both [12]. The serum concentration of calcium tends to be slightly higher in hyperthyroid patients than in normal persons, and the phosphate clearance lower [1]. These changes suggest that endogenous parathyroid secretion is decreased by the rise in serum ionized calcium which is due to the mobilization of calcium from bone in hyperthyroidism. Since parathyroid hormone accelerates the resorption of calcium from glomerular filtrate, this would account for the hypercalciuria often seen without frank hypercalcemia in hyperthyroidism.

HYPERCALCIURIA

Perhaps one-third of all patients with calcium-containing stones excrete somewhat larger amounts of calcium in the urine than the generally accepted norm of 300 mg. per day for men and 250 mg. for women. In most of these patients the serum calcium is not elevated, and there is no evidence of bone disease. It seems possible that the hypercalciuria observed in some patients with "idiopathic" renal stones is merely an example of the tendency of one "tail" of the general population to increase calcium absorption inordinately at high calcium intakes. Peacock et al. [132] found little difference between the urinary excretion of calcium of stone-forming and nonstone-forming individuals at low calcium intakes, but as the intake was raised, the urine calcium rose more steeply in some of the stone-formers than in the controls. "Hypercalciuria" was therefore detectable only at moderately high calcium intakes (800 to 1000 mg.), the characteristic feature of the syndrome being a steep regression slope of urinary on dietary calcium. This relation of urinary to dietary calcium is similar to that reported by Knapp [95] in a small proportion of normal persons. "Idiopathic" hypercalciuria may therefore be attributed to increased calcium absorption, its nature being similar to that seen in some normal persons without stones.

The renal handling of calcium in "idiopathic hypercalciuria" is influenced by the same factors that operate in healthy persons, permitting a rational approach to therapy. Thus, chronic, mild, salt depletion through the use of low-salt diets [142] and thiazide diuretics [129] are efficacious in reducing urinary calcium in hypercalciuria. (It should be emphasized that when hypercalcemia is present, the serum calcium is likely to be further elevated by salt depletion, precisely because urinary excretion of calcium is reduced.) Calcium deprivation will also reduce urinary calcium in "idiopathic" hypercalciuria, but when intestinal absorption is superefficient, as in the patient reported by Dent and Watson [39], calcium may even have to be eliminated from the drinking water. There is no evidence that reduction of milk intake is beneficial in cases of stone without hypercalciuria. Finally, oral phosphate will return urinary calcium to low levels and may reduce the incidence of stone [17, 129].

EFFECT OF RENAL DISEASE ON CALCIUM EXCRETION

Calcium excretion in the urine is greatly reduced in most patients with renal insufficiency, even when the impairment of renal function is very mild and before serum calcium has decreased [106]. The reduction in urine calcium is associated with a specific decrease in intestinal absorption of calcium and an increase in calcium appearing in the feces [38, 147]. The defect in absorption from the bowel can be reversed by large doses of vitamin D [38, 147], and it is interesting that uremic plasma has an action antagonistic to vitamin D in that it retards the calcification of rachitic cartilage in vitro [173]. Whether this is also the factor responsible for impaired intestinal absorption in uremia is not clear. An increase in the secretion of parathyroid hormone may contribute to the hypocalciuria seen early in renal decompensation, as well as to the decrease in tubular reabsorption of phosphate that helps maintain serum phosphorus at normal levels. After renal insufficiency progresses and the serum phosphorus rises above normal, a reduction in the concentration of diffusible calcium in the glomerular filtrate tends to reduce urinary calcium even further.

Patients with disease of the interstitium or medulla of the kidney tend to excrete larger amounts of calcium in the urine than patients with glomerulonephritis [18, 90]. This is not entirely referable to their tendency to waste sodium, since a difference is also apparent when urine calcium is corrected for concomitant sodium excretion. The urine of certain patients with medullary cystic disease may contain 400 to 600 mg. of calcium per day despite severe uremia.

Effects of Calcium on the Kidney

When injected directly into the renal tubule in high concentration (15 to 20 mEq. per liter), calcium has been shown to decrease sodium efflux from both proximal and distal tubules of the rat [74], and to diminish the water permeability of the distal (but not the proximal) tubule [98]. Experimental hypercalcemia also reduces reabsorption by the proximal tubule, as measured in stop-flow experiments in single nephrons by the shrinking-drop technic [63]. These actions are presumably related to the well-known ability of calcium infusions to produce a diuresis of water and sodium as well as of potassium, phosphate, and magnesium [170]. Calcium has the general property of producing a "tightening" of biologic membranes and a decrease in their permeability to water and urea, in opposition to the action of antidiuretic hormone [115, 133]. In addition, calcium is a potent inhibitor of key enzymes of intermediary metabolism like phosphofructokinase, pyruvic kinase, and pyruvic carboxylase [25], as well as of the "transport" adenosine triphosphatase of cell membranes activated by sodium and potassium [54]. A high concentration of calcium within renal cells might therefore be expected to interfere with tubular transport, and under some circumstances to lead to cellular death.

In hypercalcemia, concentrating ability is impaired out of proportion to the general reduction in renal function. The reduction in concentrating capacity is manifested both at low urine flow (U_{max}) and during mannitol diuresis ($Tm^{C}_{H_2O}$) [50]. Sodium content of the medulla is reduced [116], probably because active transport of sodium out of the thin ascending limb is inhibited. There is no evidence for disequilibrium between collecting ducts and vasa recta or thin limbs in the renal papilla of hamsters with hypercalcemic nephropathy [13]. The cause of the concentrating defect is therefore probably a defect in sodium transport by loops of Henle in the medulla rather than a change in the permeability of the collecting duct and distal tubule to water. Fluid aspirated from the distal tubules of surface nephrons of hypercalcemic rats have a normal concentration of sodium [13], implying a normal rate of sodium transport by the ascending limb of Henle's loop. Surface nephrons of the rat, however, do not have long loops of Henle dipping into the medulla and so are not accurate guides to events occurring in the depths of the renal papilla. Samples of distal tubular fluid from juxtamedullary nephrons would be more to the point, but these are impossible to obtain by conventional technics.

EFFECTS OF CALCIUM ON RENAL STRUCTURE

In the kidney, as in other organs, calcium frequently precipitates in dead or dying tissues. Occasional scattered deposits of calcium, not extensive enough to interfere with renal function, are found in the renal tubules or interstitium of 12 to 23 per cent of autopsies [8, 136]. The nephrocalcinosis seen in cases of mercury or uranium poisoning, or occasionally in chronic glomerulonephritis [11], is different in location and functional effect from that which follows hypercalcemia and hypercalciuria — for example, in parathyroid intoxication or the milk-alkali syndrome. In the former states, calcium is deposited chiefly in the cortex, in proximal tubules specifically damaged by the toxin or by nephritis. In diseases characterized by hypercalciuria, on the other hand, calcification has a tendency to occur predominantly in the medulla and in the collecting tubules. Bell [15] found in a case of hyperparathyroidism that all the calcium was in the medulla, in the shape and direction of collecting ducts. In experimental studies of vitamin D poisoning in dogs, Steck and his co-workers [149] described the earliest and most numerous lesions in the collecting tubules, where cells were injured with and without histologically demonstrable precipitates of calcium. In experimental nephrocalcinosis induced by a high intake of phosphate [112], as well as by vitamin D intoxication or parathyroid poisoning, calcification is often most prominent in a band marking the junction of the outer third with the inner two-thirds of the medulla.

Experimental hypercalcemia produced by vitamin D or injections of calcium salts leads to thickening and calcification of the basement membrane of proximal tubules, perhaps because the transport of calcium through these membranes is greatly increased [47, 48, 59]. Because calcium is concentrated in the medulla of the kidney, the early destructive lesions of hypercalcemia and hypercalciuria tend to occur here in the collecting ducts and the ascending limb of Henle's loop. With more severe or prolonged hypercalcemia, calcium deposition extends generally throughout the kidney to include the convoluted tubules as well as, in advanced cases, the glomeruli and vasculature.

In the earliest stages of the hypercalcemic lesion, degenerative and necrotic alterations are apparent in tubular epithelium in focal areas of the ascending loop of Henle, the distal convoluted tubule, and throughout the entire collecting system, where they are more severe and numerous (Fig. 24-1). Proximal convoluted tubules are generally uninvolved. Casts of calcified cellular debris obstruct some tubules, causing dilatation of the nephrons proximal to the obstruction (Figs. 24-2, 24-3). These changes are noted in microdissection studies of the kidneys of animals given parathyroid hormone [28] or vitamin D [52]. In such animals, the increase in calcium content of the medulla,

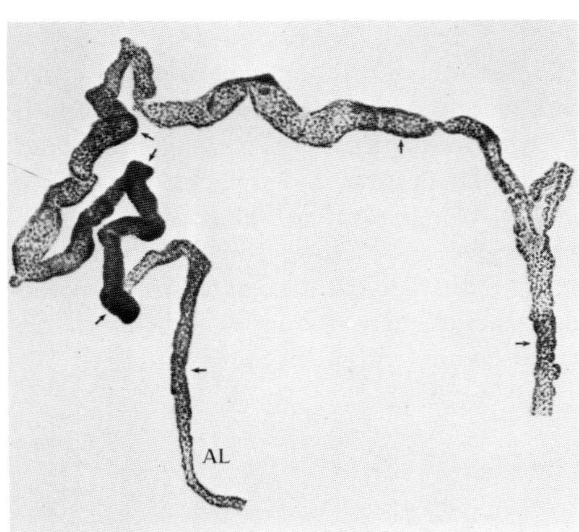

Figure 24-1. Degenerative and fatty changes (*arrows*) in an ascending limb of Henle (AL), distal convoluted segment, and cortical collecting tubule. Microdissected nephron from a dog which had received large doses of parathyroid extract for 24 hours [28].

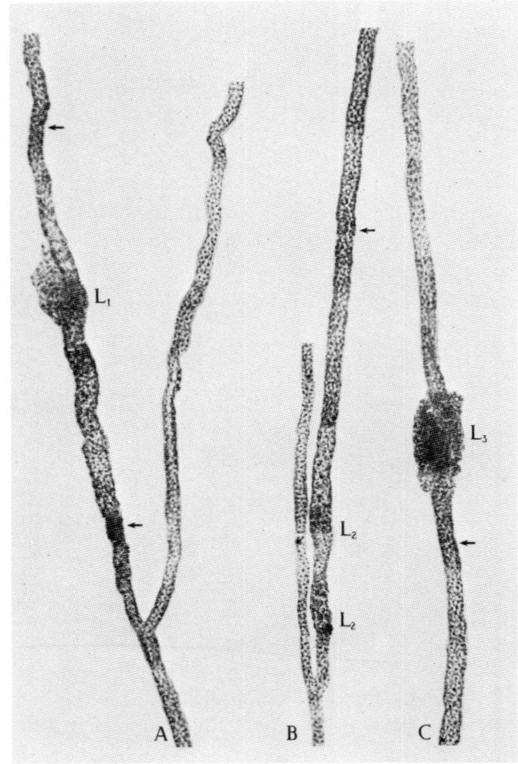

Figure 24-2. Microdissection of medullary collecting ducts from the kidney of a dog which had received large doses of parathyroid extract for 24 hours nine days before autopsy. Calcified casts with proliferation of interstitial connective tissue are apparent at L_1 and L_3. In segment B there are two obstructing casts at points labeled L_2. (See reference 28.)

by chemical analysis, is much more marked than that of the cortex.

When hypercalcemia has been of long duration, the deposits of calcium tend to assume an interstitial position. Calcification, which has initially been intratubular or intracellular, may be removed to the interstitium as regenerating epithelium grows into or around the calcified intraluminal casts in the medullary collecting ducts, or as obstructed tubules containing calcium collapse and atrophy [28, 75]. Interstitial

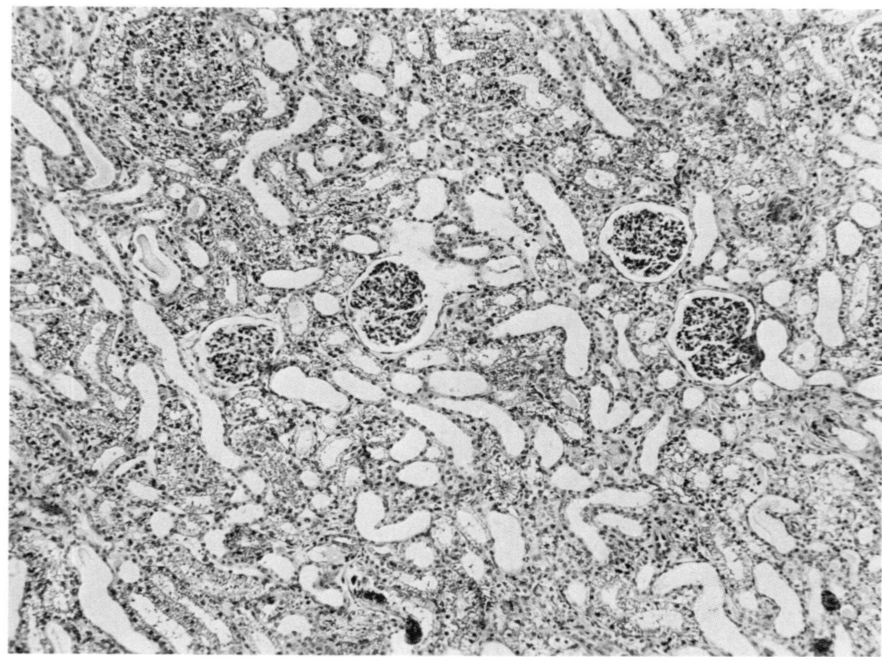

Figure 24-3. Focal dilatation of tubules in the outer cortex resulting from intrarenal obstruction by calcium deposits. Dog, 23 days after treatment with parathyroid extract.

involvement is particularly striking in patients with long-standing hyperparathyroidism [7], and is characterized by infiltration with chronic inflammatory cells and fibrous tissue. Glomeruli may be partially or completely fibrosed, but evidence of proliferative or exudative changes in glomeruli, such as are seen in glomerulonephritis, are absent. The clusters of dilated cortical tubules, the small cortical cysts, and many of the obliterations of glomeruli (Figs. 24-3, 24-4) are probably results of intrarenal obstruction.

It is clear that associated vascular disease and superimposed infection play an important role in stimulating an inflammatory reaction in the kidneys in hypercalcemic nephropathy. In certain patients, intracellular and interstitial deposits of calcium seem to evoke little or no cellular response (Fig. 24-5). Nevertheless, considerable interstitial fibrosis may be initiated by long-term treatment of growing rats with parathyroid extract alone [32]. It is probable that in many patients with nephrocalcinosis, cellular necrosis and mineral deposits secondary to high concentrations of calcium, as well as changes resulting from tubular obstruction, are themselves sufficient to evoke a pathologic picture extraordinarily difficult to distinguish from chronic pyelonephritis.

Clinical Features of Calcium Nephropathy

Regardless of the cause of hypercalcemia and hypercalciuria, calcium nephropathy is characterized by a number of distinctive features. Variations in the course of the renal disease are likely to reflect variations in the degree and duration of hypercalcemia rather than differ-

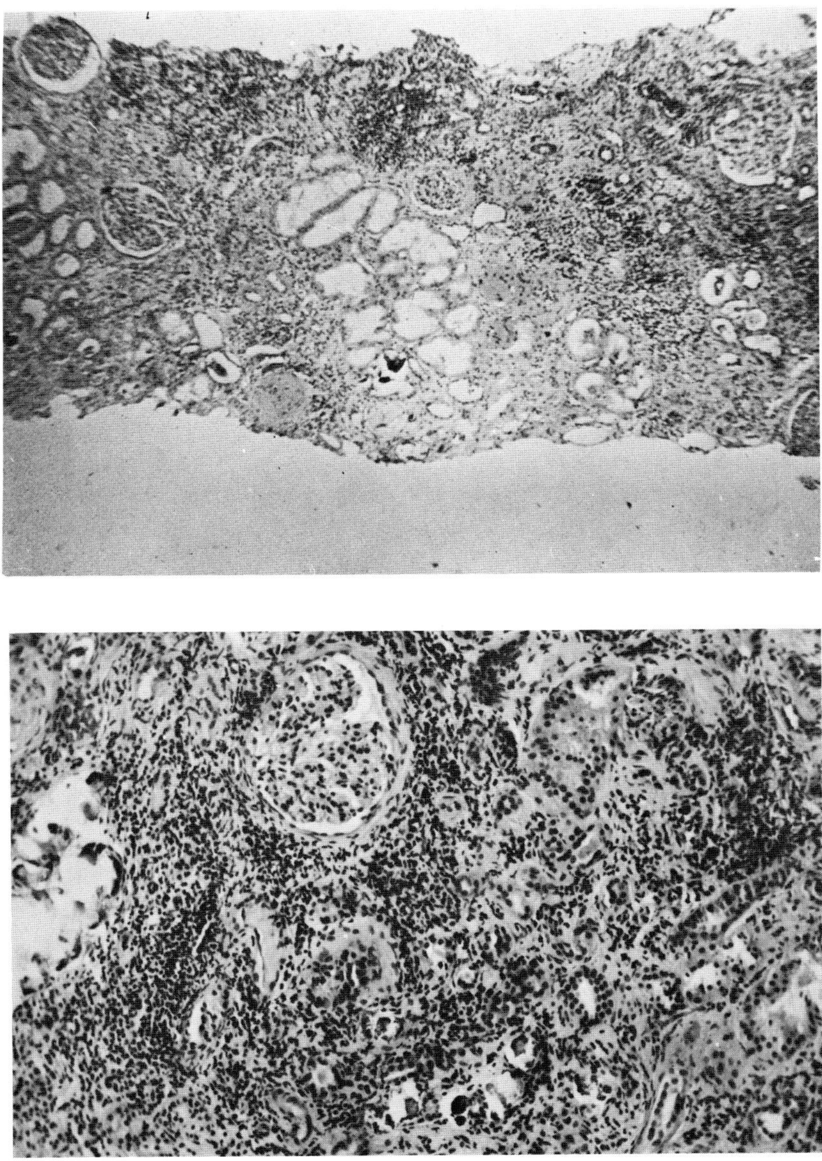

Figure 24-4. Renal biopsy specimens from a patient with hypercalcemic nephropathy resulting from hyperthyroidism. Chronic inflammatory changes are prominent, with colloid casts, periglomerular fibrosis, and clusters of dilated cortical tubules. Culture of the urine and of the biopsy needle proved negative.

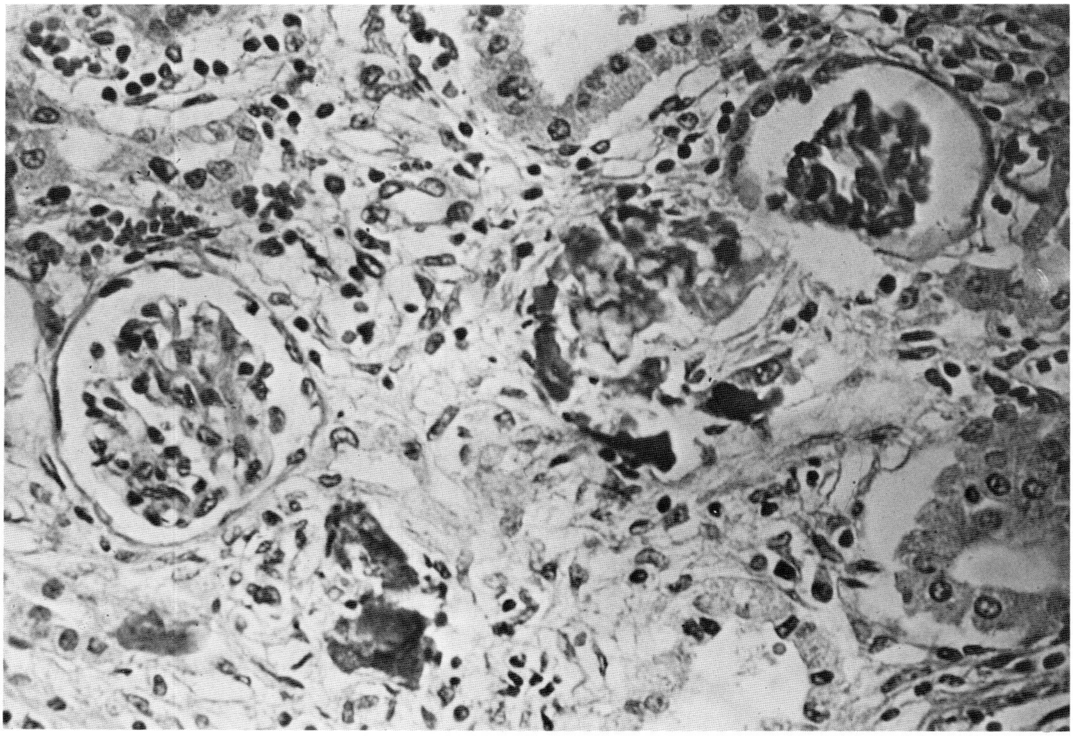

A

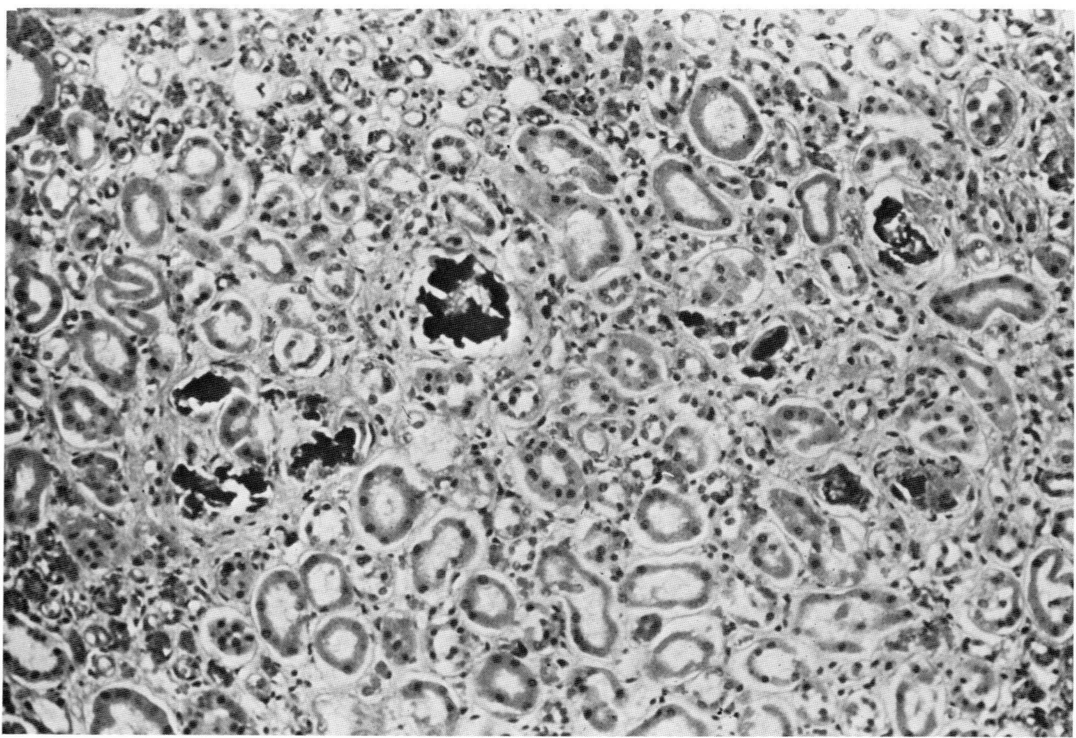

B

ences in the nature of the pathologic process which produces the hypercalcemia. These processes may be classified as follows:

Causes of Hypercalcemic Nephropathy

Dissolution of bone
- Immobilization
- Metastatic cancer
- Hyperthyroidism
- Hyperparathyroidism
- Vitamin D intoxication
- Multiple myeloma

Excessive ingestion or absorption of calcium
- Milk-alkali syndrome
- Vitamin D intoxication
- Boeck's sarcoid
- Idiopathic infantile hypercalcemia

Hypercalciuria intense enough to cause azotemia is generally associated at some time with an elevated level of serum calcium. Concentrating ability may be impaired by hypercalciuria, however, even when serum calcium remains normal. After an episode of hypercalcemia resulting in renal impairment, serum calcium may return to normal long before any improvement in renal function is apparent.

One of the earliest clinical signs is a diminished ability to concentrate the urine. Polyuria and polydipsia are often the chief complaints; they may be so striking that diabetes insipidus is suspected [5]. These symptoms are often out of proportion to the degree of azotemia. It has been suggested that in some instances hypercalcemia may cause polyuria by producing thirst [60], but in most cases in which these symptoms are prominent, the kidneys are unable to concentrate the urine much above the osmolarity of plasma, even when vasopressin is injected. Rapid improvement in concentrating capacity frequently follows successful treatment of hypercalcemia. In some cases (e.g., following removal of a parathyroid adenoma) polyuria disappears so rapidly that functional changes in the kidney secondary to hypercalcemia, rather than structural alterations of nephrocalcinosis, must be held responsible for the abnormally increased urinary flow. In other instances, improvement may occur only slowly or not at all after hypercalcemia is relieved.

Certain hypercalcemic patients seem to retain the ability to concentrate urine normally. This is especially likely to be the case, in my experience, when the serum calcium has never risen above 13 mg. per 100 ml., although an elevated serum calcium is not a prerequisite for the concentrating defect. It is unusual to encounter a patient with calcium nephropathy who is completely unable to concentrate the urine above plasma osmolarity, but in whom the blood urea nitrogen has remained normal. This combination of findings is not uncommon, by contrast, in the nephropathy of potassium deficiency.

The ability to dilute the urine and to excrete ingested water promptly may be retained early in experimental nephrocalcinosis, even when concentrating ability is severely impaired. With progressive renal damage, however, water diuresis soon becomes limited.

Prolonged hypercalcemia and hypercalciuria, resulting in diffuse nephrocalcinosis, may present as renal insufficiency, insidious in onset and only slowly progressive. Glomerular filtration rate and renal plasma flow are depressed proportionately, without a change in filtration fraction [35, 45]. These alterations are reflected in a rise in blood urea nitrogen and a decrease in the excretion of phenolsulfonphthalein. Tm_{PAH} is usually depressed out

Figure 24-5. Calcium deposition in distal convoluted tubules of the cortex (A) and in the medulla (B) of a patient with repeated recent episodes of vitamin D intoxication. In contrast to Figure 24-4, there is little cellular reaction to the deposits of calcium.

of proportion to the fall in inulin clearance [35, 45], reflecting disproportionate impairment of tubular function as compared to glomerular filtration.

In some instances of calcium nephropathy there are changes suggesting specific damage to the proximal tubule. Renal glycosuria was reported in five cases of vitamin D intoxication by Anning et al. [9], although this is not a common finding. Aminoaciduria and "renal tubular proteinuria" are frequently detected in hyperparathyroidism, and disappear when the adenoma is removed [37]. Lysozymuria has been noted in several patients with nephrocalcinosis in whom blood urea was normal [76].

Hypercalcemia produced by acute infusions of calcium stimulates the secretion of acid by the kidneys as well as by the stomach [139]. Perhaps for this reason, but also because the dissolution of bone releases buffer to the extracellular fluid, certain hypercalcemic states (e.g., carcinoma, acute vitamin D intoxication) are frequently associated with mild alkalosis [78, 158]. Paradoxically, acidosis is a feature of calcium nephropathy in other patients. The ability of the kidneys to secrete an acid urine and to manufacture ammonia in response to acidifying salts was noted to be diminished in hypercalcemic patients by Wrong and Davies [172]. In most patients with hypercalcemic nephropathy, however, acidosis does not appear to be out of proportion to azotemia. Renal bicarbonate-wasting is not a common feature of nephrocalcinosis unless the latter is caused by the congenital disorder of renal tubular acidosis. Nevertheless, it seems clear that occasionally repeated episodes of nephrocalcinosis may induce selective impairment of the ability of the kidneys to secrete hydrion and result in an acquired syndrome of systemic acidosis with alkaline urine [20, 56a].

With the appearance of azotemia, the ability to conserve sodium may be impaired. This is not a prominent accompaniment of mild calcium nephropathy in human beings, however, in contrast to the disease produced by injecting vitamin D into rats [117]. Gill and Bartter [66] found that patients with hypercalciuria of various etiologies who demonstrated definite impairment of renal-concentrating capacity all conserved sodium on a diet containing 9 mEq. of sodium per day.

The defect in potassium conservation induced by vitamin D in rats appears to have its occasional counterpart in the calcium nephropathy observed in human patients. Renal potassium-wasting probably is not often severe enough to become clinically important, however, until anorexia limits the intake of potassium in the diet. When this occurs, moderate potassium depletion may complicate the picture [20, 56, 56a].

Proteinuria may be absent and is usually slight unless congestive heart failure or malignant hypertension is present. The excretion of more than 2 gm. of protein daily should suggest the presence of another disease of the kidneys. The urinary sediment may be remarkably free of formed elements. In some cases, red blood cells, leukocytes, and white blood cell casts are seen. The last may be observed even when urine cultures are repeatedly sterile. Calcium casts may occasionally be detected in the urinary sediment [2].

It is important to appreciate that severe impairment of renal function resulting from nephrocalcinosis need not be associated with radiologic evidence of stones or of calcification in the kidneys. In fact, x-ray signs of diffuse nephrocalcinosis are commonly absent [128].

Moderate anemia often appears in association with renal impairment and may overshadow other features of the disorder because of the paucity of signs suggesting renal or metabolic disease. The anemia is normocytic and normochromic in type [144].

Pruritus is a prominent complaint of many patients with hypercalcemic nephropathy. Prompt relief of itching is observed when parathyroidectomy is performed in cases of renal insufficiency complicated by "tertiary" hyperparathyroidism. The cause of the itching is probably deposition of calcium within the skin [92].

When serum calcium is elevated, calcium tends to precipitate in the cornea and conjunctivae [159], presumably because of the relative alkalosis of these tissues, owing to the rapid loss of carbon dioxide from their surfaces [130]. Band keratopathy [33, 163] is often a useful clinical sign of hypercalcemia with metastatic calcification. The corneal deposits superficially resemble arcus senilis except that the crescentic infiltrations are most marked at the medial and lateral poles (Fig. 24-6). The diffuse, superficial opacities are concentric with the limbus but separated from it by a clear interval. Subconjunctival deposits occur as white flecks or glass-like crystals resembling clusters of fish eggs. They may produce a persistent and irritating conjunctivitis. Examination with the slit lamp is sometimes necessary to detect the corneal changes. Calcium deposits in the eye may also be detected by the use of a "bone-free" roentgenographic technic, utilizing dental films [57]. Band keratopathy and calcific conjunctival deposits tend to regress over the course of months or years after hypercalcemia is controlled. Local applications of a chelating agent have been employed successfully in the rare case of intractable conjunctivitis or interference with vision [71].

It might be expected that scarring subsequent to extensive deposition of calcium in the substance of the kidneys would result in hyper-

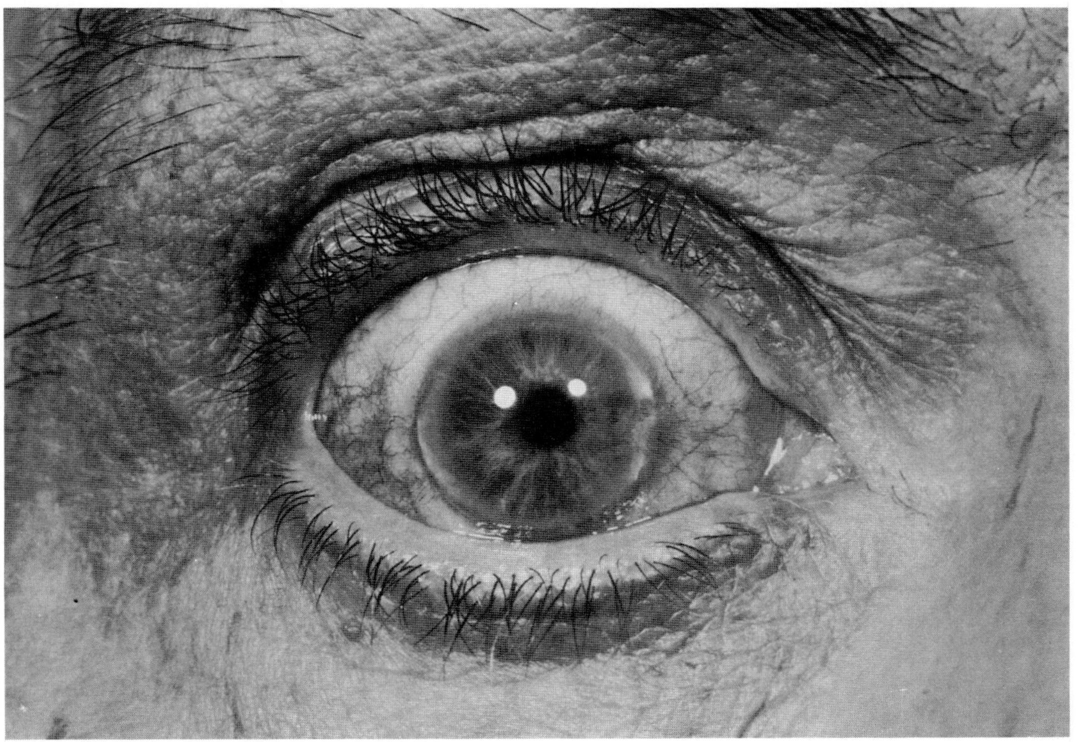

Figure 24-6. Band keratopathy in a patient with the milk-alkali syndrome. (Reproduced with the kind permission of Dr. Maurice B. Strauss.)

tension. About half of all patients with hypercalcemic nephropathy have an elevated blood pressure. In a few cases, blood pressure returns to normal when hypercalcemia is successfully treated [44]. In most, however, hypertension persists even after hypercalcemia and hypercalciuria have been eliminated. Such patients may eventually die from the effects of progressive vascular disease, although renal insufficiency may remit temporarily when the serum calcium is returned to normal.

The presence or absence of infection also influences the course of calcium nephropathy. Patients with renal stones are notoriously susceptible to resistant infections of the urinary tract. One might predict that pyelonephritis would regularly accompany diffuse nephrocalcinosis, since medullary scars can be demonstrated to predispose the kidneys to experimental bacterial infection [14]. More than half of one series of hyperparathyroid patients had infected urine [81]. Nevertheless, many patients develop progressive renal insufficiency with extensive interstitial scarring of the kidneys as a result of hypercalcemia and hypercalciuria and without clinical or bacteriologic evidence of complicating infection or hypertension.

The degree of reversibility of renal impairment induced by an excess of calcium is related to the extent of scar formation and permanent medullary obstruction by calcium precipitates as well as to the presence of vascular disease. Even after hypercalciuria is relieved, renal function may remain depressed or deteriorate slowly. On the other hand, after the disappearance of hypercalcemia and hypercalciuria, function may improve and continue to do so slowly for several months or even years. Such gradual improvement is probably related to the hypertrophy of remaining undamaged renal tissue. Though damage produced by hypercalcemia of short duration is, as a rule, more rapidly reversible, short-lived episodes of hypercalcemia may also produce scars, the residual effects of which persist long after the disturbance in calcium metabolism has disappeared.

ACUTE HYPERCALCEMIC CRISIS

Perhaps the most dramatic example of the deleterious effect of hypercalcemia on the kidneys is acute hypercalcemic crisis, where a rapid rise in serum calcium concentration, usually to levels above 15 mg. per 100 ml., is associated with striking clinical deterioration [156]. The syndrome is most frequently observed, perhaps, as a complication of hyperparathyroidism, but identical clinical manifestations may develop in a variety of other hypercalcemic states — for example, hypervitaminosis D [9], carcinoma [65], sarcoidosis [88], multiple myeloma [156], leukemia [122], Paget's disease [4], and the bone atrophy of disuse [3, 40]. Immobilization often appears to play an important role in triggering hypercalcemic crisis. Treatment of carcinomatous metastases with estrogen or androgen may precipitate acute hypercalcemia [87].

Clinical Picture. Initial polyuria followed by dehydration, oliguria, and azotemia comprise the usual sequence of events. Abdominal symptoms may dominate the clinical picture. Nausea, vomiting, and abdominal discomfort are almost universal. The resulting dehydration is exacerbated by the inability of the kidneys to concentrate the urine. In turn, dehydration reduces the ability of the kidneys to excrete calcium in the urine, producing more intense hypercalcemia and creating a vicious circle. Weakness, lethargy, drowsiness, and mental confusion are common symptoms. Occasionally a toxic psychosis may supervene. Although these symptoms most often develop with a serum calcium concentration of 18 to 20 mg. per 100 ml., some patients tolerate higher concentrations without such manifestations, while in others they may occur at lower calcium levels. If hypercalcemia is not controlled, stupor and azotemia progress, and death ensues.

Pathologic Changes. Pathologic changes, observed at postmortem, resemble those described in animals treated with large doses of parathyroid extract [96]. There is usually widespread calcification of soft tissues including kidney, heart, and lung. In addition, necrotic lesions are observed in the kidneys, pancreas, and cardiac muscle [131, 150]. Peptic ulceration and focal necrosis of the liver have also been described [126, 148]. Recently formed vascular thrombi are common [126, 150], possibly as a result of profound dehydration.

Treatment. Initial treatment must be directed at the dehydration, with infusion of generous quantities of saline and glucose solution. Expansion of the extracellular fluid accelerates calcium excretion by the kidneys and tends to lower serum calcium. Mobilization of a patient with Paget's disease or carcinoma, recently put to bed, may reverse the sequence of events which precipitated hypercalcemia. Large doses of cortisone or prednisone often lower serum calcium concentration in sarcoid, vitamin D poisoning, and multiple myeloma, though not in hyperparathyroidism [36, 154]. Infusions of sodium citrate reduce the concentration of ionized calcium in the serum and extracellular fluids by the formation of a soluble calcium-citrate complex, and greatly accelerate the excretion into the urine of calcium bound to citrate [30, 69]. Infusions of sodium sulfate [29, 162] might be expected to have the same salutary effect because of the formation of undissociated ion pairs between calcium and sulfate, though it is not much more effective than sodium chloride. Sodium ethylenediamine tetra-acetate (sodium EDTA) is a powerful chelating agent with a strong avidity for calcium, which is rapidly and almost completely excreted by the kidneys, carrying with it the bound calcium [84]. Five to 6 gm., administered intravenously over several hours to a hypercalcemic patient, causes a prompt though transient fall in serum calcium. Unfortunately, its use has been associated in some cases with severe damage to the proximal convoluted tubules of the kidney, extensive internal hemorrhages, and the appearance of large cells, stuffed with eosinophilic granules, in the reticuloendothelial system [42]. When hyperparathyroidism is the cause of hypercalcemic crisis, prompt surgical removal of the parathyroid adenoma may be lifesaving.

Hypercalcemia can be effectively treated by an isotonic solution of inorganic phosphate, given either orally or intravenously [68]. The equivalent of 1 to 3 gm. of phosphorus daily may be taken by mouth; the limiting factor is usually diarrhea. When given intravenously, care should be taken not to give more than 50 mM of phosphate (900 mg. of elemental phosphorus) in 24 hours. Phosphate should not normally be given when the serum phosphorus is already elevated, since this will tend to accelerate extraskeletal calcification. A danger of intravenous phosphate treatment for hypercalcemia is that serum calcium will fall below normal, producing tetany or heart failure.

Although in most instances of hypercalcemic nephropathy, hypertension, if present, does not disappear when the serum calcium returns to normal, in an occasional case of hypercalcemic crisis, the blood pressure may be elevated during the acute episode but become normal after a parathyroid adenoma is removed.

HYPERTHYROIDISM

Hyperthyroidism is often associated with osteoporosis [4, 97], increased urinary excretion of calcium [12], and an accelerated turnover of calcium stores [96]. Despite hypercalciuria, renal stones are extremely uncommon. Hypercalcemia may rarely complicate the hyperthyroid state, and when it does, it is usually associated with some degree of reversible renal insufficiency [51].

Anorexia, nausea, and vomiting (paradoxical in patients with hyperthyroidism) may indicate the possibility of hypercalcemia. Unexpected mental changes, anemia, thirst, and polyuria are common clinical features. The hypercalcemia and hypercalciuria are accompanied by a normal serum phosphorus and alkaline phosphatase. After hyperthyroidism is controlled, serum phosphorus may be depressed and alkaline phosphatase elevated for several months, as previously osteoporotic bone is recalcified.

In hyperthyroid patients *without* hypercalcemia, glomerular filtration rate and renal blood flow are generally normal [34]. Some diminution in maximum concentrating ability has been reported [165] and denied [52]. It is possible that transient hypercalcemia or prolonged hypercalciuria results in residual impairment of concentrating ability in some patients. In an occasional patient, nephrocalcinosis producing renal tubular acidosis and potassium-wasting may be a legacy of thyrotoxicosis [123].

Figure 24-4 depicts the biopsy findings in an instance of hypercalcemic nephropathy occurring in a 25-year-old man with hyperthyroidism. In this case, renal function improved slowly after the hyperthyroid state was controlled, but hypertension persisted. Despite the histologic resemblance to chronic pyelonephritis, several urine cultures and culture of the biopsy needle proved to be sterile.

Although losses of skeletal calcium are common in hyperthyroidism, severe and symptomatic hypercalcemia is rare. One may speculate that the few thyrotoxic patients in whom marked hypercalcemia does develop have trouble in turning off their parathyroid glands [49]. In some hypercalcemic and hyperthyroid patients, a parathyroid adenoma has been found. In other cases, a tendency to autonomy of the parathyroid glands may have been present.

MILK-ALKALI SYNDROME

In 1949 Burnett et al. [24] described a syndrome occurring in patients who had ingested several quarts of milk daily and large amounts of absorbable alkali for a prolonged time, generally to assuage symptoms of peptic ulcer. In the patients of Burnett's original report, the characteristic features were severe renal insufficiency with azotemia, hypercalcemia without hypercalciuria or hypophosphatemia, a normal serum alkaline phosphatase, alkalosis, and calcinosis, manifested chiefly by the presence of band keratopathy.

It is clear from subsequent reports that the essentials of the syndrome are a history of prolonged ingestion of calcium leading to nephrocalcinosis with impairment of renal function [137]. The disorder appears to have a strong predilection for men. Perhaps this is connected with the fact that in women, urinary calcium does not rise as much as it does in men, for a given increment in dietary calcium [132]. Hypercalcemia may be transitory or intermittent, so that the serum calcium is not necessarily high at the time of examination. The excretion of calcium is often elevated rather than normal, especially if renal function is not severely impaired. The prominence of alkalosis appears to depend on recent ingestion of alkali or concomitant deficiency of potassium; if these factors are not present, plasma bicarbonate may be normal or low. Deposits of calcium in the cornea and conjunctivae may serve to suggest the diagnosis but are not specific or invariably present. Calcium need not be ingested in the form of milk to do harm; the calcium of calcium carbonate, a frequent ingredient of proprietary antacid mixtures, is absorbed as readily from the gastrointestinal tract after neutralization by gastric hydrochloric acid [94].

Although the disease is not rare and is probably often overlooked, it occurs in only a small minority of patients with peptic ulcer. Many who ingest large amounts of calcium and alkali for years are apparently spared. It has been proposed that prior disease of the kidneys is a prerequisite to the development of the syndrome [164], but underlying renal disease has clearly *not* been present in some cases

Even if renal function has been normal before the development of ulcer symptoms, it may be depressed as a result of dehydration, sodium depletion, and potassium deficiency in patients with obstructing ulcers [23]. Urinary excretion of calcium is probably restricted in such patients, and if the intake of calcium is continued, hypercalcemia may more readily ensue. Interstitial deposition of calcium salts might then be further enhanced by episodic dehydration and low rates of the tubular flow of urine. Hypercalcemia develops more readily in certain normal persons than in others after the ingestion of calcium. Differences in the absorption of calcium from the intestine or in the responsiveness of the parathyroid glands to the level of serum calcium may be responsible for such variations.

An excess of alkali might be expected to predispose to nephrocalcinosis, since calcium phosphate precipitates more readily in alkaline urine. Gough et al. [70] found that nephrocalcinosis was indeed more pronounced when an alkaline-ash diet was fed to rats receiving calciferol. Large amounts of systemic alkali also promote urinary losses of potassium and, if intake of this ion is limited, accelerate potassium deficiency. The resulting renal injury may itself favor the development of nephrocalcinosis. Aside from these mechanisms, there is no unequivocal evidence that antacids per se injure the kidney.

Clinical Picture. Renal insufficiency is frequently detected as a subsidiary finding at the time the patient presents with intractable or recurrent ulcer symptoms. On close questioning, the symptoms of nocturia, polyuria, and polydipsia are elicited. Fatigue and asthenia are common. Mild anemia is the rule. Occasionally, intense generalized pruritus is the chief complaint.

The body content of calcium is greatly increased, as manifested by an expanded "exchangeable pool" of radioactive calcium [82]. Chalky deposits of calcium phosphate tend to localize in the joints and bursae. Metastatic calcification in the cornea and conjunctiva frequently gives rise to intense local inflammation; more often, band keratopathy is asymptomatic. Osteosclerosis has been reported [142]. Nephrocalcinosis is invariably present at postmortem or on renal biopsy. Nephrolithiasis may be present. Deposits of calcium have been noted in the alveolar septa and the walls of the bronchi of the lungs.

Treatment and Prognosis. In about half the cases, renal function improves when the intake of calcium and alkali is stopped. The rapidity with which improvement occurs bears a rough relationship to the length of time that calcium intake has been excessive. In other instances, renal insufficiency remains unchanged or progresses though serum calcium returns to normal. Because of continued mobilization of calcium from soft tissue deposits, the serum calcium may remain elevated for many months even after milk has been interdicted [82].

Differential Diagnosis. As renal function improves, calcium excretion may occasionally increase from normal or low values to the elevated levels commonly encountered in hyperparathyroidism. In such cases, the differential diagnosis may be particularly difficult and is sometimes resolved only by surgical exploration of the neck. Serum phosphorus is generally not depressed in the milk-alkali syndrome, in contradistinction to hyperparathyroidism, though occasional patients with low serum phosphorus are reported [137]. Phosphate-creatinine clearance ratios, or determinations of the tubular reabsorption of phosphorus, are usually not helpful, since tubular rejection of phosphate tends to be increased above normal in all renal diseases whenever glomerular filtration rate is depressed [67].

The response to an infusion of calcium may sometimes aid in distinguishing patients with milk-alkali syndrome from those with hyperparathyroidism. Phosphorus excretion falls following a calcium infusion in patients with normal parathyroid glands, but not in individuals with hyperparathyroidism or hypoparathyroidism [85]. Hyperparathyroidism is unlikely, therefore, in a patient whose excretion of phosphorus declines when the serum calcium is raised by infusions. It should be remembered, however, that if serum calcium is already high or if renal insufficiency is severe, the response may mimic that seen in hyperparathyroidism [155]. The following case is illustrative.

Case 1. A 53-year-old man had suffered from peptic ulcer for 18 years. For seven years he had drunk 6 to 7 quarts of milk daily and had taken large quantities of "Tums" for epigastric pain. Six months before admission severe pruritus and polyuria developed.

Band keratopathy was evident on physical examination, but there were no other signs of metastatic calcification. Blood pressure was normal. Albuminuria was present, and the blood nonprotein nitrogen was elevated. Urinary calcium was normal although hypercalcemia was present (Table 24-1). Serum sodium, potassium, bicarbonate, and chloride were normal. The urine was sterile.

Restriction of the intake of calcium was followed by marked subjective improvement and some amelioration of renal insufficiency. For about a year, however, the serum calcium remained slightly elevated and the serum phosphorus was low on several occasions, so that the diagnostic possibility of hyperparathyroidism was raised. Infusion of calcium produced a fall in phosphorus excretion (Table 24-1), a response unlike that expected in hyperparathyroidism. Under further observation, serum calcium eventually returned to normal, though renal function was permanently impaired.

SARCOIDOSIS

The serum calcium is elevated at some time in 10 to 20 per cent of patients with Boeck's sarcoid [109, 121]; the frequency of hypercalciuria is approximately twice as great [169]. When renal insufficiency occurs in this disease, it is usually a result of nephrocalcinosis associated with hypercalcemia. (Elevated levels of serum calcium have also been reported in the variety of sarcoidosis associated with beryllium poisoning [33].) It is noteworthy that even in cases of sarcoid with well-marked hypercalcemic nephropathy, hypertension appears to be rare. In other respects, however, the clinical features [6, 88] resemble those of other hypercalcemic states. Nephrolithiasis is

Table 24-1. Milk-Alkali Syndrome in a 53-Year-Old Man

Date	Nonprotein Nitrogen (mg./100 ml.)	Serum Calcium (mg./100 ml.)	Serum Phosphorus (mg./100 ml.)	Calcium Excretion (mg./24 hr.)	Phosphorus Excretion (mg./24 hr.)
11/23/54	134	12.0	7.0	90	
2/4/55	94	12.4	3.3		
4/15/55	74	11.3	3.3		
9/16/55	79	11.5	2.9		
10/28/55	74	12.2	3.7		
11/4/55	76	11.3	3.2	120	330
11/5/55[a]		14.3	3.9		193
11/6/55		11.4	3.1		225
3/12/56	65	10.2	5.0		
4/6/56	75	10.5	4.5		
2/19/57	69	9.5	4.8		

[a] Infusion 1 gm. of Ca^{++} over 4 hours.

common, as is superimposed pyelonephritis. Generalized calcinosis and band keratopathy may be noted. Alkaline phosphatase is generally normal, though it may be elevated with extensive granulomatous infiltration of the liver. Serum phosphorus is normal or occasionally low. Biopsy of the kidney may reveal granulomas characteristic of sarcoid [16], as well as deposits of calcium [145]. Perhaps because of the rarity of complicating vascular disease, there is frequently a striking and permanent improvement in renal function when hypercalcemia is controlled.

The lack of any direct correlation between the serum calcium level and the concentration of protein in the serum, the occurrence of hypercalciuria, and the well-known fact that calcium is bound principally to albumin rather than globulin, would appear to exclude hyperglobulinemia as the cause of the elevated serum calcium. Hypercalcemia does not appear to be a result of parathyroid stimulation, as there is usually no hypophosphatemia or generalized osteoporosis. In several cases normal parathyroid glands have been removed [4, 88].

Nearly all sarcoid patients with hypercalcemia or hypercalciuria appear to be abnormally susceptible to vitamin D. Exposure to the sun or treatment with small doses of calciferol [27, 121, 145] may precipitate severe hypercalcemia with consequent renal insufficiency. It is interesting that the frequency of hypercalcemia in sarcoidosis parallels the seasonal change in naturally occurring ultraviolet radiation [154]. In most instances, bone disease is not apparent on x-ray examination. Absorption of calcium from the intestine is characteristically increased [6, 79]. Urinary calcium tends to be elevated and fecal calcium diminished even in cases in which the serum calcium is normal [86, 145]. Treatment with corticosteroids (150 mg. of cortisone daily) reverses these abnormalities within days to weeks and returns the serum calcium to normal levels [6, 79, 145].

HYPERPARATHYROIDISM

Renal calculi or diffuse nephrocalcinosis often complicate primary hyperparathyroidism. Parenchymal calcification or calculus formation (more frequently the latter) occurred in 80 per cent of the cases studied by Hellstrom [80] and by Albright and Reifenstein [4] and in 62 per cent of 45 cases reported by Pyrah and Raper [136]. It is the impression of some that patients with diffuse nephrocalcinosis usually do not have nephrolithiasis and vice versa [4], but this has not been my experience. Hyperparathyroidism is variously estimated to account for less than 1 to more than 10 per cent of all cases of nephrolithiasis [7, 124, 125].

Of 50 cases of hyperparathyroidism reported by Hellstrom [81], 37 of the patients had renal impairment, as evidenced by an elevated level of blood urea nitrogen or a diminished ability to concentrate the urine. Not infrequently, maximum specific gravity is found to be somewhat depressed, even when the blood urea is not elevated. Following removal of a parathyroid adenoma, polyuria may diminish abruptly; as hypercalcemia disappears, the kidneys regain the ability to concentrate urine. Renal concentrating ability may continue to improve gradually over the course of several months.

Clearances of inulin and para-aminohippurate (PAH) were decreased in most patients with hyperparathyroidism studied preoperatively by Edvall [45]. The filtration fraction was elevated in advanced cases of renal impairment (perhaps with the development of severe hypertension?) but was normal with less marked renal insufficiency. In contrast to the improvement in concentrating ability after hypercalcemia was relieved by operation, there was little change in glomerular filtration rate or renal blood flow in patients studied from one week to 16 months after parathyroidectomy.

After ingestion of ammonium chloride, certain patients with hyperparathyroidism fail to acidify the urine in a normal fashion [61].

Fourman et al. [61] have suggested that inability to secrete a urine of sufficiently acid pH may contribute to calculus formation in the hyperparathyroid state.

Serum calcium is characteristically elevated and serum phosphorus depressed. When renal insufficiency supervenes, the concentration of phosphorus in serum may be normal or even elevated, and the serum calcium may fall toward normal. Such cases may be extremely difficult to distinguish from secondary parathyroid hyperplasia occurring in the course of a primary disease of the kidneys. Sustained hypercalcemia, however, is *not* a feature of the secondary variety of hyperparathyroidism.

Renal excretion of calcium is typically elevated if hypercalcemia is present. When the rate of glomerular filtration is depressed by hypercalcemic nephropathy, however, calcium excretion often falls to normal. In addition, urinary excretion of calcium may be normal in certain patients with unimpaired renal function, even in the presence of mildly elevated serum calcium levels. These findings are attributable to the action of parathyroid hormone in promoting the retention of calcium by the kidneys, presumably by increasing its tubular reabsorption from the glomerular filtrate [93, 153].

In 70 per cent of Hellstrom's [80] large series of patients with hyperparathyroidism hypertension either was present, or developed at varying intervals after parathyroidectomy, presumably as a result of renal scarring secondary to nephrocalcinosis or pyelonephritis [80]. As already mentioned, hypertension persists in most patients after operation. Rienhoff [140] reported that of 25 patients cured of hyperparathyroidism nine died 3 to 11 years after the operation; *deaths in all cases resulted from hypertension or renal insufficiency.*

The renal injury resulting from parathyroid intoxication is, in all likelihood, entirely a result of hypercalcemia, although it has been suggested that an excess of parathyroid hormone may be toxic of itself [26], particularly since the earliest experimental lesions in kidney and myocardium consist of cellular necrosis, often without histologically demonstrable calcification. The dissolution of bone induced by hyperparathyroidism is thought to liberate large amounts of glycoprotein into the bloodstream, which when excreted in the urine may serve as a nidus or template to facilitate crystallization of calcium phosphate in the renal tubules [22, 46].

HYPERCALCEMIA IN NEOPLASTIC DISEASE

Hypercalcemia has been reported as a complication of metastatic neoplastic disease of almost every variety; in many cases, acute hypercalcemic crisis follows immobilization or the use of hormones in treatment [87]. Moreover, hypercalcemia and consequent nephropathy may occur in association with cancer, despite the absence of demonstrable metastases to bone [73, 135]. This interesting syndrome has been encountered most frequently as a complication of carcinomas of the lung and of the kidney. Chemical findings in serum and urine may be identical with classic hyperparathyroidism, and (as in hyperparathyroidism) the elevated serum calcium often does not return to normal after treatment with corticosteroids [155]. When hypercalcemia is caused by multiple myeloma, on the other hand, the response to prednisone is usually quite prompt.

IDIOPATHIC HYPERCALCEMIA

The syndrome of "idiopathic hypercalcemia with failure to thrive" was first described by Lightwood in 1952 [107]. The disorder is usually noted in the first year of life. It is characterized by anorexia, vomiting, retarded growth, irritability, constipation, and typically "elfin" facies [21, 110]. The serum calcium is elevated, but serum phosphorus, phosphatase, bicarbonate, chloride, sodium, and potassium are generally normal. Osteosclerosis may be a feature of severe cases. The syndrome is sometimes associated with supravalvular aortic stenosis [64]. The cause of the syndrome is unknown, but it may represent an expression of hypersensitivity to vitamin D in certain infants. Nephrocalcinosis and consequent impairment of renal function are almost universally present. Hypertension, probably secondary to renal scarring, has been reported in about half the cases. Severely affected children die early from renal insufficiency. In milder cases the child may show improvement spontaneously when the intake of vitamin D is completely interrupted. Improvement in hypercalcemia has been reported to follow the administration of corticosteroids [58]. As with other forms of hypercalcemic nephropathy, renal insufficiency does not necessarily disappear, even after the serum calcium returns to normal.

VITAMIN D INTOXICATION

Vitamin D intoxication occurs chiefly in patients receiving massive doses of the vitamin prescribed as treatment for some disease such as rheumatoid arthritis or lupus vulgaris. In addition, the disorder may occur in patients taking toxic doses of vitamin D in potent vitamin preparations without medical surveillance: 1000 international units of calciferol (vitamin D_2) per kilogram per day, taken by mouth, is the smallest dose reported to cause toxic symptoms; most of the 35 patients studied by Anning et al. [9] had received between 1100 and 2300 units per kilogram per day for 1 to 21 months.* It might be expected that a high intake of calcium would enhance the toxicity of calciferol, but this relationship is not obvious, even when a large series of cases is critically reviewed [9]. Prior impairment of renal function is said to increase susceptibility to vitamin D poisoning [31].

Vitamin D produces hypercalcemia by increasing calcium absorption from the intestines and by promoting the dissolution of calcium salts from bone [138]. It does not share the action of parathyroid hormone to increase the renal threshold for calcium; hypercalciuria therefore is the rule early in vitamin D intoxication and even when serum calcium is maintained at normal levels in hypoparathyroidism by the use of vitamin D [108]. The effect of vitamin D on the renal handling of phosphorus is variable; urinary phosphorus is decreased when therapeutic doses of vitamin D are prescribed in rickets, but increased when toxic doses are given to normal subjects.

The patient with vitamin D intoxication is likely to come to the physician because of fatigue, nonspecific gastrointestinal complaints, or neuropsychiatric difficulties [9]. The earliest symptoms to appear are thirst, anorexia, and tiredness. Nausea and vomiting are common; headache and abdominal pain are frequent presenting symptoms. Radiologic findings may include generalized osteoporosis and metastatic calcification. The latter is often particularly marked in synovial cavities, bursae, tendon sheaths, and other periarticular structures and may be associated with the formation of cystic tumors. Roentgen evidence of nephrocalcinosis is usually not present. Serum calcium is elevated, while serum phosphorus is not characteristically altered. The serum alkaline phosphatase is normal. The patient is usually anemic as well as azotemic.

Much of the diffuse symptomatology of vitamin D intoxication is a reflection of the insidious progression of renal insufficiency. The latter is largely a result of nephrocalcinosis. Renal calculi are surprisingly uncommon in this disorder.

The degree of reversibility of the renal disease varies with its duration before vitamin D intake is interrupted. It should be emphasized that intermittent episodes of hypercalcemia, sustained, for example, in the course of overtreatment for hypoparathyroidism, can leave a legacy of nephrocalcinosis and impaired renal function which may persist after the serum calcium returns to normal.

* Smaller doses of vitamin D may produce hypercalcemia in sarcoid and the "idiopathic" hypercalcemic syndrome of children.

Case 2. A 6½-year-old boy with hypoparathyroidism had undergone two severe episodes of vitamin D intoxication, associated with hypercalcemia and dehydration, during the year prior to his last admission. The chemical findings were a serum sodium of 134 mEq., potassium of 1.9 mEq., carbon dioxide of 7.4 mEq., and chloride of 111 mEq. per liter; a blood urea nitrogen of 10 mg. and creatinine of 1.3 mg. per 100 ml.; and an osmolality of 304 mOsm per liter. The urinary findings were a urine flow of 2 ml. per minute, a sodium of 63 mEq. and a potassium of 19 mEq. per liter; the urine gave an alkaline reaction and had an osmolality of 250 mOsm per liter after vasopressin (Pitressin). The final admission was prompted by the appearance of a syndrome resembling diabetes insipidus, with chemical findings suggesting renal tubular acidosis and potassium-wasting nephropathy. Serum calcium was normal, but postmortem examination revealed microscopic deposits of calcium in the distal convoluted tubules and outer medulla of the kidneys (Fig. 24-5) identical to those seen in experimental calciferol poisoning in rats [56, 56a].

A more typical example of vitamin D poisoning is summarized in Table 24-2.

Case 3. A 66-year-old woman with rheumatoid arthritis had taken 150,000 units of calciferol daily for four years. For three months she had been troubled by increasing weakness, thirst, and choreiform movements of the legs and chin. The blood pressure was 180/80; only a trace of protein was present in the urine. Deposits of calcium were noted at the temporal margins of both corneas. Azotemia, acidosis, hypercalcemia, hyponatremia, and anemia were present on admission. Renal function gradually improved when vitamin D was stopped and salt intake was increased. One year later she felt well. Neurological symptoms had disappeared; band keratopathy was absent and anemia was improved, although moderate azotemia persisted.

The elevated serum calcium of vitamin D intoxication, like that of sarcoid and multiple myeloma, tends to return to normal over the course of several days when cortisone is administered [168].

Table 24-2. Vitamin D Intoxication in a 66-Year-Old Woman

Date	Calcium (mg./100 ml.)	Phosphorus (mg./100 ml.)	Nonprotein Nitrogen (mg./100 ml.)	Hemoglobin (gm./100 ml.)	Urine Protein	Urine Specific Gravity
9/54	11.5	7.0	128	9.3	trace	1.008
10/54	10.7	2.6	59	10	0	1.012
10/55	10.3	3.9	61	13.5	0	1.016

References

1. Adams, P. H., Jowsey, J., Kelley, P. J., Riggs, B. L., Kinney, V. R., and Jones, J. D. Effect of hyperthyroidism on bone and mineral metabolism in man. *Quart. J. Med.* 36:1, 1967.
2. Albright, F., and Bloomberg, E. Hyperparathyroidism and renal disease, with a note as to the formation of calcium casts in this disease. *Trans. Amer. Ass. Genitourin. Surg.* 2:195, 1934.
3. Albright, F., Burnett, C. H., Cope, O., and Parson, W. Acute atrophy of bone simulating hyperparathyroidism. *J. Clin. Endocr.* 1:711, 1941.
4. Albright, F., and Reifenstein, E. C., Jr. The parathyroid glands and metabolic bone disease. Baltimore: Williams & Wilkins, 1948.
5. Allen, F. N. A diabetes-insipidus-like syndrome in hyperthyroidism. *Proc. Mayo Clin.* 6:684, 1931.
6. Anderson, J., Dent, C. E., Harper, C., and

Philpot, G. R. Effect of cortisone on calcium metabolism in sarcoidosis with hypercalciuria: Possible antagonistic actions of cortisone and vitamin D. *Lancet* 267:720, 1954.

7. Anderson, W. A. D. Hyperparathyroidism and renal disease. *Arch. Path.* 27:753, 1939.
8. Anderson, W. D. Renal calcification in adults. *J. Urol.* 44:29, 1940.
9. Anning, S. T., Dawson, J., Dolby, D. E., and Ingram, J. T. The toxic effects of calciferol. *Quart. J. Med.* 17:203, 1948.
10. Ardaillou, R., Vuagnat, P., Milhaud, G., and Richet, G. Effects de la thyrocalcitonine sur l'excretion rénale des phosphates, du calcium, et des ions H^+ chez l'homme. *Nephron* 4:298, 1967.
11. Arons, W. L., Christensen, W. R., and Sosman, M. C. Nephrocalcinosis visible by x-ray associated with chronic glomerulonephritis. *Ann. Intern. Med.* 42:260, 1955.
12. Aub, J. C., Bauer, W., Heath, C., and Ropes, M. Studies of calcium and phosphorus metabolism: III. Effects of thyroid hormone and thyroid disease. *J. Clin. Invest.* 7:97, 1929.
13. Bank, N., and Aynedjian, H. S. On the mechanism of hyposthenuria in hypercalcemia. *J. Clin. Invest.* 44:681, 1965.
14. Beeson, P. B., Rocha, H., and Guze, L. B. Experimental pyelonephritis: Influence of localized injury in different parts of the kidney on susceptibility to hematogenous infection. *Trans. Ass. Amer. Physicians* 70:120, 1957.
15. Bell, E. T. *Renal Diseases* (2nd ed.). Philadelphia: Lea & Febiger, 1950. P. 408.
16. Berger, K. W., and Relman, A. S. Renal impairment due to sarcoid infiltration of the kidney: Report of a case proved by renal biopsies before and after treatment with cortisone. *New Eng. J. Med.* 252:44, 1955.
17. Bernstein, D. S., and Newton, R. The effect of oral sodium phosphate on the formation of renal calculi and on idiopathic hypercalciuria. *Lancet* 2:1105, 1966.
18. Bettor, O. S., Kleeman, C. R., Gonick, H. C., Varrody, P. D., and Maxwell, M. H. Renal handling of calcium magnesium and inorganic phosphate in chronic renal failure. *Israel J. Med. Sci.* 3:60, 1967.
19. Blythe, W. B., Gitelman, H. J., and Welt, L. G. Effect of expansion of the extracellular space on the rate of urinary excretion of calcium. *Amer. J. Physiol.* 214:52, 1968.
20. Boettiger, L. E. Hypopotassemia in hyperparathyroidism. *Acta Med. Scand.* 148:51, 1954.
21. Bongiovanni, A. M., Eberlein, W. R., and Jones, I. T. Idiopathic hypercalcemia of infancy, with failure to thrive: Report of three cases, with a consideration of the possible etiology. *New Eng. J. Med.* 257:951, 1957.
22. Boyce, W. H., and Garvey, F. K. The amount and nature of the organic matrix in urinary calculi: A review. *J. Urol.* 76:213, 1956.
23. Burnett, C. H., Burrows, B. A., and Commons, R. R. Studies of alkalosis: I. Renal function during and following alkalosis resulting from pyloric obstruction. *J. Clin. Invest.* 29:169, 1950.
24. Burnett, C. H., Commons, R. R., Albright, F., and Howard, J. E. Hypercalcemia without hypercalciuria or hypophosphatemia, calcinosis and renal insufficiency, a syndrome following prolonged intake of milk and absorbable alkali. *New Eng. J. Med.* 240:787, 1949.
25. Bygrave, F. L. The ionic environment and metabolic control. *Nature* (London) 214:667, 1967.
26. Cantarow, A., Stewart, H. L., and Hausel, E. I. Experimental acute hyperparathyroidism: II. Morphologic changes. *Endocrinology* 22:13, 1938.
27. Cantwell, D. F. Sarcoidosis with renal involvement. *Irish J. Med. Sci.* 6:233, 1954.
28. Carone, F. A., Epstein, F. H., Beck, D., and Levitin, H. The effects of transient hypercalcemia induced by parathyroid extract upon the kidney. *Amer. J. Path.* 36:77, 1960.
29. Chakmakjian, Z. H., and Bethune, J. E. Sodium sulfate treatment of hypercalcemia. *New Eng. J. Med.* 275:862, 1966.
30. Chang, T. S., and Freeman, S. Citric

acid and its relation to serum and urinary calcium. *Amer. J. Physiol.* 160:330, 1950.
31. Chaplin, H., Jr., Clark, L. D., and Ropes, M. W. Vitamin D intoxication. *Amer. J. Med. Sci.* 221:369, 1951.
32. Chown, B., Lee, M., and Teal, J. Studies in mineral metabolism. Calcium and the kidney: Experimental. I and II. *Canad. Med. Ass. J.* 35:513, 1936 and 36:7, 1937.
33. Cogan, D. G., Albright, F., and Bartter, F. C. Hypercalcemia and band keratopathy, report of nineteen cases. *Arch. Ophth.* 40:624, 1948.
34. Corcoran, A. C., and Page, I. H. Specific renal functions in hyperthyroidism and myxedema: Effects of treatment. *J. Clin. Endocr.* 7:801, 1947.
35. Corcoran, A. C., Taylor, R. D., and Page, I. H. Functional patterns in renal disease. *Ann. Intern. Med.* 28:560, 1948.
36. Dent, C. E. Cortisone test for hyperparathyroidism. *Brit. Med. J.* 1:230, 1956.
37. Dent, C. E. Discussion in Wolstenholme, G. E. W., and Knight, J. (Eds.), *The Balkan Nephropathy*. Ciba Foundation. Boston: Little Brown, 1967. P. 108.
38. Dent, C. E., Harper, C. M., and Philpot, G. R. The treatment of renal glomerular osteodystrophy. *Quart. J. Med.* 30:1, 1961.
39. Dent, C. E., and Watson, L. Metabolic studies in a patient with idiopathic hypercalciuria. *Brit. Med. J.* 2:449, 1965.
40. Dodd, K., Graubarth, H., and Rapoport, S. Hypercalcemia, nephropathy and encephalopathy following immobilization; case report. *Pediatrics* 6:124, 1950.
41. Duarte, C. G., and Watson, J. F. Calcium reabsorption in proximal tubule of the dog nephron. *Amer. J. Physiol.* 212:1355, 1967.
42. Dudley, H. R., Ritchie, A. C., Schilling, A., and Baker, W. H. Pathologic changes associated with the use of sodium ethylene diamine tetraacetate in the treatment of hypercalcemia. *New Eng. J. Med.* 252:331, 1955.
43. Earley, L. E., and Orloff, J. The mechanism of antidiuresis associated with the administration of hydrochlorothiazide to patients with vasopressin-resistant diabetes insipidus. *J. Clin. Invest.* 14:1988, 1962.
44. Earll, J. M., Kurtzman, N. A., and Moser, R. H. Hypercalcemia and hypertension. *Ann. Intern. Med.* 64:378, 1966.
45. Edvall, C. A. Renal function in hyperparathyroidism: A clinical study of 30 cases with special reference to selective renal clearance and renal vein catheterization. *Acta Chir. Scand.* Suppl. 229, 1958.
46. Engel, M. B. Mobilization of mucoprotein by parathyroid extract. *A.M.A. Arch. Path.* 53:339, 1952.
47. Engfeldt, B., Gardell, S., and Logergren, C. Studies of renal function and structure in experimental hyperparathyroidism. *Acta Chir. Scand.* 123:137, 1962.
48. Engfeldt, B., Rhodin, J., and Strandh, J. Studies of the kidney ultrastructure in hypervitaminosis D. *Acta Chir. Scand.* 123:145, 1962.
49. Epstein, F. H. Bone and mineral metabolism in hyperthyroidism. *Ann. Intern. Med.* 68:490, 1968.
50. Epstein, F. H., Beck, D., Carone, F. A., Levitin, H., and Manitius, A. Changes in renal concentrating ability produced by parathyroid extract. *J. Clin. Invest.* 38:1214, 1959.
51. Epstein, F. H., Freedman, L. R., and Levitin, H. Hypercalcemia, nephrocalcinosis and reversible renal insufficiency associated with hyperthyroidism. *New Eng. J. Med.* 258:872, 1958.
52. Epstein, F. H., and Rivera, M. J. Renal concentrating ability in thyrotoxicosis. *J. Clin. Endocr.* 18:1135, 1958.
53. Epstein, F. H., Rivera, M. J., and Carone, F. A. The effect of hypercalcemia induced by calciferol upon renal concentrating ability. *J. Clin. Invest.* 37:1702, 1958.
54. Epstein, F. H., and Whittam, R. The mode of inhibition by calcium of cell-membrane adenosine-triphosphatase activity. *Biochem. J.* 99:232, 1966.
55. Farquharson, R. F., Salter, W. T., and Aub, J. C. Studies of calcium and phosphorus metabolism: XIII. The effect of ingestion of phosphates on the excretion of calcium. *J. Clin. Invest.* 10:251, 1931.
56. Ferris, T. F., Levitin, H., Phillips, E. T., and Epstein, F. H. Renal potassium-wast-

ing induced by vitamin D. *J. Clin. Invest.* 41:1222, 1962.

56a. Ferris, T. F., Kashgarian, M., Levitin, H., Brandt, I., and Epstein, F. H. Renal tubular acidosis and renal potassium wasting acquired as a result of hypercalcemic nephropathy. *New Eng. J. Med.* 265:924, 1961.

57. Fleischner, F. G., and Shalek, S. R. Conjunctival and corneal calcification in hypercalcemia: Roentgenologic findings. *New Eng. J. Med.* 241:863, 1949.

58. Forfar, J. O., Balf, C. L., Maxwell, G. M., and Tompsett, S. L. Idiopathic hypercalcemia of infancy: Clinical and metabolic studies with special reference to etiological role of vitamin D. *Lancet* 1:981, 1956.

59. Fourman, J. Two distinct forms of nephrocalcinosis in the rat. *Brit. J. Exp. Path.* 40:464, 1959.

60. Fourman, P., and Leeson, P. M. Thirst and polyuria with a note on the effects of potassium deficiency and calcium excess. *Lancet* 1:268, 1959.

61. Fourman, P., McCouhey, B., and Smith, J. W. G. Defects of water reabsorption and of hydrogen-ion excretion by the renal tubules in hyperparathyroidism. *Lancet* 1:619, 1960.

62. Frick, A., Rumrich, G., Ullrich, K. J., and Lassiter, W. E. Microperfusion study of calcium transport in the proximal tubule of the rat kidney. *Pflueger Arch.* 286:109, 1965.

63. Fulgraff, G., and Heidenreich, O. Mikropunctionsuntersuchungen uber die Wirkung von Calciumionen auf die Resorptionskapazitat und auf die prozentuale Resorption im proximalen Konvolut von Ratten. *Naunyn Schmiedeberg. Arch. Pharm. Exp. Path.* 258:440, 1967.

64. Garcia, R. E., Friedman, W. F., Kaback, M. M., and Rowe, R. D. Idiopathic hypercalcemia and supravalvular aortic stenosis. *New Eng. J. Med.* 271:117, 1964.

65. Gellhorn, A., and Holland, J. F. Neoplastic diseases. *Ann. Rev. Med.* 5:187, 1954.

66. Gill, J. R., and Bartter, F. C. On the impairment of renal concentrating ability in prolonged hypercalcemia and hypercalciuria in man. *J. Clin. Invest.* 40:716, 1961.

67. Goldman, R., and Bassett, S. H. Phosphorus excretion in renal failure. *J. Clin. Invest.* 33:1623, 1954.

68. Goldsmith, R. S., and Ingbar, S. H. Inorganic phosphate treatment of hypercalcemia of diverse etiologies. *New Eng. J. Med.* 274:1, 1966.

69. Gomori, G., and Gulyas, E. Effect of parenterally administered citrate on the renal excretion of calcium. *Proc. Soc. Exp. Biol. Med.* 56:226, 1944.

70. Gough, J., Duguid, J. B., and Davies, D. R. The renal lesions in hypervitaminosis D: Observations on the urinary calcium and phosphorus excretion. *Brit. J. Exp. Path.* 14:137, 1933.

71. Grant, W. M. New treatment for calcific corneal opacities. *A.M.A. Arch. Ophthal.* 48:681, 1952.

72. Greenberg, A. J., McNamara, H., and McCrory, W. W. Metabolic balance studies in primary renal tubular acidosis: Effects of acidosis on external calcium and phosphorus balances. *J. Pediat.* 69:610, 1966.

73. Gutman, A. B., Tyson, T. L., and Gutman, E. B. Serum calcium, inorganic phosphorus and phosphatase activity in hyperparathyroidism, Paget's disease, multiple myeloma and neoplastic disease of bones. *Arch. Intern. Med.* 57:379, 1936.

74. Gutman, Y., and Gottschalk, C. W. Microinjection study of the effect of calcium on sodium transport in the rat kidney. *Israel J. Med. Sci.* 2:243, 1966.

75. Hass, G. M. Pathological Calcification. In Bourne, G. H. (Ed.), *The Biochemistry and Physiology of Bone.* New York: Academic, 1956.

76. Hayslett, J., Perillie, P., Finch, S., and Epstein, F. H. Unpublished data.

77. Heaton, F. W., and Hodgkinson, A. External factors affecting diurnal variation in electrolyte excretion with particular reference to calcium and magnesium. *Clin. Chim. Acta* 8:246, 1963.

78. Heineman, H. O. Metabolic alkalosis in patients with hypercalcemia. *Metabolism* 14:1137, 1965.

79. Heineman, P. H., Dempsey, E. F., Carroll, E. L., and Albright, F. The cause of hypercalciuria in sarcoid and its treatment with cortisone and sodium phytate. *J. Clin. Invest.* 35:1229, 1956.
80. Hellstrom, J. Experience from 105 cases of hyperparathyroidism. *Acta Chir. Scand.* 113:501, 1957.
81. Hellstrom, J. Primary hyperparathyroidism: Observations in a series of 50 cases. *Acta Endocr.* 16:30, 1954.
82. Henneman, P. H., and Baker, W. H. The mechanisms of sustained hypercalcemia following hypervitaminosis D and the milk-alkali syndrome. *J. Clin. Invest.* 36:899, 1957.
83. Hodgkinson, A., and Pyrah, L. N. The urinary excretion of calcium and inorganic phosphate in 344 patients with calcium stone of renal origin. *Brit. J. Surg.* 46:10, 1958.
84. Holland, J. F., Danielson, E., and Sahagian-Edwards, A. Use of ethylene diamine tetraacetic acid in hypercalcemic patients. *Proc. Soc. Exp. Biol. Med.* 84:359, 1953.
85. Howard, J. E., Hopkins, R. R., and Connor, T. B. On certain physiologic responses to intravenous injection of calcium salts into normal, hyperparathyroid and hypoparathyroid persons. *J. Clin. Endocr.* 13:1, 1953.
86. Jackson, W. P. U., and Dancaster, C. A consideration of the hypercalciuria in sarcoidosis, idiopathic hypercalciuria, and that produced by vitamin D: A new suggestion regarding calcium metabolism. *J. Clin. Endocr.* 19:658, 1959.
87. Kennedy, B. J., Tibbetts, D. M., Nathanson, I. T., and Aub, J. C. Hypercalcemia, a complication of hormone therapy of advanced breast cancer. *Cancer Res.* 13:445, 1953.
88. Klatskin, G., and Gordon, M. Renal complications of sarcoidosis and their relationship to hypercalcemia, with a report of two cases simulating hyperparathyroidism. *Amer. J. Med.* 15:484, 1953.
89. Kleeman, C. R., Bernstein, D., Rockney, R., Dowling, J. T., and Maxwell, M. H. Studies on the renal clearance of diffusible calcium and the role of the parathyroid glands in its regulation. *Yale J. Biol. Med.* 34:1, 1961.
90. Kleeman, C. R., Bettor, O., Massry, S. G., and Maxwell, M. H. Divalent ion metabolism and osteodystrophy in chronic renal failure. *Yale J. Biol. Med.* 40:1, 1967.
91. Kleeman, C. R., Bohannon, J., Bernstein, D., Ling, S., and Maxwell, M. H. Effect of variations in sodium intake on calcium excretion in normal humans. *Proc. Soc. Exp. Biol. Med.* 115:2932, 1964.
92. Kleeman, C. R., Massry, S. G., Popovtzer, M. D., Makoff, D. L., Maxwell, M. H., and Coburn, J. W. The disappearance of intractable pruritus after parathyroidectomy in uremic patients with secondary hyperparathyroidism. *Trans. Ass. Amer. Physicians* 81:203, 1968.
93. Kleeman, C. R., Rockney, R. E., and Maxwell, M. H. The effect of parathyroid extract (PTE) on the renal clearance of diffusible calcium. *J. Clin. Invest.* 37:907, 1958.
94. Kleeman, C. R., Rockney, R. E., Maxwell, M. H., and Grossman, M. I. Further observations on the pathogenesis of hypercalcemia secondary to calcium carbonate ($CaCO_3$) ingestion in duodenal ulcer patients. *Clin. Res.* 6:272, 1958.
95. Knapp, E. L. Factors influencing the urinary excretion of calcium: I. In normal persons. *J. Clin. Invest.* 26:182, 1946.
96. Krane, S. M., Brownell, G. L., Stanbury, J. B., and Corrigan, H. Effect of thyroid disease on calcium metabolism in man. *J. Clin. Invest.* 35:874, 1956.
97. Laake, H. Osteoporosis in association with thyrotoxicosis. *Acta Med. Scand.* 151:229, 1955.
98. Lassiter, W. E., Frick, A., Rumrich, G., and Ullrich, K. J. Influence of ionic calcium on the water permeability of proximal and distal tubules in the rat kidney. *Pflueger. Arch. Ges. Physiol.* 285:440, 1967.
99. Lassiter, W. E., Gottschalk, C. W., and Mylle, M. Micropuncture study of renal tubular reabsorption of calcium in normal rodents. *Amer. J. Physiol.* 204:771, 1963.
100. Lemann, J., Jr., Litzow, J. R., and Lennon,

E. J. Studies of the mechanism by which chronic metabolic acidosis augments urinary calcium excretion in man. *J. Clin. Invest.* 46:1318, 1967.

101. Lemann, J., Jr., Piering, W. F., and Lennon, E. J. The acute effect of aldosterone on the renal excretion of calcium and magnesium in man. *Clin. Res.* 15:362, 1967.
102. Lemann, J., Jr., Lennon, E. J., Piering, W. F., Prien, E. L., Jr., and Ricanati, E. S. Evidence that glucose ingestion inhibits net renal tubular reabsorption of calcium and magnesium in man. *J. Lab. Clin. Med.* 75:578, 1970.
103. Levinsky, N. G., and Lalone, R. C. The mechanism of sodium diuresis after saline infusion in the dog. *J. Clin. Invest.* 42:1261, 1963.
104. Levitin, H., and Epstein, F. H. Unpublished observations.
105. Lichtwitz, A., Parlier, R., de Sèze, S., Hioco, D., and Miravet, L. L'effet hypocalciurique des sulfamides diurétiques. *Sem. Hop. Paris* 37:2350, 1961.
106. Lichtwitz, A., de Sèze, S., Parlier, R., Hioco, D., and Bordier, P. L'hypocalciurie glomérulaire. *Bull. Soc. Med. Paris* 16:98, 1960.
107. Lightwood, R. Idiopathic hypercalcemia in infants with failure to thrive. *Arch. Dis. Child.* 27:302, 1952.
108. Litvak, J., Moldawer, M. P., Forbes, A. P., and Henneman, P. H. Hypocalcemic hypercalciuria during vitamin D and dihydrotachysterol therapy of hypoparathyroidism. *J. Clin. Endocr.* 18:246, 1958.
109. Longcope, W. T., and Freiman, D. G. A study of sarcoidosis based on a combined investigation of 160 cases including 30 autopsies from the Johns Hopkins Hospital and the Massachusetts General Hospital. *Medicine* (Balt.) 31:1, 1952.
110. Lowe, K. G., Henderson, J. L., Park, W. W., and McGreal, D. A. The idiopathic hypercalcemic syndromes of infancy. *Lancet* 2:101, 1954.
111. Liu, S. H., Su, C. C., Chou, S. K., Chu, H. I., Wang, C. W., and Chang, K. P. Calcium and phosphorus metabolism in osteomalacia: V. The effect of varying levels and ratios of calcium to phosphorus intake on their serum levels, paths of excretion and balances, in the presence of continuous vitamin D therapy. *J. Clin. Invest.* 16:603, 1937.
112. Mackay, E. M., and Oliver, J. Renal damage following the ingestion of a diet containing an excess of inorganic phosphate. *J. Exp. Med.* 61:319, 1935.
113. Malm, O. J. Adaptations to Alterations in Calcium Intake. In Wasserman, R. H. (Ed.), *The Transfer of Calcium and Strontium Across Biological Membranes.* New York: Academic, 1963. P. 145.
114. Malm, O. J. On phosphates and phosphoric acid as dietary factors in the calcium balance of man. *Scand. J. Clin. Lab. Invest.* 5:75, 1953.
115. Manery, J. F. Effect of Ca ions on membranes. *Fed. Proc.* 25:1804, 1966.
116. Manitius, A., Levitin, H., Beck, D., and Epstein, F. H. On the mechanism of impairment of renal concentrating ability in potassium deficiency. *J. Clin. Invest.* 39:693, 1960.
117. Manitius, A., Levitin, H., Beck, D., and Epstein, F. H. The mechanism of impairment of renal concentrating ability in hypercalcemia. *J. Clin. Invest.* 39:693, 1960.
118. Massry, S. G., Coburn, J. W., Chapman, L. W., and Kleeman, C. R. Effect of NaCl infusion on urinary Ca^{++} and Mg^{++} during reduction in their filtered loads. *Amer. J. Physiol.* 213:1218, 1967.
119. Massry, S. G., Coburn, J. W., Chapman, L. W., and Kleeman, C. R. The effect of long-term desoxycorticosterone acetate administration on the renal excretion of calcium and magnesium. *J. Lab. Clin. Med.* 71:212, 1968.
120. Massry, S. G., Coburn, J. W., and Kleeman, C. R. The acute effect of adrenal steroids on the interrelationship between the renal excretion of sodium, calcium and magnesium. *J. Lab. Clin. Med.* 70:563, 1967.
121. Mather, G. Calcium metabolism and bone changes in sarcoidosis. *Brit. Med. J.* 1:248, 1957.
122. Maudsley, C., and Holman, R. L. Hyper-

calcemia in acute leukemia. *Lancet* 1:78, 1957.

123. Mayock, R. L., and Kerr, R. M. Hyperthyroidism associated with renal tubular acidosis. Discussion of possible relationship. *Amer. J. Med.* 26:818, 1959.
124. McGeown, M. G. Normal standards of renal phosphate clearance and observations on calculus patients. *Clin. Sci.* 16:297, 1957.
125. Melick, R. A., and Henneman, P. H. Clinical and laboratory studies of 207 consecutive patients in a kidney-stone clinic. *New Eng. J. Med.* 259:307, 1958.
126. Mellgren, J. Acute fatal hyperparathyroidism. *Acta Path. Microbiol. Scand.* 20:693, 1943.
127. Moehlig, R. C., and Steinback, A. L. Cortisone interference with calcium therapy in hypoparathyroidism. *J.A.M.A.* 154:42, 1954.
128. Mortenson, J. D., Baggenstoss, A. H., Power, M. H., and Pugh, D. G. Roentgenographic demonstration of histologically identifiable renal calcification. *Radiology* 62:703, 1954.
129. Nassim, J. R., and Higgins, B. A. Control of hypercalciuria. *Brit. Med. J.* 1:675, 1965.
130. Newman, E. V., and Lawrence, A. Respiration, acid secretion and calcium deposition; the eye as a clinical and experimental example. *Trans. Ass. Amer. Physicians* 71:85, 1958.
131. Oliver, W. A. Acute hyperparathyroidism. *Lancet* 2:240, 1939.
132. Peacock, M., Hodgkinson, A., and Nordin, B. E. C. Importance of dietary calcium in the definition of hypercalciuria. *Brit. Med. J.* 3:469, 1967.
133. Petersen, M. J., and Edelman, I. S. Calcium inhibition of the action of vasopressin on the urinary bladder of the toad. *J. Clin. Invest.* 43:583, 1964.
134. Piering, W. F., Lemann, J., Jr., and Lennon, E. F. The effect of carbohydrate administration on urinary calcium and magnesium excretion. *Clin. Research* 16:393, 1968.
135. Plimpton, C. H., and Gellhorn, A. Hypercalcemia in malignant disease without evidence of bone destruction. *Amer. J. Med.* 21:750, 1956.
136. Pyrah, L. W., and Raper, F. P. Renal calcification and calculus formation. *Brit. J. Urol.* 27:333, 1955.
137. Randall, R. E., Jr., Strauss, M. B., and McNeely, W. F. The milk-alkali syndrome: I. The diversity of clinical manifestations: II. Pathogenesis. *Arch. Intern. Med.* (Chicago) 107:163, 1961.
138. Reed, C. I., Stuck, H. C., and Steck, I. E. *Vitamin D.* Chicago: University of Chicago Press, 1939.
139. Richet, G., Ardaillou, R., Amiel, C., and Lecestre, M. Acidification de l'urine par injection intraveineuse de sels de calcium. *J. Urol.* 69:373, 1963.
140. Rienhoff, W. F., Jr. The surgical treatment of hyperparathyroidism, with a report of 27 cases. *Trans. Southern Surg. A.* 61: 340, 1949.
141. Rifkind, B. M., Chasan, B. I., and Aitchison, J. D. Chronic milk-alkali syndrome with generalized osteosclerosis after prolonged excessive intake of "Rennie's" tablets. *Brit. Med. J.* 1:317, 1960.
142. Royer, P., and Balsan, S. Effet d'un régime pauvre en chlorure de sodium dans le "syndrome d'hypercalciurie idiopathique avec nanisme et troubles rénaux" de l'enfant. *Schweiz. Med. Wschr.* 96:412, 1966.
143. Schatzmann, H. J. ATP dependent Ca^{++} extrusion from human red cells. *Experientia* 22:364, 1966.
144. Scharfman, W. B., and Propp, S. Anemia associated with vitamin D intoxication. *New Eng. J. Med.* 255:1207, 1956.
145. Scholz, D. A., and Keating, F. R., Jr. Renal insufficiency, renal calculi and nephrocalcinosis in sarcoidosis: Report of eight cases. *Amer. J. Med.* 21:75, 1956.
146. Sherwood, L. M. Relative importance of parathyroid hormone and thyrocalcitonin in calcium homeostasis. *New Eng. J. Med.* 278:663, 1968.
147. Stanbury, S. W., and Lumb, G. A. Metabolic studies of renal osteodystrophy. *Medicine* (Balt.) 41:1, 1962.
148. Staub, W., Grayzel, D. M., and Rosenblatt,

P. Mediastinal parathyroid adenoma. *Arch. Intern. Med.* 85:765, 1950.

149. Steck, I. E., Deutsch, H., Reed, C. I., and Struck, H. G. Further studies on intoxication with vitamin D. *Ann. Intern. Med.* 10:951, 1937.
150. Smith, F. B., and Cooke, R. T. Acute fatal hyperparathyroidism. *Lancet* 2:650, 1940.
151. Suki, W. N., Hall, A. R., Rector, F. C., Jr., and Seldin, D. W. Mechanism of the effect of thiazide diuretics on calcium and uric acid. *Clin. Res.* 15:78, 1967.
152. Suki, W. N., Schwetmann, R. S., Rector, F. C., Jr., and Seldin, D. W. The effect of chronic mineralocorticoid administration on calcium excretion. *Clin. Res.* 15:372, 1967.
153. Talmage, R. V. Studies on the maintenance of serum calcium levels by parathyroid action on bone and kidney. *Ann. N.Y. Acad. Sci.* 64:326, 1956.
154. Taylor, R. L., Lyrich, H., Jr., and Wyson, W. G., Jr. Seasonal influence of sunlight on hypercalcemia of sarcoidosis. *Amer. J. Med.* 34:221, 1963.
155. Thomas, W. C., Jr., Connor, T. B., and Morgan, H. G. Some observations on patients with hypercalcemia exemplifying problems in differential diagnosis, especially in hyperparathyroidism. *J. Lab. Clin. Med.* 52:11, 1958.
156. Thomas, W. C., Jr., Wiswell, J. G., Connor, T. B., and Howard, J. E. Hypercalcemic crisis due to hyperparathyroidism. *Amer. J. Med.* 24:229, 1958.
157. Ullrich, K. J., and Jarausch, K. H. Untersuchungen zum Problem der Harnkonzentrierung und Harnverdunnung. *Pflueger. Arch. Ges. Physiol.* 262:537, 1956.
158. Verbanck, M. Le fonctionnement du rein dans les états d'hypercalcémie. *Acta Clin. Belg.* Suppl. 1:1, 1965.
159. Wagener, H. P. The ocular manifestations of hypercalcemia. *Amer. J. Med. Sci.* 231:218, 1956.
160. Wajchenberg, B. L., Quintao, E. R., Liberman, B., and Cintra, A. B. U. Antagonism between adrenal steroids and parathyroid hormone. *J. Clin. Endocr. Metab.* 25:1677, 1965.
161. Walser, M. Calcium clearance as a function of sodium clearance in the dog. *Amer. J. Physiol.* 200:1099, 1961.
162. Walser, M., and Browder, A. Effect of sulfate on physical state and renal excretion of divalent cations. *J. Clin. Invest.* 37:940, 1958.
163. Walsh, F. B., and Howard, J. E. Conjunctival and corneal lesions in hypercalcemia. *J. Clin. Endocr.* 7:644, 1947.
164. Wenger, J., Kirsner, J. B., and Palmer, W. L. The milk-alkali syndrome: Hypercalcemia, alkalosis and azotemia following calcium carbonate and milk therapy of peptic ulcer. *Gastroenterology* 33:745, 1957.
165. Weston, R. E., Horowitz, H. B., Grossman, J., Hanenson, I. B., and Leiter, L. Decreased antidiuretic response to beta-hypophamine in hyperthyroidism. *J. Clin. Endocr.* 16:322, 1956.
166. Widrow, S. H., and Levinsky, N. G. The effect of parathyroid extract on renal tubular calcium reabsorption in the dog. *J. Clin. Invest.* 41:2151, 1962.
167. Williamson, B. J., and Freeman, S. Effect of acute changes in acid-base balance on renal calcium excretion in dogs. *Amer. J. Physiol.* 191:384, 1957.
168. Winberg, J., and Zetterstrom, R. Cortisone treatment in vitamin D intoxication. *Acta Paediat.* 45:96, 1956.
169. Winnaker, J. L., Becker, K. L., and Katz, S. Endocrine aspects of sarcoidosis. *New Eng. J. Med.* 278:247, 1968.
170. Wolf, A. V., and Ball, S. M. Effect of intravenous calcium salts on renal excretion in the dog. *Amer. J. Physiol.* 158:205, 1949.
171. Wolf, A. V., and Ball, S. M. Effect of intravenous sodium sulfate on renal excretion in the dog. *Amer. J. Physiol.* 160:353, 1950.
172. Wrong, O., and Davies, H. E. F. The excretion of acid in renal disease. *Quart. J. Med.* 28:259, 1959.
173. Yendt, E. R., Connor, T. B., and Howard, J. E. In vitro calcification of rat cartilage in normal and pathological human sera with some observations on the pathogenesis or renal rickets. *Bull. Johns Hopkins Hosp.* 96:1, 1955.

25

Nephropathy of Potassium Depletion

Walter Hollander, Jr., and William B. Blythe

The renal disease with which this chapter deals has been recognized as a clinical entity only rather recently [202, 210, 225]. It has been the subject of many reviews [47, 117, 118, 167, 211, 212, 226, 236, 240, 241, 261]. The correction of potassium deficiency or the correction of its cause is usually not difficult, and the question of whether the nephropathy of potassium depletion is of major or minor importance in man hinges largely on whether there are any permanent or progressive (or both) structural or functional renal changes and whether kaliopenic nephropathy renders the kidney more susceptible to superimposed infectious pyelonephritis. As will be discussed later, these matters have not been settled.

Pathogenesis

Since potassium is the principal intracellular cation, it is not surprising that potassium deficiency causes widespread alterations of structure and function of many tissues and organs, including the kidney [261].

At the outset, it is important to define what is meant by potassium deficiency and depletion, since the two are not necessarily synonymous with a negative potassium balance. Scribner and Burnell [227] have developed the concept of "potassium capacity," a concept that helps to clarify the situation. Almost all the potassium of the body is in the intracellular fluids, where its quantity is closely related to the quantities of protein and glycogen. If potassium is lost from the body, but in association with an equivalent loss of potassium capacity (equivalent losses of protein or glycogen, or both), the quantity of potassium per unit of cell mass will not fall. If, on the other hand, potassium is lost without equivalent losses of protein and glycogen, intracellular potassium concentration will fall. It has also been shown that a fall occurs if the potassium capacity of a protein-depleted animal is suddenly increased by the ingestion of protein without potassium [188]. In this chapter, the terms *potassium depletion, potassium deficiency*, and *potassium deficit* will be used to mean a loss of potassium without or in excess of any loss of potassium capacity. In this circumstance, the quantity of potassium per unit of any tissue solids will ordinarily be less than normal.

There are many specific causes of potassium depletion, most of which involve inadequate intake coupled with losses from the gastrointestinal tract or excessive losses in the urine (or both). Ordinarily, a diet that is adequately nutritious in other respects is adequate in potassium. However, renal potassium conservation is considerably less efficient than renal conservation of sodium, and the ingestion of a low-potassium diet is usually accompanied by urinary excretion of potassium in excess of intake for 8 to 20 days or more, depending on the amount of potassium as well as the concomitant quantity of sodium ingested [17, 18, 81, 89, 208, 238]. This, plus the fact that small quantities of potassium continue to be excreted in the stool [65], explains the ease with which a deficit of potassium can develop when its intake is low.

One of the most common causes of potassium depletion is loss of gastrointestinal fluids. This may occur with diarrhea of any cause, including that associated with certain tumors of the colon [218], islet cell tumors of the pancreas [36], and carcinoid tumors [243]; with excessive use of laxatives [3, 43, 63, 131, 158, 210, 225]; with multiple enemas [69, 203]; in anorexia nervosa [79, 265]; with fistulous drainage; and with vomiting. Potassium depletion develops with vomiting not only because potassium is lost in vomitus, but also because persistent vomiting precludes ingestion and retention of potassium-containing foods, and because the loss of acid gastric juice induces metabolic alkalosis which, in turn, causes increased excretion of potassium by the kidneys. Another condition in which potassium depletion results from excessive renal excretion superimposed on gastrointestinal losses is ureterosigmoidostomy [51, 239].

The other principal cause of potassium depletion is an excessive excretion of potassium in the urine. Although this is a common occurrence only in those renal disorders ordinarily grouped under the terms renal tubular acidosis and the Fanconi syndrome [27, 154, 163, 175, 197], it may also occur in various types of chronic renal disease, and has even been reported to occur intermittently and concomitantly with exacerbations of urinary tract infection [138]. It is prominent in those conditions in which there is excessive secretion of adlosterone, whether primary [48, 159] or secondary [104, 152]; in addition, it also occurs in conditions involving excessive secretion of other adrenal cortical hormones and the administration of large amounts of closely related synthetic steroids. The most common cause of excessive excretion of potassium in the urine is undoubtedly the administration of oral diuretics such as the thiazides.

In addition, there is a small group of patients whose renal losses of potassium are not clearly ascribable to any of the above causes. Finally, it should be noted that potassium depletion has been reported to be a consequence of acclimatization to heat as a result of excessive losses of potassium via sweat *and* urine [42, 149].

Renal Compositional Changes

The kidneys in experimental potassium depletion are enlarged, the increase being due to more water and more solids, either without change in their relative proportions [70, 134, 235] or with a greater proportional increase in water [22, 200]. The ratio of deoxyribonucleic acid–phosphorus to fat-free dry solids appears to be the same in potassium-deficient rats as in pair-fed controls [61], which suggests that hyperplasia is the cause of the renal enlargement. Fat has been found to remain a constant percentage of kidney mass [232, 235].

Although the kidney almost certainly shares in whole-body deficits of potassium, the decrease in renal potassium concentration is often less than the simultaneous depression of muscle potassium concentration [22, 60, 129, 135, 187, 194, 268]. The largest reduction in renal potassium appears to be in the inner medulla and papilla [266]. As regards the nature of the cation replacing potassium, several groups have demonstrated increased quantities of the cationic amino acids lysine and arginine in the kidneys of potassium-depleted rats [21, 75, 133], but this has not been found in dogs [136]. No increase in sodium concentration has been demonstrated [22, 166, 187].

Structural Changes

HISTOPATHOLOGIC CHANGES IN LABORATORY ANIMALS

It has been well established that potassium depletion causes significant renal histopathologic changes in laboratory animals. In the rat, the renal structural change consists of uniform and reproducible lesions that are primarily located in collecting ducts and other cells of the medulla and papilla [54, 121, 128, 161, 167, 174, 178, 183, 192, 199, 235–237, 246, 251]. Renal histopathologic changes have also been found in other potassium-depleted rodents — for example, mice [157], hamsters [103], gerbils [236], and hibernating woodchucks (marmots) [39]. Such change has been found in only one [170] of seven studies of potassium-depleted dogs [191, 207, 232, 234, 236]. Segar and Oliver have found both the hyperplastic and droplet lesion in the collecting ducts of one potassium-depleted monkey, and although the lesions were minimal, their location was similar to that previously described for the rat [190, 191]. As noted later, however, it is now almost certain that with one or perhaps two apparent exceptions [95], potassium deficiency does not cause similar-appearing or similarly located renal structural alterations in man [59, 110, 178, 183, 190, 191, 210, 212, 226, 234, 236]. Since the most prominent renal *functional* abnormality caused by potassium depletion is the same in man as in the rat, the apparent lack of structural coincidence is, in a sense, disappointing.

The most important recent contributions to knowledge and understanding of the renal histopathology of potassium deficiency have stemmed from the application of electron microscopy and from various cytochemical technics. The reports, however, have been somewhat contradictory or differently interpreted, and they have yet to show a single prominent structural abnormality that is common to both man and laboratory animals.

Beginning in 1937 with the studies of Schrader and his associates [224], many investigators have demonstrated structural changes in the kidneys of potassium-depleted rats [54, 70, 88, 95, 99, 121, 128, 142, 143, 150, 161, 167, 174, 178, 179, 183, 192, 199, 200, 224, 235–237, 246, 251, 267]. Since the studies of Spargo in 1954 [235] and of Oliver et al. in 1957 [192], there has been generally uniform agreement that the primary structural response of the rat nephron to potassium deficiency is in cells of the collecting duct [54, 95, 99, 121, 128, 174, 183, 192, 213, 235–237, 246, 267].

The lesions of the collecting duct in potassium-depleted rats are of two quite different types: one consists of an intense hyperplasia and swelling of collecting tubular cells in the outer medulla; the other is an accumulation of intracellular granules or droplets in all cells of the inner medulla and papilla [192, 236, 267].

The hyperplastic lesion, though limited primarily to the outer medulla, is also seen in the inner cortex to a lesser extent [192, 236]. Both hyperplasia and marked swelling affect the

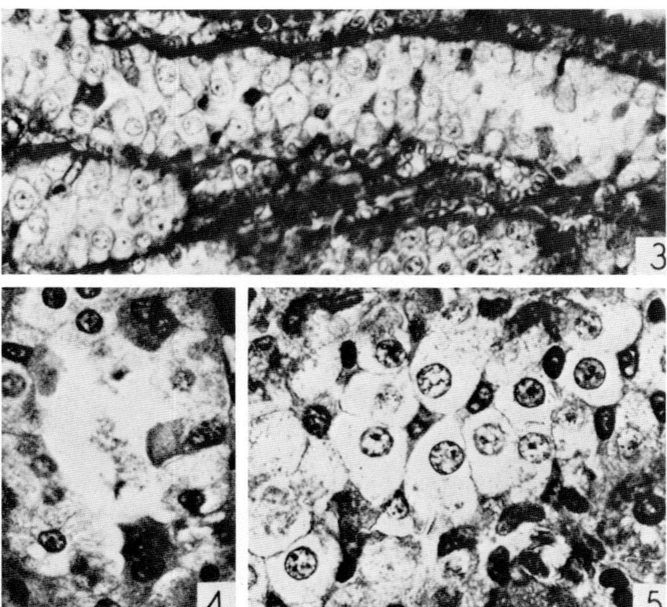

Figure 25-1. Light microscopic views of collecting tubules in the outer medulla of a potasium-depleted rat. The clear cells are significantly swollen. The dark intercalated cells are considerably more numerous than normal, and several show double nuclei. (From Oliver, J., et al. [192].)

clear cells of the collecting ducts, whereas the dark (intercalated) cells are primarily hyperplastic. These changes are shown well in Figure 25-1. There is no evidence that a similar hyperplasia affects any other cells elsewhere in the kidney in or apart from the nephron [192, 236, 237], except for proximal tubular changes now thought to be due to chloride depletion [124]. As shown in Figure 25-2, the hyperplasia may be so marked as to obstruct the tubular lumen, with consequent dilatation proximal to the lesion [161, 192]. Figure 25-3 shows the diffuse but variable degree of dilatation, particularly in the outer medulla. There appears to be some interstitial reaction in the vicinity of these lesions [192], and there are several reports of thickened basement membranes in various parts of the nephron [161, 192, 236]. It seems likely that this hyperplastic, obstructive lesion, together with the interstitial reaction adjacent to it, accounts for any scarring, fibrosis, and tubular dilatation which constitute whatever irreversible renal pathologic change occurs in the potassium-depleted rat.

The cytoplasmic droplet change found in potassium-deficient rodents was first described in mice in 1941 [157]; subsequently, it has been noted repeatedly in potassium-depleted rats [54, 179, 192, 199, 235]. In 1957, using light microscopy and nephron microdissection, Oliver et al. [192] concluded that, in the potassium-deficient rat, this granular lesion was confined to lining cells of collecting ducts in the inner medulla and papilla. In 1960, however, Spargo and his associates [236, 237, 267] showed that, with the far greater magnification provided by the electron microscope, apparently identical droplets could be identified in *all* cells of the renal medulla and papilla, but with diminished intensity as the corticomedullary junction is approached. It is therefore apparent that, to some extent, this abnormality of the potassium-depleted rat involves cells of the collecting ducts, interstitial cells, capillary endothelial cells, and cells of the loop of Henle at all levels of the renal medulla [174, 183, 236, 267]. According to Wilson et al. [267], the droplets in the collecting duct epithelial cells are larger and denser than in other cell types, which may explain their more ready visibility by light microscopy (Fig. 25-4A).

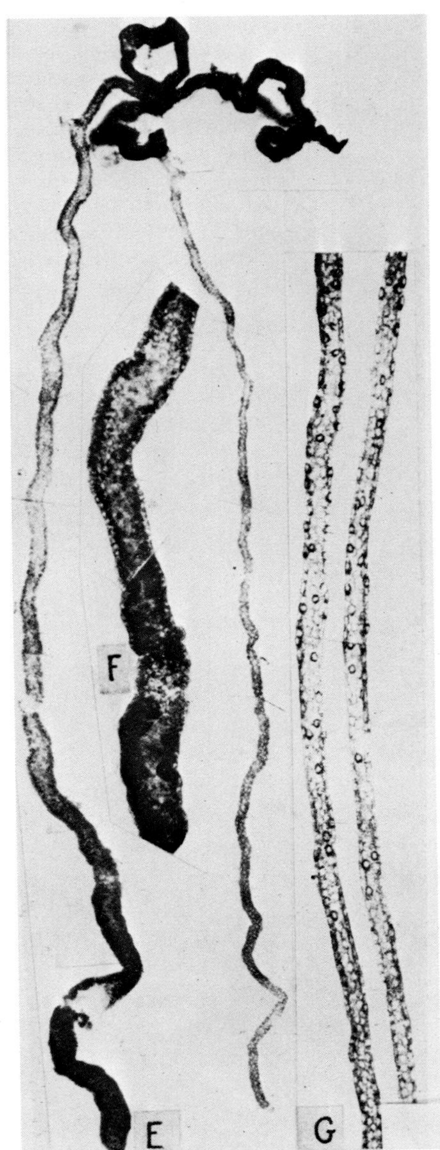

Figure 25-2. Portions of microdissected nephrons. *G.* Two normal collecting ducts from the outer medulla of a rat. *E.* Ascending limb of Henle's loop (*right*), distal convolution (*top*), and collecting duct descending through the cortex to the outer medulla (*left*) of a potasium-depleted rat. The ascending limb and the distal convolution appear normal. The collecting duct contains the characteristic hyperplastic lesion of potassium deficiency (shown at higher magnification in *F*). The collecting duct is irregularly dilated proximal to the lesion. (From Oliver, J., et al. [192].)

They are more numerous, however, in the interstitial cells and in the capillary endothelial cells, which are swollen and seem clearly to diminish the vascular lumen (Fig. 25-5). They are least numerous in cells of the loop of Henle (Fig. 25-6), but there, too, they may seem to swell the cells and narrow the lumen.

The nature and pathogenesis of these cytoplasmic droplets or granules have been the subject of several recent electron microscopic, microchemical, and cytochemical studies [95, 99, 161, 173, 174, 178, 183, 236, 237, 267]. At least four different concepts have emerged: (1) the droplets are altered or derived from mitochondria [161, 178*]; (2) the droplets are, at least in part, a consequence of increased reabsorption of protein from the lumen of collecting ducts [99, 172–174]; (3) the granules represent newly formed cytoplasmic lysosomes,† not derived from mitochondria [174, 183]; and (4) the droplets are discrete, cytoplasmic structures best characterized as multivesicular bodies, each of which encloses many membranous structures of various configurations within a single outer limiting membrane, also not derived from mitochondria [236, 267]. The electron microscopic basis for the latter view is well illustrated in Figures 25-7, 25-8, and 25-9. Although we are not competent to judge these differing views critically, we are impressed with the apparent validity of the reasons and data which Spargo and his associates use to support the last of these concepts and to tentatively refute the others [236, 267].

Using the electron microscope, MacDonald and associates [161] have concluded that the most obvious and constant visible abnormality in rats mildly depleted of potassium is a thickening (three to five times normal) of the base-

* In a more recent article, this investigator (Muehrcke) indicates serious doubts about any direct relationship to mitochondria, aside from finding what he thought were mitochondria as inclusions in some of the droplets.

† As a generality, lysosomes may be defined as cytoplasmic organelles with an outer limiting membrane, containing a number of soluble acid hydrolases, and with a fine structure which may vary from one cell type to another [62].

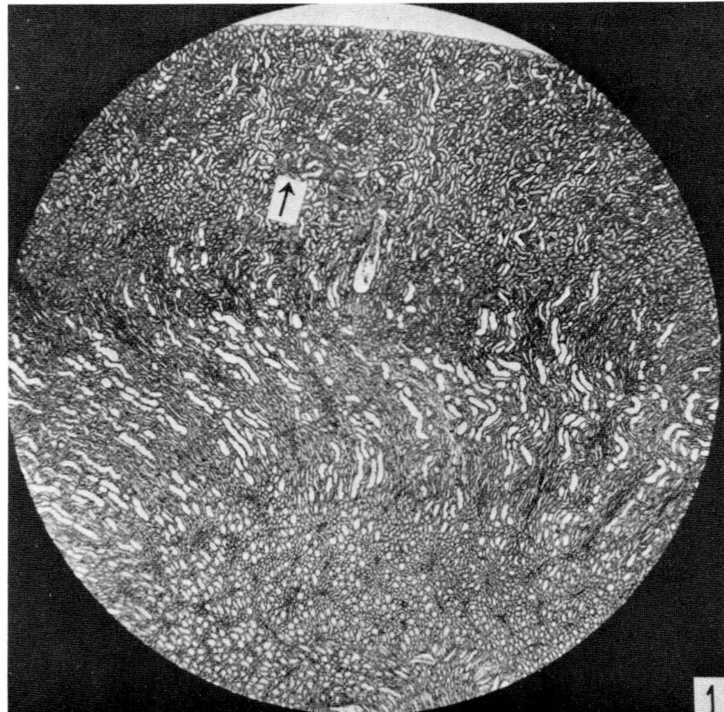

Figure 25-3. Low power view of cortex and medulla of a rat after four weeks of potassium depletion. The striking change is the dilated collecting tubules in the outer medulla. The general appearance of the cortex is not much altered, though the *arrow* points to an indefinite area of thickened tubules. (From Oliver, J., et al. [192].)

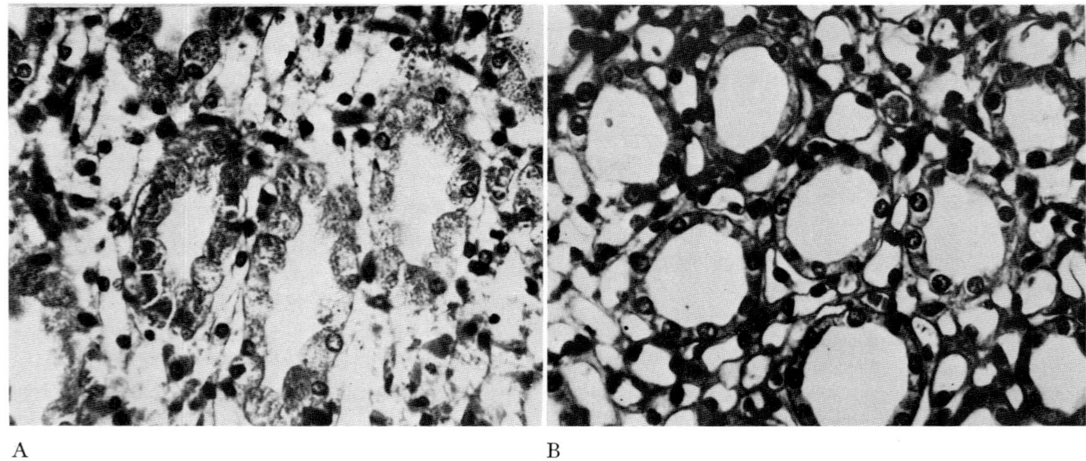

Figure 25-4. High power light microscopic view of the droplet lesion in the inner medulla of a potassium-depleted rat (A). The droplets had completely disappeared by the third days of rapid potassium repletion (B). (Reported as abstract by Hollander, W., Jr., et al. [121].)

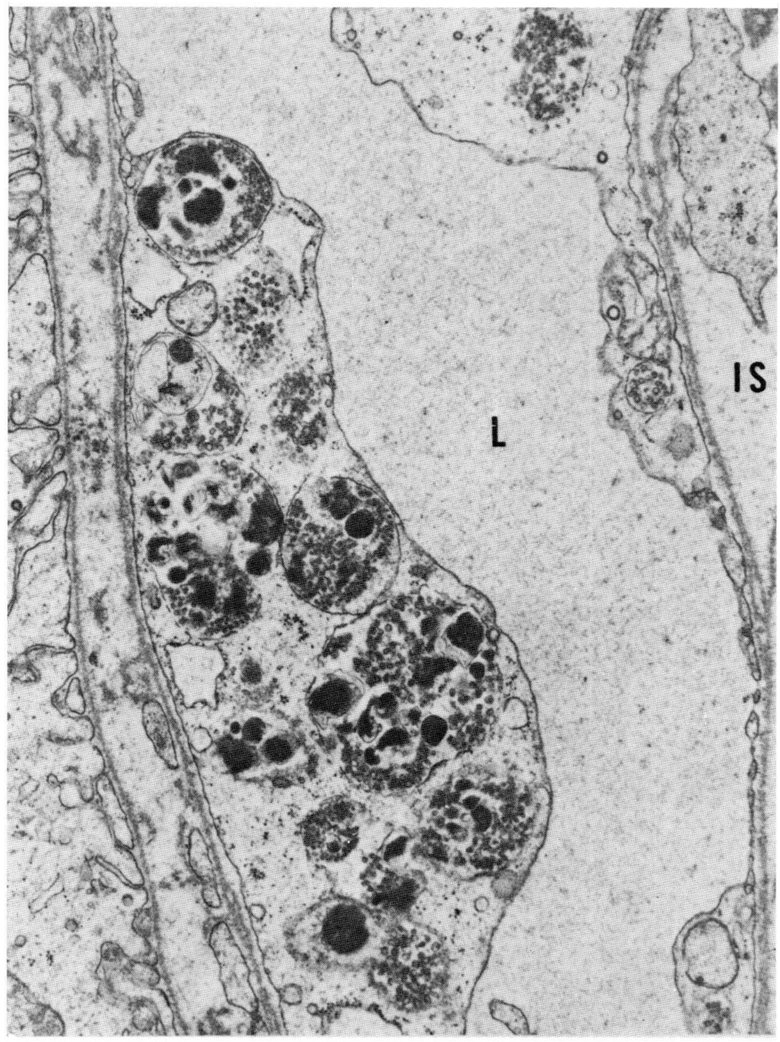

Figure 25-5. Electron microscopic view of an efferent capillary from the papillary tip of a potassium-depleted rat. Prominent "multivesicular bodies" in the epithelium appear to impinge on the vascular lumen (L). *IS* = interstitial space. (From Wilson, H., Spargo, B., and Penksa, R. [267].)

ment membrane of the thin limb of Henle's loop and of the *pars recta* of the proximal tubule. The basement membrane often appeared to become fibrillar. To our knowledge, attempts to confirm this interesting observation have been unsuccessful [183, 236]. In the same study, there was a separation of lateral borders of adjacent collecting duct lining cells, without disruption of the basement membrane [161], but this, too, has not been confirmed [174, 236].

There are no other consistent structural renal lesions in potassium-depleted rats. Nonetheless, it is important to recognize that potassium deficiency (whether experimental or clinical) is commonly complicated by other physiologic and biochemical disorders. In such situations, three questions need answering: (1) What renal lesions, if any, may the "other disorders" cause? (2) How, if at all, do the "other disorders" modify the renal lesions caused by the potassium depletion? (3) Does

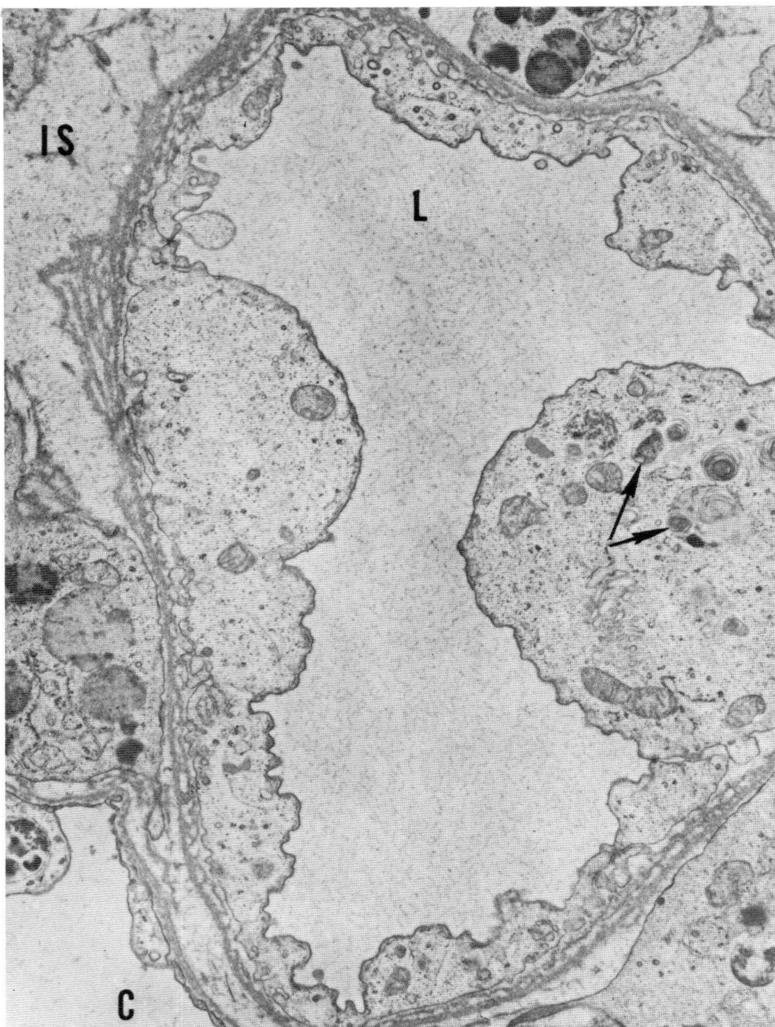

Figure 25-6. Electron microscopic view of the thin limb of the loop of Henle from the papillary tip of a potassium-depleted rat. One lining cell appears to impinge on the lumen (L). The *arrows* point to whorl-like bodies that were occasionally seen along with the "multivesicular bodies." IS = interstitial space; C = capillary. (From Wilson, H., Spargo, B., and Penksa, R. [267].)

the coexistence of potassium deficiency alter renal lesions that are essentially a consequence of the complicating disorders? These questions can be partially answered for experimental potassium depletion in rats.

Some of the common complicating electrolyte and acid-base disorders of experimentally potassium-depleted rats are chloride depletion (with or without hypochloremia), extracellular alkalosis or acidosis, a relatively large or small sodium or bicarbonate intake, hypercalcemia or hypocalcemia, magnesium deficiency, and a relatively large phosphate intake. Four of these — chloride depletion, hypercalcemia, magnesium depletion, and phosphate loading — are known to cause characteristic and distinct renal structural lesions in the rat [124, 129, 165, 193, 213, 260, 263, 264]. By light microscopy none of these — nor any of the other "complicating disorders" — visibly modify the typical renal lesions of the potassium-depleted rat [124, 129, 193, 213, 264]. On the

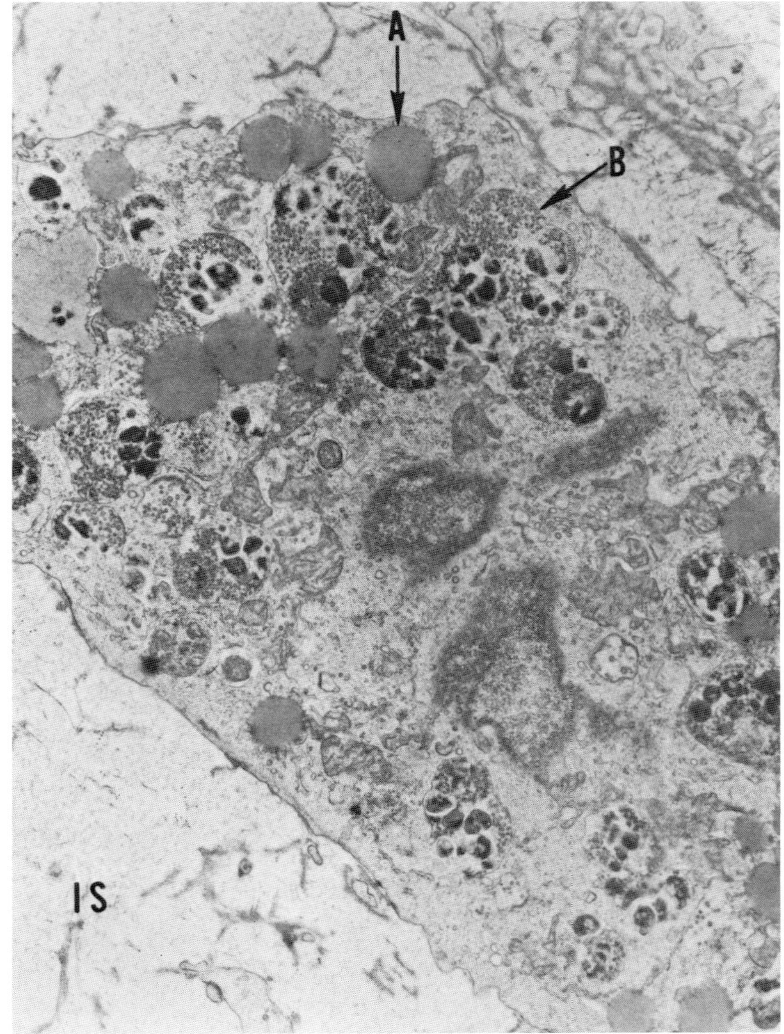

Figure 25-7. Electron microscopic view of an interstitial cell from the papillary tip of a potassium-depleted rat. Much cytoplasm seems to consist of "multivesicular bodies" (B); these are distinct from normally occurring dense droplets (A). IS = interstitial space. From Wilson, H., Spargo, B., and Penksa, R. [267].)

other hand, lesions of chloride deficiency, magnesium depletion, and phosphate loading all appear to be more severe or more readily induced by the coexistence of potassium deficiency [124, 129, 193, 263, 264]. Finally, it is reported that potassium depletion of the rat fails to cause its characteristic renal lesions if the ureters are ligated [244 as cited in reference 267].

It is important to know whether the duration or degree of potassium depletion primarily determines the intensity of consequent renal lesions. Holliday and associates have presented data supporting duration as the major factor [124, 128]. This may well be true when the duration is very short [124] or very long [47, 128, 192], since there must be minimal duration necessary for visible lesions to develop and since secondary changes, such as scarring and fibrosis, seem to develop with prolonged potassium deficiency even though the total potassium deficit is no longer chang-

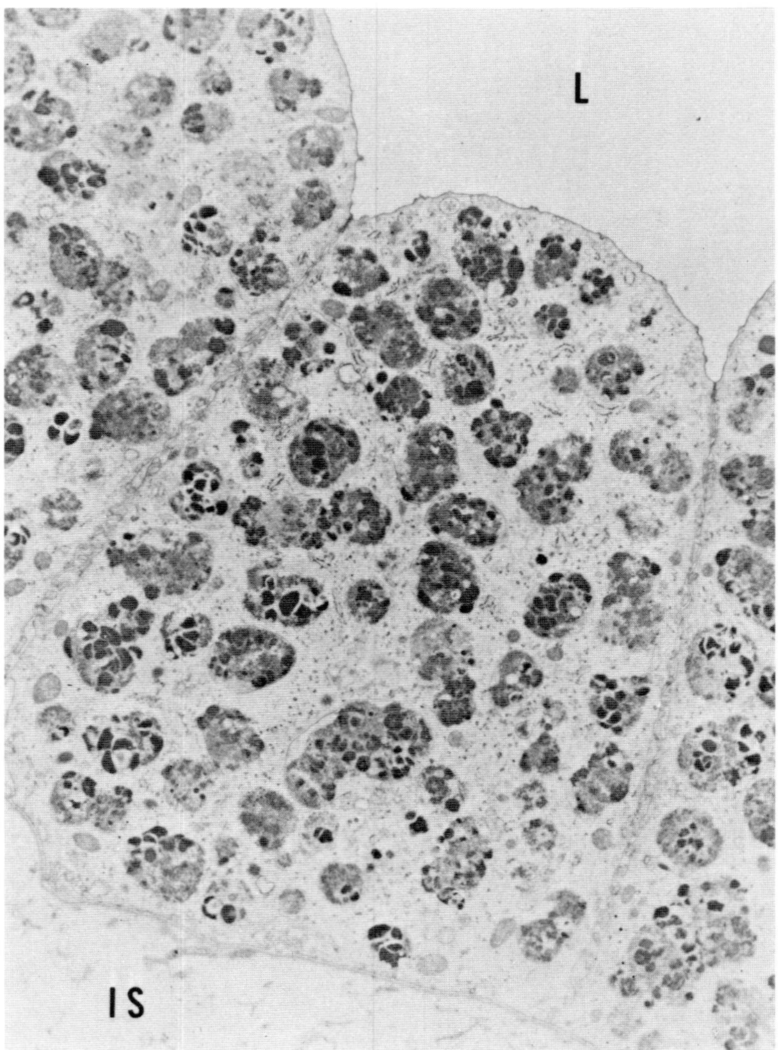

Figure 25-8. Electron microscopic view of a collecting duct cell from the papillary tip of a potassium-depleted rat. "Multivesicular bodies" are prominent. L = lumen; IS = interstitial space. From Wilson, H., Spargo, B., and Penksa, R. [267].)

ing much [128, 192]. Nonetheless, this specific matter has now been examined in rats simultaneously depleted of potassium over a wide spectrum of degree and for durations of 9, 18, and 28 days [254, 255]. The results indicate that degree rather than duration of potassium depletion is the more important variable.

As noted earlier, the kidneys of potassium-depleted rats increase in size and weight. Accordingly, renal weight may be a semiquantitative index of renal histopathology. In the experiments just cited [254, 255], there was an almost exact linearity between renal weight and the degree of potassium depletion, whether renal weight was related to initial or final body weight, and without regard to the duration of potassium deficiency.

HISTOPATHOLOGIC CHANGES IN MAN

Information about renal structure in potassium-depleted humans comes largely from two clinical situations: (1) major losses of

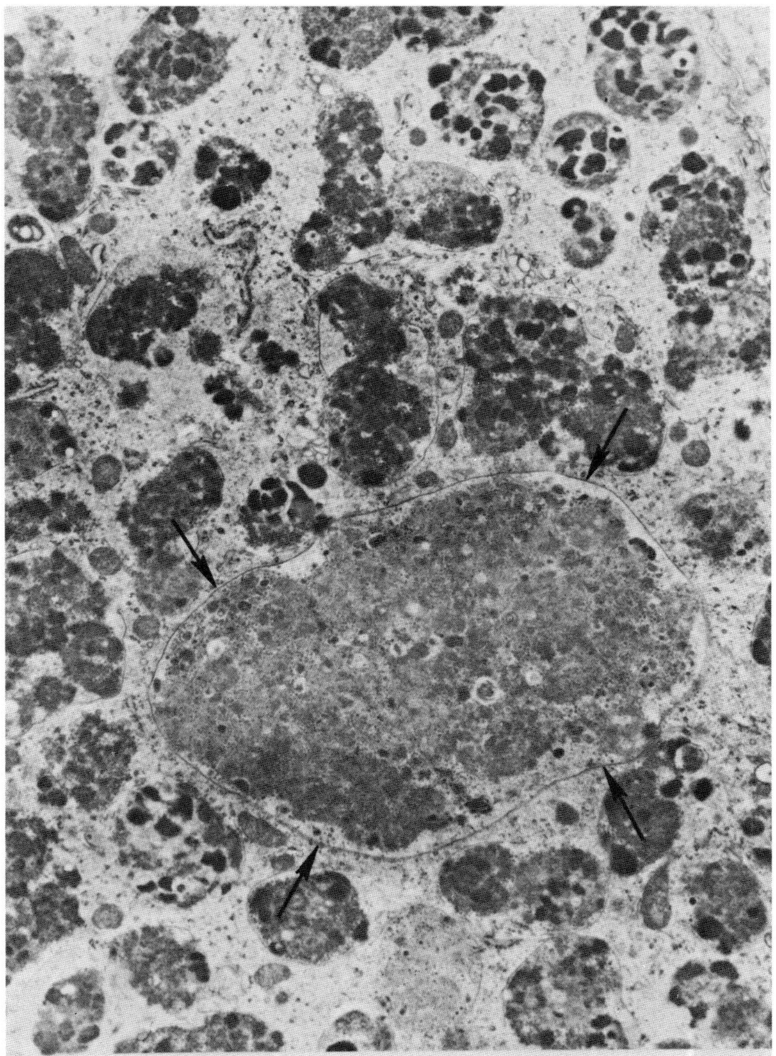

Figure 25-9. High electron magnification of one of the larger collecting tubule "multivesicular bodies." A single intact membrane (*arrows*) around the entire structure appears to enclose multiple tiny vesicles and other membranous configurations. (From Wilson, H., Spargo, B., and Penksa, R. [267].)

fluid from the digestive tract, and (2) major losses of potassium in the urine caused by steroid hormones or by diuretics. A third group, those with renal potassium-wasting apparently due to underlying renal disease may, of course, have renal damage secondary to the potassium depletion itself. Because of the known or suspected primary renal disease, however, it is particularly difficult to know to what extent the renal findings in such patients are properly attributable to potassium deficiency [23, 32, 74, 160, 163, 221, 272]. Similarly, there are many patients with renal damage and probable potassium depletion who provide only inferential evidence because neither the potassium depletion nor other possibly coexisting fluid and electrolyte disorders are documented. These are primarily a large group of patients with acute or chronic gastrointestinal losses whose body fluid and electrolyte status can be reasonably guessed but cannot be supported with appropriate data (many are in the medical literature of a time when most or all of today's commonplace laboratory methods were unavailable or rarely used). This group has been excellently reviewed by Relman and Schwartz [210, 211] and by Conn and Johnson [47].

It is now (1970) two decades since the first report in which renal damage in man was ascribed to potassium depletion [202]. The major histopathologic finding was vacuolation of what was thought to be mainly tubular epithelium of the proximal convolution. Subsequently, in 1953 and 1956, Relman and Schwartz published metabolic, renal physiologic, and renal biopsy studies from several patients with long-standing potassium deficiency due to chronic diarrhea or laxative abuse [210, 225]. The renal biopsies showed prominent vacuolation, swelling, and some degeneration of cortical tubular epithelium.

This renal vacuolar change is now a well-known, but by no means constant, feature of potassium depletion in man [59, 111, 118, 178, 183, 210–212, 226, 236]. It is usually limited to the proximal tubule, but it may also involve the distal convolutions. In some cases, vacuoles may fill and swell the cells, thereby creating a foamy appearance (Fig. 25-10). Less frequently, the vacuoles are more clearly defined and more irregular in size and shape, sometimes filling the cell, often not. It has been suggested that the latter appearance, as shown in Figure 25-11, is virtually pathognomonic of potassium depletion, except for a resemblance to mild cases of ethylene glycol poisoning and to the mildest form of renal damage caused by disodium or calcium ethylenediaminetetraacetic acid (sodium and calcium EDTA) [4, 111, 211, 212, 226]. In contrast, the foamy appearance is not generally considered pathognomonic of potassium deficiency, since it cannot be readily distinguished from tubular changes of other etiologies — for example, the "osmotic nephrosis" that may follow infusion of hypertonic solutions of sucrose or glucose [4, 212, 226, 236]. Regardless of specificity, either form of the vacuolation may distend tubular cells, which thereby appear to encroach on the lumen. Furthermore, some distinguished renal

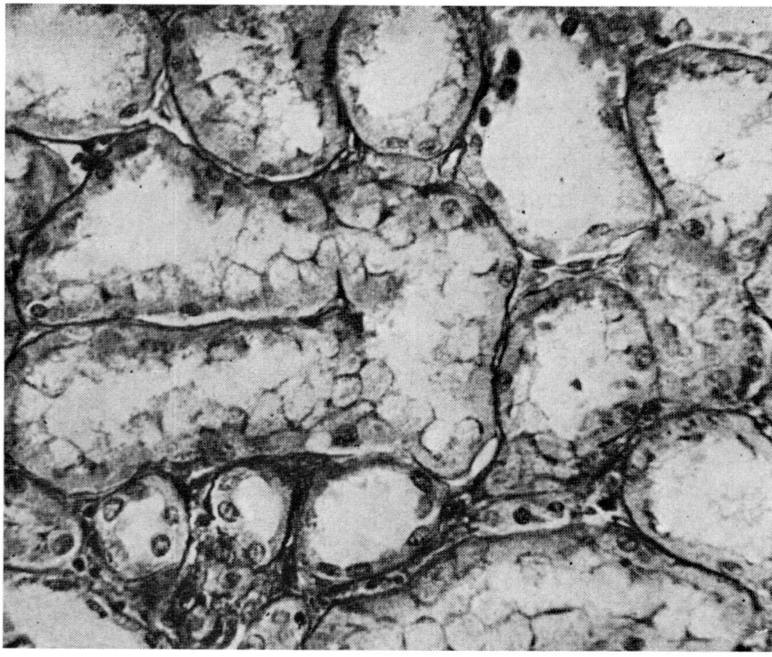

Figure 25-10. Foamy appearance of tubular epithelium from a potassium-depleted patient. Renal biopsy specimen. (From Relman, A. S., and Schwartz, W. B. [210], courtesy of *New England Journal of Medicine.*)

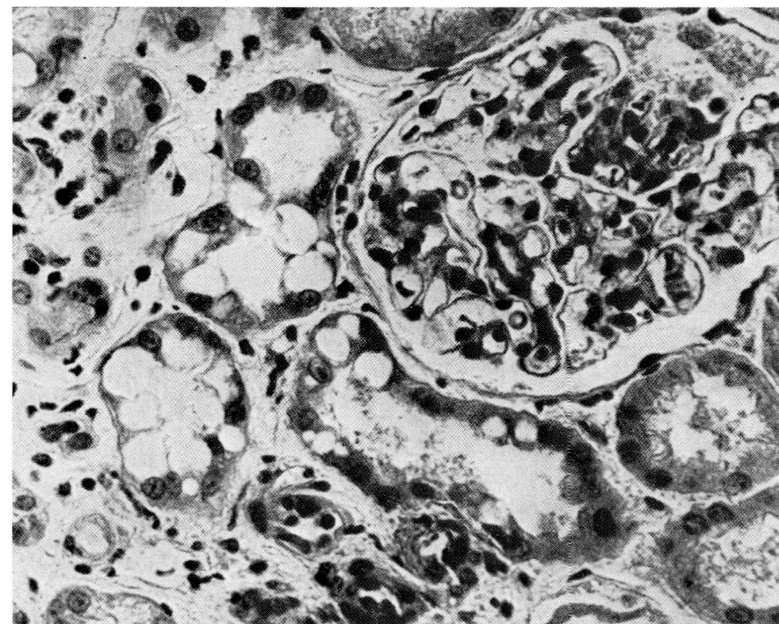

Figure 25-11. Renal biopsy specimen from same patient as in Figure 25-10. It was obtained after partial and intermittent potassium repletion over a 12-month period. It has the irregular hydropic degeneration of cortical epithelial cells thought by some to be essentially pathognomonic of potassium depletion. (From Relman, A. S., and Schwartz, W. B. [210], courtesy of *New England Journal of Medicine.*)

pathologists now express doubt that the characteristics of the tubular vacuolation are often, if ever, so distinctive as to be pathognomonic of potassium deficiency [110, 234, 236].

A vacuolar or "hydropic" lesion of the proximal and sometimes distal convoluted tubules, with a somewhat variable appearance, is now considered to be the one characteristic, albeit variable, structural alteration in the kidneys of potassium-depleted man [4, 111, 212, 226, 236]. As was documented in Chapter 21 of the previous edition of this book, however, this "characteristic" change is far from universal [118]. Specifically, it was noted in only about 60 per cent of 34 cases in which potassium depletion was reasonably certain and renal tissue was examined [9, 10, 12, 28, 29, 31, 35, 36, 45, 46, 48, 52, 59, 63, 64, 73, 83, 96, 97, 144, 145, 151, 210, 230, 239, 265]. Neither the presence nor the absence of vacuoles can be correlated with any particular underlying cause of the potassium depletion [118]. The significance of its absence, however, is sometimes difficult to evaluate because of variable and uncertain degrees of potassium repletion before renal tissue was obtained. As judged from cytochemistry, the vacuoles rarely contain fat [28, 31, 46, 144, 202] or glycogen [31, 46]. It seems possible that they are a counterpart of the proximal tubular lesions due to chloride deficiency in the rat, particularly since chloride depletion is such a frequent concomitant of potassium deficiency in humans.

With the exception of one (possibly two) patients [95], we do not know of any potassium-depleted humans with renal medullary lesions resembling those that are so characteristic of the potassium-depleted rat. Unfortunately, many negative reports are of questionable meaning, because the tissues examined were obtained by renal biopsy which, with the widely used Vim-Silverman technic, secures little if any of the renal medulla or papilla.* Nonetheless, many pathologists have looked for medullary and papillary lesions in kidneys obtained at autopsy from potassium-depleted

* Apparently this is not true for those who use the Iversen and Brun technic [206].

patients and have not found anything resembling either the hyperplastic or the droplet lesion [4, 110, 111, 191, 212, 226, 234, 236].

The one exception was a patient who died with idiopathic potassium depletion [95]. He clearly had a medullary droplet lesion [190]. The distribution and staining characteristics of the droplets appear quite similar to those of the potassium-depleted rat [95, 190, 192, 235, 236]. The other and less convincing case (the brother of the patient just described) also had potassium deficiency of unknown etiology [95]. Renal tissue obtained by open biopsy (but when partly potassium-repleted) showed a droplet lesion in cells of the medulla, but it was much less extensive than in the patient who died [95].

Although the vacuolar lesion in cortical tubular epithelium is the single most consistent renal histopathology described in potassium-deficient man, some reports indicate a striking rarity of this finding together with an equally striking frequency of interstitial fibrosis, tubular atrophy, tubular dilatation, fibrosed glomeruli, and sometimes cellular infiltrates [111, 178, 180, 182, 183] — findings that have, in the relatively recent past, been widely used as criteria for diagnosing chronic (infectious) pyelonephritis. We are now in an era of increasing skepticism about the histologic basis for diagnosing chronic pyelonephritis of infectious origin [40, 111, 112], a matter that will be discussed in more detail later. Hence, these histopathologic findings have more recently, and perhaps more correctly, been related to vascular sclerosis, without intending to implicate the potassium deficiency as a cause of the vascular disease [111, 112, 183]. Regardless, there is a marked discrepancy between the findings of different investigative groups regarding the prominence of presumably irreversible renal structural damage in potassium-depleted patients [47, 178, 180, 183, 210–212, 226]. It is probable that duration of the potassium deficiency is an important (and usually uncertain) variable, more prolonged periods of potassium depletion causing increasing degrees of irreversible change [47, 183], but this has not yet been clearly demonstrated in man.

During the past decade, electron microscopy has been used by a few investigators to define the renal ultrastructure of potassium-depleted humans [16, 178, 183, 234, 236]. Results have varied. The major renal structural changes seen by electron microscopy have been:

1. Extracellular rather than intracellular vacuolation in cortical tubular epithelium [16]. In a study of one patient with primary aldosteronism, Biava and associates [16] found that the vacuoles that were (by light microscopy) apparently within cortical epithelial cells, seemed instead to represent expansions of extracellular fluid in the space between infolded membranes at the base of tubular cells and between adjacent cells. The lateral separations, however, stopped abruptly at the terminal bars ("tight junctions"); the latter appeared intact, thereby preventing any direct connection between intraluminal and extracellular fluid. This interesting report has been confirmed in two other studies [183, 236], but in both there were intracellular, cytoplasmic vacuoles as well. In one of these the extracellular expansion and partial cell separation was associated with small vacuoles, whereas the intracellular vacuoles appeared to be large [183].

2. Thickening and focal lamination of basement membranes in various regions of the kidney [16, 183].

3. Swollen mitochondria in cortical tubular cells of four out of six patients studied [183], a finding that, to our knowledge, has not been confirmed.

4. Increased interstitial collagen in both cortex and medulla [183]. This observation by Muehrcke and Rosen fits with the previous reports of Muehrcke [178] and of Muehrcke and McMillan [180] in which interstitial fibrosis

appeared to be a prominent structural abnormality in chronically potassium-deficient patients.

Reversibility of Structural Changes

The reversibility of structural damage in the kidneys of potassium-depleted humans is of obvious clinical importance. Indeed, on it — and on the question of susceptibility to pyelonephritis — hinge a major part of a larger issue: the long-run significance of potassium deficiency in man. Unfortunately, there is a relative paucity of published information about reversibility of the renal lesions in man. There is more for the rat, and this will be examined first.

LABORATORY ANIMALS: THE RAT AND OTHER RODENTS

The droplet lesion is readily and rapidly reversible [121, 167, 179, 199, 236, 237, 246, 267]. As illustrated in Figure 25-4, if potassium repletion is accomplished quickly, even cells with full-blown, intense cytoplasmic droplet change may revert to normal appearance by light microscopy in as little as three days [121]. The electron microscope has been used in an effort to observe the stages of droplet disappearance, but it is still not clear exactly what happens. Spargo [236] states that the droplets do not seem to be extruded by the cells. Increased phospholipid content of the medullary tip falls to normal concomitant with the loss of droplets [267]. The hyperplastic collecting duct lesion in the outer medulla and inner cortex is less quickly and possibly less completely reversible [121].

Most cytochemical evidence of enzymatic changes in the kidneys of potassium-depleted rats has disappeared within one week after the start of potassium repletion [199]. The renal histopathologic changes in potassium-deficient rats will disappear (or be prevented) if rubidium is substituted for potassium [87, 211]. Potassium repletion restores renal architecture to normal rapidly in potassium-depleted mice [157]. And the droplet lesion disappears within one to three months (mainly in a few weeks) after woodchucks emerge from hibernation and begin to eat their normal spring and summer diet [39].

Despite the evidence just cited that renal damage in potassium-depleted rats is largely reversible, there are some potentially important contradictory findings. The first of these was reported in 1956 by Fourman et al. [92]. They produced severe potassium depletion in rats by combining a low-potassium diet with an ammonium-cycle, ion-exchange resin for eight weeks. After that, the rats were given a normal diet for seven months. At the end of the seven months' repletion period, the rats had severe renal damage and were azotemic. The kidneys were grossly enlarged. As shown in Figure 25-12, there was interstitial fibrosis, tubular atrophy, and gross dilatation of tubules. As can also be seen in Figure 25-12, there appeared to be an interstitial cellular reaction; if so, its cause is unknown. Quite reasonably, however, it leads to consideration of superimposed infection, a possibility that cannot be confirmed or refuted without bacteriologic cultures of urine or of renal tissue. (See the section *Effect of Potassium Deficiency on Pyelonephritis* below.)

At least five other studies suggest residual renal damage following potassium depletion [105, 121, 141, 178, 228]. In one of these, rats were repeatedly subjected to a potassium-depleting (and probably acidifying) regimen for the first four of every seven weeks during a period of nearly two years [178]. At the end of the 2-year period, there was mild but inconstant fibrosis of renal tissue. In a somewhat similar experiment, several groups of rats were placed on cyclic potassium-depleting–potassium-repleting regimens for a year [228]. The regimens were designed to produce different

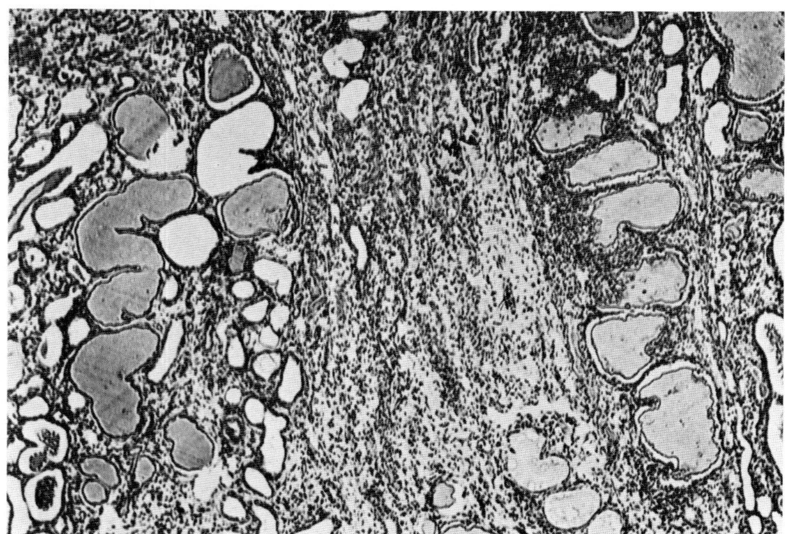

Figure 25-12. Fibrous scarring, gross tubular dilatation, and what appears to be interstitial inflammation in a rat kidney 7 months after recovery from a transient but severe episode of potassium depletion. (From Fourman, P., McCance, R. A., and Parker, R. A. [92].)

degrees of potassium deficiency (and presumably alkalosis) during a small part of each month. At the end all experimental groups showed renal tubular dilatation, and though this did not vary significantly between the experimental groups themselves, it was not found in controls. Segar and Schulz [228] state specifically that there was no interstitial fibrosis and no evidence of pyelonephritis. In still another experiment, fairly similar in design to that of Fourman et al., rats were made severely potassium deficient and alkalotic for four to five weeks, after which they received a normal diet for eight months [121]. Chemical data documented both the depleted and the repleted states. After eight months of repletion, there were occasional fibrous scars and a few rather grossly dilated tubules (Fig. 25-13), changes similar in type but far less severe than those found by Fourman et al. The rather mild histopathology was not seen in controls, however, thus excluding the possibility that it was merely the result of aging. There was no azotemia and no defect of renal concentrating ability. There were no inflammatory infiltrates. Bacterial cultures of one ground-up kidney from each rat were negative.

Thus, in five of six studies there were slight renal histopathologic changes as an apparent consequence of an earlier period of potassium depletion. The sixth study — that of Fourman et al. [92] — showed severe renal lesions and evidence of renal failure. In none had the kidneys returned wholly to normal, as judged by appropriate controls. Accordingly, it seems beyond reasonable doubt that, in the rat, potassium depletion may cause irreversible changes of renal structure. The significance of the changes cannot yet be assessed. As will be discussed in a later section, they could, even when mild, cause increased susceptibility to pyelonephritis.

REVERSIBILITY OF KALIOPENIC NEPHROPATHY IN MAN

There is, to our knowledge, no information about renal architecture following *experimental* potassium depletion in man. The little that can be said about reversibility of the structural features of kaliopenic nephropathy in humans is based on information obtained clinically. Thus, there are only a very few reports of renal biopsy specimens obtained from previously potassium-depleted patients. Also, as

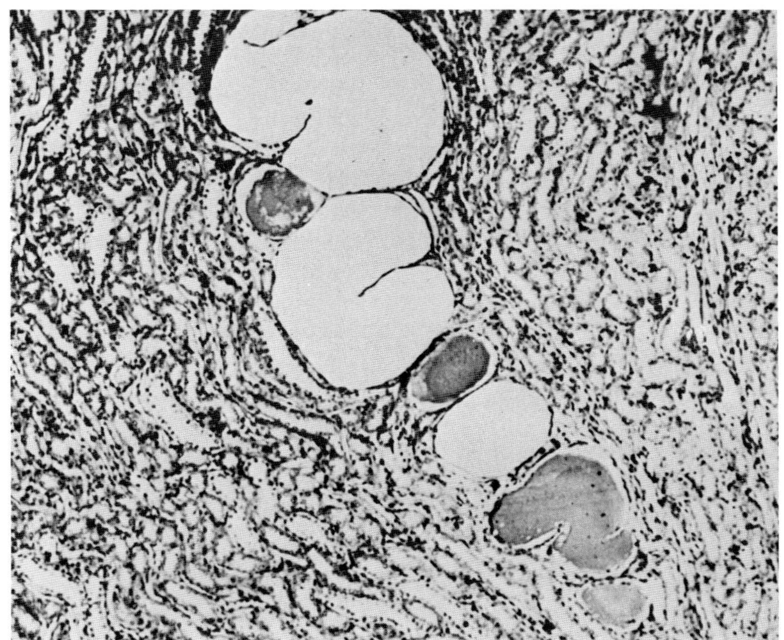

Figure 25-13. Gross dilatation of a renal tubule from a rat 8 months after a temporary period of potassium depletion had been corrected. No similar abnormalities were seen in controls. (From Hollander, W., Jr., et al. *Clin. Res.* [121].)

already discussed, there are many reports of renal tissue examined during a period of potassium depletion, which allows the renal pathologist an "educated guess" as to whether the renal structural changes found are of a sort likely to be wholly reversible and, if not, the probable nature of permanent damage. Obviously, the educated-guess approach is far from ideal.

De Graeff and Schuurs [63] have reported the interesting case of a young woman with chronic or intermittent potassium depletion as a result of taking laxatives excessively for at least eight years, at the end of which time she had severe chronic renal disease. The creatinine clearance was 10 to 15 ml. per minute, and there were renal histologic changes resembling chronic pyelonephritis despite many negative urine cultures. Seven years earlier, however, the urea clearance had been as low as 29 ml. per minute and the blood urea concentration as high as 150 mg. per 100 ml., so it is difficult to state with confidence that the patient did not have chronic pyelonephritis, or another form of chronic renal disease, in addition to potassium-depletion nephropathy. It is also of interest that, when renal insufficiency was far advanced, this patient developed renal potassium-wasting as an additional cause for potassium depletion.

We are aware of four patients from whom renal tissue was obtained and examined both during and several months following a period of potassium depletion [44, 48, 201, 210]. All specimens were obtained by biopsy. The potassium deficiency and its repair appear to have been adequately documented in all. In three, the potassium deficit was secondary to chronic losses via the gastrointestinal tract [201, 210]. One patient was the original case of primary aldosteronism described by Conn [44, 45, 48]. When the patients were potassium-depleted, the renal cortex of all four showed vacuolar changes of tubular epithelium. Some months after potassium repletion was achieved, renal cortical tissue of all four was free of vacuolation [44, 48, 201, 210]. Residual abnormalities of renal architecture, whether or not a consequence of the potassium deficiency, were seen in two of the four patients. In one of the patients whose potassium deficit was secondary to losses from the digestive tract, there were what were then (1956) called pyelonephritic scars [210]. In the renal tissue from the patient whose potassium deficiency had developed as a result of primary aldosteronism, there were some moderately advanced arteriosclerotic changes, which were thought to be essentially unchanged from that seen when the patient was potassium deficient — that is, at the time of surgery for removal of the adrenal adenoma [44]. It is important to stress two things in particular: (1) four cases are not enough; and (2) the residual changes in two of the four cannot be attributed to the earlier episode of potassium depletion but also such a causal relationship cannot be convincingly excluded.

In summary, it seems likely that the primary lesions of the renal tubular epithelium are reversbile in humans and in laboratory animals, but that secondary changes, such as fibrous scarring and tubular dilatation, may be irreversible. The rate at which the latter events occur is almost certainly dependent on the duration of potassium deficiency and probably on the degree of depletion as well; however, unequivocal evidence on these points is lacking. Whether or not potassium depletion is ever solely responsible for serious chronic renal disease and renal insufficiency in humans is not known.

Effect of Potassium Deficiency on Pyelonephritis

MAN

The possibility that potassium depletion may increase susceptibility to pyelonephritis was suggested more than a decade ago [73, 167, 181]. Since then, it has been the subject of several studies and much discussion, but its validity remains uncertain [110, 111, 178, 180, 183, 234, 236]. It is obviously important since, if true, it could be the origin of *chronic* pyelonephritis, in which case it would clearly be among the most serious consequences of potassium deficiency. Before going further, we should make it clear that by pyelonephritis we mean an inflammatory disease of the kidney *of infectious origin* [13, 40].

The major reason for continued uncertainty is that the available tools for proving or disproving this vital question are not adequate. There is increasing recognition that chronic pyelonephritis is usually very difficult to diagnose solely from histopathologic evidence [5, 13, 40, 98, 111, 112, 183, 191, 198, 206]. The difficulties have been examined recently, thoroughly, and critically, by Heptinstall [112] and by Freedman in Chapter 18 of this volume. In essence, chronic pyelonephritis cannot ordinarily be diagnosed without corroborative evidence of positive urine, renal biopsy, or renal postmortem cultures. Such evidence has not generally been reported in cases purporting to show pyelonephritis in potassium-depleted patients. This difficulty is compounded by studies (previously discussed) which suggest the possibility that potassium deficiency itself may sometimes cause nonspecific, irreversible structural changes in the human kidney resembling those commonly associated with chronic pyelonephritis [111, 112, 180, 183, 234; see also Chapter 18]. Another is the occasional instance of chronic pyelonephritis apparently causing renal potassium-wasting (discussed above under *Pathogenesis*).

A second serious deficiency of available methodology is that, even when chronic pyelonephritis and potassium depletion both seem well documented, it is rarely possible to know which came first. An example of this was noted in Chapter 21 of the previous edition of this book. On reviewing 20 cases in the literature with unequivocal potassium depletion and with at least one reason for *suspecting* pyelonephritis [9, 10, 28, 33, 63, 69, 131, 145,

146, 151, 168, 181, 204, 210, 211, 265], there was evidence in at least five of the 20 that pyelonephritis may have been present before the potassium deficiency [9, 10, 28, 131, 146].

A final obstacle, but no less important, is our inadequate knowledge of the prevalence of chronic pyelonephritis in an appropriate control population. We are in the odd position of trying to determine the frequency of pyelonephritis in potassium-deficient patients without knowing its true prevalence in similar individuals who are not potassium-depleted.

Despite these serious handicaps, there have been several attempts to study the question in man and in animals. In 1960 Muehrcke [178] reported the startling finding of chronic pyelonephritis in 12 of 18 patients with chronic potassium depletion. Although the presence of pyelonephritis was based on histopathologic evidence, an infectious etiology was clearly implied. More recently, as the inadequacy of histopathologic evidence alone has been increasingly appreciated, Muehrcke and associates [180, 183] have placed quotation marks around "pyelonephritis" and have, themselves, pointed out that it is quite possible that the histopathology commonly associated with chronic pyelonephritis in patients with prolonged potassium deficiency results from etiologies other than bacterial infection [180]. Heptinstall [111] has emphasized the same point: "Scars in the cortex may be present in which the glomeruli are sclerotic, the tubules lost or atrophic, and the interstitial tissue fibrosed with or without chronic inflammatory cells. Although these scars may represent chronic infection and are eagerly seized on by those seeking to demonstrate that potassium deficiency predisposes the kidney to infection, they are equally likely to be the result of ischemia, especially in the older age groups."

Thus, the crucial question about potassium-depleted patients with these nonspecific findings is whether it has been possible to establish renal infection as the cause or even as an associated condition of the histopathologic findings. The answer is a qualified "no." The qualification stems largely from a report by Muehrcke and McMillan [180]; the "no" stems from scattered, mostly inadequate data in the literature and from a study by Muehrcke and Rosen [183].

More than a decade ago Relman and Schwartz [211] suggested that pyelonephritis was a more common complication in potassium depletion of primary aldosteronism than in that resulting from gastrointestinal disorders. More recently, after reviewing their own data and that in the literature, these same authors [212, 226] have said that they could not find convincing evidence for an increased frequency of pyelonephritis with potassium depletion of any etiology, except possibly with primary aldosteronism, which, as they note, is commonly complicated by hypertensive vascular disease and consequent interstitial scars resembling chronic pyelonephritis. Relman and Schwartz [212, 226] conclude that the problem is simply unresolved. We agree.

LABORATORY ANIMALS — RATS

Although studies of this problem in laboratory animals do not yield an unequivocal answer, they are clearer than the data from man. Woods et al. [270, 271] have shown that, in rats, susceptibility to experimental hematogenous pyelonephritis with *Escherichia coli* is markedly increased both during and seven months after an episode of potassium depletion. In contrast, Carone et al. [30] found no increased susceptibility of potassium-depleted rats to an injection of a different strain of *E. coli.* They also showed that, using a particular strain of enterococcus, potassium-depleted rats had a general decrease in resistance to hematogenous infection that was as definite in extrarenal organs as in the kidneys [30]. Muehrcke and his colleagues have reported equivocal results [178].

We are aware of two studies in which potassium-depleted rats were shown not to have any increase in *spontaneous* renal infection.

One of these was at the end of a three-months' potassium-depleting regimen [236]; the other involved culture of one whole kidney during and many months after a four-week episode of severe potassium depletion [121].

In summary, there is equivocal evidence implicating potassium depletion as a predisposing factor to the development of infectious pyelonephritis in man. There is, moreover, some support for this concept from studies on potassium-depleted rats. Unfortunately, the latter are less meaningful because of different structural lesions. We can only conclude that there is a definite need for more studies in man, and these should be prospective and should include properly matched control patients.

Renal Physiology

URINARY CONCENTRATION

The most striking alteration of renal function resulting from potassium depletion, consistently found in all potassium-depleted species studied, is impairment of the urinary concentrating function. This has been increasingly evident since first described in 1953 [225]. In retrospect, it may well have caused the diabetes insipidus syndrome noted in DOCA-treated dogs described in 1940 and 1941 by Ferrebee [82], Ragan [207], and Mulinos [184] and their associates. However, the data they reported do not exclude — and to some extent suggest — an increased rate of water turnover that was not completely ascribable to potassium depletion [118]. Subsequently, in 1950, Smith and Lasater [233] described a similar diabetes insipidus condition in dogs eating a potassium-deficient diet and *not* receiving DOCA or any other similar steroids; however, primary polydipsia (as opposed to primary polyuria) could not be excluded. In 1953 Brokaw [22] demonstrated a markedly augmented water turnover in rats fed a potassium-deficient diet, but she also showed an apparently *normal* renal concentrating power. The latter conclusion was, from today's vantage point, almost surely wrong, perhaps because the method of testing maximal urinary concentration did not eliminate evaporation during the collection of urine [123].

Also in 1953, Schwartz and Relman [210, 225] showed a clear-cut urinary concentrating defect in humans, almost surely due to potassium depletion, and there have now been numerous well-documented studies supporting their conclusion. Impairment of urinary concentrating capacity has been shown repeatedly in rats experimentally depleted of potassium as illustrated in Figure 25-14 [7, 24, 77, 103, 123, 127, 139, 166, 167, 214, 254]. The only contrary, and unexplained, result, in the rat, known to the authors is the report of Manitius and Epstein [165] that rats with experimentally induced *magnesium* deficiency (which in turn causes *potassium* depletion) have normal urinary concentrating power despite low concentrations of potassium in skeletal muscle *and in the renal medulla.* A urinary concentrating defect has also been shown in experimentally potassium-deficient dogs [100], hamsters [103], and humans [219]. It almost surely occurs in potassium-depleted rabbits, though the evidence presented is not wholly convincing [143]. It probably is a consequence of potassium deficiency in toads, as judged by in vitro studies of the bladders from toads experimentally depleted of potassium in vivo [273]. The latter conclusion is supported by two of three other experiments in which potassium concentration was lowered in the fluid bathing the serosal surface of bladders from normal toads [14, 84, 106].

The degree to which renal concentrating capacity is impaired is probably a function of both the duration and the severity of the potassium deficit. As most studies have not been designed to separate the effects of these two normally interrelated variables, it has not generally been possible to ascertain their effects

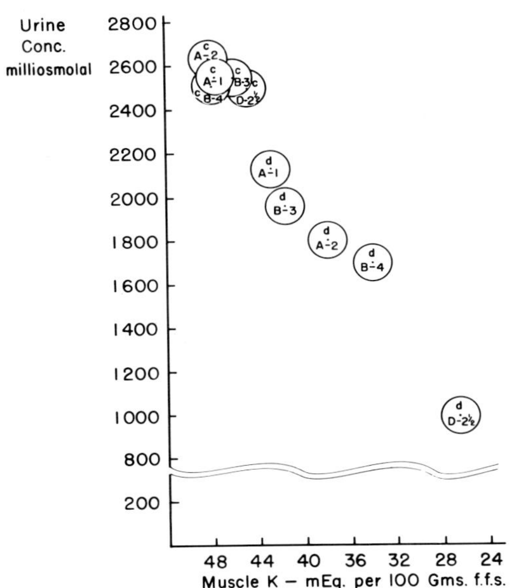

Figure 25-14. Data from several experiments in which rats were depleted of potassium and tested for maximal achievable urine concentration. Each potassium-depleted group (*d*) had a simultaneously studied control group (*c*). The large letters within the circles designate different experiments, whereas the arabic numerals indicate the number of weeks on the potassium-depleting regimen. Muscle potassium concentration is expressed as milliequivalents per 100 gm. of fat-free dry solids (f.f.s.). Maximal urine concentration was tested by freezing point determinations on urine collected under oil for 8 to 12 hours, beginning approximately 5 hours after the subcutaneous injection of 50 milliunits of vasopressin in oil. (From Hollander, W., Jr., et al. [123].)

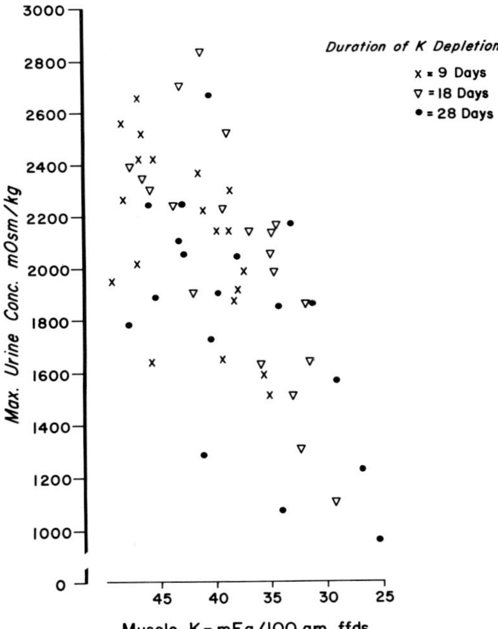

Figure 25-15. Maximal urinary concentration of rats depleted of potassium to varying degrees over 9-day (X), 18-day (▽), and 28-day (●) periods. Statistical analysis indicates that maximal urine concentration was highly correlated with degree of potassium deficiency and only slightly with the duration of the potassium-depleting regimen. (Not previously reproduced. Reported as abstract by Warner, J. F., and Hollander, W., Jr., *Clin. Res.* 10:257, 1962 [254].

independent of each other. In the rat, however, Warner and Hollander [253, 254] have performed two studies specifically designed to examine the relative importance of degree and of duration of potassium depletion on the urinary concentrating defect. The results show a clear relation of the severity of the urinary concentrating defect to the intensity but not the duration of the potassium deficit (Fig. 25-15). These results conflict with those of Holliday et al. [128].

The renal concentrating defect in rats experimentally depleted of potassium does not depend on the coexisting acid-base status [122, 123, 128]. Also, in rats, it is not merely the consequence of primary polydipsia [20], though, as discussed on page 961, primary polydipsia may occur. The renal concentrating impairment has been demonstrated by measurements of maximum urinary concentration not only at normal rates of solute excretion but also during a solute diuresis.

Urinary concentration in the toad, *Bufo marinus*, is accomplished by the antidiuretic hormone of that species acting on the urinary bladder to produce net water transport in excess of solute from the mucosal to the serosal side. The maximum concentration of urine, however, is isotonic, not hypertonic. Yount et al. [273] have shown that such vasopressin-induced net water transport is depressed in toads made potassium-deficient in vivo, as judged by in vitro studies of their urinary bladders.* In an earlier study, Bentley [14] showed a urinary concentrating defect when bladders from normal toads were studied in vitro with a low potassium concentration in the bathing solution on the serosal, but not on the mucosal, side. A similar result has been found by Finn et al. [84] using the lucite chamber technic. In addition, they showed that the decreased sodium transport, which also occurs with low serosal potassium concentration and which is also dependent on antidiuretic hormone, did not explain the diminished net water transport. The failure to link the effect of low potassium concentration on net water transport to a depressed sodium transport has also been confirmed by Bentley's method using choline rather than sodium chloride on the mucosal surface [119].

As with other animals, potassium depletion in humans causes an impairment of urinary concentrating ability as the most prominent and consistent renal physiologic defect. Among 48 patients with reasonably certain potassium deficiency in whom urinary concentrating ability was specifically tested — and who were previously cited in the first edition of this book [118] — only four [56, 83, 259, 265] had approximately normal maximal urinary concentration [3, 9–12, 23, 28, 35, 45, 46, 52, 56, 57, 72, 73, 83, 102, 108, 113, 116, 120, 130, 146, 151, 156, 162, 168, 169, 196, 204, 210, 225, 230, 248, 249, 258, 259, 265]. These were all patients with spontaneous potassium deficiency secondary to gastrointestinal losses or excess endogenous or exogenous steroids. In a separate group of seven patients with potassium depletion of less certain etiology, only one [29] had reasonably normal urinary concentrating power [23, 29, 74, 160, 163, 221, 242, 272]. In most cases, maximum specific gravity was less than 1.015. A new tabulation has not been made in view of the convincing nature of the previously cited data [118]. It is still noteworthy, however, that some of the patients mentioned may have had superimposed or preexisting pyelonephritis; if so, the impaired renal concentrating ability could have been wholly or partially secondary to that disorder.

In one case reported by Kleeman and Maxwell [146] it was suggested that potassium deficiency had caused a temporary episode of true diabetes insipidus, a possibility that has received little attention in other studies. However, in at least two investigations [123, 222], maximal achievable urinary concentration of potassium-depleted rats was approximately the same when tested by water deprivation as when tested with exogenous vasopressin.

Impaired urinary concentrating ability in humans is a completely reversible abnormality in many instances. Recent data indicate, however, that this may not always be so. Furthermore, we do not know how often the reversibility is complete; the role played by the degree or duration of the potassium deficit; the importance, if any, of other conditions concomitant with the potassium depletion; or the frequency with which superimposed pyelonephritis, not the potassium deficit itself, is the limiting factor.

The renal concentrating defect has been rapidly and completely correctable in the experimentally potassium-deficient rat [121, 167] and dog [100]. It was equally reversible in the one instance (to our knowledge) in which renal concentrating capacity has been studied in *experimentally* potassium-depleted humans [219]. In the first edition of this book [118] it was noted that 11 cases had been found in which renal concentrating ability returned to normal in from 1½ months to four years after correction of a spontaneously occurring potassium deficit. In most of these, normal maximal urinary concentration was achieved within one year following potassium repletion [11, 52, 73,

* Sequential bladder weighing method of Bentley [14].

108, 116, 120, 130, 225, 247]. It was also noted that 19 examples of a renal concentrating defect associated with potassium depletion had, at the time of the report, only partial restoration of urinary concentrating power [1, 3, 45, 46, 52, 57, 72, 113, 146, 156, 163, 196, 204, 210, 230, 258]. The follow-up period at that time was, for most of the patients, less than six months, but in one instance the interval since the documented episode of potassium deficiency was five years [1, 2]. Finally, there were three case reports indicating essentially no improvement in urinary concentrating power following potassium repletion; however, in one of these the problem appeared to be complicated by chronic pyelonephritis [168], in one the initial impairment was slight and the duration of follow-up study uncertain [9], and in the third the interval since surgical removal of an aldosterone-secreting adenoma had been only 10 weeks [35].

No effort has been made to determine initial and follow-up urinary concentrating ability in the numerous patients (particularly with primary aldosteronism) reported since the first edition. An attempt has been made, however, to obtain more recent follow-up data regarding the urinary concentrating defect in the patients previously reported. In patient one of the three patients reported by Dustan et al. [71, 72] in 1956 the maximum specific gravity 10 years after removal of an aldosterone-secreting adenoma was only 1.017, not significantly different from the preoperative and early postoperative values. Patient F. C., one of the patients originally reported by Relman and Schwartz [210] in 1956 about whom there is significantly later data regarding urinary concentrating ability, is reported as having a specific gravity of 1.021 in 1961 [155]. In one of the two patients studied by Crane et al. in 1956 and 1958 [56, 57], a recent test of renal concentrating power still showed considerable impairment [55]. The same is true for the patient reported by Chalmers et al. in 1956 [34, 35] and that of Achor and Smith [2, 231]. In contrast, several of those reported as having impaired renal concentrating capacity in the first edition of this book apparently now function normally in this regard. This is true of the case reported by Hellem [107, 108] and that of Ortuzar and associates [195, 196]. Thus, there are now at least five patients in whom some impairment of urinary concentrating power has persisted for many years after presumed potassium repletion.

The mechanism by which potassium depletion impairs the urinary concentrating mechanism is uncertain. Basically, there are two general possibilities: (1) failure of tubular fluid water to equilibrate with interstitial fluid as tubular urine courses through the collecting ducts; and (2) some aberration of or relating to the countercurrent multiplier and exchanger systems which ordinarily cause markedly elevated interstitial fluid tonicity in the renal medulla and papilla with which collecting duct urine comes into equilibrium (see Chapter 2).

In some early studies of this problem, the finding of distinct histologic lesions in the collecting ducts of potassium-depleted rats led to the suggestion that these lesions and the concentrating defect were related, specifically that the permeability of the collecting ducts to water was diminished [192]. Most subsequent studies of this subject, however, have left the matter unsettled. Furthermore, it is now well established that man also acquires a significant urinary concentrating defect as a consequence of potassium depletion, but essentially all evidence to date suggests that there are no histologic lesions in the collecting ducts of potassium-depleted humans (see above in section on *Structural Changes*).

There has been one study using potassium-depleted hamsters in which it was demonstrated that there was osmotic equilibrium between collecting duct fluid, loop of Henle fluid, and blood from the vasa recta at any particular level of the renal papilla [103]. This was true in the nondiuretic state as well as during an osmotic diuresis caused by mannitol. Thus, for the hamster, the urinary concentrating defect caused by potassium depletion is not due to impaired water permeability across the collecting ducts. For technical reasons similar experimental data are not available for other species.

The possibility of impaired water movement across the collecting duct or distal convolution (or both) of the potassium-depleted dog and man is suggested by the fact that, in these species, during maximal antidiuretic activity, a solute diuresis of only *modest* proportions causes the urine to become more dilute than plasma [100, 219]. This is in contrast to what occurs in the potassium-deficient rat and hamster in which, under similar conditions, $[U/P]_{OSM}$ approaches but never goes below one even during a marked solute diuresis [85, 103, 126, 139]. This fact, however, does not necessarily imply unusual osmotic disequilibrium in some portion of the distal nephron of potassium-deficient dogs and primates, since micropuncture data demonstrate that, in contrast to that of the rodent, tubular fluid in the distal convoluted tubule of the normal dog and subhuman primate does not reach osmotic equilibrium even in the absence of a solute diuresis and with full vasopressin activity (see Chapter 2).

Manitius and his associates [166] attempted to distinguish between the several possible explanations for the urinary concentrating defect by studying the composition of the renal papilla and medulla in potassium-depleted rats and dogs during hydropenia. The concentration of sodium in the papilla and medulla, expressed in relation to dry tissue solids as well as to tissue water, was lower than that of control animals, thereby supporting the concept of an impaired countercurrent mechanism in the loops of Henle or the vasa recta (or both). On the other hand, the ratio of urinary solute concentration to papillary sodium concentration or to *calculated* papillary solute concentration was lower than that in control animals, which is compatible with an impaired permeability of the collecting duct or distal convolution to water.

In a somewhat similar study, Eigler et al. [77] measured electrolyte concentrations in small consecutive portions (less than 2 mg. per sample) of renal tissue of potassium-depleted, hydropenic rats. Their method was based on the principle of specific activities. They found the expected decrease in maximal urinary concentration and a proportionate or slightly greater decrease of sodium concentration in the renal papilla [77]. These results strongly support the concept of a deranged countercurrent system and lend no support to the concept of impaired water diffusion across the epithelium of collecting ducts or distal convoluted tubules.

Using a quantitative histochemical technic, Wilson and Kissane [266] found a lower renal papillary sodium concentration per unit of dry tissue in potassium-depleted rats than in pair-fed controls. Interpretation is uncertain, however, because the rats had been subjected to 42 hours of water restriction, which might well have caused a disproportionate depression of glomerular filtration rate in the potassium-deficient rats, thereby causing a similarly disproportionate impaired delivery of sodium and urea to the loops of Henle. With ad libitum water intake or with an acute water load, renal papillary sodium concentration was the same in potassium-depleted as in control rats. Measurements of urinary sodium concentration or osmolality were not reported.

Studies have been performed in which the urinary diluting capacity of rats has been used to demonstrate the improbability of any failure of sodium reabsorption in the ascending limb of the loop of Henle. In general, diluting capacity of potassium-depleted rats has been essentially the same as that of controls — as judged by the osmolality of fluid taken from the early distal convolution [7, 103], or from dilution of the finally formed urine [103, 127, 128, 156]. In fact, this finding does not exclude some impairment of sodium reabsorption at an earlier portion of the ascending limb. Furthermore, there is one study by Holliday and Egan [125] in which capacity to form dilute urine was less in potassium-deficient rats than in controls (p less than 0.05). The difference disappeared when potassium depletion was corrected [125]. In addition, a definite diluting defect has been demonstrated in experimentally potassium-depleted humans, although it did not become clearly evident until impairment of the urinary concentrating mechanism was apparent [219].

There are now a number of studies that make it unlikely that the concentrating defect is caused by a solute diuresis [7, 100, 103, 123, 219]. On the contrary, there have been two studies of potassium-deficient rats which suggest a decreased delivery of solute to the loops of Henle as at least one reason for their deranged urinary concentrating function [7, 139]. In one [139], the conclusion is based on the finding of a net increase in urea reabsorption by the proximal portion of nephrons associated with prolonged urea transit times. In the other [7], the authors ascribe what they believe to be diminished delivery of solute to to loops of Henle resulting from a modest and statistically questionable decrease of glomerular filtration rate (GFR) — or to an increased proximal sodium reabsorption in some way a consequence of decreased intracellular potassium in the proximal tubular epithelium. One argument that might be used against this hypothesis is the fact that the impaired renal concentrating mechanism is not corrected when ample solute is delivered to the loops of Henle during a solute diuresis [7, 24].

There are several reports showing by use of electron microscopy that there are osmophilic bodies markedly encroaching on the lumen of capillaries deep in the medulla and papilla of potassium-depleted rats (Fig. 25-5) [161, 236, 267]. This could mean diminished blood flow in that area, but if so, one would expect increased rather than decreased interstitial osmolality. It is possible, however, that such an impairment of blood flow could lead to increased arteriovenous shunting of blood in more proximal regions of the renal medulla, thereby impairing the countercurrent exchange role of the vasa recta. In that event, diminished osmolality of the renal interstitial medulla could be explained. To our knowledge, there are as yet no adequate data to confirm or refute this concept in potassium-depleted animals, primarily because of methodological deficiencies.

In summary, then, it is well established that potassium depletion causes a decreased osmolality in the renal medulla and papilla of laboratory animals, primarily rodents. Except for one study on hamsters, there are no data that conclusively rule out impaired water reabsorption from the collecting ducts. There is a preponderance of evidence implicating an aberration of some aspect of the countercurrent concentrating mechanism, but there is also some evidence suggesting decreased water permeability across the collecting ducts.

URINARY ACIDIFICATION AND BICARBONATE EXCRETION

Impaired bicarbonate excretion in association with potassium depletion has been demonstrated experimentally in dogs [101], rats [50], and humans [17, 86, 148, 216, 217], and consequently, the kidneys of a potassium-depleted, alkalotic individual often excrete urine which is inappropriately acid. The urinary pH is frequently less than 7.0, a fact which has led to the term *paradoxical aciduria*, an expression which might more appropriately be used merely to imply that acid excretion and bicarbonate reabsorption are greater than what the extracellular acid-base status would ordinarily dictate.

Since there is evidence to support the hypothesis that the secretion of potassium and hydrogen by the distal portion of the nephron is, in some manner, competitive [15], the concept has arisen that the relatively increased excretion of acid in potassium depletion is due to a deficiency of potassium in the renal tubular cells and the resultant absolute or relative increased availability of hydrogen ions within these cells. Consistent with this idea are the observations that a large intake of sodium bicarbonate in the absence of potassium depletion may produce little or no alkalosis [50, 250] and, furthermore, that the administration of sodium chloride may not correct the alkalosis associated with potassium depletion [58].

In recent years, however, several types of observations have been reported which make it unlikely that this explanation is the entire one. First of all, it has been shown that chloride depletion plays an important role in the alkalosis of potassium deficiency [6, 140]. Kassirer and Schwartz have demonstrated that removal of hydrochloric acid by gastric drainage leads to the development of persistent metabolic alkalosis and an elevated renal threshold for bicarbonate in the absence of potassium depletion [140]. They showed further that when alkalosis is produced by gastric drainage and potassium deficiency is allowed to occur, the administration of sodium chloride results in a rise in urinary pH, a reduction in urinary acid excretion, and a fall in plasma bicarbonate concentration. It is thus clear that chloride depletion perhaps plays a more critical role in the impaired renal excretion of bicarbonate and the production of metabolic alkalosis than does deficiency of potassium per se — at least in the order of magnitude of the usual clinical situation of potassium depletion.

In primary aldosteronism and other types of steroid-induced potassium depletion, the urinary pH tends to be somewhat more alkaline than in other forms of potassium deficiency, though not consistently greater than 7.0 as has been suggested [72, 113]. This might be expected since in this situation renal excretion of potassium remains relatively high (greater than 20 mEq. per 24 hours, frequently much greater) despite potassium concentrations in serum of less than 3.0 mEq. per liter and despite presumably low levels of potassium within renal tubular cells [9, 10, 12, 23, 35, 45, 46, 52, 56, 73, 94, 102, 108, 114, 116, 130, 162, 168, 169, 196, 223, 230, 259]. This is in contrast to the generally low rate of urinary potassium excretion, usually less than 15 mEq. per 24 hours, observed in patients whose potassium depletion is due to losses of gastrointestinal fluid [3, 36, 43, 69, 131, 146, 158, 210, 225, 262, 265] and in human subjects whose potassium depletion is induced experimentally [17, 18, 41, 81, 89, 208, 269].

Despite the fact that acid excretion is greater than might be expected in patients with potassium depletion, there is evidence suggesting that there is also a limited ability to acidify the urine. This concept is derived primarily from studies by Clarke and his associates [41] in which acidosis was produced in previously potassium-depleted subjects as well as in control subjects by the administration of ammonium chloride. A lesser fall in urinary pH and a higher final urinary pH were observed in the potassium-depleted subjects. They also noted that urinary pH increased when potassium depletion was superimposed on already existing metabolic acidosis. On the basis of these observations, together with measurements of titratable acidity during an infusion of neutral sodium phosphate, the authors reasoned that potassium depletion limits the maximal hydrogen ion gradient but not the maximal rate of hydrogen ion excretion. Rubini and his co-workers [220] also administered ammonium chloride to experimentally potassium-depleted subjects and also noted a less acid urine as well as a smaller increment in titratable acidity than they observed in control subjects.

Potassium depletion is associated with a greater excretion of ammonium ions than is normally expected at the almost neutral urinary pH which is usually present. This has been noted in several studies of experimental potassium depletion in humans [41, 220, 238, 269], in two patients with potassium depletion resulting from losses of gastrointestinal fluid [225], and in primary aldosteronism [73, 168, 240]. The augmented excretion of ammonium has been ascribed to the elevated levels of glutaminase found in the kidneys of potassium-depleted animals [134].

The findings are not consistent in regard to the effect of potassium depletion on the excretion of organic acids. There is evidence suggesting that excretion of organic acids is diminished in rats and humans [41, 82, 93]. In contrast, the excretion of organic acids did not change significantly during the development or repair of potassium depletion and alkalosis in dogs [6].

SODIUM EXCRETION

Potassium depletion is generally associated with retention of sodium which exceeds the negative balance of potassium [17, 18, 78, 132, 135, 208, 209]. Some of the retained sodium replaces potassium lost from cells [49], and some is associated with an expanded extracellular volume [17, 18, 37, 38, 53, 78, 109, 135, 185, 229, 269], although frank edema is unusual [261]. The explanation for the extracellular expansion is not entirely clear. Except in cases of primary aldosteronism and other forms of steroid-induced potassium depletion it cannot be ascribed to increased secretion of aldosterone, since potassium depletion per se appears to diminish secretion of this hormone [137]. Since some, usually minor, depression of GFR is common in association with potassium depletion, the associated decrease in filtered load of sodium may be the primary cause in some instances [205]. However, recently Lennon and Lemann [153] have produced evidence suggesting that potassium depletion may cause increased fractional reabsorption of sodium, chloride, and water by the proximal tubules. These investigators produced potassium depletion and metabolic acidosis in two groups of human subjects by administering ammonium chloride. One group of subjects was allowed to recover from acidosis while eating diets containing normal amounts of potassium, and the other group recovered while eating diets with very low potassium contents. The two groups gained weight and retained sodium and chloride at the same rates during the immediate recovery period; during this time the group with normal potassium intakes restored their potassium deficits and the other group remained potassium depleted. In the subsequent recovery days, the subjects who had restored body potassium stores to normal had a diuresis and sodium and chloride balances returned to control values. In contrast, the subjects who remained potassium-depleted retained additional quantities of sodium and chloride and actually developed pitting edema in spite of the facts that the creatinine clearances increased and aldosterone excretion rates decreased. Furthermore, if the investigators used changes in the sum of urinary net acid plus potassium excretion as an index of sodium reabsorption at distal tubular sites, they concluded that the increased reabsorption of sodium, chloride, and water occurred at the proximal tubular level, since the net acid plus potassium excretion rates decreased. This latter postulation is in keeping with the finding of Bank and Aynedjian [7] of increased fractional reabsorption of solute and water in the proximal tubules of potassium-depleted rats.

As regards the effects of potassium depletion on renal sodium-conserving ability, potassium depletion does not ordinarily prevent the excretion of an essentially sodium-free urine under conditions stimulating maximal sodium conservation [10, 11, 63, 128, 225, 238]. However, it has been shown in the dog and the rat that potassium depletion is associated with small negative balances of sodium when these animals are ingesting sodium-free diets [166], and there is a report of a patient with chronic renal disease and potassium-wasting in whom intermittent impairment of sodium conservation was thought to be due to potassium depletion [163].

POTASSIUM CONSERVATION

Essentially all evidence indicates that potassium depletion does not impair renal conservation of potassium [49, 50, 69, 76, 88, 135, 148, 194, 210, 225, 235]. Indeed, renal potassium excretion apparently remains low even in the face of stimuli, such as acute bicarbonate loading, that normally cause a rise in potassium excretion [41, 50, 81]. Micropuncture studies in the dog and the rat indicate that the conservation of potassium results from large adjustments in the distal rather than the proximal portion of the nephron [164, 256, 257].

REABSORPTION OF GLUCOSE, PHOSPHATE, AND AMINO ACIDS

Renal tubular glucose reabsorption is normal in potassium-depleted dogs [100, 176], and renal glycosuria has not been a feature of potassium depletion in humans. The data concerning tubular reabsorption of phosphate are conflicting, but they mostly suggest that it is unaltered [49, 50, 88, 115, 171, 215].

Although aminoaciduria has been reported as a feature of potassium depletion in several cases [66, 242], it has not been found in many others. Urinary amino acids have been reported as normal in primary aldosteronism [73, 248, 249]. The urinary excretion of amino acids has not been well studied in potassium-depleted animals.

GLOMERULAR FILTRATION RATES AND RENAL BLOOD FLOW

Changes in the GFR usually are not striking in potassium deficiency. The GFR has been found normal in experimental potassium depletion in human subjects [90, 269], normal or slightly depressed in patients with steroid-induced potassium depletion [11, 12, 23, 29, 35, 45, 46, 64, 72, 73, 83, 102, 108, 113, 130, 162, 168, 196, 230, 248, 249] as well as in patients with gastrointestinal causes for their potassium depletion [69, 158, 210, 225, 262].

In dogs, the creatinine clearance has been reported to remain constant or fall slightly with potassium depletion [100, 177], and in rats potassium depletion appears to cause a slight reduction in creatinine clearance [186] and inulin clearance [127, 128]. However, none of these studies is conclusive since there was simultaneous protein depletion.

The clearance of para-aminohippurate (PAH) is often minimally depressed in potassium-depleted patients [35, 64, 72, 151, 162, 210, 225], but this depression is probably a reflection of the decreased excretion of organic anions, discussed earlier, or of a specific defect in the extraction and secretion of PAH [162, 225, 245]. A similar mechanism presumably explains the frequently encountered moderate suppression of phenol red excretion [31, 52, 56, 116, 156, 210, 225, 258].

URINARY SEDIMENT

When the nephropathy of potassium depletion is not complicated by other renal disease, there is usually slight or no proteinuria, and the urinary sediment is generally unremarkable except for occasional red cells, leukocytes, and/or casts.

Relation of Alkalosis to Renal Abnormalities

Inasmuch as potassium depletion is commonly associated with an extracellular alkalosis, it is pertinent to consider what, if any, role the alkalosis itself may play in the renal damage and altered renal function associated with potassium depletion. In the past, alkalosis has been thought to be a cause of impaired renal function [25, 26]. However, extracellular alkalosis is commonly, if not invariably, accompanied by a potassium deficit, and it is at least possible that potassium depletion (plus undoubted dehydration and sodium depletion in some instances) has been responsible for the diminished renal function previously attributed to alkalosis.

In a previous review [261], it was pointed out that potassium depletion with alkalosis did not seem to cause any structural changes in the rat kidney which were not also seen when potassium deficiency was associated with acidosis, and that the renal structural damage and renal functional changes in patients with potassium depletion and a prominent degree of alkalosis were not obviously different than those in patients whose potassium deficiency was accompanied by little or no alkalosis. Newton et al. [189], using rats, have produced severe metabolic alkalosis without significant potassium depletion, and the kidneys from these rats are reported as having no lesions different from those found in comparably treated nonalkalotic controls. Although this finding supports the hypothesis that alkalosis is not damaging to the kidneys, the evidence it provides relates solely to microscopic structure and does not provide any direct evidence with respect to renal function.

Polyuria and Polydipsia

Polyuria and polydipsia are frequent accompaniments of potassium depletion, and two important questions concerning their significance have arisen: (1) Is the renal concentrating defect secondary to the intake of large quantities of water? (2) Is the polydipsia a consequence of the renal concentrating defect or is it an effect of potassium depletion per se?

There is precedent for raising the first question since it has been shown that excessive water intake may diminish concentrating ability [8, 67, 80, 147]. However, it has been shown in the rat that the concentration defect of potassium depletion is not affected by restriction of water intake [20].

As has been noted by several authors [68, 91, 240, 261], there is circumstantial evidence supporting the hypothesis that the polydipsia of potassium deficiency is a primary effect of potassium depletion; however, attempts at answering the question experimentally have failed to support the hypothesis [19, 268], and the question remains open.

Acknowledgment

The authors' investigations have been supported by grants from the American Heart Association and from the National Institutes of Health, U.S. Public Health Service.

References

1. Achor, R. W. P. Personal communication, 1960, regarding case reported in reference 2.
2. Achor, R. W. P., and Smith, L. A. Nutritional deficiency syndrome with diarrhea resulting in hypopotassemia, muscle degeneration and renal insufficiency; report of a case with recovery. *Proc. Mayo Clin.* 30: 207, 1955.
3. Aitchison, J. D. Hypokalaemia following chronic diarrhoea from overuse of cascara and a deficient diet. *Lancet* 2:75, 1958.
4. Allen, A. C. *The Kidney: Medical and Surgical Diseases* (2d ed.). New York: Grune & Stratton, 1962. P. 324.
5. Angell, M. E., Relman, A. S., and Robbins, S. L. "Active" chronic pyelonephritis without evidence of bacterial infection. *New Eng. J. Med.* 278:1303, 1968.

6. Atkins, E. L., and Schwartz, W. B. Factors governing correction of the alkalosis associated with potassium deficiency; the critical role of chloride in the recovery process. *J. Clin. Invest.* 41:218, 1962.
7. Bank, N., and Aynedjian, H. S. A micropuncture study of the renal concentrating defect of potassium depletion. *Amer. J. Physiol.* 206:1347, 1964.
8. Barlow, E. D., and de Wardener, H. E. Compulsive water drinking. *Quart. J. Med.* 28:235, 1959.
9. Barrett, P. K. M., Bayliss, R. I. S., and Rees, J. R. Conn's syndrome. *Proc. Roy. Soc. Med.* 51:720, 1958.
10. Barrett, P. K. M., Rees, J. R., and Marrack, D. Case of Conn's syndrome. *Brit. Med. J.* 2:1047, 1959.
11. Bartter, F. C., and Biglieri, E. G. Primary aldosteronism. Clinical Staff Conference at the National Institutes of Health. *Ann. Intern. Med.* 48:647, 1958.
12. Baulieu, E.-E., Robel, P., Siguier, F., and Jayle, M.-F. Metabolic observations in a case of pure primary hyperaldosteronism. *J. Clin. Endocr.* 19:1081, 1959.
13. Beeson, P. B. Definition of Chronic Pyelonephritis. In Kass, E. H. (Ed.), *Progress in Pyelonephritis.* Philadelphia: Davis, 1965. P. 367.
14. Bentley, P. J. The effects of ionic changes on water transfer across the isolated urinary bladder of the toad *Bufo marinus. J. Endocr.* 18:327, 1959.
15. Berliner, R. W., Kennedy, T. J., Jr., and Orloff, J. Relationship between acidification of the urine and potassium metabolism: Effect of carbonic anhydrase inhibition on potassium excretion. *Amer. J. Med.* 11:274, 1951.
16. Biava, C. G., Dyrda, I., Genest, J., and Bencosme, S. A. Kaliopenic nephropathy: A correlated light and electron microscopic study. *Lab. Invest.* 12:443, 1963.
17. Black, D. A. K., and Milne, M. D. Experimental potassium depletion in man. *Clin. Sci.* 11:397, 1952.
18. Blahd, W. H., and Bassett, S. H. Potassium deficiency in man. *Metabolism* 2:218, 1953.
19. Blythe, W. B., Newton, M., and Welt, L. G. Personal communication, 1960 .
20. Blythe, W. B., Newton, M., Lazcano, F., and Welt, L. G. Effect of water restriction on urinary concentrating ability of K-depleted rats. *Amer. J. Physiol.* 199:912, 1960.
21. Brandt, I. K., Matalka, V. A., and Combs, J. T. Amino acids in muscle and kidney of potassium-deficient rats. *Amer. J. Physiol.* 199:39, 1960.
22. Brokaw, A. Renal hypertrophy and polydipsia in potassium-deficient rats. *Amer. J. Physiol.* 172:333, 1953.
23. Brooks, R. V., McSwiney, R. R., Prunty, F. T. G., and Wood, F. J. Y. Potassium deficiency of renal and adrenal origin. *Amer. J. Med.* 23:391, 1957.
24. Buckalew, V. M., Jr., Ramirez, M. A., and Goldberg, M. Free water reabsorption during solute diuresis in normal and potassium-depleted rats. *Amer. J. Physiol.* 212:381, 1967.
25. Burnett, C. H., Burrows, B. A., and Commons, R. R. Studies of alkalosis: I. Renal function during and following alkalosis resulting from pyloric obstruction. *J. Clin. Invest.* 29:169, 1950.
26. Burnett, C. H., Burrows, B. A., Commons, R. R., and Towery, B. T. Studies of alkalosis: II. Electrolyte abnormalities in alkalosis resulting from pyloric obstruction. *J. Clin. Invest.* 29:175, 1950.
27. Burnett, C. H., and Williams, T. F. An analysis of some features of renal tubular dysfunction. *A.M.A. Arch. Intern. Med.* 102:881, 1958.
28. Campbell, C. H., Nicolaides, N., and Steinbeck, A. W. Adrenocortical tumour with hypokalaemia and flaccid muscle paralysis. *Lancet* 2:553, 1956.
29. Capers, T. H., and Race, G. J. Primary aldosteronism without adrenal adenomata; report of a case. *A.M.A. Arch. Path.* 69:142, 1960.
30. Carone, F. A., Kashgarian, M., and Epstein, F. H. Effect of acute potassium deficiency on susceptibility to infection with particular reference to the kidney. *Yale J. Biol. Med.* 32:100, 1959.

31. Castleman, B. (Ed.). Case Records of the Massachusetts General Hospital (No. 40081). *New Eng. J. Med.* 250:334, 1954.
32. Castleman, B. (Ed.). Case Records of the Massachusetts General Hospital (No. 41171). *New Eng. J. Med.* 252:723, 1955.
33. Castleman, B. (Ed.). Case Records of the Massachusetts General Hospital (No. 44491). *New Eng. J. Med.* 259:1128, 1958.
34. Chalmers, T. M. Personal communication, 1969.
35. Chalmers, T. M., Fitzgerald, M. G., James, A. H., and Scarborough, H. Conn's syndrome with severe hypertension. *Lancet* 1:127, 1956.
36. Charles, B., and Cochrane, W. A. Islet cell tumour of the pancreas with chronic diarrhoea and hypokalaemia — a recently recognized syndrome. *Canad. Med. Ass. J.* 82:579, 1960.
37. Cheek, D. B. Total body chloride of children in potassium deficiency and under circumstances of poor nutrition. *Pediatrics* 14:193, 1954.
38. Cheek, D. B., and West, C. D. Alterations in body composition with sodium loading and potassium restriction in the rat: The total body sodium, nitrogen, magnesium, and calcium. *J. Clin. Invest.* 35:763, 1956.
39. Christian, J. J. Potassium deficiency in marmots during hibernation. *Science* 134: 390, 1961.
40. Chronic "active" pyelonephritis. (Editorial.) *New Eng. J. Med.* 278:1346, 1968.
41. Clarke, E., Evans, B. M., MacIntyre, I., and Milne, M. D. Acidosis in experimental electrolyte depletion. *Clin. Sci.* 14:421, 1955.
42. Coburn, J. W., and Reba, R. C. Potassium depletion in heat stroke: A possible etiologic factor. *Milit. Med.* 131:678, 1966.
43. Coghill, N. F., McAllen, P. M., and Edwards, F. Electrolyte losses associated with the taking of purges investigated with aid of sodium and potassium radioisotopes. *Brit. Med. J.* 1:14, 1959.
44. Conn, J. W. Personal communication, 1968.
45. Conn, J. W. Primary aldosteronism, a new clinical syndrome. *J. Lab. Clin. Med.* 45:3, 1955.
46. Conn, J. W., and Louis, L. H. Primary aldosteronism, a new clinical entity. *Ann. Intern. Med.* 44:1, 1956.
47. Conn, J. W., and Johnson, R. D. Kaliopenic nephropathy. *Amer. J. Clin. Nutr.* 4:523, 1956.
48. Conn, J. W., and Conn, E. S. Primary aldosteronism versus hypertensive disease with secondary aldosteronism. *Recent Progr. Hormone Res.* 17:389, 1961.
49. Cooke, R. E., Segar, W. E., Cheek, D. B., Coville, F. E., and Darrow, D. C. The extrarenal correction of alkalosis associated with potassium deficiency. *J. Clin. Invest.* 31:798, 1952.
50. Cooke, R. E., Segar, W. E., Reed, C., Etzwiler, D. D., Vita, M., Brusilow, S., and Darrow, D. C. The role of potassium in the prevention of alkalosis. *Amer. J. Med.* 17:180, 1954.
51. Cooperstein, I. L., and Brockman, S. K. The electrical potential difference generated by the large intestine: Its relation to electrolyte and water transfer. *J. Clin. Invest.* 38:435, 1959.
52. Cortes, F., Shuman, C. R., and Channick, B. J. Primary aldosteronism, observations on 2 cases. *Amer. J. Med. Sci.* 239:324, 1960.
53. Cotlove, E., Holliday, M. A., Schwartz, R., and Wallace, W. M. Effects of electrolyte depletion and acid-base disturbance on muscle cations. *Amer. J. Physiol.* 167:665, 1951.
54. Craig, J. M., and Schwartz, R. Histochemical study of the kidney of rats fed diets deficient in potassium. *A.M.A. Arch. Path.* 64:245, 1957.
55. Crane, M. G. Personal communication, 1969.
56. Crane, M. G., Vogel, P. J., and Richland, K. J. Observations on a presumptive case of primary aldosteronism. *J. Lab. Clin. Med.* 48:1, 1956.
57. Crane, M. G., Short, G., and Peterson, J. E. Observations on a case of primary aldosteronism. *Amer. J. Med.* 24:313, 1958.
58. Danowski, T. S., Austin, A. C., Gow, R. C., Mateer, F. M., Weigand, F. A., Peters, J. H., and Greeman, L. Electrolyte and ni-

trogen balance studies in infants following cessation of vomiting. *Pediatrics* 5:57, 1950.
59. Darmady, E. M., and Stranack, F. Microdissection of the nephron in disease. *Brit. Med. Bull.* 13:21, 1957.
60. Darrow, D. C., Cooke, R. E., and Coville, F. E. Kidney electrolyte in rats with alkalosis associated with potassium deficiency. *Amer. J. Physiol.* 172:55, 1953.
61. Davis, R. P. Enzyme adaptation in potassium depletion: Pyruvate kinase in renal cortex and medulla. (Abstract.) *Fed. Proc.* 19:361, 1960.
62. de Duve, C. The Lysosome Concept. In de Reuck, A. V. S., and Cameron, M. P. (Eds.), *Lysosomes.* Ciba Foundation Symposium. Boston: Little, Brown, 1963. P. 1.
63. de Graeff, J., and Schuurs, M. A. M. Severe potassium depletion caused by the abuse of laxatives: One patient followed for 8 years. *Acta Med. Scand.* 166:407, 1960.
64. Delorme, P., and Genest, J. Primary aldosteronism: A review of medical literature from 1955 to June 1958. *Canad. Med. Ass. J.* 81:893, 1959.
65. Dempsey, E. F., Carroll, E. L., Albright, F., and Henneman, P. H. A. A study of factors determining fecal electrolyte excretion. *Metabolism* 7:108, 1958.
66. Denton, D. A., Wynn, V., McDonald, I. R., and Simon, S. Renal regulation of the extracellular fluid: II. Renal physiology in electrolyte subtraction. *Acta Med. Scand.* Suppl. 261, 1951.
67. de Wardener, H. E., and Herxheimer, A. The effect of a high water intake on the kidney's ability to concentrate the urine in man. *J. Physiol.* (London) 139:42, 1957.
68. de Wardener, H. E. Polyuria. *J. Chronic Dis.* 11:199, 1960.
69. Dunning, M. F., and Plum, F. Potassium depletion by enemas. *Amer. J. Med.* 20:789, 1956.
70. Durlacher, S. H., Darrow, D. C., and Winternitz, M. C. The effect of low potassium diet and of desoxycorticosterone acetate upon renal size. *Amer. J. Physiol.* 136:346, 1942.
71. Dustan, H. P. Personal communication, 1968.
72. Dustan, H. P., Corcoran, A. C., and Page, I. H. Renal function in primary aldosteronism. *J. Clin. Invest.* 35:1357, 1956.
73. Eales, L., and Linder, G. C. Primary aldosteronism: Some observations on a case in a Cape coloured woman. *Quart. J. Med.* 25:539, 1956.
74. Earle, D. P., Sherry, S., Eichna, L. W., and Conan, N. J. Low potassium syndrome due to defective renal tubular mechanisms for handling potassium. *Amer. J. Med.* 11:283, 1951.
75. Eckel, R. E., Norris, J. E. C., and Pope, C. E., II. Basic amino acids as intracellular cations in K deficiency. *Amer. J. Physiol.* 193:644, 1958.
76. Eckel, R. E., Pope, C. E., II, and Norris, J. E. C. Influence of lysine and ammonium chloride feeding on the electrolytes of normal and K-deficient rats. *Amer. J. Physiol.* 193:653, 1958.
77. Eigler, J. O. C., Salassa, R. M., Bahn, R. C., and Owen, C. A., Jr. Renal distribution of sodium in potassium-depleted and vitamin D-intoxicated rats. *Amer. J. Physiol.* 202:1115, 1962.
78. Elkinton, J. R., Squires, R. D., and Crosley, A. P., Jr. Intracellular cation exchanges in metabolic alkalosis. *J. Clin. Invest.* 30:369, 1951.
79. Elkinton, J. R., and Huth, E. J. Body fluid abnormalities in anorexia nervosa and undernutrition. *Metabolism* 8:376, 1959.
80. Epstein, F. H., Kleeman, C. R., and Hendriks, A. The influence of bodily hydration on the renal concentrating process. *J. Clin. Invest.* 36:629, 1957.
81. Evans, B. M., Hughes-Jones, N. C., Milne, M. D., and Steiner, S. Electrolyte excretion during experimental potassium depletion in man. *Clin. Sci.* 13:305, 1954.
82. Ferrebee, J. W., Parker, D., Carnes, W. H., Gerity, M. K., Atchley, D. W., and Loeb, R. F. Certain effects of desoxycorticosterone; the development of "diabetes insipidus" and the replacement of muscle potassium by sodium in normal dogs. *Amer. J. Physiol.* 135:230, 1941.
83. Fine, D., Meiselas, L. E., Colsky, J., and Oxenhorn, S. Primary aldosteronism: Report

of a case and discussion on the pathogenesis. *New Eng. J. Med.* 256:147, 1957.

84. Finn, A. L., Handler, J. S., and Orloff, J. Relation between toad bladder potassium content and permeability response to vasopressin. *Amer. J. Physiol.* 210:1279, 1966.
85. Finn, A. L., and Welt, L. G. Urea excretion in the potassium-deficient rat. *Proc. Soc. Exp. Biol. Med.* 124:724, 1967.
86. Fitzgerald, M. G., and Fourman, P. The renal factor in the alkalosis of potassium deficiency. *Lancet* 2:848, 1955.
87. Follis, R. H., Jr. Histological effects in rats resulting from adding rubidium or cesium to a diet deficient in potassium. *Amer. J. Physiol.* 138:246, 1943.
88. Follis, R. H., Jr., Orent-Keiles, E., and McCollum, E. V. The production of cardiac and renal lesions in rats by a diet extremely deficient in potassium. *Amer. J. Path.* 18: 29, 1942.
89. Fourman, P. Depletion of potassium induced in man with an exchange resin. *Clin. Sci.* 13:93, 1954.
90. Fourman, P., and Hervey, G. R. An experimental study of oedema in potassium deficiency. *Clin. Sci.* 14:75, 1955.
91. Fourman, P., and Leeson, P. M. Thirst and polyuria with a note on the effects of potassium deficiency and calcium excess. *Lancet* 1:268, 1959.
92. Fourman, P., McCance, R. A., and Parker, R. A. Chronic renal disease in rats following a temporary deficiency of potassium. *Brit. J. Exp. Path.* 37:40, 1956.
93. Fourman, P., and Robinson, J. R. Diminished urinary excretion of citrate during deficiencies of potassium in man. *Lancet* 2:656, 1953.
94. Foye, L. V., Jr., and Feichtmeir, T. V. Adrenal cortical carcinoma producing solely mineralocorticoid effect. *Amer. J. Med.* 19:966, 1955.
95. France, R. Intracellular granules of the renal medulla in potassium depletion. *Trans. Amer. Clin. Climat. Ass.* 74:211, 1962.
96. France, R., Merrill, J. M., Norris, J. L., and Tolleson, W. J. Further studies in a case of potassium depletion of undetermined cause. *Trans. Amer. Clin. Climat. Ass.* 71:45, 1959.
97. France, R., and Tolleson, W. J. Potassium depletion of undetermined origin in two brothers. *Trans. Amer. Clin. Climat. Ass.* 69:106, 1957.
98. Freedman, L. R. Chronic pyelonephritis at autopsy. *Ann. Intern. Med.* 66:697, 1967.
99. Gasic, G., and Morrison, A. B. Mucopolysaccharides of renal collecting tubule cells in potassium deficient rats. *Proc. Soc. Exp. Biol. Med.* 112:871, 1963.
100. Giebish, G., and Lozano, R. The effects of adrenal steroids and potassium depletion on the elaboration of an osmotically concentrated urine. *J. Clin. Invest.* 38:843, 1959.
101. Giebisch, G., MacLeod, M. B., and Pitts, R. F. Effect of adrenal steroids on renal tubular reabsorption of bicarbonate. *Amer. J. Physiol.* 183:377, 1955.
102. Goldsmith, R. S., Meroney, W. H., and Bartter, F. C. Prominent peripheral edema associated with primary aldosteronism due to an adrenocortical adenoma. *J. Clin. Endocr.* 20:1168, 1960.
103. Gottschalk, C. W., Mylle, M., Jones, N. F., Winters, R. W., and Welt, L. G. Osmolality of renal tubular fluids in potassium-depleted rodents. *Clin. Sci.* 29:249, 1965.
104. Gowenlock, A. H., and Wrong, O. Hyperaldosteronism secondary to renal ischaemia. *Quart. J. Med.* 31:323, 1962.
105. Grollman, A., and White, F. N. Induction of renal hypertension in rats and dogs by potassium or choline deficiency. *Amer. J. Physiol.* 193:144, 1958.
106. Hays, R. M., and Leaf, A. The problem of clinical vasopressin resistance: *In vitro* studies. *Ann. Intern. Med.* 54:700, 1961.
107. Hellem, A. J. Personal communication, 1968.
108. Hellem, A. J. Primary aldosteronism (report of a case). *Acta Med. Scand.* 155:271, 1956.
109. Heppel, L. A. The electrolytes of muscle and liver in potassium-depleted rats. *Amer. J. Physiol.* 127:385, 1939.
110. Heptinstall, R. H. Personal communication, 1969.

111. Heptinstall, R. H. Sundry Conditions Affecting the Renal Tubules. In *Pathology of the Kidney*. Boston: Little, Brown, 1966. P. 679.
112. Heptinstall, R. H. The Limitations of the Pathological Diagnosis of Chronic Pyelonephritis. In Black, D. A. K. (Ed.), *Renal Disease* (2d ed.). Philadelphia: Davis, 1967. P. 350.
113. Hewlett, J. S., McCullagh, E. P., Farrell, G. L., Dustan, H. P., Poutasse, E. F., and Proudfit, W. L. Aldosterone-producing tumors of the adrenal gland: Report of three cases. *J.A.M.A.* 164:719, 1957.
114. Hill, S. R., Jr., Nickerson, J. F., Chenault, S. B., McNeil, J. H., Starnes, W. R., and Gautney, M. C. Studies in man on hyper- and hypo-aldosteronism. *A.M.A. Arch. Intern. Med.* 104:982, 1959.
115. Hogben, C. A., and Bollman, J. L. Renal reabsorption of phosphate: Normal and thyroparathyroidectomized dog. *Amer. J. Physiol.* 164:670, 1951.
116. Hollander, W., Jr. The effect of potassium depletion on the kidneys. *North Carolina Med. J.* 18:505, 1957.
117. Hollander, W., Jr. The Effects of Potassium Deficiency on Renal Function. In Moyer, J. H., and Fuchs, M. (Eds.), *Edema, Mechanisms, and Management.* Philadelphia: Saunders, 1960. P. 522.
118. Hollander, W., Jr. The Nephropathy of Potassium Depletion. In Strauss, M. B., and Welt, L. G. (Eds.), *Diseases of the Kidney.* Boston: Little, Brown, 1963.
119. Hollander, W., Jr., and Shrauger, C. Unpublished observations, 1965.
120. Hollander, W., Jr., and Welt, L. G. Unpublished observations on a case of proved primary aldosteronism, 1961.
121. Hollander, W., Jr., Winters, R. W., Bradley, J., Williams, T. F., Loring, W. E., Oliver, J., and Welt, L. G. The effect of potassium repletion on the renal concentrating defect, the renal structural changes, and the cardiac and skeletal muscle lesions produced by potassium depletion in rats. (Abstract.) *Clin. Res.* 6:287, 1958.
122. Hollander, W., Jr., Winters, R. W., and Welt, L. . G. Unpublished observations, 1957.
123. Hollander, W., Jr., Winters, R. W., Williams, T. F., Bradley, J., Oliver, J., and Welt, L. G. Defect in the renal tubular reabsorption of water associated with potassium depletion in rats. *Amer. J. Physiol.* 189:557, 1957.
124. Holliday, M. A., Bright, N. H., Schulz, D., and Oliver, J. The renal lesions of electrolyte imbalance: III. The effect of acute chloride depletion and alkalosis on the renal cortex. *J. Exp. Med.* 113:971, 1961.
125. Holliday, M. A., and Egan, T. J. Changes in GFR and C_{H_2O} before and after repair of K deficiency in rats. *Amer. J. Physiol.* 202:773, 1962.
126. Holliday, M. A., Egan, T. J., Morris, C. R., Jarrah, A. S., and Harrah, J. L. Pitressin-resistant hyposthenuria in chronic renal disease. *Amer. J. Med.* 42:378, 1967.
127. Holliday, M., Egan, T., and Wirth, P. Inulin and free water clearance studies in potassium-deficient rats. *A.M.A. Amer. J. Dis. Child.* 96:524, 1958.
128. Holliday, M. A., Segar, W. E., Bright, N. H., and Egan, T. The effect of potassium deficiency on the kidney. *Pediatrics* 26:950, 1960.
129. Holliday, M. A., Winters, R. W., Welt, L. G., MacDowell, M., and Oliver, J. The renal lesions of electrolyte imbalance: II. The combined effect on renal architecture of phosphate loading and potassium depletion. *J. Exp. Med.* 110:161, 1959.
130. Holten, C., and Petersen, V. P. Malignant hypertension with increased secretion of aldosterone and depletion of potassium. *Lancet* 2:918, 1956.
131. Houghton, B. J., and Pears, M. A. Chronic potassium depletion due to purgation with cascara. *Brit. Med. J.* 1:1328, 1958.
132. Huth, E. J., Squires, R. D., and Elkinton, J. R. Experimental potassium depletion in normal human subjects: II. Renal and hormonal factors in the development of extracellular alkalosis during depletion. *J. Clin. Invest.* 38:1149, 1959.
133. Iacobellis, M., Muntwyler, E., and Dodgen, C. L. Free amino acid patterns of certain

tissues from potassium and/or protein-deficient rats. *Amer. J. Physiol.* 185:275, 1956.

134. Iacobellis, M., Muntwyler, E., and Griffin, G. E. Enzyme concentration changes in the kidneys of protein- and/or potassium-deficient rats. *Amer. J. Physiol.* 178:477, 1954.
135. Iacobellis, M., Muntwyler, E., and Griffin, G. E. Kidney glutaminase and carbonic anhydrase activity and tissue electrolyte composition in potassium-deficient dogs. *Amer. J. Physiol.* 183:395, 1955.
136. Iacobellis, M., Griffin, G. E., and Muntwyler, E. Free amino acid patterns of certain tissues from potassium-deficient dogs. *Proc. Soc. Exp. Biol. Med.* 96:64, 1957.
137. Johnson, B. B., Lieberman, A. H., and Mulrow, P. J. Aldosterone excretion in normal subjects depleted of sodium and potassium. *J. Clin. Invest.* 36:757, 1957.
138. Jones, N. F., and Mills, I. H. Reversible renal potassium loss with urinary tract infection. *Amer. J. Med.* 37:305, 1964.
139. Jones, N. F., Mylle, M., and Gottschalk, C. W. Renal tubular microinjection studies in normal and potassium-depleted rats. *Clin. Sci.* 29:261, 1965.
140. Kassirer, J. P., and Schwartz, W. B. Correction of metabolic alkalosis in man without repair of potassium deficiency. *Amer. J. Med.* 40:19, 1966.
141. Kennedy, G. C., Flear, C. T. G., and Parker, R. A. Renal disease and secondary potassium depletion in ageing rats. *Quart. J. Exp. Physiol.* 45:82, 1960.
142. Kennedy, G. C., and Parker, R. A. The influence of age on the acute renal effects of cortexone and of dietary potassium depletion in the rat. *Quart. J. Exp. Physiol.* 45:77, 1960.
143. Kerpel-Fronius, E., Romhanyi, G., Gati, B., and Dobak, E. Influences of depletion of potassium, of sodium, or of water on function and structure of the kidney. *Pediatrics* 26:939, 1960.
144. Keye, J. D., Jr. Death in potassium deficiency; report of a case including morphologic findings. *Circulation* 5:766, 1952.
145. Kistler, H., and Frawley, T. F. Effects of a spirolactone (Sc-8109) in primary mineralocorticoid excess. *J. Clin. Endocr.* 20:1158, 1960.
146. Kleeman, C. R., and Maxwell, M. H. Contributory role of extrarenal factors in the polyuria of potassium depletion. *New Eng. J. Med.* 260:268, 1959.
147. Kleeman, C. R. Maxwell, M. H., and Witlin, S. Functional isosthenuria. *A.M.A. Arch. Intern. Med.* 101:1023, 1958.
148. Kleeman, C. R., Rubini, M. E., Lamdin, E., Kiley, R. F., and Bennett, I. L., Jr. Interrelationship of acute alkalosis and potassium metabolism. *Metabolism* 4:238, 1955.
149. Knochel, J. P., Beisel, W. R., Herndon, E. G., Jr., Gerard, E. S., and Barry, K. G. The renal, cardiovascular, hematologic and serum electrolyte abnormalities of heat stroke. *Amer. J. Med.* 30:299, 1961.
150. Kornberg, A., and Endicott, K. M. Potassium deficiency in the rat. *Amer. J. Physiol.* 145:291, 1946.
151. Kretchmer, N., Dickinson, A., and Karl, R. Aldosteronism in a nine-year-old child. *A.M.A. Amer. J. Dis. Child.* 94:452, 1957.
152. Laragh, J. H., Ulick, S., Januszewicz, V., Kelly, W. G., and Lieberman, S. Electrolyte metabolism and aldosterone secretion in benign and malignant hypertension. *Ann. Intern. Med.* 53:259, 1960.
153. Lennon, E. J., and Lemann, J., Jr. The effect of a potassium-deficient diet on the pattern of recovery from experimental metabolic acidosis. *Clin. Sci.* 34:365, 1968.
154. Lerner, B. A., and Brickner, P. W. Renal tubular acidosis and potassium loss. *Amer. J. Med.* 27:664, 1959.
155. Levinsky, N. G. Personal communication, 1968.
156. Levitin, H., Manitius, A., and Epstein, F. H. Urinary dilution in potassium deficiency. *Yale J. Biol. Med.* 32:390, 1960.
157. Liebow, A. A., McFarland, W. J., and Tennant, R. The effects of potassium deficiency on tumor-bearing mice. *Yale J. Biol. Med.* 13:523, 1941.
158. Litchfield, J. A. Low potassium syndrome resulting from the use of purgative drugs. *Gastroenterology* 37:483, 1959.
159. Luetscher, J. A. Primary aldosteronism:

Observations in six cases and review of diagnostic procedures. *Medicine* (Balt.) 43:437, 1964.

160. Luft, R., Ringertz, N., and Sjøgren, B. Two cases of cryptogenetic hypokalemia with pathological anatomical findings. *Acta Endocr.* (Kobenhavn) 7:196, 1951.
161. MacDonald, M. K., Sabour, M. S., Lambie, A. T., and Robson, J. S. The nephropathy of experimental potassium deficiency: An electron microscopic study. *Quart. J. Exp. Physiol.* 47:262, 1962.
162. Mader, I. J., and Iseri, L. T. Spontaneous hypopotassemia, hypomagnesemia, alkalosis and tetany due to hypersecretion of corticosterone-like mineralocorticoid. *Amer. J. Med.* 19:976, 1955.
163. Mahler, R. F., and Stanbury, S. W. Potassium-losing renal disease; renal and metabolic observations on a patient sustaining renal wastage of potassium. *Quart. J. Med.* 25:21, 1956.
164. Malnic, G., Klose, R. M., and Giebisch, G. Micropuncture study of renal potassium excretion in the rat. *Amer. J. Physiol.* 206: 674, 1964.
165. Manitius, A., and Epstein, F. H. Some observations on the influence of a magnesium-deficient diet on rats, with special reference to renal concentrating ability. *J. Clin. Invest.* 42:208, 1963.
166. Manitius, A., Levitin, H., Beck, D., and Epstein, F. H. On the mechanism of impairment of renal concentrating ability in potassium deficiency. *J. Clin. Invest.* 39: 684, 1960.
167. Milne, M. D., and Muehrcke, R. C. Potassium deficiency and the kidney. *Brit. Med. Bull.* 13:15, 1957.
168. Milne, M. D., Muehrcke, R. C., and Aird, I. Primary aldosteronism. *Quart. J. Med.* 26:317, 1957.
169. Moran, W., Goetz, F. C., Melby, J., Zimmerman, B., and Kennedy, B. J. Primary hyperaldosteronism without adrenal tumor. *Amer. J. Med.* 28:638, 1960.
170. Morrison, A. B. Personal communications, 1960, 1968.
171. Morrison, A. B., Buckalew, V. M., Jr., Miller, R., and Lewis, J. D. The reabsorption of phosphate by the kidney in potassium-deficient dogs. *J. Clin. Invest.* 39:1014, 1960.
172. Morrison, A. B., and Gardner, K. D., Jr. Detection of serum proteins within the renal collecting tubule cells of the potassium-deficient rat. *Nature* (London) 190: 96, 1961.
173. Morrison, A. B., and Gardner, K. D., Jr. The effect of potassium deficiency on the reabsorption of protein in the renal tubule of the rat. *J. Exp. Med.* 118:479, 1963.
174. Morrison, A. B., and Panner, B. J. Lysosome induction in experimental potassium deficiency. *Amer. J. Path.* 45:295, 1964.
175. Mudge, G. H. Clinical patterns of tubular dysfunction. *Amer. J. Med.* 24:785, 1958.
176. Mudge, G. H., and Beskind, H. Effect of potassium deficiency on renal tubular reabsorption and assimilation of glucose. *Bull. Johns Hopkins Hosp.* 104:252, 1959.
177. Mudge, G. H., and Hardin, B. Response to mercurial diuretics during alkalosis: A comparison of acute metabolic and chronic hypokalemic alkalosis in the dog. *J. Clin. Invest.* 35:155, 1956.
178. Muehrcke, R. C. Prolonged Potassium Deficiency and Chronic Pyelonephritis in Man and Animals. In Quinn, E. L., and Kass, E. H. (Eds.), *Biology of Pyelonephritis*. Boston: Little, Brown, 1960. P. 581.
179. Muehrcke, R. C., and Bonting, S. L. Electronmicroscopic and ultramicrobiochemical studies of the potassium-depleted kidney. (Abstract.) *Clin. Res.* 6:413, 1958.
180. Muehrcke, R. C., and McMillan, J. C. The relationship of "chronic pyelonephritis" to chronic potassium deficiency. *Ann. Intern. Med.* 59:427, 1963.
181. Muehrcke, R. C., and Milne, M. D. Primary hyperaldosteronism, long-standing potassium depletion and pyelonephritis. (Abstract.) *Clin. Res. Proc.* 5:190, 1957.
182. Muehrcke, R. C., and Pirani, C. L. Percutaneous Renal Biopsy. In Black, D. A. K. (Ed.), *Renal Disease* (2d ed.). Philadelphia: Davis, 1967. P. 170.
183. Muehrcke, R. C., and Rosen, S. Hypokalemic nephropathy in rat and man: A

light and electron miscroscopic study. *Lab. Invest.* 13:1359, 1964.

184. Mulinos, M. G., Spingarn, C. L., and Lojkin, M. E. A diabetes insipidus-like condition produced by small doses of desoxycorticosterone acetate in dogs. *Amer. J. Physiol.* 135:102, 1941.
185. Muntwyler, E., and Griffin, G. E. Effect of potassium on electrolytes of rat plasma and muscle. *J. Biol. Chem.* 193:563, 1951.
186. Muntwyler, E., and Griffin, G. E. Creatinine clearance in normal and potassium deficient rats. *Amer. J. Physiol.* 173:145, 1953.
187. Muntwyler, E., and Griffin, G. E. Tissue electrolyte content of potassium and protein-deficient rats. *Proc. Soc. Exp. Biol. Med.* 89:349, 1955.
188. Muntwyler, E., Griffin, G. E., and Arends, R. L. Muscle electrolyte composition and balances of nitrogen and potassium in potassium-deficient rats. *Amer. J. Physiol.* 174:283, 1953.
189. Newton, M., Welt, L. G., and Oliver, J. Metabolic alkalosis without potassium depletion. (Abstract.) *Clin. Res.* 9:207, 1961.
190. Oliver, J. Personal communications, 1960, 1968.
191. Oliver, J. Discussion. In Quinn, E. L., and Kass, E. H. (Eds.), *Biology of Pyelonephritis.* Boston: Little, Brown, 1960. P. 604.
192. Oliver, J., MacDowell, M., Welt, L. G., Holliday, M. A., Hollander, W., Jr., Winters, R. W., Williams, T. F., and Segar, W. E. The renal lesions of electrolyte inbalance: I. The structural alterations in potassium-depleted rats. *J. Exp. Med.* 106: 563, 1957.
193. Oliver, J., MacDowell, M., Whang, R., and Welt, L. G. The renal lesions of electrolyte imbalance: IV. The intranephronic calculosis of experimental magnesium depletion. *J. Exp. Med.* 124:263, 1966.
194. Orent-Keiles, E., and McCollum, E. V. Potassium in animal nutrition. *J. Biol. Chem.* 140:337, 1941.
195. Ortuzar, R. Personal communication, 1968.
196. Ortuzar, R., Croxatto, R., Thomsen, P., and Gonzalez, J. Effects of an acute salt load in a case of primary hyperaldosteronism before and nine months after surgical cure. *J. Lab. Clin. Med.* 54:712, 1959.
197. Owen, E. E., and Verner, J. V., Jr. Renal tubular disease with muscle paralysis and hypokalemia. *Amer. J. Med.* 28:8, 1960.
198. Pawlowski, J. M., Bloxdorf, J. W., and Kimmelstiel, P. Chronic pyelonephritis: A morphologic and bacteriologic study. *New Eng. J. Med.* 268:965, 1963.
199. Pearse, A. G. E., and MacPherson, C. R. Renal histochemistry in potassium depletion. *J. Path. Bact.* 75:69, 1958.
200. Perdue, H. S., and Phillips, P. H. Effect of high fat diet on the potassium deficiency syndrome in the rat. *Proc. Soc. Exp. Biol. Med.* 81:405, 1952.
201. Pereira, V. G., Wajchenberg, B. L., Quintao, E. R., and Machado, M. M. Electrolyte and renal changes in severe potassium depletion. *Metabolism* 14:800, 1965.
202. Perkins, J. G., Petersen, A. B., and Riley, J. A. Renal and cardiac lesions in potassium deficiency due to chronic diarrhea. *Amer. J. Med.* 8:115, 1950.
203. Plum, F., and Dunning, M. F. Enema-induced potassium loss in patients with diseases of spinal cord roots. *Trans. Amer. Neurol. Ass.* 80:219, 1955.
204. Pollak, V. E., Flagg, G. W., Muehrcke, R. C., and Kark, R. M. Potassium depletion following self-induced diarrhea and vomiting, treated by prolonged psychotherapy. (Abstract.) *Clin. Res. Proc.* 5:194, 1957.
205. Poutsiaka, J. W., Nasveschuk, M., and Millstein, L. G. Effects of steroid induced potassium depletion on renal control of sodium. *Proc. Soc. Exp. Biol. Med.* 102: 506, 1959.
206. Raaschou, F. Definition of Chronic Pyelonephritis. In Kass, E. H. (Ed.), *Progress in Pyelonephritis.* Philadelphia: Davis, 1965. P. 373.
207. Ragan, C., Ferrebee, J. W., Phyfe, P., Atchley, D. W., and Loeb, R. F. A syndrome of polydipsia and polyuria induced in normal animals by desoxycorticosterone acetate. *Amer. J. Physiol.* 131:73, 1940.

208. Reimer, A., Schoch, H. K., and Newburgh, L. H. Certain aspects of potassium metabolism. *J. Amer. Diet. Ass.* 27:1042, 1951.
209. Relman, A. S., and Schwartz, W. B. The effect of DOCA on electrolyte balance in normal man and its relation to sodium chloride intake. *Yale J. Biol. Med.* 24:540, 1951–1952.
210. Relman, A. S., and Schwartz, W. B. The nephropathy of potassium depletion: A clinical and pathological entity. *New Eng. J. Med.* 255:195, 1956.
211. Relman, A. S., and Schwartz, W. B. The kidney in potassium depletion. *Amer. J. Med.* 24:764, 1958.
212. Relman, A. S., and Schwartz, W. B. Effects of Electrolyte Disorders on Renal Structure and Function. In Black, D. A. K. (Ed.), *Renal Disease* (2d ed.). Philadelphia: Davis, 1967. P. 754.
213. Richardson, J. A., Huffines, W. D., and Welt, L. G. The effect of coincident hypercalcemia and potassium depletion on the rat kidney. *Metabolism* 12:560, 1963.
214. Richter, H. S. Action of antidiuretic hormone in potassium-depleted rats; relation to aldosteronism. *Proc. Soc. Exp. Biol. Med.* 97:141, 1958.
215. Roberts, K. E., and Pitts, R. F. The effects of cortisone and desoxycorticosterone on the renal tubular reabsorption of phosphate and the excretion of titratable acid and potassium in dogs. *Endocrinology* 52: 324, 1953.
216. Roberts, K. E., Randall, H. T., Philbin, P., and Lipton, R. Changes in extracellular water and electrolytes and the renal compensations in chronic alkalosis as compared to those occurring in acute alkalosis. *Surgery* 36:599, 1954.
217. Roberts, K. E., Randall, H. T., Sanders, H. L., and Hood, M. Effects of potassium on renal tubular reabsorption of bicarbonate. *J. Clin. Invest.* 34:666, 1955.
218. Roy, A. D., and Ellis, H. Potassium-secreting tumours of the large intestine. *Lancet* 1:759, 1959.
219. Rubini, M. E. Water excretion in potassium-deficient man. *J. Clin. Invest.* 40:2215, 1961.
220. Rubini, M. E., Blythe, W. B., Herndon, E. G., and Meroney, W. H. Influence of potassium deficiency on response to an acidifying salt. (Abstract.) *Clin. Res. Proc.* 5:193, 1957.
221. Russell, G. F. M., Marshall, J., and Stanton, J. B. Potassium-losing nephritis: A clinical investigation. *Scot. Med. J.* 1:122, 1956.
222. Salassa, R. M. Personal communication, 1961.
223. Salassa, R. M., Mattox, V. R., and Power, M. H. Effect of an aldosterone antagonist on sodium and potassium excretion in primary hyperaldosteronism. *J. Clin. Endocr.* 18:787, 1958.
224. Schrader, G. A., Prickett, C. O., and Salmon, W. D. Symptomatology and pathology of potassium and magnesium deficiencies in the rat. *J. Nutr.* 14:85, 1937.
225. Schwartz, W. B., and Relman, A. S. Metabolic and renal studies in chronic potassium depletion resulting from overuse of laxatives. *J. Clin. Invest.* 32:258, 1953.
226. Schwartz, W. B., and Relman, A. S. Effects of electrolyte disorders on renal structure and function. *New Eng. J. Med.* 276: 383, 1967.
227. Scribner, B. H., and Burnell, J. M. Interpretation of the serum potassium concentration. *Metabolism* 5:468, 1956.
228. Segar, W. E., and Schulz, D. M. Multiple episodes of potassium deficiency. *Amer. J. Dis. Child.* 109:295, 1965.
229. Seldin, D. W., Welt, L. G., and Cort, J. H. The role of sodium salts and adrenal steroids in the production of hypokalemic alkalosis. *Yale J. Biol. Med.* 29:229, 1956.
230. Skanse, B., Moller, F., Gydell, K., Johansson, S., and Wulff, H. B. Observations on primary aldosteronism. *Acta Med. Scand.* 158:181, 1957.
231. Smith, L. A. Personal communication, 1969.
232. Smith, S. G., Black-Schaffer, B., and Lasater, T. E. Potassium deficiency syndrome in the rat and the dog. *Arch. Path.* 49:185, 1950.
233. Smith, S. G., and Lasater, T. E. A diabetes insipidus-like condition produced in

dogs by a potassium deficient diet. *Proc. Soc. Exp. Biol. Med.* 74:427, 1950.

234. Spargo, B. H. Personal communication, 1968.
235. Spargo, B. Kidney changes in hypokalemic alkalosis in the rat. *J. Lab. Clin. Med.* 43:802, 1954.
236. Spargo, B. H. Renal Changes with Potassium Depletion. In Becker, E. L. (Ed.), *Structural Basis of Renal Disease.* New York: Harper & Row, 1968. P. 565.
237. Spargo, B., Straus, F., and Fitch, F. Zonal renal papillary droplet change with potassium depletion. *Arch. Path.* (Chicago) 70:599, 1960.
238. Squires, R. D., and Huth, E. J. Experimental potassium depletion in normal human subjects: I. Relation of ionic intakes to the renal conservation of potassium. *J. Clin. Invest.* 38:1134, 1959.
239. Stamey, T. A. The pathogenesis and implications of the electrolyte imbalance in ureterosigmoidostomy. *Surg. Gynec. Obstet.* 103:736, 1956.
240. Stanbury, S. W. Some aspects of disordered renal tubular function. *Advances Intern. Med.* 9:231, 1958.
241. Stanbury, S. W., Gowenlock, A. H., and Mahler, R. F. Interrelationships of Potassium Deficiency and Renal Disease. In Muller, A. F., and O'Connor, C. M. (Eds.), *An International Symposium on Aldosterone.* Boston: Little, Brown, 1958. P. 155.
242. Stanbury, S. W., and Macaulay, D. Defects of renal tubular function in the nephrotic syndrome. *Quart. J. Med.* 26:7, 1957.
243. Steele, C. W. Malignant carcinoid: Metastasis to skin and production of carcinoid syndrome, hypertension, diarrhea, dementia, and hypopotassemia: A case report. *Arch. Intern. Med.* (Chicago) 110:763, 1962.
244. Strauss, F. Ureteral ligation: A method of inhibiting the formation of acidophilic droplets in the renal papilla of potassium deficient rats. M.S. Thesis, Chicago (1964), as cited in reference 267.
245. Taggert, J. V., Silverman, L., and Trayner, E. M. Influence of renal electrolyte composition on the tubular excretion of p-aminohippurate. *Amer. J. Physiol.* 173:345, 1953.
246. Tauxe, W. N., Wakim, K. G., and Baggenstos, A. H. The renal lesions in experimental deficiency of potassium. *Amer. J. Clin. Path.* 28:221, 1957.
247. van Buchem, F. S. P. Personal communication, 1960, regarding case reported in references 248 and 249.
248. van Buchem, F. S. P., Doorenbos, H., and Elings, H. S. Conn's syndrome caused by adrenocortical hyperplasia: Pathogenesis of the signs and symptoms. *Acta Endocr.* (Kobenhavn) 23:313, 1956.
249. van Buchem, F. S. P., Doorenbos, H., and Elings, H. S. Primary aldosteronism due to adrenocortical hyperplasia. *Lancet* 2:335, 1956.
250. van Goidsenhoven, G. M.-T., Gray, O. V., Price, A. V., and Sanderson, P. H. The effect of prolonged administration of large doses of sodium bicarbonate in man. *Clin. Sci.* 13:383, 1954.
251. Wachstein, M., and Meisel, E. Enzymatic staining reactions in the kidneys of potassium-depleted rats. *Amer. J. Path.* 35:1189, 1959.
252. Warner, J. F., and Hollander, W., Jr. Unpublished observations, 1962.
253. Warner, J. F., and Hollander, W., Jr. The effect of altering magnitude but not duration of potassium deficit on the renal concentrating defect of potassium depleted rats. (Abstract.) *Clin. Res.* 9:37, 1961.
254. Warner, J. F., and Hollander, W., Jr. Duration and intensity of potassium deficit as factors in the renal concentrating defect of potassium depleted rats. (Abstract.) *Clin. Res.* 10:257, 1962.
255. Warner, J. F., Huffines, W. D., and Hollander, W., Jr., Unpublished observations, 1962.
256. Watson, J. F. Potassium reabsorption in the proximal tubule of the dog nephron. *J. Clin. Invest.* 45:1341, 1966.
257. Watson, J. F., Clapp, J. R., and Berliner, R. W. Micropuncture study of potassium

concentration in proximal tubule of dog, rat, and necturus. *J. Clin. Invest.* 43:595, 1964.

258. Watson, J. F., and Katz, F. H. Hypokalemic nephropathy in an adrenalectomized patient. *Amer. J. Med.* 27:844, 1959.
259. Webster, G. D., Jr., Touchstone, J. C., and Suzuki, M. Adrenocortical hyperplasia occurring with metastatic carcinoma of the prostate: Report of a case exhibiting increased urinary aldosterone and glucocorticoid excretion. *J. Clin. Endocr.* 19:967, 1959.
260. Welt, L. G. Experimental magnesium depletion. *Yale J. Biol. Med.* 36:325, 1964.
261. Welt, L. G., Hollander, W., Jr., and Blythe, W. B. The consequences of potassium depletion. *J. Chronic Dis.* 11:213, 1960.
262. Welt, L. G., Hollander, W., Jr., Williams, T. F., and Winters, R. W. Unpublished observations, 1955–1958.
263. Whang, R., Oliver, J., McDowell, M., and Welt, L. G. The renal lesion of magnesium depletion. (Abstract.) *Clin. Res.* 10:257, 1962.
264. Whang, R., and Welt, L. G. Observations in experimental magnesium depletion. *J. Clin. Invest.* 42:305, 1963.
265. Wigley, R. D. Potassium deficiency in anorexia nervosa, with reference to renal tubular vacuolation. *Brit. Med. J.* 2:110, 1960.
266. Wilson, D. M., and Kissane, J. M. Quantitative histochemistry of the kidney: The distribution of electrolytes in the kidneys of potassium-deficient and normal rats in varying states of hydration. *Lab. Invest.* 2:45, 1962.
267. Wilson, H., Spargo, B., and Penksa, R. An Experimental System for the Study of a Specific Pattern of Cytoplasmic Change. In Bajusz, E., and Jasmin, G. (Eds.), *Meth. Achievm. Exp. Path.* Basel/New York: Karger, 1969. Vol. 4, p. 92.
268. Winters, R. W., and Welt, L. G. Unpublished observations, 1958.
269. Womersley, R. A., and Darragh, J. H. Potassium and sodium restriction in the normal human. *J. Clin. Invest.* 34:456, 1955.
270. Woods, J. W., Welt, L. G., Hollander, W., Jr., and Newton, M. Susceptibility of rats to experimental pyelonephritis following recovery from potassium depletion. *J. Clin. Invest.* 39:28, 1960.
271. Woods, J. W., Welt, L. G., and Hollander, W., Jr. Susceptibility of rats to experimental pyelonephritis during potassium depletion. *J. Clin. Invest.* 40:599, 1961.
272. Wyngaarden, J. B., Keitel, H. G., and Isselbacher, K. Potassium depletion and alkalosis: Their association with hypertension and renal insufficiency. *New Eng. J. Med.* 250:579, 1954.
273. Yount, J. A., Shrauger, C. R., and Hollander, W., Jr. Impaired vasopressin-induced net water transport across the urinary bladder of potassium (K) depleted toads. (Abstract.) *Clin. Res.* 13:81, 1965.

26

Kidney Stones

Lloyd H. Smith, Jr., and Hibbard E. Williams

Kidney stones are frequent and important causes of morbidity and occasionally of mortality. It has been estimated that approximately 1 in every 1000 inhabitants of the United States requires hospitalization each year because of stones [12]. This figure, based on a questionnaire survey, probably represents an underestimation and, furthermore, does not include stones passed spontaneously in nonhospitalized patients. A similar prevalence has been reported from Czechoslovakia [58]. As another index of incidence, kidney stones were found in 1.12 per cent of 25,000 autopsies in the United States [6], again with similar figures from Czechoslovakia [58]. Stones occurred in antiquity, as reflected in the Hippocratic injunction not to "cut persons laboring under the stone" and the finding of stones in archeological studies in Egypt [79] and the United States [5].

The epidemiology of stones has been intriguing but not particularly illuminating of pathogenesis. Less than 1 per cent of stones occur in children; in adults the sex incidence is roughly equal, or perhaps with a slight preponderance in males. Stones are less common in Negroes than in Caucasians and are less frequent in manual than in sedentary workers. In the thorough studies from Czechoslovakia, an administrative worker was found to be 20 times more likely to develop a kidney stone than an agricultural worker [58]. Stone belts have been described, as have stone epidemics. The geographical distribution of stones in the United States, based on figures from 20 years ago, is shown in Figure 26-1. The frequency of stones in the South and Southeast was previously noted in examinations for military service in World War I and also in a survey directed to members of the American Urological Association [14]. Even more remarkable have been the well-documented stone epidemics. The records of the Norfolk and Norwich Hospital in England reveal that 1 in every 38 patients admitted between 1772 and 1816 had a bladder stone, a disorder soon virtually to disappear in Europe [58]. There are similar epidemics of bladder stone disease now in Thailand, India, and Turkey, with greatest prevalence in male children [40]. In the Ubol Hospital in northeast Thailand in the early 1960's, one boy patient in

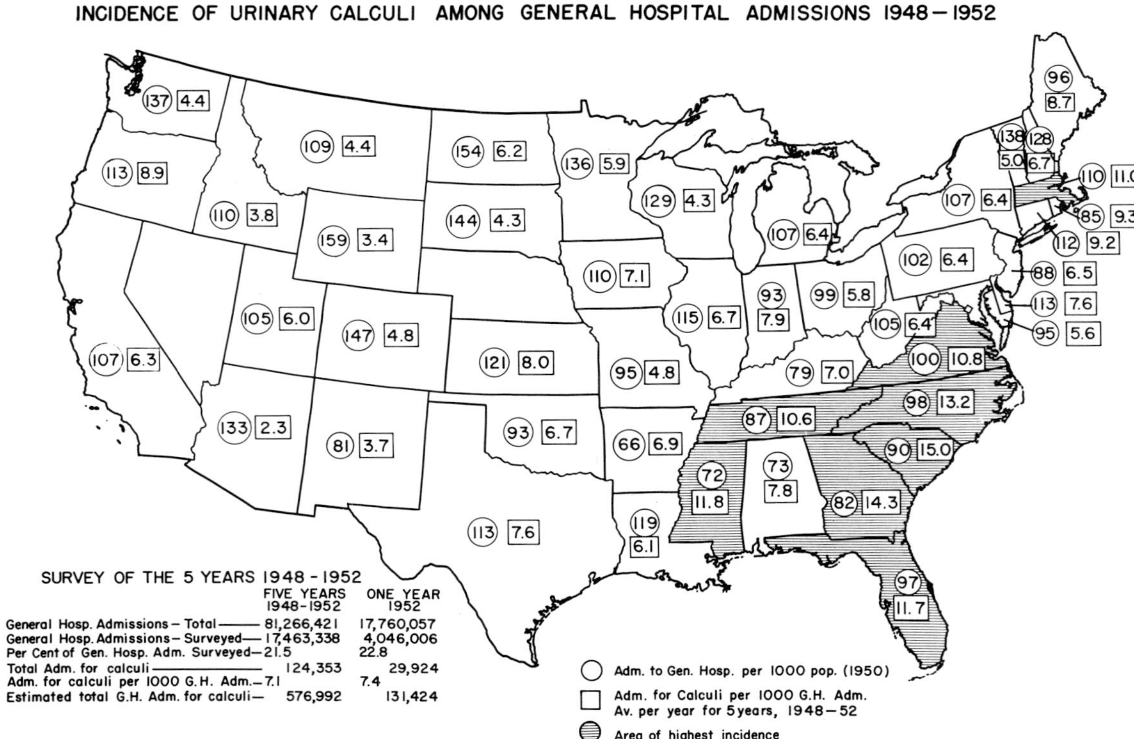

Figure 26-1. Geographical survey of the incidence of urinary calculi in hospitalized patients in the United States. (From Boyce, W. H., Garvey, F. K., and Strawcutter, H. E. Incidence of urinary calculi among patients in general hospitals, 1948–1952. *J.A.M.A.* 161:1437, 1956.)

three had a bladder stone. Less dramatic regional and temporal variations in other types of stones have been reported.

Familial stone diathesis has long been noted. The mechanism is clear in specific genetic disorders such as cystinuria, metabolic (overproduction) gout, primary hyperoxaluria, and familial renal tubular acidosis. In addition, several large studies have indicated a familial, presumably genetic, predisposition to form calcium oxalate stones in the absence of hyperoxaluria [37, 59, 75]. The mode of inheritance has been interpreted as polygenic [75], but in the absence of a reliable biochemical marker this is difficult to establish. Curiously, calcium oxalate stones have also been described in association with hyperglycinuria [23]. Uric acid stone diathesis may also be inherited in the absence of gout [22].

In this chapter attention is directed to stone pathogenesis and how knowledge of this may guide medical management — that is, the prevention of recurrence. The differential diagnosis of renal colic and the complications of stones — pain, obstruction, bleeding, infection, loss of renal parenchyma — are not discussed. Similarly, indication and methods of surgical intervention are not presented. In the oath of Hippocrates we are enjoined to "leave this to be done by men who are practitioners of this work."

Composition and Structure of Stones

Kidney stones represent a heterogeneous group of concretions, the composition and structure of which may be indicative of pathogenesis. The first approach of the physician should be to obtain the stone for analysis. This may be only a simple qualitative analysis of the crystalloids present. It is preferable, however, to employ some of the more sophisticated methods in crystallography (x-ray diffraction, polarizing microscopy) which will reveal architectural structure as well as composition [70]. All stones contain complex mucoproteins called matrix. Conversely stated, kidney stones are not composed solely of agglutinated masses of inorganic or organic crystals. The protein content comprises, on the average, about 2.5 per cent of the dry weight of the stone [11]. This section, therefore, is concerned with the crystalloid and matrix content of stones and the interrelation of the two.

CRYSTALLOID COMPOSITION

The composition of stones varies with age, geographical area, frequency of infection, economic status, and even the date of the study. The figures given are, of necessity, of general statistical value only. Table 26-1 illustrates two of the largest studies available in the United States [60, 70]. Similar figures have been reported from Sweden [57]. From this information, certain simplifications can be derived. Approximately 90 per cent of stones contain calcium; two-thirds contain oxalate. Uric acid stones constitute 5 to 10 per cent; cystine 2 to 3 per cent (except in childhood where the relative incidence is higher). Many stones are mixed in crystalloid composition. Magnesium ammonium phosphate stones, for practical purposes, reflect the frequency of infection with urea-splitting organisms, although prolonged excessive use of alkali may occasionally produce such a stone.

STONE MATRIX

The biochemical composition of stone matrix is similar in all kidney stones that have been studied, being predominantly mucoprotein [11]. Average analytical figures of lyophilized matrix are: protein, 64 per cent; nonamino sugars (galactose, glucose, mannose, rhamnose, and fucose), 9.6 per cent; glucosamine, 5 per cent; and bound water, 10 per cent [9]. The remainder represents residual inorganic ash, especially calcium and phosphate. The protein contains no hydroxyproline and less than 2 per cent proline, clearly distinguishing it from collagen and elastin. No sialic acid, ketohexose, or hexuronic acid has been detected [53]. Matrix recovered from decrystallized calculi has been highly insoluble, making further studies difficult. Using primarily immunologic technics, Boyce and his associates have described a small protein (molecular weight of 30,000 to 40,000) termed ma-

Table 26-1. Crystalloid Composition of Stones

Composition	% Total No. of Stones: Collection of 1000 Stones [70]	% Total No. of Stones: Stones Analyzed from 155 Patients [60]
Calcium oxalate	33	23
Calcium phosphate — hydroxyapatite	3	17
hydrogen phosphate dihydrate	2	
Calcium oxalate and calcium phosphate	34	26
Magnesium ammonium phosphate with either calcium oxalate or calcium phosphate	19	13
Uric acid (including stones with calcium oxalate)	6	11
Cystine	3	2

trix substance A, which appears to represent the major protein, certainly the major antigenic substance in stones [9, 10]. Other minor components of matrix may include albumin, alpha globulin, some gamma globulins, and uromucoid.

STONE STRUCTURE

The relationship in a stone between crystalloid and matrix may vary widely, from a regular, highly organized, interwoven pattern to a disordered intermixture without discernible architecture [11, 70]. Concentric laminations may be grossly visible, seeming to represent "growth rings" between which the matrix is arranged in dense, parallel fibrils. Some stones, especially those high in uric acid, have marked radial striations containing fibrous matrix at right angles to the concentric laminations. These matrix radial striations may be simulated by crystals of calcium hydrogen phosphate monohydrate of similar orientation. Another characteristic configuration, especially of calcium oxalate stones, is that of frond formation, the knobs of "jack-stone calculi." These stones have continuous concentric laminations of fibrous matrix over the body and the knobs, as described above. The knobs are formed by additional accretions of amorphous matrix between these laminations. The mechanism of this type of stone growth is not understood. The spherule, another frequently encountered architectural unit, is a very small (1 mm. or less) rounded concretion found on many stones, containing concentric fibrous laminations and often poorly crystallized centers [9]. Rarely, renal concretions may be largely composed of matrix, so called "matrix stones" or "matrix concretions" [63, 90]. Depending upon the amount of calcium phosphate present, they may be radiolucent or only faintly radiopaque.

Stone structure may vary not only in the type of crystalloid found, and its relationship to matrix, but also in radial structure. This is particularly true for mixed stones whose natural history may be frozen in the radial crystal sequence. A calcium oxalate center may be surrounded by a shell of magnesium ammonium phosphate, reflecting the time sequence of superimposed urinary infection. Uric acid may serve as a nidus for calcium oxalate. Some of the structural characteristics of stones are illustrated in Figure 26-2.

Pathogenesis of Stones

The physician charged with the care of a patient with a kidney stone faces first the immediate problem of the treatment of renal colic and the determination of whether surgical treatment is required. His second responsibility is to try to find out the pathogenesis of the stone in order to plan for prevention of recurrence. In addition, a stone may be the first clinical manifestation of an important systemic disease (hyperparathyroidism, for example).

It is convenient to think of the pathogenesis of kidney stones under two general headings [30, 81]:

1. Changes which increase the urinary concentration of constituent crystalloids:
   - Reduction in urine volume
   - Increased excretion of calcium, oxalate, cystine, uric acid, xanthine, ammonia (phosphate)
2. Physicochemical changes conducive to stone formation at normal concentration of crystalloids:
   - pH
   - Stone matrix
   - Stasis
   - Foreign bodies
   - Presence of protective substances—Mg^{++}, pyrophosphate, citrate, inhibitor peptides, & other normal constituents

Factors affecting the urinary concentration of calcium, oxalate, cystine, uric acid, and xanthine have been studied more extensively and are consequently much better understood.

Phosphaturia has not been demonstrated as a cause of stones, and, in fact, orthophosphate is widely used in stone prevention. The variables listed under the second heading, especially the normal protective substances in the control of crystallization, are probably of greatest importance, as noted below. This classification of stone pathogenesis is both self-evident and oversimplified but will serve until further work allows a more rational approach.

Before the discussion of individual factors in stone pathogenesis, it should be noted that the elementary point of where stones begin has not been finally established. Do they begin as crystal foci or matrix precipitates within pelvic urine, most being harmlessly washed out in the urinary stream? Do they begin as plaques on the papillary epithelium, or "milk patches" as described by Randall 34 years ago [72]? Is the initial nidus that of crystal-laden macrophages beneath the urinary tract epithelium? In a study of experimental kidney stones in the rat, induced with oxamide or ethylene glycol, Vermeulen and Lyon [89] have presented convincing evidence that stone embryogenesis, as they describe it, occurs in the terminal papillary ducts where maximal crystalloid concentration is found. This allows attachment of the microstone to prevent its abortion and also exposure of its crystal surface to pelvic urine to allow for further growth. This promising work in the rat should stimulate more thorough studies of the pathology of kidneys from human stone formers.

INCREASED URINARY CONCENTRATION OF CRYSTALLOIDS

The concentration of crystal constituents in urine depends on the urine volume, the absolute rate of excretion of the substance, and the presence of agents in urine which decrease chemical activity (ion association of calcium, for example). The latter variable is considered in the section on *Physiocochemical Changes in the Urine or Urinary Tract.* Concentration is obviously not a fixed function but will vary widely with changes in urine water and diurnal patterns in renal excretion. Fluid intake, like other food habits, exhibits marked individual and cultural differences. It is curious that no systematic study has been made of fluid ingestion or urine volumes, particularly nocturnal urine volumes, in habitual stone formers. Extrarenal loss of water may lead to persistently concentrated urines with increased frequency of stones. Stones seemingly related to dehydration may be nearly epidemic in troops recently arrived in tropical areas [8]. Manipulation of water intake is basic in the treatment of most stones (see below). Most attention has been directed to the excretion of individual components of stones.

Calcium. Ninety per cent of all kidney stones contain calcium [70]. These stones consist of calcium oxalate, calcium phosphate (in one or more of its crystal forms), or mixtures of the two. The majority of patients with calcium-containing stones excrete normal amounts of calcium, the abnormality presumably being one of the factors listed under the heading *Physicochemical Changes in the Urine or Urinary Tract.* Hypercalciuria, however, is the most frequent metabolic abnormality demonstrable in patients with stones [25]. Some aspects of calcium excretion are described here briefly. A more complete discussion of calcium and the kidney is presented in Chapter 24.

Approximately 60 to 70 per cent of calcium is not bound by plasma proteins and is therefore filterable at the glomerulus. Of the 9000 to 10,000 mg. of calcium filtered per 24 hours, about 98 per cent is reabsorbed by the renal tubule. A number of factors influence the amount of calcium excreted by the kidney. Urinary excretion will usually vary in the direction of the amount of calcium in the glomerular filtrate; hypercalcemia (specifically an increase in nonprotein-bound calcium) leading to hypercalciuria and diminished renal function will tend to reduce urinary excretion of calcium. It should be noted that in uremia

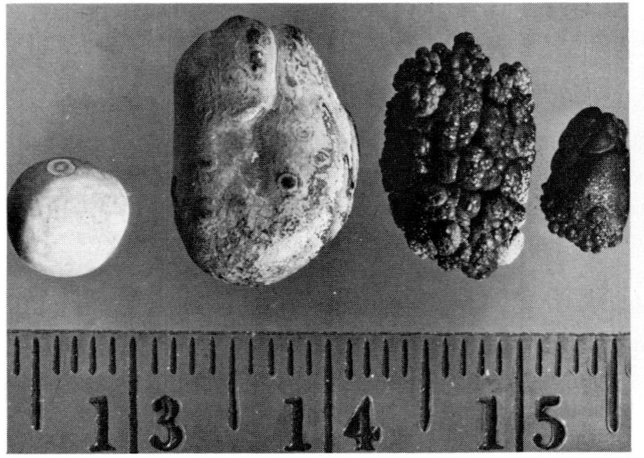

A

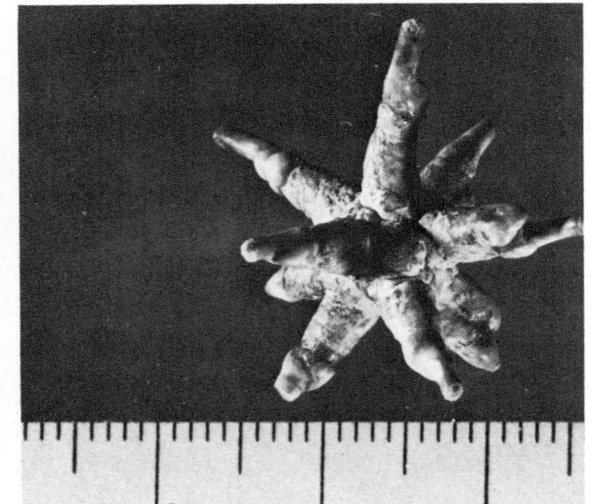

B

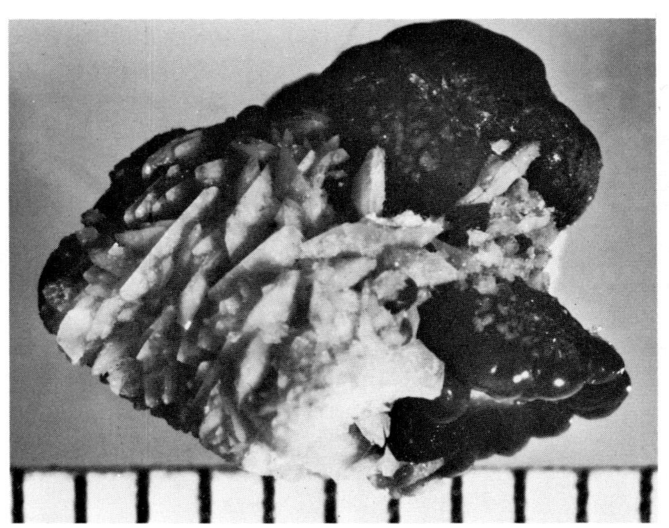

C

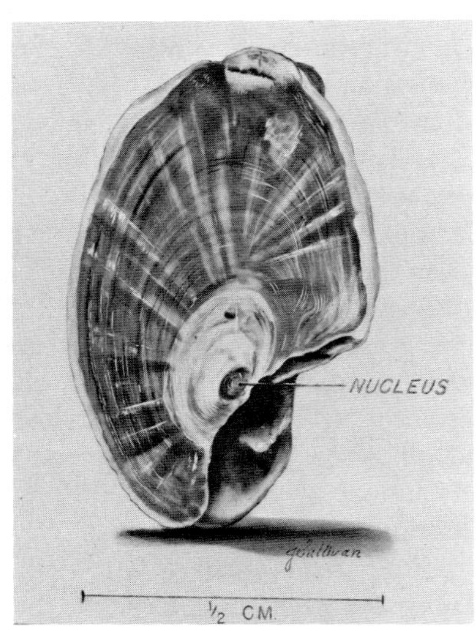

D

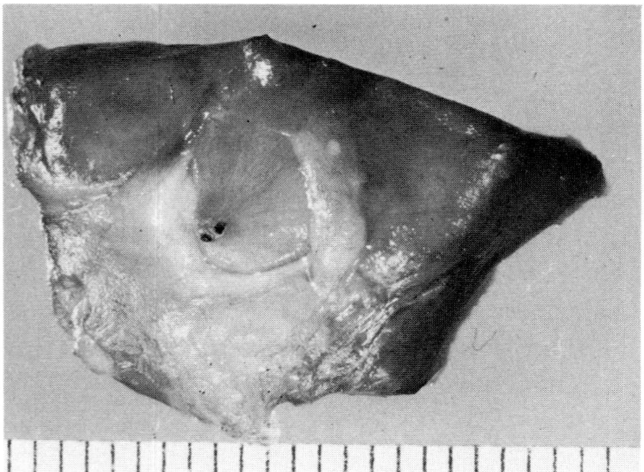

E

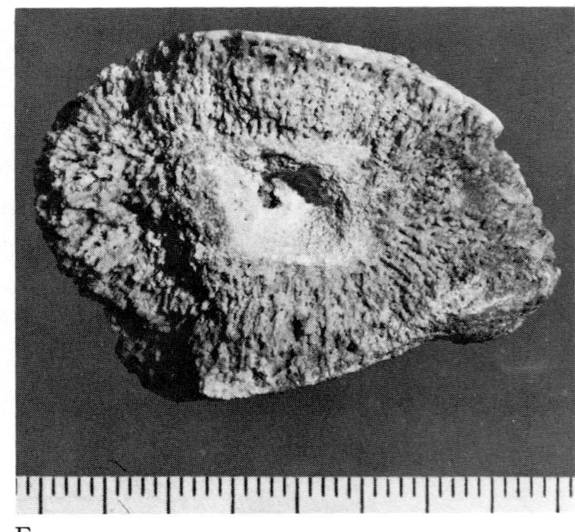

F

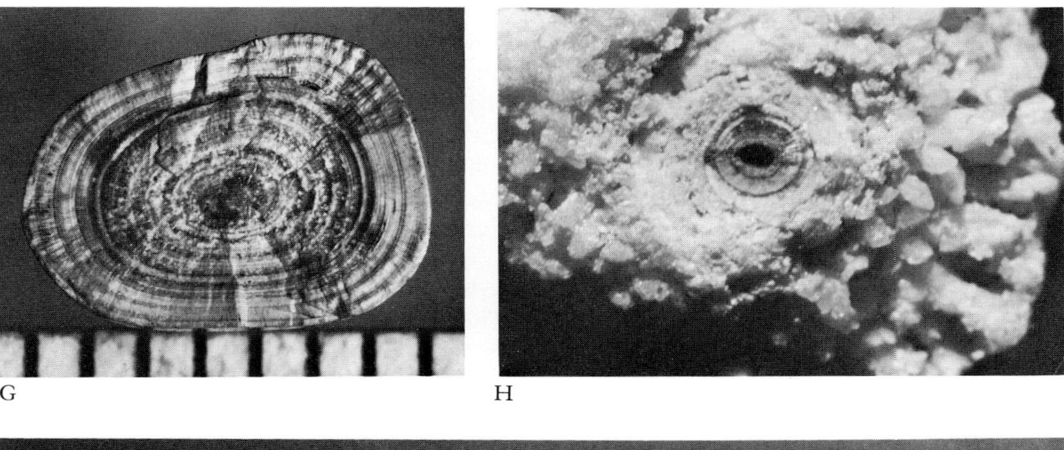

G H

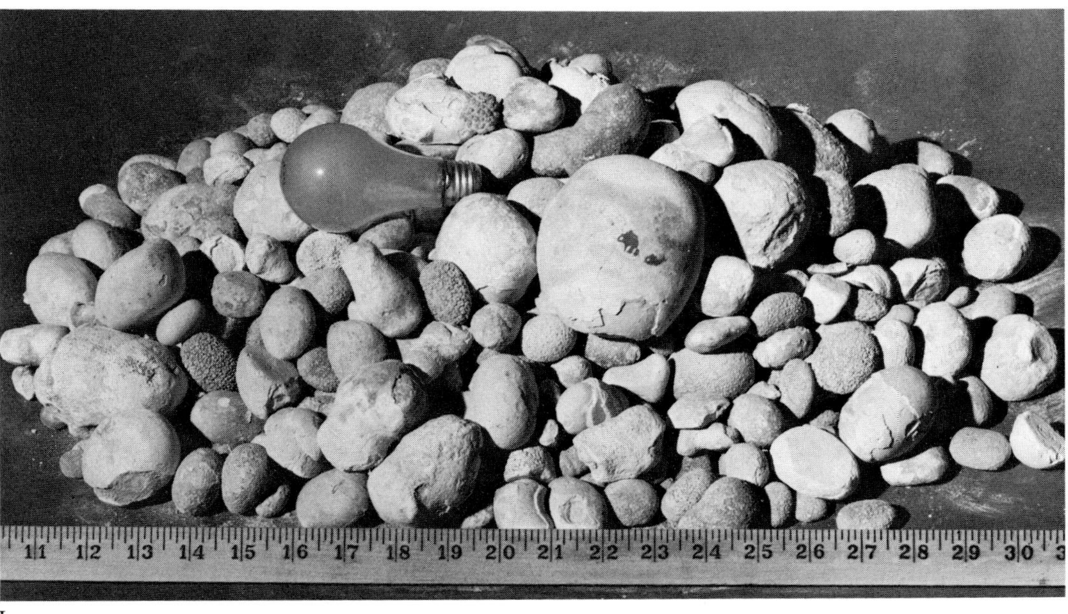

I

Figure 26-2. Various types of renal calculi. A. Calcium oxalate monohydrate calculi. The two on the left are "hempseed" types; the two on the right "mulberry" types. Scale in millimeters. B. Calcium oxalate monohydrate calculus, "jackstone" type. Scale in millimeters. C. Calcium oxalate calculus. Deposition of calcium oxalate dihydrate crystals (*white*) upon calcium oxalate monohydrate (*black*) which forms the bulk of the stone. Scale in millimeters. D. Calcium oxalate calculus which developed from a nucleus originating as a Randall's plaque upon the surface of the renal papilla. E. Two small calcium oxalate monohydrate calculi, developing upon apatite nuclei which are adherent to the summit of an excised human renal papilla. Scale in millimeters. F. Fractured surface of phosphatic "staghorn" calculus. Central nucleus of apatite is surrounded by columnar structure of $MgNH_4PO_4$. Intercolumnar spaces filled with apatite. Scale in millimeters. G. Uric acid calculus. Alternating dark and light layers and central nucleus all of pure uric acid. Dark layers are composed of coarser crystal grains than light layers. Scale in millimeters. H. Calculus of mixed composition. Central rounded nucleus of calcium oxalate monohydrate (nucleolus [*black*] has fallen out), intermediate zone of mixed calcium oxalate monohydrate and apatite, outer coarse crystals of magnesium ammonium phosphate. Scale — central black nucleolus 1 mm. across. I. Calculi from bladders of children in northern Thailand. Numbered divisions on scale are inches. Light bulb is standard 60 watt size. (Prien, E. L., and Prien, E. L., Jr. Composition and structure of urinary stone. *Amer. J. Med.* 45:654, 1968.)

there is, in addition, impairment of calcium absorption from the gut [20]. Parathyroid hormone increases renal tubular reabsorption of calcium [51, 85], its effect on calcium excretion representing a balance of increased filtration (hypercalcemia from osteolysis) and enhanced reabsorption. Of particular interest and importance has been the demonstration that calcium clearance tends to parallel that of sodium. Sodium restriction or the use of thiazide diuretics to deplete sodium stores (and increase its absorption in the proximal tubule) will reduce calcium excretion. Ingestion of excess sodium will increase calcium excretion. On occasion, this relationship of sodium and calcium is of considerable therapeutic importance. Calcium excretion exhibits a diurnal variation, being greatest by day [42]. This is fortunate in that urine is more concentrated normally during the night. The diurnal variation seems to be caused by the interesting effects of glucose and protein to enhance calcium excretion [69]. Metabolic, but not respiratory, acidosis increases urinary calcium, probably by bone dissolution [25]. The hypercalciuria associated with glucocorticoid excess and with thyrotoxicosis is presumed to be similarly secondary to bone dissolution. Calcium excretion tends to vary inversely with ingestion of orthophosphate. This effect is not through reduced intestinal absorption of calcium but through enhanced deposition in bone and decreased osteolysis. Finally, excessive ingestion of calcium will increase urinary calcium, probably by a slight increase of serum calcium with reduced secretion of parathyroid hormone. The response is not a striking one, however, as demonstrated in Figure 26-3, which compares calcium intake and urinary calcium in 25 patients on dietary intakes between 100 and 2000 mg per day.

Hypercalciuria may be difficult to define because of the number of variables listed above. Generally speaking, urinary calcium of greater than 300 mg. per 24 hours for a man and 250 mg. for a woman on a diet without added milk or milk products would be considered abnormal. Some would place the upper normal daily excretion of calcium for an active adult at not greater than 200 mg. [1]. The major clinical causes of hypercalciuria can be classified as [25]:

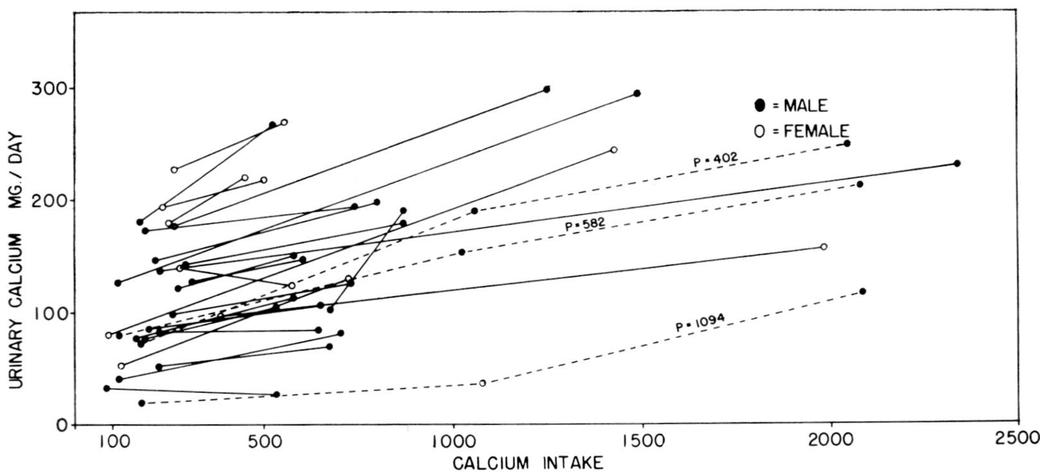

Figure 26-3. Calcium intake and urinary calcium. Subjects studied at multiple levels of intake. (Courtesy of Dr. Anne P. Forbes.)

1. Dissolution of bone:
   - Hyperparathyroidism
   - Metastatic cancer
   - Multiple myeloma
   - Progressive "senile" osteoporosis
   - Cushing's syndrome and the administration of adrenal steroids
   - Immobilization
   - Renal tubular acidosis
   - Hyperthyroidism
   - Fanconi's syndrome
2. Excessive ingestion or absorption of calcium:
   - Milk-alkali syndrome (initially)
   - Vitamin D intoxication
   - Boeck's sarcoid and beryllium poisoning
   - "Idiopathic" hypercalciuria
   - Idiopathic infantile hypercalcemia

The causes of hypercalciuria most frequently found in patients with kidney stones are hyperparathyroidism, renal tubular acidosis, excessive ingestion of calcium, and idiopathic hypercalciuria.

It is axiomatic that all patients with calcium-containing stones must be studied for the presence of hyperparathyroidism. Renal manifestations of primary hyperparathyroidism (stones or nephrocalcinosis, or both) are those most frequently encountered, occurring in 49 to 78 per cent of patients in large series [1, 44]. Clinical bone involvement, as judged by radiographic changes or elevation of serum alkaline phosphatase, is much less frequently found (in approximately 20 to 25 per cent of patients). Of patients seen with nephrolithiasis in a hospital setting, about 5 to 10 per cent are found to have primary hyperparathyroidism on subsequent investigation. Patients with hyperparathyroidism do not necessarily exhibit hypercalciuria at the time of study, because of the opposing effects of hypercalcemia and the hormonal enhancement of calcium reabsorption and the effect of variations in dietary phosphate on calcium excretion. It is beyond the scope of this chapter to review the differential diagnosis of hyperparathyroidism and the tests now available to study patients suspected of having this disorder. In our opinion, the diagnosis now rests on otherwise unexplained hypercalcemia, perhaps unmasked by a low-phosphate diet, with the various parameters for measuring a renal "phosphate leak" being of less importance. At this time, early reports give promise that measurement of circulating parathyroid hormone by a radioimmunoassay, perhaps coupled with calcium infusion to demonstrate autonomy of secretion, will allow more accurate diagnosis in the future [74].

Renal tubular acidosis not infrequently results in hypercalciuria, stones, and nephrocalcinosis, presumably from dissolution of bone secondary to metabolic acidosis. The pathophysiology of the various forms of renal tubular acidosis, that of an inability to maintain a normal hydrogen ion gradient in the distal tubule, is discussed in Chapter 30. A few patients with calcium-containing stones give a history of drinking large amounts of milk and ingesting calcium-containing antacids over long periods. As noted above (and in Figure 26-3), the increase of urinary calcium through this mechanism is rarely large, but it may suffice to result in stone formation.

When other known causes of hypercalciuria have been excluded, there remains a group of patients who have persistent normocalcemic hypercalciuria in the absence of demonstrable bone disease. This abnormality, known for more than 30 years as that most frequently found in patients with stone diathesis [29], has been called idiopathic hypercalciuria [45]. It tends to occur in middle life and is more frequent in men than in women. Recent studies indicate that these patients reduce urine calcium normally (conserve calcium) at very low levels of ingestion, but show excessive absorption and excretion of calcium at normal and increased levels of intake. The primary abnormality — that of excessive gut absorption of calcium — differs from that of sarcoid and of vitamin D toxicity in not being suppressed by glucocorticoid administration. Hyperparathyroidism has been well ruled out in a number of these patients, not only by the absence of hypercalcemia but also by neck exploration. This particular condition, or group of conditions, warrants further investigation because of its frequent association with recurrent kidney stones. Methods of treatment are described in a later section.

Oxalate. After calcium, oxalate is the most frequent crystalloid in kidney stones, being found in approximately two-thirds of stones in the United States (see Table 26-1). These may be essentially pure calcium oxalate stones, or calcium oxalate in combination with other constituents (calcium phosphate, uric acid, magnesium ammonium phosphate). The great majority of patients with calcium oxalate stones have no detectable abnormality of oxalate metabolism. They either have some disorder of calcium metabolism leading to hypercalciuria, or more frequently must be presumed to have some alteration in the factors listed in the section on physicochemical changes in the urine or urinary tract conducive to stone formation.

Normal excretion of oxalic acid in the adult is 20 to 55 mg. per 24 hours (Fig. 26-4). Oxalate is a nonmetabolizable end product, virtually all of that synthesized being excreted by the kidney. Although an area of some controversy, it seems most likely that clearance of oxalate equals or exceeds that of inulin, as measured by constant infusion of ^{14}C-labeled oxalate in man [91]. At the present time there are five known conditions which result in excessive renal excretion of oxalate [92]: (1) ingestion of large amounts of oxalate or oxalate precursors (glycolate, ethylene glycol, glyoxylate, not glycine), (2) pyridoxine (vitamin B_6) deficiency, (3) primary hyperoxaluria with glycolic aciduria, (4) primary hyperoxaluria with L-glyceric aciduria, and (5) inflammatory bowel disease with excessive bacterial conversion of bile salt glycine to oxalate. Oxalate is poorly absorbed, 3 to 5 per cent of that ingested [2], so that overindulgence in high oxalate foods (such as "rhubarb gluttony") is seldom found as a cause of hyperoxaluria. None of the oxalate precursors listed above except glycine is found in high concentrations in food. Increased ingestion of glycine does not significantly enhance oxalate excretion. Pyridoxine is

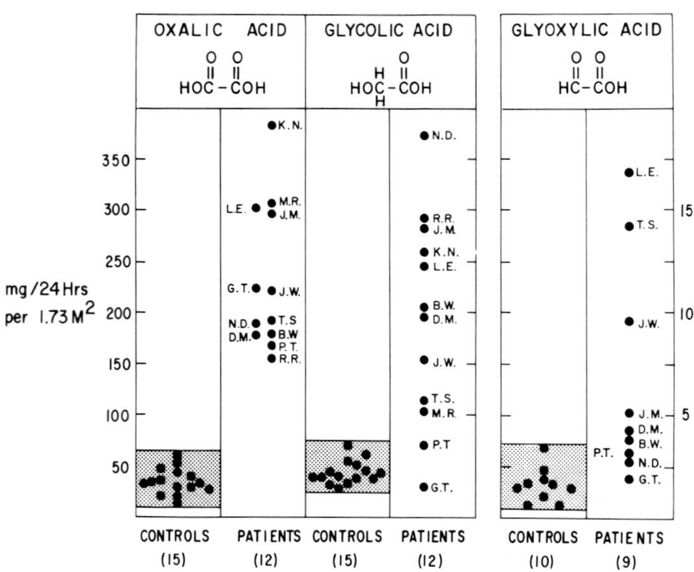

Figure 26-4. Urinary excretion of oxalic, glycolic, and glyoxylic acids by normal control subjects and by patients with primary hyperoxaluria. Patients P.T. and G.T., with normal excretions of glycolic acid, were later found to have glyceric aciduria. (From Hockaday, T. D. R., Frederick, E. W., Clayton, J. E., and Smith, L. H., Jr. Studies on primary hyperoxaluria: II. Urinary oxalate, glycolate, and glyoxylate measurement by isotope dilution methods. *J. Lab. Clin. Med.* 65: 677, 1965.)

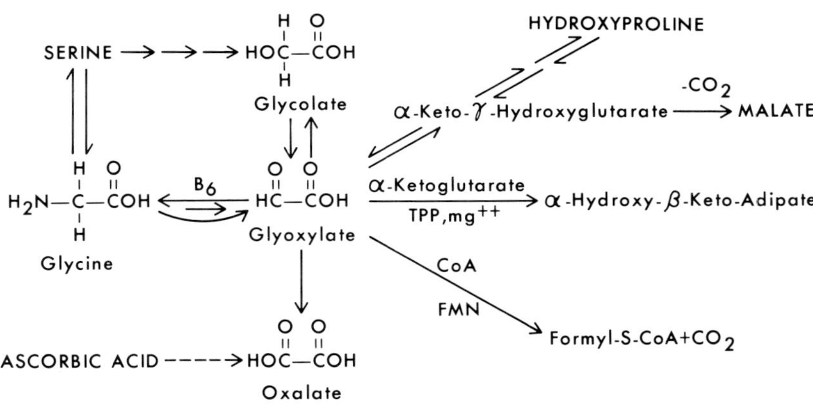

Figure 26-5. Pathways of oxalate synthesis and the metabolism of glyoxylate in man. TPP, thiaminpyrophosphate; FMN, flavinmononucleotide; CoA, coenzyme A.

a cofactor in the reaction or reactions by which glyoxylate is transaminated to glycine [95] (Fig. 26-5). Pyridoxine deficiency in man [26] and in laboratory animals [35] leads to increased oxalate excretion, probably through a partial block in this pathway of glyoxylate metabolism. A few patients have been described in whom hyperoxaluria and resulting calcium oxalate nephrolithiasis were most likely secondary to spontaneous pyridoxine deficiency [24]. Most attention has been directed to the two genetic diseases which lead to increased oxalate synthesis and excretion [47, 94].

The two variants of primary hyperoxaluria cannot be distinguished clinically and so are discussed together. The typical manifestations are those of early onset of recurrent calcium oxalate stones and nephrocalcinosis which, often complicated by superimposed pyelonephritis, lead to progressive loss of renal function and early death in uremia [47]. At postmortem examination widespread deposition of calcium oxalate may be found in many organs, a condition known as oxalosis. An increasing number of milder cases are now being discovered in adults, who do not exhibit the inexorable course of the usual childhood disease.

Primary hyperoxaluria is diagnosed by demonstrating excessive urinary excretion of oxalate (usually more than 120 to 150 mg. per 24 hours; see also Fig. 26-4) in the absence of pyridoxine deficiency. Although pyridoxine (50 to 100 mg. per day) may diminish oxalate excretion somewhat in primary hyperoxaluria, it will not return it to normal. Oxalate excretion falls with the onset of renal failure, so that it may be impossible to diagnose the disease by current technics during the uremic phase. The reliability of reported methods for measuring plasma oxalate remains to be established [98]. Primary hyperoxaluria type I is diagnosed by the measurement of an associated excessive excretion of glycolic acid, greater than the normal excretion rate of 20 to 60 mg. per 24 hours (Fig. 26-4) [48, 92]. In recently discovered primary hyperoxaluria type II there is excretion of large amounts (225 to 638 mg. per 24 hours) of L-glyceric acid, a compound that cannot be detected in normal urine [93]. The enzyme defect in type I disease is that of soluble alpha-ketoglutarate:glyoxylate carboligase, demonstrated in preparations from liver, kidney, and spleen [55]. The resulting accumulation of glyoxylate leads to its enhanced oxidation to oxalate and reduction to glycolate (Fig. 26-5), both of which appear in increased amounts with glyoxylate in urine. In primary

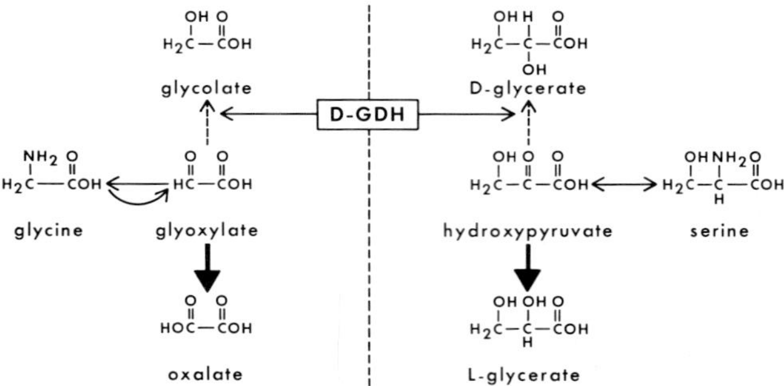

Figure 26-6. Pathways of glyoxylate and hydroxypyruvate metabolism. The enzyme D-glyceric dehydrogenase (D-GDH) has a catalytic function in both pathways. (From Williams, H. E., and Smith, L. H., Jr. L-glyceric aciduria: A new genetic variant of primary hyperoxaluria. *New Eng. J. Med.* 278:233, 1968.)

hyperoxaluria type II, there is deficient activity of D-glyceric dehydrogenase, an enzyme in the pathway of serine metabolism [94]. The reduction of hydroxypyruvate by lactic dehydrogenase appears to be coupled to LDH catalyzed oxidation of glyoxylate to oxalate (Fig. 26-6). D-glyceric dehydrogenase can be assayed in leukocyte preparations, and therefore a direct measurement of its activity can be conveniently carried out for diagnostic purposes.

Both types of primary hyperoxaluria appear to be transmitted as autosomal recessive traits. No increased excretion of oxalate is usually found in presumed heterozygotes (parents of affected children). The frequency of genetic hyperoxaluria has not been established. More widespread use of reliable methods of measuring oxalate excretion will probably continue to detect other mild cases in adults with calcium oxalate stone diathesis.

Cystine. A cystine kidney stone is diagnostic of cystinuria, a genetic disorder characterized by continued excessive excretion of cystine, lysine, arginine, and ornithine (Fig. 26-7). Excessive urinary excretion of cystine may occur in other generalized aminoacidurias (in the Fanconi syndrome, for example), but in none of these conditions does its concentration reach levels associated with stone formation (about 350 mg. per liter of urine). Cystinuria has a long history of investigation since cystine was first discovered as a bladder stone constituent (hence its name) and since it represented one of Garrod's original four "inborn errors of metabolism." Recent advances in the study of cystinuria have been extensively reviewed elsewhere [51, 52].

In cystinuria there is defective renal tubular reabsorption of the amino acids shown in Figure 26-7, as well as the mixed disulfide of cysteine and homocysteine [53] as shown by clearance technics. The clearance of cystine not infrequently exceeds that of inulin, indicating net tubular secretion [54, 55]. Tissue-slice preparations from cystinuric kidneys

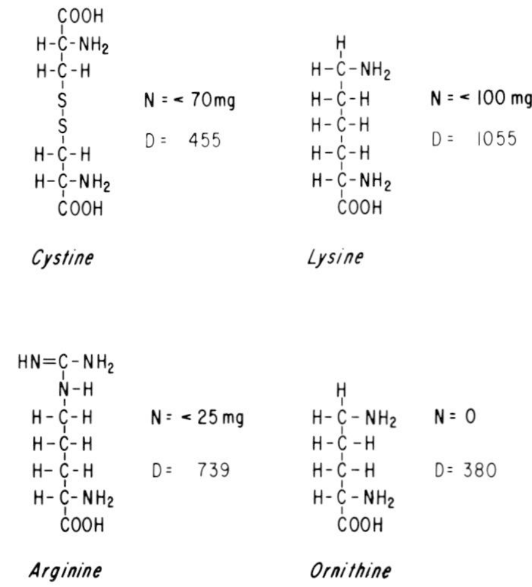

Figure 26-7. Formulas of the major amino acids excreted in excess in cystinuria as described by Harris et al. [41]. N, normal; D, cystinurics.

have confirmed impaired transport of lysine, ornithine, and arginine [56]. So far it has not been possible to demonstrate any renal abnormality of cystine or cysteine transport in vitro. Defective transport of the specific amino acids may also occur in the gut, as shown by oral tolerance tests [57] and by in vitro studies of preparations from intestinal mucosa [58]. There is no evidence that active transport of these amino acids is altered in other cells or tissues. The study of active transport of amino acids is still primarily at the descriptive level. It can be anticipated that future work will be directed to the binding protein (or proteins) or receptor sites required for this process and which are presumably altered in cystinuria.

The frequency of homozygous cystinuria has been estimated to be of the order 1:20,000 (England) to 1:100,000 (Sweden) [18]. As noted, cystine stones constitute 1 to 2 per cent of all stones. Cystinuria occurs equally in men and women, but tends to be clinically more severe in men. The transmission of cystinuria is autosomal recessive in pattern, but the work of several groups of investigators has clearly established the presence of heterogeneity in the disease. In important early work based on extensive family studies, Harris and his colleagues [41] presented a classification of "completely recessive" and "incompletely recessive" cystinuria representing about two-thirds and one-third of cases, respectively. In the former group heterozygotes exhibited no aminoaciduria. Incompletely recessive heterozygotes of cystinuria, on the other hand, excreted increased amounts of the amino acids, in particular cystine and lysine. In vitro studies of biopsies from gut mucosa have been interpreted as being consistent with three patterns in cystinuria, representing a further subdivision of the Harris incompletely recessive group (Table 26-2) [76]. This work has also suggested that a patient doubly heterozygous for two forms of cystinuria may be indistinguishable from a homozygous patient in phenotypic expression, indicating allelism of the defects [77].

Except for some statistical evidence for reduced stature, the only clinical manifestation of cystinuria is that of recurrent cystine stones. The gut defect is not clinically important (unless lysine deficiency is related to short stature). It does lead to increased bacterial degradation of the amino acids to putrescine

Table 26-2. Classification of Cystinuria

Classification[a]	Amino Acid Excretion in Heterozygotes[a]	In Vitro Gut Transport Studies[b]	Response of Plasma Cystine to an Oral Load[b]
Completely recessive [41] Type I [76]	Normal	No transport of cystine, lysine, or arginine	None
Incompletely recessive [41] or:			
Type II [76]	Cystine & lysine increased	No transport of lysine; very reduced cystine transport	Slight rise
Type III [76]	Cystine & lysine increased	Transport of cystine & lysine present but generally less than in normal controls	Subnormal rate of rise to a normal final concentration

[a] According to Harris et al. [41].
[b] According to Rosenberg et al. [76].
SOURCE: Crawhall, J. C., and Watts, R. W. E. [18].

and cadaverine, and the excessive urinary excretion of these diamines and their cyclic products pyrrolidine and piperidine. The upper limit of normal cystine excretion is about 18 mg. per gram of creatinine. Patients with cystine stones generally excrete more than 350 to 400 mg. of cystine per 24 hours. The disease can be diagnosed by analysis of a stone (which may occasionally be mixed in composition) or by measurement of excess urinary cystine. The nonspecific but sensitive nitroprusside test reveals the presence of excess disulfide groups in the urine, and can be made semiquantitative. It is preferable to demonstrate the specific pattern of aminoaciduria using paper or column chromatography. The typical cystine "benzene ring" crystals can usually be found in concentrated, acidified (glacial acetic acid), chilled urine specimens. Variants of the typical patterns of aminoaciduria and the occurrence of a similar typical pattern in the rare disorder hereditary pancreatitis are discussed elsewhere [18, 38].

Uric Acid. Uric acid is the major constituent in about 5 to 10 per cent of kidney stones in the United States (see Table 26-1). It may also be the nidus of a superimposed radiopaque calcium oxalate, calcium phosphate, or magnesium ammonium phosphate stone. Uric acid stones occur in approximately 10 to 25 per cent of patients with primary gout and 30 to 40 per cent of those with gout secondary to proliferative disorders, such as myeloid metaplasia and polycythemia vera [39]. On the other hand, most patients with uric acid nephrolithiasis do not have clinical gout or essential hyperuricemia. In general there are two conditions conducive to uric acid stones: (1) increased excretion of urate, and (2) increased urine acidity.

In a sense, uric acid stones represent an error in evolution for primates in that the enzyme uricase has been deleted. This enzyme catalyzes the conversion of relatively insoluble uric acid to highly soluble allantoin. The presence of uric acid, of use to the bird and reptile in forming a cloacal paste with water conservation, is a constant hazard to the primate kidney with concentrated, often highly acidified urine. In the adult on a low-purine diet the normal rate of synthesis of uric acid is in the range of 600 to 1000 mg. per 24 hours. Of this amount approximately one-quarter to one-third is excreted into the gut where it is destroyed by bacterial action [84]. The remainder is excreted in the urine, amounting to 250 to 550 mg. per day on a low-protein diet. Plasma urate is completely filtrable at the glomerulus, with a net reabsorption of approximately 92 per cent. Urine urate represents the net balance of that filtered and that reabsorbed and actively secreted by the renal tubule. An increased concentration of urinary urate could result from a reduction in urine water (dehydration), increased synthesis of urate from endogenous purines, excessive ingestion of purines in the diet, or a partial diversion of secretion from the gut to the kidney (not yet demonstrated). Temporarily it may result from the use of a uricosuric agent, but after depletion of urate stores renal excretion will again be a function of urate synthesis. Pathways of purine synthesis, their control in man, and the disorders in the various forms of gout have been described elsewhere and are not reviewed here [96]. On investigation it is found that most patients with uric acid stones excrete normal amounts of urinary urate. A few patients exhibit significant hyperuricosuria in the absence of an elevated serum uric acid.

The solubility of uric acid is much less than that of its salts with sodium or potassium. The result is that stones are uric acid rather than a urate salt. As a consequence, urine pH is the major determinant of the fraction of urate excreted in its poorly soluble undissociated form. The pK of the N-9 position of uric acid, which largely accounts for its acidic qualities in the physiologic range, is 5.75. At this pH uric acid is half ionized and half undissociated. The titration curve is such that the undissociated uric acid increases to 85 per cent at pH 5.0, and at this pH only 6 to 8 mg. of urate is soluble per 100 ml. of urine, so that supersaturation is required to excrete an average uric acid load in a normal urine volume. The solubility of urate rises to 158 mg. per 100 ml. of urine at pH 7.0 [68]. This twentyfold change over a physiologic pH range is the major determinant of urinary urate solubility. Any condition that enhances the acidity of urine therefore increases the chance of uric acid stone formation, including acidifying medications, chronic diarrhea, and an overactive ileostomy. It has been reported that many patients with recurrent uric acid stones, with or without associated primary gout, demonstrate a renal defect in that they excrete urines of increased acidity at the expense of urinary ammonia [39, 46]. The hypothesis has been set forward that a defect in renal tubular production of ammonia is primary, so that excretion of a more acid urine is necessary in the face of a normal metabolic acid load. The observations on which this hypothesis rest have been repeated in a number of laboratories with both confirmation [73] and failure of confirmation [61]. A review of the conflicting evidence is published elsewhere [39].

Many patients with recurrent uric acid stones have not demonstrated excessive urate excretion or any gross derangement in urinary acidification. It is possible that they may have blunting or loss of normal "alkaline tides" in urine. Since normal urine is often supersaturated with uric acid, they may have diminished ability to maintain such a metastable state. Uric acid stone diathesis in the absence of hyperuricemia has been described as a familial disorder, seemingly transmitted as a dominant trait [22].

Xanthine. Xanthine is an extremely rare component of stones, only about 40 such stones having been described in the past 150 years [78]. Xanthine stones are the only clinical manifestation of xanthinuria, a rare genetic disorder with marked reduction in, to absent activity of, xanthine oxidase, which normally catalyzes the oxidation of hypoxanthine to xanthine and of xanthine to uric acid. In its absence the purine excretory load is excreted as xanthine and hypoxanthine (roughly two-thirds and one-third, respectively), with only trace amounts of uric acid. Only three of the seven described patients with this disease have had xanthine stones [78]. The occurrence in the past of other patients with xanthine stones may have represented heterozygotes with xanthinuria although this requires confirmation. Xanthine is a normal constituent of urine, but is present in an amount of only 5 to 20 mg. per day. In urine it is even less soluble than uric acid. The use of allopurinol to inhibit uric acid synthesis in gout produces reversible xanthinuria. So far this has not resulted in stone formation.

Ammonia. Ammonia is a constituent of stones as magnesium ammonium phosphate, its frequency varying with the incidence of urinary tract infection with urea-splitting organisms. Urinary ammonia may derive from two sources: (1) from the tubule in defense of acid-base balance (primarily released from glutamine by glutaminase) and (2) from urea by the action of urease from certain bacteria. Excessive urinary ammonia, always of bacterial origin, produces both increase in concentration of ammonium ion and pathologic alkalinization of urine, favoring the precipitation of calcium phosphate and magnesium ammonium phosphate. The percentage of stones attributed to infection has varied markedly in different series. Often it has been difficult to determine whether infection was primary, or occurred as a complication of stones. Topographical analyses of the stone may help resolve this if the core is of different composition. In a large Swedish series, 22 per cent of stones were thought to originate with infection [43]. In sharp contrast, only 3 of 207 patients in a Boston clinic were thought to have had infection as the origin of stone pathogenesis, although an additional 31 of these patients had urinary tract infection judged to be secondary to the presence of stones [60].

PHYSICOCHEMICAL CHANGES IN THE URINE OR URINARY TRACT

Thorough investigation of a patient with a kidney stone often — in fact, probably most often — fails to reveal any gross abnormality in the urinary excretion or concentration of calcium, oxalate, cystine, urate, xanthine, or ammonia. It is possible that such abnormalities may not be constant, but they may have produced triggering of embryonic stones in the past [89]. It is more likely that some of the variables involved in physicochemical changes in the urine or urinary tract are responsible. Some of these factors, in general much less well understood than those of crystalloid excretion, are reviewed briefly.

pH. Urine acidity affects the solubility of several constituents of stones, as outlined in Figure 26-8. The effect is most striking for uric acid, as noted above, since the actual concentration of the undissociated acid varies with the point on its titration curve fixed by urine pH. The solubility of cystine also increases with alkalinity, but unfortunately the sharp upswing of the curve occurs at pH 7.2 to 7.4, a range difficult to maintain without hazard. Calcium phosphate stones are more apt to form at this pH, and magnesium ammonium phosphate stones form only in alkaline urines. The solubility of calcium oxalate does not change appreciably over the pH range of urine.

Matrix. A previous part of this chapter contains a brief description of matrix as a structural component of stones, constituting about 2.5 per cent of the dry weight. The role which this mucoprotein may play in stone genesis, growth, and form is not clear, although evidence for a matrix influence on growth and cohesiveness is perhaps more likely than its serving as the initial nucleating event. This evidence, reviewed in detail elsewhere [11], is summarized briefly here.

The architecture of stones (laminations, radial striations, frond formation, spherules) appears to depend upon the structural organization of contained matrix. Matrix "stones" or concretions have been described, resembling staghorn calculi in gross structure and matrix laminations, but so very poorly mineralized that they are generally radiolucent (calcium phosphate, 28 to 42 per cent of the dry weight) [63, 90]. Rapid mineralization of calculus matrix in vivo has occurred in a few patients with cystinuria adequately treated previously with D-penicillamine [13]. The assumption is that

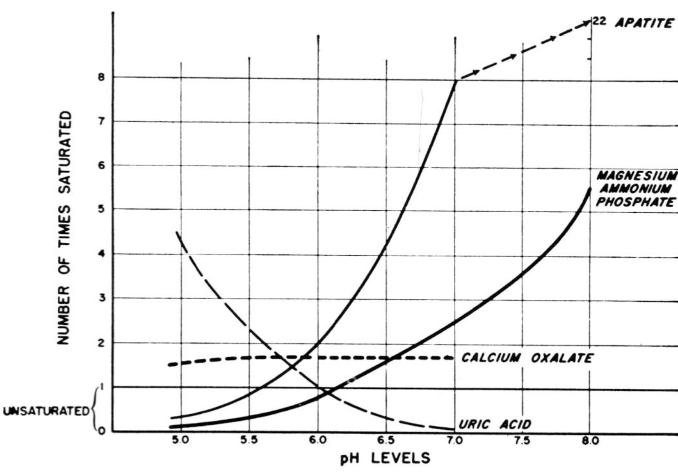

Figure 26-8. Saturation of urine with crystalloids at different pH levels. (Courtesy of Dr. Anne P. Forbes.)

residual matrix, from which cystine had been reabsorbed, serves to nucleate a calcific stone. The matrix composition of stones is quite constant in the face of wide differences in crystalloid content, suggesting specificity rather than adventitious absorption. Finally, it has been reported that matrix substance A is present in the urine and kidney extracts from patients with stone diathesis but not in controls. The statement has been made, "Its presence in urine is generally directly proportional to the clinical predisposition to frequency and size of renal calculus formation" [11]. These provocative observations should be further pursued. It should be noted that experimental concretions can be produced in vitro in the absence of matrix proteins [89].

Stasis. "Stagnation in any place along the urinary stream probably favors crystallization just as projecting stones allow ice to form behind them in a cold running brook" [30]. This simple statement summarizes the extent of current knowledge about the role of stasis in stone genesis. It probably contributes time for crystallization to occur in urine which is often normally supersaturated and prevents the rapid abortion of embryonic stones. An anatomic cause should be suspected when repeated stone formation is limited to one kidney.

Foreign Body. Insertion of a foreign body is one of the most effective means of inducing experimental stone formation. This rarely pertains clinically, unless one considers the presence of one stone as a foreign body on which a stone of different composition may be deposited.

Diminished Activity of Protective Substances. It is quite possible that this is the most important category of stone pathogenesis, but it is the one about which least is known. It is apparent that substances protective against crystallization must exist in urine, because it is impossible to maintain the crystalloids of urine in simple solution in water. Some of the factors thought to be of importance are citrate [71], magnesium [50a], pyrophosphate [28], and inhibitor polypeptides [49]. In addition there may be nonspecific "salting-in effects" from electrolytes (sodium, potassium, chloride, etc.) and from certain organic components such as urea and amino acids.

Citrate is an effective chelator of calcium, but there is little evidence that reduced urine citrate plays any role in stone formation [52]. The excretion of citrate varies with urine pH. Extensive studies have been carried out on the possible role of magnesium deficiency in stone pathogenesis [50a]. Magnesium deficiency in the rat leads to reproducible renal tubular degeneration and calcification, which has been termed "intranephronic calculosis" [66]. The addition of magnesium in vitro will inhibit the calcification of rachitic rat cartilage [64]. Magnesium gives partial protection against experimental calcium oxalate deposition in the rat [34], and has been reported to reduce the recurrence of oxalate stones in man [36]. It has been reported, and denied, that the ratio of magnesium to calcium is reduced in the urine of some patients with recurrent stones [52]. At the present time magnesium deficiency is unproved as a cause of stones in man.

Pyrophosphate is released in a number of biosynthetic processes, but the majority of it is quickly hydrolyzed in the presence of pyrophosphatase. Pyrophosphate is an effective inhibitor of calcium phosphate crystallization and of bone salt deposition in osteoid [56]. About 1 to 4 mg. of pyrophosphate is excreted per 24 hours in normal urine, this amount increasing twofold to threefold on treatment with large amounts of orthophosphate [56]. It also increases in conditions associated with excessive osteolysis [3]. It has not been established that patients with stones have a deficiency of pyrophosphate [65], but this substance may contribute to the normal protective barrier against crystallization. Particular interest relates to the work of Howard and Thomas and their colleagues [49, 50] in their description and partial purification from urine of low-molecular-weight polypeptides which seem to inhibit crystallization of calcium phosphate and perhaps also calcium oxalate. The deposition of bone salts in rachitic rat cartilage incubated in urine was introduced as a biologic test of the crystallization potential of urine, the assumption being made that this, beyond its intrinsic interest, might bear some relationship to the propensity toward stone formation. Normal urine does not support deposition of bone salts in rachitic cartilage despite a high calcium × phosphate product.

Urine from patients with stone diathesis often, although not in every specimen, does calcify rachitic cartilage. In a few instances "calcifying urine" found in a seemingly normal subject has been predictive of subsequent stone formation. Using the cartilage test, extensive but as yet incomplete studies have been carried out in an attempt to isolate and identify the substance or substances in urine which exert this control of crystallization [49]. Chromatography of urine has yielded two fractions of high potency as measured in the rachitic cartilage test or by simple inhibition of hydroxyapatite crystal formation on incubation of calcium phosphate solutions. These fractions will also retard the crystallization of calcium oxalate. Initial studies indicate that these are small polypeptides. No methods for measuring the amounts of inhibitor peptides excreted has been reported, due to large and variable losses during the purification procedure. It is not yet possible to state, therefore, that such peptides are reduced in concentration in the urine (from stone formers) which calcifies rachitic cartilage. This approach appears to be of particular promise in the study of the processes that restrain crystallization in urine.

Treatment of Stones

The treatment of stones divides itself between urologic management of the anatomic problem of the stone lodged in kidney, ureter, or bladder and measures to prevent stone growth or recurrence. Urologic aspects of treatment are not presented here. The prevention of stone recurrence is in part empirical and in part based on the information available about pathogenesis, as reviewed above. By and large it is directed toward decreasing the concentration of urinary crystalloids. More recently measures to control crystallization in urine have been introduced. It is remarkably difficult to evaluate the efficacy of stone prophylaxis programs. Recurrence rates are unpredictable in the individual as well as in groups of patients. Few of the recommendations below rest on firm statistical proof of effectiveness.

CALCIUM-CONTAINING STONES

Most frequently such stones are calcium oxalate or mixed calcium oxalate and calcium phosphate (see Table 26-1). Such patients may or may not have hypercalciuria. Those with hyperoxaluria are described below. If a cause of hypercalciuria can be determined (e.g., hyperparathyroidism, sarcoid, renal tubular acidosis), specific treatment is directed toward the basic disorder. If there is no hypercalciuria or if the diagnosis is by exclusion idiopathic hypercalciuria, the object of treatment is to reduce the concentration of urinary calcium and to control the crystallization potential of urine.

A cornerstone of treatment of all patients with stone diathesis of any pathogenesis is to increase urine volume by *forcing fluids.* It is particularly important to blunt the physiologic concentration of urine which occurs at night. Simple injunctions to "drink more water" are rarely effective. Specific directions concerning fluid intake at meals should be given as well as water by the glass at bedtime sufficient, as a rule of thumb, to induce nocturia. Occasional checks of 24-hour urine volumes or morning urine specific gravities may be of help in monitoring compliance.

Patients with calcium-containing stones

should generally reduce calcium intake by avoiding milk as a beverage and high-calcium foods. Such dietary measures rarely lead to a major reduction in urine calcium, but the slope of calcium absorbed to that ingested has been reported increased in idiopathic hypercalciuria [67]. Except in the treatment of sarcoid or vitamin D intoxication, attempts to diminish calcium absorption are not in general use now.

Three other measures may reduce urinary calcium. The ingestion of large amounts of orthophosphate, as described below, reduces urine calcium [88]; the mechanism of this effect has not been well studied, but does not seem to occur by impairment of absorption from the gut. As previously described, the clearance of calcium tends to parallel that of sodium [25]. A strict low-sodium diet may lower urine calcium. Some patients are particularly sensitive to this effect. Finally, certain diuretic agents, particularly the chlorothiazides, have been shown to reduce urine calcium in normal subjects and patients with idiopathic hypercalciuria, presumably through the mechanism of sodium depletion [97]. Their use, now under investigation, may represent an important advance in the treatment of idiopathic hypercalciuria.

A brief description of substances controlling crystallization has been given above. Urine pH has no significant effect on calcium oxalate crystallization, but acidification may reduce the tendency for calcium phosphate stone formation. Orthophosphates, given in amounts of 1 to 2 gm. of phosphorus daily, have been reported to reduce stone recurrence [88]. The mechanism of action, beyond its effect in reducing urine calcium, has not been established. This regimen will increase the rate of excretion of pyrophosphate twofold or threefold. It will also change calcifying urine to noncalcifying, as measured in the rachitic rat cartilage assay [87]. It has not been possible to determine whether the excretion of inhibitor peptides is increased. This form of treatment is described in more detail elsewhere [7, 88]. The demonstration that magnesium will inhibit crystallization of calcium phosphate in vitro [64] and will protect against experimental oxalosis [34] has led to its use in stone prophylaxis. A regimen of magnesium oxide (200 mg. per day) has been reported to give partial protection against recurrence of calcium oxalate stones [36]. As noted, it is very difficult to evaluate such therapy, but there is enough background of information to warrant careful trials of magnesium supplementation.

CALCIUM OXALATE STONES WITH HYPEROXALURIA

In the absence of specific measures to reduce oxalate synthesis and excretion, the treatment of primary hyperoxaluria is largely the same as that described for other calcium-containing stones [82]. In the rare instance of pyridoxine deficiency, supplementation with the vitamin will lower oxalate excretion to normal. In primary hyperoxaluria, large amounts of pyridoxine (100 to 200 mg. per day) may cause modest reductions in oxalate excretion, perhaps by enhancing transamination of glyoxylate to glycine [82]. Calcium carbimide has been introduced as an inhibitor of oxalate synthesis [83], but its effectiveness has not been confirmed in other studies [99]. Childhood primary hyperoxaluria usually leads to early death in uremia. An effective inhibitor of oxalate synthesis would represent the most rational treatment of this serious disorder and might have additional usefulness in the treatment of the much more frequent patient with calcium oxalate stones in the absence of hyperoxaluria.

URIC ACID STONES

Hydration should be stressed in the treatment of uric acid stones, as described above. The most important approach, however, is to raise urine pH to take advantage of the remarkable increase of urate solubility which occurs [39]. No attempt should be made to alkalinize the urine because of the excess of alkali required and the dangers of producing calcium phosphate stones. A pH range of 6.0 to 6.5 usually suffices. Any convenient form of supplementary alkali can be used, monitored by the use of nitrazine paper to ensure that the proper pH range is attained. This is particularly important for the overnight concentrated, usually highly acidic specimen. In the few patients who fail to respond to these simple measures, allopurinol may be added to the regimen (200 to 400 mg. per day) to inhibit partially the synthesis of uric acid from hypoxanthine and xanthine. The rare xanthine stones are also treated by forcing fluids and alkalinization of urine [78].

HOOC—C(NH₂)(H)—C(H)(H)—SH
CYSTEINE
+
HOOC—C(NH₂)(H)—C(CH₃)(CH₃)—SH
PENICILLAMINE
→
HOOC—C(NH₂)(H)—C(H)(H)—S
HOOC—C(NH₂)(H)—C(CH₃)(CH₃)—S
MIXED DISULFIDE
50 X Solubility of Cystine

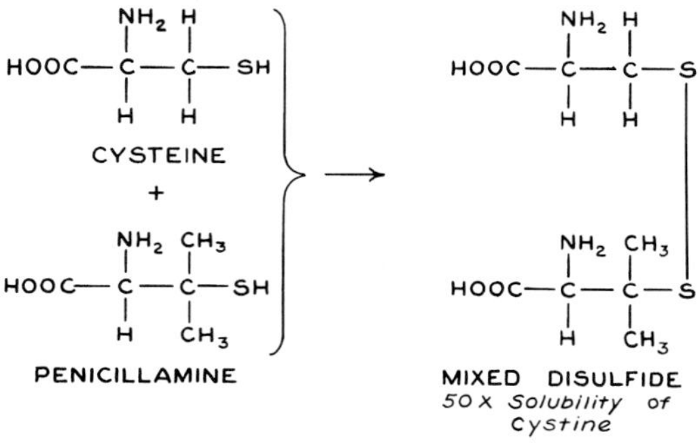

Figure 26-9. The therapeutic use of D-penicillamine as a sulfhydryl trap to form a mixed disulfide of cysteine of enhanced solubility.

CYSTINE STONES

Cystine stones may be frequent or rare despite the continuation of cystinuria. Forcing fluids is particularly important in the treatment of cystinuria, as well documented by Dent and his colleagues [21]. They have emphasized the hazards of nocturnal urine concentration in patients with cystinuria. Methionine is the major precursor of cystine, and a diet low in methionine has been reported to reduce urinary cystine significantly in cystinuria [80]. Others have failed to confirm a useful reduction in urinary cystine in patients on diets that are practical for long-term therapy [100]. Dietary treatment does not have a major role now in most patients. Some increase in the solubility of cystine can be attained by raising urine pH to 7.0, but unfortunately, the major increment in solubility comes at pH's greater than 7.4 and therefore higher than can be safely maintained [19, 21].

An important advance in the treatment of cystinuria was the introduction of D-penicillamine to form mixed disulfides of cysteine and penicillamine ($\beta\beta$ dimethylcysteine) of enhanced solubility (Fig. 26-9) [17]. Through the use of this agent, approximately 1 to 2 grams per day, the excretion of free cystine can be regularly reduced below the level associated with stone formation [4, 16]. Its use is now limited by a wide variety of toxic reactions, some of which occur in one-third to one-half of all patients (serum sickness type reaction, dermatitis, leukopenia, gastrointestinal disturbances, nephrotic syndrome, etc.). Other cysteine analogues, such as N-acetyl-D-penicillamine, are now being explored in an effort to obtain less toxic substances equally capable of sulfhydryl coupling [18].

Acknowledgment

This work was supported by Grant AM 5846, National Institute of Arthritis and Metabolic Diseases.

References

1. Albright, F., and Reifenstein, E. C. *Parathyroid Glands and Metabolic Bone Disease.* Baltimore: Williams & Wilkins, 1948.
2. Archer, H. E., Dormer, A. E., Scowen, E. F., and Watts, R. W. E. Studies on the urinary excretion of oxalate by normal subjects. *Clin. Sci.* 16:405, 1957.
3. Avioli, L. V., McDonald, J. E., and Singer,

R. A. Excretion of pyrophosphate in disorders of bone metabolism. *J. Clin. Endocr.* 25:912, 1965.

4. Bartter, F. C., Lotz, M., Thier, S., Rosenberg, L. E., and Potts, J. T. Cystinuria: Combined clinical staff conference at the National Institutes of Health. *Ann. Intern. Med.* 62:796, 1965.
5. Beck, C. W., and Mulvaney, W. P. Apatitic urinary calculi from early American Indians. *J.A.M.A.* 195:1044, 1966.
6. Bell, E. T. Renal Calculi. In Bell, E. T. (Ed.), *Renal Diseases* (2d ed.). Philadelphia: Lea & Febiger, 1950. P. 414.
7. Bernstein, D. S., and Newton, R. The effect of oral sodium phosphate on the formation of renal calculi and on idiopathic hypercalciuria. *Lancet* 2:1105, 1966.
8. Block, J. M. Oxaluria in British troops in India. *Brit. Med. J.* 1:590, 1945.
9. Boyce, W. H. Kidney Stone, In Budy, A. M. (Ed.), *Biology of Hard Tissue, Proceedings of the First Conference, Princeton, N.J., 1965.* New York: Academy of Sciences Interdisciplinary Communications Program, 1967. Pp. 196–254.
10. Boyce, W. H. Macromolecular Components of Kidney Calculi in Urine. In Hodgkinson, A., and Nordin, B. E. C. (Eds.), *Proceedings of the Renal Stone Research Symposium Held at Leeds, April 1968.* London: Churchill, 1969. Pp. 181–189.
11. Boyce, W. H. Organic matrix of human urinary concretions. *Amer. J. Med.* 45:673, 1968.
12. Boyce, W. H., Garvey, F. K., and Strawcutter, H. E. Incidence of urinary calculi among patients in general hospitals, 1948–1952. *J.A.M.A.* 161:1437, 1956.
13. Boyce, W. H., Smith, M. J. V., and King, J. S., Jr. Some observations on the use of D-penicillamine in the treatment of cystinuria. *Urol. Dig.* 7:19, 1968.
14. Burkland, C. E., and Rosenberg, M. Survey of urolithiasis in the United States. *J. Urol.* 73:198, 1955.
15. Crawhall, J. C., Scowen, E. F., Thompson, C. J., and Watts, R. W. E. The renal clearance of amino acids in cystinuria. *J. Clin. Invest.* 46:1162, 1967.
16. Crawhall, J. C., Scowen, E. F., and Watts, R. W. E. Further observations on the use of D-penicillamine in cystinuria. *Brit. Med. J.* 1:1411, 1964.
17. Crawhall, J. C., Scowen, E. F., and Watts, R. W. E. Effect of penicillamine on cystinuria. *Brit. Med. J.* 1:585, 1965.
18. Crawhall, J. C., and Watts, R. W. E. Cystinuria. *Amer. J. Med.* 45:736, 1968.
19. Dent, C. E., Friedmann, M., Green, H., and Watson, L. C. A. Treatment of cystinuria. *Brit. Med. J.* 1:403, 1965.
20. Dent, C. E., Harper, C. M., and Philpot, G. R. The treatment of renal glomerular osteodystrophy. *Quart. J. Med.* 30:1, 1961.
21. Dent, C. E., and Senior, B. Studies on the treatment of cystinuria. *Brit. J. Urol.* 27: 317, 1955.
22. DeVries, A., Frank, M., and Atsmon, A. Inherited uric acid lithiasis. *Amer. J. Med.* 33:880, 1962.
23. DeVries, A., Kochwa, S., Lazebnik, J., Frank, M., and Djaldetti, M. Glycinuria, a hereditary disorder associated with nephrolithiasis. *Amer. J. Med.* 23:408, 1957.
24. Elder, T. D., and Wyngaarden, J. B. The biosynthesis and turnover of oxalate in normal and hyperoxaluric subjects. *J. Clin. Invest.* 39:1337, 1960.
25. Epstein, F. H. Calcium and the kidney. *Amer. J. Med.* 45:700, 1968.
26. Faber, S. R., Feitler, W. W., Bleiler, R. E., Ohlson, M. A., and Hodges, R. E. The effects of an induced pyridoxine and pantothenic acid deficiency on excretions of oxalic and xanthurenic acids in the urine. *Amer. J. Clin. Nutr.* 12:406, 1963.
27. Fariss, B. L., and Kolb, F. O. Factors involved in crystal formation in cystinuria: Reduction of cystine crystaluria with chlordiazepoxide and during nephrotic syndrome. *J.A.M.A.* 205:846, 1968.
28. Russell, R. G. G., and Fleisch, H. Pyrophosphate and Stone Formation. In *Hodgkinson*, A., and Nordin, B. E. C. (Eds.), *Proceedings of the Renal Stone Research Symposium Held at Leeds, April 1968.* London: Churchill, 1969. Pp. 165–180.
29. Flocks, R. H. Prophylaxis and medical management of calcium urolithiasis: Role of quantity and precipitability of urinary calcium. *J. Urol.* 44:183, 1940.

30. Forbes, A. P., and Dempsey, E. Nephrolithiasis. In Strauss, M. B., and Welt, L. G. (Eds.), *Diseases of the Kidney*. Boston: Little, Brown, 1963. P. 712.
31. Fox, M., Thier, S., Rosenberg, L. E., Kiser, W., and Segal, S. Evidence against a single renal transport defect in cystinuria. *New Eng. J. Med.* 270:556, 1964.
32. Frimpter, G. W. Cystinuria: Metabolism of the disulfide of cysteine and homocysteine. *J. Clin. Invest.* 42:1956, 1963.
33. Frimpter, G. W., Horwith, M., Furth, E., Fellows, R. E., and Thompson, D. D. Inulin and endogenous amino acid renal clearances in cystinuria: Evidence for tubular secretion. *J. Clin. Invest.* 41:281, 1962.
34. Gershoff, S. N., and Andrus, S. B. Effect of vitamin B_6 and magnesium on renal deposition of calcium oxalate induced by ethylene glycol administration. *Proc. Soc. Exp. Biol. Med.* 109:99, 1962.
35. Gershoff, S. N., Faragalla, F. F., Nelson, D. A., and Andrus, S. B. Vitamin B_6 deficiency and oxalate nephrocalcinosis in the cat. *Amer. J. Med.* 27:72, 1959.
36. Gershoff, S. N., and Prien, E. L. Effect of daily MgO and vitamin B_6 administration to patients with recurring calcium oxalate kidney stones. *Amer. J. Clin. Nutr.* 20:393, 1967.
37. Gram, H. C. Heredity of oxalic urinary calculi. *Acta Med. Scand.* 78:268, 1932.
38. Gross, J. B., Ulrich, J. A., and Jones, J. D. Urinary excretion of amino acids in a kindred with hereditary pancreatitis and amino aciduria. *Gastroenterology* 47:41, 1964.
39. Gutman, A. B., and Yü, T. F. Uric acid nephrolithiasis. *Amer. J. Med.* 45:756, 1968.
40. Halstead, S. B., and Valyasevi, A. Studies of bladder stone disease in Thailand: I. Introduction and description of area studies. *Amer. J. Clin. Nutr.* 20:1312, 1967.
41. Harris, H., Mittwoch, U., Robson, E. B., and Warren, F. L. Phenotypes and genotypes in cystinuria. *Ann. Hum. Genet.* 20: 57, 1955.
42. Heaton, F. W., and Hodgkinson, A. Extrarenal factors affecting diurnal variation in electrolyte excretion with particular reference to calcium and magnesium. *Clin. Chim. Acta* 8:246, 1963.
43. Hellstrom, J. Staphylococcus stones: A clinical study of 90 cases. *Acta Chir. Scand.* Suppl. 46, 1936.
44. Hellstrom, J., and Ivemark, B. I. Primary hyperparathyroidism. *Acta Chir. Scand.* Suppl. 294, 1962.
45. Henneman, P. H., Benedict, P. H., Forbes, A. P., and Dudley, H. R. Idiopathic hypercalciuria. *New Eng. J. Med.* 259:802, 1958.
46. Henneman, P. H., Wallach, S., and Dempsey, E. F. Metabolic defect responsible for uric acid renal stone formation. *J. Clin. Invest.* 37:901, 1958.
47. Hockaday, T. D. R., Clayton, J. E., Frederick, E. W., and Smith, L. H., Jr. Primary hyperoxaluria. *Medicine* 43:315, 1964.
48. Hockaday, T. D. R., Frederick, E. W., Clayton, J. E., and Smith, L. H., Jr. Studies on primary hyperoxaluria: II. Urinary oxalate, glycolate, and glyoxylate measurement by isotope dilution methods. *J. Lab. Clin. Med.* 65:677, 1965.
49. Howard, J. E., and Thomas, W. C., Jr. Control of crystallization in urine. *Amer. J. Med.* 45:693, 1968.
50. Howard, J. E., Thomas, W. C., Jr., Barker, L. M., Smith, L. H., and Wadkins, C. L. The recognition and isolation from urine and serum of a peptide inhibitor to calcification. *Johns Hopkins Med. J.* 120:119, 1967.
50a. Human renal calculus formation and magnesium. *Nutr. Rev.* 24:43, 1966.
51. Kleeman, C. R., Bernstein, D., Rockney, R., Dowling, J. T., and Maxwell, M. H. Studies on the renal clearance of diffusible calcium and the role of the parathyroid glands in its regulation. *Yale J. Biol. Med.* 34:1, 1961.
52. King, J. S., Jr. Etiologic factors involved in urolithiasis: A review of recent research. *J. Urol.* 97:583, 1967.
53. King, J. S., Jr., and Boyce, W. H. Analysis of renal calculous matrix compared with some other matrix materials and with uromucoid. *Arch. Biochem. Biophys.* 82: 455, 1959.

54. Knox, W. E. Cystinuria. In Stanbury, J. B., Wyngaarden, J. B., and Fredrickson, D. S. (Eds.), *The Metabolic Basis of Inherited Disease*. New York: McGraw-Hill, 1966. P. 1262.
55. Koch, J., Stokstad, E. L. R., Williams, H. E., and Smith, L. H., Jr. Deficiency of 2-oxo-glutarate:glyoxylate carboligase activity in primary hyperoxaluria. *Proc. Nat. Acad. Sci. USA* 57:1123, 1967.
56. Lewis, A. M., Thomas, W. C., Jr., and Tomita, A. Pyrophosphate and the mineralizing potential of urine. *Clin. Sci.* 30: 389, 1966.
57. Logergren, C. Biophysical investigations of urinary calculi. *Acta Radiol.* Suppl. 133:1, 1956.
58. Lonsdale, K. Human stones. *Science* 159: 1199, 1968.
59. McGeown, M. G. Heredity in renal stone disease. *Clin. Sci.* 19:465, 1960.
60. Melick, R. A., and Henneman, P. H. Clinical and laboratory studies of 207 consecutive patients in a kidney-stone clinic. *New Eng. J. Med.* 259:307, 1958.
61. Metcalfe-Gibson, A., McCallum, F. M., Morrison, R. B. I., and Wrong, O. Urinary excretion of hydrogen ion in patients with uric acid calculi. *Clin. Sci.* 28:325, 1965.
62. Milne, M. D., Asatoor, A. M., Edwards, K. D. G., and Loughridge, L. W. The intestinal absorption defect in cystinuria. *Gut* 2:323, 1961.
63. Mogg, R. A. Matrix calculi. *Proc. Roy. Soc. Med.* 57:935, 1964.
64. Mukai, T., and Howard, J. E. Some observations on the calcification of rachitic cartilage by urine. *Bull. Johns Hopkins Hosp.* 112:279, 1963.
65. O'Brien, M. M., Uhlemann, I., and McIntosh, H. W. Urinary pyrophosphate in normal subjects and in stone formers. *Canad. Med. Ass. J.* 96:100, 1967.
66. Oliver, J., MacDowell, M., Whang, R., and Welt, L. G. The renal lesions of electrolyte imbalance: IV. The intranephronic calculosis of experimental magnesium depletion. *J. Exp. Med.* 124:263, 1966.
67. Peacock, M., Hodgkinson, A., and Nordin, B. E. C. Importance of dietary calcium in the definition of hypercalciuria. *Brit. Med. J.* 3:469, 1967.
68. Peters, J. P., and Van Slyke, D. D. *Quantitative Clinical Chemistry* (2d ed.). Baltimore: Williams & Wilkins, 1946. Vol. 1.
69. Piering, W. F., Lemann, J., Jr., and Lennon, E. F. The effect of carbohydrate administration on urinary calcium and magnesium excretion. *Clin. Res.* 16:393, 1968.
70. Prien, E. L., and Prien, E. L., Jr. Composition and structure of urinary stone. *Amer. J. Med.* 45:654, 1968.
71. Raaflaub, J. On the relationships between the total content of calcium and the calcium ion concentration in the urine. *Helv. Physiol. Pharmacol. Acta* 18:87, 1960.
72. Randall, A. The origin and growth of renal calculi. *Ann. Surg.* 105:1009, 1937.
73. Rapoport, A., Crassweller, P. O., Husdan, H., From, G. L. A., Zweig, M., and Johnson, M. D. The renal excretion of hydrogen ion in uric acid stone formers. *Metabolism* 16:176, 1967.
74. Reiss, E., and Canterbury, J. M. A radioimmunoassay for parathyroid hormone in man. *Proc. Soc. Exp. Biol. Med.* 128:501, 1968.
75. Resnick, M., Pridgen, D. B., and Goodman, H. O. Genetic predisposition to formation of calcium oxalate renal calculi. *New Eng. J. Med.* 278:1313, 1968.
76. Rosenberg, L. E., Downing, S., Durant, J. L., and Segal, S. Cystinuria: Biochemical evidence for three genetically distinct diseases. *J. Clin. Invest.* 45:365, 1966.
77. Rosenberg, L. E., Durant, J. L., and Albrecht, I. Genetic heterogeneity in cystinuria: Evidence for allelism. *Trans. Ass. Amer. Physicians* 79:284, 1966.
78. Seegmiller, J. E. Xanthine stone formation. *Amer. J. Med.* 45:780, 1968.
79. Shattock, S. G. Prehistoric or predynastic Egyptian calculus. *Trans. Path. Sci.* (London) 56:275, 1905.
80. Smith, D. R., Kolb, F. O., and Harper, H. A. Management of cystinuria and cystine-stone disease. *J. Urol.* 81:61, 1959.
81. Smith, L. H., Jr. Introduction: "Books in

the running brooks; sermons in stone." *Amer. J. Med.* 45:649, 1968.

82. Smith, L. H., Jr., and Williams, H. E. Treatment of primary hyperoxaluria. *Mod. Treatm.* 4:522, 1967.
83. Solomons, C. C., Goodman, S. I., and Riley, C. M. Calcium carbide in treatment of primary hyperoxaluria. *New Eng. J. Med.* 276:207, 1967.
84. Sorensen, L. B. Degradation of uric acid in man. *Metabolism* 8:687, 1959.
85. Talmage, R. V., and Kraintz, F. W. Progressive changes in renal phosphate and calcium excretion in rats following parathyroidectomy or parathyroid administration. *Proc. Soc. Exp. Biol. Med.* 87:263, 1954.
86. Thier, S., Fox, M., Segal, S., and Rosenberg, L. E. Cystinuria: *In vitro* demonstration of an intestinal transport defect. *Science* 143:482, 1964.
87. Thomas, W. C., Jr., and Howard, J. E. Studies on the mineralizing propensity of urine from patient with and without renal calculi. *Trans. Ass. Amer. Physicians* 72: 181, 1959.
88. Thomas, W. C., Jr., and Miller, G. H., Jr. Inorganic phosphates in the treatment of renal calculi. *Mod. Treatm.* 4:494, 1967.
89. Vermeulen, C. W., and Lyon, E. S. Mechanisms of genesis and growth of calculi. *Amer. J. Med.* 45:684, 1968.
90. Williams, D. I. Matrix calculi. *Brit. J. Urol.* 35:411, 1963.
91. Williams, H. E., Morris, R. C., and Smith, L. H., Jr. To be published.
92. Williams, H. E., and Smith, L. H., Jr. Disorders of oxalate metabolism. *Amer. J. Med.* 45:715, 1968.
93. Williams, H. E., and Smith, L. H., Jr. Identification and determination of glyceric acid in human urine. *J. Lab. Clin. Med.* 71:495, 1968.
94. Williams, H. E., and Smith, L. H., Jr. L-glyceric aciduria: A new genetic variant of primary hyperoxaluria. *New Eng. J. Med.* 278:233, 1968.
95. Williams, H. E., Wilson, K. M., and Smith, L. H., Jr. Studies on primary hyperoxaluria: III. Transamination reactions of glyoxylate in human tissue preparations. *J. Lab. Clin. Med.* 70:494, 1967.
96. Wyngaarden, J. B. Gout. In Stanbury, J. B., Wyngaarden, J. B., and Fredrickson, D. S. (Eds.), *The Metabolic Basis of Inherited Disease* (2d ed.). New York: McGraw-Hill, 1966. P. 667.
97. Yendt, E. R., Gagne, R. J. A., and Cohanim, M. Effects of thiazides in idiopathic hypercalciuria. *Amer. J. Med. Sci.* 251:451, 1966.
98. Zaremski, P. M., and Hodgkinson, A. Fluorimetric determination of oxalic acid in blood and other biological material. *Biochem. J.* 96:717, 1965.
99. Zarembski, P. M., Hodgkinson, A., and Cochran, M. Treatment of primary hyperoxaluria with calcium carbimide. *New Eng. J. Med.* 277:1000, 1967.
100. Zinneman, H. H., and Jones, J. E. Dietary methionine and its influence on cystine excretion in cystinuric patients. *Metabolism* 15:915, 1966.

27

Obstructive Nephropathy

Neal S. Bricker and Saulo Klahr

Urinary tract obstruction may have far-reaching effects on the structure and function of the human kidney. Some of these effects relate to the direct and indirect consequences of the obstructing process; others undoubtedly reflect continuing imperfections in technics of clinical management.

It has become evident in recent years that urinary tract obstruction occurs with considerable frequency. It also has been established that the stigmata of obstruction may vary from abrupt and complete impairment of renal function to slow, progressive destruction of the renal parenchyma evolving over many years. On the other hand, it is neither as well known nor as widely accepted that urinary tract obstruction may persist indefinitely without modifying the integrity of kidney.

Both the propensity for nephron destruction and the potential benignity of some obstructing lesions emphasize the need for effective and comprehensive principles of management. It is essential that deleterious forms of urinary tract obstruction be recognized early and treated before irreversible kidney damage ensues. But it is of equal importance that nonprogressive forms of obstruction be managed with the utmost conservatism. In both situations, the complexities of diagnosis and therapy must be approached with one goal uppermost in mind: assurance of the long-range survival of a maximal number of nephrons.

Such an approach requires that the natural history of urinary tract obstruction and all factors, including iatrogenic, which may influence the natural history be clearly and succinctly defined. Unfortunately, existing knowledge does not permit such exact definition. Although certain aspects of the overall problem have been studied intensively, a number of critical areas remain virtually unexplored. It is somewhat paradoxical, for example, that while ureteral obstruction has been employed by physiologists for several decades to investigate normal mechanisms of renal function, extension of their interests to the clinical level has been slow in developing. To date, the great bulk of clinical literature is concerned more with structural changes in the conduit system than with the immediate and long-term effects of obstruction (and its treatment) on nephron survival. Moreover, a disquieting number of reported observations are based upon evidence that has not been subjected to rigorous scientific analysis. Finally, many of the technics widely employed for diagnosis and management of urinary tract obstruction are capable of introducing infection into the urinary tract above the site of the obstructing process; and with few exceptions, the potential detrimental effects of these procedures versus their potential benefits have not been examined in long-term carefully controlled studies.

Despite the many gaps in knowledge, there is an increasing need for periodic critical review of the available data. By collecting the cumulative observations, it may be possible to segregate established principles from speculative hypotheses. It may also be possible to delimit those areas wherein knowledge is incomplete or seemingly inexact.

Prospectus

Obstruction to the free flow of urine may ultimately impair renal function through a combination of events. It will be helpful to specify these events at the outset of this discussion.

Functional Decrease in Glomerular Filtration Rate. It is inherent in the filtration-reabsorption-secretion system of urine formation that a continuing pressure gradient is maintained between glomerular capillaries and tubular lumina. This gradient is initiated by the transmission of hydrostatic pressure from the left ventricle to the glomeruli; however, it must be preserved by the uninhibited flow of urine through the length of the nephron, the calyces, the renal pelvis, the ureters, and the bladder. When the free flow of urine is inhibited at any point in the urinary tract, the intraluminal pressures proximal to the site of the obstruction may increase progressively, approaching the glomerular capillary filtration pressure* as an upper limit. Owing to its distensibility and valvular components, the conduit system has some capacity to protect the nephrons from pressure abnormalities. However, this is limited in degree, and in sustained or very severe obstruction intratubular pressures may also rise. When this occurs, the pressure gradient across the glomeruli may decrease, and in turn the rate of formation of new glomerular filtrate will fall. All other things being equal, the greater the rise in intratubular pressure, the greater will be the impairment of the filtration process.

Pressure-Induced Parenchymal Damage. The persistence of abnormally high pressures within the renal pelvis may result in permanent anatomic deformation of the renal parenchyma. Initially, this is most evident in the region of the renal papillae; but pathologic changes may eventually extend throughout the structure of the kidney, resulting in massive nephron destruction.

Pyelonephritis. Pyelonephritis occurs with great frequency in obstructive nephropathy, and in many instances represents the major factor in renal structural and functional deterioration. The interrelationships between urinary tract obstruction and renal infection are considered in detail in the discussion to follow.

Renal Papillary Necrosis. The coexistence of obstruction and infection may occasionally be complicated by renal papillary necrosis. This potentially grave abnormality often heralds the early demise of the patient.

Semantic Considerations

Three terms are used to designate the consequences of urinary tract obstruction: *obstructive uropathy, hydronephrosis,* and *obstructive nephropathy.* Although the expres-

* Glomerular capillary blood pressure minus colloid oncotic pressure.

sions are frequently used interchangeably, each has its specific connotations; it is conceptually important to distinguish among them.

Obstructive uropathy is a general expression used to describe the structural changes that occur at any point in the urinary tract proximal to the site of the lesion. In its usual and presently accepted context, this terms tends to focus on the anatomic changes in the *urinary tract* without specific regard for the structure or function of the involved kidney. Obstructive uropathy therefore may exist in the absence of renal disease, or it may be associated with advancing nephropathy. Under any condition, however, it must be regarded as a potential forerunner of intrinsic renal disease.

Hydronephrosis is defined as dilatation of the renal pelvis. When employed in this restricted sense, the term is unambiguous and serves a useful purpose. Thus the presence of pelvic dilatation provides *presumptive* evidence of urinary tract obstruction, and the degree of dilatation may be an important clue in the overall assessment of the consequences and natural history of an obstructing lesion.

The term *hydronephrosis* is frequently used to characterize the composite effects of urinary tract obstruction not only on the renal pelvis but on the kidney. It is perhaps an outgrowth of this practice that the pyelographic appearance of the renal pelvis is widely accepted as an adequate means of following the function of a chronically obstructed kidney. But a given degree of hydronephrosis may produce highly variable changes in renal function; hence the magnitude of pelvic dilatation can at best provide only indirect and limited information about the functional capacity of the involved kidney. For example, marked dilatation of a pelvis that lies predominantly extrinsic to the hilum of the kidney (extrarenal pelvis) may occur without significant functional or structural changes in the kidney, whereas more modest degrees of dilatation in an intrarenal pelvis may be associated with severe nephron destruction. Moreover the anatomic variation in size and configuration of the normal renal pelvis is sufficiently great that moderate degrees of dilatation may not be accepted as valid evidence of an obstructing lesion.

Obstructive nephropathy will be used in this chapter to describe the renal lesion that occurs as a consequence of urinary tract obstruction. Hence this expression, in contrast to the other two terms, attaches primacy to the anatomic and functional integrity of the *kidney*. Obstructive nephropathy occurs less frequently than either obstructive uropathy or hydronephrosis; its incidence and severity depend upon a number of interrelated phenomena including the nature, site, and duration of the obstructing lesion, the severity of pressure abnormalities, and the extent of pyelonephritis. The selection of this term for the title of this chapter reflects the view that central attention must be given to the existing and projected effects of urinary tract obstruction upon the nephron population.

Physiology of the Urinary Tract

By virtue of the convergence of distal tubules in the renal cortex and the subsequent convergence of collecting ducts in the medulla, the million nephrons in the human kidney ultimately discharge their contents through a relatively small number of papillary orifices. The fluid emanating from these orifices represents the final product of the interaction between glomerular filtration and tubular transport, and it must be conducted freely and unidirectionally to the exterior. The conduit system subserving this function begins at the tips of the renal papillae and continues through the urethral meatus. A consideration of certain properties of this system may facilitate interpretation of pathologic states interfering with its effective operation.

The major force for urine propulsion is provided by contraction of the muscle bundles in the walls of the urinary tract. Unidirectional flow is facilitated by an integrated and rhythmic pattern of contraction of these muscles coupled with strategically placed sphincters (or sphincter-like areas).

Because the tips of the papillae descend into the cups of the calyces, the urine emerging from the papillary orifices enters immediately into the calyceal system. The calyces in turn eject the urine into the renal pelvis, presumably intermittently. Narath [76] has suggested that calyceal filling is associated with relaxation of proximal circular muscle fibers surrounding the calyces at the level of the tips of the papillae; contraction of distal circular fibers lying at the junction of the calyces and pelvis; and contraction of a third set of fibers oriented longitudinally along the neck of the calyces. The third set of fibers is thought to shorten and widen the calyceal lumina. Narath conceives of these events as producing a negative pressure within the calyces which serves to draw urine from the papillae.

With the onset of calyceal emptying, the proximal circular fibers are thought to contract, thereby protecting the papillary orifices from reflux. The longitudinal muscles and distal circular fibers simultaneously relax, thereby promoting the flow of urine into the pelvic cavity.

The muscle fibers of the renal pelvis are oriented longitudinally, obliquely, and in transverse directions, and contraction is associated with a "squeezing effect" on the entire structure [76]. The ejection of urine from the pelvis generally occurs intermittently, and reflux back into the calyces is prevented by contraction of the calycopelvic circular fibers.

The junction of the pelvis and ureter (i.e., the *ureteropelvic junction*) generally occurs several centimeters below the hilum of the kidney and is a site of particular importance because of the frequency with which luminal narrowing is encountered. There apparently is no true anatomic sphincter at the ureteropelvic junction; however, the intermittency of pelvic emptying suggests a sphincter-like action.

The ureters are well endowed with muscle fibers throughout their length, but possess no sphincters. Urine is propelled through the ureters by sequential muscular contractions, and significant reflux back into the pelvis is thought not to occur normally. Each ureter enters the bladder near its base, penetrating the successive layers of the bladder wall tangentially before terminating in the ureterovesical opening. No true anatomic sphincter exists at this site either, but during bladder contraction the intramural portion of the ureter is normally compressed and a sphincter-like effect is provided.

The ureterovesical "sphincter" may not be highly efficient during infancy and childhood, and recent anatomic studies may provide a partial explanation [23]. During the first 12 years of life, there appears to be a continuous increase in the number of smooth muscle fibers in the ureteral wall. This anatomic transformation occurs throughout the length of the ureter and includes the portion residing within the structure of the bladder. In addition, the intravesical portion of the ureter tends to elongate. The combination of more smooth muscle plus the elongation of the intravesical segment may contribute to an increase in efficiency of the sphincter-like effect obtained during bladder contraction. The anatomic changes therefore would provide an explanation for the spontaneous cessation of reflux which often occurs in children with increasing age.

The urinary bladder is a flexible reservoir with a considerable degree of distensibility. It has muscular walls throughout, but the muscle bundles of particular importance in initiating micturition are found in the trigone, the triangular area bordered by the two ureteral orifices and the urethra. The bladder is richly supplied with both sympathetic and parasympathetic fibers, and it is the latter which stimulate contraction.* Abnormalities in innervation may be associated with ineffectual bladder emptying which in turn may contribute to the development of obstructive nephropathy. Bladder contraction and simultaneous relaxation of the internal sphincter are initiated by an increase in intraluminal pressure, but bladder emptying does not occur until the external sphincter, which is subject to voluntary control, relaxes. Normally, there is virtually no residual urine at the end of micturition. When the bladder is markedly or chronically distended (or both), the force of muscular contraction may diminish appreciably, and in the laboratory animal the instillation of large volumes of fluid into the urinary bladder will increase intravesical pressure acutely, but thereafter a progressive and sustained decrease in pressure will occur without any change in the urine volume [59]. As has been noted above, when the bladder contracts during micturition the most distal portion of the ureter, which lies within the wall of the bladder, is compressed and reflux normally is prevented. This valve-like effect may not be universally efficient, and the possibility has already been noted that some degree of reflux may occur — particularly in infants and children — in the absence of any pathologic process.

The urethra in the female is a short, relatively uncomplicated structure. In the male, the proximal portion of the urethra is surrounded by the prostate gland, and in the adult, encroachment upon the urethral lumen by prostatic enlargement represents a common cause of urinary tract obstruction.

* An extensive review dealing with the innervation of the bladder and the control of micturition has been published [58].

NATURE OF URETERAL CONTRACTION

Clarification of the functional mechanisms of the urinary tract is an important requisite to an understanding of obstructive nephropathy. Although the existing information still is incomplete, studies on both dog and man have served to elucidate certain aspects of ureteral function [17, 18, 71]. These studies are reviewed briefly.

Ureteral Action Potentials. Peristaltic waves in the ureters were consistently preceded by action potentials. The duration of the action potentials was found to correlate with the strength of ureteral contractions; moreover, experimental events that influenced the shape of the action potentials modified the propagation speed of the peristaltic waves.

Peristaltic Waves. The period of time for a single peristaltic wave to pass through the length of the ureter was such that the front of the wave reached the bladder at approximately the same time that the pelvic region finished its recovery phase. Spontaneous waves, however, were found to occur in series such that three peaks could frequently be discerned in a ureter simultaneously. The latter finding is consistent with the observation of Narath [76] that urine appears to be propelled through the ureter a third of its length at a time.

Ureteral Pressure. When a peristaltic wave approached any point in the ureter, the intraluminal pressure rose to approximately 20 to 40 cm. of water above the resting level; as the wave receded, the pressure frequently became subnormal, dropping to approximately 10 to 20 cm. of water below the resting level.

Initiation and Modifications of Peristalsis. Ureteral distention was found to be the most effective means of initiating peristalsis. When the urine was diverted through a small incision in the renal pelvis, the ureter remained quiescent for periods as long as one minute, and spontaneous waves were few. Cooling of the ureter was also associated with a decrease in conduction, but it is of some interest that a number of drugs, including Prostigmine (neostigmine), acetylcholine, atropine, and epinephrine produced no change in either the velocity of conduction or the shape of the action potentials. Furthermore, temporary denervation, produced by injecting the periureteral tissue with Xylocaine (lidocaine) or procaine, paralyzed conduction for only a brief interval (approximately 8 to 12 minutes), following which conduction resumed despite the fact that the pharmacologic denervation was assumed still to be in effect.

Effects of Hydronephrosis. In hydronephrosis which followed severing and subsequent reanastomosis of the ureter, it was found that the greater the degree of dilatation of the ureters and pelvis, the longer peristaltic wave conduction was delayed and the slower was the velocity of waves. Contraction waves were also found to pass in a retrograde direction toward the kidney after they arrived at the anastomotic site.

Nature of Ureteral Conduction. On the basis of their experimental observations, Butcher and Sleator [17, 18] concluded that the conduction of peristalsis through the ureters is primarily influenced by physical forces and that neural elements are not responsible for conduction. It was postulated that ureteral conduction may relate to the direct firing of a cell by the "electrical breakdown" of contiguous cells or to the release by a contracting cell of "some substance" which activates contiguous cells.

However, in the last few years Boyarsky and Labay [11] have presented evidence for the presence of sympathetic nerves in the ureters. In addition, they have demonstrated an area in the renal pedicle which when stimulated mechanically dramatically altered the peristaltic rhythm of the ureters. This effect was observed at both low and high rates of urine flow. Electrical stimulation of this area also increased the frequency of peristalsis. After alpha-adrenergic blockade, however, electrical stimulation slowed peristalsis. Topical 1% nicotine applied to these trigger areas also reduced peristaltic acceleration following electrical stimulation. These observations suggest an additional neuromuscular mechanism in ureteral contraction, and raise the possibility of the presence of a "pacemaker" high in the ureter or in the renal pelvis.

In summary, it may be reiterated that the pattern of muscular contraction throughout the length of the conduit system is designed for efficient propulsion of urine and that strategically situated valves, or valve-like areas, function to prevent retrograde flow. However, when obstruction to free urine flow exists, (1) the propulsive forces may diminish because of a decrease in the frequency and strength of muscular contraction; (2) some retrograde peristalsis may occur; and (3) continued retention of urine will lead to interference with effective sphincter action between the successive segments of the urinary tract.

Obstructing Lesions of the Urinary Tract

Because of length and relative complexity of the conduit system, a large variety of pathologic processes may interfere with the efficient transport of urine from the renal papillae to the external environment. Urinary tract obstruction may occur at any age and in either sex. When the obstructing process is above the bladder, it usually, but not invariably, is unilateral; when the lesion is at the level of the bladder or below, untoward effects may be manifested bilaterally. Obstruction is frequently of a mechanical nature, in which case the pathologic process may be intraluminal, intramural, or extrinsic to the conduit system. Occasionally, however, there may be no evident mechanical obstruction. In the latter instance, impairment of urine transit may be idiopathic, and presumably congenital, or it may be secondary to abnormalities in bladder innervation.

FREQUENCY

Urinary tract obstruction is a relatively common disorder. Bell [4], in an analysis of 32,360 autopsies, found 1226 cases of hydronephrosis, an overall frequency of 3.8 per cent. Although these data do not reveal the prevalence of structural or functional abnormalities in the kidney, it is probable that an appreciable percentage of patients had at least some degree of obstructive nephropathy. For all age groups combined, the frequency of urinary tract obstruction in males and females was approximately the same, and before the age of 20 years no striking differences were found between the sexes. However, between 20 and 60 years of age, hydronephrosis was considerably more frequent in females, principally, according to Bell, due to pregnancy and carcinoma of the uterus. Over the age of 60 years the great majority of cases was found in males, and this preponderance was related to the frequency of prostatic enlargement.

ETIOLOGIC FACTORS

A detailed discussion of the multiple events that may produce urinary tract obstruction will not be undertaken. However, certain of the etiologic factors may be surveyed briefly.

Infants and Children. CONGENITAL ANOMALIES. Urinary tract obstruction in infants and children usually is the result of congenital lesions. Hydronephrosis may be present at birth (particularly in the male) as a consequence of stenosis of the external urethral meatus or of congenital urethral valves. Hydronephrosis may also develop in infancy and early childhood in association with partial obstruction at the level of the ureteropelvic junction. According to Ostling [78], this site in the urinary tract is normally narrowed in the newborn infant.

NEUROMUSCULAR DEFECTS. Dilatation of the ureter or renal pelvis (or both) may be observed in infants and children in the absence of a focal area of obstruction, and in some instances the degree of dilatation is quite remarkable. Although the underlying abnormalities are traditionally attributed to "neuromuscular defects," their precise nature remains obscure. The possibility has been entertained that in idiopathic hydronephrosis and ureteral dilatation (i.e., megaureter) there may be a failure of development of ganglion cells in the bladder. The abnormality has been likened to Hirschsprung's disease [98]. To date, however, this concept has not been documented.* It is worthy of emphasis that idiopathic dilatation of the urinary tract in infants and children does not invariably lead to progressive obstructive nephropathy. Thus Williams [101], in a study of a large number of patients with megaureter, found that a significant percentage of persons responded favorably to long-term conservative therapy directed principally toward eradication of urinary tract infection. Williams also emphasized the fact that the degree of ureteral dilatation may remain unchanged and symptomless for many years in the absence of any therapy.

INFECTION. Urinary tract obstruction in children may also follow in the wake of longstanding infection. Obstructing lesions of the bladder neck and at the ureterovesical junctions may result from inflammatory changes in these areas; hence infection may precede rather than follow a mechanical obstruction.

Adults. The majority of causes of obstructive nephropathy in the adult may be grouped into several categories.

BENIGN AND MALIGNANT TUMORS. A wide

* Williams [101], in a series of 90 cases of Hirschsprung's disease, failed to discover any cases of idiopathic urinary tract obstruction.

variety of neoplastic processes may interfere with effective urine drainage. Obstruction may result from extrinsic pressure on the lower urinary tract by expanding tumor masses; invasion of the ureters; infiltration of the bladder in the region of the ureterovesical junction; or rarely mechanical plugging of the ureterovesical openings by flaps of tumor tissue originating within the urinary bladder. Enlargement of the prostate gland in the male due either to hypertrophy or to carcinoma will produce obstruction at the level of the bladder neck.

The damage sustained by the kidneys when obstruction is secondary to tumors depends upon a number of general factors such as the site of the lesion in the urinary tract, the degree of luminal narrowing, and the presence or absence of infection. In addition, however, the intrinsic properties of the neoplastic process are of fundamental importance in the pattern of evolution of obstructive nephropathy. In benign tumors such as uterine fibromas and hypertrophy of the prostate, the chronicity of the underlying process may be associated with slow progression of renal damage over a long period. When the obstruction is due to metastatic invasion of the ureters, on the other hand, high-grade obstruction may occur with alarming rapidity. In the latter instance, the malignancy represents a limiting factor in survival; nevertheless, when the obstruction is bilateral, ureteral transplantation or other surgical procedures for urine diversion frequently prolong life.

CALCULI. Intraluminal obstruction of the urinary tract not infrequently results from calculus formation. Calculi in the renal pelvis may ultimately obstruct one or more papillae, and when a calculus becomes lodged in a ureter, it produces partial to complete obstruction of the involved conduit system. A detailed discussion of nephrolithiasis is presented in Chapter 26; for our purposes, only two special considerations concerning the development and progress of renal damage are noted: (1) Nephrolithiasis may represent a chronic and recurring process; hence the kidney may be subjected to repeated insults — for this reason, the duration of obstruction in any given instance should be rendered as short as possible; and (2) nephron destruction is accelerated by pyelonephritis, and the frequency of elective diagnostic procedures involving urethral instrumentation must be minimized. To accomplish both goals may require a high level of expertise.

URETEROPELVIC OBSTRUCTION. The ureteropelvic junction is a common site of obstruction in adults as well as children, and neither a well-defined organic lesion nor an obvious etiologic factor may be demonstrable. Although extrinsic bands of fibrous tissue or aberrant blood vessels may overlie the area of luminal narrowing, it is not clear whether these structures initiate the obstruction or impinge upon the pelvis only after it dilates. The prevailing opinion appears to be that the obstruction, in most instances, is congenital and that extrinsic bands represent the initiating process in only a small percentage of patients [65, 83].

Because at least some forms of ureteropelvic obstruction are congenital, hydronephrosis, when first discovered in the adult, may have been present for many years; moreover, it may remain unchanged for many more years [47]. But pelvic dilatation and nephron destruction may also be progressive, particularly when pyelonephritis is present.

CHRONIC URINARY TRACT INFECTION. That chronic infection may produce luminal narrowing at the level of the ureterovesical junction or bladder neck has already been indicated. In addition, Talbot [100] and his associates have suggested that dilatation and a diminished capacity of the pelvis and ureters to project urine through muscular contraction may occur from infection in the absence of mechanical obstruction.

NEUROMUSCULAR ABNORMALITIES. Functional disturbances in the mechanical emptying of the bladder may be present in the adult without obvious cause, or they may follow several different forms of primary disease of the spinal cord including transection and other traumatic injuries, spina bifida, tabes dorsalis, and diabetic neuropathy. When voluntary emptying of the bladder is impaired, large volumes of residual urine may result in increased pressure in the proximal portions of the conduit system, and the increased pressure in turn may lead to the development of varying degrees of obstructive nephropathy.

PREGNANCY. During the course of normal uncomplicated pregnancy some degree of ureteral dilatation frequently occurs [10]. This generally is more marked on the right side than on the left, and although the factors underlying the ureteral changes are largely unknown, the mechanical presence of a dextroverted uterus is considered to play at least a contributory role. Unless complicating factors, including pyelonephritis, develop, the limited degree of obstruction seen during pregnancy does not appear to initiate progressive destruction of the renal parenchyma.

MISCELLANEOUS CAUSES. Among the miscellaneous causes of urinary tract obstruction are ureteral ligation during pelvic surgery, edema of the terminal portion of the ureter after retrograde pyelography [90], kinking of the ureters by retroperitoneal hemorrhage following complicated deliveries and uterine rupture, and retroperitoneal fibrosis. Retroperitoneal fibrosis is an entity of unknown cause which has been described with increasing frequency in recent medical literature [38, 57, 72]. The lesion is characterized by retroperitoneal fibrous tissue that surrounds the ureters and fixes them to contiguous structures. The progression of the pathologic process, which some investigators consider to be of a chronic inflammatory nature, may eventually lead to a marked decrease in the caliber of one or both ureters. The symptoms often are nonspecific until ureteral obstruction is high grade. Retroperitoneal fibrosis has been associated with the use of methysergicide in high dosage for headaches [35].

Pathology

The onset, extent, and rate of progression of pathologic changes in obstructive nephropathy vary considerably from patient to patient. It is evident that the greater the degree of luminal narrowing at the site of obstruction, the greater will be the resistance to the free flow of urine, and in general the more destructive will be the effects upon the renal parenchyma. Similarly, the longer the obstruction persists, the more likely it is that the pathologic consequences will be severe. However, with a given degree of luminal narrowing and a specified duration, at least two other factors will be of major importance in determining the course of the nephropathy.

The first and more important is the severity of pyelonephritis. The second is the level of the urinary tract at which the lesion occurs. Thus there frequently is a direct relationship between the proximity of the obstruction to the kidney and the progress of nephron destruction. For example, when the lesion is at the ureteropelvic junction (and the pelvis is predominantly intrarenal), the degree to which pelvic dilatation can minimize untoward pressure effects upon the renal papillae is limited; whereas in a bladder neck lesion the bladder, serving as a reservoir, as well as the ureters and renal pelvis may buffer the kidney for a prolonged period of time from the adverse effects of increasing hydrostatic pressure.

Despite the variability in the natural history of the pathologic changes, the morphologic details of these changes tend to follow a common pattern. In the early phases of obstructive nephropathy, the kidney appears edematous and hemorrhagic, and the renal papillae are soft and friable [92]. With persisting high-grade obstruction, the kidney may gradually enlarge because of progressive dilatation of the renal pelvis; however, the encroachment of the pelvic space upon the renal medulla results in thinning of the parenchymal mass. Flattening of the papillae and narrowing of the medulla may be particularly striking, but the renal cortex will also be affected, and in the later stages of obstructive nephropathy the large dilated pelvis is surrounded by only a thin rim of renal parenchyma.

Histologically a prominent and early change consists of marked tubular dilatation. Initially this may be confined to the collecting ducts, but distal and proximal convolutions will eventually share in the dilatation [41]; indeed, Strong [94] has noted that a marked degree of dilatation occurs in the proximal tubules. The epithelial cells lining dilated tubules acquire a flattened appearance and ultimately become atrophic [41, 94].

In addition to the changes in the nephron, marked alterations have been described in the renal arterioles [2, 45]. In the laboratory animal with unilateral ureteral ligation, postmortem perfusion of the renal vasculature using various dyes reveals a striking and progressive decrease in the number of visible arterioles. Moreover, those vessels that do admit a dye are very distorted. The interlobar arteries and the arcuate vessels appear narrowed and elongated, and the interlobular arteries are extremely tortuous. The elastica interna of the intrarenal vessels appears torn, and Altschul and Fedor [2] have described changes in this region similar to those seen in permanently ligated vessels.

In advanced obstructive nephropathy, the kidney may be virtually destroyed [1, 4, 42]. Dilated tubules collapse and are replaced by fibrous tissue. Glomeruli may also appear fibrotic. The distribution of fibrosis, though characteristically patchy, may nevertheless be extensive. In many instances, the pathologic stigmata of pyelonephritis will contribute decisively to the composite structural abnormalities. Finally, when renal papillary necrosis develops, the unique anatomic changes of this process will be superimposed upon all other abnormalities.

Pyelonephritis in Obstructive Nephropathy

Clinically, urinary tract infection is observed so frequently in long-standing obstruction that it often is accepted as an invariable complication. Although the precise incidence of pyelonephritis at different stages of the various types of urinary tract obstruction is not yet known, pathologic evidence of pyelonephritis was found in 60 per cent of 1229 cases of unselected hydronephrosis studied at autopsy by Bell [4]. Bell also demonstrated that pyelonephritis is found with far greater frequency (more than a tenfold difference) at autopsy in patients with than in those without obstruction [3]. It is of some interest, however, that Bell's data indicate that pyelonephritis occurs approximately twice as often when the site of obstruction is in the urethra or bladder as when it is in the ureters. The the pathogenesis of pyelonephritis will be possible implications of this observation in considered later.

Experimentally, it has long been recognized that ureteral obstruction greatly increases the susceptibility of animals to pyelonephritis. In 1921 Lepper [61] found that the susceptibility to hematogenous pyelonephritis (following the injection of coliform bacteria) was increased when the ureter was occluded for a period as short as 15 minutes. Urinary tract obstruction also greatly increases the susceptibility to ascending pyelonephritis in the laboratory animal when bacteria are introduced into the urinary tract above the site of obstruction. Finally, renal infection has been found to occur spontaneously in rats with one ureter ligated [36].

Unfortunately, the mechanisms by which obstruction predisposes a kidney to the development of pyelonephritis remain largely unknown. It has generally been held that the pooling of urine in the renal pelvis and in dilated tubules in some way decreases host resistance to renal infection. This thesis, however, has been challenged by Guze and Beeson [37] on the basis of studies on animals with partial ureteral obstruction induced by irradiation of the ureters. It was found that chronic partial obstruction did not predispose animals to pyelonephritis following intravenous inoculation with either *Escherichia coli* or *Staphylococcus aureus*. It is important to note that an experimental model with partial ureteral obstruction simulates more closely the situation found in the great majority of patients with chronic urinary tract obstruction than does the animal with a completely ligated ureter. If the observations of Guze and Beeson are extended and confirmed, the thesis that pyelonephritis is essentially an unavoidable and almost inevitable complication of obstructive nephropathy may require major revision.

The fact that pyelonephritis was found by Bell [4] in 60 per cent of patients with hydronephrosis must not obscure the fact that the remaining 40 per cent did not develop this lesion. It seems reasonable, therefore, at the present stage of knowledge, to accept as a working hypothesis the view that pyelonephritis is a preventable complication of urinary tract obstruction. From the point of view of prevention, the finding that renal infection is considerably more common in patients in whom obstructing lesions are at the level of the bladder or urethra than in those with supravesical lesions [3] is of particular interest. The fact that the former group are more often subjected to catheterization and related urologic procedures raises the possibility that the iatrogenic introduction of bacteria above the site of obstruction may be a potent factor in initiating infection of the kidney.

Mechanisms of Nephron Destruction

It might be presumed that, in the absence of infection, a sustained elevation of intratubular pressures could mechanically decrease the glomerular filtration rate, but that the involved nephrons might survive indefinitely. Indeed, when obstruction to urine flow is low grade and nonprogressive, there is some evidence to indicate that this concept may be valid [46]. However, when the obstruction is high grade or complete, nephron destruction will occur, often in a relentless fashion.

In addition to the adverse effects of pyelonephritis, other mechanisms must be invoked in explanation of the structural derangements of obstructive nephropathy. The mechanical effects of abnormally high pressures brought to bear on the renal papillae may well contribute to the anatomic deformation of these segments of the parenchyma. Certainly high pressures are associated with structural changes in the lower urinary tract, and the friable, almost mushy appearance of the renal papillae in early obstruction and the flattening and virtual loss of the papillae in sustained obstruction are consistent with an untoward effect of elevated pressure.

Alteration in blood flow through the kidney may represent a contributing factor in the evolution of nephron destruction. Total renal blood flow is diminished in the laboratory animal with sustained ureteral ligation [48, 53, 64]. Moreover, the anatomic studies of the renal vasculature which have already been described reveal a marked decrease in the number and caliber of arterioles as well as distortion of the persisting vessels. Direct measurements of pressures in peritubular capillaries of the rat demonstrate that elevation of ureteral pressure evokes not only a rise in intratubular pressure but also a corresponding rise in capillary pressure [33]. The latter data suggest that urinary tract obstruction may markedly increase the resistance to postglomerular capillary blood flow. It is also possible that increased pressure within the renal pelvis may preferentially depress vasa recta blood flow through the inner medulla, an area that is relatively poorly perfused in the normal state.

The possibility that decreased renal blood flow may contribute in some manner to parenchymal destruction is supported by studies of Hepler [39] and Hinman and Hepler [43] in animals with ureteral ligation in which renal blood flow to the involved kidneys was decreased mechanically by chronically constricting the renal artery. This procedure might be expected to diminish the rate of nephron destruction by decreasing hydrostatic pressure in the glomerular capillaries and thereby decreasing the rate at which hydronephrosis develops from the accession of new urine. The observed effects on the kidney, however, were just the reverse: Arterial compression was associated with an increase in the rate at which the obstructed kidney was destroyed.

Although both the direct effects of abnormally high pressures and the indirect effects of altered perfusion of the kidney may contribute to the pathologic changes, the intimate mechanisms of nephron destruction in obstructive nephropathy remain obscure. It is often stated that nutritional abnormalities develop in the tubular epithelial cells, but neither the definition of nor the biochemical basis for such abnormalities has been demonstrated. Wilmer [103] and others have described the early disappearance of alkaline phosphatase from the epithelial cells of the proximal convolutions in the hydronephrotic kidney, and Levy and his co-workers [64] found that total oxygen consumption by the obstructed kidney decreases; however, the significance of the former remains to be established and the latter could relate simply to a decrease in the rate of net sodium transport. To date, the details of cellular metabolism and the possibility that specific substrates may be deficient, or noxious metabolites retained, as a consequence of urinary tract obstruction must await future investigation.

Pathogenesis of Hydronephrosis

Obstruction of the urinary tract may lead to extreme dilatation of the renal pelvis. There are numerous cases in the literature in which volumes of fluid in excess of 3 liters (and in rare instances as much as 10 to 15 liters) [1] have been recovered from hydronephrotic kidneys. The accumulation of fluid proximal to the site of obstruction furnishes provisional evidence that glomerular filtration and flow of tubular fluid throughout the length of at least some nephrons continue despite the absolute obstruction to outflow through the conduit system.

Because glomerular filtration must cease when intrapelvic pressure equals the filtration pressure in the glomerular capillaries (i.e., capillary blood pressure minus colloid oncotic pressure), the acquisition of new urine in a hydronephrotic renal pelvis suggests that a pressure gradient across the glomerular capillaries is reestablished, at least intermittently, in the face of continuing outflow obstruction. Several mechanisms exist which may permit this.

FLOW OF URINE BEYOND THE SITE OF OBSTRUCTION

When obstruction is partial, flow of urine through the area of luminal narrowing acts to drain the pelvic pool and to permit continued filtration. The greater the degree of obstruction, the less effective is this mechanism of decompression.

ALTERATIONS IN THE GROSS STRUCTURE AND FUNCTION OF THE CONDUIT SYSTEM

Were the renal pelvis to remain rigid and indistensible, intrapelvic pressure would rise pari passu with the volume of retained urine. However, when the pressure in the obstructed pelvis of the laboratory animal is measured serially, it is found to decrease with time, despite the fact that the volume of sequestered urine remains constant or increases [104]. This phenomenon appears to relate to two changes that occur in the urinary tract: (1) Muscular tone in the wall of the pelvis diminishes, and areas above the site of obstruction undergo progressive dilatation; and (2) there is a decrease in the force and amplitude of peristaltic contraction.

The combination of these events serves to decrease intrapelvic pressure and to restore pressure relationships that favor the formation of new glomerular filtrate. As new urine enters the obstructed pelvis, intrapelvic pressures rise again, and the entire cycle may then be repeated.

EGRESS OF URINE FROM THE RENAL PELVIS

It is very likely that, even in the presence of total obstruction, the urine contained in the conduit system represents a labile pool characterized by continuing turnover of solutes and water. To whatever extent this turnover is associated with the net removal of water from the pool, intrapelvic pressures would decrease (irrespective of anatomic changes) and new urine could be delivered from surviving nephrons.

Direct evidence that certain solutes may leave an obstructed renal pelvis has been obtained from several sources. Hinman and Vecki [46] injected phenol red into the renal pelvis of rabbits with ligated ureters. They found that the concentration of dye diminished appreciably in aspirated pelvic urine within 24 hours of injection, and generally no dye was detectable after 48 hours. Magoun [68] found in the dog that phenol red introduced into a normal renal pelvis which then was acutely obstructed could be recovered from the urine of the contralateral kidney within 20 minutes. Further evidence suggesting that solutes may escape from the renal pelvis exists in the observation that contrast materials may occasionally be seen radiographically in the superficial vessels about the hilum of the kidney following instillation of these compounds in the course of retrograde pyelography [42]. Finally, Persky et al. [82] and Risholm and Obrink [85] have detected radioactivity in the systemic blood following the introduction of ^{131}I and ^{131}I-labeled albumin into the renal pelvis of man.

Although the efflux of dyes and radioactive materials generally has been demonstrated following acute injection under pressures that exceed those spontaneously occurring in urinary tract obstruction, Hinman and Lee-Brown [44] noted that the pressure required to produce efflux of dye from the obstructed pelvis of laboratory animals decreased progressively over a period of several weeks.

That water as well as solute may escape from the totally obstructed renal pelvis is suggested by the fact that the volume of pooled urine proximal to a ligated ureter increases progressively for only a limited period, following which it decreases. On theoretical grounds, it may be assumed that whatever route solute particles take in leaving the renal pelvis, water molecules may follow in at least isosmotic quantities (unless the pooled urine is hyperosmotic). The possible mechanisms which would account for the egress of solutes and water merit brief consideration.

Diffusion. It has been widely believed that the epithelial cells lining the normal pelvis, ureters, and bladder provide an absolute barrier to the diffusion of major urinary solutes and water. However, Levinsky and Berliner [63] have demonstrated that urea, sodium potassium, chloride, creatinine, hydrogen ions, and water all will diffuse across the ureter and bladder of normal dogs. It also is established that irrigation of the urinary bladder with hypotonic solutions during transurethral prostatectomy may be attended by the translocation of large quantities of water into the systemic circulation. Presumably at least some of this water moves across the intact bladder mucosa.

In the presence of hydronephrosis, it is conceivable that there may be greatly augmented exchange of solutes and water between the pooled urine in the renal pelvis and contiguous fluid compartments. Two such compartments might participate in this exchange: (1) the plasma and interstitial fluid of the pelvic wall; and (2) the tubular fluid, urine, plasma, and interstitial fluid within the inner medulla and papillae of the obstructed kidney.

Pelvic Extracellular Fluid. Both the stagnancy of the pooled urine and the alterations in membrane characteristics of a dilated and distended pelvic wall could enhance passive transport across the epithelial cells lining the renal pelvis. The stagnancy would increase the time available for diffusion; the membrane alterations might diminish the impedance to passive movements of certain ionic and molecular species. Freely diffusible substances, such as urea, which enter the pelvic urine in concentrations greater than those in systemic plasma may well diffuse out of the pelvis in the direction of their chemical concentration gradients. Loss of solute by this means would increase the chemical potential of water molecules in the urine (i.e., the osmolality would diminish), and the efflux of an isosmotic equivalent of water would thereby be promoted.

The extent to which ions, particularly sodium and chloride, diffuse across the dilated pelvic wall is unknown. However, because the sodium concentration of newly formed urine may well be less than the concurrent plasma concentration, despite the presence of obstructive nephropathy, the chemical concentration gradients should favor the net diffusion of sodium ions into the pooled urine. The accession of sodium (and chloride) in this manner would ultimately serve to increase rather than decrease the volume of the hydronephrotic pool.

Although the occurrence of this phenomenon cannot be excluded, one physical force exists which might minimize its importance and could in fact reverse the direction of net sodium flow. The relatively stagnant pool of urine having a low protein concentration is surrounded by a constant stream of protein-rich plasma. To the extent that the negatively charged plasma protein molecules are nondiffusible across the pelvic membrane and monovalent ions more freely diffusible, it is theoretically possible, on the basis of the Gibbs-Donnan equilibrium, to account for continuing removal of salt (and water) from the renal pelvis.

The net direction of migration of water molecules across the pelvic mucosa will be influenced by the respective osmotic pressures of pooled urine and extracellular fluid within the wall of the renal pelvis. If the newly formed urine is hypo-osmotic or efflux of solute particles exceeds influx (or both), water moves out of the pool. If intrapelvic pressures exceed the hydrostatic pressure of the surrounding capillaries, the chemical potential of water molecules in the pool is increased further and net outward diffusion promoted. On the other hand, if the newly formed urine is hyperosmotic, or if influx of osmotically active particles predominates, there can be accession of water in the pool.

Exchange with Renal Medullary Fluids. In the presence of hydronephrosis, the renal papillae may actually be immersed in pooled urine. Conceivably, therefore, the vasa recta blood might provide a route of escape for solutes and water from the pool. Urea molecules are known to diffuse out of the collecting ducts into the medullary interstitium and thereafter into the ascending limbs of the loops of Henle [32]. Urea also would be expected to diffuse freely into the vasa recta capillary blood. Hence, in urinary tract obstruction associated with limited formation of new filtrate and sluggish movement of fluid through the tubules, a continuing migration of urea molecules might occur from pooled urine into collecting duct fluid, then into medullary interstitial fluid, and finally into vasa recta capillary plasma. It also is possible that direct exchange could occur between pooled urine and the interstitial fluid. These events could serve further to dissipate the contribution of urea molecules to the osmolality of the pelvic urine, and water diffusion might then occur more freely across the pelvic mucosa. Furthermore, to whatever degree the concentrating mechanism engenders a hyperosmotic medullary interstitium in the presence of urinary tract obstruction, water molecules might diffuse into the inner medulla. Any movement of sodium in the opposite direction (i.e., into the pelvic pool) would of course oppose this decompression influence.

Although the interplay of these various factors could explain pelvic decompression, the key formulations remain theoretical, and their validity must await the measurements of appropriate chemical and electrochemical potential gradients, as well as solute and water fluxes across the obstructed renal pelvis. The acquisition of at least a portion of the critical data should be entirely possible with existing experimental technics.

Tubular Reflux. It is widely held that urine may escape from a hydronephrotic pool by reflux into collecting ducts [39, 85]. Two lines of evidence are cited in support of this concept: (1) Contrast material introduced into the renal pelvis above the site of an obstruction may occasionally be visualized roentgenographically in the substance of the renal parenchyma as radiating streaks which are thought to correspond to the distribution of collecting ducts; and (2) dyes such as Berlin blue introduced into the hydronephrotic pool of urine in laboratory animals have been found at autopsy to extend into the lumina of collecting ducts and in some instances into more proximal portions of nephrons [39]. That retrograde flow of urine constitutes a significant source of solute and water removal, however, remains to be established. It is conceivable that the recycling of pelvic urine back into functioning units could be attended by additional sodium and chloride reabsorption by the collecting ducts; water, particularly in the presence of antidiuretic hormone, could diffuse across the tubular cell membranes into the medullary interstitium. However, if this mechanism is to be made theoretically sound, it is necessary to invoke a number of supporting ad hoc hypotheses. The nephrons which dilate sufficiently to permit reflux must remain functional. In addition, if free reflux occurs, a pressure gradient in the collecting ducts must exist which is opposite in direction to the normal one, and this would virtually preclude the continued formation of filtrate in the involved units (unless filtration and reflux occurred in an alternating fashion).

At the present time, it seems reasonable to attribute the movement of a foreign dye into collecting ducts to diffusion from a region of high concentration (i.e., the pelvic urine where the dye is injected) into adjacent columns of relatively motionless intratubular urine. The possibility that endogenous solutes may escape from the pool in a similar manner has already been considered.

Pyelovenous Outflow. The observation that contrast materials may move out of the renal pelvis and into renal veins led Hinman and Lee-Brown [44] to postulate the existence of "direct communications" between the pelvis in the region of the fornices and the venous system of the kidney. However, it seems more likely that pyelovenous outflow simply reflects diffusion from the pelvic urine to vasa recta capillary blood, and it is questionable whether a special term should be preserved.

Lymphatic Drainage. The lymphatics may well contribute to egress of urine from a hydronephrotic renal pelvis. Ureteral ligation in the laboratory animal is attended by a marked increase in lymphatic drainage [75], and presumably intrapelvic urine could enter lymphatic vessels in much the same way that it enters capillaries. The relative contributions of lymphatic and venous drainage of the obstructed renal pelvis remain unknown.

A third mechanism exists that could facilitate the continued formation of glomerular filtrate in the presence of urinary tract obstruction. Gottschalk and Myelle [33] found in the rat that an increase in intratublar pressure led to a corresponding increase in peritubular capillary pressure. Rising intratubular pressures may therefore increase the resistance to venous flow on the efferent side of the glomerulus, and for any given level of afferent arteriolar blood pressure a rise in efferent resistance could increase filtration pressure within the glomerular capillaries. Such a physical feedback mechanism could help to maintain filtration pressures in excess of intratubular pressures until the latter exceeds a critical level.

In summary, the evolution of progressive hydronephrosis in all probability depends upon several interrelated events. Whether the obstruction is partial or complete, the volume of pooled urine may increase with time. It is presumed, therefore, that new urine is formed despite conditions which in theory might abolish the effective filtration pressure. Three factors appear to contribute to the continuing ability of the surviving nephrons of the obstructed kidney to form urine: (1) dilatation and loss of tone of the pelvic wall; (2) removal of sequestered urine from the pelvis; and (3) an increase in filtration pressure occurring as a consequence of a readjustment of intrarenal vascular pressures.

Effects of Urinary Tract Obstruction on Renal Function

OBSERVATIONS ON THE LABORATORY ANIMAL

Short-Term Obstruction. The acute effects of urinary tract obstruction are better characterized than are the effects of sustained obstruction. Gottschalk and Myelle [33] studied the pressure changes in individual nephrons and peritubular capillaries of the rat, using micropuncture technics. When the ureter was occluded during brisk diuresis, intratubular pressures rose to levels as high as 88 mm. Hg; yet in most instances intratubular pressures remained slightly greater than those in the ureter. Peritubular capillary pressures were found to approximate intratubular pressures closely. Dye injected directly into tubular lumina tended to remain stagnant or to move sluggishly down the nephron. Thus the formation of new glomerular filtrate presumably was suppressed.

A considerable amount of information about the influence of short-term ureteral obstruction on renal function has been obtained by use of the "stop-flow" technic [70]. This procedure is based upon the thesis that sudden occlusion of the ureters during a brisk diuresis will result in virtual cessation of filtration, but the columns of urine which remain stationary in the tubular lumina will be subjected to continuing modification by tubular transport systems. Although the stop-flow technic has been used primarily to study normal renal function, the data also may be examined to obtain further insight into the influence of short-term ureteral obstruction on renal function. The results of stop-flow experiments corroborate the micropuncture evidence that filtration almost ceases within a very short time (probably less than a minute) after ureteral occlusion and remains limited during occlusion lasting for as long as six to eight minutes. In addition, it has been well documented that a number of tubular functions persist during ureteral occlusion. Thus analysis of urine samples obtained immediately after release of the occlusion provides evidence for continued tubular transport of glucose, para-aminohippurate, sodium, potassium, calcium, magnesium, and a number of other substances.

Jaenike and Bray [49] have used a modified stop-flow technic to investigate the effects of high intrapelvic pressures on renal concentrating ability. In anesthetized, hydropenic dogs, both ureters were catheterized through flank incisions. One of three solutions (isotonic saline, urine, and mineral oil) was then injected into the pelvis, and a hydrostatic pressure of 100 to 120 mm. Hg was maintained for five to six minutes. The opposite kidney was used as a control. After release of the obstruction, the osmolality of the urine from the experimental kidney was found to be considerably less than that of the control organ. This effect was most prominent immediately after release of the obstruction, but in two experiments it persisted for more than four hours. No consistent changes were noted in the patterns of solute excretion, and the glomerular filtration rate (GFR) either remained constant or decreased transiently. When GFR did decrease, the concentrating impairment persisted after the GFR had returned to a level approximating that of the contralateral kidney. Analyses of slices of the papilla and inner medulla demonstrated a decrease in the concentration of urea and sodium in the obstructed kidney as compared with the control organ. These decrements were evident whether the values were expressed per gram of dry weight of kidney tissue or per gram of tissue water. Slices from the obstructed kidney also had a higher water content in the papilla. The slice data, however, while of interest, do not clarify the mechanisms underlying the self-limited concentrating defect.

The influence of increased ureteral pressure on renal function has also been studied in the intact animal by means of clearance technics. Share [88] observed a modest decrease in filtration rate when ureteral pressures were elevated to a range of 20 to 30 mm. Hg in anesthetized dogs. Selkurt et al. [87] also studied the effects of elevated ureteral pressures in acute experiments on dogs. Polyethylene catheters were secured within both ureters and functions of the separate kidneys were measured. When the ureteral pressure was elevated unilaterally to 52 cm. of water by raising the level of the inlying polyethylene catheter, filtration rate decreased by approximately 15 per cent in comparison with the contralateral kidney. In the studies of both Share and Selkurt, a decrease in sodium excretion and in urine flow accompanied the fall in filtration rate.

Suki et al. [96] performed clearance studies on dogs in which the ureter to one kidney was obstructed acutely while the contralateral kidney was left unaltered to serve as a control. Simultaneous evaluation thus could be obtained of the function of an obstructed and a control kidney in the same animal. To induce obstruction, a polyethylene catheter was inserted into the ureter of the experimental kidney and the intraureteral pressure was elevated to 60 to 80 cm. of water by varying the height of the catheter. Glomerular filtration rate and urine flow diminished on the obstructed side in relation to the contralateral kidney. Under conditions of water diuresis, with dilute urine bilaterally, urinary osmolality from the obstructed kidney was higher than that of the contralateral organ, and the sodium concentration was lower. This pattern is the same as that observed when GFR per nephron is reduced in one kidney by constricting its renal artery and the values of the constricted kidney are compared with those of the contralateral kidney. Thus, *acute* obstruction appears to result in a decrease in GFR per nephron and an increase in fractional sodium (and water) reabsorption. As will be noted below, the pattern observed by Suki et al. in *chronic* unilateral obstruction is quite different. Using micropuncture technics, Rector et al. [84] and Brenner et al. [13] found that acute obstruction leads to an increased diameter of the proximal tubule and that the time required for a dye (lissamine green) injected intravenously to move through the nephron is increased. Although initially it was thought that the net rate of sodium reabsorption increased with the increment in tubular diameter [16], subsequent studies have not confirmed this [13]. But neither was there any defect in sodium reabsorption observed during acute obstruction despite the increase in tubular diameter and the increase in intratubular pressure.

Sustained Obstruction. Most studies of the effects of chronic obstruction on animals have been done by completely obstructing a ureter and then making measurements either during the period of obstruction or after release of the obstruction. Relatively little information has been obtained in animals with persisting *partial* obstruction.

Idbohrn and Muren [48] measured renal blood flow in both kidneys of rabbits from 1 to 17 weeks after one ureter was occluded. Values for the obstructed kidney were found to be markedly decreased after one week of occlusion and further decrements were noted in the animals studied through the fourth week of occlusion. It is of interest, however, that values obtained after 6, 8, and 17 weeks of total obstruction were approximately the same as those after 4 weeks. The values for the unobstructed kidneys increased compensatorily within a week and were still elevated after 17 weeks. After the fourth week of obstruction, renal blood flow values in the obstructed kidneys were approximately one-third of those for the contralateral organs.

Measurements of renal blood flow have also been made in the dog by Levy and his coworkers [64]. Control studies were performed before obstruction, and repeat measurements were obtained three to four days after both ureters were occluded. The decrease in values from control levels ranged from 23 to 66 per cent (mean, 44 per cent). Studies of oxygen consumption were also performed in these experiments. It was found that the arteriovenous oxygen difference remained unchanged in the obstructed kidney, but because of the marked decrease in renal blood flow, total oxygen consumption diminished considerably. This presumably relates to the decrease in sodium transport by the tubular epithelial cells which in turn is secondary to the decrease in glomerular filtration rate.

Kerr [53] investigated the long-term effects of ureteral ligation on renal function in dogs. One ureter was ligated for seven days, the ligature was then removed, and serial studies were performed over a period varying from two months to over a year. An estimate of the function of the individual kidneys was obtained prior to unilateral ureteral ligation by studying both kidneys and assuming that each kidney contributed one-half of renal function. After the ureteral obstruction was released, both kidneys were studied serially. Immediately after the release of obstruction, the glomerular filtration rate for the obstructed kidneys averaged 25 per cent of their own control values and 16 per cent of the concurrent values for the contralateral kidneys, the latter having undergone some compensatory increase in function. In follow-up studies, the GFR rose in the obstructed kidneys and decreased in the normal kidneys; however, both organs tended to stabilize within two months, and in no instance did complete functional recovery occur in the obstructed organ. In five dogs followed for from 49 to 442 days after release of obstruction, the GFR of the experimental kidneys remained approximately 50 per cent below the simultaneous values for the contralateral organs.

The percentage decrease in effective renal plasma flow (as estimated by PAH clearance) closely approximated the corresponding fall in filtration rate, and filtration fractions remained essentially equal bilaterally. Ratios of GFR to Tm_{PAH} also remained equal bilaterally. A limited number of studies on acidifying and alkalinizing ability demonstrated comparable patterns for the experimental and control kidneys. In three animals, maximal urinary osmolalities were measured following water deprivation and in each instance the experimental kidney demonstrated the capacity to concentrate the urine, although not to the same degree as the contralateral kidney.

The results of Kerr's studies indicate that permanent nephron destruction occurs after seven days of total ureteral obstruction. This is attested not only by the failure of clearance values to return to control levels in long-term follow-up studies but also by the fact that in three dogs studied at autopsy, the weights of the experimental kidneys were from 26 to 49 per cent less than those of the contralateral organs. The data on filtration fractions, GFR-Tm_{PAH} ratios, and acidifying and alkalinizing capacity suggest that those nephrons that survived the obstruction retained qualitatively normal functional characteristics.*

Berlyne and Macken [8] have studied the effects of ureteral obstruction on the concentrating capacity of the laboratory animal. As in the studies of Kerr, one kidney was obstructed for seven days and the contralateral kidney used as a control. The experiments were performed immediately after release of the obstruction. The osmolality of the urine from the obstructed kidney was always less than that from the contralateral organs, although in most instances the experimental organs continued to elaborate hypertonic urine. Analysis of tissue slices revealed an increase in the concentration of sodium and urea as the papilla was approached in the normal kidneys, whereas these gradients were markedly attenuated in the hydronephrotic organs. The estimated osmolality of tissue slices also was lower in the obstructed kidneys. These data are of interest although they do not indicate the mechanisms underlying the concentrating defect. Moreover, they have the disadvantage of reflecting the patterns of function immediately after release of sustained obstruction and cannot be safely extrapolated to the functional status of the kidney with chronic partial obstruction or the kidney which has recovered from complete obstruction.

The functional patterns of chronic persisting obstruction have been studied by Suki et al. [96] in the dog. One ureter was constricted at the level of the ureteropelvic junction, and studies were performed from one week to four months after induction of the lesion. Hydronephrosis developed in each of the animals. The contralateral kidney was maintained intact as a control organ. The functional pattern differed quite strikingly from those observed by the same authors in dogs with acute obstruction (see above). The glomerular filtration rate in the obstructed kidneys was decreased in chronic as in acute obstruction. However, the urinary sodium concentration was *greater* from the obstructed than from the contralateral control organs. The obstructed kidneys also excreted a greater fraction of filtered salt and water than did the control organs. Free water clearance (C_{H_2O}) values were similar in the obstructed and normal kidneys when comparable rates of solute delivery were used in the calculations. Thus in contrast to the pattern observed in acute obstruction, which suggested a decrease in GFR per nephron and a decrease in fractional salt and water reabsorption, the picture in chronic obstruction resembles closely that observed in animals with chronic nonobstructive experimental renal disease [15]. Suki et al. [96] suggested that chronic hydronephrosis resulted in a decreased nephron population and that glomerular filtration rate per nephron in the surviving units might be increased. Another possibility which would obviate the necessity of postulating an increased GFR per nephron in the presence of elevated intratubular pressures is that glomerulotubular balance in the obstructed kidney was such that rela-

* In a subsequent study, Kerr [54] extended his observations to the effects of complete unilateral obstruction for periods up to four weeks in duration. Only a limited number of animals were studied, but the data are similar to those in the animals with seven days of obstruction, except that the permanent decrease in GFR was more marked with longer periods of total obstruction.

tive glomerular preponderance prevailed. This could occur with a decrease in GFR per nephron but a proportionately greater reduction in fractional reabsorption of salt and water.

Summary of Experimental Data. The immediate effects of urinary tract obstruction include an increase in intratubular pressure and a corresponding rise in peritubular capillary pressure, a decrease in glomerular filtration rate per nephron, and a prolonged transit time for the flow of tubular fluid through the nephron. There is no obvious impairment in sodium and water reabsorption in the proximal tubule, and transepithelial transport for many other solutes continues throughout the nephron. When total obstruction is maintained even for a short period of time, a defect in concentrating ability develops. This is associated with an attenuation of the normal concentration gradient in kidney slices from cortex toward papilla for sodium, osmolality, and urea. Clearance data in acute obstruction reveal a pattern of function similar to that seen with constriction of the renal artery. Thus there is a decrease in GFR per nephron and an increase in fractional sodium and water reabsorption. When the obstruction is sustained, certain of the changes are the same as, whereas others are different from, those seen with acute obstruction. When obstruction is complete (e.g., by ligating the ureter), renal blood flow measured during the period of obstruction decreases, but after a period of several weeks there still is roughly 25 per cent of the original blood flow persisting. Total obstruction leads to a permanent reduction in renal function, suggesting that nephron destruction occurs. For example, seven days of total obstruction of one ureter in the dog produces loss of an estimated 50 per cent of the nephron population in the involved kidney. A concentrating defect also follows total obstruction. Clearance data performed in the presence of persisting partial obstruction suggest glomerular preponderance rather than a decrease in GFR per nephron. The explanation for this could be an increase in GFR per nephron despite the elevated intratubular pressure, or a *reduction* in GFR per nephron with a *greater reduction* in fractional reabsorption of salt and water. Either alteration could explain the increase in the fraction of filtered sodium and water excreted by the obstructed kidney and the fact that the overall pattern of function resembles that observed in the kidney with chronic nonobstructive renal disease.

OBSERVATIONS IN MAN

Unfortunately, few systematic attempts have been made to investigate either the intricacies of renal function during continuing obstruction or the long-term changes in function which occur after relief of obstruction. The majority of detailed studies have been performed on single patients who presented unusual clinical or biochemical features.

Several facts, however, about the effects of obstruction on renal function in man seem clear. When the luminal occlusion is complete or almost complete, the glomerular filtration rate decreases markedly; and if the process is bilateral, progressive renal failure results. When the obstruction is relieved, some degree of restoration of renal function may be expected unless the nephron population has been totally destroyed.

A few studies are available on certain aspects of renal function in patients with continuing obstruction. Olbrick et al. [77] studied 60 males with bladder neck obstruction due to prostatic enlargement. The average age of the patients was 72 years, and the criteria for inclusion in the study were limited to symptoms of frequency and difficulty of urination. The glomerular filtration rate and renal plasma flow were estimated in each patient, using single-injection technics. In 32 patients bacteriuria was absent; in 28 the urine was infected. The filtration rate and renal plasma flow were found to be decreased by approximately 30 per cent in the uninfected group and by approximately 50 per cent in the infected group when compared with values obtained by the same clearance methods from patients without renal disease in the same age group. Twelve patients were restudied from 10 to 90 days after prostatectomy. In six, the filtration rate increased, in five it decreased, and in one it remained unchanged. The mean change in GFR from the preoperative values was not statistically significant; however, renal plasma flow did show a statistically significant rise for the group data.

Edvall [27] studied 10 patients with hydronephrosis due to calculi or strictures. Values for the filtration rate and renal plasma flow were generally decreased although in one patient supernormal values were found. Filtration fractions tended to be low, whereas in the majority of patients GFR-Tm_{PAH} ratios were either normal or slightly increased. However, in bilateral renal disease (in contrast to unilateral disease with a contralateral control organ), both numerator and denominator of such clearance ratios are variables without any standard for comparison; thus, the values of the ratios have very limited meaning. PAH extraction generally was normal in Edvall's patients.

Studies on seven patients with chronic hydronephrosis have also been reported by Berlyne [7]. These subjects ranged in age from 11 to 67 years, and the filtration rates (uncorrected for body surface area) ranged from 9 to 64 ml. per minute. Data were described on both the concentrating and the acidifying abilities. Maximal urinary osmolality was measured over a period of four to six hours following the intramuscular injection of 5 units of vasopressin (Pitressin) tannate in oil. In six of the seven patients values were low, and in three of the seven the urinary osmolality was less than that of the plasma. Unfortunately no data were included about the prior state of hydration of the patients or their rates of solute excretion. In six patients mannitol and Pitressin were infused and values for solute-free water abstraction ($T^{c}_{H_2O}$) were measured. In the three patients with Pitressin-unresponsive urinary hypotonicity, values for $T^{c}_{H_2O}$ were negative. In the other four patients values were positive and, when expressed as milliliters of $T^{c}_{H_2O}$ per 100 ml. of glomerular filtrate, fell within the range observed in normal subjects. Acidifying ability was measured in the presence of either ammonium chloride-induced or spontaneous acidosis. In two patients minimal urinary pH values were less than 5.5; in two they were between 5.5 and 6.0; in two they fell between 6.0 and 6.38; in one the minimum value was 7.04. For the group, values for ammonium excretion per 100 ml. of glomerular filtrate were normal. In one patient titratable acid excretion was low, in another it was normal.

Two of Berlyne's patients were restudied following prostatectomy and relief of urinary tract obstruction. In one, hypotonic urine had been excreted initially, but four weeks after surgery the urinary osmolality (486 mOsm per kilogram of water) was distinctly greater than that of the plasma. In the same patient the minimal urinary pH following acid loading diminished from a preoperative value of 6.1 to a value of 5.06 after repair of the obstruction. In the other patient the initial urinary pH was 5.46 and two months after surgery 5.3. Creatinine clearance measured before and after surgery in one of these two patients increased from 13.7 to 65 ml. per minute.

The existence of polyuria in patients with persisting obstruction has been noted by a number of investigators [25, 26, 29, 30, 57, 95, 107]. In the majority of instances, the large urine volumes appeared to relate to a Pitressin-unresponsive concentrating defect. To date, however, neither the nature nor the consistency of this abnormality in obstructive nephropathy has been delineated.

The extent to which solute diuresis contributes to the polyuria and the inability to concentrate the urine in obstructive nephropathy is not known. Franklin and Merrill [30] have suggested that an exaggerated salt-losing state may occur in patients with hydronephrosis, but detailed information about the patterns of sodium excretion at varying stages of obstructive nephropathy is not yet available.

Acidosis out of proportion to the degree of azotemia also has been described in urinary tract obstruction [29, 30, 107], but the frequency of this abnormality and the mechanism underlying its development must be added to the list of unknown quantities.

Clinical Manifestations of Obstructive Nephropathy

The symptoms and signs of obstructive nephropathy are very often nonspecific, and the clinical abnormalities may be dominated by the degree of renal functional impairment, by the severity of urinary tract infection, and by any extrarenal manifestations of the underlying pathologic process (for example, local and distant effects of a malignant process when the obstruction is due to ureteral invasion). Some clinical features of obstructive nephropathy, however, are sufficiently distinctive to point attention to the proper diagnosis, when they exist.

Pain and Renal Enlargement. Pain may occasionally be a prominent symptom. In the presence of acute ureteral obstruction this may be colicky in nature and have a characteristic pattern of reference. On the other hand, it must be emphasized that some patients experience no pain even when obstruction is acute in onset, complete, and bilateral. When the obstruction is of long duration, renal colic is relatively infrequent, but vague and often ill-defined, nonradiating back pain or flank pain may occur. When the obstruction is intermittent (i.e., in so-called intermittent hydronephrosis), pain patterns may exhibit a corresponding intermittency. This is most characteristically seen in recurrent ureteral lithiasis, but it may also be observed in obstruction of the ureteropelvic junction due to extrinsic bands. Covington and Reeser [22] have described a patient in whom symptoms and pyelographic evidence of pelvic dilatation were present only during high rates of urine flow.

The size of the kidney may occasionally increase sufficiently in long-standing obstruction for the patient to note increased abdominal girth or a palpable flank mass. Campbell [20] has suggested that in children, hydronephrosis is the commonest cause of abdominal tumor.

Anuria and Polyuria. If the obstruction is complete and bilateral (or complete and unilateral in a patient with only one functional kidney), total anuria results. *However, if the obstruction is partial, urine volume may be greater than normal,* and when polyuria is marked, thirst becomes a prominent symptom. A finding which is highly characteristic of intermittent total obstruction is the sequential occurrence of total anuria and brisk polyuria. The sequence may occur in either direction and may be repetitive. The onset of polyuria coincides with dislodgement of the obstructing lesion; if anuria supervenes again, the obstructing lesion may be assumed to have become reimplanted. Aside from plugging of a bladder catheter, intermittent obstruction with alternating anuria and polyuria is perhaps most often seen when the offending lesion is a stone or a pedunculated malignancy.

"Bladder Symptoms." In obstructing lesions situated at the bladder neck, difficulties in the mechanics of micturition such as narrowing and decrease in the force of the urinary stream may develop. In addition, if there is a large volume of residual urine in the bladder, frequency of urination may be marked, even in the absence of infection, and the patient will present with a history of frequent voiding of small volumes of urine. In severe bladder neck obstruction, the bladder may become markedly distended, and incontinent

dribbling of urine (overflow incontinence) may occur.

Recurrent or Refractory Urinary Tract Infection. Infection of the urinary tract is a frequent complication of chronic urinary tract obstruction. Moreover, as long as the obstruction persists, eradication of the infection may prove exceedingly difficult. Therefore, in any patient with a history of repeated urinary tract infections or with a sustained infection that is refractory to antibiotic therapy, urinary tract obstruction must be considered and a detailed investigation to exclude an obstructing lesion is indicated.

Deterioration of Renal Function Without Apparent Cause. Unrecognized urinary tract obstruction may occasionally present as far-advanced uremia without overt manifestations ascribable to the urinary tract. This is most likely to occur when the cause of the obstruction is itself insidious, such as retroperitoneal fibrosis where symptoms may be nonspecific, seldom relating to the urinary tract until late in the course of the disease. Perhaps more common than the induction of far-advanced uremia in patients with no preexisting renal disease is the intensification of uremia in patients with bilateral renal parenchymal disease of a nonobstructive nature. The added complication of urinary tract obstruction can lead to a serious and in some instances life-threatening exacerbation of renal failure if GFR is already markedly reduced. Two special circumstances serve to predispose the uremic patient to obstruction: (1) parasympatholytic drugs which may be prescribed for the control of nausea and vomiting can lead to bladder atony; and (2) if the uremic patient becomes overtly symptomatic, he may fail to respond appropriately to bladder distention. Partial bladder neck obstruction due to an enlarged prostate may enhance the predisposition to urinary tract obstruction in a uremic patient as in any other patient.

Urinary tract obstruction must be considered in any patient who presents with severe renal insufficiency without an adequate history or in any patient who has sustained recent deterioration of renal function. Once the possibility is considered, all the clinical data must be considered including the presence of a palpably enlarged bladder. It is by no means justifiable, however, to instrument all patients with uremia of unknown cause or with recent exacerbation of uremia; many other causes besides obstruction exist for both, and these often may be defined without recourse to instrumentation.

Polycythemia. Several cases have been recorded in the literature in which polycythemia was found in association with hydronephrosis. In some instances, the polycythemia remitted following surgery [50]. The relation of increased urinary tract pressure to increased erythropoietin production in human beings is not clear. In most of the cases reported erythropoietin assays were not carried out, and in two cases in which erythropoietin was measured, none was detected [50]. However, unilateral hydronephrosis has been shown to produce erythrocytosis in rabbits, and in some animals an elevation of plasma erythropoietin was observed before the increase in hemoglobin levels occurred.

Hypertension. Hypertension has been described in association with hydronephrosis (especially unilateral), and its reversal has been observed with the amelioration of the hydronephrosis [60]. Braasch et al. [12] reported on 73 patients with hydronephrosis, 29 of whom were hypertensive before surgery. Ten of the 29 patients became normotensive after surgery, with follow-up periods extending from one to five years. Nephrectomy was performed in most, and repair of the obstruction in two. In a case of unilateral hydronephrosis with hypertension reported recently [5], increased renin activity was found in the renal vein draining the hydronephrotic kidney. The mechanism by which ureteral obstruction is associated with renin release is not clearly defined, although a decrease in renal blood flow secondary to obstruction has been a favorite explanation. In the laboratory animal, hypertension has been observed after induction of obstruction at the ureteropelvic junction [89], and distention of the bladder has been observed to result in an increase in blood pressure in anesthetized dogs and cats and in patients with spinal cord injuries [99].

Diagnostic Considerations

The recognition of urinary tract obstruction is often complicated by the fact that few or none of the manifestations described in the foregoing paragraphs (flank pain, colic, polyuria of unexplained origin, frequent small voidings, overflow incontinence, etc.) may be present.

Physical examination may in some instances aid in the diagnosis of obstructive nephropathy. As mentioned previously, in infants and children a hydronephrotic kidney may become sufficiently enlarged to be detected on palpation of the abdomen, and in patients of all age groups, but especially in the very young, the very old, and the debilitated, high-grade bladder neck or urethral obstruction may be associated with a palpable urinary bladder. Lesser degrees of enlargement of the bladder may be detected by careful percussion. Flank tenderness and occasionally abdominal tenderness also may be found in obstructive nephropathy and, in most instances, presumably reflect the presence of active pyelonephritis.

Although the approach to diagnosis must be highly individualized, certain procedures have general applicability. A flat film of the abdomen is important in the preliminary examination. Enlargement of one or both kidneys or a discrepancy in size between the two kidneys may occur with urinary tract obstruction. A standard PSP test will indicate pooling of urine if the volume of dye recovered in the urine during the first 15 minutes following injection is less than that recovered during any subsequent 15-minute period. The presence of residual urine should also be checked routinely, and several technics have been introduced that permit accurate measurement of residual urine without recourse to bladder catheterization [21, 40, 74].

Bacteriologic examination of the urine is essential in the evaluation of patients with suspected obstructive nephropathy. Under most circumstances urine samples for cultures may be obtained from clean-voided midstream specimens, and the cultures optimally should be performed using quantitative technics [51].

In patients with adequate renal function, intravenous pyelography may be decisive in establishing the diagnosis of obstruction. Technically satisfactory pyelograms may reveal not only the presence of pooling of urine in the pelvis and ureters but also the morphologic details of the calyceal system and the renal pelvis. It must be emphasized, however, that correct interpretation of the pyelogram may be extremely difficult. Thus, rounding and dilatation of the renal pelvis may be present in normal individuals, and pathologic dilatation of the renal pelvis may be a consequence of infection without mechanical obstruction. Distortion of the calyceal cups, with blunting of the forniceal angles and flattening of the papillae, is a fairly consistent finding in hydronephrosis; but these changes too are not entirely unambiguous, since similar abnormalities may be found in nonobstructive pyelonephritis.

When satisfactory visualization of the conduit system cannot be accomplished by intravenous urography, retrograde pyelography may be of considerable value. It must be acknowledged, however, that this procedure carries the risk either of introducing bacteria into the urinary tract or, if the urine is already infected, of disseminating bacteria into the systemic circulation. During retrograde pyelography, it frequently is possible to obtain quantitative urine collections from the individual kidneys for renal function studies and bacteriologic analysis. Useful collateral information may also be obtained in retrograde pyelography by determining the so-called distention volume of the renal pelvis. Normally the renal pelvis of an adult has a capacity of less than 10 ml., and the ability of a pelvis to accept volumes in excess of this suggests dilatation or decrease in tone (or both).

When the obstruction is not severe and the intravenous pyelograms are technically adequate, considerable information may be deduced about anatomic deformation of the renal pelvis, calyces, and papillary regions. However any effort to extrapolate from the intravenous pyelogram to the level of renal function in a quantitative sense is fraught with major error. Retrograde pyelograms also cannot provide information about the level of renal function unless hydronephrosis is so advanced as to demonstrate virtual complete obliteration of the renal parenchyma.

Because renal blood flow may be relatively well maintained even in the presence of high-grade obstruction, the opportunity for demonstrating opacification of the renal vasculature is good in obstructive nephropathy. If a patient is totally anuric, therefore, an arteriogram will help to exclude the diagnosis of bilateral arterial occlusion. However, whether the arteriogram has any value in differentiating between acute renal failure due to acute tubular necrosis and high-grade obstruction remains to be determined.

In some instances, the complete evaluation of the patient requires endoscopic visualization of the ureter or bladder lumen (or both). While the importance of these procedures in selected patients cannot be minimized, their inherent risks must also be considered. At the present time it seems quite likely that more nephrons are destroyed through inappropriate instrumentation than are salvaged by the correct application of these procedures.

Postobstructive Diuresis

An intriguing abnormality in renal function may develop following the relief of severe urinary tract obstruction. This state is characterized by a dramatic and often life-threatening, temporarily unremitting, but self-limited polyuria. The diuresis involves high rates of excretion of both solutes and water and generally does not serve the preservation of the integrity of body fluids. Indeed, it may result in rapid depletion of extracellular fluid volume, peripheral vascular collapse, and death.

Although it may be assumed that postobstructive diuretic states have complicated the therapy of urinary tract obstruction since the introduction of urethral catheterization centuries ago, specific reference to this abnormality prior to the last decade has not been discovered.* In 1951 Wilson et al. [105] noted that large losses of salt and water may ensue following the relief of urinary tract obstruction, and several additional reports have since been published [14, 28, 80, 81, 106].

The precise incidence of the postobstructive diuresis and the conditions predisposing to it are not yet clearly defined. However, Eiseman and his co-workers [28] found some degree of negative water balance in each of 24 patients who were studied following the relief of acute urinary tract obstruction. In each instance the acute obstruction was superimposed upon some degree of chronic obstruction. In 16 patients, negative water balance of 1500 ml. or greater was found during at least one 24-hour

* However, in 1917 Keith [52], in a study on experimental hydronephrosis in dogs, included observations on one animal that died within 72 hours after removal of bilateral ureteral ligatures. The level of the blood urea nitrogen, which rose from 11 to 64 mg. per 100 ml. during the five-day period of total obstruction, increased to 111 mg. per 100 ml. on the day before death. This occurred despite large urine volumes on the two days following removal of the ureteral ligatures. Balance data included in the report indicate that the animal was in markedly negative fluid balance.

period, and four patients lost 9 pounds or more during the 72-hour interval following relief of obstruction. Persky and his co-workers [81] studied six patients with acute urinary retention. Following institution of indwelling catheterization, the patients were maintained on a standard diet containing approximately 90 mEq. of sodium, and although fluid intake was unrestricted, no supplementary fluids were administered. Each of the patients developed negative salt and water balance. The cumulative negative balances during the first four days ranged from 50 to 470 mEq. for sodium and from 50 to 525 mEq. for potassium. In four patients appreciable decreases in plasma volume developed. In all but one of the patients studied, the diuresis was relatively short-lived, and salt and water balance was reestablished spontaneously within three days without supplementary fluid therapy. In one patient, however, the cumulative water loss approximated 4 liters in three days, and sodium and potassium depletion were equally marked.

Some evidence exists about the mechanisms of the postobstructive diuresis [14]. Studies were performed on patients in whom urine volumes following the relief of obstruction ranged from 4.5 to 15.0 liters per day, and sodium excretion ranged from 250 to 1900 mEq. per day. In each case, outflow obstruction had been virtually complete, and at the time of initial observation (i.e., prior to relief of the obstruction) manifestations of acute renal failure were present. Renal function studies performed during the diuretic phase revealed variable decreases in glomerular filtration rate and PAH clearance. The most striking feature of the abnormality, however, related to the patterns of solute and water excretion. During the clearance studies, maximal urine flows ranged from 15 to 31 per cent of the filtered water, and from 6.3 to 20.0 per cent of the filtered sodium was excreted. Analysis of the solute composition of the urine indicated that electrolytes (sodium, chloride, and potassium) rather than urea were principally responsible for the high rates of urine flow. The characteristics of the diuresis closely resembled those seen in normal individuals subjected to the infusion of an osmotically active, essentially nonreabsorbed solute such as mannitol; however, since no exogenous loading solute was employed, it was concluded that the primary abnormality related to an intrinsic tubular defect in sodium reabsorption. It was also suggested that the principal site of impaired salt and water reabsorption was in the proximal convoluted tubules. This was based upon two observations: (1) The magnitude of the natriuresis in some patients was so great that complete cessation of distal sodium reabsorption theoretically could not have accounted for it; and (2) during the height of diuresis, the capacity to dilute the urine (as determined by the ratio of free water clearance to filtration rate) persisted. In view of the evidence that urinary dilution results from the reabsorption of sodium from the tubular fluid in the ascending limb of the loop of Henle [6], the presence of essentially intact diluting ability during brisk natriuresis supports the view that extensive suppression of sodium reabsorption did not extend to the diluting segments of the nephron. Moreover, in three of four patients, the amount of potassium excreted approached or exceeded the amount filtered, suggesting that the distal sites wherein potassium is secreted, presumably in exchange for sodium, were functional.

The foregoing observations imply that the postobstructive diuresis is solute-mediated, and that the underlying abnormality relates to the inappropriately low rates of net sodium and chloride reabsorption primarily in the proximal tubules. If net sodium transport across the proximal tubular epithelial cells is suppressed selectively, it would be of considerable importance to define the underlying mechanisms. Because the proximal tubules make the greatest quantitative contribution to the total reabsorption of sodium from the tubular fluid, it is conceivable that dilatation of this segment of the nephron may, by compressing the microvilli, decrease the total luminal surface area of the epithelial cells which make contact with the tubular fluid. It is of interest, in this connection, that in experimental obstruction the epithelial cells of the proximal tubules appear to be flattened against the basement membranes [94]. Attention also is directed to the proximal tubular epithelial cells by Wilmer's [103] observations that alkaline phosphatase is selectively decreased in this area following ureteral ligation. These observations have recently been confirmed by Kissane and Heptinstall [55], who found that in rats, after two days of complete ureteral obstruction, alkaline phosphatase activity in the proximal tubules was greatly reduced. A further decrease in enzyme activity was noted after seven days. Recovery of alkaline phosphatase activity was observed two days following release of the obstruction and after six days values were comparable to those observed preceding obstruction. No changes in acid phosphatase were observed with obstruction, but acid phosphatase activity increased significantly early in the course of recovery from obstruction and decreased toward control levels after six days of recovery. Kissane and Heptinstall [56] have also found that glucose 6-phosphate dehydrogenase and 6-phosphogluconic dehydrogenase activity increased in the proximal tubules of obstructed kidneys. Following release of the obstruction, these enzyme activities remained elevated during the initial 48 hours but returned to normal after 6 days of recovery. To date, however, the role of these enzymes (acid and alkaline phosphatases, glucose 6-phosphate dehydrogenase, and 6-phosphogluconic dehydrogenase) in active sodium transport has not been established.

Recent experiments [102] have suggested another possible explanation for the natriuresis. It has been demonstrated that ureteral ligation causes a decrease in the sodium-potassium activated adenosine triphosphatase (ATPase) of the involved kidney. Magnesium ATPase and sodium plus potassium ATPase activities were assayed on microsomal fractions from hydronephrotic and contralateral normal kidneys of female rats before and at one, two, and five days following ureteral ligation. No changes in magnesium ATPase were observed with obstruction. On the other hand, there was a steady decrease in sodium plus potassium ATPase activity with longer periods of obstruction. Sodium plus potassium activated ATPase activity is closely associated with the active transport of sodium, and it is tempting to speculate that the sodium diuresis which may follow the release of obstruction could be related to decreased ATPase activity in the epithelial cells of the proximal tubules.

A third mechanism for the natriuresis also may be considered. As a consequence of the pressure and volume alterations of the proximal tubules, passive sodium influx back into the tubular fluid (the sodium leak) could be greatly augmented. Under these conditions, net sodium reabsorption would be decreased whether or not a decrement in active transport occurred. Correlation of the rates of net sodium reabsorption with renal oxygen consumption could very well provide considerable insight into this problem.

Still another factor that could contribute to the natriuresis is the presence of high concentrations of urea in the glomerular filtrate. Urea is an osmotically active solute that is only partially reabsorbed, and high filtered loads of urea will decrease the net reabsorption of solutes and water in the proximal tubule. Maher et al. [69] have presented evidence in one patient with postobstructive diuresis for a role of urea (as an osmotic diuretic) in the development of the diuretic state. However, in other patients described in the literature [14, 106] the continuing diuresis could not be explained on the basis of the osmotic effect of urea.

A final factor that could contribute in some instances to an inappropriate natriuresis is an increased blood level of a natriuretic substance. If there is a natriuretic hormone, as many observers presently believe, chronic obstruction followed by acute urinary suppression could lead to high rates of its secretion; and the high activity might persist for variable periods after relief of the obstruction. Future studies will establish the validity of this concept.

That the sodium diuresis following relief of urinary tract obstruction represents a salutary response and not an abnormal one has recently been argued by Muldowney et al. [73]. In 14 patients with urinary tract obstruction they measured the changes in total exchangeable sodium following relief of the obstruction. Only patients with chronic obstruction showed increased values for total exchangeable sodium. In patients with acute obstruction total exchangeable sodium was found to be within normal limits. Sodium balance studies in 9 of the 14 subjects disclosed prolonged negative sodium balance that was more marked in the cases with chronic obstruction. During the period that followed the release of obstruction there was a decrease to normal levels of total exchangeable sodium in the group with chronic obstruction. No consistent change was observed in patients with acute obstruction. Muldowney et al. suggested that chronic urinary obstruction gives rise to sodium retention and increased total body sodium; relief of obstruction will be followed by sodium diuresis and a reduction in body sodium content to normal limits. These observations suggest not so much an abnormal sodium loss following relief of obstruction as a physiologic excretion of excess body sodium that had accumulated during the period of urinary tract obstruction.

The possibility that in some instances the postobstructive diuresis is secondary to, or at least potentiated by, preexisting expansion of the extracellular fluid volume seems reasonable. However, that this cannot be the universal explanation, and indeed may not be the usual basis for the natriuresis, is suggested by several observations. First, when obstruction is unilateral, the natriuretic response may be observed from the involved kidney (but not the unobstructed organ) after the relief of the obstruction. Second, some patients with postobstructive diuresis will continue to lose salt and water until hypotension supervenes unless replacement is adequate. Third, rarely the postobstructive diuresis will persist for weeks to months [67] and repeated attempts to reduce the volume of fluid used in replacement therapy to levels below the contemporaneous losses are unsuccessful in aborting the diuresis.

Whatever the mechanism for the sodium diuresis may be, the abnormality appears to be triggered by high-grade urinary tract obstruction followed by restitution of pressure relationships in the conduit system toward normal. Why the diuretic state appears in an overt form in a relatively small percentage of patients with total obstruction and whether it occurs in the presence of persisting incomplete obstruction are unknown.

Clinically, several important aspects of the postobstructive diuresis warrant emphasis. It already has been pointed out that the antecedent obstruction is generally high grade and often complete, and in most instances it is superimposed on some degree of chronic obstruction. At the initial examination, the majority of patients present evidence of renal insufficiency, and frequently this is manifested as severe acute renal failure. The onset of the diuresis usually begins within the first few hours after decompression, but in rare instances it may be delayed for 24 hours or more. As we have already noted, an expanded extracellular fluid volume prior to relief of obstruction does not appear to be an essential requisite for the development of the diuresis; yet an excessively high rate of fluid administration during the period of diuresis may potentiate the losses of salt and water [14].

The basis of effective therapy consists of

adequate and continued replacement of both prior and contemporaneous urinary losses of sodium, chloride, potassium, and water. Because of the unremitting (albeit self-limited) nature of the diuresis, fluid restriction can be disastrous. Salt-retaining mineralocorticoids do not appear to have any detectable salutary effects. Spontaneous improvement generally occurs within several days, although recovery may occasionally be delayed for weeks to months. When improvement does occur, the kidneys regain the ability to regulate the volume and composition of extracellular fluid in a manner commensurate with the population of surviving nephrons.

Evaluation of Renal Function in the Presence of Obstructive Nephropathy

Evaluation of the functional capacity of the obstructed kidney may present certain difficulties not ordinarily encountered in other forms of renal disease. These relate to the pooling of urine in the conduit system and to the fact that the renal disease is frequently unilateral.

BILATERAL OBSTRUCTION

When obstructive nephropathy is bilateral, an estimate of the composite function of both kidneys may be obtained using conventional criteria.

Urea and Creatinine Concentrations in Body Fluids. The levels of blood urea nitrogen (BUN) and serum (or plasma) creatinine provide a rough index of the glomerular filtration rate, and serial measurements serve to indicate changes in GFR with time. Theoretically, however, pooling of urine may interfere with the relationship between GFR and body fluid levels of urea and creatinine. Thus urea and, to a limited degree, creatinine may diffuse out of the urine pooled above the site of obstruction into the systemic blood in greater than normal amounts. Hence, it is conceivable that measured values in the blood, especially of urea, may be disproportionately high for any given level of GFR.

Urea and Endogenous Creatinine Clearances. Serial measurement of clearance values is the most reliable of the clinically applicable means of following GFR in a patient with progressive renal disease.* In obstructive nephropathy, however, pooling of urine may render interpretation difficult. Not only may there be augmented diffusion of the reference substances out of the urine, but the increased dead space in the conduit system introduces a major and often indeterminable variable. In the performance of clearance tests, two maneuvers will help to minimize the dead space error: (1) The rate of urine flow should be maintained as brisk as the clinical condition and renal function permit (if water loading will suffice to evoke a copious water diuresis, this procedure should be employed; otherwise urine flows may be increased by using an osmotically active non-reabsorbable solute such as mannitol); and (2) the time allowed between the onset of the diuresis and the beginning of clearance measurements should be lengthy, and individual urine collections should generally be maintained for periods of at least one hour.†

Phenol Red Excretion. The use of the phenolsulfonphthalein (PSP) test in the assessment of renal function in obstructive nephropathy is subject to the same limitations as are clearance studies; the test has the further disadvantage of being more empiric and less amenable to precise interpretation. In per-

* The endogenous creatinine clearance provides a close approximation of GFR in patients with normal or modestly compromised renal function; however, in patients with bilateral nephropathy and GFRs below 20 ml. per minute, the true filtration rate approximates the mean of the endogenous creatinine clearance and the urea clearance [66].

† If mannitol infusion is employed, careful observation of the patients is required when the duration of the infusion is lengthy.

forming this test, high rates of urine flow are desirable. Individual collection periods, however, cannot be prolonged beyond the predetermined intervals if any attempt at quantitation is to be made.

The pattern of PSP excretion may provide a certain amount of information about the degree of urine pooling. Because of the single-injection technic which is routinely employed in this test, the plasma concentration of dye is maximal immediately after injection and the quantity of PSP excreted by the *kidneys* during the first 15 minutes must exceed that excreted during any subsequent interval. Therefore, if the amount of dye recovered in the *urine* is greater during the second or third 15-minute period than during the first, evidence is provided for pooling of urine beyond the level of the nephron.

Maximal Urinary Concentrating Ability. To date, detailed investigation of the concentrating ability at successive stages of obstructive nephropathy is not available. There is reason to believe that the concentrating mechanism may be impaired relatively early in the course of urinary tract obstruction, and the degree of suppression of the maximal achievable urinary osmolality (or specific gravity) may probably not be accepted as an index of the severity of the renal lesions or of the extent of nephron destruction.

Intravenous and Retrograde Pyelography. Most compounds currently used for intravenous pyelography are excreted primarily by filtration (i.e., they are excreted as if they were filtered completely, not reabsorbed, and not secreted). The dyes are then concentrated as they move down the nephron by virtue of the reabsorption of water. The success of an intravenous pyelogram depends, therefore, first upon the amount of dye filtered and second upon the degree of concentration of the dye. The amount of dye filtered in bilateral obstruction will depend upon how markedly GFR is diminished. If the obstruction is only partial, GFR may not be markedly decreased, and filtration of dye may permit adequate visualization. The ultimate success of the intravenous pyelogram will therefore depend upon concentration of dye en route down the tubular lumina which is a function of the fractional reabsorption of water. If the obstruction is high grade or complete, new glomerular filtrate occurs only as tubular fluid is reabsorbed from the blocked nephrons and as fluid diffuses out of the renal pelvis. These combined processes may be slow, and thus it may take hours before sufficient dye enters the tubular lumina to permit any roentgenographic visualization. However, if the population of surviving nephrons is substantial, a delayed "nephrogram" may be obtained even in the presence of high-grade bilateral obstruction.

Renogram and Isotopic Scanning. A radioisotope renogram is a grossly qualitative technic that is of primary value in demonstrating gross differences between the function of the two kidneys. It thus is of very restricted value in bilateral urinary tract obstruction. Isotopic scanning technics involving the intravenous injection of a radioactive compound which is concentrated by the renal tubular epithelial cells will allow the demonstration of the respective patterns of isotope accumulation in the separate kidneys and may give some indication as to the size of the kidneys. Scanning has no specific attributes, however, beyond these relatively nonspecific contributions in obstructive nephropathy.

Urinary Sediment. The urinary sediment is of considerable value in judging the activity of pathologic changes in nephrons which contribute to urine formation. But, aside from changes that may point to pyelonephritis (bacteria, white cells, white cell casts, etc.), there is nothing specific about the sediment in obstructive nephropathy. One exception to the lack of specificity may be found in an occasional patient with renal papillary necrosis, in which case some fragments of papillary tissue occasionally may be observed in the urine.

UNILATERAL OBSTRUCTION

When urinary tract obstruction is unilateral, the difficulties in quantitating the level of function of the diseased kidney are greatly magnified. As the function of the involved kidney decreases, that of the contralateral kidney increases compensatorily, and values for composite (i.e., bilateral) renal function may obscure the true extent of unilateral damage. Body fluid levels of substances that are excreted primarily by filtration such as urea and creatinine may therefore remain close to normal even in the presence of advanced unilateral obstructive nephropathy. To evaluate the function of the unilaterally diseased kidney quantitatively, separate urine samples must be obtained from the diseased and the contralateral control organ. This ordinarily requires catheterization of both ureters, a technic that for many reasons is not applicable to the systematic evaluation of the natural history of obstructive disease. Bernstein and Hamby [9] have introduced a technic that involves external abdominal compression designed to occlude each ureter separately and thus to permit collection of urine from the individual kidneys. While this procedure has the advantage of being relatively simple and does not require ureteral instrumentation, the validity of the technic requires confirmation.

The radioisotope renogram, as suggested above, is not a quantitative test of renal function, but it will demonstrate a difference in pattern between an obstructed and a contralateral nonobstructed kidney. Nevertheless, the technic is of primary value in screening and in our opinion does not permit the quantitative and ongoing assessment of renal function in unilateral obstruction. Neither does the intravenous pyelogram provide the necessary information. Yet for lack of anything better, the intravenous pyelogram may be employed in the long-term follow-up evaluation of patients with unilateral urinary tract obstruction on the assumption that the structural changes of the pelvis and calyceal system will correlate grossly with changes in function. If the evaluation of renal function in an obstructed kidney becomes essential to the design of therapy — for example, if nephrectomy is contemplated because the obstructed kidney is believed to be contributing very little to total renal function — ureteral catheterization with divided renal function studies is unquestionably indicated. Separate urine samples will permit the measurement of respective levels of GFR as well as the concentrating abilities and patterns of salt and water excretion by the two kidneys. If divided function studies are performed, it is essential that GFR, either as endogenous creatinine clearance or preferably as inulin clearance, be measured and that renal function not be estimated on the basis of the comparative rates of urine flow, for the obstructed kidney may excrete an inordinately high fraction of its filtered water. Thus the urine flow rate may be disproportionately high for the level of GFR, and urine flow rates from the damaged kidney may be equal to or even greater than those from a contralateral intact organ.

Approach to Therapy

There is no question that a focal obstructing lesion of the lower urinary tract which is responsible for progressive renal functional impairment should be removed if that is technically feasible. If, however, the preservation of nephrons is to represent the principal goal underlying the therapy of urinary tract obstruction, a direct attack upon the obstructing process cannot invariably dominate therapeutic formulations. Reference has been made to the fact that hydronephrosis may persist indefinitely without compromising renal function. In such patients, serial renal function studies, intravenous pyelograms, and urine cultures constitute the most rational program of management. Certainly, major surgery is contraindicated, and any procedures that may introduce pyelonephritis should be avoided if possible. If urinary tract obstruction is the *result* of pyelonephritis, therapy should consist of vigorous and sustained attempts to eradicate the infection, and surgery should be considered only if medical management proves unsuccessful in improving the function of the conduit system. Finally, when mechanical obstruction is responsible for deterioration of renal function, major attention must still be given to the problem of pyelonephritis. Thus, prior to attempts at definitive surgery, strenuous efforts should be made to decrease the bacterial population of the urine; during and immediately following surgery, every precaution should be taken to minimize the introduction of new pathogenic organisms; and after correction of the defect, long-term follow-up care replete with periodic urine cultures must be maintained to detect the persistence of infection and to prevent, if possible, the progression of pyelonephritis.

The specific details of surgical correction of urinary tract obstruction are not considered in this discussion. However, certain general principles of therapy will be reviewed.

NEPHRECTOMY

It frequently has been contended that nephrectomy is the procedure of choice for an obstructed kidney that has sustained a mild decrease in functional capacity. Proponents of this thesis have maintained that the residual nephrons of a severely damaged kidney are unable to exhibit functional recovery if the contralateral kidney has undergone compensatory hypertrophy [42]. *Strong objections must be raised to this thesis.* There is no evidence to support the contention that surviving nephrons of a diseased kidney are functionally inhibited by the presence of a contralateral normal organ, and in the laboratory animal with chronic nonobstructive unilateral renal disease the functioning units of the diseased organ appear to make essentially the same quantitative contribution to overall renal function as do a comparable number of nephrons in the contralateral kidney [15]. There are other compelling reasons why a diseased kidney should not be removed in the absence of very specific indications. For example, if the obstructed kidney is infected, the possibility must always be considered that bacteria from the bladder urine may have reached the unobstructed kidney by retrograde dissemination. Hence, the allegedly normal organ may be afflicted with potentially progressive pyelonephritis. The unnecessary removal of nephrons in this case could foreshorten the life of the patient. It appears at the present stage of knowledge, therefore, that unless damage is very far advanced the long-range interests of the patient may best be subserved by attempting to salvage nephrons by instituting sustained treatment of infection and correcting the obstruction if possible. One major exception to this rule exists: If the obstructed kidney is extensively damaged and is the seat of florid and refractory infection which continually threatens the integrity of the contralateral kidney, or if it is responsible for repeated episodes of bacteremia, nephrectomy may represent the most rational therapeutic procedure.

URETEROPELVIC OBSTRUCTION

When hydronephrosis exists in association with narrowing of the ureteropelvic junction, the initial therapeutic efforts should, in most instances, be directed along conservative lines. Surgical attempts at correcting the abnormality should be considered, however, if there is evidence of progression of the hydronephrosis, decrease in renal function, or advancing and refractory pyelonephritis.

URETERAL OBSTRUCTION

Because of the narrow cross-sectional diameter of the ureter, acquired mechanical lesions frequently produce high-grade obstruction. For example, relatively small calculi which become wedged in the ureter may seriously interfere with effective draining of urine, and in some instances may produce total obstruction after edema of the mucosal wall and spasm of the ureter occur. Similarly, extraluminal processes such as invading neoplasms may rapidly occlude the ureter.

Kerr's demonstration [53] that ureteral ligation for a period of only seven days produced a permanent and appreciable decrease in renal function dictates that, in high-grade obstruction, definitive therapy be initiated as expeditiously as possible. Thus, in a patient with recurrent stone formation, repeated individual insults may lead to progressive renal damage, and undue delay in relieving the obstruction may accelerate the cumulative loss of nephrons. Accordingly, the time allowed for a calculus which completely occludes the ureter to pass spontaneously should probably not exceed a week. On the other hand, if the obstruction is only partial, and particularly if the urine is sterile, it may be wise to extend the interval of conservative management in order to avoid premature instrumentation. When ureteral narrowing occurs from an extraluminal process, the decision as to the wisdom and time of surgical intervention must depend not only upon the effects of the involved urinary tract and kidney but also upon the nature, natural history, and stigmata of the underlying disease process.

BLADDER NECK OBSTRUCTION

In the presence of bladder neck obstruction due to enlargement of the prostate gland, the advisability of prostatectomy must be established on the basis of the status of renal function, the presence or absence of infection, and the volume of residual urine.

If renal function is not impaired (as judged by a normal glomerular filtration rate) and the urine is sterile, both diagnostic catheterization and surgical removal of the prostate gland should be deferred unless the symptoms prove incapacitating. Reevaluation must be performed, however, at frequent intervals. If infection is present at the initial examination, but renal function is unimpaired, vigorous attempts to correct the bacteriuria should be made in advance of definitive procedures. If the urine can be made sterile, conservative management again represents the course of choice. On the other hand, if bacteriuria persists and a significant volume of residual urine is found, prostatectomy may be indicated.

When bladder neck obstruction is associated with impairment of renal function, surgery should probably be performed at the earliest opportunity and with minimal preliminary instrumentation. There is a growing belief among urologists that the initial preoperative cystoscopy can be performed in the operating room and prostatectomy accomplished immediately thereafter if indications exist.

In a patient with azotemia, it is conventionally deemed advisable to employ an indwelling bladder catheter for several days to several weeks before undertaking prostatectomy. This procedure is intended to provide maximal recovery of renal function before the patient is subjected to surgery. The obvious hazard of chronic indwelling catheterization is the initiation or exacerbation of urinary tract infection. Thus, immediate prostatectomy, with close postoperative supervision of salt and water balance, and the use of dialysis as a therapeutic adjunct may be more rational and beneficial than the conventional approach. At least, this approach is deserving of critical evaluation.

BLADDER OUTFLOW OBSTRUCTION IN THE FEMALE

Increasing attention has recently been focused on lesions that are presumed to produce bladder outlet obstruction in the female, especially the young female with chronic bacteriuria. However, when the diagnostic criteria for bladder neck obstruction and the response to therapy are analyzed critically, the data are difficult to interpret. For example, a number of studies have pointed out that neither bladder voiding pressures nor urine flow dynamics during micturition are sufficiently distinctive to be diagnostic in patients believed to have bladder outflow obstruction [24]. Other diagnostic criteria have yielded equally ambiguous results [31]. In studies by Scott et al. [86] in girls with clinical bladder neck obstruction, the urethral luminal pressure tracings were not different from those obtained in children with no symptoms referable to outflow tract obstruction. The presence of a fibrous ring in the distal urethra has been suggested as a cause of outflow obstruction and urinary infection in female children, and dilatation of the urethra has been advocated as a therapeutic procedure for this condition. However, measurements of urethral caliber in such patients have failed to show evidence of a significant narrowing or obstruction [34]. Thus cumulative data fail to provide a firm basis for the view that bladder outlet obstruction is either a common or a clearly definable entity in females. And as long as the diagnostic criteria for an abnormality are poorly defined, it will remain extremely difficult to assess the response to therapy. It seems quite likely that fewer women and children have true anatomic bladder outlet obstruction than are treated for it.

RESIDUAL URINE

The larger the volume of residual urine, the greater the propensity for the development of obstructive nephropathy from untoward pressure relationships. If, in addition, the urine is infected, a constant pool of urine in the bladder will (in the absence of therapy) support bacterial multiplication. In theory, therefore, the presence of residual urine is both unphysiologic and potentially dangerous. However, the approach to treatment is not simple. If the urine is sterile, the use of an indwelling catheter in an effort to restore bladder tone, or of transurethral resection designed to restore a more favorable ratio between projectile force of the bladder and outflow resistance, may have the net effect of initiating bacteriuria without producing sustained improvement in the capacity to empty the bladder completely.

For this reason, a less direct approach to treatment may in many instances be the most effective. Multiple voiding technics may be of considerable value. Because untoward pressure relationships develop only when the bladder is overextended, frequent voiding and special maneuvers such as double voiding [93] may obviate bladder distention despite the constant presence of a moderate volume of residual urine. In the absence of a high-grade mechanical block, attempts may also be made to improve the efficiency of bladder function pharmacologically by the use of a parasympathomimetic drug such as bethanechol (Urecholine). When the volume of residual urine is large (greater than 100 ml.) and there is an associated decrease in the glomerular filtration rate, cystoscopy and appropriate corrective procedures must be undertaken.

REFLUX OF URINE

Reflux of urine from the bladder to the ureters, particularly if the urine is infected represents another potentially harmful situation. When the reflux relates to primary anatomic abnormalities in the bladder, bladder neck, or urethra, removal of the offending lesion or transplantation of the ureters (or both) is often indicated. In some instances, however, the reflux may occur secondary to obstruction or ureteral dilatation resulting from persisting infection [62, 93]. If there is uncertainty as to the cause of the reflux, it seems advisable to initiate a period of conservative management involving vigorous treatment of the infection and special voiding technics before subjecting the patient to formidable operative procedures.

URINARY DIVERSION

"Urinary diversion" refers to the anastomosis of the ureters to some portion of either the large or the small bowel. The procedure is used in treatment of a variety of pathologic states involving the lower urinary tract. Carcinoma of the bladder and neurogenic bladder with refractory infection are among the common conditions for urinary diversion [79]. Diversion is also used for severe reflux that is refractory to sustained conservative therapy and that is attended by progressive deterioration of renal function. Anastomosis of the ureters to the sigmoid colon (ureterosigmoidostomy), formerly a popular procedure, is now being used infrequently because of the multiple complications that can attend the procedure. These include: ascending infection, which may be severe and contribute to progressive impairment of renal function; metabolic acidosis, which occurs in 50 to 75 per cent of patients; ureteral reflux, which may be accompanied by gas in the ureters and renal pelvis; and progressive dilatation of the ureters and pelvis.

Because of the unfavorable course that frequently attends ureterosigmoidostomy, efforts have been made to develop more effective technics of urinary diversion. The most satisfactory of these involves the anastomosis of the ureters to a segment of ileum. An isolated loop of ileum is produced surgically, and its blood supply is retained. The proximal end of the isolated loop is usually closed and infolded, and the lower or distal end is brought up to the surface of the abdomen as an ileostomy. The ureters drain into the lumen of the loop. The ileal conduit offers major advantages over the ureterosigmoidostomy. The conduit has a limited capacity, and the urine is evacuated frequently. Thus the reservoir is limited in size, and the period of urinary stasis is short; both events will serve to reduce the hazards or intensity (or both) of infection. The rapid evacuation of urine also minimizes the formation of ammonia by urea-splitting bacteria and thus decreases the rate at which ammonium ions enter the systemic circulation. Consequently, the incidence of hyperchloremic metabolic acidosis is markedly decreased. The separation of the ileal conduit from the lumen of the bowel also provides a separate route of excretion for urine and feces.

Despite the advantages of the uretero-ileostomy, a number of complications have been noted. Postoperatively ileus, peritonitis, and fistulas have been described, and late complications include hydroureter, hydronephrosis, severe pyelonephritis, and obstruction and narrowing of the ileal cutaneous stoma. Cinefluorographic studies have recently revealed that there may be a lack of coordination between the contractions of the conduit and ureteral peristalsis [19]. When this occurs, a considerable degree of reflux may develop. To obviate the reflux, with its hazards of ascending infection, ureteral dilatation, etc., a tunneling uretero-ileal anastomosis has been proposed [71]. When the ureters are damaged or functionless, the renal pelvis may be anastomosed directly to the ileum [97].

POSTOPERATIVE TREATMENT

No attempt will be made to discuss the general principles of postoperative therapy. Rather, three specific situations are considered that are of particular importance in patients with urinary tract obstruction.

1. Following surgical modification of any segment of the conduit system, it often is necessary to maintain indwelling catheters at least until wound healing has occurred. However, the period for which a catheter is left in either the bladder or the ureter should be as short as possible, and every effort should be directed toward safeguarding the patient from the effects of infection. Although no technics currently exist which will uniformly prevent the introduction of bacteria into the urinary tract of a patient with an indwelling catheter, rigid asepsis during the insertion of the catheter, use of an antibiotic ointment to lubricate urethral catheters and to coat the junction between the urethral meatus and the catheters, the use of closed systems which do

not expose the urine to contaminating bacteria, and in some instances the use of tidal drainage and urinary acidifiers may all decrease the population of bacteria in the urine. The routine treatment of patients with potent antibiotics during the period of catheterization is probably inadvisable in view of increasing evidence that the organisms which remain in the urinary tract after discontinuation of the drugs may be resistant to the agents employed in attempted prophylaxis.

2. A second problem that may develop during the postoperative period in patients with urinary tract obstruction is unremitting diuresis. Although this abnormality in renal function is uncommon, its possible occurrence must be anticipated in order to prevent major derangements of body fluid economy. The basic therapy of the post-obstructive diuresis consists of quantitative replacement of salt and water losses until spontaneous recovery occurs. If treatment is initiated at the onset of diuresis, replacement therapy need be designed only to prevent negative balances of sodium, potassium, chloride, and water and the evolution of severe metabolic acidosis. On the other hand, if extracellular fluid depletion has occurred before therapy is begun, fluid replacement must include replacement not only of current urine losses but of the estimated deficits. In practice the estimated losses are most effectively replaced by using a synthetic solution having the composition of extracellular fluid; the continuing losses must be determined by analyzing the composition of the urine.

3. Because of the limitation in present knowledge regarding effective methods of treating pyelonephritis, serial observations of the patient must be performed for a lengthy period even after the successful removal of a focal obstruction lesion. Once a patient has sustained the combined effects of urinary tract obstruction and pyelonephritis, urine cultures should be performed routinely until the urine has been sterile for a period of at least six months.

Conclusions

Any contemporary discussion of obstructive nephropathy must of necessity be incomplete and in many respects speculative. Although the understanding of renal physiology and the extension of this knowledge to the pathologic physiology of many forms of renal disease have increased impressively in recent years, the information relevant to the numerous problems associated with urinary tract obstruction has not enjoyed the same rate of progress. This is the result of a number of factors. First, most of the experimental observations have been obtained from animals subjected to short-term total ureteral ligation, whereas in human beings luminal occlusion is generally of long duration and is only rarely complete. Second, controlled, comprehensive, long-term experiments on human beings with urinary tract obstruction are virtually nonexistent. In part this lack is due to the great difficulties in designing prospective studies in a population of patients in which natural history is modified by multiple variables. Third, and of great importance, the problems of obstructive nephropathy have failed to stimulate the interest of investigators principally concerned with the functional integrity of the nephron. Consequently, a mechanistic approach has been taken to clinical management, and critical evaluation of therapeutic and diagnostic technics with particular regard to their inherent long-term hazards is incomplete.

The discussion of obstructive nephropathy in this chapter is based upon the thesis that nephron survival, in the final analysis, is the goal of supreme importance both to the patient and to the physician. Therefore, the concepts which have been presented cannot be considered to be free of bias. Emphasis on the hazards of urethral instrumentation is evident throughout the discussion, and it may well be that the preoccupation with this aspect of the overall problem has been overextended. Nevertheless, some swing of the pendulum from its present position is necessary, and it is hoped that these comments may at least serve to stimulate the acquisition of vitally needed new information.

References

1. Allen, A. C. *The Kidney: Medical and Surgical Diseases.* New York: Grune & Stratton, 1951.
2. Altschul, R., and Fedor, S. Vascular changes in hydronephrosis. *Amer. Heart J.* 46:291, 1953.
3. Bell, E. T. Exudative interstitial nephritis (pyelonephritis). *Surgery* 11:261, 1942.
4. Bell, E. T. *Renal Diseases.* Philadelphia: Lea & Febiger, 1946.
5. Belman, A. B., Kropp, K. A., and Simin, N. M. Renal-pressor hypertension secondary to unilateral hydronephrosis. *New Eng. J. Med.* 278:1133, 1968.
6. Berliner, R. W., Levinsky, N. G., Davidson, D. G., and Eden, M. Dilution and concentration of the urine and the action of antidiuretic hormone. *Amer. J. Med.* 24:730, 1958.
7. Berlyne, G. M. Distal tubular function in chronic hydronephrosis. *Quart. J. Med.* 30: 339, 1961.
8. Berlyne, G. M., and Macken, A. On the mechanism of renal inability to produce a concentrated urine in chronic hydronephrosis. *Clin. Sci.* 22:315, 1962.
9. Bernstein, L. M., and Hamby, W. M. Unilateral urine sampling utilizing external ureteral compression. *New Eng. J. Med.* 268:1093, 1963.
10. Bligh, A. S. Pyelographic changes in pregnancy. *Brit. J. Radiol.* 30:489, 1957.
11. Boyarsky, A., and Labay, P. Stimulation of ureteral peristalsis through the renal nerves. *Invest. Urol.* 5:200, 1967.
12. Braasch, W. F., Walters, W., and Hammer, H. J. Hypertension and the surgical kidney. *J.A.M.A.* 115:1837, 1940.
13. Brenner, B. M., Bennett, C. M., and Berliner, R. W. The relationship between glomerular filtration rate and sodium reabsorption by the proximal tubule of the rat nephron. *J. Clin. Invest.* 47:1358, 1968.
14. Bricker, N. S., Shwayri, E. D., Reardan, J. B., Kellogg, D., Merrill, J. P., and Holmes, J. H. An abnormality in renal function resulting from urinary tract obstruction. *Amer. J. Med.* 23:554, 1957.
15. Bricker, N. S., Klahr, S., Lubowitz, H., and Rieselbach, R. E. Renal function in chronic renal disease. *Medicine* (Balt.) 44: 263, 1965.
16. Brenner, F. P., Rector, F. C., Jr., and Seldin, D. W. Mechanism of glomerulotubular balance: II. Regulation of proximal tubular reabsorption by tubular volume, as studied by stopped-flow microperfusion. *J. Clin. Invest.* 45:603, 1966.
17. Butcher, H. R., Jr., and Sleator, W., Jr. Effect of ureteral anastomosis upon conduction of peristaltic waves: Electroureterographic study. *J. Urol.* 75:650, 1956.
18. Butcher, H. R., Jr., Sleator, W., Jr., and Schmandt, W. P. A study of the peristaltic conduction mechanism in the canine ureter. *J. Urol.* 78:221, 1957.
19. Campbell, J. E., Oliver, J. A., and McKay, D. E. Dynamics of ileal conduits. *Radiology* 85:338, 1965.
20. Campbell, M. Hydronephrosis in infants and children. *J. Urol.* 65:734, 1951.
21. Cotran, R. S., and Kass, E. H. Determination of the volume of residual urine in the bladder without catheterization. *New Eng. J. Med.* 259:337, 1958.
22. Covington, T., Jr., and Reeser, W. Hydronephrosis associated with overhydration. *J. Urol.* 63:438, 1950.

23. Cussen, L. J. The structure of the normal human ureter in infancy and childhood. *Invest. Urol.* 5:179, 1967.
24. Donohue, J. P., and Leadbetter, G. W., Jr. An evaluation of voiding cystometry as a diagnostic test for bladder outlet obstruction. *J. Urol.* 92:464, 1964.
25. Dorhout Mees, E. J. Reversible water-losing state, caused by incomplete ureteric obstruction. *Acta Med. Scand.* 168:193, 1960.
26. Earley, L. E. Extreme polyuria in obstructive uropathy: Report of a case of "water-losing nephritis" in an infant with a discussion of polyuria. *New Eng. J. Med.* 255: 660, 1956.
27. Edvall, C. A. Influence of ureteral obstruction (hydronephrosis) on renal function in man. *J. Appl. Physiol.* 14:855, 1959.
28. Eiseman, B., Vivion, C., and Vivian, J. Fluid and electrolyte changes following the relief of urinary obstruction. *J. Urol.* 74: 222, 1955.
29. Ericsson, N. O., Winberg, J., and Zetterstrom, R. Renal function in infantile obstructive uropathy. *Acta Paediat.* 44:444, 1955.
30. Franklin, S., and Merrill, J. P. The kidney in health; the nephron in disease. *Amer. J. Med.* 28:1, 1960.
31. Gleason, D. M., Bottaccini, M. R., Perling, D., and Lattimer, J. K. A challenge to current urodynamic thought. *J. Urol.* 97: 935, 1967.
32. Gottschalk, C. W. Micropuncture studies of tubular function in the mammalian kidney. *Physiologist* 4:35, 1960.
33. Gottschalk, C. W., and Mylle, M. Micropuncture study of pressures in proximal tubules and peritubular capillaries of the rat kidney and their relation to ureteral and renal venous pressures. *Amer. J. Physiol.* 185:430, 1956.
34. Graham, J. B., King, L. R., Kropp, K. A., and Vehling, D. T. The significance of distal urethral narrowing in young girls. *J. Urol.* 97:1045, 1967.
35. Graham, J. R., Suby, H. I., LeCompte, P. R., and Sadowsky, N. L. Fibrotic disorders associated with methysergicide therapy for headache. *New Eng. J. Med.* 274: 359, 1966.
36. Guze, L. R., and Beeson, P. B. Experimental pyelonephritis: I. Effect of ureteral ligation on the course of bacterial infection in the kidney of the rat. *J. Exp. Med.* 104: 803, 1956.
37. Guze, L. R., and Beeson, P. B. Experimental pyelonephritis: II. Effect of partial ureteral obstruction on the course of the bacterial infection in the kidney of the rat and the rabbit. *Yale J. Biol. Med.* 30:315, 1958.
38. Hellstrom, H. R., and Perez-Stable, E. C. Retroperitoneal fibrosis with disseminated vasculitis and intrahepatic sclerosing cholangiitis. *Amer. J. Med.* 40:184, 1966.
39. Hepler, A. B. Intrarenal changes in hydronephrosis. *J. Urol.* 38:593, 1937.
40. Hershman, H. A. New method of determining bladder residual urine volume. *J. Urol.* 83:283, 1960.
41. Hinman, F. Hydronephrosis: I. The structural changes. *Surgery* 17:816, 1945.
42. Hinman, F. *Principles and Practice of Urology*. Philadelphia: Saunders, 1955.
43. Hinman, F., and Hepler, A. B. Experimental hydronephrosis: The effect of changes in blood pressure and in blood flow on its rate of development. Partial obstruction of renal artery. *Arch. Surg.* 11:649, 1925.
44. Hinman, F., and Lee-Brown, R. K. Pyelovenous backflow; its relation to pelvic reabsorption, to hydronephrosis and to accidents of pyelography. *J.A.M.A.* 82:607, 1924.
45. Hinman, F., and Morison, D. M. Comparative study of circulatory changes in hydronephrosis, caseo-cavernous tuberculosis, and polycystic kidney. A preliminary report. *J. Urol.* 11:131, 1924.
46. Hinman, F., and Vecki, M. Pyelovenous back flow: The fate of phenolsulphonepthalein in a normal renal pelvis with the ureter tied. *J. Urol.* 15:267, 1926.
47. Hoyt, H. S. Equilibrium in hydronephrosis. *Stanford M. Bull.* 12:71, 1954.
48. Idbohrn, H., and Muren, A. Renal blood

flow in experimental hydronephrosis. *Acta Physiol. Scand.* 38:200, 1957.

49. Jaenike, J. R., and Bray, G. A. Effects of acute transitory urinary obstruction in the dog. *Amer. J. Physiol.* 199:1219, 1960.
50. Jaworski, Z. F., and Wolan, C. T. Hydronephrosis and polycythemia. *Amer. J. Med.* 34:523, 1963.
51. Kass, E. H. Bacteriuria and the diagnosis of infections of the urinary tract, with observations on the use of methionine as urinary antiseptic. *A.M.A. Arch. Intern. Med.* 100:709, 1957.
52. Keith, N. M. Experimental hydronephrosis. *Arch. Intern. Med.* 20:853, 1917.
53. Kerr, W. S., Jr. Effect of complete ureteral obstruction for one week on kidney function. *J. Appl. Physiol.* 6:762, 1953–1954.
54. Kerr, W. S., Jr. Effects of complete ureteral obstruction in dogs on kidney function. *Amer. J. Physiol.* 184:521, 1956.
55. Kissane, J. M., and Heptinstall, R. H. Experimental hydronephrosis; morphologic and enzymatic studies of renal tubules in ureteric obstruction and recovery in the rat: I. Alkaline and acid phosphatases. *Lab. Invest.* 13:539, 1964.
56. Kissane, J. M., and Heptinstall, R. H. Experimental hydronephrosis; morphologic and enzymatic studies of renal tubules in ureteral obstruction and recovery in the rat: II. Pentose phosphate pathway. *Lab. Invest.* 13:547, 1964.
57. Knowlan, D., Corrado, M., Schreiner, G. E., and Baker, R. Periureteral fibrosis, with a diabetes insipidus-like syndrome occurring with progressive partial obstruction of a ureter unilaterally. *Amer. J. Med.* 28:22, 1960.
58. Kuru, M. Nervous control of micturition. *Physiol. Rev.* 45:425, 1965.
59. Lawson, J. D., and Tomlinson, W. B. Observation on the dynamics of acute urinary retention in the dog. *J. Urol.* 66:678, 1951.
60. Legrain, M., Bitker, M., and Küss, R. Obstructive Nephropathy in Adults. *Proceedings of Third International Congress of Nephrology,* Vol. 2, page 336. Karger: Basel, New York, 1967.
61. Lepper, M. H. The production of coliform infection of the urinary tract of rabbits. *J. Path. Bact.* 24:192, 1921.
62. Leuzinger, D. E., Lattimer, J. K., and McCoy, C. B. Reflux is dangerous but not always disastrous: Conservative therapy often effective. *J. Urol.* 82:294, 1959.
63. Levinsky, N. G., and Berliner, R. W. Changes in composition of the urine in ureter and bladder at low urine flow. *Amer. J. Physiol.* 196:549, 1959.
64. Levy, S. E., Mason, M. F., Harrison, T. R., and Blalock, A. The effects of ureteral occlusion on the blood flow and oxygen consumption of the kidneys of unanesthetized dogs. *Surgery* 1:238, 1937.
65. Lich, R., Jr. The obstructed ureteropelvic junction. *Radiology* 68:337, 1957.
66. Lubowitz, H., Slatopolsky, E., Shankel, S., Rieselbach, R. E., and Bricker, N. S. Glomerular filtration rate: Determination in patients with chronic renal disease. *J.A.M.A.* 199:252, 1967.
67. Luton, E. F., and Dietrich, F. S. Postobstructive saluresis. *J. Urol.* 98:402, 1967.
68. Magoun, J. A. H., Jr. Absorption from the urinary tract. *J. Urol.* 10:67, 1923.
69. Maher, J. F., Schreiner, G. E., and Water, T. J. Osmotic diuresis due to retained urea after release of obstructive nephropathy. *New Eng. J. Med.* 268:1099, 1963.
70. Malvin, R. L., Sullivan, L. P., and Wilde, W. S. Stop-flow analysis of renal tubule localization. *Physiologist* 1:1, 1957.
71. Minton, J. P., Kiser, W. S., and Ketcham, A. S. A study of the functional dynamics of ileal conduit urinary diversion with relationship to urinary infection. *Surg. Gynec. Obstet.* 119:541, 1964.
72. Morgan, A. D., Loughridge, L., and Calne, R. Y. Combined mediastinal and retroperitoneal fibrosis. *Lancet* 1:67, 1966.
73. Muldowney, F. P., Duffy, G. J., Kelly, D. G., Duff, F. A., Harrington, C., and Freaney, R. Sodium diuresis after relief of obstructive nephropathy. *New Eng. J. Med.* 274:1294, 1966.
74. Mulrow, P. J., Huvos, A., and Buchanan, D. L. Measurement of residual urine with I^{131}-labeled Diodrast. *J. Lab. Clin. Med.* 57:109, 1961.

75. Myint, M. K., and Murphy, J. J. The renal lymphatics: I. The effects of diuresis and acute ureteral obstruction upon the rate of flow and composition of thoracic duct lymph. *Surg. Forum* 7:656, 1957.
76. Narath, P. A. The Physiology of the Renal Pelvis and the Ureter. In Campbell, M. (Ed.), *Urology,* Vol. I. Philadelphia: Saunders, 1954.
77. Olbrick, O., Woodford-Williams, E., Irvine, R. E., and Webster, D. Renal function in prostatism. *Lancet* 1:1322, 1957.
78. Ostling, K. Genesis of hydronephrosis, particularly with regard to changes at ureteropelvic juncture. *Acta Chir. Scand.* 86 (Suppl. 72):10, 1942.
79. Parkhurst, E. C. Experience with more than 500 ileal conduit diversions in a 12-year period. *J. Urol.* 99:434, 1968.
80. Parsons, F. M. Chemical imbalance occurring in chronic prostatic obstruction: A preliminary survey. *Brit. J. Urol.* 26:7, 1954.
81. Persky, L., Benson, J. W., Levey, S., and Abbott, W. E. Metabolic alterations in surgical patients: X. The benign course of the average patient with acute urinary retention. *Surgery* 42:290, 1957.
82. Persky, L., Bonte, F. J., and Austen, G., Jr. Mechanisms of hydronephrosis: Radioautographic backflow patterns. *J. Urol.* 75: 190, 1956.
83. Prather, G. C. Hydronephrosis. *New Eng. J. Med.* 250:944, 1954.
84. Rector, F. C., Jr., Brunner, F. P., and Seldin, D. W. Mechanism of glomerular balance: I. Effect of aortic constriction and elevated ureteropelvic pressure on glomerular filtration rate, fractional reabsorption, transit time, and tubular size in the proximal tubule of the rat. *J. Clin. Invest.* 45: 590, 1966.
85. Risholm, L., and Obrink, K. J. Pyelorenal backflow in man. *Acta Chir. Scand.* 115: 144, 1958.
86. Scott, J. E. S., Clayton, C. B., Dee, P. M., and Simpson, W. A. Study of the hemodynamics of the female urethra. Parts I and II. *J. Urol.* 96:763 and 770, 1966.
87. Selkurt, E. E., Brandfonbrener, M., and Geller, H. M. Effects of ureteral pressure increase on renal hemodynamics and the handling of electrolytes and water. *Amer. J. Physiol.* 170:61, 1952.
88. Share, L. Effect of increased ureteral pressure on renal function. *Amer. J. Physiol.* 168:97, 1952.
89. Silk, M. R. Hypertension secondary to hydronephrosis in adult and young animals. *Invest. Urol.* 5:30, 1967.
90. Sirota, J. H., and Narrins, L. Acute urinary suppression after ureteral catheterization: The pathogenesis of "reflex anuria." *New Eng. J. Med.* 257:1111, 1957.
91. Sleator, W., Jr., and Butcher, H. R., Jr. Action potentials and pressure changes in ureteral peristaltic waves. *Amer. J. Physiol.* 180:261, 1955.
92. Smith, H. W. *The Kidney. Structure and Function in Health and Disease.* New York: Oxford University Press, 1951.
93. Straffon, R. A., and Engel, W. J. The diagnosis and treatment of urinary tract obstruction in children. *J.A.M.A.* 174:1377, 1960.
94. Strong, K. C. Plastic studies in abnormal renal architecture: V. The parenchymal alterations in experimental hydronephrosis. *Arch. Path.* 29:77, 1940.
95. Sturtz, G. S., and Burke, E. C. Obstructive water-losing uropathy. *J.A.M.A.* 166: 45, 1958.
96. Suki, W., Eknoyan, G., Rector, F. C., Jr., and Seldin, D. W. Patterns of nephron perfusion in acute and chronic hydronephrosis. *J. Clin. Invest.* 45:122, 1966.
97. Sunshine, H., Cordonnier, J. J., and Butcher, H. Bilateral pyeloileostomy. *J. Urol.* 92:358, 1964.
98. Swenson, O., MacMahon, H. E., Jaques, W. E., and Campbell, J. S. New concept of etiology of megaloureters. *New Eng. J. Med.* 246:41, 1952.
99. Szasz, J. J. G., and Whyte, H. M. Effect of distension of the bladder and of contraction of the sphincters on blood pressure. *Brit. Med. J.* 2:208, 1967.

100. Talbot, H. S. Role of ureter in pathogenesis of ascending pyelonephritis. *J.A.M.A.* 168:1595, 1958.
101. Williams, D. I. Chronically dilated ureter. *Ann. Roy. Coll. Surg. Eng.* 14:107, 1954.
102. Williams, R. D., and Fanestil, D. D. Na + K-ATPase deficit in hydronephrotic rats. *Clin. Res.* 15:437, 1967.
103. Wilmer, H. Disappearance of phosphatase from the hydronephrotic kidney. *J. Exp. Med.* 78:225, 1943.
104. Wilmer, H. Static intrapelvic pressure of hydronephrotic kidney. *Proc. Soc. Exp. Biol. Med.* 56:52, 1944.
105. Wilson, B., Riseman, D. D., and Moyer, C. A. Fluid balance in the urological patient: Disturbances in the renal regulation of the excretion of water and sodium salts following decompression of the urinary bladder. *J. Urol.* 66:805, 1951.
106. Witte, M. H., Short, F. A., and Hollander, W., Jr. Massive polyuria and natriuresis following relief of urinary tract obstruction. *Amer. J. Med.* 37:320, 1964.
107. Zetterstrom, R., Ericcson, N. O., and Winberg, J. Separate renal function studies in predominantly unilateral hydronephrosis. *Acta Paediat.* 47:540, 1958.

28

Atheroembolic Renal Disease

Jerome P. Kassirer

A clinical picture of either acute or chronic renal failure may occur when atheromatous material, dislodged from a severely atherosclerotic aorta, obstructs small renal arteries. Only a limited number of patients with atheroembolic renal disease and renal failure have been described, but it seems likely that the disorder will be met with greater frequency in the future. This view is based on the observations that an increasing number of elderly patients with severe atherosclerosis of the aorta enlarges the population at risk, and that procedures known to induce atheroembolism such as abdominal aortic surgery and abdominal aortography are being accepted as routine practices in many hospitals. Patients with extensive atheroembolism of the kidney often have, in addition to renal failure, a variety of clinical manifestations including hypertension, gastrointestinal bleeding, pancreatitis, and ischemic extremities. The renal involvement, however, appears to be the major factor limiting their prognostic outlook.

Pathology

Consideration of the changes induced by atheroembolism in the kidney is critical to understanding the clinical manifestations. The essential lesion of atheroembolic renal disease is extensive occlusion of the lumina of small renal arteries by atheromatous material. Initially the lumina of involved vessels contain cholesterol crystals and amorphous debris; later foreign body giant cells appear, and finally concentric fibrosis dominates. The lesions are frequently found at bifurcations of arteries; they are usually focal accumulations, but occasionally they extend throughout a major vessel and its branches [31]. Arcuate, intralobular, and terminal arteries are most frequently affected [8, 13, 30, 31], and involvement is most notable in vessels 150 to 200 microns in diameter [31]. Occlusion of vessels of this size can account in full for the changes in the renal parenchyma, described in detail in a later section.

MORPHOLOGY OF CHOLESTEROL CRYSTALS

Microemboli of atheromatous material are readily identified by the characteristic appearance of the cholesterol crystal inclusions which appear in a biconvex needle-shaped form (Figs. 28-1, 28-2). In routine paraffin-embedded histologic sections, the cholesterol is not seen because the methods used in preparing sections dissolve the crystals [6, 11];

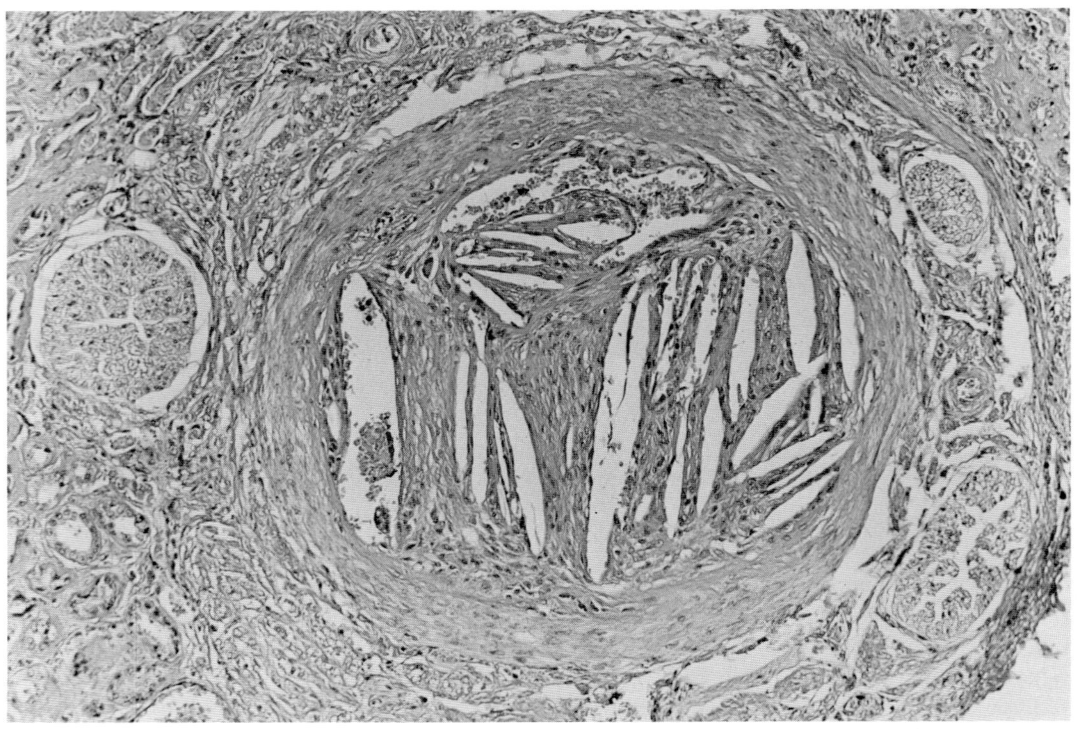

Figure 28-1. A branch of the renal artery, 500 microns in diameter, at the corticomedullary junction is mostly occluded by needle-shaped clefts containing embolized cholesterol crystals and other atheromatous debris. There is fibrous organization and marginal recanalization. Small nerves are shown in the periarterial fibrous tissue. The specimen was taken from a patient with atheroembolic renal disease and severe renal failure [18]. Hematoxylin and eosin. ×200, before 16% reduction.

nevertheless, the characteristic biconvex cleft in the lumen persists, thus permitting easy identification. The crystals can also be recognized by their birefringence when sections of frozen fresh tissue or wet formalin-fixed tissue are examined under polarized light [3, 7, 13, 27, 30]. Definitive identification of cholesterol crystals can be accomplished on frozen sections by a histochemical method for detecting sterols (the Schultz modification of the Liebermann-Burchardt reaction [13, 30, 32]. The crystals* are sometimes found singly in a vessel but are more often in clusters which, along with amorphous eosinophilic material, entirely occlude the lumen. There is no characteristic orientation of the crystals to the wall of the lumen, though crystals tend to lie parallel to one another in a given cluster [31] (Fig. 28-2). On occasion, the sharp crystals have been observed to pierce the intima of an artery and, less often, to penetrate the entire wall of the vessel [12, 28]. Although the crystals almost invariably involve the small intrarenal arteries, they have rarely been found in afferent arterioles or glomeruli [9, 28].

* For convenience, the clefts remaining after dissolution of cholesterol during tissue processing will be considered to represent actual crystals.

EVOLUTION OF THE ARTERIAL LESIONS

Observations in patients with atheroembolism and in animals with experimental atheroembolism provide a clear picture of the

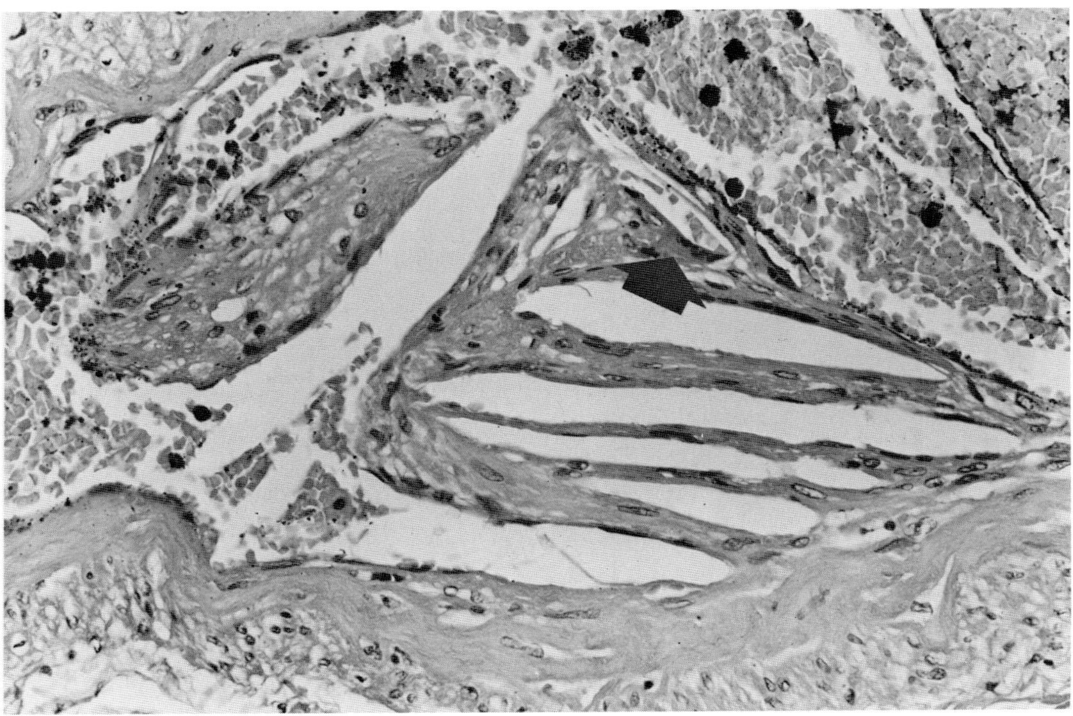

Figure 28-2. Foreign body giant cell (*arrow*) surrounds the cholesterol crystal clefts that are impacted in the renal arterial lumina. From the same specimen shown in Figure 28-1. Hematoxylin and eosin. ×500, before 16% reduction.

evolving vascular lesions. In patients the earliest lesion consists of crystals surrounded by eosinophilic material; the endothelial cells have not yet reacted to the presence of the foreign body [30, 31]. In older lesions, connective tissue is seen surrounding the embolic debris, the intima is thickened, and macrophages and multinucleated foreign body giant cells (Fig. 28-2) appear in the lumen [8, 11, 13, 31]. In the lesions generally considered to be the "latest" manifestations of atheroembolism the intima is markedly thickened by concentric fibrosis, and this dense collagenous tissue with its crystalline inclusions entirely occupies the lumen except for small areas of recanalization [13, 31] (Fig. 28-1). Although the foreign body leads to a striking tissue reaction in the intima, overt necrosis and acute inflammatory reaction in the arterial wall are not seen; arteriolitis has been reported in atheroembolism involving the heart [32] and skeletal muscle [1], but has not been observed in the kidney.

The sequential changes in the lesions in *experimental atheroembolism* in animals closely mimic those of atheroembolic disease in man. One to two days after injection of pure cholesterol crystals or atheromatous material, the predominant findings in the lumen* include needle-shaped crystals surrounded by leukocytes; the wall of the artery appears unaffected [8, 10, 22, 29]. In three to five days macrophages and multinucleated

* It should be noted that the lung has been evaluated in virtually all of the animal experiments; the kidney has not yet been studied.

foreign body giant cells appear regularly in the lesions, and the number of leukocytes is reduced [10, 22, 29]. Seven to ten days after injection, endothelial overgrowth has become prominent, and at that time the crystals, giant cells, and marked intimal fibrosis entirely occlude the lumen [8, 10, 29]. Beyond this time few changes take place, although increasing fibrosis has sometimes been observed [10, 22, 29].

The long-term fate of the crystalline material has not been settled. In two studies the crystals have become less prominent, possibly because some have been extruded through the wall of the affected vessel [10, 22]. An apparent reduction in the quantity of crystals in the kidney vessels has also been seen in man, but this observation has been made in only one patient and requires confirmation [14].

RENAL PARENCHYMAL CHANGES IN ATHEROEMBOLISM

Multiple occlusions of small arteries lead to patchy ischemic degeneration of the kidney. Spotty atrophy of the parenchyma is the most striking and most frequent finding; even in the presence of extensive embolism atrophy predominates over acute infarctions [8, 9, 12, 13, 31]. Atrophy is often confined to wedge-shaped incompletely or completely infarcted zones separated by relatively unaffected tissue [8, 12, 13, 26, 31], and in the affected area all structures appear to be involved to the same extent. Glomeruli and tubules are ischemic and atrophic, and the glomeruli are partly hyalinized [8, 12, 13, 26, 31]. Careful sectioning of the involved areas often demonstrates an occluded artery at the apex of the involved wedge of tissue [12]. The findings on gross examination of the kidneys reflect these parenchymal changes, but atheromatous embolism is rarely diagnosed from the gross examination alone because other renal diseases produce a similar appearance [28]. The kidneys are usually reduced in size [11, 12, 27, 31] and have a rough granular surface, corresponding to the wedge-shaped scars; irregular narrowing of the cortex can be appreciated when the kidneys are cut [8, 11–13, 18, 21, 25, 27, 31]. Acute infarcts are occasionally seen grossly [3a, 18]. Although these changes are not specific, a diagnosis of atheroembolic renal disease should be suspected when wedge-shaped scars and acute infarcts are accompanied by severe atheromatous disease of the abdominal aorta.

Pathogenesis

THE AORTA IN ATHEROEMBOLIC DISEASE

It is apparent from the appearance of the abdominal aorta in patients with atheroembolic renal disease that little or no trauma is required to dislodge embolic material. Typically the internal lining of the aorta is irregularly ulcerated and extensively covered by masses of shaggy red thrombi that are soft, mushy, and easily brushed off [3a, 8, 11, 13, 14, 18, 21, 26, 27, 31, 32]. In many areas the intima is eroded, and ruptured soft yellow atheromas communicate with the aortic lumen [8, 13, 14, 18, 32]. Closer examination of the thickened, distorted intima reveals amorphous eosinophilic material containing cholesterol crystals, findings identical to those in the renal arteries [6, 8, 25, 27]. The thrombi, loosely attached to the ulcerated intima, also contain this material. In patients with severe erosive disease of the aorta, the frequency of atheroembolic renal disease is approximately 15 to 30 per cent [8, 28, 30]; by contrast, in patients with atherosclerosis but with only slight to moderate erosions peripheral embolism has only a 1 per cent frequency [8].

INCITING FACTORS

In many patients with atheroembolic renal disease, no antecedent history of trauma has been elicited, and although minor disturbances such as coughing have occasionally been implicated, this relationship is only circumstantial. Approximately 20 patients with *"spontaneous"* atheroembolism and azotemia have been reported; two had fallen and sustained fractured hips prior to their hospitalization [12, 18], but the remainder had no history of trauma. On the other hand, atheroembolism to the kidneys commonly occurs as a result of operative trauma during *aortic surgery* for aneurysm or severe occlusive atherosclerosis. In one report the frequency of emboli in the kidneys of patients dying after surgery for severe atherosclerosis of the aorta was 77 per cent [30]. It should be noted, of course, that although atheroembolism is frequent in such patients, serious renal complications occur in only a minority. In one series, for example, approximately one-fifth of patients with atheroembolic involvement of the kidneys following aortic surgery developed acute renal failure. Many of these patients had undergone elective surgery, became oliguric or anuric postoperatively without having experienced a hypotensive episode, and died in uremia a few days after surgery [30]. Recently, several patients with fatal atheroembolic renal disease have been described in whom the trauma of *renal arteriography* seems to have been responsible for dislodging embolic material [3a, 14]. It has been suggested that the relatively stiff catheters utilized during selective arteriography, and the high pressure generated near the tip of the catheters during forced injection [19] may be important factors in the rupture of soft plaques [14]. The role of *anticoagulants* in initiating renal atheroembolism is unsettled. The observation [21] that many patients with ischemia of the lower extremities secondary to atheroembolism had received anticoagulants has suggested the possibility that prevention of thrombus formation over ulcerated aortic plaques might favor release of cholesterol-laden material. Data on the frequency of atheroembolic renal disease in patients treated with anticoagulants are not available.

GENESIS OF THE VASCULAR LESIONS

Although there is little uncertainty about the embolic origin of the arterial lesions (and in the above discussion this pathogenesis has been assumed), notice should be given to the thought that an intrarenal local accumulation of atheromatous material could explain the findings instead. From clinical observations alone, the embolic origin is on firm grounds. Thus, the finding of extensive lesions in the small renal arteries of patients with acute renal failure after aortic surgery is most readily explained on the basis of acute atheroembolism; local deposition of the material in arteries could not be expected to develop acutely, and furthermore it seems unlikely that the widespread arterial lesions could have antedated surgery without inducing a marked disturbance in renal function in the preoperative period. Aside from the observation that local atheroma formation is extremely rare in arteries as small as those usually involved in atheroembolic renal disease [7], other convincing arguments favor embolism. These include the identity of the crystalline material in the wall of the aorta and the renal arteries [6, 8, 25, 27], and as described above, the striking correlation between the severity of the atheromatous lesions of the abdominal aorta and the frequency of crystalline material in peripheral arteries [8, 30]. These many observations coupled with the close resemblance of the lesions seen in patients and those in laboratory animals [8, 10, 22, 29] leave little doubt that the crysalline lesions described in detail above are embolic in origin.

Clinical Features

RENAL FAILURE

Extensive obstruction of small renal arteries by atheromatous material induces a marked impairment of renal function. As mentioned earlier, the massive acute atheroembolism typically seen after aortic surgery usually leads to oliguria or anuria, and in these patients uremia has often been the cause of death [3, 15, 30]. The influence of repeated dialysis on the outcome of such patients has not yet been reported; in the longest survivor reported on, no diuresis was observed as long as three weeks after the onset of acute renal failure. A clinical picture of acute renal failure has been occasionally reported in patients with "spontaneous" atheroembolic renal disease [18, 24], but this pattern is the exception. More often, such patients are found to be azotemic when they first come under observation, and in many of these, progressive renal failure ensues without a concomitant decrease in urine volume.

In the great majority of reported patients with spontaneous atheroembolism and azotemia, uremia was an important contributory factor to the patient's death, and in most of these patients death occurred within two weeks of the time that azotemia was first discovered [12, 13, 18, 24, 27, 31, 32]. On the other hand, a small number of patients with spontaneous atheroembolism and atheroembolism following arteriography have survived for several months [1, 3, 14, 26]. In most patients with spontaneous atheroembolic renal disease it has not been possible to determine the duration of renal failure because most were already azotemic when they first came under observation and the exact onset of embolism could not be dated. However, the initiation of embolism is reasonably well defined in patients with atheroembolism following arteriography, and in these patients a clinical picture of progressive chronic renal failure has culminated in a fatal outcome one to four months after renal function began to deteriorate [3a, 14]. None of the reported patients with atheroembolic renal disease and advanced renal insufficiency has recovered, and none has regained normal renal function even transiently. However, the occasional finding of fluctuant azotemia [1, 12] — in one patient over a nine-month period [1] — raises the possibility that the disorder may not be uniformly fatal. Repeated dialysis of biopsy-proved cases may ultimately determine whether there is any significant degree of reversibility.

HYPERTENSION

At the present time, most of the data regarding hypertension are available in patients with spontaneous atheroembolism, and in these individuals it is often not clear whether the blood pressure elevation — which frequently antedated the development of renal failure — changed in severity following atheroembolism. Most patients with spontaneous atheroembolism and renal failure are hypertensive; many have had diastolic blood pressures of 120 mm. Hg or higher [3, 12, 13, 18, 20, 24–26], and a few patients have had severe diastolic hypertension with blurred disc margins or papilledema [12, 21, 24]. In a small number of patients with atheroembolic renal disease with previously normal or slightly elevated blood pressures, a substantial rise in blood pressure was associated with the onset of renal atheroembolism [24, 25]. The course of one such patient is of particular interest. In this patient, hypertension was alleviated after removal of a nonfunctioning kidney which on examination showed extensive atheroembolism and widespread parenchymal atrophy. Two years later hypertension recurred, accompanied by progressive azotemia, when atheroembolism involved the remaining kidney [9].

It seems likely that renal atheroembolism itself can lead to hypertension, or at least that it can induce an acceleration of existing hypertension. If nothing more, the location of the obstructing emboli in the renal arterial tree proximal to the juxtaglomerular apparatus suggests that activation of the renin-angiotensin mechanism may be responsible for the blood pressure elevation. Although no direct evidence is yet available to support this view (i.e., no measurements of plasma enzyme activity or histologic descriptions of the juxtaglomerular apparatus), the frequent finding of wedge-shaped atrophic areas in the kidney, without overt infarction, and the scattered clinical observations described above favor the view that the hypertension in patients with renal atheroembolism may occasionally be a "renovascular" type. On the other hand, certain aspects such as the persistence of a normal blood pressure in some patients with atheroembolic renal disease [11, 26] have yet to be explained.

RELATED CLINICAL FINDINGS

Acute pancreatitis and gastrointestinal bleeding secondary to atheroembolism in the vessels of the pancreas and gastrointestinal tract have often been recognized clinically in patients with atheroembolic renal disease [1, 3, 3a, 12, 14, 21, 24, 32] but have only infrequently been correctly diagnosed during the patient's life. Involvement of small blood vessels of the lower extremities may result in livedo reticularis [3, 14, 15, 20, 25, 26, 27], painful muscle nodules [3, 15], or to overt gangrene [1, 3, 24, 26, 31]. Although frequently other organs such as the spleen, prostate, and adrenal glands and less often the thyroid, liver, and testes are found on postmortem examination to be involved by atheroembolism, no clinical manifestations have yet been attributed to such involvement. The findings in patients with atheroembolism to the retinal vessels are discussed below.

Diagnosis

The great majority of patients with atheroembolic renal disease have been over the age of 60 years, and, in fact, none has been younger than 50. Atheroembolism should be considered in any elderly patient with unexplained renal failure, especially when the patient is known to have an abdominal aortic aneurysm or a history of some complication of atherosclerosis; all but a few of the patients with spontaneous atheroembolism were known to have had coronary heart disease, a stroke, or ischemia of the lower extremities. Other complications of atheroembolism such as acute pancreatitis, gastrointestinal bleeding, or retinal embolism should also raise the level of suspicion. Embolism of atheromatous material in the retinal vessels is readily recognizable clinically. The patient may complain of sudden monocular blindness, but more often there are no visual symptoms. On funduscopic examination single or multiple bright yellow crystalline plaques, often lodged at bifurcations of retinal arterioles, are easily seen [3a, 5, 16, 23]. In some instances it is possible to observe their downstream movement or even their disappearance from the retinal vessels when external pressure is applied to the eye [16].

No characteristic urinary abnormalities have been found in patients with atheroembolic renal disease. Patients with spontaneous atheroembolism usually have at most a slight increase in red blood cells and a modest increase in white blood cells in the urinary sediment [3a, 11, 12, 14, 18, 21]. Occasional hyaline and granular casts have also been reported [3a, 12, 14, 18, 21, 27, 32]. Proteinuria has rarely been quantified, but qualitative tests usually show a 1 + to 3 + reaction [1, 3, 3a, 12, 14, 18, 21, 25, 32]. There are no reports of urinalyses in patients with the postoperative variety of acute renal failure secondary to atheroembolism. When patients with acute renal failure following surgery for aortic aneurysm are found to have a large number of narrow hyaline and granular casts and renal tubular cells in the urinary sediment, the renal disease is usually considered potentially reversible, but the possibility should not be overlooked that acute atheroembolism could lead to the same urinary findings.

Except when multiple complications of atheroembolism are present concurrently, a diagnosis of atheroembolic renal disease can be made only by examination of excised tissue. Renal biopsy offers a definitive means of establishing the diagnosis and has been carried out in a limited number of patients [14, 24]. It should be emphasized that renal insufficiency should not be ascribed to atheroembolism unless the involvement of the arterial tree is extensive; some patients with potentially reversible acute tubular necrosis have been found to have a few emboli in their kidneys as an incidental finding. A needle biopsy may not provide a specimen large enough to allow an adequate assessment of the extent of arterial involvement, and therefore open biopsy is to be preferred; careful observation of all arteries in the specimen is, of course, mandatory.

In a number of instances a tentative diagnosis of polyarteritis or vasculitis has been made in patients with widespread atheroembolism because of the diverse nature of the organ involvement in association with hypertension and renal failure [1, 25]. The absence of fever, neuropathy, pulmonary lesions, or joint findings in patients with atheroembolism should be helpful in distinguishing between these disorders. In some of these patients the correct diagnosis will be established when changes of atheroembolism, rather than vasculitis, are found in a muscle biopsy [1–3, 15] or amputated toes [17]. Probably of most help in differential diagnosis is an examination of the urinary sediment; hematuria and red blood cell casts are rare among patients with atheroembolism but are found regularly among patients with an acute glomerulitis secondary to an inflammatory disease of small blood vessels. A diagnosis of subacute bacterial endocarditis might also occasionally be entertained in these patients, but ordinarily there should be little difficulty in distinguishing this disorder from atheroembolism.

Prevention and Treatment

It appears that certain types of atheroembolic renal disease can be prevented. Thus, recent experience with a large number of patients subjected to aortic surgery for atherosclerosis [4] suggests that the frequency of acute renal failure secondary to atheroembolism is far lower than that described from the same group in an earlier report [30]. This reduction can probably be attributed to the introduction of certain surgical technics (outlined below) aimed at minimizing the likelihood of atheroembolism at the time of arterial repair [4]. During the operative removal of a severely atherosclerotic aorta, an attempt is made to apply occluding clamps well below the renal arteries. If it becomes necessary, however, to apply such clamps near the origin of the renal arteries and if the aorta in this region is severely arteriosclerotic, the renal arteries are gently freed up and clamped while atheromatous debris is flushed out of the opened aorta [4]. It may also be possible to prevent the renal involvement following aortography by reducing to a minimum the manipulations during the procedure, particularly with the rigid catheters used in selective arterial visualization [14]. Unfortunately there is currently no regularly effective means of preventing atherosclerosis and avoiding spontaneous atheromatous embolism.

At the present time no therapeutic measure has improved renal function. Patients have been given adrenal steroids [25], low-molecular-weight dextran [14], anticoagulants [14, 25], intraarterial vasodilators [25], and have also been subjected to sympathetic blocks [14], all without effect. Hypertension should, of course, be controlled medically; a resistance to antihypertensive therapy has been described [13], but experience is too limited to determine if this finding is typical. Repeated dialysis has not been utilized, but it is uncertain whether renal function would spontaneously improve in time, since, as mentioned above, some patients who have survived for as long as several months have failed to show significant improvement.

References

1. Anderson, W. R. Necrotizing angiitis associated with embolization of cholesterol: Case report, with emphasis on the use of the muscle biopsy as a diagnostic aid. *Amer. J. Clin. Path.* 43:65, 1965.
2. Anderson, W. R., and Richards, A. M. Evaluation of lower extremity muscle biopsies in the diagnosis of atheroembolism. *Arch. Path.* (Chicago) 86:535, 1968.
3. Carvajal, J. A., Anderson, W. R., Weiss, L., Grismer, J., and Berman, R. Atheroembolism: An etiologic factor in renal insufficiency, gastrointestinal hemorrhages, and peripheral vascular diseases. *Arch. Intern. Med.* (Chicago) 119:593, 1967.

3a. Case records of the Massachusetts General Hospital (Case 25-1967). *New Eng. J. Med.* 276:1368, 1967.

4. Darling, R. C. Personal communication.
5. David, N. J., Klintworth, G. K., Friedberg, S. J., and Dillon, M. Fatal atheromatous cerebral embolism associated with bright plaques in the retinal arterioles: Report of a case. *Neurology* 13:708, 1963.
6. Eliot, R. S., Kanjuh, V. I., and Edwards, J. E. Atheromatous embolism. *Circulation* 30:611, 1964.
7. Fisher, E. R., Hellstrom, H. R., and Myers, J. D. Disseminated atheromatous emboli. *Amer. J. Med.* 29:176, 1960.
8. Flory, C. M. Arterial occlusions produced by emboli from eroded aortic atheromatous plaques. *Amer. J. Path.* 21:549, 1945.
9. Gore, I., and Collins, D. P. Spontaneous atheromatous embolization: Review of the literature and a report of 16 additional cases. *Amer. J. Clin. Path.* 33:416, 1960.
10. Gore, I., McCombs, H. L., and Lindquist, R. L. Observations on the fate of cholesterol emboli. *J. Atheroscler. Res.* 4:527, 1964.
11. Goulet, Y., and MacKay, C. G. Atheromatous embolism: An entity with a polymorphous symptomatology. *Canad. Med. Ass. J.* 88:1067, 1963.
12. Greendyke, R. M., and Akamatsu, Y. Atheromatous embolism as a cause of renal failure. *J. Urol.* 83:231, 1960.
13. Handler, F. P. Clinical and pathologic significance of atheromatous embolization, with emphasis on an etiology of renal hypertension. *Amer. J. Med.* 20:366, 1956.
14. Harrington, J. T., Sommers, S. C., and Kassirer, J. P. Atheromatous emboli with progressive renal failure: Renal arteriography as the probable inciting factor. *Ann. Intern. Med.* 68:152, 1968.
15. Haygood, T. A., Fessel, W. J., and Strange, D. A. Atheromatous microembolism stimulating polymyositis. *J.A.M.A.* 203:135, 1968.
16. Hollenhorst, R. W. Significance of bright plaques in the retinal arterioles. *J.A.M.A.* 178:123, 1961.
17. Hoye, S. J., Teitelbaum, S., Gore, I., and Warren, R. Atheromatous embolization: A factor in peripheral gangrene. *New Eng. J. Med.* 261:128, 1959.
18. Kaplan, K., Millar, J. D., and Cancilla, P. A. "Spontaneous" atheroembolic renal failure. *Arch. Intern. Med.* (Chicago) 110:218, 1962.
19. Lim, T. P. K., and Cadwallader, J. A., III. Delivery pressure at the catheter tip in selective angiocardiography. *J.A.M.A.* 199:69, 1967.
20. Maurizi, C. P., Barker, A. E., and Trueheart, R. E. Atheromatous emboli. *Arch. Path.* (Chicago) 86:528, 1968.
21. Moldveen-Geronimus, M., and Merriam, J. C., Jr. Cholesterol embolization: From pathological curiosity to clinical entity. *Circulation* 35:946, 1967.
22. Otken, L. B., Jr. Experimental production of atheromatous embolization. *A.M.A. Arch. Path.* 68:685, 1959.
23. Pribram, H. F. W., and Couves, C. M. Retinal embolism as a complication of angiography: The possible role of platelet and cholesterol emboli. *Neurology* 15:188, 1965.
24. Retan, J. W., and Miller, R. E. Microembolic complications of atherosclerosis. *Arch. Intern. Med.* (Chicago) 118:534, 1966.
25. Richards, A. M., Eliot, R. S., Kanjuh, V. I., Bloemendaal, R. D., and Edwards, J. E. Cholesterol embolism: A multiple-system disease masquerading as polyarteritis nodosa. *Amer. J. Cardiol.* 15:696, 1965.
26. Roujeau, J., Albahary, C., Guillaume, J., and

Galian, A. Embolies atheromateuses diffuses avec insuffisance renale. *Sem. Hop. Paris* 41:1161, 1965.

27. Sayre, G. P., and Campbell, D. C. Multiple peripheral emboli in atherosclerosis of the aorta. *A.M.A. Arch. Intern. Med.* 103:799, 1959.
28. Schnornagel, H. E. Emboli of cholesterol crystals. *J. Path. Bact.* 81:119, 1961.
29. Snyder, H. E., and Shapiro, J. L. A correlative study of atheromatous embolism in human beings and experimental animals. *Surgery* 49:195, 1961.
30. Thurlbeck, W. M., and Castleman, B. Atheromatous emboli to the kidneys after aortic surgery. *New Eng. J. Med.* 257:442, 1957.
31. Uys, C. J., and Watson, C. E. The effects of atheromatous embolization on small arteries and arterioles. *S. Afr. Med. J.* 37:69, 1963.
32. Zak, F. G., and Elias, K. Embolization with material from atheromata. *Amer. J. Med. Sci.* 218:510, 1949.

29

Effects of Irradiation on the Kidney

Reginald William Luxton

Radiation nephritis may result when the kidneys are included within therapeutic fields of deep x-rays. Other sources of ionizing radiations, such as atomic explosion [44], radioactive isotopes, and diagnostic x-rays, have not produced clinical nephritis in human beings, although renal changes have been described in animals after whole-body irradiation [1, 3, 21], intravenous radiophosphorus [47], and nuclear detonation [45].

In 1952 Kunkler et al. [24] showed that when the whole of both kidneys is irradiated to a dose exceeding 2300 R (in five weeks or less) there is real danger of clinical nephritis. Before this fact was generally appreciated, radiation nephritis arose in relation to four main radiotherapeutic procedures:

1. Routine abdominal irradiation, therapeutic or prophylactic, after unilateral orchidectomy for seminoma testis. This highly malignant tumor produces metastases in the abdominal lymph nodes, not readily detected clinically, which are extremely sensitive to x-irradiation. Statistics show a considerable improvement in the five-year survival rate (as regards the malignant tumor) when abdominal irradiation is added to orchidectomy [6]. Radiation nephritis ceased to be a problem in this condition when the importance of protecting the kidneys from exposure to this radiation therapy was appreciated and renal screening became routine.

2. Treatment of ovarian carcinoma, in which condition seedling metastases may be implanted on the peritoneum [11, 50]. (This procedure has now become one of the most frequent sources of x-ray injury to the kidney.)

3. Irradiation of malignant masses in or near the kidneys [13].

4. Irradiation of the lower thoracic and lumbar spine for lesions such as osteogenic sarcoma or metastatic carcinoma [12, 27]. I know of no authoritative report on radiation nephritis resulting from the x-ray treatment of ankylosing spondylitis; indeed, the association is unlikely, since the x-ray dose is low and the spinal strip commonly irradiated is

narrow. The nephropathy associated with ankylosing spondylitis is commonly due to amyloid disease.

Clinical Types of Radiation Nephritis

Although previously placed in four categories (Luxton [27]) for the purpose of clinical description, cases of radiation nephritis are now classified into five main groups: acute radiation nephritis, chronic radiation nephritis, asymptomatic proteinuria, benign essential hypertension, and late malignant hypertension. Generalized edema with serous effusions may occur in severe acute radiation nephritis, but there is no clear evidence that a chronic nephrotic syndrome results from renal irradiation in man.

As will be seen later, individual cases may pass through several clinical phases, presenting initially in one group and evolving into another. The clinical features of the five groups will now be considered.

ACUTE RADIATION NEPHRITIS

Symptoms of renal involvement do not appear until several months after the commencement of radiotherapy. In adults the limits of this latent period are 6 to 13 months (average, 8½ months), but in children the latent period may be shorter [11, 40, 43, 51]. Clinical examination of the patient during the prodromal phase, however, may reveal evidence of renal damage long before symptoms are first encountered, the most frequent signs being proteinuria, increase in blood pressure, anemia, and cardiac enlargement (best detected in chest x-ray films). Although the development of symptoms is gradual, most patients are incapacitated within one month after their onset. There is no preceding sore throat. The commonest early symptoms are edema and dyspnea on exertion, but hypertensive headache or nocturia may be the first complaint. In brief, the main symptoms are dyspnea, headache, nocturia, nausea and vomiting, drenching sweats, and lassitude; and the main signs are edema, hypertension, abnormalities in the urine, anemia, retinitis, and cardiac enlargement. The syndromes of left ventricular failure, hypertensive encephalopathy, congestive heart failure, and chronic uremia may develop singly or together.

Edema. Edema is not invariably a feature of acute radiation nephritis, although it is found in the majority of patients. The edema may be confined to the legs, but is more generalized in the more severe cases, in which it may be associated with pleural and peritoneal effusions. Edema of the face is seen occasionally.

Hypertension and Malignant Hypertension. Hypertension is always present at some stage but varies in degree and duration from case to case. In most patients the systolic pressure is 170 mm. Hg or more at the first clinical examination, the diastolic pressure being raised in proportion. In a few patients, however, the blood pressure may not be raised until several weeks after the first indications of renal damage. Usually the blood pressure reaches its highest level within six months of the first symptom. In half the patients who survive the acute phase of the disease the blood pressure returns to near-normal levels within two years of the onset of symptoms.

Malignant hypertension may be a striking feature of acute radiation nephritis and may resolve spontaneously within a few months, as is illustrated in the following case:

A man aged 32 years was submitted to abdominal radiotherapy following unilateral orchidectomy for seminoma testis. Commencing in May, 1948, 3250 R was administered in 32 days. There was no preceding proteinuria. In January, 1949, he complained of headache and dyspnea; cardiac enlargement was found on chest x-ray, and anemia was present (hemoglobin of 44 per cent). In March, 1949, headache, nausea, vomiting, blurring of vision, and lassitude were so severe that he was first considered to have cerebral metastases. The observation of hypertension (blood pressure of 205/125 mm. Hg), heavy proteinuria, and bilateral papilledema with retinal hemorrhages and exudates established the correct diagnosis of malignant hypertension and raised the question of x-ray damage to the kidneys. Renal failure was present, the blood urea being 85 mg. per 100 ml. and the urea clearance 25 per cent of normal. There was no edema, oliguria, or hematuria. In May, 1949, the retinitis became severe enough to cause transient blindness, and the blood pressure was 210/140 mm. Hg. A month later, however, clinical improvement was sufficient to permit discharge from hospital after a stay of 4 months. No specific treatment had been given for hypertension, but complete rest was enforced and anemia treated by blood transfusions.

In September, 1949, the blood pressure had fallen to 195/125 mm. Hg, the blood urea was 36 mg. per 100 ml., the hemoglobin was 62 per cent, and both retinas showed clear-cut nodular exudates. In February, 1950, the patient was well enough to return to work, his blood pressure being 180/115 mm. Hg. By January, 1951, the blood pressure had fallen to 170/110 mm. Hg and the blood urea to 25 mg. per 100 ml.; the hemoglobin had increased to 76 per cent. A year later the blood pressure was 150/100 mm. Hg, the urea clearance 61 per cent of normal, and the hemoglobin 76 per cent. Over the next 8 years this man was examined at intervals of 1 to 3 months; during this period he remained well and active, with normal blood pressure and blood count but with the blood urea ranging between 35 and 75 mg. per 100 ml. In 1959 the blood pressure was 120/80 mm. Hg, and the urea clearance was 76 per cent of normal. Proteinuria has persisted throughout, but at times has been barely detectable by the usual clinical tests. In 1968 the patient is living a normal life. He has a moderate degree of chronic renal failure, with proteinuria, a serum urea of 81 mg. per 100 ml., and a blood pressure 160/100 mm. Hg. Since 1963 he has had three attacks of acute gout in the feet, the serum uric acid ranging between 8 and 11 mg. per 100 ml.

Anemia. A severe normochromic, normocytic anemia occurs, refractory to all forms of therapy except blood transfusion. The leukocyte count, coagulation time, bleeding time, serum bilirubin, and reticulocyte counts are normal, but thrombocytopenia and purpura may arise in the later stages. The sternal bone marrow is active, as is marrow taken from vertebrae within the field of irradiation. Although the anemia is regarded as being due to the concomitant renal failure, there may be some additional and unknown factor at work, for the anemia is usually more severe than the associated rise in blood urea would warrant [33, 36]. It is possible that x-irradiation of the kidney interferes with the production of renal erythropoietin.

Urinary Changes. Proteinuria is always marked, varying between 0.5 and 4.0 gm. per liter. Some patients show no serious limitation of urinary concentration, but in most the urinary specific gravity is less than 1.012. Macroscopic hematuria does not occur; microscopy may reveal a few red blood corpuscles along with epithelial, hyaline, or granular casts.

Renal Function Tests. Impairment of renal function is variable, about one-third of patients having a urea clearance below 25 per cent of normal when first examined. With clinical recovery the test shows corresponding improvement.

Blood Urea. A moderate increase in the blood urea is usual, being over 80 mg. per 100 ml. in two-thirds of patients when first seen. As the phase of acute nephritis subsides, the blood urea tends to fall but may be sharply elevated for a time by intercurrent infection or after blood transfusion.

Clinical Course and Prognosis. The immediate prognosis depends largely on whether or not the syndrome of malignant hypertension arises during acute radiation nephritis. Of the 22 patients in my personal care, nine had malignant hypertension; of these nine six died within 3 to 12 months and one (treated with modern hypotensive drugs) died five years later of uremia. The remaining 2 patients recovered spontaneously from the malignant phase of hypertension, but one of the two died 6 years later with chronic renal failure. The fatal cases showed combinations of the syndromes of hypertensive encephalopathy, left ventricular failure, congestive heart failure, and uremia.

In patients who have survived acute radiation nephritis, improvement has usually begun within six months after the first symptom. As early prognostic signs, generalized edema and serous effusions are ominous, and a blood urea figure over 100 mg. per 100 ml. during the first three months after the onset of symptoms is a serious though not necessarily fatal portent. The blood pressure alone is not a good guide, but increasing hypertension, progressive anemia, and a rising blood urea form a dangerous combination. Retinitis is a disturbing sign, being largely an effect of hypertension and anemia. Factors of little prognostic value are the latent period before the onset of symptoms, the age of the patient, the blood pressure in the early stages, and renal function tests during the first five months.

An assessment of the ultimate prognosis in acute radiation nephritis is now possible [28]. Of my 22 patients 12 have died from the effects of renal irradiation. Of these, six died from malignant hypertension within 12 months of the commencement of symptoms, and five died of chronic uremia 5 to 12 years after radiotherapy. One died of a hypertensive cerebrovascular lesion after four years. Of the patients who have not died from the effects of renal irradiation, one has died of recurrent ovarian malignant neoplasm. Nine patients are alive at an average interval of 16 years after radiotherapy; all are at work but most have now some degree of chronic renal failure and hypertension. Proteinuria has persisted in all cases, though sometimes in very small quantity: it is the only evidence of renal injury in four patients. Worthy of note is the long period during which some patients have lived active lives despite chronic renal failure, a feature seen in chronic pyelonephritis but not common in chronic glomerulonephritis; for four years the blood urea level of three patients remained between 100 and 200 mg. per 100 ml.

Treatment. In one sense acute radiation nephritis is a self-limiting disease and every effort must be made to help the patient through the few months which constitute its natural course. The patient's interest in food is limited by nausea and malaise; in general, the diet should be light and easily digestible and should avoid an excess of protein. Symptomatic treatment is useful for edema, pulmonary edema, and cardiac complications. Modern hypotensive drugs may be life-saving in the phase of malignant hypertension and have proved valuable in preventing this dreaded complication. Hemodialysis or peritoneal dialysis are to be considered. Stress must be laid on two factors in treatment: rest in bed and blood transfusion. Lessening of dyspnea, edema, and headache, with some reduction in blood pressure and retinal improvement, may result from bed rest alone, which may be required continuously for many weeks. The anemia is refractory to intravenous iron, vitamin B_{12}, folic acid, proteolyzed liver, intramuscular liver extract, vitamins A, B, C, and D, and ACTH. Blood transfusion seems to be the only way to sustain the patient's hemoglobin level and thereby reduce his liability to congestive heart failure. Cross matching and administration of blood need particular care, for reactions to transfusion are readily evoked and may be severe when several transfusions are needed over a relatively short period.

CHRONIC RADIATION NEPHRITIS

Chronic radiation nephritis originates in two ways.

1. *Primary chronic radiation nephritis.* Routine examination of patients who have been subjected to x-irradiation involving the

whole of both kidneys to a dose above 2300 R but who may have had no symptoms of nephritis, acute or chronic, frequently reveals the readily discovered signs of chronic nephritis.

2. *Secondary chronic radiation nephritis.* In patients surviving acute radiation nephritis the kidneys remain permanently damaged; in this sense the chronic radiation nephritis is secondary or consecutive.

The syndrome of chronic radiation nephritis comprises proteinuria, anemia, hyposthenuria, and impairment of renal function revealed by standard tests. In a given patient the blood urea may be at times normal, at other times moderately increased. Granular, epithelial, and hyaline casts may be found in the urine. It is noteworthy that only about half the patients with secondary chronic radiation nephritis have hypertension, usually of moderate degree.

The distinction between primary and secondary chronic radiation nephritis relates to their mode of development. In a review of patients up to 1960 the impression was gained that secondary radiation nephritis offered a somewhat better prognosis than the primary type. More prolonged clinical observation has not confirmed this view, for duration of survival shows little difference in the two groups. Of 13 patients with primary chronic radiation nephritis seven have died in an average period of 10 years after radiotherapy, and six are alive and reasonably well at an average of 16 years after their renal irradiation.

Treatment. In a disorder with so protracted a course the patient's general health must be maintained at a high level. His way of life should be reviewed and appropriate advice offered on occupation, general activities, rest, and recreations. Prompt treatment of intercurrent infections is essential. As previously mentioned, a moderate but slowly increasing azotemia may persist for several years during which the patient can live in a reasonably normal way. His main problem arises from anemia which causes fatigue and may predispose to effort angina. Blood transfusions at intervals of several months usually help such patients and should be considered when the hemoglobin falls below 8.5 gm. per 100 ml. A modified Giovannetti [41] diet helps to control the azotemia, and there is naturally scope for renal dialysis procedures in the later stages. A renal transplant operation has not yet been recorded in radiation nephritis. Gout is a not infrequent complication of chronic radiation nephritis and responds well to standard treatments. It should be remembered that certain drugs used in treatment of hypertension may predispose to gout.

ASYMPTOMATIC PROTEINURIA

Twelve patients with asymptomatic proteinuria have now been under clinical observation for from 12 to 26 years (average period, 17 years) after radiotherapy. The degree of proteinuria has at times been slight and in seven patients intermittent. For many years standard renal function tests were normal, but these patients seemed to have an impaired renal reserve, indicated by occasional elevation of the blood urea level for no obvious reason and by a liability to temporary renal failure after relatively minor stress such as the systemic disturbance associated with an abdominal operation. Of the 12 patients eight have remained well, two have died of coronary disease 14 years after renal irradiation, and two, though clinically well, give evidence of minor renal impairment (mild hypertension and serum urea levels over 60 mg. per 100 ml.) 14 and 15 years, respectively, after radiotherapy. It is of interest that one such patient shows definite reduction in renal size in tomograms taken 15 years after irradiation.

Some individuals are more susceptible to irradiation than others, just as are some tumors. It appears that renal irradiation within the "therapeutic" range may provoke nephritis or may produce permanent renal injury without overt nephritis. The ultimate prognosis is therefore to be assessed only in terms of decades.

BENIGN ESSENTIAL HYPERTENSION

After renal irradiation, a few patients show the clinical picture of benign essential hypertension, the main findings being hypertension and a variable degree of proteinuria. In these cases symptomless hypertension seems to develop within 6 to 12 months after the start of radiotherapy. This clinical syndrome of essential hypertension may persist for several years without obvious deterioration, but patients may succumb to cardiovascular complications, or malignant hypertension may supervene.

LATE MALIGNANT HYPERTENSION

Apart from the frequent occurrence in acute radiation nephritis of malignant hypertension (which might then be termed *early malignant hypertension*), this complication has been seen at a later stage in three circumstances:

1. Well beyond the known latent period of acute radiation nephritis, malignant hypertension may arise and prove fatal within a few weeks. Two such cases have been observed in which the intervals between radiotherapy and the first evidence of renal injury were 18 months and 46 months, respectively. In both cases the kidneys were of normal size.

2. Patients with known chronic radiation nephritis or with the syndrome of benign hypertension have developed malignant hypertension after a period of years. Renal contraction, if present, has involved the kidneys equally. In the clinical management of such patients, hypotensive drugs have been valuable.

3. After one kidney has been given an unusually high dose of x-rays (because of its proximity to neoplastic tissue receiving radiotherapy or its malposition in the x-ray field), malignant hypertension has been observed years later and has been cured or relieved by removal of the sclerosed kidney. This group of cases is particularly important from the therapeutic standpoint and requires more detailed consideration.

In 1944 Dean and Abels [13] described a girl aged 20 who received 4600 R in 25 days, directed to the left renal area because of a local tumor thought to be a lymphosarcoma, the blood pressure and urine being then normal. Six and one-half years later the blood pressure was 150/100 mm. Hg and within 6 months rose to 184/125 mm. Hg. The total renal function was within the normal range and, in the belief that the rapidly rising blood pressure was due to a radiation lesion of one kidney, a study of the separate function of each kidney was made. This indicated a gross defect in the irradiated kidney. After nephrectomy the blood pressure fell promptly to normal and remained normal. The upper half of the excised kidney was normal, but the lower third was grossly sclerosed and showed extreme obliterative arteritis.

In 1956 Levitt and Oram [26] recorded the relief of malignant hypertension by left nephrectomy in a man who had been given radiotherapy for seminoma metastases in the upper abdomen and who developed malignant hypertension 11 years later. They estimated that the left renal area received 3000 R, the right 2000 R. After divided renal function studies, the left kidney was removed; it weighed 84 gm.

The following is an abbreviated account of a somewhat similar case.

A man aged 50 years was given 3000 R in 34 days to the abdomen after unilateral orchidectomy for seminoma testis. Forty-six months after radiotherapy malignant hypertension developed (blood pressure 260/130 mm. Hg, gross retinitis, and bilateral papilledema). During the investigation hy-

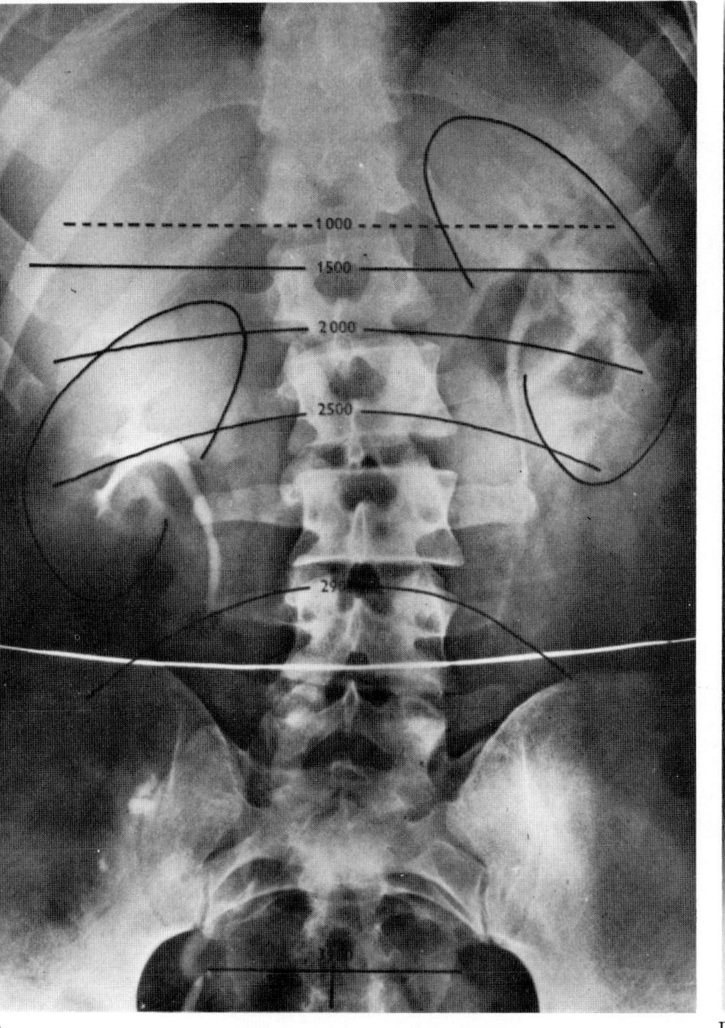

A

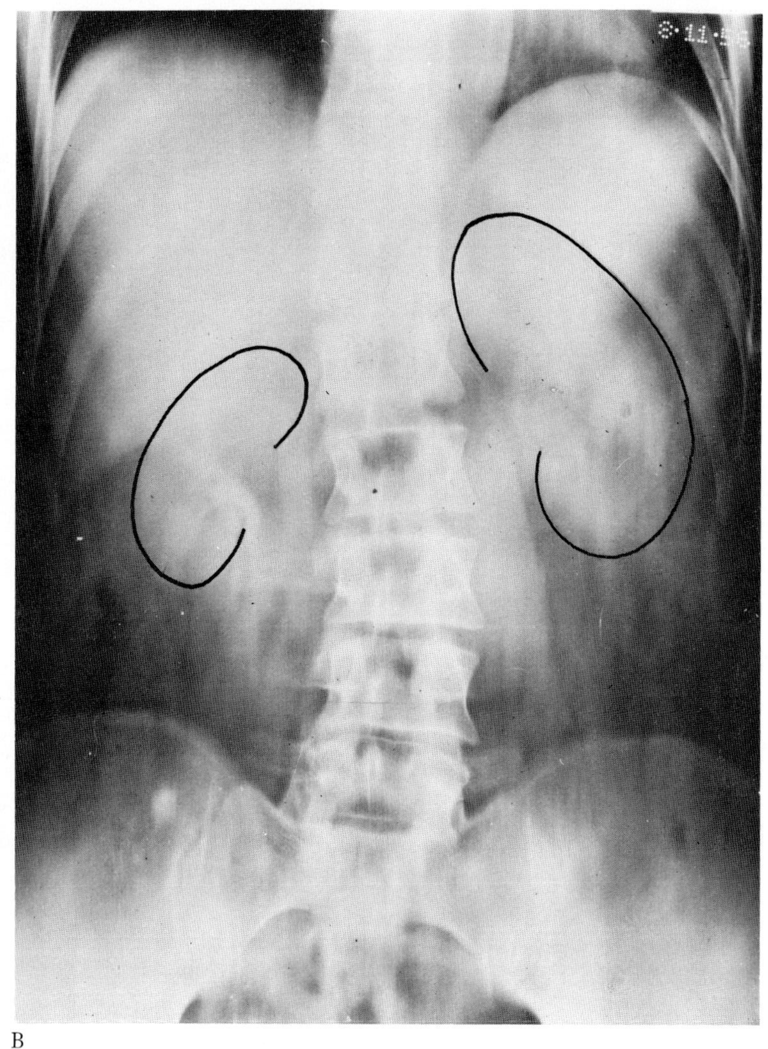

B

Figure 29-1. Late malignant hypertension. A. Intravenous pyelogram before radiotherapy. Blood pressure and urine normal. Right kidney low in position. Note the dosage isobars which explain why the upper half of the left kidney escaped serious radiation injury. B. Tomogram and intravenous pyelogram of same patient, 4 years after radiotherapy, showing contraction of the right kidney. Malignant hypertension now present.

potensive drugs were used for 3 months with benefit. Tomographic technics combined with intravenous pyelography showed a considerable relative reduction in size of the right kidney compared with the left, and an absolute reduction when compared with a pyelogram made prior to radiotherapy, at which time it was noted that the right kidney was abnormally low in position (Fig. 29-1A, B). At laparotomy (Mr. J. Tasker) the right kidney, obviously small and fibrosed, was excised, and a biopsy of the lower pole of the left kidney was taken. The right kidney (Fig. 29-2A, B) weighed 80 gm. and showed the histologic picture typical of chronic radiation nephritis without, however, histologic evidence of malignant hypertension (Fig. 29-3A). The biopsy specimen of the left kidney (Fig. 29-3B) was histologically indistinguishable from that of the right. (This patient's survival depends on the upper part of the left kidney, which received a smaller dose of x-rays.) No hypotensive drugs have been given since nephrectomy. One month after operation the blood pressure was 185/125 mm. Hg, 6 months after operation 170/110 mm. Hg, and 10 months after operation 150/95 mm. Hg. Five years after operation, the patient had no symptoms and required no treatment; the blood pressure was 160/85 mm. Hg, the serum was 45 mg. per 100 ml., and proteinuria persisted.

Unilateral nephrectomy may be of great benefit in hypertension resulting from radiation damage to one kidney, and as Levitt [25] remarks, "It is important that the possibility of unilateral damage should be considered in every case of radiation malignant hypertension with a view to possible surgical treatment." It is evident that in many patients with radiation malignant hypertension both kidneys are implicated, and careful assessment of the size and function of the kidneys separately is essential. When serious doubt

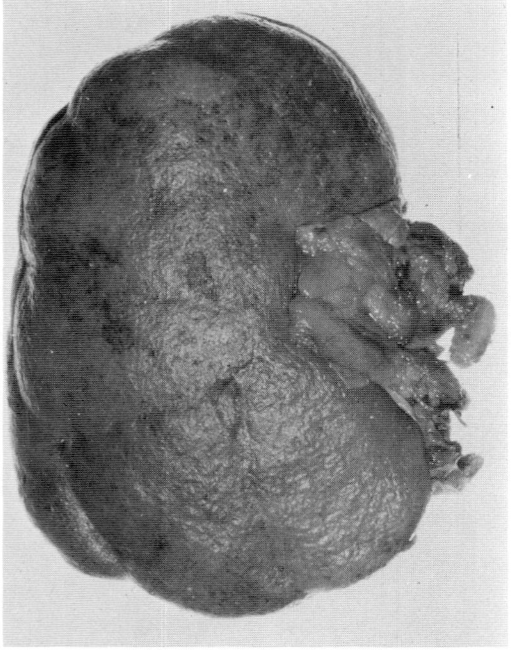

A

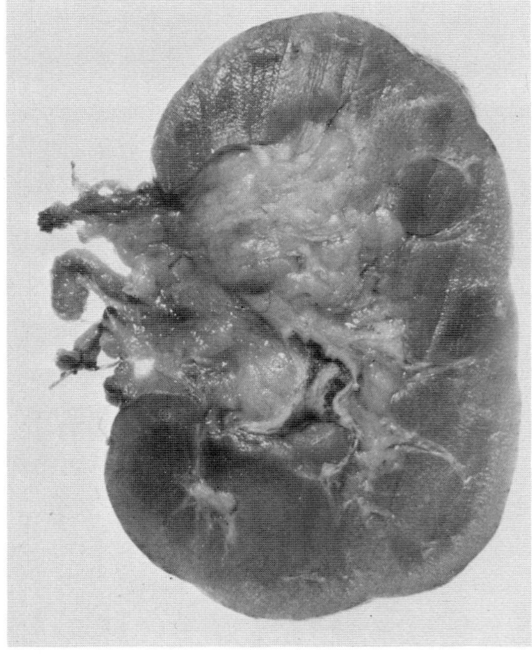

B

Figure 29-2. Late malignant hypertension. A. The excised kidney, which weighed 80 gm., had pale, mainly smooth surface with a few linear scars. B. Cut surface showing thin cortex well demarcated from the medulla.

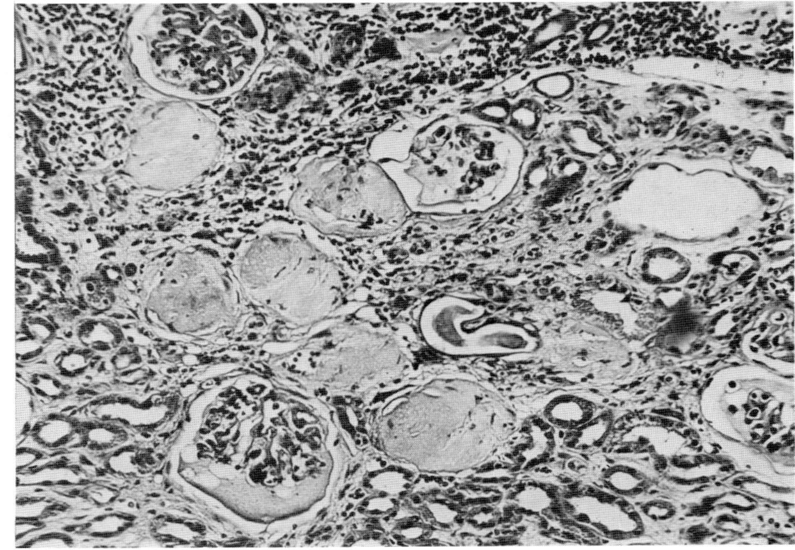

A

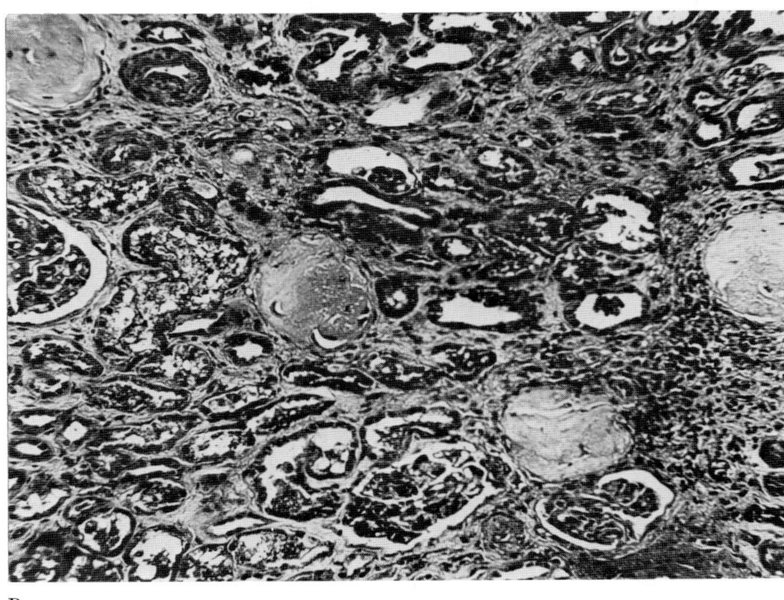

B

Figure 29-3. Late malignant hypertension. A. The excised right kidney. Many glomeruli are completely hyalinized, others show contraction or distortion. The tubules are small and there is diffuse intertubular fibrosis. Hyalinization of the media is pronounced in some intralobular arteries. Hematoxylin and eosin. ×160. B. Biopsy of the lower pole of the left kidney — the histologic picture is very similar to that of the excised kidney. Hematoxylin and eosin. ×160.

about nephrectomy arises, hypotensive drugs may be useful either until the doubt is resolved or permanently. That difficulties could arise in deciding the best line of treatment is illustrated by brief reports on cases in which one kidney was slightly smaller than the other but both organs showed severe radiation damage.

In 1950 a 44-year-old man presented with malignant hypertension and renal failure. Two years previously he had been given 3000 R in 25 days to the abdomen after unilateral orchidectomy for seminoma. At autopsy the right kidney weighed 125 gm., the left kidney 170 gm. Histologically both kidneys showed severe hypertensive nephrosclerosis, more marked in the right kidney.

Kincaid-Smith et al. [23] have referred to a man given abdominal radiotherapy for seminoma testis, whose blood pressure before treatment was 120/75 mm. Hg. Six years after radiotherapy the patient was uremic and had bilateral papilledema. At autopsy one kidney weighed 167 gm., the other 134 gm., and histologically both showed malignant nephrosclerosis. Interstitial fibrosis was more marked in the smaller kidney.

Pathology

There is considerable literature on the pathology of renal irradiation lesions produced experimentally in animals, but few observations in humans have been recorded. The latter fall into two main groups — those in children who have been given abdominal irradiation combined with nephrectomy in treatment of a Wilms's tumor [11, 15, 19, 43, 51], and those in adults treated either prophylactically for seminoma of the testis or for known malignant lesions near the kidney [12, 13, 25].

In children the histologic changes of acute radiation nephritis have been considered in detail by Zuelzer et al. [51], confirming and expanding the observations of Domagk (1927) [15], who was probably the first to describe fatal renal lesions in humans caused by exposure to x-rays. Dr. Helen Russell [39], former consultant pathologist at the Christie Hospital and Holt Radium Institute, Manchester, England, has described the macroscopic and microscopic features in five adults who died of acute radiation nephritis between 5 and 16 months after irradiation; similar descriptions of isolated cases are given by others [40, 49].

In acute radiation nephritis the kidneys are of normal size and weight (Fig. 29-4); in

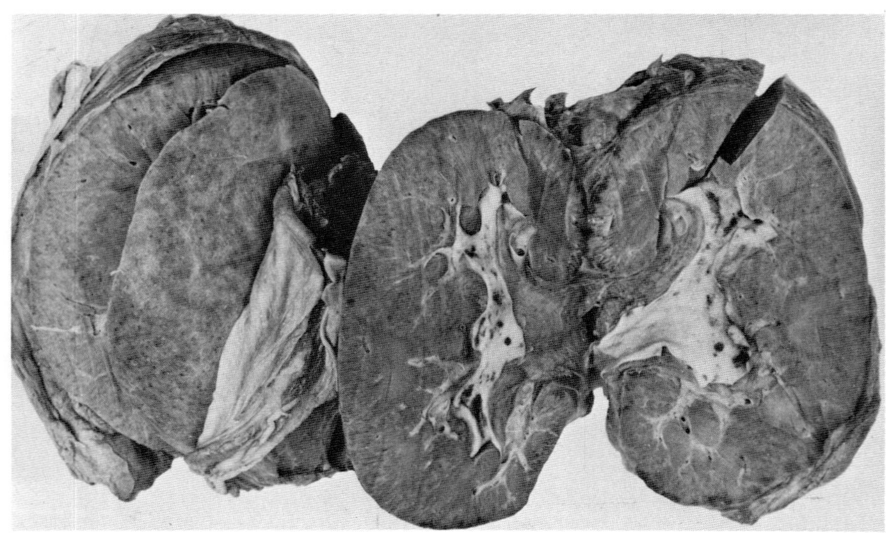

Figure 29-4. Acute radiation nephritis. The kidneys are of normal size and weight. The renal capsule is somewhat thickened, and subcapsular petechiae are visible. (Reproduced by courtesy of the *Scottish Medical Journal.*)

children treated for Wilms's tumor by nephrectomy and radiotherapy, however, the remaining kidney may be somewhat enlarged. In some cases there is a layer of moderately dense fibrous tissue separating kidneys and suprarenals from peritoneum — a perirenal fibrosis. (In no case were the kidneys obviously compressed by fibrous tissue, and the hypertension is not produced by the fibrous perinephritis described by Page [32].) The renal pelves, ureters, and bladder are normal. The kidney capsule may or may not be thickened and adherent. Subcapsular petechiae may be scattered on the renal surface. The cut surface has no characteristic feature, but engorged glomeruli are sometimes visible and the normal cortical architecture may be obliterated. The main histologic findings in adults, as described by Russell [39] and by others [40, 49], comprise thickening of the renal capsule (Fig. 29-5), widespread glomerular damage (in the form of hyaline obliteration of capillary loops, necrosis of fibrinoid or of hemorrhagic type with, in places, proliferation of capsular epithelium and early capsular fibrosis), extensive tubular degeneration and atrophy (Fig. 29-6), diffuse intertubular fibrosis, and fibrinoid necrosis of arterioles (Fig. 29-7) and interlobular arteries. In children the histologic changes are essentially similar; for a careful description thereof, the paper by Zuelzer et al. [51] should be consulted. Apart from renal changes there are commonly serous effusions in peritoneum, pleura, and pericardium, and the heart is much enlarged.

This description applies to the fully developed picture seen at autopsy in patients dying of the renal lesion, but the histologic changes of earlier stages have also been described. In a man who died of pulmonary embolism five weeks after the start of abdominal radiotherapy, Russell [39] records that the kidney showed "some degree of interstitial edema and general capillary dilatation tending to separate the capillaries and tubules from one another, and also dilatation of the glomerular

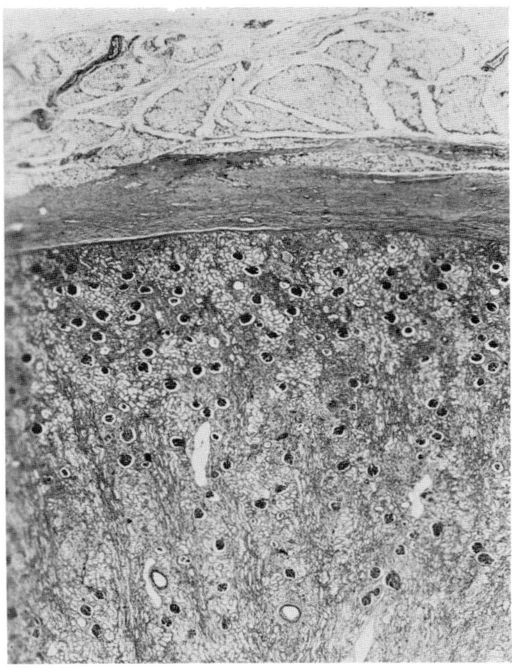

Figure 29-5. Acute radiation nephritis. Kidney cortex. ×10. Perirenal fibrous tissue. (Reproduced by courtesy of the *British Journal of Radiology.*)

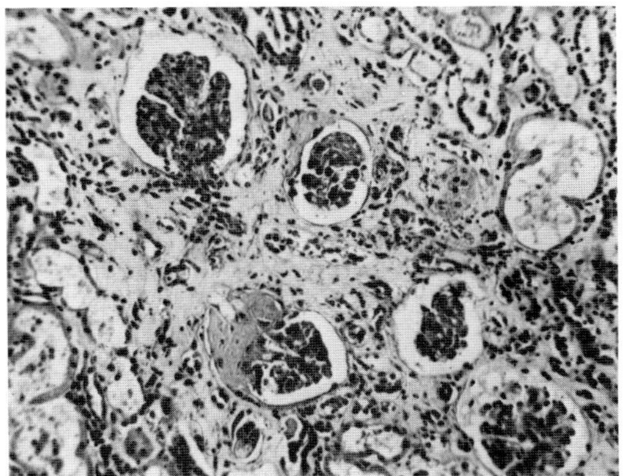

Figure 29-6. Acute radiation nephritis. The glomeruli show varying degrees of hyalinization and ischemic collapse. Fibrosis of the interstitial tissue is pronounced and tubules are grossly atrophic. Hematoxylin and eosin. ×116, before 32% reduction. (Reproduced by courtesy of the *British Journal of Radiology.*)

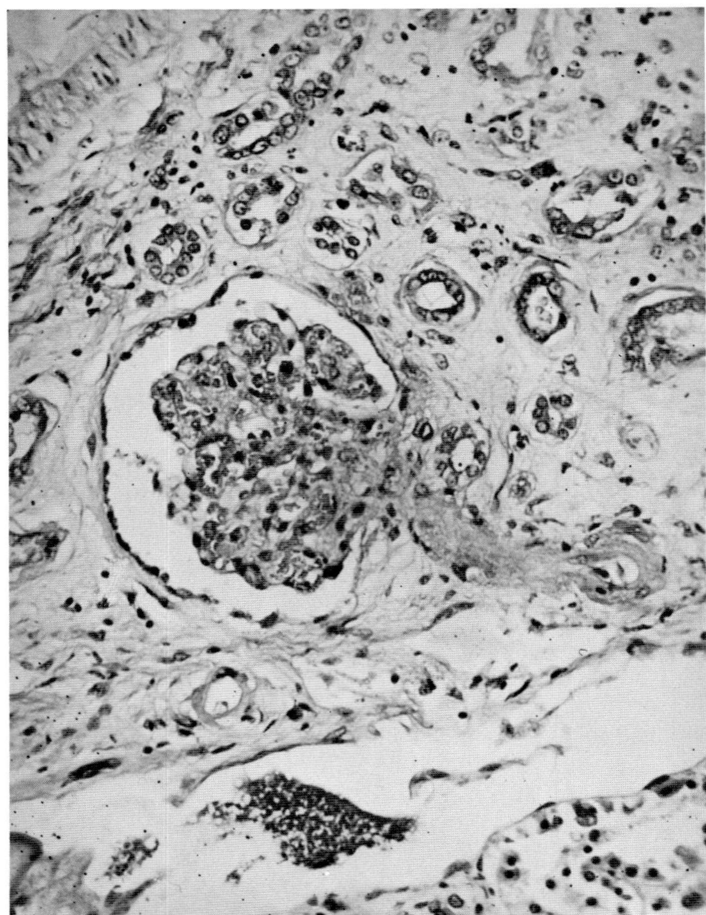

Figure 29-7. Acute radiation nephritis. Fibrinoid necrosis of an afferent arteriole is well shown. The glomerulus shows ischemic collapse. Intertubular fibrosis is pronounced and the tubules are atrophied. Hematoxylin and eosin. ×116. (Reproduced by courtesy of the *British Journal of Radiology*.)

vessels and widening of the whole glomerular structure." Cogan et al. [11] record the renal histology (obtained by percutaneous renal biopsy) in a 49-year-old woman 14 weeks after the start of radiotherapy, and also in a child of 14 months whose kidney was removed surgically 16 weeks after the start of radiotherapy. The abnormalities seen were "mainly in the glomerulus with thickening of tufts, degenerative cellular changes and a few areas of inter-tubular fibrosis." They suggest that the glomerulus is the primarily affected portion of the kidney and that tubular atrophy is secondary, and they agree with Zuelzer et al. [51] that these findings differ from those of glomerulonephritis in the lack of inflammatory cellular infiltrate, glomerular adhesions, and epithelial proliferation. It should be added that the initial site of x-ray injury in the kidney is debatable. Some authors [5, 7, 8, 15, 48] have regarded the tubules as more sensitive than the glomeruli. The view now firmly held by other authors [11, 29, 35, 49] is that the arterial structures of the kidney, including the glomeruli, are the elements most sensitive to x-irradiation, a view supported by electron microscopy [37]. X-ray injury to small- and medium-sized arteries such as were described by Sheehan [42] may influence the clinical course of radiation nephritis, a view supported by Rubenstone and Fitch [38].

In certain patients who have survived acute radiation nephritis a process aptly described by Dr. Helen Russell as "the shrinking kidney" may be found (Figs. 29-8, 29-9). Figure 29-10 illustrates the shriveled organs in a man aged 40 who died of chronic uremia eight years after renal irradiation. Each kidney weighed 45 gm. They were densely sclerosed and granular: histologically there was advanced interstitial fibrosis with loss of parenchyma. Surviving glomeruli appeared hypertrophic, and although some afferent arterioles were hyalinized, arteriolar necrosis within the tufts was not seen. Very few tubules appeared healthy. The renal capsule was much thickened and the arteries of all sizes sclerosed.

The tabulation shown below indicates how, in course of time, the kidneys tend to "shrink" after irradiation. The data, obtained from autopsy information in patients initially treated at the Holt Radium Institute, Manchester, England, relates the total weight of kidney tissue to the time interval between the commencement of radiotherapy and the death of the patient.

Renal Contraction Resulting From Renal Irradiation

Interval (months) Between X-ray Therapy and Autopsy	Total Kidney Tissue (normal = 300 gm.)
13	360
15	"normal"
16	280
25	295
38	200
43	190
46	205
49	180
88	90
102	155
135	180
159	195
228	80

Radiologic evidence of this process of renal contraction is obtainable during life. Figure 29-11 shows comparable intravenous pyelograms taken in the same patient before radiotherapy and 9 years later.

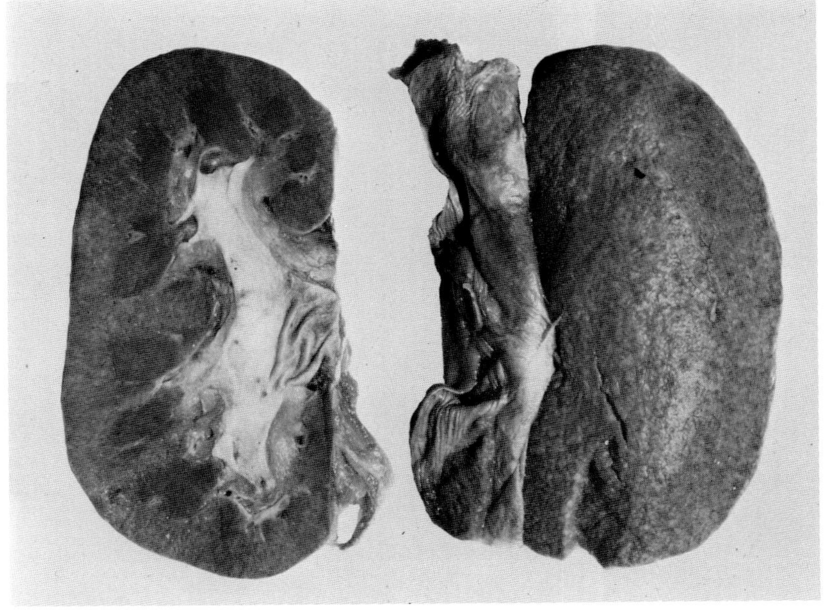

Figure 29-8. Chronic radiation nephritis. The patient died of intercurrent disease 3 years after renal irradiation. Both kidneys are moderately contracted (each weighed 100 gm.).

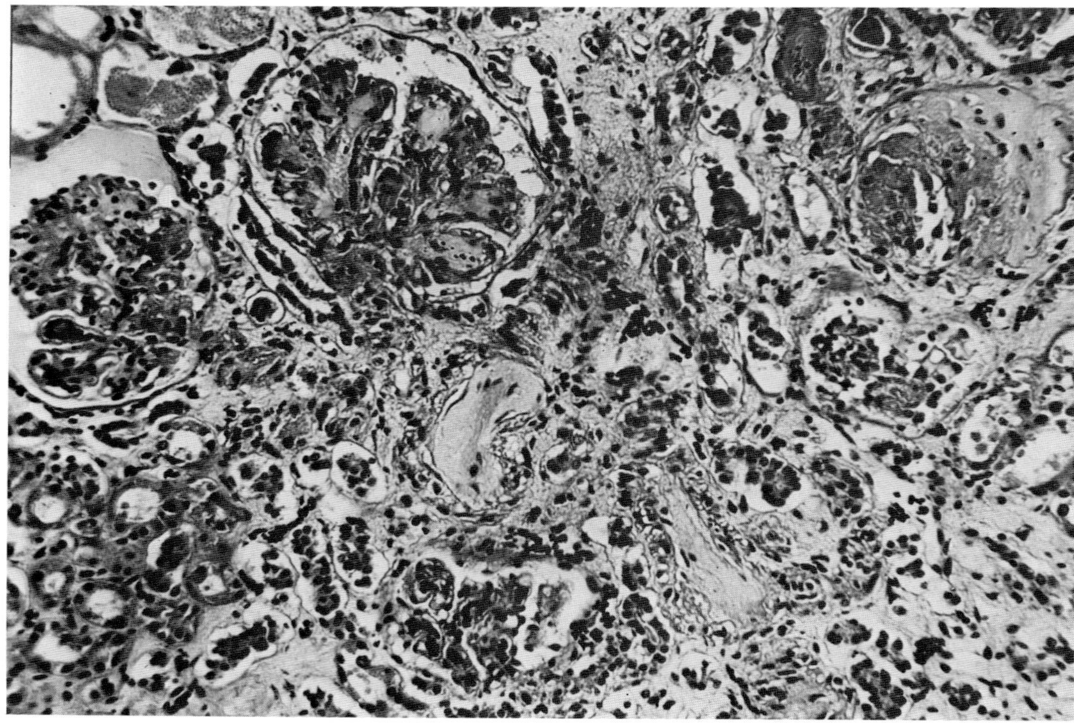

Figure 29-9. Chronic radiation nephritis. Histology of kidney in Figure 29-8. Some of the glomeruli are hyalinized, some have thickened basement membrane. The tubules show dilatation or atrophy. Endarteritis fibrosa of intralobular arteries is present. Hematoxylin and eosin. ×160, before 10% reduction.

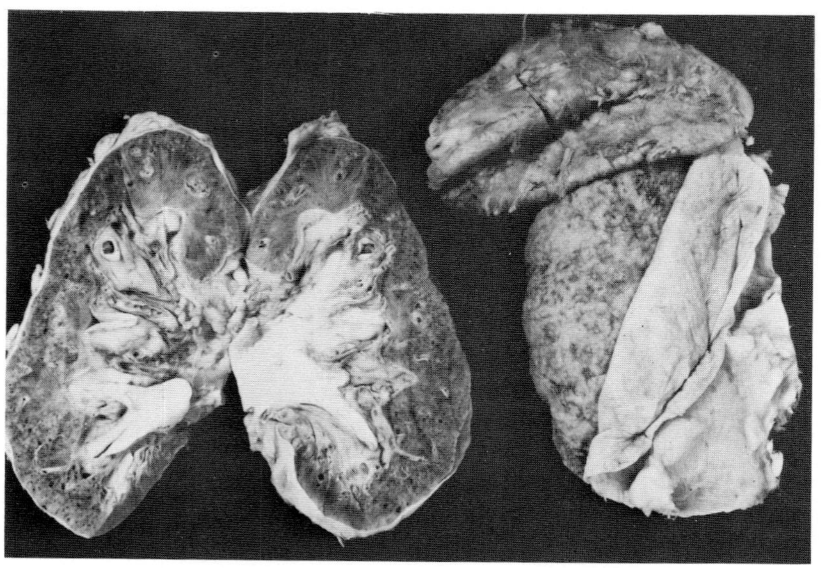

Figure 29-10. Chronic radiation nephritis. The patient died of chronic renal failure 8 years after irradiation. The kidneys were densely sclerosed; each weighed 45 gm. The attached adrenal gland weighed 12 gm.

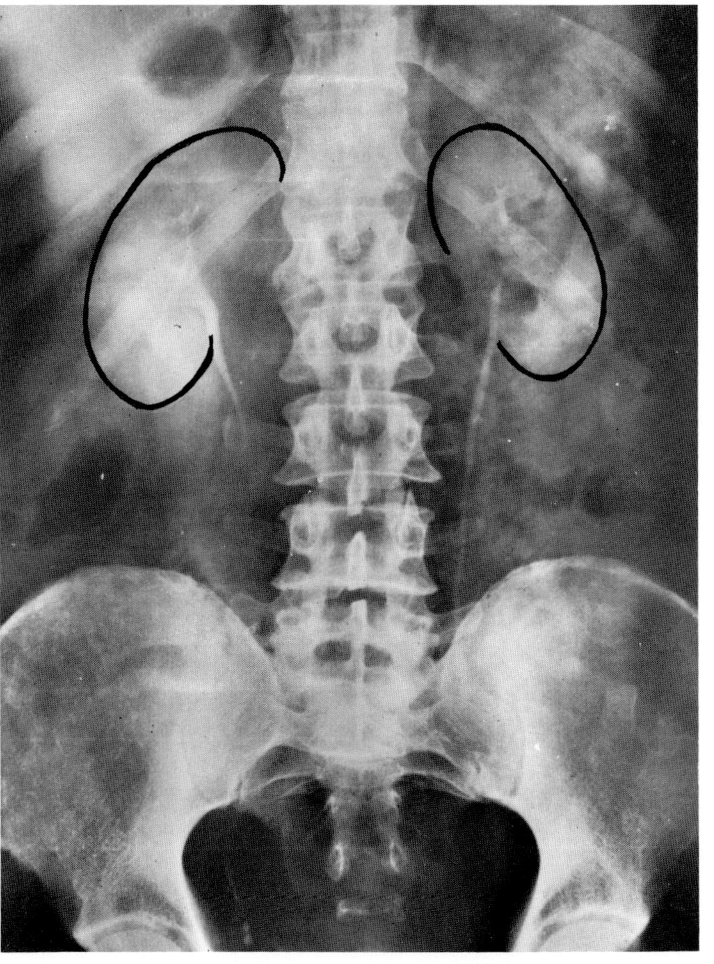

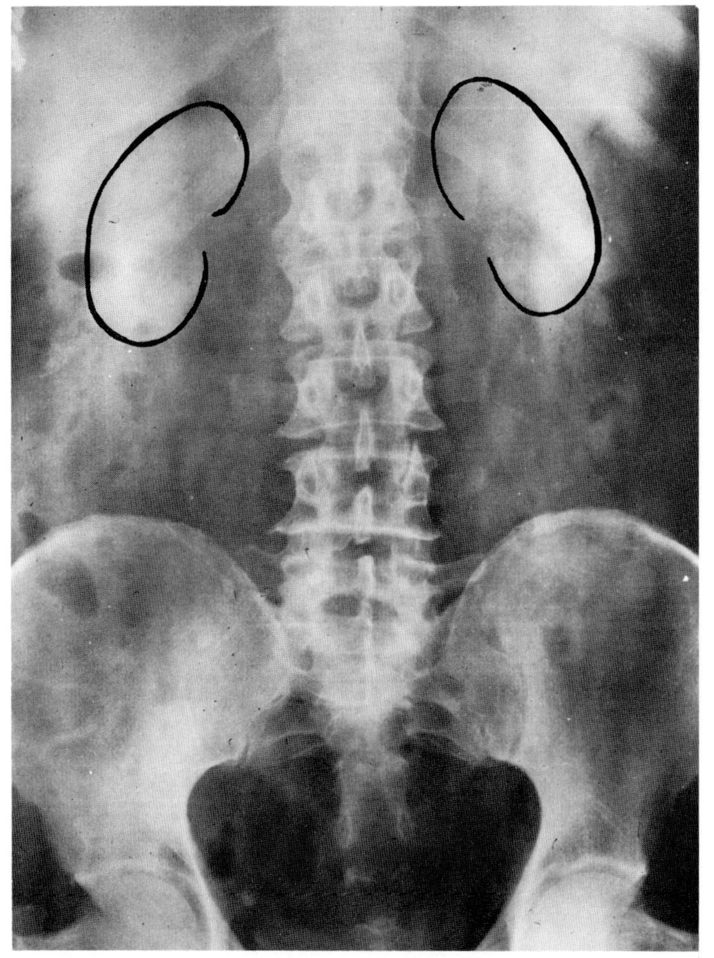

Figure 29-11. Chronic radiation nephritis. The process of renal contraction after irradiation shown by intravenous pyelography. A. Kidney outlines before radiotherapy. B. Kidney outlines 9 years after radiotherapy.

Animal Experiments and Pathogenesis

In what is essentially a clinical text it is not necessary to review the extensive literature on radiation nephritis induced experimentally in animals; such reviews have been made by Grossman [19] and by Redd [35]. A perusal of the literature does, however, emphasize the hazards of inadequate clinical study of patients before, and for a long period after, the use of a potent therapy. For many years radiotherapists regarded kidney tissue as relatively radioresistant, following the comments of Hall and Whipple [20], who wrote in 1919, after their experiments on dogs, "Careful examination of the kidneys of our series of animals at autopsy and of the microscopic sections has convinced us that if there is renal injury it is of a relatively slight grade and is not a constant finding"; and of McQuarrie and Whipple [30], who stated, in 1922, after similar animal studies, "We feel confident that the clinician may use the x-rays over the kidney areas with confidence that renal tissue is resistant to the hard Roentgen rays." This view was disputed two years later by Desjardins [14] and subsequently by Doub et al. [16]. Ultimately Elward and Belair [17], in 1939, and Warren [46], in 1942, came to regard the kidney as moderately responsive to x-irradiation — that is, as less sensitive than lymphoid tissue, skin, lung, or liver, but more sensitive than muscle, nervous tissue, endothelial cells, or connective tissue cells.

Although in this connection animal experiment had confused the clinical situation, its clarifying value is also evident. Wilson et al. [49], working at the London Hospital, observed that in a patient who developed malignant hypertension after abdominal irradiation (a fatal case of acute radiation nephritis) histologic study of the kidneys revealed a picture indistinguishable from malignant essential hypertension. They therefore planned a series of experiments in which they observed the effect of suitable measured doses of x-rays on the blood pressure and on the renal histology of rats which had one or both kidneys exposed to irradiation, taking full precautions to ensure that what they were studying was the result of irradiation of kidney tissue only. In some experiments the kidneys were drawn out onto the rats' flanks during irradiation; in others the kidneys were irradiated in situ.

Four relevant conclusions emerge from these experiments:

1. Irradiation of both exteriorized kidneys in rats causes hypertension after a latent period corresponding with that in man.
2. The irradiation has two distinct and independent biologic effects, hypertension and interstitial fibrosis; these two effects have different time relations and may develop together or separately.
3. Irradiation sclerosis of the kidney is a composite picture of structural damage due to the two separate processes.
4. There is no evidence that the hypertension which follows irradiation is due to constriction of the kidney by fibrosis of its capsule, or to constriction of the renal artery by fibrosis at the kidney hilus.

The experimental work of Wilson et al. offers a neat explanation of the main features of radiation nephritis in man, for the concept of two independent biologic effects, hypertension and interstitial fibrosis, would account for the pathologic and histologic changes seen at various stages of the disorder. Moreover, the clinical syndromes seen during and after acute radiation nephritis (Table 29-1) lend support to this concept.

One aspect of the experimental work of Wilson et al. [49] is of special interest to physicians and may prove helpful in elucidating the mechanism of primary essential hypertension. If both kidneys in the rat are irradiated in situ, hypertension and renal structural changes develop after the latent period of 9 to 12 months, as in man. Wilson

Table 29-1. Acute Radiation Nephritis — Clinical Syndromes Seen in 20 Cases to Year 1961

	Clinical Syndrome	Cases
During acute phase	Malignant hypertension[a]	8
Sequel to acute phase	Chronic renal failure with hypertension	6
	Chronic renal failure without hypertension	3
	Chronic hypertension without renal failure	1
	No residual hypertension or obvious renal failure	4

[a] Two patients with malignant hypertension recovered from acute radiation nephritis but developed other syndromes later.

et al. found that if the rat's kidney is excised at the very onset of hypertension, it may appear histologically normal. In essential hypertension in human beings there is much doubt as to whether the source of hypertension is *renal* or *nonrenal.* This rat experiment demonstrates that hypertension which is certainly of renal origin can arise without any recognizable histologic change in the kidney. (Studies of such kidneys with the electron microscope would be valuable.) Asscher et al. [2] have shown that x-irradiation increases the susceptibility of arteries in the mesentery to hypertensive vascular damage. They suggest that x-irradiation similarly sensitizes the arterial structures of the kidney to hypertension, subsequently resulting in abnormal vasoconstriction therein as a response to physiologic changes in systemic blood pressure. In a personal communication, Wilson states that serial studies of the histologic changes caused by varying doses of x-rays suggest a primary glomerular lesion closely resembling the ischemic glomerular damage occurring in benign essential hypertension, or as part of the aging process.

Some Clinicopathologic Features

Recently consideration has been given by Luxton and Baker [29] to certain clinicopathologic aspects of the disease.

LATENT PERIOD

The potential tissue changes due to ionizing radiation must be present from the moment the electron gives up its excess energy. Despite the long latent period before symptoms are apparent, the injury is irrevocable from the time of irradiation. An important effect of irradiation is interference with cell division. In tissues with a rapid turnover of cells this effect is soon obvious, but in tissues in which the normal turnover is slower the current population of cells takes longer to become obsolescent, resulting in a greater interval before changes are manifest. Apart from the gradual tissue changes in the kidney, the latent period between renal irradiation and the onset of symptoms is extended because the normal kidney has considerable functional reserve. Thus, although signs of renal injury are present earlier, symptoms may not occur until the onset of renal failure many weeks or months later.

EVOLUTION OF ACUTE RADIATION NEPHRITIS INTO CHRONIC

In most patients who survive acute radiation nephritis there is a general improvement which may last many years, although all these patients have chronic nephritis and impaired renal reserve. This improvement in function is difficult to explain when the kidney appears to be undergoing steady destruction. I can only suggest that the functional improvement is related to the reduction of interstitial edema which could be brought about by the obliteration of the more severely damaged intertubular capillaries. This would parallel the changes seen in the glomerular tuft in which obliteration of severely damaged capillaries may lead to a reduction in proteinuria.

The histologic changes responsible for the final progressive renal failure are difficult to define. As with many chronic renal diseases the final picture is a sclerosed kidney in which it is impossible to say what was the primary and what a secondary change. There seems little doubt from our observations that vascular damage (including glomeruli) is the most widespread and probably the most significant feature in acute radiation nephritis.

Is the final sclerosis of the kidney secondary to glomerular damage or to arterial change? Both are commonly seen in patients dying of renal failure. It is of note that intrarenal arterial changes are prominent in symptom-free patients whose glomeruli, although not normal, are not severely affected. This leads us to suspect that glomerular damage is the more important as a cause of severe renal failure. In proliferative glomerulonephritis the importance of obliteration of the capsular space has been stressed [4]. Obliteration by crescent formation is indeed the characteristic feature of cases of glomerulonephritis with a poor prognosis. In all the fatal cases of chronic radiation nephritis reduction and final obliteration of Bowman's space is widespread, often without marked periglomerular fibrosis. Sclerosis of glomeruli is, of course, seen in many forms of chronic renal disease and is frequently the final stage in the process of glomerular destruction. Radiation nephritis appears to differ from these other cases in two ways: (1) A very large proportion of glomeruli show obliteration of the capsular space, and (2) obliteration can be seen to start in glomeruli when the tuft is not very severely diseased. Hence, I believe that this capsular change is important.

FIBROSIS

The degree of fibrosis differs considerably from case to case, ranging from marked increase of fibrosis tissue separating the renal tubules to what can only be considered as a condensation of the preexisting stroma. In trying to assess the reasons for the variations the following factors should be considered. Chronic edema and infection undoubtedly promote fibrosis. Ischemia, provided it is produced slowly and does not lead to frank infarction, probably causes disappearance of tubules and consequent collapse of the kidney, with approximation of glomeruli. High doses of irradiation may have a similar effect. Destruction of glomeruli, tubules, and vascular bed leads to marked shrinkage without excessive fibrosis, the size of the kidney and the degree of fibrosis therefore being dependent on two opposing processes — that is, edema, primarily active in the acute stage, and ischemia during the chronic stage. The hypothesis is supported to some extent by the finding of the steady reduction of renal size with increasing length of survival. The periphery of the kidney frequently shows greater shrinkage than the juxtamedullary region. This, we suggest, is due to damage to the intrarenal vessels. For practical purposes, all the arteries receive the same dose of irradiation. The lesions tend to be patchy, however, and the longer the vessel, the greater the chance that it will develop a serious occlusion. One may thus expect ischemic lesions to arise more readily at the periphery of the kidney.

HYPERTENSION

The pathogenesis of hypertension in renal disease is not understood. In radiation nephritis the pathogenesis is likely to be even more complicated than in other renal disorders because changes may arise in many relevant structures — for example, the glomeruli, the juxtaglomerular apparatus, and the blood vessels. The differences detectable between patients with and those without hypertension, are probably due to the hypertension itself. It is of interest that hypertension in radiation nephritis follows much the same pattern as in other renal diseases having two distinct phases — for example, poststreptococcal nephritis. In the acute state, affecting mainly the glomeruli, hypertension is common, but the blood pressure may return to normal as the patient improves. If chronic nephritis follows, hypertension is likely to reappear in association with kidney contraction.

MALIGNANT HYPERTENSION

Renal irradiation has a remarkable tendency to cause malignant hypertension. Of my own personal series of 58 patients, malignant hypertension developed sooner or later in 16 (28 per cent). It is conceivable that further study of the effects of renal irradiation may shed light not only on essential hypertension but also on the pathogenesis of malignant hypertension.

Diagnosis

A history of exposure of kidney tissue to therapeutic x-irradiation in relevant dosage affords a fundamental clue to diagnosis. The clinical picture presented or the known development of proteinuria and hypertension after radiotherapy offer further evidence. Renal biopsy may help but may be unfruitful in chronic radiation nephritis, in which the renal tissue is sclerotic and difficult to retain in the aspirating needle.

Three main mistakes in diagnosis have been observed:

1. The symptoms of acute radiation nephritis may be attributed to metastases, the anemia, ascites, and debility to abdominal metastases, and the headache, vomiting, and papilledema of malignant hypertension to cerebral metastases. The history of radiotherapy and the presence of hypertension and proteinuria should prevent this serious clinical error.

2. Renal disease or hypertension of benign essential or malignant type arising months or years after abdominal radiotherapy may be attributed to other causes or, contrariwise, may be attributed wrongly to the radiotherapy.

3. Idiopathic periureteric fibrosis [9, 10, 31, 34] may be associated with renal fibrosis and contraction [Raper, personal communication], and as some patients with periureteric fibrosis have been treated by abdominal radiotherapy the differential diagnosis from chronic radiation nephritis may be difficult, as in the following case:

In April 1959, a man aged 52 years complained of anginal pain and dyspnea on effort. He was anemic (hemoglobin, 42 per cent; red blood cell count, 2,300,000 per cubic millimeter), had proteinuria, hypertension (blood pressure 170/90 mm. Hg), normal retinas, and a little cardiac enlargement. The blood urea was 140 mg. per 100 ml., and urea clearance 25 per cent of normal.

He had been given abdominal radiotherapy (3000 R in 29 days) after laparotomy in 1952, and it was at first considered that the present symptoms and signs were due to chronic radiation nephritis. A more detailed history revealed that in 1952 low back pain radiating into groins and scrotum had been associated with loss of weight. Four months later a firm, slightly uneven fixed mass, of 6 inches vertical extent, was felt to the left of the lumbar spine, and a similar but less marked mass was detectable to the right of the spine.

At laparotomy (Mr. Alan Nicholson) the following observation was made: "The peritoneum was stripped up and the retroperitoneal mass was exposed. The mass was firm, almost hard, and extended from the promontory of the sacrum upwards into the upper abdomen beyond reach of the finger. The mass appeared to be in one piece, and the common iliac vessels and abdominal aorta were so intimately involved in it that surgical removal was impracticable. A representative piece was taken for biopsy." Histologically the mass consisted of fibrous and fatty tissue containing scattered foci of lymphoid cells. After radiotherapy the mass became impalpable and the patient was well until 1959. Radiologic examination (Dr. J. Blair Hartley) now revealed bilateral hydronephrosis, and ureteric catheterization (Mr. D. S. Poole-Wilson) showed obstruction of the left ureter 4.5 cm. from the bladder. Subsequent percutaneous renal biopsy showed that many glomeruli were replaced by hyaline fibrotic tissue, and there was extensive tubular atrophy. It was impossible to say how much of the renal injury was due to x-irradiation.

In the diagnosis of radiation nephritis it is important to know the state of the kidneys before radiotherapy. A patient who is to be given deep x-ray treatment by fields which for some reason must include part or all of one or both kidneys should have the blood pressure determined, a careful examination of the urine for protein, an intravenous pyelogram, and, if necessary, renal function tests. The elementary examinations of blood pressure and of urine for protein are highly valuable and should be clearly and permanently recorded for, though so simple, they are of the utmost importance if, after radiotherapy, suspicious renal symptoms arise. More detailed accounts of the histologic diagnosis of radiation nephritis are given by Luxton and Baker [29], Rubenstone and Fitch [38], and Heptinstall [22].

Prevention

Clinical radiation nephritis can be prevented to a large extent but not entirely. Although it seems to depend on the irradiation of both kidneys to a homogeneous dose above 2300 R in five weeks (or an equivalent dose in other periods), the absence of renal signs and symptoms in patients irradiated to this level, or even to a smaller dose, does not mean that the kidneys have escaped damage, for the renal reserve is considerable. In such patients a follow-up in terms of decades might be revealing.

Factors that may predispose to radiation nephritis in the individual patient require consideration when his radiotherapy is being prescribed. Such factors include congenital renal lesions such as horseshoe kidney or cysts, malposition of one or both kidneys, tumor masses adjacent to the kidney which could interfere with its blood supply [25], preceding chronic nephritis, and infection within the urinary tract.

Until recently it has not been easy to screen the kidneys from radiation injury and at the same time give a therapeutic dose of x-rays to adjacent malignant tissue. However, the advent of megavoltage machines permits homogeneous radiation of a treated volume without regard to its shape. Upper abdominal metastases from seminoma testis are commonly located in lymph nodes close to the midline (the para-aortic nodes), which can now be given the relatively low dose of x-rays required, with the kidneys effectively shielded. (For the technic involved and for the precautions taken to avoid renal injury by x-rays, modern radiotherapeutic literature should be consulted; the method current at the Holt Radium Institute, Manchester, England, has been described by Gibb [18].) Ovarian carcinoma is less radiosensitive than seminoma, and a higher x-ray dosage is necessary. Moreover, besides involving the abdominal lymph nodes, metastasis from ovarian carcinoma can occur at any point in the peritoneal cavity, so that shielding of the kidneys, though practiced, may lead to the protection of peritoneal secondary deposits from irradiation. Consequently, for some of these patients, and for others in whom malignant tissue in or near the kidney is efficiently irradiated, the risk of radiation nephritis remains.

Acknowledgments

I wish to thank my colleagues at the Christie Hospital and Holt Radium Institute, Manchester, for their cooperation, especially Dr. Helen Russell, Professor J. Ralston Paterson, Dr. J. Blair Hartley, and Dr. J. L. Dobbie; also Dr. James Davson, pathologist at Crumpsall Hospital, Manchester. The illustrations were prepared in the Departments of Medical Illustration at the Christie Hospital (by Mr. R. Schofield) and at Crumpsall Hospital (by Miss Jean Perry).

References

1. Anapole, W., and Glaubeck, S. Renal lesions in mice receiving 600r whole body radiation. *Fed. Proc.* 15:505, 1956.
2. Asscher, A. W., Wilson, C., and Anson, S. G. Sensitisation of blood vessels to hypertensive damage by x-irradiation. *Lancet* 1:580, 1961.
3. Bennett, L. R., Chastian, S. M., Flint, J. S., Hansen, R. A., and Lewis, A. E. Late effects of roentgen irradiation; studies on rats irradiated under anoxia. *Radiology* 61:411, 1953.
4. Berlyne, G. M., and Baker, S. B. de C. Acute anuric glomerulonephritis. *Quart. J. Med.* 33:105, 1964.
5. Bianchi, L. Zur Morphologie und Funktion experimentell erzeugter Röntgennieren. *Virchow. Arch.* [Path. Anat.] 334:206, 1961.
6. Boden, G., and Gibb, R. Radiotherapy and testicular neoplasms. *Lancet* 2:1195, 1951.
7. Bolliger, A., and Earlam, M. S. S. Experimental renal disease produced by x-rays: Production and functional study of standardized lesion. *Med. J. Aust.* 1:340, 1930.
8. Buschke, A., and Schmidt, H. E. Über die Wirkung der Röntgenstrahlen auf Drüsen. *Deutsch. Med. Wschr.* 31:495, 1905.
9. Case Records of the Massachusetts General Hospital. *New Eng. J. Med.* 255:90, 1956.
10. Case Records of the Massachusetts General Hospital. *New Eng. J. Med.* 256:1198, 1957.
11. Cogan, S. R., and Ritter, I. Radiation nephritis; a clinicopathologic correlation of three surviving cases. *Amer. J. Med.* 24:530, 1958.
12. Davey, P. W., Hamilton, J. D., and Steele, H. D. Radiation injury of kidney. *Canad. Med. Ass. J.* 67:648, 1952.
13. Dean, A. L., and Abels, J. C. Study by newer renal function tests of an unusual case of hypertension following irradiation of one kidney and the relief of the patient by nephrectomy. *J. Urol.* 52:497, 1944.
14. Desjardins, A. U. Reaction of abdominal tumours to radiation. *J.A.M.A.* 83:109, 1924.
15. Domagk, G. Röntgenstrahlen Schädigungen der Niere beim Menschen. *Med. Klin.* 23:345, 1927.
16. Doub, H. P., Bolliger, A., and Hartman, F. W. The relative sensitivity of the kidney to irradiation. *Radiology* 8:142, 1927.
17. Elward, J. F., and Belair, J. F. Relative degrees of radiosensitivity of tissue. *Radiology* 33:450, 1939.
18. Gibb, R. Some clinical aspects of megavoltage. *Proc. Roy. Soc. Med.* 53:235, 1960.
19. Grossman, B. J. Radiation nephritis. *J. Pediat.* 47:424, 1955.
20. Hall, C. C., and Whipple, G. H. Roentgen-ray intoxication: Disturbances in metabolism produced by deep massive doses of the hard roentgen rays. *Amer. J. Med. Sci.* 157:453, 1919.
21. Hallcraft, J., Lorenz, E., Millar, E., Congdon, C. C., Schweisthal, R., and Uphoff, D. Delayed effects in mice following acute total body x-irradiation: Modification by experimental treatment. *J. Nat. Cancer Inst.* 18:615, 1957.
22. Heptinstall, R. H. *Pathology of the Kidney.* Boston: Little, Brown, 1966.
23. Kincaid-Smith, P., McMichael, J., and Murphy, E. A. The clinical course and pathology of hypertension with papilloedema (malignant hypertension). *Quart. J. Med.* 27:117, 1958.
24. Kunkler, P. B., Farr, R. F., and Luxton, R. W. The limit of renal tolerance to x-rays: An investigation into renal damage occurring following the treatment of tumours of the

testis by abdominal baths. *Brit. J. Radiol.* 25: 190, 1952.
25. Levitt, W. M. Radiation nephritis. *Brit. J. Urol.* 29:381, 1957.
26. Levitt, W. M., and Oram, S. Irradiation-induced malignant hypertension: Cured by nephrectomy. *Brit. Med. J.* 2:910, 1956.
27. Luxton, R. W. Radiation nephritis. *Quart. J. Med.* 22:215, 1953.
28. Luxton, R. W. Radiation nephritis: A long-term study of fifty-four patients. *Lancet* 2: 1221, 1961.
29. Luxton, R. W., and Baker, S. B. de C. Radiation Nephritis. In Becker, E. L. (Ed.), *Structural Basis of Renal Disease*. Harper & Row, Publishers, 1969.
30. McQuarrie, I., and Whipple, G. H. Study of renal function in roentgen ray intoxication; resistance of renal epithelium to direct radiation. *J. Exp. Med.* 35:225, 1922.
31. Ormand, J. K. Bilateral ureteral obstruction due to envelopment and compression by an inflammatory retroperitoneal process. *J. Urol.* 59:1072, 1948.
32. Page, I. H. Production of persistent arterial hypertension by cellophane perinephritis. *J.A.M.A.* 113:2046, 1939.
33. Platt, R. Structural and functional adaptation in renal failure. *Brit. Med. J.* 1:1372, 1952.
34. Raper, F. P. Idiopathic retroperitoneal fibrosis involving the ureters. *Brit. J. Urol.* 28: 436, 1956.
35. Redd, B. J. Radiation nephritis; review, case report and animal study. *Amer. J. Roentgen.* 83:88, 1960.
36. Roscoe, M. H. Anaemia and nitrogen retention in patients with chronic renal failure. *Lancet* 1:444, 1952.
37. Rosen, S., Swerdlow, M. A., Meuhrcke, R. C., and Pirani, C. L. Radiation nephritis: Light and electron microscopic observations. *Amer. J. Clin. Path.* 41:487, 1964.
38. Rubenstone, A. I., and Fitch, L. B. Radiation nephritis: A clinicopathologic study. *Amer. J. Med.* 33:545, 1962.
39. Russell, H. Renal sclerosis, "post radiation nephritis" following irradiation of the upper abdomen. *Edinb. Med. J.* 60:474, 1953.
40. Schreiner, B. F., and Greendyke, R. M. Radiation nephritis; report of a fatal case. *Amer. J. Med.* 26:146, 1959.
41. Shaw, A. B., Bazzard, F. J., Booth, E. M., Nilwarangkur, S., and Berlyne, G. M. The treatment of chronic renal failure by a modified Giovannetti diet. *Quart. J. Med.* 34:134, 1965.
42. Sheehan, J. F. Foam cell plaques in the intima of irradiated small arteries (one hundred to five hundred microns in external diameter). *Arch. Path.* 37:297, 1944.
43. Smith, W. G., and Williams, A. W. Irradiation nephritis. *Lancet* 2:175, 1955.
44. Sullivan, M. P., and Takahashi, Y. Incidence of abnormal urinary findings in children exposed to the atomic bomb in Hiroshima. *Pediatrics* 19:607, 1957.
45. Upton, A. C., and Furth, J. Nephrosclerosis induced in mice by total body irradiation. *Fed. Proc.* 13:445, 1954.
46. Warren, S. Effects of radiation on normal tissues. *Arch. Path.* 34:1070, 1942.
47. Warren, S., MacMillan, J. C., and Dixon, F. J. Effects of internal irradiation of mice with P32: II. Gonads, kidneys, adrenal glands, digestive tract, spinal cord, lungs, and liver. *Radiology* 55:557, 1950.
48. Willis, D. A., and Bachem, A. The effects of roentgen rays upon the kidney. *Amer. J. Roentgen.* 18:334, 1927.
49. Wilson, C., Ledingham, J. M., and Cohen, M. Hypertension following x-irradiation of the kidneys. *Lancet* 1:9, 1958.
50. Ziegerman, J. H., Tulsky, E. G., and Makler, P. Post-radiation nephritic syndrome; report of a case. *Obstet. Gynec.* 9:542, 1957.
51. Zuelzer, W. W., Palmer, H. D., and Newton, W. A., Jr. Unusual glomerulonephritis in young children: Probably radiation nephritis; report of three cases. *Amer. J. Path.* 26:1019, 1950.

30

Renal Tubular Dysfunction

Malcolm D. Milne

Renal tubular disorders may be defined as conditions in which, early in the course of the disease, there is specialized or generalized impairment of tubular function with little or no evidence of glomerular deficiency. It is essential to include the qualifying phrase "early in the course of the disease," because, in the later stages, tubular damage may cause secondary glomerular impairment—for example, the effects of calculous hydronephrosis in cystinuria, secondary renal fibrosis from cystinosis in the Lignac-Fanconi syndrome or from nephrocalcinosis in renal tubular acidosis, and the increased susceptibility to chronic pyelonephritis in many chronic tubular syndromes.

The two main effects of glomerular damage are a fall in the glomerular filtration rate causing increase of the blood urea and plasma nonprotein nitrogen, and increased permeability of the glomerular basement membrane leading to proteinuria. In this type of proteinuria the smaller-molecular-weight proteins are preferentially excreted in the urine. Albumin is present in highest concentration, but globulins, chiefly consisting of alpha globulin, the metal-carrying proteins, siderophilin and caeruloplasmin, and some gamma globulin, are also to be found. Early in the course of renal tubular syndromes the glomerular filtration rate is normal or only slightly reduced, and therefore there is no significant increase of blood urea or plasma nonprotein nitrogen. In tubular diseases due to highly specialized defects of a single transport system (e.g., cystinuria and Hartnup disease) there is no proteinuria in the early stages. By contrast, in conditions due to more generalized tubular damage (e.g., Fanconi syndrome and renal tubular acidosis) there is frequently proteinuria of a completely different type from the more familiar variety secondary to increased glomerular permeability. Electrophoresis shows that the proteins mainly consist of a mixture of globulins [43], with a pattern quite different from that of glomerulonephritis or of the nephrotic syndrome. In addition, the protein loss is quantitatively much less than in the nephrotic syndrome.

The renal tubules are primarily concerned with transport of substances from the tubular lumen into the renal capillary blood (i.e., renal tubular reabsorption) and less commonly with transport in the reverse direction (i.e., renal tubular secretion). A tubular defect therefore results either in excretion of substances which are not present in normal urine, or in excretion in abnormal amounts, or with abnormal renal clearances, of substances which are normal urinary constituents.

There are three main varieties of increased excretion of a substance:

1. The overflow type of increased excretion. This is due to an extrarenal metabolic disturbance which increases the concentration of the substance concerned in the plasma. The kidney is behaving normally in an abnormal environment. This therefore is not strictly an example of a renal tubular disorder, but it must be considered in differential diagnosis. Typical examples are diabetes mellitus involving glucose, and phenylketonuria and maple syrup urine disease involving specific amino acids.

2. Increase in renal clearance with increase in total excretion of the substance in unit time. This type of defect is obviously most easily recognized by finding abnormal amounts of the substance in urine, while the plasma concentration is either normal or only slightly reduced. The defect will directly cause symptoms only if there is undue urinary loss of an essential substance (e.g., the severe glycosuria of phlorizin poisoning), or if the excess excretion causes secondary effects on the kidney (e.g., cystine calculous disease in severe cystinuria).

3. Increase in renal clearance with normal excretion of the substance in unit time. This type of tubular defect is recognized by analysis of the plasma, the plasma concentration of the substance being abnormally low. Symptoms occur only if the low plasma levels are directly harmful — for example, reduced plasma phosphate in many proximal tubular syndromes causing rickets or osteomalacia, and reduced plasma potassium causing muscular weakness or periodic paralysis. Occasionally the reduced plasma level may be advantageous to the patient (e.g., the abnormally low plasma uric acid in many cases of the Fanconi syndrome).

Obviously, determination of plasma concentration of the substance is of crucial importance in assessment of the type of defect. This may be technically difficult if the plasma concentration is very low (e.g., β-aminoisobutyric acid), and in such cases administration of the substance concerned, preferably parenterally, may help in differential diagnosis.

Cause of Renal Tubular Disorders

In many cases the cause of renal tubular disorders is unknown. There are, however, two important known causes: toxic effects produced either by exogenous or by endogenous poisons, and hereditary defects. Poisons often affect other tissues besides the renal tubules, but the kidney is often unduly susceptible because poisons may be concentrated in renal cells or in the urine during their excretion. Many nephrotoxic drugs or poisons in high dosage produce severe proximal tubular necrosis with acute oliguric renal failure (e.g., mercuric chloride, carbon tetrachloride, and ethylene glycol). Less severe damage, however, often causes multiple defects of tubular function (e.g., those due to metallic poisons, uranium, lead or cadmium, and maleic acid). Poisons which particularly affect sulfhydryl enzyme systems (e.g., dehydrogenases) seem especially liable to cause proximal tubular damage. Examples of endogenous poisons are copper deposits in hepatolenticular degeneration, galactose 1-phosphate in galactosemia, and probably Bence Jones proteose in some cases of multiple myelomatosis.

Most of the hereditary defects causing renal tubular syndromes are pure mendelian recessive characters, but occasionally dominant inheritance occurs. Modern concepts of hereditary defects involving a single gene suggest that there is usually no or deficient synthesis of a single protein, which is often an enzyme. In a few hereditary diseases, proof of deficiency of a known enzyme has been obtained — for example, phenylketonuria is due to absence of phenylalanine hydroxylase, alkaptonuria to absence of homogentisic acid oxidase, and galactosemia to absence of galactose 1-phosphate uridyl transferase. The clinical symptoms and signs of the disease often involve organs which are not the site of the enzymatic defect. Thus, in phenylketonuria the enzyme concerned is normally present only in the liver, and therefore strictly the condition is a hereditary disease of the liver. Clinically the effects of the biochemical disorder are recognized by disturbances of the central nervous system and by the excretion of abnormal metabolic products in the urine. In hereditary diseases of the renal tubules we have as yet no knowledge of which enzyme or enzymes are deficient, and are equally ignorant of the enzymatic processes concerned in active transport mechanisms. By analogy, however, it is reasonable to postulate absence of some unknown enzyme, which Knox [144] has whimsically termed a "here-to-there -ase."

Mudge [204] has suggested that there are five separate ways in which a genetic variant may cause an abnormality of urinary excretion:

1. There may be a block in an extrarenal metabolic chain causing an increase in the concentration of a metabolite in body fluids and plasma, which is therefore excreted in excess. This is an example of the overflow type of increased urinary excretion of a substance. Typical substances are glucose in diabetes mellitus, L-xylulose in essential pentosuria, phenylalanine in phenylketonuria, argininosuccinic acid in argininosuccinuria, and branched-chain amino acids in maple syrup urine disease.

2. The defect may have a direct and specific effect on renal tubular transport of the substance in the absence of any defect elsewhere in the body. Obviously, until the enzymatic defect is known, it is a dangerous assumption that it is confined to the kidney. Mudge [204] suggests that cystinuria is an example of this type of defect, but evidence is given later in this chapter that there is an associated defect in jejunal transport of amino acids in this disease. There is, in fact, no certain example of this type of hereditary tubular lesion.

3. There may be a specific defect of transport systems both in the renal tubules and in other organs. The jejunum has certain analogies to the renal tubule, since glucose and amino acids are transported from the lumen to the capillary blood. Most examples of cystinuria, Hartnup disease, and some cases of prolinuria are examples of this type of defect. There is evidence of defective amino acid transport both in the renal tubules and in the jejunum.

4. The genetic defect may involve an enzyme which is not directly concerned with tubular transport but alters normal cellular function so that damage occurs which is shown by histopathologic changes and by multiple tubular transport defects. The functional defect is both more diffuse and more variable from case to case than the highly specific type described in (3). There is often proteinuria of the tubular type with predominant excretion of globulin. The disturbance of tubular function may resemble that due to poisons, and associated disturbances may occur from cellular damage in other organs than the kidney. The specific type of defect should be termed a renal tubular "disease," but this variety is better described as a renal tubular "syndrome" until more detailed information is available on the primary enzymatic defect. Typical examples of this type of renal tubular disorder are the Lignac-Fanconi syndrome, the adult Fanconi syndrome, Lowe's syndrome, and the hereditary variety of renal tubular acidosis.

5. The hereditary trait may cause a block in an extrarenal metabolic chain which in turn leads either to increased concentration of a substance in plasma or in renal tissue, or to its increased excretion in the urine. This in turn

exerts a toxic influence on tubular transport systems, and in fact acts as an endogenous tubular poison. The defect obviously is nonspecific and variable, similar to that produced by exogenous poisons. Typical examples are the tubular defects of galactosemia, in which the toxic metabolite is galactose 1-phosphate, and of Wilson's disease, probably due to the effect of excess copper within proximal tubular cells on tubular enzyme systems.

FUNCTIONAL DIVISIONS OF THE NEPHRON IN RELATION TO RENAL TUBULAR DISORDERS

Division of tubular function into actions of the proximal and of the distal tubules should not be too rigid, and there may well be continuous gradation of function along the length of the tubule. Nevertheless, it is convenient to classify renal tubular disorders into those primarily affecting the proximal tubule and those causing distal tubular defects. There may be considerable overlap, however, as in the Fanconi syndrome, which is primarily a proximal tubular defect but often shows abnormalities usually attributed to disordered function of the distal tubule. Water, sodium, and chloride are reabsorbed throughout the length of the nephron, whereas potassium is reabsorbed proximally and secreted distally. The proximal tubule reabsorbs almost all the glucose and amino acids and a large fraction of the phosphate and uric acid filtered at the glomerulus. Proximal tubular syndromes are therefore characterized by various combinations of renal glycosuria, aminoaciduria, increased renal clearance of phosphate causing rickets and osteomalacia, and a high uric acid clearance causing an abnormally low plasma urate. Owing to the large number of different amino acids, aminoaciduria has a disproportionate importance in the classification of proximal tubular defects and is discussed first and in greatest detail.

Hydrogen ion is secreted into the tubular lumen throughout the length of the nephron [116], with consequent bicarbonate reabsorption and progressive fall of pH of tubular fluid. The distal tubule, however, is of major importance in the final adjustment of urinary pH; consequently, renal tubular acidosis is classified as a distal tubular syndrome. Similarly, sodium-losing renal lesions and nephrogenic diabetes insipidus are disorders of the lower segments of the nephron.

Proximal Tubular Syndromes

AMINOACIDURIA

The majority of proximal tubular syndromes involve abnormalities of urinary amino acids, and this fact is of especial importance in classification.

Normal Physiology of Amino Acid Excretion. With the single exception of tryptophan [181], amino acids are not bound to plasma proteins and therefore are in identical concentration in the glomerular filtrate and in plasma. Normally they are almost completely reabsorbed by the proximal tubular cells, urine containing only about 1 per cent of the filtered amino nitrogen. In the case of the majority of amino acids more than 99 per cent of the amount filtered is reabsorbed. The chief exceptions are glycine, of which 95 to 98 per cent is reabsorbed, and histidine, 90 to 95 per cent reabsorbed [60]. In general, essential amino acids are more completely reabsorbed than the physiologically less important nonessential amino acids. Reabsorption of amino acids which are not normal constituents of body proteins is more variable. Thus, ornithine derived from arginine is almost completely reabsorbed, but taurine reabsorption ranges from 88 to 99 per cent. The clearance of other amino acids of this group is often much higher, and may approximate the glomerular filtration rate — for example, β-aminoisobutyric acid derived from thymine metabolism, 1-methylhistidine from anserine, a peptide in muscle fibers, and 3-methylhistidine all have a clearance of this order. Some substances giving a positive Ninhydrin reaction are normally confined to the intracellular compartment, and therefore are not normally present in urine. In certain metabolic disorders, however, they may occur in plasma, and are then excreted with a clearance approximately equal to the glomerular filtration rate — for example, argininosuccinic acid in argininosuccinuria, phosphoethanolamine in hypophosphatasia, and cystathionine in cystathioninuria.

The amino acid pattern of normal adult urine is obviously dependent on the plasma level of amino acids and the proportion reabsorbed by the proximal tubule cells. Three normal variants occur:

1. Glycine is by far the most prominent Ninhydrin-positive substance.
2. Taurine is in equal or even greater concentration than glycine.
3. β-Aminoisobutyric acid is excreted in equivalent amounts to glycine. This variant is an interesting hereditary metabolic anomaly and is described in more detail later.

In addition, histidine, serine, glutamine, and alanine are often present in sufficient quantity to give a positive reaction by paper chromatography, and the methylhistidines are also frequently excreted in considerable quantity. Smaller amounts of other amino acids — for example, lysine, tryptophan, tyrosine, cystine, leucine, valine, and phenylalanine — are normally present in urine, but not in quantity sufficient to give a positive reaction by paper chromatography.

Variation in diet has much less effect on amino acid output than on urea or uric acid excretion. However, a high-protein diet slightly increases urinary amino nitrogen, and in particular a diet rich in meat causes increase of urinary histidine, probably derived from the peptide carnosine, and of 1-methylhistidine from anserine. Occasionally, unusual Ninhydrin-reacting compounds in urine may be derived from specific articles of diet — for example, 5-hydroxypipecolic acid after ingestion of large amounts of dates [117]. Increased metabolism of thymine, as in fasting or after breakdown of large numbers of nucleated cells (e.g., during treatment of leukemia or cellular new growths) leads to excess output of β-aminoisobutyric acid [20]. Pregnancy causes a slight increase of urinary amino acids because of a rise in glomerular filtration rate and reduced tubular reabsorption [270]. There is some increase of urinary tyrosine, arginine, phenylalanine, serine, threonine, and tryptophan, but in particular there is a large rise of urinary histidine. This histidinuria persists throughout pregnancy, but disappears early in the puerperium [209].

Reabsorption of amino acids by the proximal tubule cells is less complete in infancy and childhood. Many discrete renal functions are less efficient in early life than in the adult, but amino acid transport remains relatively poor for a longer period, until late childhood or adolescence. In addition, there is more variation between individual infants and children than between adults, making interpretation of aminoaciduria more difficult in early life. Expression of amino acid output in relation to urinary creatinine is probably the most satisfactory method of comparing excretion rates. Normal values from infancy to adult life are given in Table 30-1. Usually the four most prominent amino acid spots in a chromatogram from adult urine are glycine, taurine, histidine, and methylhistidine. These four amino acids account for over 70 per cent of the

Table 30-1. Normal Excretion of Amino Nitrogen in Infants, Children, and Adults

Subject	α-amino Nitrogen (mg./day)	Mg. α-amino Nitrogen/mg. Creatinine
Premature infants	20–40	0.40–1.40
Full-term infants	15–40	0.35–0.50
Children	60–120	0.10–0.20
Adults	130–230	0.07–0.14

total urinary amino nitrogen in adults, but only about 50 per cent of that in the urine of a full-term newborn infant and about 35 per cent of that in a premature infant. In addition, in urine from infants, there may be appreciable quantities of the essential amino acids threonine, leucine, phenylalanine, and lysine, as well as of the nonessential amino acids serine, alanine, cystine, tyrosine, proline, and hydroxyproline.

Although nothing is known of the actual mechanisms of amino acid transport, important information is available on inhibitory interrelationships among different amino acids by reason of their competition for the available transport system.

Important earlier experimental studies were reported by Beyer et al. [29] and Kamin and Handler [140]. Evidence from human hereditary disease and from clearance studies in the dog now suggest that amino acids may be divided into at least five separate transport groups:

1. The basic amino acids lysine, ornithine, and arginine. Cystine, which is not basic, is included in a less specific manner. Transport of this group is involved in cystinuria [68, 194].
2. The acidic amino acids, glutamic and aspartic acids. These are not involved in any known human disease but specifically compete for proximal tubular transport in the dog kidney [271].
3. The iminoglycine group, proline, hydroxyproline, and glycine. Transport is defective in cases of iminoglycinuria [238].
4. The other mono-amino monocarboxylic acids of protein. Renal transport of these is specifically deficient in Hartnup disease [22, 195].
5. The β-amino acids, β-alanine, β-aminoisobutyric acid, and taurine. Excretion of this group is abnormal in β-alaninemia [240].

In all these conditions, although renal transport is reduced as compared to the normal, it is by no means completely absent, suggesting that there are two or more separate mechanisms involved in amino acid reabsorption [238].

Specific Disorders of Amino Acid Transport

There are three specific disorders of amino acid transport in man which differ fundamentally from cases of generalized tubular damage with multiple proximal tubular functional defects — that is, cystinuria, Hartnup disease, and iminoprolinuria. In particular, the defect is present from birth and is not progressive. No other renal abnormality is present in the uncomplicated disease, and there is no proteinuria of the tubular type.

CYSTINURIA

Cystinuria is a disorder of proximal tubular transport of the dibasic amino acids, cystine, lysine, arginine, and ornithine, without any other primary defect of renal tubular function, but associated with a similar defect of jejunal transport of the same amino acids. Cystinuria is therefore comparable to Hartnup disease, in which there is also conclusive evidence of *both* proximal tubular and jejunal defects of amino acid transport. All other functions of the proximal tubule are normal in cystinuria early in the course of the disease. In particular there is no glycosuria, no phosphate leak, no increase of uric acid clearance, and no proteinuria. With available technics there is no histopathologic abnormality of the tubules, although presumably an unknown enzyme or enzyme system involved in the transport of the four amino acids is deficient.

History. This condition has the longest history of any renal tubular disorder, but it is only recently that the true nature of the disease has been recognized. Wollaston [278] first described a cystine calculus from the urinary bladder 150 years ago, and for many years cystine calculi were the only available source of cystine for chemical purposes. The stones were at first thought to be formed within the bladder, but renal cystine calculi were described by Marcet [184] eight years later, and hexagonal cystine crystals in the urine of cystinurics were recognized by Prout [214]. For many years diagnosis rested on the analysis of calculi removed at operation or on detection of cystine crystals in urine, methods which are inadequate in many milder examples of the disease.

Technical methods improved at the beginning of the present century when Friedmann [96] established the correct chemical formula of cystine, and analytical methods dependent on the determination of urinary "neutral sulphur" were developed by Alsberg and Folin [8]. About this time cystinuria was described by Garrod [105] as one of the four original "inborn errors of metabolism," and its hereditary nature was clearly determined. Modern views of cystinuria date from the recognition by Yeh et al. [283], using microbiologic technics, of an abnormally high urinary output of lysine and arginine as well as cystine. Dent and his colleagues [68, 70] conclusively proved the disease to be due to a tubular amino acid transport defect rather than to a disorder of amino acid metabolism. There is still, however, much to be learned regarding this interesting condition which has been the subject of detailed medical research for the past 150 years.

Heredity. The hereditary aspects of cystinuria have been investigated by Harris and his colleagues [120–124]. Cystinuric families can be divided into two distinct groups. In the first type only two classes of individuals are found: completely normal individuals and affected subjects excreting grossly abnormal amounts of the four amino acids, cystine, lysine, arginine, and ornithine. The heredity is typical of a mendelian recessive character, the homozygotes being examples of the disease and the heterozygotes showing no detectable abnormality. There is an increased frequency of consanguinity in the parents, the disease is not passed on from generation to generation, and the incidence in siblings is typical of a recessive hereditary trait. In the second type of family, which is rather less common than the first, there are three different types of individual: (1) severe cystinurics with increased excretion of the four amino acids are homozygotes for the abnormal gene; (2) mild cystinurics with a moderately increased output of cystine and lysine but with normal or very slightly increased output of arginine and ornithine are heterozygotes; and (3) unaffected individuals are homozygotes for the normal gene. Segregation between the three groups is not so clear-cut as the sharp distinction between the two groups in the first type of family. Obviously in the second type of family the condition can be passed from generation to generation, and the severely affected homozygote occurs only from the mating of two heterozygotes who show the disease in a mild degree. The two types of cystinuria have been termed the *recessive type* and the *incompletely recessive type*. Calculus formation is likely to occur only in the severely affected homozygotes of both family types. Cystinuria is one of the more common hereditary traits. Lewis [156] found an incidence of about 1 per 600 of the population. Stone formation only occurs in about 3 per cent of cystinuric patients, an incidence of about 1 in 18,000 individuals. Rosenberg et al. [220], from simultaneous studies of the intestinal transport defect, have more recently shown that there are at least three varieties of the disease. Type I corresponds to the "recessive type," and is characterized by absent or diminished jejunal uptake of all the affected amino acids. Types II and III correspond to the "incompletely recessive type." In the former, jejunal uptake of the basic amino acids is deficient, but that of cystine is normal; in the latter, uptake of all these amino acids is normal. Rosenberg et al. [221] have shown that double heterozygotes for types I and III are clinically indistinguishable from homozygous cystinuric patients, but on functional studies fall midway between the two types. This suggests that the abnormal genes for the three types are allelic mutations at the same locus on the affected chromosome.

Urinary Abnormalities. All patients with cystinuria excrete abnormal amounts of cystine and lysine. Lysine is more sensitive to bacterial breakdown than cystine, however, and an occasional cystinuric patient with a gross urinary infection may pass urine containing little or no lysine, this having been converted to cadaverine by the bacterial enzyme lysine decarboxylase. In the absence of infection there is a close correlation between the amounts of cystine and lysine excreted, the amount of cystine being roughly half the amount of lysine. This is similar to the proportionate concentrations of the two amino acids in plasma. Arginine and ornithine are excreted in abnormal quantities only in patients with severe cystinuria in whom the lysine output is more than 400 mg. per gram of urinary creatinine, and the cystine output is more than 200 mg. per gram of urinary creatinine. These figures correspond to an average daily output in the adult subject of 640 mg. of lysine and 320 mg. of cystine. There is always less ornithine excreted than any of the other three amino acids, but in severe cases arginine output may exceed that of cystine. Thus Stein [254], in a series of five adult patients with severe cystinuria, found an average excretion of 1.8 gm. of lysine, 0.83 gm. of arginine, 0.73 gm. of cystine, and 0.37 gm. of ornithine. Cusworth and Dent [60] found an average normal plasma level of the four amino acids of lysine, 2.3 mg. per 100 ml., arginine 1.5 mg. per 100 ml., cystine 0.80 mg. per 100 ml., and ornithine 0.92 mg. per 100 ml. The plasma concentrations of the amino acids in cystinuric patients are either normal or very slightly reduced [14, 70].

The clearances of the four amino acids are grossly increased above normal values. Cystine clearance approximates the glomerular filtration rate, and in some instances even exceeds it, indicating net tubular secretion [57, 100], whereas that of the other three amino acids is somewhat less. Doolan et al. [73] reported an average lysine clearance of 55 ml. per minute, about 45 per cent of the amount filtered being reabsorbed by the renal tubules. This shows that the defect in amino acid transport is not absolutely complete, although it is grossly abnormal when compared with clearance in normal subjects. The four amino acids show a mutual competition for the available transport system. Thus infusions of lysine or of arginine [219] in normal subjects increase the excretion of the other three amino acids of the system as well as of the amino acid infused. In particular there is a gross increase of urinary cystine, whereas in patients with cystinuria there is little or no increase in urinary cystine because the cystine clearance is already maximal and approximating the glomerular filtration rate. This roughly corresponds to the observations of Beyer et al. [29] in dogs. Arginine and lysine show mutual competition for tubular reabsorption, and ornithine would be expected to be equally involved since it is structurally very similar to lysine. The association of cystine with the more basic amino acids is, however, more surprising. The connection cannot be related to the acid-base properties of the amino acids, as the isoelectric point of cystine is in fact more acidic than that of most monoamino-monocarboxylic amino acids; e.g. the isoelectric points of arginine, lysine, and cystine are 10.76, 9.74, and 4.80, respectively. The best available hypothesis is that of Dent and Rose [68], who suggested that all four amino acids have two positively charged amino- or guanido-groups which are separated by a chain of four to six atoms (Fig. 30-1) involving a spatial separation of the basic radicles of about 9A. Transport might conceivably involve temporary combination with two acidic groupings, separated by a similar distance in the transport carrier substance.

More recent investigations suggest that cystine transport, although connected with that of the three dibasic amino acids, has separate distinctive features. Rosenberg et al. [220a]

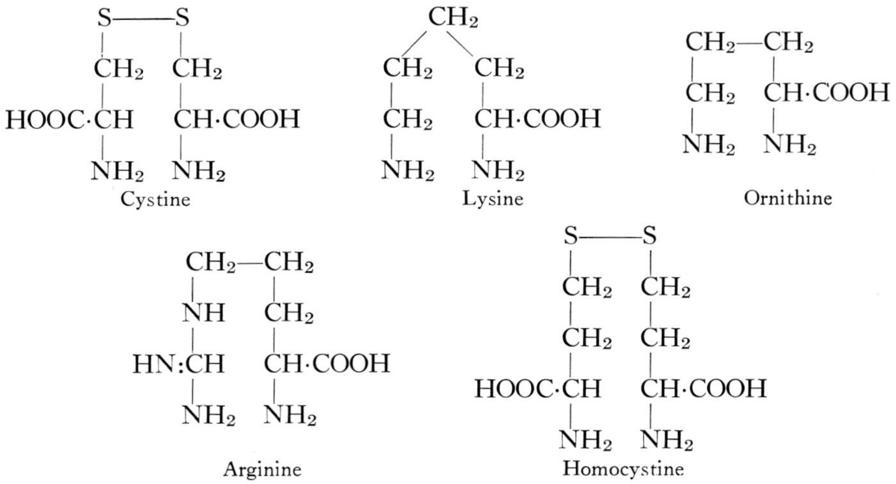

```
S———S
|        |
CH2  CH2
|        |
HOOC·CH    CH·COOH
|        |
NH2  NH2
Cystine
```

```
      CH2
     /   \
CH2      CH2
|          |
CH2      CH·COOH
|          |
NH2      NH2
Lysine
```

```
CH2—CH2
|        |
CH2   CH·COOH
|        |
NH2   NH2
Ornithine
```

```
CH2—CH2
|        |
NH     CH2
|        |
HN:CH    CH·COOH
|        |
NH2   NH2
Arginine
```

```
S———S
|        |
CH2  CH2
|        |
CH2  CH2
|        |
HOOC·CH    CH·COOH
|        |
NH2  NH2
Homocystine
```

Figure 30-1. Formulas of the dibasic amino acids cystine, lysine, ornithine, arginine, and homocystine. These amino acids are probably transported by an identical transport mechanism both in the proximal renal tubules of the kidney and in the jejunum. The mechanism is defective in both sites in cystinuria.

found that the dibasic amino acids were concentrated in rat kidney slices, whereas cystine was not. Identical results were later obtained by Fox et al. [92] using human tissue obtained at nephrectomy. In addition, in type II cystinuria, cystine is normally concentrated by jejunal epithelium, whereas the dibasic amino acids are not [220]. Spencer et al. [251] describe an important study of the transport of sulfur-containing amino acids by hamster intestinal epithelium. They showed that the disulfide linkage of cystine and of homocystine was essential for active transport to occur. Replacement of sulfur by selenium, or separation of the two sulfur atoms by one or more carbon atoms, prevented active transport. Further support for the view of a rather nonspecific association between cystine and dibasic amino acid transport is provided by a recent report of a patient in whom proximal tubular reabsorption of cystine was reduced, whereas that of the dibasic amino acids was completely normal [38].

Frimpter [97, 98] discovered that a fifth amino acid, the mixed disulfide of cysteine and homocysteine — $COOH \cdot CH(NH_2) \cdot CH_2 \cdot S \cdot S \cdot CH_2 \cdot CH_2CH(NH_2)COOH$ — was invariably present in cystinuric urine at a concentration of about one-tenth that of cystine. Solubility of sulfur-containing amino acids is related to molecular symmetry. The asymmetrical mixed disulfides, including that of cysteine + homocysteine, and that of cysteine + penicillamine (dimethylcysteine), are much more water soluble than the completely symmetrical cystine and homocystine. Therefore, the concentration of cysteine-homocysteine mixed disulfide is very low in cystine calculi, being only about 1 per cent of cystine itself.

Evidence for a Similar Jejunal Transport Defect in Cystinuria. Two series of observations in the older literature of cystinuria support a defect of amino acid transport in the jejunum. In 1889 Von Udransky and Baumann [266] found that cystinuric patients excreted increased amounts of diamines in both feces and urine, and postulated that cystinuria was due to "intestinal autointoxication." Their findings, which were later confirmed by many other workers [105], could equally well have been explained by reduced jejunal absorption of lysine and arginine which was then converted by colonic bacteria to the diamines cadaverine and putrescine. The diamines are then partially absorbed, and the fraction escaping oxidation by diamine oxidase is excreted in the urine. Moreigne [200] ten years later doubted the intestinal autointoxication theory because there was no clinical evidence of prolonged intestinal infection, and because, although confirming excess diamine output, he found that the urinary output of indican derived from bacterial degradation of tryptophan and of phenols from tyrosine and phenylalanine was within normal limits. He failed, however, to suggest the obvious explanation that lysine and arginine and not tyrosine, phenylalanine, and tryptophan were exposed to excess bacterial breakdown in the colon. Thiele [260] showed that diamine excretion in cystinuric patients was increased by a high-protein diet, and Loewy and Neuberg [165] found that feeding lysine increased urinary cadaverine, and similarly arginine increased putrescine output.

Brand et al. [35, 36] reported observations which strongly support defective cystine absorption in the jejunum. They found that feeding cystine or homocystine did not increase urinary cystine in cystinuric patients, whereas methionine, cysteine, homocysteine, and cystothionine increased cystine output. Brand interpreted these results as indicating a defect of metabolism of sulfur-containing amino acids, whereas in retrospect they suggest poor absorption from the gut of the diamino acids, cystine and homocystine, with normal transport of the monoamino acids.

A reexamination of amino acid absorption [194] in cystinuric patients has shown that lysine is poorly absorbed from the gut in cystinuria. After feeding 20 gm. of lysine to cystinuric patients, large amounts of both lysine and cadaverine can be isolated from the feces, whereas there is virtually complete absorption of lysine in normal controls. This dose of lysine increases urinary amine output in both cystinuric and normal persons, but there is evidence that the jejunal transport system is saturated in the patients but not in controls. In cystinuric patients there is an increase of urinary piperidine derived from cadaverine and of pyrrolidine from putrescine (Fig. 30-2), whereas in normal persons there is a smaller increase of urinary piperidine only. This suggests that the large dose of lysine has competed with arginine for intestinal absorption, and that increased amounts of arginine from the diet are reaching the colon. These experiments show that there is a jejunal as well as a renal tubular transport defect in cystinuria and that the condition is closely allied to Hartnup disease, in which a dual transport defect has been conclusively proved [195].

Asatoor et al. [18] obtained similar results after arginine ingestion, and London and Foley [166] showed that plasma cystine rose less after oral cystine in cystinuric patients than in normal controls. By contrast, the absorption of cysteine was completely normal [87]. Jejunal mucosa obtained by peroral biopsy from type I cystinuric patients failed to concentrate ^{14}C-labeled lysine, ornithine, arginine, and cystine [177, 261]. Similar cells from normal controls maintain a high concentration gradient of the amino acids between the tissue and the ambient fluid.

Symptoms and Signs of the Disease. As in most conditions involving increased amino acid excretion, the urinary loss of amino acids in cystinuria is of negligible nutritional significance. Lysine is the only essential amino acid excreted, although arginine has also been thought to be essential in the growing infant and child. The minimum daily requirement of lysine for the average adult has been estimated as 1.6 gm., more than that which may be lost in the urine in a patient with severe cystinuria. A good protein diet, however, provides about 6.7 gm. of lysine daily, and therefore the average loss in cystinuric patients is insufficient to cause lysine deficiency. Pos-

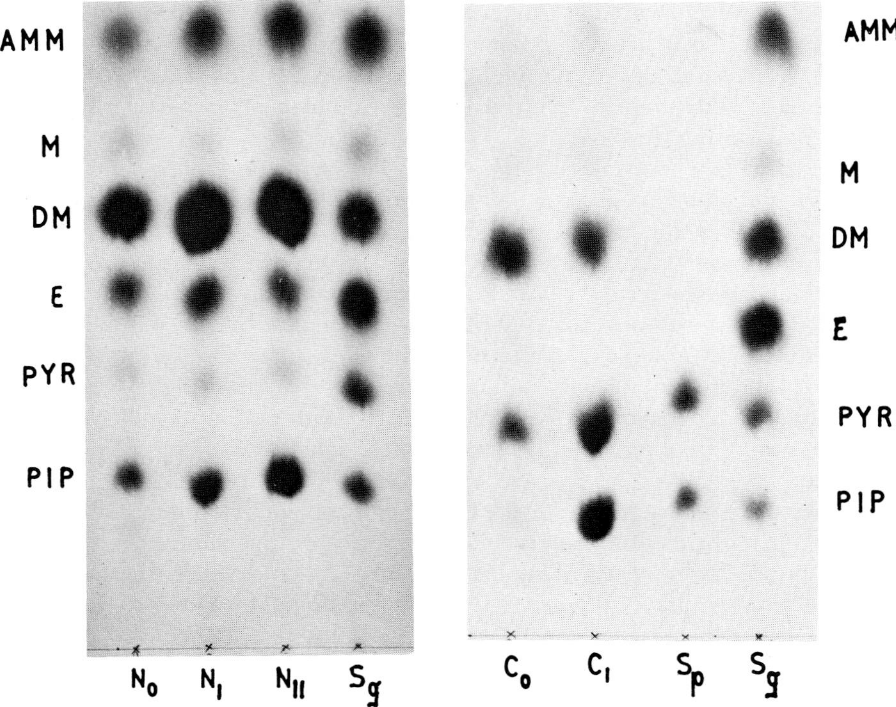

Figure 30-2. Chromatograms of urine from a normal subject and a cystinuric patient before and after ingestion of lysine by mouth. One-way chromatography of the dinitrophenyl derivatives of urinary amines; chromatogram photographed in ultraviolet light. DNP derivatives of six substances are found in normal urine by this technic: piperidine (PIP), pyrrolidine (PYR), ethylamine (E), dimethylamine (DM), methylamine (M), and ammonia (AMM). The recovery of ammonia is low by this method. N_0, normal subject before lysine; N_I and N_{II}, 10 to 12 hours and 12 to 24 hours after lysine, respectively. C_0, cystinuric patient before lysine; C_I, 10 to 12 hours after lysine. S_g is a mixed standard of the six DNP derivatives; S_p is a mixed standard of the derivatives of piperidine and pyrrolidine only. In the normal, there is a slight increase of piperidine excretion, whereas in the cystinuric patient there is a great increase of both piperidine and pyrrolidine.

sibly cystinuria might be of nutritional importance in individuals consuming unsatisfactory low-protein diets. The aminoaciduria is of major clinical importance because of the insolubility of cystine and the consequent liability to form cystine calculi. Calculi occur in about 3 per cent of cystinuric patients, and probably the majority of the homozygotes of either the "recessive" or the "incompletely recessive" types of the disease are liable to form calculi. Cystine calculi comprise about 1 per cent of all urinary stones, but the proportion is certainly much higher in children.

The solubility of cystine is dependent on pH, and is about 300 mg. per liter in acid solution. Solubility changes very little from pH 4.5 to 7.0, but increases to about 500 mg. per liter at pH 7.5, and is much higher at pH 8.0. The solubility in urine is higher than in water, and most concentrated urine samples will dissolve about 150 mg. per liter more cystine than the figures just mentioned. Cystine stones are therefore unlikely to form in heterozygotes, who usually excrete less than 300 mg. of cystine daily. (The normal daily output of cystine is 40 to 80 mg. in adults.)

In homozygotes, however, with their higher excretion rates, the urine is liable to become supersaturated with cystine during the night [69], when urine is both more concentrated and more acid than during the day.

In cystinuric patients who eventually form stones the initial symptoms of lithiasis occur most commonly between the ages of 20 and 25 years. The range is wide, however, and cases in infancy and in senility have been recorded [217]. Renal stones are bilateral in about 25 per cent of cases. Cystine calculi form a considerable proportion of urinary stones occurring in childhood, and large vesical calculi in this age group are especially likely to be cystine stones.

Cystine stones are radiopaque, the opacity to x-rays being due to their sulfur content and not to calcium present as impurity. Many cystine calculi are almost pure cystine, the ash value often being less than 1 per cent. Large vesical calculi, however, may become coated with calcium phosphate, and then the ash value may be as high as 25 per cent [217]. The roentgenologic density is less than that of most renal stones, pure cystine calculi being about 2.7 times as opaque to x-rays as an equal thickness of water, in contrast with figures of 3.2 for magnesium ammonium phosphate stones and 5.7 for calcium phosphate stones. Small cystine calculi, therefore, may occasionally be undetected by x-ray examination, the proportion not diagnosable being about 10 per cent. These are almost always in the ureters, a situation where more radiopaque stones, also, may easily be missed by radiologic examination. Very occasionally urinary stones in known cystinuric patients may contain no cystine [217].

All urinary stones should be tested routinely for cystine by use of the cyanide-nitroprusside reaction. The stone should be powdered and a small quantity of the fine powder placed in a test tube. One drop of concentrated ammonia solution should be added, followed by one drop of 5% sodium cyanide. After an interval of five minutes, three drops of 5% sodium nitroprusside are added. The presence of cystine is shown by the immediate development of a characteristic deep cherry-red color.

The symptoms of cystine urolithiasis are similar to those of other types of calculous disease of the urinary tract except for increased tendency to recurrent calculi. Men and women are equally liable to be affected by cystinuria, but, as is usual in urolithiasis, the effects are more serious in men. The average age at death before 1960 in males afflicted with cystine calculi was only 37 years [217], whereas the life span of female patients was only slightly reduced.

Boström and Hambraeus [34] have recently reported on the clinical aspects of 80 Swedish cases of homozygous cystinuria. The initial symptom in 70 per cent of the cases was lumbar pain or renal colic, and symptoms due to pyelonephritis in 25 per cent. Presentation due to hematuria or to retention of urine was unusual. The first symptom occurred in the majority of patients in the third decade, but a substantial number of the cases presented in childhood; in a minority symptoms occurred for the first time in old age. The average age at death was 51.7 years in males and 64.4 years in females.

Treatment. It is easier to prevent the formation of cystine calculi than to treat established cases. However, most cases of cystinuria require no treatment, as 97 per cent of cystinuric persons are heterozygotes with a harmless and symptomless biochemical anomaly. All homozygotes should be treated whether or not stones are present. Homozygotes can be recognized by biochemical and family studies. These individuals excrete large amounts of cystine as well as of the other three amino acids involved in the transport defect. Cystine output in adults is more than 300 mg. per day, and at all age groups is more than 200 mg. of cystine per gram of creatinine output. Reduction of protein intake has to be extreme before excretion of cystine is significantly lowered [69], and therefore is not recommended as a practical therapeutic measure.

The most important aspect of treatment is the maintenance of a high urine volume by a large fluid intake. This is especially important at night. Two pints of fluid should be taken before retiring, and the same amount repeated when the patient is awakened by the stimulus of a full bladder or by an alarm in the small hours of the morning. The value of alkalinization is more controversial. Alkalinization is probably of no value unless the night urine can be kept at a pH higher than 7.5. This can be accomplished with the use of sodium bicarbonate only if the intake is large, generally more than 10 gm. daily. Patients can more easily take large doses of alkaline sodium salts without adverse cardiac effects if there is simultaneous restriction of intake of sodium chloride. Obviously, ingestion of large amounts of sodium bicarbonate is less liable to cause serious side effects in younger cystinuric patients. In older patients the development of edema, congestive heart failure, or hypertension may make effective alkalinization therapy undesirable or even impossible.

Cystine stones may form very rapidly; there may be change from a negative x-ray to a positive in as short a period as six months. It is therefore probably desirable that routine abdominal x-ray examination should be repeated at about yearly intervals, but pyelography should be reserved for patients showing clinical evidence of urolithiasis or having doubtful shadows on routine x-ray. Known heterozygotes in families afflicted with the "incompletely recessive" type of the disease should be advised to marry individuals who are normal in this respect. The chance of marrying another known heterozygous carrier is usually about 1 in 600, but is much higher in a consanguineous union.

In cases where the high fluid regimen has failed, D-penicillamine therapy is indicated [58, 59]. Penicillamine is dimethylcysteine which reacts with cystine to form a soluble mixed disulfide and cysteine:

$$\begin{aligned}&SH\cdot C(CH_3)_2\cdot CH(NH_2)\cdot COOH\\&+(COOH\cdot CH[NH_2]\cdot CH_2\cdot S)_2\\&\rightarrow COOH\cdot CH\cdot(NH_2)\cdot CH_2\cdot SH\\&+COOH\cdot CH(NH_2)\cdot C(CH_3)_2\cdot\\&S\cdot S\cdot CH_2\cdot CH(NH_2)\cdot COOH\end{aligned}$$

At a dosage of about 2 gm. of D-penicillamine daily, the reaction is in favor of formation of the mixed disulfide and only small amounts of insoluble cystine are excreted. Unfortunately, D-penicillamine, although much less toxic than the L-isomer, frequently causes severe side effects. Rashes and fever are common, and occasionally severe blood dyscrasias have been reported. The drug causes a pyridoxal deficiency by formation of a thiazolidine derivative of the vitamin and the drug [15, 131], but this rarely results in obvious symptoms. Glomerular damage, with severe proteinuria and a nephrotic syndrome, is comparatively frequent, but is fortunately reversible on stopping the drug. Loss of taste occurs in almost all treated patients. Toxic effects from D-penicillamine are more severe in patients with cystinuria than in those with hepatolenticular degeneration. There is some evidence that the large stores of copper in the latter condition reduce toxic effects. Acetylpenicillamine [255] is equally effective and is probably somewhat less toxic, as it does not cause pyridoxal deficiency and is less liable to cause trace-metal deficiency, because it is a less potent chelating agent.

HARTNUP DISEASE

Hartnup disease was first described in 1956 by Baron et al. [22], the name being derived from the surname of the first family studied, four individuals from a sibship of nine being affected. Since then, over 20 patients have been recognized [132]. The disease, however, has an interest and importance out of all proportion to its apparent rarity. The condition is due to a recessive mendelian hereditary factor and therefore is not passed from generation to generation, and there is an increased incidence in consanguineous unions.

Hartnup disease is characterized by two apparently unrelated clinical features, a pellagrous rash and attacks of cerebellar ataxia, together with typical biochemical abnormalities. The primary disorder is an amino acid transport defect involving the proximal renal tubule and the jejunum, of which the latter is clinically the more important site. Unlike most hereditary disorders, the disease shows a succession of exacerbations and remissions, and becomes less serious in adolescence and adult life.

Clinical Signs and Symptoms. The pellagra clinically resembles the dietary type. There is a pigmented rash of the face and extremities, where it shows a typical "glove and stocking" distribution. There is usually a sharp line of demarcation between affected and unaffected skin, and the rash is made worse by exposure to sunshine. In severe cases there is a moist eczematous type of rash, with serous exudate and a tendency to crust formation. Later the skin becomes dry, scaly, and deeply pigmented. The rash responds to treatment with nicotinamide, and probably as rapidly as in pellagra due to dietary deficiency.

The neurologic signs and symptoms are remarkable for their variability over comparatively short intervals of time, and for the completeness of the patient's recovery. They consist of short-lived attacks, rarely lasting more than a few days or at the most a few weeks, of cerebellar ataxia. There is unsteadiness of the gait, shakiness of the hands, and a general clumsiness and ataxia which becomes worse if the patient tries to perform delicate coordinated movements. There may be involuntary choreiform movements of the limbs, and marked tremor of the outstretched hands. There is often diplopia and particularly poor power of convergence of the eyes, combined with a coarse nystagmus both horizontally and vertically. An especially characteristic feature is a tendency to "falling attacks" — that is, the patient suddenly loses all power in the limbs and falls to the ground without any disturbance of consciousness. After these attacks the limbs feel stiff and weak, and the patient is unable to resume walking until he has had a considerable period of rest.

Usually the physical signs are characteristic of disturbance of cerebellar function, but in the more severe attacks pyramidal signs may be found. There is then spasticity of all limbs, with exaggeration of tendon reflexes, extensor plantar response, and bilateral ankle clonus. The cerebrospinal fluid is usually normal, but there may be some increase of protein content during the height of a severe attack. During the attacks the patient is often irritable and depressed, and occasionally there may even be suicidal tendencies. There is diminution of power of concentration and headache, but usually no delusions, hallucinations, or disorientation. Between attacks there are no abnormal neurologic or psychiatric symptoms or signs. Intelligence is little, if at all, impaired, and possibly physicians who have reported intellectual impairment in this disease have too high a standard of reference. In some of the families the least intelligent member has been unaffected by the disease [22].

Biochemical Abnormalities. The bizarre symptoms and signs of Hartnup disease can be completely explained by the known amino acid transport defect in the proximal tubular cells and the jejunum. Related defects elsewhere in the body may, however, be discovered by future investigation. The renal defect is similar to that of cystinuria except that a completely different amino acid group is involved. It is a specific amino acid defect, and, as in cystinuria, there is no other defect of either proximal or distal tubular function. In particular there is no glycosuria, no phosphate leak, no increase of uric acid clearance, and no proteinuria. There is thus a specific defect of amino acid transport of genetic origin, which corresponds to Beyer's group 2 amino acids in tubular transport in the dog, just as the defect in cystinuria corresponds to Beyer's group 1.

Plasma amino acid concentrations are normal except for slight reduction of threonine, serine, glutamine, and asparagine [60], probably secondary to abnormal losses of these substances in the urine. The clearance and excretion of most amino acids, with a few important exceptions, is greatly increased. The exceptions are the amino acids concerned in the transport defect of cystinuria — that is, cystine, lysine, arginine, and ornithine, together with proline and glycine. In particular, there is gross increase of urinary glutamine, asparagine, histidine, serine, and threonine, with less marked but still very abnormal outputs of phenylalanine, tyrosine, and tryptophan. The renal clearances of the affected amino acids are correspondingly high, tubular reabsorption of the amino acids most prominently involved being about 30 to 50 per cent of the amount filtered. In most aminoacidurias, despite a gross loss of amino acids in the urine, the defect is of diagnostic and theoretical interest only, and is of insignificant nutritional or direct clinical importance. This general rule may be inapplicable in patients consuming inadequate protein diets, and, as previously stated, a striking exception occurs in some persons with cystinuria because of the insolubility of cystine. Tryptophan loss in the urine in Hartnup disease is another exception, since this contributes to the pellagra of the disease. The urine in Hartnup disease also contains increased quantities of indolic substances, but this abnormality has been proved to be secondary to the jejunal defect of the disease.

The jejunal defect in Hartnup disease is of greater clinical importance than the renal defect, but the latter is more easily recognized and therefore of greater value in diagnosis. There is probably a generalized defect of amino acid transport in the jejunum similar to that in the proximal tubule, but as yet this has been proved to occur only in the case of tryptophan.

Evidence of defective tryptophan absorption in the jejunum is based on four separate but related observations [195]:

1. After large doses of L-tryptophan by mouth, unchanged tryptophan can be detected in the feces of patients suffering from Hartnup disease but not in the feces of normal controls.

2. Plasma tryptophan levels after ingestion of the amino acid are raised to a lesser extent but remain higher for a longer period in persons with Hartnup disease than in normal subjects.

3. Following tryptophan ingestion, patients with Hartnup disease excrete abnormally large amounts of products of bacterial breakdown of tryptophan in the urine since increased quantities of the amino acid escape absorption in the jejunum and reach the colon (Figs. 30-3, 30-4). Some cases may show a high excretion of indolic substances on a normal diet, while in less severe cases the excretion without excess tryptophan ingestion is in the high normal range.

There are probably three different routes of bacterial degradation of tryptophan, all leading to characteristic urinary end products. (1) The most important is breakdown to indole by the enzyme tryptophanase. The indole is then absorbed, hydroxylated in liver cells to indoxyl, and finally converted to indoxyl sulfate or indican. (2) A smaller amount is converted to indolyl-3-acetic acid by oxidative deamination. This is absorbed and excreted partly as the free acid and partly as the glutamine conjugate. The bacterial side of this series of reactions is conversion to tryptamine by decarboxylation, followed by oxidation to indolylacetic acid by monoaminoxidase within body cells. (3) A small amount of tryptophan is converted by bacteria to indolyl-3-propionic

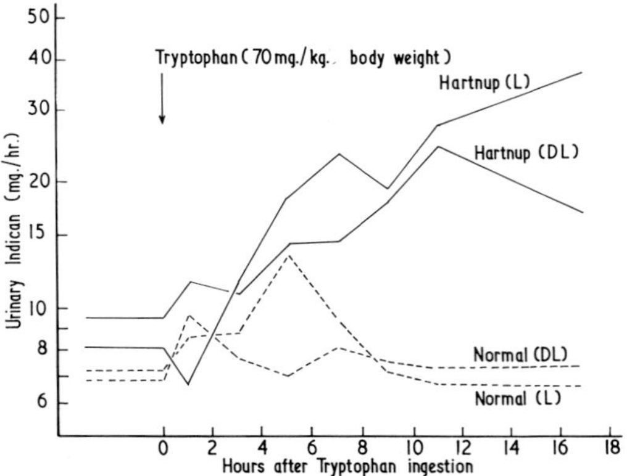

Figure 30-3. Mean excretion of indican in patients with Hartnup disease and in normal subjects after ingestion of either L-tryptophan or DL-tryptophan (70 mg. per kilogram of body weight) by mouth. In Hartnup disease, indican excretion is both abnormally high and abnormally prolonged owing to unabsorbed tryptophan reaching the colon and being degraded by colonic bacteria to indole.

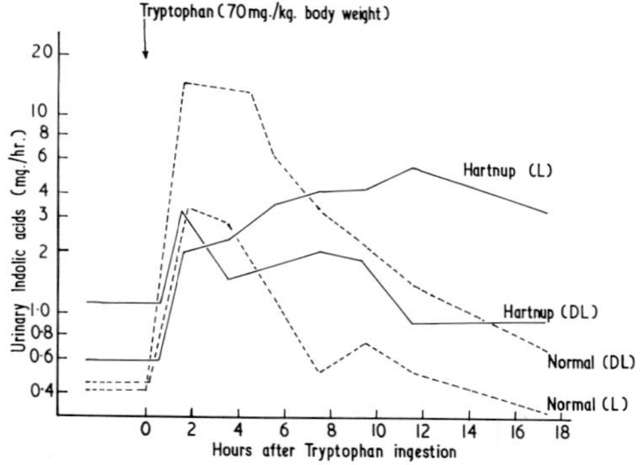

Figure 30-4. Mean excretion of indolic acids in patients with Hartnup disease and in normal subjects after ingestion of either L-tryptophan or DL-tryptophan (70 mg. per kilogram of body weight). In normal subjects there is a much greater output of indolic acids after DL- than after L-tryptophan because absorbed D-tryptophan is chiefly metabolized to indolyllactic and indolylacetic acids. In Hartnup disease, excretion of indolic acids is abnormally high and abnormally prolonged after L-tryptophan because of bacterial degradation of unabsorbed tryptophan in the colon. By contrast, after DL-tryptophan, excretion of indolic acids is below that in normal subjects because D-tryptophan is not absorbed from the jejunum in cases of Hartnup disease and is passed unchanged in the feces.

acid. After absorption this acid is partially oxidized within body cells to indolyl-3-acrylic acid, which is excreted partly unchanged and partly as the conjugate, indolylacrylylglycine.

Most patients with Hartnup disease excrete abnormally large amounts of indican, indolyl-3-acetic acid and indolylacetylglutamine. After tryptophan ingestion they excrete still larger amounts of these indolic substances for at least 24 hours (Figs. 30-3, 30-4) and also considerable quantities of indolyl-3-acrylic acid and indolylacrylylglycine. Pretreatment with chlortetracycline (Aureomycin), which is a somewhat ineffective intestinal antibiotic, causes a marked fall in indican excretion [22] but has little effect on output of indolic acids and their conjugates. By contrast, the more effective antibiotic, oral neomycin, almost completely inhibits the excretion of all the abnormal indolic compounds, but naturally has no effect on the aminoaciduria.

4. The final proof of abnormal tryptophan absorption in the jejunum in Hartnup disease is of especial theoretical interest with respect to the mechanisms of amino acid transport. There is good evidence that the abnormal enantiomorph D-tryptophan is almost completely unabsorbed in Hartnup disease. When this amino acid is ingested by normal subjects, there is considerable excretion of indolyl-3-lactic acid derived from indolyl-3-pyruvic acid, which is produced by action of D-amino acid oxidase. In Hartnup disease no indolyl-3-lactic acid is formed and large amounts of D-tryptophan appear unchanged in the feces. This suggests that D-tryptophan normally combines with the carrier substance responsible for transport of the L-amino acid, agreeing with the results of animal experiments in which it has been shown there is competition for jejunal transport between L-histidine and D-methionine, and between D-histidine and L-methionine [133, 134].

Absorption of other amino acids has not been investigated in detail. Patients with

Hartnup disease excrete large quantities of phenols and of phenolic acids in the urine, and the excretion is still further increased after tyrosine ingestion [195]. However, the variation in normal subjects is so large that cases of Hartnup disease often fall within the upper limits of the normal range. Chromatography of fecal extracts from cases of Hartnup disease shows considerable excess of other amino acids besides tryptophan [16, 237]. There is thus considerable presumptive evidence of a more generalized jejunal transport defect, exactly similar to that present in the proximal tubule.

Causation of the Signs and Symptoms. A normal adult requires about 20 mg. daily of nicotinamide, and about half of this is derived from intake of the vitamin in the diet and half from dietary tryptophan. Dietary pellagra is therefore particularly liable to occur when there is deficient intake both of nicotinamide and of tryptophan.

There are three known metabolic causes of pellagra unassociated with dietary deficits; in each of these types there is reduced conversion of tryptophan to nicotinamide.

1. In severe cases of the carcinoid syndrome, pellagra occurs [37, 249] because a large amount of dietary tryptophan is hydroxylated to 5-hydroxytryptophan and is therefore unavailable to the kynurenine-nicotinamide pathway.

2. After prolonged treatment with large doses of isoniazid [126, 178, 280], pellagra may occur because of inhibition of pyridoxin, which is a coenzyme in the kynurenine-nicotinamide pathway.

3. Pellagra may occur in Hartnup disease because of deviation of tryptophan from the kynurenine-nicotinamide pathway from three separate causes: tryptophan is excreted in excess in urine, a considerable proportion is unabsorbed by the jejunum and escapes unchanged in the feces, and finally part is degraded by colonic bacteria to indole and indolic acids.

The cause of the cerebellar attacks is less certain and is the subject of active current research. The phasic and temporary nature of the disorder without permanent sequelae strongly suggests an intoxication of the central nervous system. In some cases the attacks have been precipitated by diarrhea, which would increase bacterial degradation of amino acids by colonic bacteria. The exact nature of the toxic substance produced can only be speculative at present. Possible toxic compounds formed by bacterial degradation of amino acids include indole, tryptamine, phenylethylamine, tyramine, histamine, and other toxic amines produced by bacterial decarboxylases.

Treatment. Hartnup disease is fortunately not serious unless the patient is in relapse, and appears to improve with advancing age. The attacks are most frequent in childhood and become less severe and occur at longer intervals in adolescence and adult life. The patients should be advised to avoid undue exposure to sunshine, as this undoubtedly causes exacerbations of the rash. If pellagra occurs, the patients should be treated by supplements of nicotinamide as in dietary pellagra. In the past the attacks of cerebellar ataxia have been allowed to cease spontaneously, but now that the jejunal abnormalities of the disease have been elucidated, treatment to reduce bacterial degradation of amino acids in the colon should be tried. A regimen similar to that used in the treatment of hepatic coma [245] may be of benefit. The patient is given nothing except water or sweetened fruit drinks by mouth, and nutrition is maintained by parenteral glucose infusions. In severe cases the stomach and colon should be washed out and the colonic contents temporarily sterilized by administration of 5 gm. of neomycin daily by mouth. Oral sodium bicarbonate in solution would probably be beneficial because alkalosis increases the rate of excretion of some indolic acids [196], and an acid reaction within the colonic contents favors bacterial decarboxylation. Obviously, certain drugs would theoretically be unusually toxic in Hartnup disease and should be avoided if possible. Iproniazid would be especially toxic for two reasons: it is a potent monoaminoxidase inhibitor and it also reduces the rate of detoxication reactions by interference with microsomal enzyme systems in the liver [39]. In particular, it delays hydroxylation of indole to indoxyl [192]. Other monoaminoxidase inhibitors, which might conceivably be prescribed for the mental depression occurring in the exacerbations of the disease, should be avoided, and prolonged use of isoniazid for intercurrent tuberculous infection should be combined with supplements both of pyridoxine and of nicotinamide.

Unsolved Problems. Research on the pathophysiology of this interesting disease, which occupies a key position in disorders of amino acid transport, has been hampered by the rarity of the condition and the undesirability of subjecting clinically well subjects to prolonged and repeated periods of investigation. Future research which should be particularly rewarding would be a more thorough examination of heterozygous parents of patients with the disease, further exploration of the amino acid transport defects, and clarification of the causes of the neurologic symptoms and signs. In particular, it would be of especial importance to know whether the affected neutral amino acids are concentrated by intestinal mucosa obtained by peroral biopsy. It is as yet unknown whether active transport is defective, similar to that proved to exist for the dibasic acids and cystine in type I cases of cystinuria.

IMINOGLYCINURIA

This renal tubular anomaly seems to cause no clinical disability [114, 238, 258] but is of great physiological interest. Plasma concentrations of proline, hydroxyproline, and glycine are normal, but the clearances and urinary output of all three amino acids are greatly increased. More than 60 per cent of the filtered load of the three amino acids is, however, reabsorbed by the proximal tubule cells, suggesting that there is a dual reabsorptive mechanism, and that only the quantitatively less important one is absent in the affected individuals. In heterozygotes the clearances and output of proline and hydroxyproline are normal, while those of glycine are intermediate between the homozygotes and normal controls. Some of the families showed a similar jejunal transport defect of the affected amino acids [114, 201], others did not [238]. It now seems probable that the affected members of the family described by de Vries et al. [71] in which dominant heredity for hyperglycinuria was described, were in fact heterozygotes for iminoglycinuria.

Nonspecific Hereditary Disorders of Amino Acid Transport

Diseases classified under this heading are the Lignac-Fanconi syndrome, the adult Fanconi syndrome, and Lowe's syndrome.

LIGNAC-FANCONI SYNDROME

This syndrome is a disease of childhood due to a recessive autosomal gene. It is characterized by deposits of cystine in various organs including the kidney, by renal tubular defects of a generalized and nonspecific character, by dwarfism, infantilism, and rickets, and usually by death from renal failure.

History. The association of rickets with abnormalities of renal function was recognized by Lucas [169] about 80 years ago. Although Abderhalden [2], at the beginning of the present century, described the first example of cystine storage disease, the earliest detailed account was given about 20 years later by Lignac [160–162], who clearly recognized the hereditary nature of the condition. Fanconi [83] differentiated the condition from classic renal rickets or azotemic renal osteodystrophy. Since then many excellent reviews have been made available [30, 75, 180].

Hereditary Aspects, Incidence, and Prognosis. The disease is a typical example of a recessive hereditary disease of metabolism. It is approximately as common a condition as phenylketonuria, being found in about 1 in every 40,000 births [30]. This suggests that about 1 in every 100 individuals is a heterozygous carrier of the gene, with the proportion greatly increased among children from consanguineous unions. The disease is seldom recognized before the child is 6 months old, and carries a poor prognosis, death occurring in childhood or adolescence. Since infantilism is a feature of adolescent survivors, all cases are probably derived from the union of heterozygous carriers. The patient described by Cogan [51, 52] is almost certainly an example of a type of cystinosis quite different from that of the Lignac-Fanconi syndrome. This patient was a healthy male, aged 23, in whom cystine deposits in the conjunctivae were found at routine ophthalmic examination. Cystine deposits were later found in the bone marrow, but there were no other features of the Lignac-Fanconi syndrome.

Pathogenesis. The pure recessive heredity of the Lignac-Fanconi syndrome suggests deficiency or absence of a single protein, probably an enzyme. The exact nature of this deficiency, however, remains unknown.

The tubular defects are quite different from those of cystinuria or Hartnup disease. They are much more generalized and more variable from case to case, and therefore are more likely to be due to nonspecific tubular damage. In contrast to cystinuria, in which there is no known histopathologic abnormality, there are two pathologic changes in the tubules in cases of Lignac-Fanconi syndrome: a "swan-neck" deformity of the juxtaglomerular portion of the proximal tubule [49] and cystinosis. The "swan-neck" deformity is probably a secondary change since it is not pathognomonic of Lignac-Fanconi syndrome but also occurs in the separate conditions of adult Fanconi syndrome and the proximal tubular lesion associated with congenital nephrotic syndrome [112].

There has been considerable controversy regarding the precise connection between cystinosis and the proximal tubular lesion, some authorities having considered them to be separate, unrelated abnormalities. A complete spectrum of cases exists, however, ranging from patients with apparently pure cystinosis and without prominent defects of proximal tubular function, through the more common variety, in which there is a combination of the two lesions, to patients in whom proximal tubular damage occurs alone and cystine deposits are not detected even at autopsy. This variation could be explained by the variable manifestations of a gene which causes nonspecific cellular damage and has effects on various organs which differ from patient to patient. This unified view of the disease regards cystinosis as the only known manifestation in the affected cells of a hereditary defect which produces anomalies of transport in the highly specialized renal tubular cells. An abnormality of transport of amino acids across the cell membrane would alter the concentration of amino acids within intracellular water. Cystine in high concentration might easily precipitate from the intracellular fluid, which is more acidic than plasma, but obviously the extent and distribution of the precipitation would vary from patient to patient.

Clinical Symptoms and Signs. The course of the disease is variable, and cases may conveniently be divided into acute and chronic types. The two types, however, are not fundamentally different disorders, and an analogy occurs in another recessive hereditary disease of metabolism, hepatolenticular degeneration, which is also best described as having an acute or a chronic clinical course.

Children with acute cases of Lignac-Fanconi syndrome are usually first recognized as abnormal between the ages of six months and one year. The commonest presenting symptoms are vomiting, refusal of food, constipation, and failure to gain weight. These are nonspecific symptoms of a variety of infantile conditions which are characterized by "a failure to thrive." The infant is usually excessively thirsty and takes water greedily, whereas more nutritious fluids are obstinately refused. There is thus polyuria, which at first is probably secondary to the polydipsia. On examination the infant is found to be undersized and underweight, and often shows clinical evidence of rickets. Routine urine testing suggests the correct diagnosis at this early stage of the disease. There is glycosuria, and usually slight proteinuria and pyuria. More detailed examination shows the characteristic aminoaciduria of the syndrome.

Signs of dehydration from vomiting and insufficient fluid intake are common. The skin may lose its normal elasticity and the extremities are cold and sometimes cyanosed. An increase of blood urea or plasma nonprotein nitrogen at this early stage is never due to permanent glomerular damage, but is a secondary reversible manifestation of reduced renal circulation from salt deficiency and dehydration. There is often fever due to the intercurrent infections to which patients with acute cases of Lignac-Fanconi syndrome are abnormally susceptible. Starvation ketosis from vomiting and refusal of food is extremely common. This, in combination with the glycosuria, may result in a mistaken first diagnosis of infantile diabetes mellitus. Photophobia due to the ocular manifestations of the disease is a common early symptom. In summary, the child with acute Lignac-Fanconi syndrome is usually a puny, wizened, and unattractive infant, showing clinical evidence of rickets and dehydration; it is usually irritable and has a weak, plaintive cry, resenting interference and burying its head under the bedclothes from severe photophobia.

Death from chronic uremia is much less common in the acute than in the chronic type of Lignac-Fanconi syndrome. The child more often dies from intercurrent infections or metabolic upsets unassociated with uremia — for example, acidosis, dehydration, or hypokalemia — and occurring before renal destruction or fibrosis has become clinically important. Whatever the exact cause of death, the prognosis is always very poor, and the child usually dies before the age of 10 years.

The chronic form of the syndrome is not usually diagnosed until about the age of 2 years. The severe constitutional symptoms which are so prominent in the acute form are rarely seen until the terminal stages of the condition. The patient usually presents as a problem of rickets resistant to vitamin D, easily distinguished from the more common pure vitamin-D-resistant rickets by examination of the urine. Dwarfing is a constant clinical sign, and overt rickets is common before treatment is commenced. Genu valgum is the most common skeletal deformity, but genu varum, coxa vara, saber tibia, a rickety rosary of the ribs, and kyphoscoliosis of the thoracic spine may often occur.

Photophobia, due to cystine deposits in the conjunctivae and cornea, occurs in about half the patients. A peripheral retinopathy has recently been described, and seems to occur in all cases of the disease [279]. There are areas of depigmentation, with a superimposed deposition of fine pigment clumps. The abnormality does not seem to impair visual acuity or cause restriction of the visual fields. The retinal pigmentary abnormality precedes the corneal changes and therefore is of especial diagnostic importance in early infancy.

The liver and spleen are often easily palpable from the changes associated with cystine deposits. Urinary abnormalities are less extreme than in the acute form of the syndrome — proteinuria, glycosuria, and aminoaciduria all being less prominent but usually easily detectable on careful analysis. Starvation ketosis is rare until the terminal stages of the condition, when uremic vomiting and anorexia occur.

Uremic symptoms and signs are prominent in the last year or two of life, usually when the child is between 10 and 14 years of age. Vomiting, diarrhea, and hemorrhagic manifestations (e.g., epistaxis, bruising, and purpura) are usually present, and there is often associated hypertension, causing retinopathy and left ventricular failure. Severe uremic acidosis, with hyperpnea and deepening stupor and coma, occurs immediately before death. With progressive fall of the glomerular filtration rate in the last year or two of life, glycosuria and aminoaciduria steadily decrease and may, in fact, be completely absent in the terminal stages of the syndrome.

Biochemical Abnormalities and Diagnosis. CYSTINOSIS. The intracellular fluid of cells in which there are cystine deposits must presumably be saturated with cystine. There must obviously be either excess transport of cystine into the cell, or diminished transport from the cell into the extracellular fluid, or increased intracellular production of cystine from other amino acids (e.g., methionine) or diminished utilization or degradation of intracellular cystine. By analogy with the renal tubular abnormality, it is likely that other amino acids are involved in the cellular defect, cystine being prominent clinically because of its insolubility in relatively acidic intracellular fluid.

Research has been hampered by the difficulties of biopsy of affected tissue in sufficient quantity. Muscle, the tissue most available for bulk biopsy, is invariably unaffected in Lignac-Fanconi syndrome. The demonstration that white cells in the peripheral blood [146] are sometimes involved may be of great value in future research. The eye, lymph nodes, bone marrow, and the peripheral blood are the most available tissues in life to confirm the presence of cystinosis. A complaint of photophobia should lead to careful examination of the eye by the slit lamp, and in doubtful cases conjunctival biopsy may be useful. Cystine deposits in the eye may occasionally occur without a complaint of photophobia. Gross deposits are revealed by use of a hand lens combined with oblique illumination. Less severe cases require careful slit-lamp examination, and in young children adequate sedation or even anesthesia is usually necessary. Biopsies of lymph nodes and of bone marrow are useful diagnostic procedures. Renal biopsy has been used less often because of the difficulty of percutaneous renal biopsy in uncooperative children.

At autopsy, cystine crystals are found particularly in cells of the reticuloendothelial system. There is never any tissue reaction around naturally occurring cystine deposits in the disease, although injection of crystals experimentally produces a conspicuous reaction. The difference is probably explained by the intracellular localization of the crystals in the disease. In the liver the Kupffer cells are chiefly affected; the parenchymal cells more usually show fatty infiltration, but occasionally early signs of cirrhosis are present. Crystals are prominent in the spleen, lymph nodes, and red bone marrow.

Lymph node biopsy is the single most helpful method of diagnosing cystinosis in life. Most of the crystals occur in reticulum cells around lymph sinuses. Bone marrow trephine biopsy is much more reliable than aspiration biopsy as a diagnostic procedure, possibly because the latter method removes tissue admixed with excess blood in which cystine crystals are soluble. Cystine crystals are much less obvious in the kidneys than in the liver, spleen, lymph nodes, or bone marrow, and are more commonly found in the medulla than in the cortex. The characteristic lesion in the later stages of the chronic form of the disease is a diffuse interstitial fibrosis with associated tubular atrophy and glomerular changes. Severe hypertensive changes may occur in the renal vessels. Nephrocalcinosis is unusual, but occasionally may be a prominent feature [21]. The central nervous system is normal except for occasional cystine deposits in the choroidal plexuses.

Cystine crystals are birefringent to polarized light, a property which greatly helps their recognition in tissues or urine. Small crystals dissolve easily in distilled water, and therefore tissue suspected of containing cystine crystals should be fixed in absolute alcohol and stained with basic fuchsin in 50 per cent alcohol. Crystals in tissues rarely show the classic hexagonal plates characteristic of pure cystine. Recognition may require chromatography of deproteinized tissue extracts, or differential solubility tests. Although suspected crystals disappear from tissue on treatment with distilled water, they should be completely insoluble in water previously saturated with pure cystine.

In extracellular fluid and plasma, cystine predominates over cysteine, whereas in normal cells very little, if any, free cystine exists. The high intracellular cysteine-cystine ratio in normal cells reflects a strong intracellular reduction potential. Glutathione reacts with cystine by action of the enzyme cystine-glutathione-transhydrogenase to maintain the cystine-cysteine complex in the reduced form. The enzyme is not significantly reduced in cases of cystinosis [243]. Cystine crystals are only occasionally found in the leukocytes of peripheral blood, but the content of free cystine is about 80 times the normal value in homozygotes and six times the normal in heterozygotes [233]. Cystinotic leukocytes take up twice as much ^{35}S-labeled cysteine as control leukocytes [233]. Similar results were found in cultured fibroblasts from cases of the disease.

In summary no enzymatic defect has been found in this disease, and the basic abnormality seems likely to be a fault in the subcellular compartmentalization of cystine [243]. This hypothesis explains why cystinotic cells can remain viable despite a high intracellular content of cystine, a substance that is toxic and inhibitory to many enzyme systems.

RENAL TUBULAR DEFECTS. The abnormalities of renal tubular function are much more diffuse and variable than in cystinuria or Hartnup disease, and often involve distal as well as proximal tubular function. The excretion of most amino acids is moderately raised, especially that of alanine, valine, and cystine. Serine, glycine, proline, ornithine, glutamine, and asparagine are also excreted in considerable quantity. Involvement of the basic amino acids, and of glycine, cystine, and proline, distinguishes the aminoaciduria from the more specific type found in Hartnup disease. The plasma concentrations of amino acids are usually somewhat reduced because of the excessive urinary loss. Bickel and Smellie [31] originally thought that the aminoaciduria was partly due to increase of plasma levels, but later reports of Bickel [32] indicate some modification of his original opinion. Most investigators consider that the aminoaciduria of Lignac-Fanconi syndrome is entirely of renal origin and not of the overflow type. The clearances of the affected amino acids are correspondingly increased, but with diminution of the filtered load of amino acids in the later stages of terminal renal failure, amino acid excretion becomes much less prominent and may virtually disappear.

Renal glycosuria has been proved to be due to reduction of the total tubular reabsorptive capacity for glucose, rather than to heterogeneity of tubular function, which is usual when renal glycosuria is an isolated defect [148, 218]. It is of especial importance in diagnosis because urine is routinely tested for reducing substances, whereas tests for amino acids are performed only in more specialized circumstances. The frequent association of ketosis has led to erroneous diagnoses of diabetes mellitus. Renal phosphate leak and increase of uric acid clearance are diagnosed more by the finding of reduced plasma concentrations than by any increase of urinary excretion. The high phosphate clearance which is of especial importance in causation of the rickets is reduced to normal by appropriate therapy with calciferol.

In addition to proximal tubular defects, distal tubular damage is common, possibly because of the localization of renal cystine deposits in the renal medulla. There may be reduction of urinary concentrating power at a time when the blood urea is normal and the glomerular filtration rate is little reduced. This leads to the thirst and polyuria which are prominent features of the early stages of the acute type of the disease. Failure of excretion of hydrogen ion with inability to acidify the urine below pH 6.0 or 5.5 despite a systemic acidosis is common. Acid-base balance may be maintained by excess excretion of ammonia, but usually only with a sustained acidosis and with considerable reduction of arterial blood bicarbonate and pH. With progressive renal fibrosis in the more advanced stages there is progressive inability to synthesize and excrete ammonia in the urine. In these cases acidosis becomes extreme unless it is treated with appropriate supplements of sodium bicarbonate. Excess urinary potassium loss is common, and presumably the mechanisms are similar to those discussed in the section on renal tubular acidosis. There is associated hypokalemia with muscular weakness and electrocardiographic changes. Frank hypokalemic paralysis is comparatively rare in Lignac-Fanconi syndrome, but may occur when renal potassium loss is augmented by loss in vomit and in fluid stools. Sodium deficiency in the early stages is probably due more to gastrointestinal loss than to failure of the kidneys to conserve sodium. However, in the stage of renal failure, sodium loss in the urine becomes more prominent, and further reduction of the glomerular filtration rate by salt deficiency may augment the uremia primarily due to progressive renal fibrosis and destruction.

Treatment. Treatment is unfortunately symptomatic and does not in any way influence the poor prognosis of the disease. The rickets usually responds dramatically to calciferol therapy, although much larger doses than the physiologic amounts effective in dietary rickets are required. The dose should be large enough to produce healing that can be demonstrated radiologically and an increase of plasma phosphate to normal, with corresponding reduction of renal phosphate clearance, but should not be so large that it produces hypercalcemia. This dose may vary from 50,000 to 500,000 units of calciferol daily. Acidosis should be treated by appropriate supplements of sodium bicarbonate or sodium citrate. A modified Albright's solution [5] consisting of sodium citrate, 100 gm., and citric acid, 60 gm., made up to 1 liter with water is a popular prescription for alkaline salts. From 10 to 50 ml. four or five times daily will be required in most cases. While it is imperative to restore the plasma bicarbonate to normal in the early stages when the blood urea is normal, only partial correction should be used in the stage of terminal renal failure, owing to the risk of production of uremic tetany or convulsions. If there is hypokalemia or other evidence of potassium depletion, potassium bicarbonate or potassium citrate supplements should be substituted for an equivalent amount of sodium salts. In view of thirst and anorexia, special diets may be required during acute exacerbations, and sweetened citrated milk is especially valuable.

In the terminal uremic stages of the disease, azotemic renal osteodystrophy may replace the pure rachitic pathology of the skeleton of the earlier stages. Calciferol treatment is often still of value, but owing to greater risk of ectopic calcification as the plasma phosphate rises, the dose may have to be decreased and controlled with even greater care. The usual symptomatic treatment for uremia, including a reduced protein intake, will prolong life and give some relief of symptoms. Treatment will remain unsatisfactory, however, until measures that will delay or prevent the progressive cystine deposition in various tissues including the kidneys are available.

Few useful advances in therapy of the

Lignac-Fanconi disease have been made. Clayton and Patrick [50] advocated the use of penicillamine, which was claimed to reduce the high plasma pyruvate found in many cases of the condition and to improve the growth rate of the patients. In addition, it seemed possible, by analogy with the undoubted benefit of this drug in cystinuria, that it would reduce intracellular cystine deposits. A recent careful trial, both of pencillamine therapy and of the use of a diet low in cystine and methionine [56], has shown that neither procedure leads to any significant improvement. Plasma cystine concentration fell, but there was no effect on intracellular cystine and no clinical benefit.

A type of cystinosis has been described [51, 52, 158] in which there are no renal abnormalities but substantial deposits of cystine occur in other sites. This is a relatively benign condition, with no severe symptoms and no evidence to date that it will cause a significant reduction in life expectancy. Patients with the Lignac-Fanconi syndrome in terminal uremia might therefore be very suitable candidates for renal transplantation, and possibly the extensive cystine deposits in many body cells could reduce the intensity of the immune response to homotransplants. The disease is certainly due to an intracellular defect rather than to a circulating toxic factor, and therefore homotransplants would be unlikely to be involved in the disease process. In this respect the Lignac-Fanconi disease differs fundamentally from hyperoxaluria, where there is a generalized metabolic abnormality, and the high plasma oxalate results in damage to the transplanted organ equivalent to that which previously occurred in the patient's own kidneys.

ADULT FANCONI SYNDROME

This condition is quite different from the Lignac-Fanconi syndrome. Some of the cases have been shown to be due to a recessive hereditary factor, but there is no record of cases of adult Fanconi syndrome and of Lignac-Fanconi syndrome in the same family. Cystinosis does not occur in the adult Fanconi syndrome, and the prognosis with adequate treatment is excellent, the patients being rendered free of symptoms and showing no evidence of progressive deterioration.

Causation, Incidence, and Pathology. The cause of adult Fanconi syndrome is unknown, and, unlike the Lignac-Fanconi syndrome, which always seems to be due to a recessive gene, the condition may be due to other causes than a hereditary renal tubular defect. Cases associated with multiple myelomatosis will be considered separately since they are probably examples of toxic damage to the tubular cells. Dent [67] has published the most convincing example of recessive heredity in the adult Fanconi syndrome — namely, occurrence of the condition in three siblings. Adult Fanconi syndrome is very rare; Wallis and Engle [269], reviewing the cases described before 1957, were able to list only 18 cases. Hunt et al. [129] have now listed more than 40 acceptable cases, excluding patients in whom proximal tubular damage was clearly due to a known exogenous toxic agent; however, there was clear evidence of a hereditary cause in only 15 per cent of the total. They report a further family in which the inheritance was thought to be of the dominant type, as the abnormal urinary amino acid loss was transmitted through three generations. The occurrence of both recessive and dominant heredity suggests that there is more than one single gene defect involved in the causation of the syndrome, and the unknown cellular abnormality may not necessarily be identical in all hereditary examples of the condition.

Cystine deposits in tissues have never been found, and possibly the cellular damage is confined to the renal tubular cells. Clay et al. [49] described a "swan-neck" deformity of the proximal tubules in one case. Presumably this is not the primary lesion, as it also occurs in other proximal tubular syndromes, but is a secondary manifestation of cellular damage. There are generalized and variable defects of function both of the proximal and distal tubules, so presumably the hereditary cases are not due to absence of an enzyme specifically concerned with tubular transport systems.

Symptoms and Signs. The onset of the disease is in adult life, the mean age being 30 years. The usual presenting symptom is bone pain, usually in the back, hips, thighs, and legs. This is often accompanied by muscular weakness and the waddling gait typical of osteomalacia. Examination of asymptomatic siblings has occasionally shown that the typical urinary abnormalities may precede the clinical manifestations of the syndrome [67]. Radiologic examination of the skeleton shows changes typical of osteomalacia: reduced density of bone, biconcavity of vertebral bodies, pseudofractures (first described in a case of this syndrome by Milkman [190]), and sometimes a triradiate pelvis. In doubtful cases the diagnosis of osteomalacia can be confirmed by trephine biopsy of the iliac crest. Hypokalemic paralysis of muscle occasionally occurs, but is not so common or so severe as in renal tubular acidosis [198].

Biochemical Abnormalities. The biochemical abnormalities are typical of a generalized tubular defect, and include proteinuria of the tubular type [43], renal glycosuria, generalized aminoaciduria, high phosphate and uric acid clearances with reduced plasma levels of these two substances, reduced urinary concentrating power, reduced powers of acidification of the urine, and abnormal urinary potassium loss. Various combinations of these defects may occur in different cases, and nothing is gained by subdivision of this rare syndrome if some of the defects are absent. The glycosuria is due to reduction of the tubular maximal reabsorptive capacity for glucose, and not due to heterogeneity of nephrons, which is more common in pure renal glycosuria [149]. There may occasionally be excess excretion of acetoacetic acid due to a defect in reabsorption of this organic acid [198], which in combination with glycosuria may lead to a mistaken diagnosis of diabetes mellitus. There is usually reduction of tubular maximal secretory capacity for para-aminohippurate. Plasma amino acid concentration is normal, but there is a gross generalized aminoaciduria, with corresponding increase in amino acid clearance and reduction of tubular reabsorption. Glutamine, asparagine, alanine, proline, and glycine are usually the most prominent chromatographic spots [60]. Serine, cystine, valine, leucine, ornithine, lysine, tyrosine, and phenylalanine are also excreted in considerable quantity, and in general the chromatogram resembles that of a plasma ultrafiltrate. The clearance of many of the amino acids is only slightly less than the glomerular filtration rate. Defects of distal tubular function are especially variable, and when present are similar to those described under *Primary Renal Tubular Acidosis* (page 1121).

Treatment and Prognosis. The principles of treatment are similar to those described in the section on Lignac-Fanconi syndrome. The results of therapy are excellent, the osteomalacia responding dramatically as soon as calciferol therapy has increased plasma phosphate and reduced urinary phosphate clearance. Dosage must be controlled by the biochemical response. There is usually no evidence of progressive deterioration of renal function. Occasionally patients become resistant to calciferol therapy [60], but usually still respond to dihydrotachysterol. There is no tendency to nephrocalcinosis as in renal tubular acidosis, possibly because the continued aminoaciduria chelates calcium and prevents precipitation of calcium phosphate.

Presumably the unknown hereditary defect in the adult Fanconi syndrome only slowly produces proximal tubular damage. The defect causes no disability in childhood, and there is no evidence of infantile rickets in the history given by adult patients. The skeleton of the adult is more resistant to decalcification than the growing skeleton of the child, so presumably the abnormality is present for several years in the adult before clinical osteomalacia occurs. Fortunately the cellular damage is nonprogressive when the skeletal lesions are adequately treated. The progressive deterioration in Lignac-Fanconi syndrome is presumably due to the cystinosis, which fortunately is never seen in the adult syndrome.

LOWE'S SYNDROME (CEREBRO-OCULO-RENAL DYSTROPHY)

A few cases have been described of the association of renal tubular defects with mental retardation and severe congenital anomalies of the eyes. Although there is considerable variation from case to case, this is probably another separate nonspecific hereditary disorder of renal function with renal aminoaciduria. The first example was described by Lowe et al. [168] and in the succeeding eight years other instances were recorded [65, 175, 223]. The syndrome is probably due to a sex-linked recessive gene. The clinical symptoms and signs are more severe than in the Lignac-Fanconi syndrome, the abnormalities often being obvious at birth. There is frequently congenital glaucoma, sometimes referred to as buphthalmos. This has been shown to be due to anomalies of the canal of Schlemm or to synechia between the iris and the lens. The cornea is semiopaque and there is often a congenital cataract of both lenses. Naturally vision is usually seriously affected, the infant being totally blind or merely able to distinguish light from dark. If vision is less seriously affected, a coarse nystagmus and photophobia occurs. There is gross muscular hypotonia, sometimes associated with increase of body fat. There may be gross weakness and separation of the recti muscles with a severe umbilical hernia. After a few months, evidence of severe mental retardation becomes obvious. There is anorexia and general failure to thrive, the infant being considerably below the normal weight. Severe rickets which responds to calciferol therapy is usually present.

Biochemical Abnormalities. The tubular defects are characteristic of nonspecific damage, being both diffuse and variable. There is proteinuria of the tubular type, renal glycosuria, aminoaciduria, increased phosphate clearance with a reduction of plasma phosphate, and varied defects of distal tubular function including failure to concentrate and acidify the urine. The aminoaciduria resembles that of Lignac-Fanconi syndrome, but there is an especial increase of lysine and tyrosine.

A special feature that has not yet been satisfactorily investigated is a claim of an abnormal organic aciduria not accounted for by increase of urinary amino acids. This is somewhat difficult to investigate since the usual organic acid titration originally described by Van Slyke and Palmer [210, 265] becomes grossly inaccurate and misleading in the presence of an abnormal amino acid excretion. Urinary organic acids can be divided into several groups and these should always be investigated separately before a claim of an abnormal organic aciduria is made.

These groups include: (1) amino acids, most simply investigated by paper chromatography; (2) acetoacetic and β-hydroxybutyric acids, for which several simple methods of estimation are available; (3) nonketonic acids of the Krebs cycle, best investigated by paper chromatography [206] after column purification; (4) keto acids of the Krebs cycle and other keto acids, most simply investigated by paper chromatography of the dinitrophenylhydrazones [172]; (5) phenolic acids, which may be separated by paper chromatography after purification by extraction or absorption methods [12, 17]; and (6) indolic acids, for which several biochemical and chromatographic methods of investigation are available [62].

Interpretation is made more difficult by variation of excretion with acid-base balance [197] and by variation in diet and production of acids or their precursors by bacteria in the colon. The most convincing investigation supporting an abnormal organic aciduria in Lowe's syndrome is a report by Debré et al. [65] that one patient excreted a grossly increased amount of pyruvic acid, far in excess of the output of α-ketoglutaric acid. Normally the latter acid is in higher concentration than pyruvic acid in urine, although the reverse applies in plasma [172].

An informative review of Lowe's syndrome has recently been published [1]. A total of 70 acceptable cases has been recorded. Cataract formation is almost invariable, and nystagmus is found in most cases. Proteinuria of the tubular type with excretion particularly of a beta globulin occurs, the protein loss being variable from 50 to 4000 mg. per day. There are usually red cells, white cells, and granular casts in the urinary sediment. Hyperchloremic acidosis with a urinary defect typical of renal tubular acidosis is frequently found, but urinary concentrative ability is less often impaired. Urinary calcium is either normal or increased, and the skeletal defects include both osteoporosis and true rickets. Although there is almost always a severe generalized aminoaciduria, renal glycosuria is unusual.

There are no obvious pathologic changes in the kidneys during the first three months of life, but later the tubules are found to be abnormally dilated and contain proteinaceous casts, and after the age of 5 years there is progressive tubular atrophy. Glomerular changes are absent below the age of 5 years, but later some glomeruli were either fibrotic or hyalinized with thickening of the basement membrane. The brain shows atrophic changes with hydrocephalus and ventricular dilatation.

The prognosis of Lowe's syndrome is poor and treatment is unrewarding, as the patients are usually blind and stunted aments. The principles of treatment outlined for the Lignac-Fanconi syndrome may be of value in relieving symptoms and especially in curing the rickets. The children usually die in childhood of intercurrent infections or of progressive renal failure. In two cases recently described by McCance et al. [175] there was no aminoaciduria, but there was nephrocalcinosis and severe progressive renal failure.

Renal Aminoaciduria

TUBULAR DEFECTS DUE TO ENDOGENOUS POISONS

These syndromes include the tubular defects in galactosemia, Wilson's disease, nephrotic syndrome, multiple myeloma, and tyrosinemia.

Galactosemia. This is a recessive hereditary disease due to lack of the enzyme galactose 1-phosphate uridyl transferase in many tissues, including the liver, erythrocytes, and crystalline lens. The disease is rare; only about 75 cases have been reported. When on a milk diet, affected infants show an abnormally high plasma galactose concentration and gross galactosuria of the overflow type. The clinical effects are rather variable but include failure to thrive, anorexia, stunting of growth, mental retardation, enlargement of the liver, and cataract formation. There is a characteristic disorder of renal tubular function of the nonspecific type.

Rapid and dramatic improvement on a galactose- and lactose-free diet occurs, but symptoms recur if the child is given either of these sugars. There is an immediate galactosuria and increase of plasma galactose, with a slow and progressive development of aminoaciduria, which in one case [61] was still increasing after two weeks. Similarly the high amino acid output persists for several days after galactose is discontinued [61], whereas the galactosuria disappears more rapidly. There is especial increase of the small-molecular-weight amino acids, serine, glycine, alanine, and threonine, with less increase in glutamine, valine, leucine, isoleucine, and tyrosine. The increase in excretion of the branched-chain amino acids is less than in the Lignac-Fanconi and Lowe's syndromes. Plasma amino acids slightly increase during clinical relapse but not usually to above normal limits. The rise may possibly be due to temporary liver damage. Proteinuria of the tubular type is usually present but clears on treatment. The reducing substance in the urine is entirely galactose, renal glycosuria not being found, possibly because the high plasma concentrations of galactose cause a reduction of blood glucose with corresponding reduction of the amount in the glomerular filtrate.

The toxic compound producing the tubular damage is almost certainly galactose 1-phosphate rather than galactose itself. The slow increase of this substance within body cells accounts for the delay in development of the aminoaciduria although plasma concentrations of galactose have previously become stable at grossly high values. Galactose 1-phosphate interferes with metabolism of glucose within body cells by inhibiting phosphoglucomutase [153, 234, 247], which is essential for the interconversion of glucose 1-phosphate and glucose 6-phosphate.

Similar proximal tubular defects occur in hereditary fructose intolerance after fructose or sucrose ingestion [102, 152, 154]. There is a severe generalized aminoaciduria with a tubular type of proteinuria. The condition is due to lack of fructose 1-phosphate aldolase in many body cells, including those of the intestinal mucosa, liver, and renal tubules. The proximal tubular damage is probably due to accumulation of fructose 1-phosphate within tubule cells. As there is also considerable hepatic damage, increase of plasma amino acids may be found, leading to a mixed type of aminoaciduria, with both renal and overflow components. The renal abnormalities and other more serious effects rapidly respond to withdrawal of fructose and sucrose from the diet.

Wilson's Disease (Hepatolenticular Degeneration). This is a rare recessive hereditary disease of metabolism causing neurologic symptoms and signs, cirrhosis of the liver, and defects of renal tubular function. Bearn [24] has estimated the incidence to be 1 per 4,000,000 births, but it is more common in areas with a high consanguinity rate. The condition is probably due to abnormalities of synthesis of the copper-containing plasma protein ceruloplasmin. Most patients with Wilson's disease have less than 25 per cent of the normal content of ceruloplasmin, which is an active oxidase [25, 230]. A few, however, have a normal plasma copper, plasma ceruloplasmin, and serum oxidase activity [226]. The basic disorder seems to be a reduced ability to incorporate ingested copper into plasma ceruloplasmin rather than an actual deficiency of the protein [226]. The defect leads to increased absorption of copper by the gut, with excess deposition of copper in the liver, brain, cornea, and kidneys. This causes secondary cirrhosis, extrapyramidal neurologic symptoms and signs, Kayser-Fleischer rings in the cornea, and characteristic but variable defects of renal tubular function.

The most common defect is a renal aminoaciduria, plasma amino acids being normal unless there is liver failure, when they may be increased. Threonine and cystine output is markedly elevated, and there is a smaller but definite increase in the urinary excretion of proline, citrulline, serine, glycine, asparagine, valine, tyrosine, and lysine. Histidine, ornithine, and phenylalanine are also somewhat increased. There is no rise of taurine or of the methylhistidines. Urinary cystine is in sufficient concentration to give a positive reaction by the cyanide-nitroprusside test but not sufficient to form cystine calculi. Plasma uric acid is usually very low, owing to increase of uric acid clearance [33], and probenecid does not produce any further rise of uric acid output. Renal glycosuria sometimes occurs but is less frequent than aminoaciduria. Increase of phosphate clearance and osteomalacia are also unusual but occasionally occur. There may be osteoporosis as well as osteomalacia, associated with disuse atrophy of the skeleton and hypercalciuria [27, 164]. The coincidence of hypercalciuria with increased phosphate clearance may cause nephrocalcinosis or renal stone formation [164] despite the chelating effect of the urinary amino acids. Urinary concentrating and acidification power may be reduced.

Uzman [263, 264] has claimed that there is excessive urinary output of peptide as well as of free amino acids. Urinary copper is greatly increased and is probably excreted in combination with urinary peptide [264]. Both urinary amino acid and copper content increase in parallel with high-protein diets [26] or after ingestion of glycine or alanine [187]. Chelating agents such as dimercaprol (BAL) greatly increase copper output without producing any rise of urinary amino acids [187]. The newer chelating agent penicillamine increases urinary copper and has the advantage of being absorbed from the gut, and therefore active when taken by mouth. A recent report [103] shows that prolonged penicillamine therapy usually improves the renal acidification defect, and in some cases reduces amino acid loss.

There are excess deposits of copper throughout the renal parenchyma but especially in proximal tubular cells. In view of the known effects of heavy metals in producing renal tubular defects, it is probable that the rather variable and nonspecific abnormalities of tubular function are due to copper toxicity. It has proved impossible, however, to produce similar renal lesions experimentally by copper feeding. Efficient treatment by chelating agents and oral sodium sulfide produces considerable improvement in the neurologic and hepatic signs and symptoms, but improvement in the renal tubular defects is less obvious. Fortunately these are clinically of less importance. If bone lesions are prominent, calciferol therapy may be beneficial, but this therapy should be avoided in patients with hypercalciuria and stone formation.

Nephrotic Syndrome. In most cases of the nephrotic syndrome there are no discrete anomalies of renal tubular function [281]. The disease is due to increased glomerular permeability to macromolecules, especially plasma albumin and the smaller-molecular-weight globulins. In a few cases in childhood, however, there are features, including renal aminoaciduria and glycosuria, suggestive of the tubular defects of the Fanconi syndrome. Although these defects are very unusual in adult patients and uncommon in children with the nephrotic syndrome, they occur more frequently in congenital nephrotic syndrome. In this condition [112, 207] the infant either shows massive proteinuria and edema at birth or develops these abnormalities during the first month of life. Darmady [112] has recorded a "swan-neck" deformity of the proximal renal tubule in this type of nephrotic syndrome. The tubular defects may possibly be due to cellular damage from reabsorption of excess albumin and small-molecular-weight globulins from the tubular lumen. The maximal incidence of tubular damage occurs when there is relative immaturity of proximal tubular function, as shown by the physiologic aminoaciduria characteristic of the kidney of the infant.

Multiple Myelomatosis. A syndrome analogous to the Fanconi syndrome [81, 248] occurring in cases of multiple myelomatosis is probably a similar defect. In this disease there is tubular damage from reabsorption of Bence Jones protein, and there is cast formation within the tubular lumen throughout a greater length of the tubule than in any other renal disease. Nevertheless, the development of discrete abnormalities of tubular function in multiple myelomatosis is a great rarity, few examples having been described despite the screening of many cases of myeloma. There is aminoaciduria and renal glycosuria, but bony lesions typical of osteomalacia with prominent pseudofractures are the major source of disability. The osteomalacia usually precedes the development of skeletal lesions directly due to the plasmacytomas within the bone marrow. Treatment is obviously limited by the severity of the associated disease, but calciferol may be of temporary benefit in relieving symptoms.

Tyrosinemia. Proximal tubular damage always occurs in the rare hereditary disease tyrosinemia [108, 259], due to lack of *p*-hydroxyphenylpyruvate oxidase [147, 259].

This causes a nodular cirrhosis of the liver in infancy, associated with portal hypertension and congestive splenomegaly. There are also multiple tubular absorptive defects, and a high phosphate clearance leading to typical rickets. Biochemically there is increase of plasma tyrosine and many tyrosyl metabolites, especially *p*-hydroxyphenyllactic acid. In addition, there is sometimes hypermethioninemia attributed by some investigators to the effects of liver damage [239], but by others [107] to inhibition of enzymes involved in methionine metabolism. The proximal tubular damage is presumably due to the toxic effects of the high plasma tyrosine, or possibly to those of tyrosyl metabolites, as it rapidly responds to therapy with a diet low in both tyrosine and phenylalanine [13, 119]. The severe liver damage, however, is more resistant to dietary measures unless these are started immediately after birth. Hepatoma seems to be a more common complication than in other more usual types of hepatic cirrhosis. The aminoaciduria is of a mixed type due to overflow of tyrosine and sometimes of methionine resulting from the high plasma levels of these amino acids, and of a renal type secondary to proximal tubular damage.

TUBULAR DAMAGE DUE TO EXOGENOUS POISONS

Proximal tubular damage may occur from ingestion of many nephrotoxic drugs and poisons. The damage is often severe enough to cause proximal tubular necrosis and acute oliguric renal failure, but less severe damage may cause discrete but generalized defects in proximal tubular function. Drugs and poisons that have caused renal aminoaciduria and glycosuria include lead [276], uranium [222], cadmium [48], Lysol [250], oxalic acid [80], and maleic acid in the experimental animal [125]. The heavy metal poisons are inhibitors of sulfhydryl enzymes, especially dehydrogenases, and presumably are comparable to copper in hepatolenticular degeneration. Maleic acid is also a potent dehydrogenase inhibitor.

An interesting and detailed study of the effects of industrial cadmium poisoning on proximal tubular function has been published by Kazantzis et al. [143]. The degree and pattern of the proximal tubular damage was very variable from case to case, and illustrates the lack of uniformity of the damage to tubular function produced by a known exogenous toxic agent.

Similar effects from a degradation product of tetracycline have also been studied in detail [101, 118]. The effects have been attributed to the formation of anhydrotetracycline and of epianhydrotetracycline which arise from exposure of the drug to air, moisture, and heat over a prolonged period. This effect will probably not occur in the future, as tetracycline is now produced in a formulation which resists spontaneous degradation. The cases are of especial importance, however, in illustrating the constant care that must be applied in the introduction of new drugs to ensure lack of toxicity under all possible circumstances to specialized bodily functions.

TUBULAR DAMAGE FROM VITAMIN DEFICIENCY

Similar nonspecific proximal tubular hypofunction may occur in dietary rickets in infancy [137, 139]. There is an aminoaciduria involving the smaller-molecular-weight amino acids. The defect is extremely variable and presumably depends on the severity of the vitamin deficiency. The abnormal amino acid loss does not respond as promptly to treatment with vitamin D as do the high phosphate clearance and low plasma phosphate of untreated rickets. Complete recovery of tubular function occurs after about one month of adequate vitamin D therapy. Adult cases of dietary osteomalacia usually show no evidence of abnormal proximal tubular function except for the high phosphate clearance characteristic of the condition. The difference in the response of the infantile and adult kidney to vitamin D deficiency is similar to that seen in the nephrotic syndrome, and presumably is related to the physiologic hyperaminoaciduria of infancy.

Renal aminoaciduria also occasionally occurs in infantile scurvy [138]. This defect is unconnected with the excess excretion of phenolic acids [155, 242], especially *p*-hydroxyphenyllactic and *p*-hydroxyphenylacetic acids, which occurs after tyrosine ingestion in the disease. This is a much more constant defect in scurvy than is aminoaciduria, and is of metabolic and not of renal origin.

Overflow Aminoaciduria

The overflow aminoacidurias are not strictly renal diseases, except that the kidney may be involved in a whole-body enzymatic defect. However, they are often diagnosed by urinary abnormalities, and therefore a short account of the principal types is included.

β-AMINOISOBUTYRIC ACID EXCRETION

β-aminoisobutyric acid is one of the normal variants of amino acid excretion and is genetically determined, probably by a mendelian recessive factor [66, 120]. About 5 to 10 per cent of white subjects excrete from 50 to 200 mg. of this amino acid daily, whereas other individuals excrete only trace amounts. Some other races show a much higher incidence of this completely harmless anomaly [66, 106]. Experiments in rats, both in vivo and by the tissue slice technic [84–86], suggest that the amino acid is derived from thymine by the reactions shown in Figure 30-5.

The clearance of the amino acid is very high and approximates the glomerular filtration rate. Plasma levels are therefore low and difficult to estimate both in high and low excretors. Presumably, low excretors are able to metabolize the amino acid, whereas high excretors cannot. This amino acid is excreted in increased amounts in all subjects if nucleoprotein breakdown is increased, as in the treatment of leukemia [106] or in starvation [225].

A detailed study of the metabolism and excretion of β-aminoisobutyric acid has been published by Armstrong et al. [11]. Affected individuals are homozygotes with deficiency of β-aminoisobutyrate transaminase. The renal clearance exceeds that of inulin indicating net tubular secretion, which is depressed after administration of probenecid.

Metabolic Disorders of Amino Acids Causing Overflow Aminoaciduria

Hereditary disease involving absence of an enzyme necessary in the metabolism of amino acids causes increase of plasma concentration of the affected amino acid and an overflow aminoaciduria. In some cases this may be sufficient to saturate the relevant transport system, and to cause a secondary renal aminoaciduria of the other amino acids in the transport group. This has been described in hypermethioninemia [211], in citrullinemia [181a],

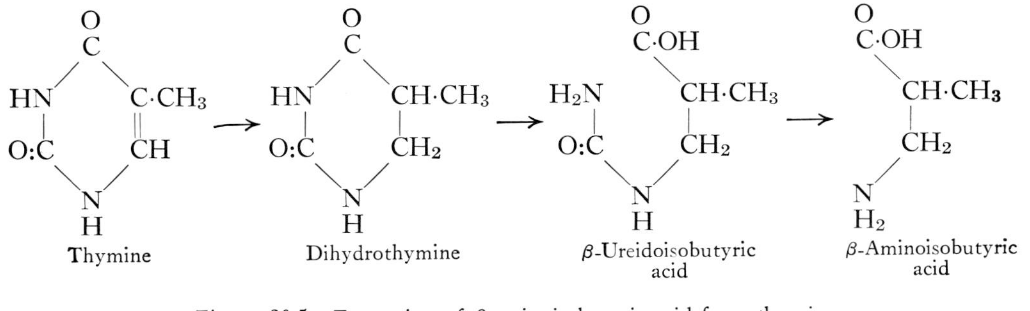

Thymine → Dihydrothymine → β-Ureidoisobutyric acid → β-Aminoisobutyric acid

Figure 30-5. Formation of β-aminoisobutyric acid from thymine.

Table 30-2. Disorders of Amino Acid Metabolism Causing an "Overflow" Type of Aminoaciduria

Disease	Abnormalities of Plasma Amino Acids	Abnormalities of Urinary Amino Acids	Type of Aminoaciduria	Enzyme Deficiency	References
Phenylketonuria	Phenylalanine	Phenylalanine	Pure overflow	Phenylalanine hydroxylase	Følhing [89], Jervis [136], Lyman [170], Mitoma et al. [199], & Wallace et al. [268]
Tyrosinemia	Tyrosine; sometimes methionine	Generalized aminoaciduria; tyrosine predominant	Mixed	*p*-Hydroxy-phenyl-pyruvate oxidase	Gentz et al. [108], LaDu [147], & Tani-guchi & Gjessing [259]
Tryptophanemia	Tryptophan	Tryptophan	Pure overflow	Possibly tryptophan pyrrolase	Tada et al. [257]
Hypervalinemia	Valine	Valine	Pure overflow	Valine transaminase	Wada et al. [267]
Branched chain ketoaciduria (maple syrup urine disease)	Leucine, isoleucine, valine, allo-isoleucine	Same amino acids; occasion-ally other neutral amino acids	Usually pure overflow; sometimes mixed	Branched chain α-keto-acid decarboxylase	Dancis et al. [63], & Menkes et al. [189]
Histidinemia	Histidine	Histidine	Pure overflow	Histidase	Auerbach et al. [19], & Ghadimi et al. [111]
Methioninemia	Methionine, & some-times tyrosine	General aminoaciduria; methionine & tyrosine predominant	Mixed	Unknown	Perry et al. [211]
Homocystinuria	Homocystine & some-times methionine	Homocystine & sometimes methionine	Pure overflow	Cystathionine synthetase	Mudd et al. [203], & Schinke et al. [232]
Cystathioninuria	Cystathionine	Cystathionine	Pure overflow	Cystathioninase	Frimpter et al. [99], & Harris et al. [122]
Hyperlysinemia	Lysine, arginine, & glutamine	Same amino acids	Pure overflow	Lysine:NAD oxido-reductase	Colombo et al. [54], & Ghadimi et al. [110]
Citrullinemia	Citrulline	Citrulline & other neutral amino acids	Mixed	Argininosuccinic acid synthetase	McMurray et al. [181a]
Argininosuccinic aciduria	Argininosuccinic acid	Same amino acid	Pure overflow	Argininosuccinase	Allan et al. [7], & Westall [274]

Hyperglycinemia					
Type 1	Glycine; lesser increase of threonine, valine, & isoleucine	Same amino acids; glycine prominent with only slight increase of the others	Pure overflow	Unknown	Childs et al. [45], & Menkes [188]
Type 2	Glycine	Glycine	Pure overflow	Probably glycine oxidase	Mabry & Karam [171]
Sarcosinemia	Sarcosine; ethanolamine	Same	Pure overflow	Probably sarcosine oxidase	Gerritsen & Waisman [109]
Prolinemia					
Type 1	Proline	Proline, hydroxyproline, & glycine	Mixed	Proline oxidase	Schafer et al. [229]
Type 2	Proline	Proline, hydroxyproline, & glycine	Mixed	Δ^1-Pyrroline-5-carboxylate dehydrogenase	Efron [76]
Hydroxyprolinemia	Hydroxyproline	Hydroxyproline predominant; sometimes increase of proline & glycine	Mainly overflow; may be of the mixed type	Hydroxyproline oxidase	Efron [76], & Efron et al. [77]
β-Alaninemia	β-Alanine	β-Alanine, β-aminoisobutyric acid, taurine, & γ-aminobutyric acid	Mixed	β-Alanine transaminase	Scriver et al. [240]

and in some cases of maple syrup urine disease (branched-chain aminoacidemia) with a secondary excess urinary excretion of other neutral amino acids. Similarly, in hyperprolinemia [229] there is an overflow excretion of proline and a renal type excretion of hydroxyproline and glycine, and in β-alaninemia there is excess excretion not only of the involved beta amino acid but of β-aminoisobutyric acid and of taurine as well [240]. In most examples of these conditions, however, including the two most common, phenylketonuria and homocystinuria, the excess amino acid output is not sufficient to saturate the appropriate amino acid transport system, and therefore a secondary renal aminoaciduria does not occur. A list of these conditions, with information regarding the amino acids increased in plasma and urine, respectively, is given in Table 30-2. The effects of tyrosinemia are exceptional, as in this disease there is actual proximal tubular damage, leading to a generalized aminoaciduria including many members of different transport groups. Although there is no renal aminoaciduria in the most common of these conditions, phenylketonuria, renal function in this disease is not completely normal. A large quantity of abnormal organic acids is excreted in the urine, especially phenylacetylglutamine. This partially saturates the proximal tubular secretory mechanism for organic acids with less efficient excretion of these compounds. The secretory mechanism is not, however, fully inhibited [135], as it is still further depressed by administration of probenecid.

Renal Glycosuria

Spontaneous renal glycosuria is a relatively common disorder of proximal tubular function. The natural disease is harmless except for the possibility of mistaken diagnosis as diabetes mellitus and consequent prescription of dangerous medicaments or dietary restrictions. The experimental glycosuria of phlorizin poisoning is a much more severe and eventually fatal disorder. The incidence of spontaneous renal glycosuria depends on the definition of the condition. There is, in fact, a gradation in severity from the more severe cases which fulfill the most rigid criteria of diagnosis to those that have only postprandial glycosuria. Various investigators have therefore recorded an incidence varying from 0.1 to 2 per cent of the general population [88, 183].

Marble's criteria of diagnosis [183] are as follows:

1. Presence of glycosuria in all urine specimens, unaccompanied by abnormal increase of blood glucose and independent of diet.
2. A fasting blood sugar less than 120 mg. per 100 ml. (older nonspecific methods for blood sugar).
3. A normal glucose tolerance with no values of blood sugar greater than 170 mg. per 100 ml. after intake of 50 gm. of glucose, and return to control values within two hours.
4. Proof that the reducing substance in urine is in fact glucose.
5. No progression in later life to true diabetes mellitus.
6. A positive family history of the disease.

A condition fulfilling these criteria of diagnosis would undoubtedly be a true case of renal glycosuria. However, such rigid criteria exclude from the diagnosis individuals in whom proximal tubular reabsorption of glucose is subnormal. For example, cases in which there is a combination of renal glycosuria and diabetes mellitus are excluded, and also cases in which glucose is not present in the urine while the patient is fasting, but yet is excreted at blood sugar values which would not cause glycosuria in normal subjects. An accurate diagnosis must therefore include the criteria of recognition and some description of the severity of the defect.

Other melliturias which may be wrongly

diagnosed as renal glycosuria include fructosuria, pentosuria, and galactosemia. Use of the specific glucose-oxidase test paper will differentiate these from true glycosuria. Lactose may appear in the urine of the pregnant and lactating woman, and noncarbohydrate reducing substances such as homogentisic acid in alkaptonuria may cause confusion. The presence of glucose in urine may be confirmed by the glucose-oxidase test as well as by a combination of paper chromatography, preparation of the osazone and fermentation tests. Sucrosuria will not cause confusion since sucrose is not a reducing sugar. Renal glycosuria is often a hereditary anomaly, inheritance being of the mendelian dominant type. A family has been recorded in which renal glycosuria occurred in seven successive generations [128].

NATURE OF THE TUBULAR DEFECT

There are two separate varieties of renal glycosuria. The less common variety is due to a reduced capability of the proximal tubular cells to transport, and therefore reabsorb, glucose from the glomerular filtrate into the renal capillary blood. In this variety the tubular maximal reabsorptive capacity for glucose (Tm_G) is reduced out of proportion to reduction of the glomerular filtration rate. Glucose reabsorption by the tubules is subnormal at all levels of blood sugar, including the abnormally high levels produced by the glucose infusions which are necessary to measure the Tm_G. This type of glycosuria is found in diseases involving nonspecific proximal tubular damage, and is often associated with other defects of proximal tubular function — for example, in the Lignac-Fanconi and adult Fanconi syndromes, Lowe's syndrome, some cases of Wilson's disease, and heavy-metal poisoning.

The more common variety, in which renal glycosuria is usually an isolated proximal tubular defect, is due to abnormal heterogeneity of the individual nephrons with respect to their capacity for glucose reabsorption. In this type of renal glycosuria, reabsorption of glucose is abnormal at blood sugar levels below that at which there is maximal glucose transport, but is completely normal at higher levels. The difference is best described by mathematical and graphical methods:

Let P_G and U_G be the concentrations of glucose in plasma and urine, respectively, V the urinary volume in milliliters per minute, C_{IN} the glomerular filtration rate, and Tm_G the amount of glucose reabsorbed from the glomerular filtrate.

The amount of glucose excreted equals the amount filtered at the glomeruli less the amount reabsorbed.

$$U_GV = P_GC_{IN} - Tm_G \qquad (1)$$

Since C_{IN} and Tm_G are constants, the graph relating glucose excretion to the plasma level of glucose is a straight line AB of gradient C_{IN} (Fig. 30-6). In this equation, when U_GV is zero, $P_G = Tm_G/C_{IN}$. This is the true mathematical expression of the *mean threshold* value of glucose, and is a measure of the plasma level of glucose at which glycosuria would occur if there were no heterogeneity of nephrons.

If equation (1) is divided throughout by P_G:

$$\frac{U_GV}{P_G} = C_{IN} - \frac{Tm_G}{P_G} \qquad (2)$$

The expression on the left is the glucose clearance C_G, and therefore the graph relating C_G to P_G is a rectangular hyperbola AB with the line $y = C_{IN}$ as one asymptote (Fig. 30-7).

In actual fact there is normally considerable heterogeneity of nephrons, and the observed relationship is given by the curves CDB in Figures 30-6 and 30-7. Some nephrons have a lower value of the ratio Tm_G/C_{IN} than the mean, and therefore there is appreciable glycosuria at lower plasma levels of glucose than the mean threshold value of 245 mg. per 100 ml. (Fig. 30-6). The plasma level of glucose at which glycosuria can first be detected in the urine may be termed the *appearance threshold* (point C in Figures 30-6 and 30-7). Conversely, some nephrons with an unusually high value of Tm_G/C_{IN} will not reabsorb glucose to a maximal degree until the

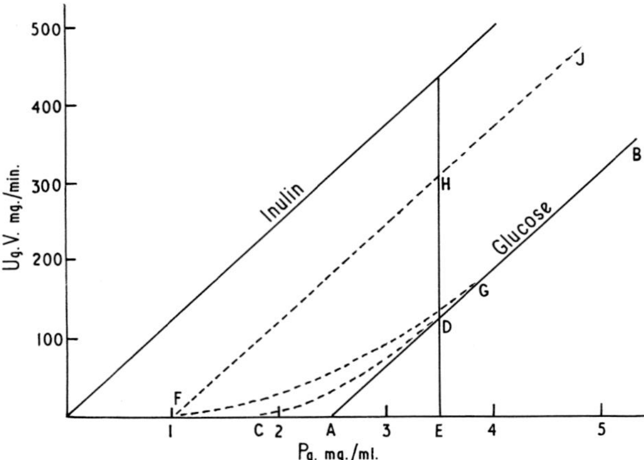

Figure 30-6. Excretion of glucose at varying plasma levels in patients with renal glycosuria and in normal subjects. The line CDB represents the normal subject; no glucose is excreted if the plasma level is below 1.8 mg. per milliliter. The line FGB represents the excretion in the common type of renal glycosuria due to increased heterogenicity of the nephron population. Glucose excretion is abnormal at low but normal at high plasma glucose levels. The line FHJ represents the state in renal glycosuria due to proximal tubular damage as in the Fanconi syndrome. Glucose excretion is abnormally high both at low and at high plasma glucose values.

plasma concentration of glucose is considerably above the mean threshold value. The value when all nephrons are reabsorbing glucose maximally may be termed the *maximal threshold* (point E in Figures 30-6 and 30-7). The separation between C and E gives a measure of heterogeneity of nephrons in relation to capacity for glucose reabsorption.

The line FGB represents the type of renal glycosuria due to increased heterogeneity of nephrons, while the line FHJ represents the less common and more serious variety, in which there is actual reduction of Tm_G. In both cases the appearance threshold F is abnormally low at a value of 100 mg. per 100 ml. instead of the average normal of 170 mg. per 100 ml. Glucose reabsorption at higher plasma levels is, however, widely different in the two types of tubular defect.

The amount of glucose lost in the urine in clinical cases of renal glycosuria is always a small fraction of the daily carbohydrate intake, being usually less than 30 gm. per day. By contrast, the glucoside phlorizin causes a severe defect of proximal tubular glucose reabsorption with marked reduction of Tm_G. The large amount of glucose in the urine may cause starvation ketosis and severe weight loss. The glucoside also inhibits glucose transport in the jejunum and the erythrocyte. The available evidence suggests [46] that the effect is not connected with the action of phlorizin in inhibiting the enzyme phosphorylase, but rather with the binding of an unknown glucose carrier on the cell membrane.

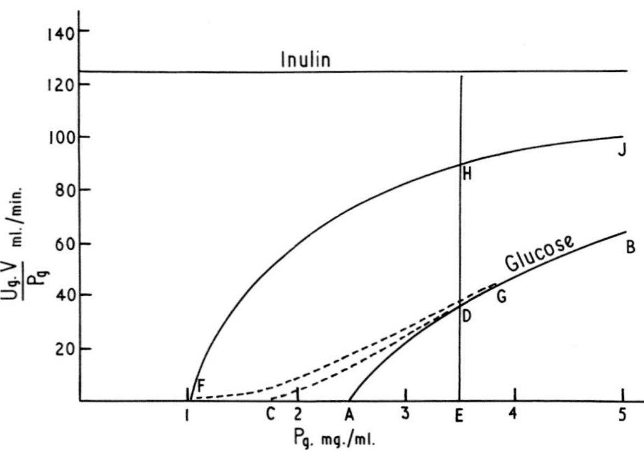

Figure 30-7. Clearances of glucose at varying plasma levels in a normal subject, CDB; in a patient with renal glycosuria due to increased heterogeneity of the nephron population, FGB; and in a case of the Fanconi syndrome, FHJ. In the first type of glycosuria, clearance is abnormally high at low plasma levels but normal at high plasma levels of glucose. In the Fanconi syndrome, the clearance is abnormally high at all plasma levels.

Causation and Clinical Types. The most common type of renal glycosuria is due to unusual heterogeneity of proximal tubular function in relation to glucose reabsorption. This is inherited as an autosomal mendelian dominant defect [128], there being no demonstrable abnormality in the heterozygotes. A variant of this condition is found in the less common condition of glucoglycinuria [141], also inherited as an autosomal dominant defect. In this condition excess urinary glycine without any increase of plasma levels occurs in addition to glycosuria. Most cases of renal glycosuria due to decrease of maximal reabsorptive capacity for glucose are due to generalized proximal tubular defects — for example, Lignac-Fanconi disease, the adult Fanconi syndrome, and Wilson's disease.

An interesting and important variant is the glycosuria associated with glucose-galactose malabsorption by the jejunum [150, 163]. In this condition, inherited as a mendelian recessive, there is severe fermentative diarrhea and failure to thrive starting immediately after birth. The infant is unable to absorb both glucose and galactose which share an intestinal transport system. The infant remains severely ill as long as there is glucose, lactose, maltose, or sucrose in the diet, but responds dramatically to a diet containing fructose as the sole carbohydrate. There is always a severe renal glycosuria, owing to fall of tubular maximal reabsorptive capacity. Galactose is not excreted in the urine since plasma levels are zero or negligible. This condition shows either that, similar to amino acid transport, reabsorption of glucose is by an identical mechanism in the jejunum and proximal renal tubule, or that at least one essential step in the process is identical in both sites.

Disorders of Phosphate Transport

Proximal tubular transport of phosphate is under the control of circulating parathyroid hormone, which inhibits phosphate reabsorption and therefore increases phosphate clearance [3]. Changes in phosphate clearance have a greater effect on plasma phosphate levels than on the amount excreted, which accounts for the high plasma phosphate of hypoparathyroidism and the low plasma phosphate of hyperparathyroidism. In man and the dog [212, 231], phosphate reabsorption increases with the amount filtered at the glomerulus up to a point considerably higher than normal plasma phosphate levels, where a maximal reabsorption rate, Tm_P, is reached. Phosphate clearance therefore increases with rising plasma phosphate values, and in normal subjects the clearance is zero at abnormally low plasma phosphate concentrations of less than 2 mg. per 100 ml. Phosphate clearance values should therefore always be interpreted from graphs [198] giving the relationship of the clearance to plasma concentrations.

The abnormally low phosphate clearance of hypoparathyroidism is increased to normal values by injected parathyroid hormone or by ingestion of calciferol or dihydrotachysterol. Conversely, the abnormally high phosphate clearance of primary hyperparathyroidism is reduced to normal values after excision of the causative parathyroid adenoma. Proximal tubular abnormalities of phosphate transport usually involve a high phosphate clearance due to reduced reabsorption from the glomerular filtrate. This causes an abnormally low plasma phosphate concentration and the bony lesions of rickets or osteomalacia. The high clearance is reduced to normal values, and the plasma phosphate is correspondingly raised by appropriate therapy with calciferol or dihydrotachysterol, possibly as a result of inhibition of secondary hyperparathyroidism. Therefore, unlike proximal tubular defects of transport of glucose and amino acids, abnormalities of phosphate transport are amenable to appropriate therapy and do not necessarily imply an innate tubular transport defect.

The evidence suggests that the abnormal phosphate transport is imposed on the tubule cells by hormonal influences, especially excess circulating parathyroid hormone. In one tubular disorder of phosphate transport, pseudohypoparathyroidism, the reverse effect occurs. The clearance of phosphate is abnormally low from innate insensitivity of the tubule cells to parathyroid hormone; consequently, the plasma phosphate is abnormally high. The hereditary condition of hypophosphatasia, in which there is diminished concentration of alkaline phosphatase in many tissues, including the kidney, will for convenience be included in this section.

DISORDERS ASSOCIATED WITH RICKETS OR OSTEOMALACIA

Almost all types of rickets and osteomalacia are associated with a reduced plasma phosphate and a high phosphate clearance. This generalization includes dietary rickets, the rickets of celiac disease, osteomalacia complicating idiopathic steatorrhea, and the various types of osteodystrophy due to renal tubular defects. The single exception is the rickets or osteomalacia of azotemic renal osteodystrophy [90, 91, 252]. Here the bony lesion is of mixed pathology, some parts of the skeleton showing osteitis fibrosa from secondary hyperparathyroidism, some areas being characteristic of rickets or osteomalacia, and others showing osteosclerotic lesions [55, 142]. In this type of osteodystrophy the plasma phosphate is above normal values, and the phosphate clearance is usually reduced in absolute figures but is high in relation to the grossly reduced glomerular filtration rate. Many types of renal tubular syndrome may cause a nonazotemic, hypophosphatemic renal osteodystrophy, including the Lignac-Fanconi syndrome, the adult Fanconi syndrome, Lowe's syndrome, renal tubular acidosis, some cases of ureterosigmoidostomy, and vitamin D resistance. The last type, which involves an almost pure phosphate transport defect, will now be described.

HEREDITARY VITAMIN-D-RESISTANT RICKETS

Now that dietary rickets is almost unknown in most civilized communities, hereditary vitamin-D-resistant rickets is the most important cause of infantile rickets. Strictly, the phrase "raised resistance to vitamin D" is more accurate, since resistance to vitamin D action is by no means absolute. It may be defined as a hereditary disease characterized by hypophosphatemia and increased phosphate clearance, without evidence of other obvious tubular defects and without evidence of celiac disease, leading to rickets which responds to large doses of vitamin D but is unaffected by small physiologic doses of the vitamin.

Symptoms and Signs. The disease presents as clinical rickets which is usually first noted when the infant attempts to stand or first begins to walk — that is, between the ages of 6 and 18 months. The most common deformities are either genu varum or genu valgum, and clear-cut evidence of rickets is found on x-ray of the epiphyses. There is rarely any marked muscular weakness or atony such as occurs in dietary rickets or acquired vitamin D resistance in adolescent patients. Tetany is uncommon, again a contrast with dietary rickets. Unless the disease is adequately treated the rachitic symptoms and deformities are maximal in mid-childhood, when there is obviously active rickets with dwarfism and severe skeletal deformities. In adult life the skeletal lesions are much less severe. There is dwarfism and residual skeletal deformity, but evidence of active osteomalacia may be either absent or slight. In the more severe cases bone pain may persist, and an occasional pseudofracture may be found on x-ray examination. Bone biopsy in such cases shows evidence of osteomalacia with uncalcified osteoid seams covering bone trabeculae. Adult female patients often have pelvic contraction necessitating delivery of babies by cesarean section.

Hereditary Aspects. This disease is transmitted as a sex-linked dominant disorder, an unusual mode of inheritance [277]. If the defect is transmitted by a female, there should be approximately equal numbers of affected and unaffected sons and daughters. In contrast, if it is passed on by a male parent, all the sons will be normal and all the daughters will have the disease. Affected males are virtually homozygous, as they do not possess a normal X chromosome; affected females with an affected and a normal X chromosome are heterozygotes. A homozygous female is a theoretical possibility but has not yet been described, as such a case could be derived only from a union in which both parents were affected by the disease. As would be expected, the virtually homozygous male patient is more severely affected than the heterozygous female patient. The skeletal lesions are more severe and the plasma phosphate concentration is lower in affected males than in affected females.

Biochemical Abnormalities. The most constant abnormality is a low plasma phosphate, which in the untreated case remains low throughout life [277]. Plasma alkaline phosphatase is increased in childhood when the rickets is active but may be within normal limits in adult life as the bony lesions become more quiescent. The plasma levels of calcium are either normal or only slightly reduced, accounting for the rarity of tetany in this type of rickets. Loss of phosphate in the urine remains normal despite the grossly reduced filtered load of phosphate. There is therefore increased phosphate clearance, with reduction of Tm_P to about half the normal value [277]. After calciferol therapy the plasma phosphate usually rises without any significant change in urinary phosphate output, and therefore there is a fall in phosphate clearance. Many patients, however, will show satisfactory healing of the rickets without restoration of plasma phosphate to normal levels. There is often a poor correlation between the calcium phosphate solubility product of plasma and the severity of the skeletal lesions.

Intestinal absorption defects of calcium and phosphorus similar to those in dietary rickets are usually present. Fecal calcium constitutes an abnormally high fraction of the dietary intake, urinary calcium output being very low. Fecal phosphate is either normal or only slightly increased, but oral loading tests [277] suggest that intestinal absorption is impaired. Some of the phosphate in the feces may escape absorption because of excess precipitation as insoluble calcium phosphate. After adequate therapy with calciferol there is a positive balance of both calcium and phosphate, almost entirely due to reduction of fecal loss.

Although vitamin-D-resistant rickets shows obvious transport defects of phosphate in the renal tubules and probably in the jejunum, there is no proof that the disease is due to a primary disorder of the proximal renal tubules. Probably the vitamin D resistance is the underlying primary abnormality. As in other types of rickets or osteomalacia, it causes secondary hyperparathyroidism with resultant increase of renal phosphate clearance. The reversibility of the tubular transport defect when it is treated with calciferol is quite unlike the irreversibility of defects of amino acid and glucose transport.

Therapy. Although there is considerable resistance to the action of vitamin D, the disease responds completely to calciferol in large doses. The degree of resistance varies from case to case, the effective dose of calciferol being between 150,000 and 1,500,000 units per day. Obviously it is essential to start treatment as early as possible to avoid permanent skeletal deformity. The dosage of calciferol often requires very careful and exact adjustment, the correct dose being that which restores plasma phosphate and phosphate clearance to normal, or almost normal, values without producing hypercalcemia. The effective dose usually varies from year to year, often having to be increased with the growth of the child and later reduced as the disease becomes less active in adolescence and adult life.

ACQUIRED VITAMIN D RESISTANCE

This type of vitamin-D-resistant rickets and osteomalacia is a much rarer disease, and is not hereditary [67]. The patient is quite normal until the middle of the second decade, when severe muscular weakness occurs. Later there is frank rickets or osteomalacia leading to severe skeletal deformities. There is a reduced plasma phosphate and an increased renal phosphate clearance as in the hereditary type. No other disorder of renal tubular function occurs except glycinuria [60, 67] due to a tubular defect of glycine reabsorption. About 90 to 92 per cent of the glycine filtered at the glomeruli is reabsorbed, compared with a normal of 95 to 98 per cent [60]. The daily urinary output of glycine is 260 to 340 mg., with a clearance of about 10 to 17 ml. per minute. The defective reabsorption of glycine is therefore much less severe than in cases of hereditary glycinuria, in which the daily glycine output is about three times as great. The condition responds to high dosage of calciferol, and careful control of therapy is required as in that of vitamin D resistance of the hereditary type The reason for the presence of muscular weakness in acquired vitamin D resistance and its absence in the hereditary disease has not been explained. Most of the patients retain their abnormal resistance to vitamin D, and therefore prolonged continuous therapy is essential. One patient, however, made a spontaneous recovery years after the first onset of the disease [67, 173].

PSEUDOHYPOPARATHYROIDISM

There are three varieties of hypoparathyroidism causing hypocalcemic tetany: post-thyroidectomy hypoparathyroidism, idiopathic hypoparathyroidism [74] with absent or atrophic parathyroid glands, and pseudohypoparathyroidism [4] with apparently normal parathyroids. The first two are parathyroid disorders, whereas the third is due to resistance of the renal tubules to the action of parathyroid hormone, and is therefore a disease of the kidneys. Idiopathic hypoparathyroidism is diagnosed by a low serum calcium and a high serum inorganic phosphate concentration, associated with chronic tetany in the absence of radiologically demonstrable abnormalities of rickets or osteomalacia, and in the absence of steatorrhea, renal insufficiency, or alkalosis [40]. Pseudohypoparathyroidism shows the same abnormalities, but in addition there are characteristic features of brachydactyly, roundness of the face and a stocky build, resistance to intravenous injections of a potent parathyroid hormone preparation, subcutaneous bone formation, and normal parathyroid glands [40].

The response to the Ellsworth-Howard test [79] using an intravenous injection of parathyroid hormone is of crucial importance in the differential diagnosis. In both idiopathic hypoparathyroidism and pseudohypoparathyroidism there is an abnormally high plasma phosphate concentration with a normal urinary phosphate output, resulting in an abnormally low phosphate clearance due to excessive renal tubular phosphate reabsorption. Patients with idiopathic hypoparathyroidism exhibit an exaggerated response to parathyroid hormone [3, 40], increase of urinary phosphate being much greater than in normal subjects. In pseudohypoparathyroidism, either the hormone has no effect or the phosphaturia is less than in normal controls. An increment in the hourly excretion of phosphate exceeding the basal levels by 40 mg. of phosphate per hour or by 250 per cent is regarded as an exaggerated response to intravenous parathyroid hormone [40].

The frequency of idiopathic hypoparathyroidism is equal in males and females, and the onset of tetany usually occurs in late adolescence. Twice as many females as males are affected by pseudohypoparathyroidism, and the mean age at onset is before puberty, although some cases start in the second decade.

Tetany, epileptic fits, muscle cramps, paresthesia, and laryngeal spasms occur with equal frequency in both types. Papilledema, cataract formation, ectodermal defects, and monilia infections are more commonly associated with idiopathic hypoparathyroidism. Calcification of basal ganglia (Fig. 30-8) is more common in pseudohypoparathyrodism, whereas subcutaneous deposits of calcium and shortening of metacarpal bones, particularly the fourth and fifth metacarpals, are features of pseudohypoparathyroidism alone. Mental retardation is common in both types, but is more frequent in pseudohypoparathyroidism, probably because of the earlier average age at onset in this disease.

There appear to be four, apparently unrelated, effects of the abnormal gene: unresponsiveness of the renal tubules to injected and endogenous parathyroid hormone, calcification of basal ganglia, subcutaneous calcifications, and dyschondroplasia usually causing shortening of metacarpal bones. Any permutation of these separate abnormalities can be found in an individual case. The disease of patients showing other manifestations of the syndrome without clinical or biochemical evidence of hypoparathyroidism has been termed "pseudo-pseudohypoparathyroidism" [6]. A better term would be "forme fruste of pseudohypoparathyroidism." Cases with and without evidence of hypoparathyroidism but with other signs of the condition may occur within the same family [72]. Some cases without any biochemical abnormalities in the plasma and without tetany may nevertheless show unresponsiveness to injected parathyroid hormone [186]. Possibly the extrarenal manifestations are due to transport defects of phosphate in other tissue cells. If this is so, the anomaly is somewhat analogous to the Lignac-Fanconi syndrome, in which the two defects of renal tubular damage and generalized cystinosis may vary considerably in their relative severity from case to case.

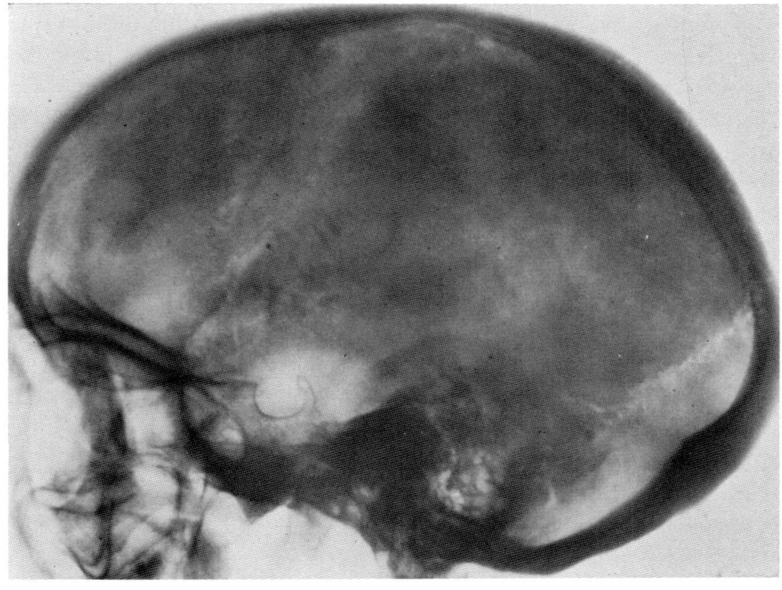

Figure 30-8. Lateral x-ray of skull in a case of chronic hypoparathyroidism showing calcification of the basal ganglia. This was a case of idiopathic hypoparathyroidism.

Hereditary Aspects and Prognosis. Mann et al. [182] have reviewed the evidence that pseudohypoparathyroidism is transmitted in a sex-linked manner, the abnormal gene being carried by the X chromosome. The disease is less severe in females than in males, but females are affected roughly twice as frequently. Male-to-male transmission has not been recorded in families showing the renal tubular defect and suffering from hypocalcemic tetany.

Four families, however, have been described [23, 113, 127] in which there seems to be a related but distinct type of gene defect. Here there was no reduction of intelligence quotient, no tetany or renal tubular defect, and no metastatic calcification. The clinical features were restricted to calcification of basal ganglia, and the typical short metacarpal bones. All the affected patients were thus cases of pseudo-pseudohypoparathyroidism.

With adequate treatment the disease carries a good prognosis with a normal life expectancy. Mental changes and the tendency to cataract formation are irreversible but may be prevented or greatly reduced in severity by early diagnosis and effective therapy.

Therapy. Fortunately, although there may be complete resistance to the phosphaturic effect of parathyroid hormone, there is no insensitivity to the phosphaturic action of calciferol or dihydrotachysterol. Patients respond rapidly to large daily doses of calciferol, usually between 50,000 and 300,000 units. Extra dietary calcium may be prescribed with advantage. Therapy should be controlled by frequent determinations of serum calcium and phosphate, the ideal dose being the smallest amount that restores serum values to normal. The development of hypercalcemia is an urgent indication to reduce the dose. Rough estimation of urinary calcium by use of the Sulkowitch reagent is sufficient for short-term control, but serum calcium determinations at about monthly intervals should be carried out routinely in all cases.

HYPOPHOSPHATASIA

Hypophosphatasia is a recessive hereditary disease characterized by skeletal abnormalities and lack or absence of alkaline phosphatase throughout the body. Although it is not primarily a renal disease, the kidney shares in the generalized enzymatic defect, and secondary renal abnormalities are frequent and important aspects of the disease. The condition was first accurately described by Rathbun [215] in 1948, but patients who were probably examples of the condition had previously been reported [93].

Clinical Signs and Symptoms. The disease is rare, the frequency having been estimated as 1 case per 100,000 live births [93]. There is great variation in the age at which symptoms and signs first occur, and usually the severity of the disease is greater the earlier the age at onset.

In the most severe cases the skeletal abnormalities may develop in utero, and always within the first six months of life. The signs are similar to those of severe rickets, particularly the marked costochondral beading and expansions of the epiphyses of long bones. Bone tenderness and kyphosis occurring soon after attempts at sitting up or standing are common. Unlike rickets, in hypophosphatasia there is a high frequency of fractures from slight degrees of trauma which result in bony angulations and severe deformity of limbs. Longitudinal growth of bone is delayed, with consequent dwarfism. Radiologic examination shows the changes at the epiphyses to be more severe than in rickets. There are gross defects in metaphyseal calcification, with an abrupt transition to a relatively normal diaphysis. There is often tilting of the epiphyseal plate and subperiosteal calcification. The skull x-ray shows an appearance suggestive of widening of the sutures with an expanded and bulging anterior fontanelle. The translucent areas are, in fact, uncalcified osteoid matrix and not bands of fibrous tissue as in normal suture lines in the skull [93, 174]. The prognosis of this severe form of the disease is poor, most of the affected babies dying in the first year of life. If the child survives the first two or three years of life the disease usually passes into a stage of partial remission.

In less severe cases the first evidence of skeletal abnormality occurs after the age of six months and in most instances the lesions are present by the age of two years. The most common deformity is genu valgum, which is sometimes severe enough to warrant surgery. Dwarfism usually occurs, but some patients are of normal height. The changes seen radiologically are similar to those in the infantile form of the disease, but are less severe. There is usually gradual improvement in the skeletal lesions in later childhood, and life expectancy is probably little reduced. In the least severe or "adult" type of the disease, the patient shows no abnormalities during childhood but presents with excess fragility of bones and liability to fractures in adult life. Radiologic examination shows a generalized skeletal osteoporosis, and the diagnosis depends on the typical abnormal biochemistry of the disease.

Biochemical Abnormalities and Renal Aspects. There is considerable reduction of serum alkaline phosphatase, but the values should always be interpreted in relation to the normal for the patient's age. In the infantile form the serum alkaline phosphatase is less than 4 Bodansky units or 10 King-Armstrong units per 100 ml., and in the less severe condition in childhood, less than 1 Bodansky or 5 King-Armstrong units per 100 ml. The amount varies from zero to about 40 per cent of the average normal value. Histochemical and other enzymatic methods have shown a reduced phosphatase content of bone, liver, intestinal mucosa (see below), and renal tubular cells [93, 174]. Although previous descriptions of the disease claimed that intestinal alkaline phosphatase was absent, this was based on unreliable analysis of postmortem specimens. Doubt was first cast when it was found that an abnormally high fraction of the reduced content of plasma phosphatase had the properties of the intestinal enzyme [205]. In addition, it was found that the alkaline phosphatase content of duodenal juice was within normal limits [228]. Danovitch et al. [64] have recently reported that the phosphatase content of mucosa obtained at peroral biopsy was within normal limits or was even on occasions abnormally high. This shows that diseases involving an enzymatic deficiency are unlikely to affect all the many isoenzymes within body cells, as these may be proteins of widely different amino acid sequence and therefore controlled by separate gene loci. There is no consistent abnormality of serum phosphate concentration, but serum calcium is abnormally high in many of the severe infantile examples of the disease.

There is invariably an abnormal output of phosphoethanolamine in the urine [95, 176]. This compound reacts with Ninhydrin and may therefore be confused with an amino acid. It is almost undetectable in plasma, as the renal clearance of the substance is high and approximates the glomerular filtration rate [60]. Normally this substance is found only within cells, but it leaks into extracellular fluid when alkaline phosphatase is reduced in hypophosphatasia and occasionally in other conditions associated with reduction of alkaline phosphatase (e.g., celiac disease, infantile scurvy, and hypothyroidism). Patients with hypophosphatasia may excrete up to 200 mg. of phosphoethanolamine daily [93, 176]. Other phosphate esters may sometimes be detected in urine from patients with phosphatasia; probably one of these is adenosine monophosphate [174]. Heterozygotes from affected families also excrete small amounts of phosphoethanolamine. This abnormality is more constant in symptomless carriers than is reduction of serum alkaline phosphatase [94].

Russell [224] found that urinary pyrophosphate was substantially elevated in cases of hypophosphatosis. He obtained excretion rates averaging 144 micromoles per 24 hours compared to a normal mean of 40 micromoles per 24 hours. In addition, the ratio of pyrophosphate to orthophosphate in urine was always greater than 0.4 per cent in the patients and always less than this figure in controls. Pyrophosphate is a known inhibitor of calcification of bone, and Russell suggests that one of the normal functions of alkaline phosphatase is removal of potentially toxic pyrophosphate from body fluids.

Evidence of impaired renal function is frequent in the more severe infantile cases [94]. There is proteinuria and increase of blood urea, and secondary hypertension is often found. These changes, however, may be secondary to nephrocalcinosis from the hypercalcemia of the disease. Although nephrocalcinosis is rarely severe enough to be demonstrated by radiology during life, deposits of calcium in the renal tubular cells and the interstitial tissue of the kidney are often found at autopsy.

Therapy. Calciferol therapy is ineffective and in fact is contraindicated because it often precipitates severe hypercalcemia [93]. Fraser [93, 94] has reported favorably on the use of cortisone in severe cases. When hypercalcemia is severe, a low calcium diet is indicated. In assessment of therapy it must be remembered that the clinical but not the biochemical abnormalities of the disease usually remit a few years after the peak severity of the condition.

Distal Tubular Syndromes

The nephropathy of potassium deficiency and that associated with hypercalcemia are discussed in other chapters. Nephrogenic diabetes insipidus is described in detail in Chapter 38. The syndromes of "salt-losing nephritis," renal tubular acidosis, and primary oxalosis will be described in this section.

SALT-LOSING NEPHRITIS

Abnormal loss of sodium in the urine is common in most cases of uremia. Normally less than 1 per cent of the sodium filtered at the glomeruli is excreted in the urine, the remainder being reabsorbed by both the proximal and the distal tubule cells. In chronic renal failure with a gross reduction of the amount of sodium filtered, there is a proportionate reduction of the fraction reabsorbed and thus sodium balance is maintained [213].

In most cases of chronic renal failure the tubules become unresponsive to aldosterone, but occasionally sensitivity to aldosterone is preserved, causing a combination of the signs and symptoms of uremia and of nephrotic edema. Under normal conditions, therefore, patients with uremia do not lose excessive amounts of sodium in the urine, but the normal reaction of the kidney to salt deficiency is lost. Normal subjects in states of sodium deficit secrete excess aldosterone and as a result the urine is virtually sodium-free. Uremic subjects insensitive to secreted aldosterone continue to excrete sodium in the urine despite salt deficiency from uremic vomiting or diarrhea. They therefore show rapid clinical deterioration unless appropriate therapy is given when salt is lost in vomit and feces. Secondary reduction of the glomerular filtration rate takes place with rapid rise of the blood urea. Death often occurs unless the vicious circle is broken by infusions of saline or sodium lactate.

Salt-losing nephritis may be defined as a nephropathy in which there is glomerulotubular imbalance with respect to sodium, with excess sodium excretion in the urine despite a normal sodium intake. It has not been proved whether there is a sharp dividing line between the familiar tendency to salt wastage in uremia and the gross urinary sodium loss in the extreme cases of salt-losing nephritis. Possibly there is a continuous spectrum of tubular insufficiency and only the most extreme cases have been termed salt-losing nephritis. The practical clinical distinction is that patients with chronic uremia are able to maintain salt balance unless there is dietary sodium restriction or an abnormal sodium loss in gastrointestinal secretions, whereas patients with salt-losing nephritis cannot maintain sodium balance unless an amount of sodium far in excess of the normal intake is given. All cases of salt-losing nephritis reported to date have shown irreversible chronic uremia. Acute exacerbation in the degree of nitrogen retention is due often to reduced glomerular filtration rate from salt deficiency added to irreversible glomerular damage. An increase of the glomerular filtration rate with a corresponding fall of blood urea occurs when appropriate supplements of saline or of sodium lactate are given. Salt-losing nephritis is in some respects analogous to pseudohypoparathyroidism since both diseases are due to insensitivity of tubular cells to a secreted hormone. The former disorder, however, although commonly encountered in medullary cystic disease (a condition believed to be congenital — see Chapter 36), may also occur as an acquired abnormality, whereas the latter is always an hereditary condition.

Clinical Signs and Symptoms. True salt-losing nephritis is rare, fewer than 20 cases having been reported since the condition was first described by Thorn et al. [262] in 1944. The clinical signs and symptoms are very similar to those of primary Addison's disease. An analogy may be drawn to spontaneous hypoparathyroidism, one type of which is due to absence or hypofunction of the endocrine gland, whereas in the other the disease is due to insensitivity of the renal tubular cells to secreted hormone. The clinical picture is dominated by signs of sodium deficiency. There is circulatory collapse with a weak rapid pulse and gross fall in arterial blood pressure, often associated with postural hypotension and syncope. The peripheral veins are collapsed, the skin loses its normal elasticity, and the eyeballs are sunken. There is gross muscle weakness and evidence of weight loss with profound anorexia, nausea, and vomiting. Severe muscle cramps from sodium deficiency are common. In relapse, the patient often seems to be moribund, and death may in fact occur unless appropriate treatment with infusions of saline or sodium lactate is urgently given. The serum sodium and chloride concentrations are reduced, and there is some rise of serum potassium. There is gross oliguria and a rapidly rising blood urea. There is usually uremic acidosis with fall of plasma bicarbonate and arterial blood pH. Pigmentation of the skin is frequent and increases the difficulty of differential diagnosis from primary adrenal cortical failure. Areas of pigmentation of the buccal mucosa are rarely, if ever, present in salt-losing nephritis.

Differential Diagnosis. Differential diagnosis from Addison's disease is of great importance because treatment with adrenal cortical hormones is valueless in salt-losing nephritis. The distribution of pigmentation is of great significance. In salt-losing nephritis the pigmentation is more diffuse than in Addison's disease, in which the pigmentation is characteristically in the mucous membrane of the mouth, at pressure points, in the axillary folds, and in the creases of the palms of the hands. Adrenal steroids — for example, cortisol and its derivatives, aldosterone, desoxycorticosterone, or fluorhydrocortisone — have no effect on the abnormal urinary sodium loss in salt-losing nephritis. Excretion of adrenal steroids and their metabolic products — for example, cortisol, cortisone and their tetrahydro derivatives, and aldosterone — is greatly reduced in Addison's disease but is normal or increased in salt-losing nephritis. Cases of salt-losing nephritis do not show the disorders of carbohydrate metabolism often seen in Addison's disease, such as hypoglycemia and abnormal sensitivity to insulin. Injection of corticotropin has no effect on urinary steroids in Addison's disease, but increases the output of ketogenic steroids, 17-hydroxycorticoids, cortisol, cortisone, and their tetrahydro derivatives in salt-losing nephritis. Excretion of a large water load is subnormal in both diseases. Cortisone increases the amount excreted in Addison's disease but has no effect in salt-losing nephritis.

Cases of salt-losing nephritis often show severe secondary hypersecretion of aldosterone. The continued loss of salt in the urine reduces the extracellular fluid and plasma volumes and stimulates aldosterone secretion. Aldosterone output in the urine is increased above normal values, and is usually much higher than in cases of primary aldosteronism. Stanbury and Mahler [253] have shown that the stimulus to increased aldosterone output may persist long after appropriate therapy has restored extracellular fluid and plasma volumes to normal. An output of aldosterone 10 times the average normal was found at a time when the patient had no deficiency of sodium and had been adequately treated for a whole year. They suggest that long-continued stimulus to excess production of aldosterone may lead to autonomy of hormone production. The excess aldosterone is ineffective in preventing renal sodium loss because of insensitivity of the tubules to the action of the hormone. The extrarenal effects of the hormone result in reduced sodium in sweat and feces and in a low ratio of sodium to potassium in saliva, as in other types of hyperaldosteronism. At autopsy the adrenal cortex is found to be hypertrophied, and sometimes there is secondary formation of adenomas [253].

Causation. Cases of this syndrome have commonly been ascribed to chronic pyelonephritis [82], but many cases have been recorded in cystic disease of the renal medulla (see Chapter 36), and one in polycystic disease presumably of the hereditary type. Pyelonephritis superimposed on old nephrocalcinosis from excessive intake of milk and alkali in treatment of peptic ulcer seems especially liable to cause salt-wasting nephropathy.

Treatment. Patients with salt-losing nephropathy require a considerably larger sodium intake than normal persons. This may be given as sodium chloride if there is no uremic acidosis, or as a mixture of sodium chloride and bicarbonate if acidosis is present. The proportion should be adjusted to keep the plasma bicarbonate and arterial blood pH in the low-normal range, as overcorrection of acidosis may cause convulsions or tetany. In the acute stages of the illness, when there is usually severe nausea or vomiting, fluid must be given by intravenous injection. Patients with salt-losing nephritis are very liable to develop water intoxication if hypotonic fluids are given by injection. All intravenous fluids at this stage should be either normal saline or one-sixth molar sodium lactate. If the sodium deficiency is especially severe, the intravenous fluids should preferably be hypertonic and contain greater amounts of sodium.

Many patients with salt-losing nephritis are unable to excrete very large amounts of sodium, and their daily dose of sodium must be defined within very narrow limits. Some patients oscillate precariously between states of sodium deficit, in which there is circulatory collapse, oliguria, and a rising blood urea, and states of sodium excess with congestive heart failure, edema, and increasing arterial blood pressure. Probably the ideal dose in most cases is the maximal amount of sodium that the patient can take without developing edema or arterial hypertension. Patients with salt-losing nephritis do not usually develop a craving for salt, since there is no instinctive reflex in relation to sodium comparable to thirst for the correction of water deficits. These patients therefore need constant expert supervision, but therapy is rewarding, the patients often being able to live normal and useful lives until terminal irreversible renal failure occurs.

RENAL TUBULAR ACIDOSIS: GENERAL CONSIDERATIONS

Physiologic Aspects. One of the most important functions of the kidney is the secretion of hydrogen ion from the tubular cells into the tubular lumen, thus eliminating the excess hydrogen ion derived from metabolism of sulfur-containing amino acids and from phospholipids. Micropuncture and stop-flow technics have proved that this transfer of hydrogen ion takes place throughout the nephron, but that final urinary acidification occurs in the distal and collecting tubule. About two-thirds of the excreted hydrogen ion is combined with ammonia as ammonium ion (NH_4^+) and one-third as free ion, which is measured by the urinary titratable acidity. Free ammonia is a diffusible base, and therefore its excretion obeys the laws of ion-trapping or non-ionic diffusion [197, 208]. More ammonium ion is excreted in acid urine and correspondingly less in alkaline urine. Graphs have been published [47, 282] giving the limits of the relationship between the ammonium output in microequivalents per minute and the urinary pH. If ammonium excretion is excessive in relation to urinary pH, there is supernormal synthesis of ammonia by distal tubular cells from glutamine and certain amino acids in the arterial blood. This occurs in chronic metabolic acidosis and in potassium deficiency. The exact stimulus to excess ammonia synthesis is unknown. It is not dependent on the intracellular pH of renal tubular cells, since there is no excess ammonia synthesis in respiratory acidosis. Deficient ammonia synthesis leads to a subnormal excretion of ammonium as related to urinary pH. This occurs only if there is gross reduction of renal tubular mass as in chronic renal failure with uremia.

Titratable acidity depends on the urinary pH and the amount of urinary buffer substances. At ordinary urinary pH values, from 5.6 to 6.6, phosphate is the only effective urinary buffer substance; therefore, excreted acid phosphate accounts for almost all urinary titratable acidity [193]. If the urine is more acid, organic acids become progressively more important, and in maximally acid urine, phosphate may account for less than half of the titratable acid. Total hydrogen ion excretion is measured by the sum of ammonia excretion and titratable acid less urinary bicarbonate. If the patient is in acid-base balance, the amount excreted must equal the acid-ash value of the diet. Another important aspect of the ability of the kidney to excrete hydrogen ion, the production of a high gradient of hydrogen ion between urine and plasma, is only indirectly related to total hydrogen ion excretion. If the urine cannot be acidified below pH values of 6.0 or 5.5, ammonium excretion is automatically less than in more acid urine, as smaller quantities of ammonia diffuse into the tubular lumen, and the kidney loses the ability to excrete hydrogen ion as free organic acid. Acid-base balance may be maintained, however, by excretion of sufficient ammonia and of acid phosphate.

Inability to maintain a normal maximal hydrogen ion gradient is the fundamental abnormality in renal tubular acidosis. In normal subjects the maximal hydrogen ion gradient between urine and plasma is dependent on the stimulus used to produce a highly acid urine. The usual method is ingestion of ammonium chloride, a daily intake of 12 gm. for three days in adults being sufficient to produce a maximal effect on hydrogen ion gradient. The urine pH will normally fall below pH 5.0 and often to pH 4.4, indicating a hydrogen ion gradient between urine and plasma of 1000:1. Other stimuli, however, are more potent in stimulating exchange of hydrogen ion for sodium in the distal tubule. Adrenal steroids increase sodium reabsorption and also the exchange of potassium and hydrogen ion for sodium. Aldosterone potentiates both potassium and hydrogen-ion exchange, but cortisol has no effect on hydrogen-ion exchange [191].

The primary effect of aldosterone on the tubule cell is probably an increased transfer of sodium from the tubular lumen into the renal capillary blood. This produces an electrochemical gradient across the tubular wall, and if sodium is chiefly accompanied by a diffusible anion, such as chloride, the gradient is neutralized by corresponding transfer of anion. If, however, sodium is accompanied by a nondiffusible anion such as sulfate, para-aminohippurate, or phosphate, the gradient can be neutralized only by exchange of hydrogen ion and potassium for the sodium reabsorbed. The result will be a highly acid urine containing large amounts of potassium. If normal subjects are infused with sodium sulfate in states of hyperaldosteronism, urine as acid as pH 4.0 may be excreted, the resultant hydrogen-ion gradient between urine and plasma being 2500 [235]. The hyperaldosteronism may be produced either by salt depletion or by injections of aldosterone or desoxycorticosterone. These physiologic considerations are essential in forming a clear conception of the defects in renal tubular acidosis.

Definition. The only way to define renal tubular acidosis is in relation to functional tests of maximal renal acidification. Under the stimulus of ammonium chloride ingestion or of spontaneous metabolic acidosis a normal subject can acidify the urine at least to pH 5.0 and often to pH 4.4. Some arbitrary level of minimum urinary pH has to be adopted in any definition of renal tubular acidosis. Probably the most useful definition: Renal tubular acidosis is an inability to acidify the urine, under the stimulus of ammonium chloride ingestion or of spontaneous metabolic acidosis, below a pH of 5.4. This leaves a group of intermediate cases in which the minimal urinary pH is from 5.0 to 5.4, emphasizing that renal tubular acidosis is not a strictly definable entity any more than is hypertension in relation to variations in arterial blood pressure, or obesity in relation to variation in body weight.

In the definition of renal tubular acidosis it is essential to include the stimulus to urinary acidification. Under the more potent stimulus of hyperaldosteronism combined with infusion of the sodium salt of a nondiffusible anion, patients with renal tubular acidosis may produce a lower urinary pH than under the stimulus of ammonium chloride, like normal subjects. The maximal hydrogen ion gradient, however, will still be below that in all normal subjects under identical experimental conditions.

Systemic acidosis in cases of renal tubular acidosis is therefore due to inability to acidify urine, which reduces ammonium excretion by lowering diffusion of ammonia into acid urine, and reduces the titratable acid fraction excreted as organic acids. In contrast, acidosis in chronic renal failure with uremia is due to reduction of the total tubular mass with corresponding reduction in the amount of ammonia synthesis. The ability to produce a high hydrogen-ion gradient between urine and plasma is usually well preserved in uremia, and the urine is therefore highly acid [282].

These physiologic differences explain the contrasts in plasma electrolyte chemistry in renal tubular acidosis and uremic acidosis. In both, there is acidosis with fall in arterial blood pH and a corresponding fall in plasma bicarbonate. The acidosis stimulates the respiratory center, and therefore there is hyperventilation with some reduction of pCO_2. In uremia, however, there is a reduced clearance of phosphate and sulfate as well as of urea and creatinine, and therefore plasma sulfate and phosphate increase. This increase is often greater than the decrease of plasma bicarbonate; consequently, plasma chloride is usually low. In renal tubular acidosis the clearances of urea, creatinine, phosphate, and sulfate are normal, and therefore plasma phosphate and sulfate concentrations remain within normal limits. The plasma phosphate is, in fact, often somewhat reduced, owing to high phosphate clearance from secondary hyperparathyroidism and systemic acidosis. A low plasma bicarbonate in renal tubular acidosis must therefore inevitably be associated with increase of plasma chloride.

The high plasma chloride of the disease has led to use of the term *hyperchloremic acidosis* to describe the abnormalities of plasma biochemistry. This is a bad term since it gives the impression that increase of plasma chloride is a primary abnormality, whereas in fact it is a secondary effect of acidosis not associated with increase of plasma phosphate and sulfate.

Causes. The foregoing definition of renal tubular acidosis as a functional defect of hydrogen-ion transfer includes cases in which there is no significant acidosis, plasma pH and bicarbonate being within the normal range. In such instances, however, the patients have a potential tendency to acidosis and always have reduced ability to excrete acid loads in comparison with normal subjects.

The principal known causes of renal tubular acidosis are various renal tubular diseases, potassium-deficient nephropathy, and inhibition of renal carbonic anhydrase. Many diseases causing renal tubular damage can interfere with distal tubular transfer of hydrogen ion. These include chronic pyelonephritis and various tubular diseases usually classified as proximal tubular disorders. Many proximal tubular disorders are due to nonspecific damage of tubular function — for example, Lignac-Fanconi syndrome, adult Fanconi syndrome, Lowe's syndrome, Wilson's disease, and poisoning with nephrotoxic drugs. Although the damage is greatest in the more sensitive proximal tubule, distal functional defects are frequent — for example, loss of urinary concentrating power and renal tubular acidosis. Inhibition of carbonic anhydrase by administration of acetazolamide, or in lesser degree by the benzothiadiazine group of diuretics, produces a renal functional defect typical of renal tubular acidosis. There is systemic acidosis with reduced ability to acidify the urine. This does not prove that other types of renal tubular acidosis are due to carbonic anhydrase deficiency, and in fact most cases of renal tubular acidosis respond normally to renal carbonic anhydrase inhibition by acetazolamide. The temporary defect produced by acetazolamide is presumably due to reduced ability to produce hydrogen ion from carbonic acid, with a reduction of hydrogen-ion transfer from the tubular cell into the tubular lumen. Renal tubular acidosis also occurs in potassium deficiency [47], although failure of concentrating power is a more characteristic and constant defect. In potassium depletion there is often an extracellular alkalosis, which makes "renal tubular acidosis" apparently an unsuitable term. However, this extracellular alkalosis is accompanied by increased hydrogen ion concentration in voluntary muscle [104, 227], and in fact gain of hydrogen ion by the intracellular compartment is often greater than loss from the extracellular fluid. There is thus a total body acidosis despite an alkalosis of the extracellular compartment. The renal functional defects both in carbonic anhydrase inhibition and in potassium deficiency are usually fully reversible after withdrawal of the inhibitor or repletion with potassium salts.

In the absence of a known cause for renal tubular acidosis it is termed *primary,* and can be divided into an infantile and an adult form. These are described separately.

PRIMARY RENAL TUBULAR ACIDOSIS IN INFANTS

This is one of a group of metabolic disorders of infants which are characterized by the general description of "failure to thrive," a term which seems to have replaced the older "marasmus." It occurs principally during the first 18 months of life and exhibits the typical biochemical abnormalities of renal tubular acidosis — that is, reduced plasma bicarbonate and arterial blood pH with a corresponding rise of plasma chloride and with an alkaline, neutral, or only faintly acid urine. There is sometimes radiologic evidence of diffuse calcification in the medulla of the kidneys. The condition was first described by Lightwood in 1935 [157] and 87 cases have been recorded since [130].

Infantile renal tubular acidosis is not considered to be hereditary, and apparently is not due to the effects of any known drug or toxin on the kidney. Males are affected more often than females in a ratio of about 2:1 [130]. There is no satisfactory evidence that the functional defect is due to deficiency of renal carbonic anhydrase.

Symptoms and Signs. The average age at onset is about 8 months, with a range of 1 to 18 months. The most common presenting symptoms are constipation, anorexia, vomiting, and failure to thrive. Apathy, irritability, thirst, and polyuria are less common in the early stages of the disease. The important clinical signs of the disease are evidence of wasting, the presence of fecal masses in the abdomen, hypotonia of muscle, and signs of dehydration. The diagnosis, however, depends on the typical abnormal biochemical findings of the disease. Plasma chloride ranges from 105 to 135 mEq. per liter, and plasma bicarbonate from 5 to 25 mEq. per liter, depending on the severity of the acidosis [159]. The urinary pH on admission to hospital is usually between 6.0 and 7.1. The blood urea is increased in about 50 per cent of cases, but this is a reversible azotemia from salt deficiency and dehydration and rapidly responds to intravenous fluid replacement. There is often a trace of protein in the urine, and secondary urinary infection with pyuria is common. The specific gravity of the urine is usually between 1.005 and 1.010.

Calcification of both kidneys can be demonstrated radiologically in about one-third of cases and is more common in the older infants. It varies in severity from particulate calcific deposits in the renal medulla to a faint ground-glass opacity of the kidneys due to minute diffuse deposits. Probably cases in which calcium cannot be demonstrated radiologically would show an increased calcium content of renal tissue if analysis could be performed. Rickets is not usually present in infantile renal tubular acidosis, and plasma potassium and phosphate are usually normal, unlike the values in the adult form of the disease.

Differential Diagnosis. The differential diagnosis is from other conditions of infancy causing failure to thrive. The biochemical findings should always give the correct diagnosis. Probably the condition which is most often confused with the disease is pyelonephritis, because of the secondary infection of the urine so often present in infantile renal tubular acidosis. Lignac-Fanconi syndrome, nephrogenic diabetes insipidus, and infantile hypercalcemia may resemble the disease clinically, but the biochemical abnormalities are completely different.

Abnormal Physiology and Biochemistry. The most important biochemical abnormalities are sodium deficiency and acidosis. Sodium deficiency causes the wasting and gastrointestinal symptoms so typical of the disease, and results in secondary hyperaldosteronism. Latner and Burnard [151] found that infusions of sodium phosphate caused a temporarily increased ability to form an acid urine. This was interpreted as a temporary improvement in renal function due to excess phosphate, but is now explained by a more potent stimulus to renal acidification due to infusion of a sodium salt of a nondiffusible anion in states of hyperaldosteronism. The tendency to nephrocalcinosis occurs in both the infantile and the adult types of primary renal tubular acidosis and is discussed in more detail in the account of the adult form of the condition. The distal tubules in renal tubular acidosis are defective in renal concentrating power, transfer of hydrogen ion, and reabsorption of sodium. Loss of sodium in the urine cannot entirely be explained by failure of exchange of hydrogen ion for sodium, since there is an additional primary defect of sodium transport possibly due to insensitivity to secreted aldosterone. Sodium loss and dehydration are naturally more severe in infants with severe vomiting.

Treatment and Prognosis. Renal tubular acidosis of infancy responds well to treatment and is a completely reversible condition provided the infant does not die in the acute stages of the disease. If dehydration is severe, treatment should be started by intravenous infusion of isotonic sodium lactate. Infants do not tolerate the high content of citric acid in the formula of Shohl and Butler [246] and Albright et al. [5]. A suitable modification is sodium citrate, 10 gm., and citric acid, 6 gm., in 100 ml. of water. An initial prescription should be 15 ml. of this mixture four times daily. After two weeks the plasma chemistry is reassessed and the dose adjusted according to the level of plasma bicarbonate which should be maintained, at values from 18 to 22 mEq. per liter. There is usually very rapid symptomatic improvement, with disappearance of the symptoms of anorexia and vomiting and rapid gain in weight. Retention in the hospital is unnecessary after the infant has started to gain weight normally. Treatment should be continued for about one year, after which the dose of alkali can be cautiously reduced. If acidosis does not recur, the alkali can be slowly reduced to zero and the infant can be regarded as cured. Some cases, however, require longer periods of therapy before spontaneous improvement in distal tubular function occurs. Some infants suffer from diarrhea on treatment and may tolerate similar doses of sodium bicarbonate better than the citrate-citric acid mixture. A follow-up study [41] has shown that renal tubular acidosis of infancy is a completely reversible condition; distal tubular function becomes completely normal after some years, and the infants show no permanent defects as a result of this severe but fortunately curable renal tubular disease.

PRIMARY RENAL TUBULAR ACIDOSIS IN ADULTS

This disease may be discovered in four ways: (1) the presenting symptom may be a periodic paralysis similar to familial periodic paralysis except that there is a chronic persistent hypokalemia between the attacks of paralysis; (2) there may be bone pain and a characteristic waddling gait found on investigation to be due to rickets or osteomalacia; (3) the patient may present with typical renal colic; or (4) the condition may be discovered entirely by accident if the abdomen is x-rayed for other unrelated conditions. Unlike renal tubular acidosis in infants, the adult form has a chronic and prolonged clinical course, and treatment with citrates or other alkalinizing salts produces symptomatic and clinical improvement but not cure. The first symptoms and signs usually occur in adolescence or early adult life but occasionally in children between 3 and 10 years old [130]. About 75 cases have been reported [130] since the first description by Albright et al. [5] in 1940. Two-thirds of the patients are females, a sex incidence completely opposite to that of the infantile type of the disease.

In the fully developed disease the diagnosis is made by finding a chronic acidosis with an abnormally low plasma bicarbonate and arterial blood pH, associated with an alkaline, neutral, or only slightly acid urine. A typical case might have a plasma bicarbonate before therapy of 16 mEq. per liter, an arterial blood pH of 7.30, and a urinary pH varying from 5.8 to 7.4. In such a case it is unnecessary to give ammonium chloride as a diagnostic procedure. This intensifies the systemic acidosis but does not cause any fall in urinary pH. About 50 per cent of cases show bilateral nephrocalcinosis, the calcification being in the medullary portion of the kidney (Fig. 30-9). Renal tubular acidosis is the third most common cause of bilateral nephrocalcinosis, being exceeded in number of cases only by primary hyperparathyroidism and chronic pyelonephritis.

There is also a less complete type or "forme fruste" of renal tubular acidosis, which is more difficult to recognize [282]. This condi-

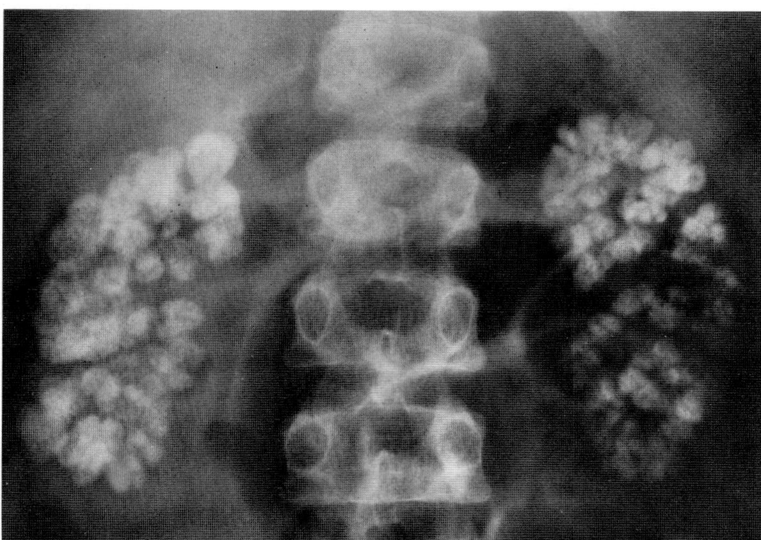

Figure 30-9. X-ray of kidneys in a case of renal tubular acidosis with severe bilateral nephrocalcinosis.

tion would be suspected and recognized only if there was unexplained nephrocalcinosis, but presumably incomplete cases without nephrocalcinosis must occasionally occur. The condition might possibly be termed *renal tubular acidosis sine acidosis*. In this type of the disease there is no systemic acidosis, plasma bicarbonate and arterial blood pH being normal. Hydrogen-ion excretion by the kidney is therefore quantitatively normal, but it is qualitatively abnormal. The amount of hydrogen ion excreted is equal to that excreted by a normal control, but a proportionately greater fraction is excreted as ammonia and less as titratable acidity. The ammonia output is abnormally high when related to urinary pH, which indicates that ammonia synthesis from glutamine and amino acids is above normal. The diagnosis is confirmed by giving ammonium chloride, 6 to 12 gm. by mouth. This causes a systemic acidosis, and normally the urinary pH should fall below 5.0. In the incomplete form of renal tubular acidosis the urinary pH does not fall below 5.4, although ammonia synthesis and excretion increase as in normal subjects.

The periodic paralysis of renal tubular acidosis may closely simulate familial periodic paralysis, in which recurrent attacks of paralysis occur in the morning on awakening or are precipitated by a large intake of carbohydrate. Unlike the familial condition, however, the periodic paralysis of renal tubular acidosis is characterized by chronic hypokalemia between attacks, and the other diagnostic biochemical signs of renal tubular acidosis are present. The condition is due to chronic increased urinary loss of potassium, the daily output of potassium in the urine being above 30 mEq. despite a plasma concentration below 3.5 mEq. per liter. The high potassium output may partly be due to decreased secretion of hydrogen ion into the tubular lumen, since normally there is competition between potassium and hydrogen ion for exchange with sodium in the tubular fluid [28]. Possibly there is in addition some secondary hyperaldosteronism from chronic sodium deficiency, which would intensify urinary potassium loss.

The rickets or osteomalacia of the condition is radiologically and clinically similar to that due to other causes (e.g., dietary vitamin D deficiency, or vitamin D resistance).

In doubtful cases a trephine biopsy of bone from the iliac crest will confirm the diagnosis. The classic biochemical signs of a reduced plasma phosphate with a normal or high urinary output of phosphate, and therefore an increased phosphate clearance, are usually present. The increased phosphate clearance is probably chiefly due to secondary hyperparathyroidism, although the chronic acidosis of the condition may have a minor influence in increasing phosphate output.

The first presenting symptom is often renal colic due to passage of a small calcium phosphate calculus down one ureter. In other cases, sudden hematuria or an attack of pyelonephritis may be the first evidence of renal disease. The calculi are usually small enough to pass down the ureters, but can cause recurrent disabling attacks of severe pain and hematuria. Female patients with renal tubular acidosis are able to have normal pregnancies, usually without complications other than increased susceptibility to secondary acute pyelonephritis. During pregnancy the ureters are often dilated and the patients frequently pass small calculi, often with little or no discomfort. The liability of patients with renal tubular acidosis to nephrocalcinosis and formation of urinary calculi is possibly due to the effect of the disease on urinary citrate output. Urinary citrate is increased in alkalosis and reduced in acidosis. These changes are not due to changes in urinary pH but are secondary to the alteration in systemic acid-base balance [197]. Calcium phosphate would precipitate to a much greater extent in alkaline urine were it not for the simultaneous increase of urinary citrate, which has an important effect of chelating calcium and increasing its solubility, despite an alkaline urinary pH. In renal tubular acidosis, urinary citrate is almost nonexistent as a result of the effects of chronic acidosis, but the urine may be neutral or frankly alkaline, favoring precipitation of calcium phosphate. Efficient therapy with alkalinizing salts increases urinary citrate and may sometimes reduce existing nephrocalcinosis.

There is always loss of normal urinary concentrating power in renal tubular acidosis. The patient passes large volumes of urine, usually of specific gravity 1.010, and suffers from a corresponding degree of thirst and nocturnal polyuria with disturbance of sleep. This is in fact a fortunate accompaniment, despite the inconvenience to the patient, because the dilute urine reduces precipitation of calcium phosphate and the tendency to nephrocalcinosis and formation of renal calculi. There is excess loss of sodium in the urine, but this is not so severe as in salt-losing nephritis and usually inconveniences the patient only when there is gastrointestinal loss of sodium from vomiting or diarrhea. In such cases, excessive salt loss may cause circulatory collapse and necessitate prompt therapy with intravenous saline or sodium lactate. The chronic potassium deficiency may cause muscular weakness and apathy even if it is not sufficiently severe to produce frank hypokalemic periodic paralysis. There is often hypokalemic nephropathy which may predispose to pyelonephritis [273], and the potassium deficiency may intensify the typical renal functional defect of inability to maintain a normal high gradient of hydrogen ion between urine and plasma [47]. The ability to acidify the urine should preferably be tested both before and after correction of the potassium deficit with potassium salts.

Secondary pyelonephritis is liable to occur in any renal disease complicated by nephrocalcinosis, since there is secondary fibrosis around the calcium deposits, predisposing to infection. In addition, there may be episodes of ureteric obstruction and secondary hydronephrosis during the passage of a renal calculus. There is no evidence, however, that pyelonephritis is the cause of the condition; it is merely a common complication both of nephrocalcinosis and of potassium deficiency.

Pathogenesis. The pathogenesis of primary renal tubular acidosis remains obscure. A similar defect of renal tubular function can be produced by administration of carbonic anhydrase inhibitors (e.g., acetazolamide) which leads to systemic acidosis with a neutral or alkaline urine and diminution of urinary citrate [47]. After administration of acetazolamide for prolonged periods, there may be an increased tendency to renal calculus formation [115]. There is no proof, however, that renal tubular acidosis is due to lack of renal carbonic anhydrase. Administration of acetazolamide to patients with the disease causes alkalinization of the urine with increase of urinary bicarbonate and intensification of the existing systemic acidosis [272]. It is perhaps more likely that the abnormality of secretion of hydrogen ion rests on the fraction which is not dependent on renal carbonic anhydrase. An alternative hypothesis — that the defect is in the collecting tubule distal to the site of acidification of tubular fluid — has never been disproved. Normally the collecting tubule is impermeable to hydrogen ion, and therefore the high gradient of hydrogen ion between tubular fluid and plasma remains constant. Increased permeability of the collecting ducts to hydrogen ion would produce the functional defect of renal tubular acidosis although secretion and exchange of hydrogen ion in the more proximal portions of the nephron remained normal.

At least 14 families with multiple cases have been reported [130, 244], suggesting that the disease is due to a dominant hereditary factor with incomplete penetrance. The unequal sex ratio can only be explained by greater penetrance in females. A suggestion that injudicious and chronic use of carbonic anhydrase inhibitors might produce irreversible enzyme inhibition remains completely unconfirmed, and there is no evidence that acetazolamide produces irreversible renal damage other than that due to nephrocalcinosis and renal calculi.

An interesting acquired type of renal tubular acidosis has been described by McCurdy et al. [179]. After administration of amphotericin B, there is almost always renal damage, the clinical picture being very similar to primary renal tubular acidosis. The drug causes a severe urinary acidification defect, usually with systemic acidosis, secondary potassium depletion, and nephrocalcinosis.

The functional defect of renal tubular acidosis is often found in conditions causing severe hyperglobulinemia [202]. Multiple myelomatosis may cause a condition resembling the Fanconi syndrome, but other types of hyperglobulinemia may produce a pure renal tubular acidosis without aminoaciduria or other disorders of proximal tubular reabsorption. Renal tubular acidosis has been described associated with cryoglobulinemia [167], hyperglobulinemic purpura [53], and the "juvenile" type of cirrhosis of the liver [216]. Morris and Fudenberg [202] studied 22 hyperglobulinemic patients, and found defective acidification in over 50 per cent of the cases, and demonstrable nephrocalcinosis in two patients. The defect is unconnected with tubular protein reabsorption, as none of the patients had severe proteinuria. It was thought that the lesion was due to impaired blood supply to the renal medulla, possibly related to the increased plasma viscosity from the elevated plasma gamma globulin level.

Treatment and Prognosis. Renal tubular acidosis responds well to therapy with sodium citrate or other alkalinizing salts. An appropriate mixture of sodium citrate, sodium bicarbonate, and potassium citrate in amounts of from 2 to 8 gm. daily is usually adequate. Dosage should be sufficient to restore the previously low plasma potassium and bicarbonate to normal values. Even if calcium deposits are not visible by x-ray examination, it should be assumed that there are microscopic calcific deposits in the renal medulla. Calciferol increases urinary calcium output and predisposes to nephrocalcinosis. It is therefore contraindicated unless rickets or osteomalacia is severe. It should not be employed in the usual case, in which skeletal lesions are clinically absent or minimal in degree.

Ammonium chloride or carbonic anhydrase inhibitors are contraindicated in renal tubular acidosis because they intensify the systemic acidosis and hypercalciuria of the disease. Pyelonephritis should be treated with long courses of the appropriate antibiotic or sulfonamide drug according to the sensitivity of the bacteria causing the infection. Although sulfanilamide itself is contraindicated as a carbonic anhydrase inhibitor, other antibacterial sulfonamide drugs have no tendency to inhibit the enzyme and may safely be used.

The exact prognosis is unknown because cases have not yet been treated for adequate periods. It is certain that the disease is only slowly progressive, renal function remaining apparently unchanged for long periods. The main hazard in the well-controlled patient is progressive renal damage from fibrosis secondary to nephrocalcinosis and to resistant pyelonephritis. In most cases of renal tubular acidosis the glomerular filtration rate is only slightly reduced and the blood urea is normal. Damage from nephrocalcinosis and chronic pyelonephritis may later cause progressive rise of blood urea and death from uremia with or without secondary hypertension.

PRIMARY HYPEROXALURIA

This is a metabolic disease causing nephrocalcinosis, formation of calcium oxalate calculi, and renal failure. It is characterized by increased urinary excretion of oxalates, usually from 100 to 400 mg. daily, as compared with the normal output of less than 45 mg. per day. The condition usually starts in childhood with symptoms of urinary calculous disease. The calculi are wholly or predominantly composed of calcium oxalate. Most patients with calcium oxalate calculi, however, do not excrete excess oxalate and therefore are not examples of primary hyperoxaluria. The prognosis of the disease is unfavorable, death usually occurring in later childhood from uremia caused by progressive renal fibrosis, secondary pyelonephritis, secondary hypertension, or hydronephrosis from ureteric obstruction. At autopsy widespread destruction of renal tubular cells with secondary fibrosis is found, and deposits of calcium oxalate are present throughout both kidneys (Fig. 30-10). Similar deposits of calcium oxalate are present in small arteries, at the growing ends of long bones, and in the myocardium and testes [42, 236]. The condition is inherited as an autosomal recessive disorder [9]. Oxalate has a high renal clearance, and therefore plasma levels are low and difficult to analyze with present biochemical technics.

The large amount of oxalate in the urine of the patients is not derived from dietary oxalate. The increase in urinary oxalate after ingestion of sodium oxalate is identical in normal subjects and patients with primary hyperoxaluria, and is only a small fraction of the ingested dose [10]. It has recently been proved that the oxalate is derived from glycine [10, 185]. This amino acid is converted by oxidative deamination to glyoxylic acid, which may be converted to formate, or reconverted to glycine by transamination. The precise enzymatic defect in primary hyperoxaluria is still unknown, but must involve one of the pathways of metabolism of glyoxylate. If glyoxylate is present in abnormally high concentration, it is converted by aldehyde oxidase or by a mutase to oxalate. Deviation of glycine from this metabolic path, as in feeding excess benzoate with conversion of some glycine to benzoylglycine (hippuric acid), depresses oxalate output in hyperoxaluria [10].

The metabolic defect in primary hyperoxaluria has recently been clarified, but no advances in treatment have been made. There are two distinct types of the disease, which cannot be distinguished on clinical grounds

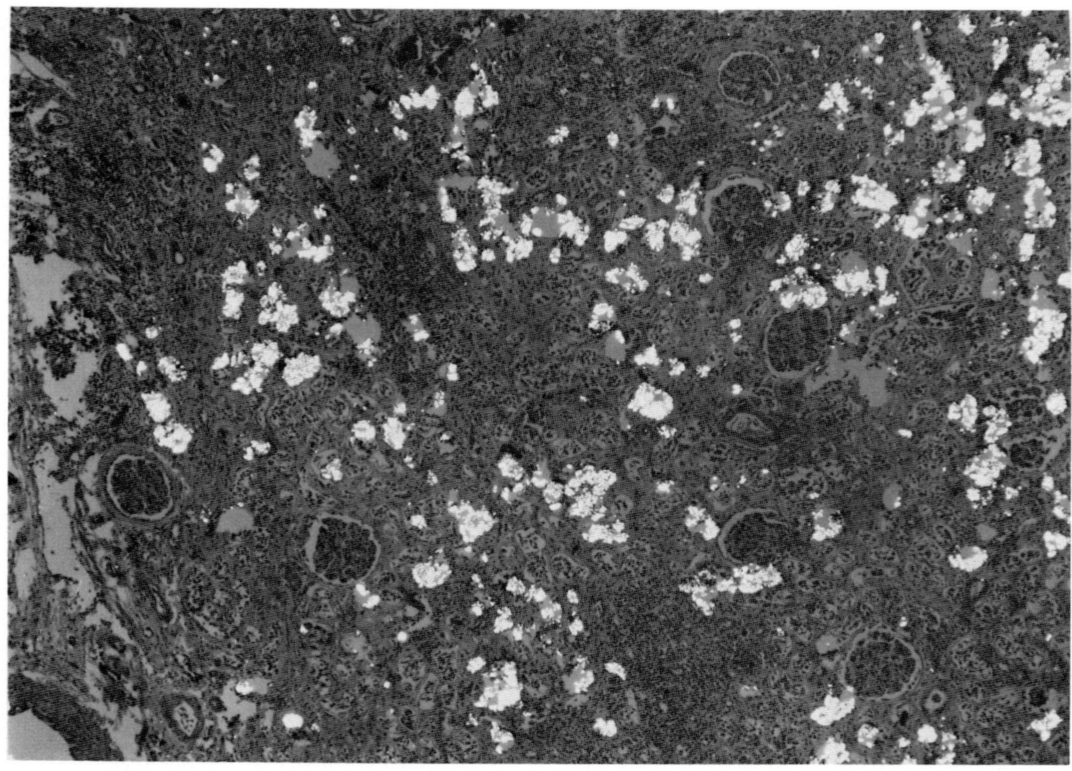

Figure 30-10. Section of kidney in a case of generalized oxalosis. Photographed in polarized light to show the birefringent calcium oxalate crystals in the renal cortex. ×60.

alone [275]. The type I variety is due to absence of the enzyme 2-oxo-glutarate:glyoxylate carboligase in liver, kidney, and spleen [145]. In this condition the urinary oxalate averages 250 mg. per 24 hours per 1.73 square meters of body surface area, and the urinary glycolic acid 250 mg. per 24 hours per 1.73 square meters surface area (normal, below 50 and 60 mg., respectively). The type II disease is due to absence of D-glyceric dehydrogenase [275]. In this disorder urinary oxalate averages 150 mg. and urinary L-glyceric acid 400 mg. per 24 hours per 1.73 square meters of body surface area. By contrast, only small amounts of L-glyceric acid occur in normal urine. In type II oxaluria, glycolate output is below normal values, indicating a reduced conversion of glyoxylate to glycolate. The reason for the increased urinary excretion of oxalate in the type II disease is not certain, but probably D-glyceric dehydrogenase and the enzyme involved in the reduction of glyoxylate to glycolic acid are identical, and therefore more glyoxylate is available for conversion to oxalate. As would be expected in a generalized metabolic disorder, transplanted kidneys in patients with terminal renal failure from hyperoxaluria are affected by the disease process, and deposition of calcium oxalate crystals rapidly occurs.

Treatment and Prognosis. The prognosis is uniformly poor, and death occurs from renal failure in late childhood or early adult life. No treatment is known which will influence the unfavorable course of the disease. In the terminal uremic stages with gross fall of the glomerular filtration rate, there is progressive fall of urinary oxalate output to normal levels. Diagnosis is therefore difficult in life in cases first investigated during the terminal uremic stage of the disease.

References

1. Abbassi, V., Lowe, C. U., and Callagno, P. L. Oculo-cerebro-renal syndrome: A review. *Amer. J. Dis. Child.* 115:145, 1968.
2. Abderhalden, E. Familiäre Cystindiathese. *Z. Physiol. Chem.* 38:557, 1903.
3. Albright, F., Bauer, W., Ropes, M., and Aub, J. C. Studies of calcium and phosphorus metabolism; the effect of the parathyroid hormone. *J. Clin. Invest.* 7:139, 1929.
4. Albright, F., Burnett, C. H., Smith, P. H., and Parson, W. Pseudo-hypoparathyroidism — example of "Seabright-bantam syndrome"; report of 3 cases. *Endocrinology* 30: 922, 1942.
5. Albright, F., Consolazio, W. V., Coombs, F. S., Sulkowitch, H. W., and Talbott, J. H. Metabolic studies and therapy in case of nephrocalcinosis with rickets and dwarfism. *Bull. Johns Hopkins Hosp.* 66:7, 1940.
6. Albright, F., Forbes, A. P., and Henneman, P. H. Pseudo-pseudohypoparathyroidism. *Trans. Ass. Amer. Physicians* 65:337, 1952.
7. Allan, J. D., Cusworth, D. C., Dent, C. E., and Wilson, V. K. A disease, probably hereditary, characterized by severe mental deficiency and a constant gross abnormality of aminoacid metabolism. *Lancet* 1:182, 1958.
8. Alsberg, C., and Folin, O. Protein metabolism in cystinuria. *Amer. J. Physiol.* 14:54, 1905.
9. Archer, H. E., Dormer, A. E., Scowen, E. F., and Watts, R. W. E. Observations on the possible genetic basis of primary hyperoxaluria. *Ann. Hum. Genet.* 22:373, 1958.
10. Archer, H. E., Dormer, A. E., Scowen, E. F., and Watts, R. W. E. The aetiology of primary hyperoxaluria. *Brit. Med. J.* 1:175, 1958.
11. Armstrong, M. D., Yates, K., Kakimoto, Y., Taniguchi, K., and Kappe, T. Excretion of β-aminoisobutyric acid by man. *J. Biol. Chem.* 238:1447, 1963.
12. Armstrong, M. D., Shaw, K. N. F., and Wall, P. E. The phenolic acids of human urine; paper chromatography of phenolic acids. *J. Biol. Chem.* 218:293, 1956.
13. Aronsson, S., Engleson, G., Jagenburg, R., and Palmgren, B. Long-term dietary treatment of tyrosinosis. *J. Pediat.* 72:620, 1968.
14. Arrow, V. K., and Westall, R. G. Amino acid clearances in cystinuria. *J. Physiol.* 142: 141, 1958.
15. Asatoor, A. M. Pyridoxine deficiency in the rat produced by D-penicillamine. *Nature* (London) 203:1382, 1964.
16. Asatoor, A. M., Craske, J., London, D. R., and Milne, M. D. Indole production in Hartnup disease. *Lancet* 1:126, 1963.
17. Asatoor, A., and Dalgliesh, C. E. The use of deactivated charcoals for the isolation of aromatic substances. *J. Chem. Soc.* (London) 1956: 2291, 1956.
18. Asatoor, A. M., Lacey, B. W., London, D. R., and Milne, M. D. Amino acid metabolism in cystinuria. *Clin. Sci.* 23:285, 1962.
19. Auerbach, V. H., Di George, A. M., Baldridge, R. C., Tourtellotte, C. D., and Brigham, M. P. Histidinemia: A deficiency in histidase resulting in the urinary excretion of histidine and imidazolepyruvic acid. *J. Pediat.* 60:487, 1962.
20. Awapara, J., and Sato, Y. Paper chromatography of urinary amino acids. *Clin. Chim. Acta* 1:75, 1956.
21. Baar, H. S., and Bickel, H. Morbid anatomy, histology and pathogenesis of Lignac-Fanconi disease (cystine storage disease with aminoaciduria). *Acta Paediat.* (Stockholm) 42(Suppl. 90):171, 1952.
22. Baron, D. N., Dent, C. E., Harris, H., Hart, E. W., and Jepson, J. B. Hereditary pella-

gra-like skin rash with temporary cerebellar ataxia, constant renal aminoaciduria, and other bizarre biochemical features. *Lancet* 2:421, 1956.

23. Bartter, F. C. Pseudohypoparathyroidism and Pseudo-pseudohypoparathyroidism. In Stanbury, J. B., Wyngaarden, J. B., and Fredrickson, D. S. (Eds.), *The Metabolic Basis of Inherited Disease* (2d ed.). New York: McGraw-Hill, 1966.
24. Bearn, A. G. Genetic and biochemical aspects of Wilson's disease. *Amer. J. Med.* 15: 442, 1953.
25. Bearn, A. G., and Kunkel, H. G. Biochemical abnormalities in Wilson's disease. *J. Clin. Invest.* 31:616, 1952.
26. Bearn, A. G., and Kunkel, H. G. Abnormalities of copper metabolism in Wilson's disease and their relationship to the aminoaciduria. *J. Clin. Invest.* 33:400, 1954.
27. Bearn, A. G., Yü, T. F., and Gutman, A. B. Renal function in Wilson's disease. *J. Clin. Invest.* 36:1107, 1957.
28. Berliner, R. W., Kennedy, T. J., Jr., and Orloff, J. Relationship between acidification of the urine and potassium metabolism; effect of carbonic anhydrase inhibition on potassium excretion. *Amer. J. Med.* 11:274, 1951.
29. Beyer, K. H., Wright, L. D., Skeggs, H. R., Russo, H. F., and Shaner, G. A. Renal clearance of essential amino acids: Their competition for reabsorption by the renal tubules. *Amer. J. Physiol.* 151:202, 1947.
30. Bickel, H., Smallwood, W. C., Smellie, J. M., and Hickmans, E. M. Clinical description, factual analysis, prognosis and treatment of Lignac-Fanconi disease. *Acta Paediat.* (Stockholm) 42(Suppl. 90):27, 1952.
31. Bickel, H., and Smellie, J. M. Cystine storage disease with amino-aciduria. *Lancet* 1: 1093, 1952.
32. Bickel, H., and Souchon, F. Die Papierchromatographie in der Kinderheilkunde. *Arch. Kinderheilk.* (Suppl. 31):1, 1955.
33. Bishop, C., Zimdahl, W. T., and Talbott, J. H. Uric acid in two patients with Wilson's disease (hepatolenticular degeneration). *Proc. Soc. Exp. Biol. Med.* 86:440, 1954.
34. Boström, H., and Hambraeus, L. Cystinuria in Sweden: VII. Clinical, histo-pathological and medico-social aspects of the disease. *Acta Med. Scand.* 175(Suppl. 411):1, 1964.
35. Brand, E., and Cahill, G. F. Further studies on metabolism of sulfur compounds in cystinuria. *Proc. Soc. Exp. Biol. Med.* 31: 1247, 1934.
36. Brand, E., Cahill, G. F., and Harris, M. M. Cystinuria; metabolism of cystine, cysteine, methionine, and glutathione. *J. Biol. Chem.* 109:69, 1935.
37. Bridges, J. M., Gibson, J. B., Loughridge, L. W., and Montgomery, D. A. D. Carcinoid syndrome with pellagrous dermatitis. *Brit. J. Surg.* 45:117, 1957.
38. Brodehl, J., Gellisen, K., and Kowalewski, S. Isolierter defekt der tubulären Cystin-Rückensorption in einer familie mit idiopathischen hypoparathyroidismus. *Klin. Wschr.* 45:38, 1967.
39. Brodie, B. B., Gillette, J. R., and La Du, B. N. Enzymatic metabolism of drugs and other foreign compounds. *Ann. Rev. Biochem.* 27:427, 1958.
40. Bronsky, D., Kushner, D. S., Dubin, A., and Snapper, I. Idiopathic hypoparathyroidism and pseudohypoparathyroidism: Case reports and review of the literature. *Medicine* (Balt.) 37:317, 1958.
41. Buchanan, E. U., and Komrower, G. M. The prognosis of idiopathic renal acidosis in infancy with observations on urine acidification and ammonia production in children. *Arch. Dis. Child.* 33:532, 1958.
42. Burke, E. C., Baggenstoss, A. H., Owen, C. A., Power, M. H., and Lohr, O. W. Oxalosis. *Pediatrics* 15:383, 1955.
43. Butler, E. A., and Flynn, F. V. The proteinuria of renal tubular disorders. *Lancet* 2:978, 1958.
44. Carson, N. A. J., Cusworth, D. C., Dent, C. E., Field, C. M. B., Neill, D. W., and Westall, R. G. Homocystinuria: A new inborn error of metabolism associated with mental deficiency. *Arch. Dis. Child.* 38:425, 1963.

45. Childs, B., Nyhan, W. L., Borden, M., Bard, L., and Cooke, R. E. Idiopathic hyperglycinemia and hyperglycinuria: A new disorder of amino acid metabolism. *Pediatrics* 27:522, 1961.
46. Chinard, F. P., Taylor, R. W., Nolan, M. F., and Enns, T. Transport of glucose by the renal tubule cells of anesthetized dogs. *Science* 125:736, 1957.
47. Clarke, E., Evans, B. M., MacIntyre, I., and Milne, M. D. Acidosis in experimental electrolyte depletion. *Clin. Sci.* 14:421, 1955.
48. Clarkson, T. W., and Kench, J. E. Urinary excretion of amino acids by men absorbing heavy metals. *Biochem. J.* 62:361, 1956.
49. Clay, R. D., Darmady, E. M., and Hawkins, M. The nature of the renal lesion in the Fanconi syndrome. *J. Path. Bact.* 65:551, 1953.
50. Clayton, B. E., and Patrick, A. D. Use of dimercaprol or penicillamine in the treatment of cystinosis. *Lancet* 2:909, 1961.
51. Cogan, D. G., Kuwabara, T., Hurlbut, C. S., Jr., and McMurray, V. Further observations on cystinosis in the adult. *J.A.M.A.* 166:1725, 1958.
52. Cogan, D. G., Kuwabara, T., Kinoshita, J., Sheehan, L., and Merola, L. Cystinosis in an adult. *J.A.M.A.* 164:394, 1957.
53. Cohen, A., and Way, B. J. The association of renal tubular acidosis with hyperglobulinaemic purpura. *Aust. Ann. Med.* 11:189, 1962.
54. Colombo, J. P., Bungi, W., Richterich, R., and Rossi, E. Congenital lysine intolerance with periodic ammonia intoxication: A defect of L-lysine degradation. *Metabolism* 16:910, 1967.
55. Crawford, T., Dent, C. E., Lucas, P., Martin, N. H., and Nassim, J. R. Osteosclerosis associated with chronic renal failure. *Lancet* 2:981, 1954.
56. Crawhall, J. C., Lietman, P. S., Schneider, J. A., and Seegmiller, J. E. Cystinosis: Plasma cystine and cysteine concentrations and the effect of D-penicillamine and dietary treatments. *Amer. J. Med.* 44:330, 1968.
57. Crawhall, J. C., Scowen, E. F., Thompson, C. J., and Watts, R. W. E. The renal clearances of amino acids in cystinuria. *J. Clin. Invest.* 46:1162, 1967.
58. Crawhall, J. C., Scowen, E. F., and Watts, R. W. E. Effect of penicillamine on cystinuria. *Brit. Med. J.* 1:588, 1963.
59. Crawhall, J. C., Scowen, E. F., and Watts, R. W. E. Further observations on the use of D-penicillamine in cystinuria. *Brit. Med. J.* 1:1411, 1964.
60. Cusworth, D. C., and Dent, C. E. Renal clearances of amino acids in normal adults and in patients with aminoaciduria. *Biochem. J.* 74:550, 1960.
61. Cusworth, D. C., Dent, C. E., and Flynn, F. V. Amino-aciduria in galactosaemia. *Arch. Dis. Child.* 30:150, 1955.
62. Dalgliesh, C. E. Two-dimensional paper chromatography of urinary indoles and related substances. *Biochem. J.* 64:481, 1956.
63. Dancis, J., Levitz, M., Miller, S., and Westall, R. G. "Maple syrup urine disease." *Brit. Med. J.* 1:91, 1959.
64. Danovitch, S. H., Baer, P. N., and Laster, L. Intestinal alkaline phosphatase activity in familial hypophosphatasia. *New Eng. J. Med.* 278:1353, 1968.
65. Debré, R., Royer, P., Lestradet, H., and Straub, W. L'insuffisance tubulaire congénitale avec arriération mentale, cataracte et glaucome. *Arch. Franc. Pediat.* 12:337, 1955.
66. de Grouchy, J., and Sutton, H. E. A genetic study of β-aminoisobutyric acid excretion. *Amer. J. Hum. Genet.* 9:76, 1957.
67. Dent, C. E., and Harris, H. Hereditary forms of rickets and osteomalacia. *J. Bone Joint Surg.* [Brit.] 38:204, 1956.
68. Dent, C. E., and Rose, G. A. Aminoacid metabolism in cystinuria. *Quart. J. Med.* 20:205, 1951.
69. Dent, C. E., and Senior, B. Studies on the treatment of cystinuria. *Brit. J. Urol.* 27:317, 1955.
70. Dent, C. E., Senior, B., and Walshe, J. M. The pathogenesis of cystinuria; polarographic studies of the metabolism of sulphur-containing amino-acids. *J. Clin. Invest.* 36:1216, 1954.
71. de Vries, A., Kochwa, S., Lazebnik, J., Frank, M., and Djaldetti, M. Glycinuria,

a hereditary disorder associated with nephrolithiasis. *Amer. J. Med.* 23:408, 1957.

72. Dickson, L. G., Morita, Y., Cowsert, E. J., Graves, J., and Meyer, J. S. Neurological, electroencephalographic, and heredo-familial aspects of pseudohypoparathyroidism and pseudo-pseudohypoparathyroidism. *J. Neurol. Neurosurg. Psychiat.* 23:33, 1960.
73. Doolan, P. D., Harper, H. A., Hutchin, M. E., and Alpen, E. L. Renal clearance of lysine in cystinuria; pathogenesis and management of this abnormality. *Amer. J. Med.* 23:416, 1957.
74. Drake, T. G., Albright, F., Bauer, W., and Castleman, B. Chronic idiopathic hypoparathyroidism; report of six cases with autopsy findings in one. *Ann. Intern Med.* 12: 1751, 1939.
75. Eberlein, W. R. Aminoaciduria in childhood: Cystinuria and cystinosis. *Amer. J. Med. Sci.* 225:677, 1953.
76. Efron, M. L. Familial hyperprolinemia. *New Eng. J. Med.* 272:1243, 1965.
77. Efron, M. L., Bixby, E. M., Pallattao, L. G., and Pryles, C. V. Hydroxyprolinemia associated with mental deficiency. *New Eng. J. Med.* 267:1195, 1962.
78. Efron, M. L., Bixby, E. M., and Pryles, C. V. Hydroxyprolinemia: II. A rare metabolic disease due to a deficiency of the enzyme "hydroxyproline oxidase." *New Eng. J. Med.* 272:1299, 1965.
79. Ellsworth, R., and Howard, J. E. Studies on physiology of parathyroid glands; some responses of normal human kidneys and blood to intravenous parathyroid extract. *Bull. Johns Hopkins Hosp.* 55:296, 1934.
80. Emslie-Smith, D., Johnstone, J. H., Thomson, M. B., and Lowe, K. G. Amino-aciduria in acute tubular necrosis. *Clin. Sci.* 15: 171, 1956.
81. Engle, R. L., Jr., and Wallis, L. A. Multiple myeloma and the adult Fanconi syndrome; report of a case with crystal-like deposits in the tumor cells and in the epithelial cells of the kidney. *Amer. J. Med.* 22:5, 1957.
82. Enticknap, J. B. The condition of the kidneys in salt-losing nephritis. *Lancet* 2:458, 1952.
83. Fanconi, G. Der frühinfantile nephrotisch-glykosurische Zwergwuchs mit hypophosphatämischer Rachitis. *Jahrb. Kinderheilk.* 147:299, 1936.
84. Fink, K. Excretion of pyrimidine reduction products by the rat. *J. Biol. Chem.* 218: 9, 1956.
85. Fink, K., Cline, R. E., Henderson, R. B., and Fink, R. M. Metabolism of thymine (methyl-C^{14} or -2-C^{14}) by rat liver in vitro. *J. Biol. Chem.* 221:425, 1956.
86. Fink, R. M., McGaughy, C., Cline, R. E., and Fink, K. Metabolism of intermediate pyrimidine reduction products in vitro. *J. Biol. Chem.* 218:1, 1956.
87. Foley, T. H., and London, D. R. Cysteine metabolism in cystinuria. *Clin. Sci.* 29:549, 1965.
88. Folin, O., and Berglund, M. Some new observations and interpretations with reference to transportation, retention, and excretion of carbohydrates. *J. Biol. Chem.* 51: 213, 1922.
89. Følling, A. Uber ausscheidung von phenylbrenztraubensäure in den harn als stoffwechsel anomalie in verbindung mit imbezellität. *Z. Physiol. Chem.* 227:169, 1934.
90. Follis, R. H., Jr. Renal rickets and osteitis fibrosa in children and adolescents. *Bull. Johns Hopkins Hosp.* 87:593, 1950.
91. Follis, R. H., Jr., and Jackson, D. A. Renal osteomalacia and osteitis fibrosa in adults. *Bull. Johns Hopkins Hosp.* 72:232, 1943.
92. Fox, M., Thier, S., Rosenberg, L., Kiser, W., and Segal, S. Evidence against a single renal transport defect in cystinuria. *New Eng. J. Med.* 270:556, 1964.
93. Fraser, D. Hypophosphatasia. *Amer. J. Med.* 22:730, 1957.
94. Fraser, D., and Laidlaw, J. C. Treatment of hypophosphatasia with cortisone. *Lancet* 1:553, 1956.
95. Fraser, D., Yendt, E. R., and Christie, F. H. E. Metabolic abnormalities in hypophosphatasia. *Lancet* 1:286, 1955.
96. Friedmann, E. Der Kreislauf des Schwefels in der organischen Natur; über die Bindung des Schwefels im Eiweiss. *Ergebn. Physiol.* 1:15, 1902.
97. Frimpter, G. W. The disulfide of L-cysteine and L-homocysteine in urine of pa-

tients with cystinuria. *J. Biol. Chem.* 236:PC 51, 1961.

98. Frimpter, G. W. Cystinuria: Metabolism of the disulfide of cysteine and homocysteine. *J. Clin. Invest.* 42:1956, 1965.
99. Frimpter, G. W., Haymovitz, A., and Horwith, M. Cystathioninuria. *New Eng. J. Med.* 268:333, 1963.
100. Frimpter, G. W., Horwith, M., Furth, E., Fellows, R. E., and Thompson, D. D. Inulin and endogenous amino acid renal clearances in cystinuria: Evidence for tubular secretion. *J. Clin. Invest.* 41:281, 1962.
101. Frimpter, G. W., Timpanelli, A. E., Eisenmenger, W. J., Stein, H. S., and Ehrlich, L. I. Reversible "Fanconi syndrome" caused by degraded tetracycline. *J.A.M.A.* 184:111, 1963.
102. Froesch, E. R., Prader, A., Labhart, A., Stuber, H. W., and Wolf, H. P. Die hereditäre fructoseintolerancz eine bisher nicht bekannte kongenitale stoffweschselstörung. *Schweiz. Med. Wschr.* 87:1168, 1957.
103. Fulop, M., Sternlieb, I., and Scheinberg, I. H. Defective urinary acidification in Wilson's disease. *Ann. Intern. Med.* 68:770, 1968.
104. Gardner, L. I., MacLachlan, E. A., and Berman, H. Effect of potassium deficiency on carbon dioxide, cation, and phosphate content of muscle, with note on carbon dioxide content of human muscle. *J. Gen. Physiol.* 36:153, 1952.
105. Garrod, A. E. The Croonian lectures on inborn errors of metabolism. *Lancet* 2:1, 73, 142, 214, 1908.
106. Gartler, S. M., Firschein, I. L., and Gidaspow, T. Some genetical and anthropological considerations of urinary β-aminoisobutyric acid excretion. *Acta Genet.* (Basel) 6:435, 1956–57.
107. Gaull, G. H., Rassin, D. K., and Sturman, J. A. Significance of hypermethioninaemia in acute tryrosinosis. *Lancet* 1:1318, 1968.
108. Gentz, J., Jagenburg, R., and Zetterström, R. Tyrosinemia: An inborn error of tyrosine metabolism with cirrhosis of the liver and multiple renal tubular defects (de Toni-Debré-Fanconi syndrome). *J. Pediat.* 66: 670, 1965.
109. Gerritsen, T., and Waisman, H. A. Hypersarcosinemia: An inborn error of metabolism. *New Eng. J. Med.* 275:66, 1966.
110. Ghadimi, H., Binnington, V. I., and Pecora, P. Hyperlysinemia associated with retardation. *New Eng. J. Med.* 273:723, 1965.
111. Ghadimi, H., Partington, M. N., and Hunter, A. A familial disturbance of histidine metabolism. *New Eng. J. Med.* 265: 221, 1961.
112. Giles, H. M., Pugh, R. C., Darmady, E. M., Stranack, F., and Woolf, L. I. The nephrotic syndrome in early infancy: A report of three cases. *Arch. Dis. Child.* 32:167, 1957.
113. Goeminne, L. Albright's Hereditary Polyosteo-chondroplasia (Pseudo-pseudohypoparathyroidism). *Proceeding of the Eleventh International Congress of Genetics,* Vol. 1. New York: Pergamon Press, 1963.
114. Goodman, S. I., McIntyre, C. A., Jr., and O'Brien, D. Impaired intestinal transport of proline in a patient with familial iminoaciduria. *J. Pediat.* 71:246, 1967.
115. Gordon, E. E., and Sheps, S. G. Effect of acetazolamide on citrate excretion and formation of renal calculi; reoprt of a case and study of five normal subjects. *New Eng. J. Med.* 256:1215, 1957.
116. Gottschalk, C. W., Mylle, M., and Lassiter, W. E. Micropuncture evidence for proximal acidification of the urine. *Fed. Proc.* 18: 58, 1959.
117. Grobbelaar, N., Pollard, J. K., and Steward, F. C. Soluble nitrogen compounds (amino and imino acids and amides) in plants. *Nature* (London) 175:703, 1955.
118. Gross, J. M. Fanconi syndrome (adult type) developing secondary to the ingestion of outdated tetracycline. *Ann. Intern. Med.* 58:523, 1963.
119. Halvorsen, S., and Gjessing, L. R. Studies on tyrosinosis: I. Effect of low-tyrosine and low-phenylalanine diet. *Brit. Med. J.* 2:1171, 1964.
120. Harris, H. Family studies on the urinary excretion of β-aminoisobutyric acid. *Ann. Eugen.* 18:43, 1953.
121. Harris, H., Mittwoch, U., Robson, E. B., and Warren, F. L. The pattern of amino

acid excretion in cystinuria. *Ann. Hum. Genet.* 19:196, 1955.

122. Harris, H., Penrose, L. S., and Thomas, D. H. Cystathioninuria. *Ann. Hum. Genet.* 23:442, 1959.
123. Harris, H., and Robson, E. B. Variation in homozygous cystinuria. *Acta Genet.* (Basel) 5:381, 1955.
124. Harris, H., and Warren, F. L. Quantitative studies on the urinary cystine in patients with cystine stone formation and in their relatives. *Ann. Eugen.* 18:125, 1953.
125. Harrison, H. E. Mechanisms of action of vitamin D. *Pediatrics* 14:285, 1954.
126. Harrison, R. J., and Feiwel, M. Pellagra caused by isoniazid. *Brit. Med. J.* 2:852, 1956.
127. Hermans, P. E., Gorman, C. A., Martin, W. J., and Kelly, P. J. Pseudo-pseudohypoparathyroidism (Albright's hereditary osteodystrophy): A family study. *Mayo Clin. Proc.* 39:81, 1964.
128. Hjärne, U. Study of orthoglycaemic glycosuria with particular reference to its hereditability. *Acta Med. Scand.* 67:422, 1927.
129. Hunt, D. D., Stearns, G., McKinley, J. B., Froning, E., Hicks, P., and Bonfiglio, M. Long-term study of family with Fanconi syndrome without cystinosis (de Toni-Debré-Fanconi syndrome). *Amer. J. Med.* 40:492, 1966.
130. Huth, E. J., Webster, G. D., Jr., and Elkinton, J. R. The renal excretion of hydrogen ion in renal tubular acidosis: III. An attempt to detect latent cases in a family; comments on nosology, genetics and etiology of the primary disease. *Amer. J. Med.* 29:586, 1960.
131. Jaffe, I. A., Altman, K., and Merryman, P. The antipyridoxine effect of penicillamine in man. *J. Clin. Invest.* 43:1869, 1964.
132. Jepson, J. B. Hartnup Disease. In Stanbury, J. B., Wyngaarden, J. B., and Fredrickson, D. S. (Eds.), *The Metabolic Basis of Inherited Disease.* (2d ed.). New York: McGraw-Hill, 1966.
133. Jervis, E. L., and Smyth, D. H. The effect of concentrations of amino acids on their rate of absorption from the intestine. *J. Physiol.* (London) 149:433, 1959.
134. Jervis, E. L., and Smyth, D. H. The active transfer of D-methionine by the rat intestine in vitro. *J. Physiol.* (London) 151:51, 1960.
135. Jervis, G. A. Studies on phenylpyruvic oligophrenia: Phenylpyruvic acid content of blood. *Proc. Soc. Exp. Biol. Med.* 81:715, 1952.
136. Jervis, G. A. Phenylpyruvic oligophrenia deficiency of phenylalanine-oxidizing system. *Proc. Soc. Exp. Biol. Med.* 82:514, 1953.
137. Jonxis, J. H. P., and Huisman, T. H. J. Amino-aciduria in rachitic children. *Lancet* 2:428, 1953.
138. Jonxis, J. H. P., and Huisman, T. H. J. Amino aciduria and ascorbic acid deficiency. *Pediatrics* 14:238, 1954.
139. Jonxis, J. H. P., Smith, P. A., and Huisman, T. H. J. Rickets and amino-aciduria. *Lancet* 2:1015, 1952.
140. Kamin, H., and Handler, P. Effect of infusion of single amino acids upon excretion of other amino acids. *Amer. J. Physiol.* 164:654, 1951.
141. Kaser, H., Cottier, P., and Antener, I. Glucoglycinuria, a new familial syndrome. *J. Pediat.* 61:386, 1962.
142. Kaye, M., Pritchard, J. E., Halpenny, G. W., and Light, W. Bone disease in chronic renal failure with particular reference to osteosclerosis. *Medicine* (Balt.) 39:157, 1960.
143. Kazantzis, G., Flynn, F. V., Spowage, J. S., and Trott, D. G. Renal tubular malfunction and pulmonary emphysema in cadmium pigment workers. *Quart. J. Med.* n.s. 32:165, 1963.
144. Knox, W. E. Sir Archibald Garrod's inborn errors of metabolism: I. Cystinuria. *Amer. J. Hum. Genet.* 10:3, 1958.
145. Koch, J., Stokstad, E. I. R., Williams, H. E., and Smith, I. H., Jr. Deficiency of 2-oxoglutarate:glyoxylate carboligase in primary hyperoxaluria. *Proc. Nat. Acad. Sci. U.S.A.* 57:1123, 1967.
146. Korn, D. Demonstration of cystine crystals in peripheral white blood cells in a patient with cystinosis. *New Eng. J. Med.* 262:545, 1960.
147. La Du, B. N. The enzymatic deficiency in

tyrosinemia. *Amer. J. Dis. Child.* 113:54, 1967.

148. Lambert, P. P. A study of the mechanism by which toxic tubular damage changes the renal threshold for glucose. In Lewis, A. A. G., and Wolstenholme, G. E. W. (Eds.), *Ciba Foundation Symposium on the Kidney*. London: Churchill, 1954. P. 79.
149. Lambert, P. P., and de Heinzelin de Braucourt, C. Syndrome de Fanconi; un cas chez l'adulte. *Acta Clin. Belg.* 6:13, 1951.
150. Laplane, R., Polonovski, C., Etienne, M., Debray, P., Lods, J. C., and Pissaro, B. L'intolérance aux sucres à transfert intestinal actif. Les rapports avec l'intolérance au lactose et le syndrome coeliaque. *Arch. Franc. Pediat.* 19:895, 1962.
151. Latner, A. L., and Burnard, E. D. Idiopathic hyperchloraemic renal acidosis of infants (nephrocalcinosis infantum); observations on the site and nature of the lesion. *Quart. J. Med.* 19:285, 1950.
152. Lelong, M., Alagille, D., Gentil, C., Colin, J., Tupin, J., and Bouquier, J. Cirrhose hépatique et tubulopathie par absence congénitale de l'aldolase hépatique: Intolérance héréditaire au fructose. *Bull. Soc. Med. Hop. Paris* 113:58, 1963.
153. Lerman, S. Enzymatic factors in experimental galactose cataract. *Science* 130:1473, 1959.
154. Levin, B., Oberholzer, V. G., Snodgrass, G. J. A. I., Stimmler, L., and Wilmers, M. J. Fructosemia: An inborn error of fructose metabolism. *Arch. Dis. Child.* 38:220, 1963.
155. Levine, S. Z., Gordon, H. H., and Marples, E. A defect in the metabolism of tyrosine and phenylalanine in premature infants: II. Spontaneous occurrence and eradication by vitamin C. *J. Clin. Invest.* 20:209, 1941.
156. Lewis, H. B. Occurrence of cystinuria in healthy young men and women. *Ann. Intern. Med.* 6:183, 1932.
157. Lightwood, R. Calcium infarction of the kidneys in infants. *Arch. Dis. Child.* 10:205, 1935.
158. Lietman, P. S., Frazier, P. D., Wong, V. G., Shotton, D., and Seegmiller, J. E. Adult cystinosis — a benign disorder. *Amer. J. Med.* 40:511, 1966.
159. Lightwood, R., Payne, W. W., and Black, J. A. Infantile renal acidosis. *Pediatrics* 12:628, 1953.
160. Lignac, G. O. E. Ueber Störung des Cystinstoffwechsels bei Kindern. *Deutsch. Arch. Klin. Med.* 145:139, 1924.
161. Lignac, G. O. E. Über Erkrankungen (u. a. Nephrose und Nephritis) mit und durch Zystinablagerungen in verschiedene Organe. *Krankheit.* 2:43, 1926.
162. Lignac, G. O. E. Zystinbefunde bei einer bestimmten Kinderkrankheit. *Verh. Deutsch. Ges. Path.* 21:303, 1926.
163. Lindquist, B., and Meeuwisse, G. W. Chronic diarrhoea caused by monosaccharide malabsorption. *Acta Paediat.* (Stockholm) 51:674, 1962.
164. Litin, R. B., Randall, R. V., Goldstein, N. P., Power, M. H., and Diessner, G. R. Hypercalciuria in hepatolenticular degeneration (Wilson's disease). *Amer. J. Med. Sci.* 238:614, 1959.
165. Loewy, A., and Neuberg, C. Zur Kenntnis der Diamine. Z. *Physiol. Chem.* 43:355, 1904.
166. London, D. R., and Foley, T. H. Cystine metabolism in cystinuria. *Clin. Sci.* 29:129, 1965.
167. Lospalluto, J., Dorward, B., Miller, W., Jr., and Ziff, M. Cryoglobulinemia based on interaction between a gamma macroglobulin and 7S gamma globulin. *Amer. J. Med.* 32:142, 1962.
168. Lowe, C. U., Terrey, M., and MacLachlan, E. A. Organic-aciduria, decreased renal ammonia production, hydrophthalmos, and mental retardation; a clinical entity. *A.M.A. Amer. J. Dis. Child.* 83:164, 1952.
169. Lucas, R. C. On a form of late rickets associated with albuminuria, rickets of adolescents. *Lancet* 1:993, 1883.
170. Lyman, F. L. *Phenylketonuria.* Springfield, Ill.: Thomas, 1963.
171. Mabry, C. C., and Karam, E. A. Idiopathic hyperglycinemia and hyperglycinuria. *Southern Med. J.* 56:1444, 1963.
172. McArdle, B. The quantitative estimation of pyruvic and α-oxoglutaric acids by paper chromatography in blood, urine and cerebrospinal fluid. *Biochem. J.* 66:144, 1947.

173. McCance, R. A. Osteomalacia with Looser's nodes (Milkman's syndrome) due to a raised resistance to vitamin D acquired about the age of 15 years. *Quart. J. Med.* 16: 33, 1947.
174. McCance, R. A., Fairweather, D. V. I., Barrett, A. M., and Morrison, A. B. Genetic, clinical, biochemical, and pathological features of hypophosphatasia; based on the study of a family. *Quart. J. Med.* 25:523, 1956.
175. McCance, R. A., Matheson, W. J., Gresham, G. A., and Elkinton, J. R. The cerebro-ocular-renal dystrophies: A new variant. *Arch. Dis. Child.* 35:240, 1960.
176. McCance, R. A., Morrison, A. B., and Dent, C. E. The excretion of phosphoethanolamine and hypophosphatasia. *Lancet* 1:131, 1955.
177. McCarthy, C. F., Borland, J. L., Jr., Lynch, H. J., Jr., Owen, E. E., and Tyor, M. P. Defective uptake of basic amino acids and L-cystine by intestinal mucosa of patients with cystinuria. *J. Clin. Invest.* 43:1518, 1964.
178. McConnell, R. B., and Cheetham, H. D. Acute pellagra during isoniazid therapy. *Lancet* 2:959, 1952.
179. McCurdy, D. K., Frederic, M., and Elkinton, J. R. Renal tubular acidosis due to amphotericin B. *New Eng. J. Med.* 278:124, 1968.
180. McCune, D. J., Mason, H. H., and Clarke, H. T. Intractable hypophosphatemic rickets with renal glycosuria and acidosis (Fanconi syndrome); report of case in which increased urinary organic acids were detected and identified, with review of literature. *Amer. J. Dis. Child.* 65:81, 1943.
181. McMenamy, R. H., Lund, C. C., and Oncley, J. L. Unbound amino acid concentrations in human blood plasmas. *J. Clin. Invest.* 36:1672, 1957.
181a. McMurray, W. C., Rathburn, J. C., Mohyuddin, F., and Koegler, S. J. Citrullinuria. *Pediatrics* 32:347, 1963.
182. Mann, J. B., Alterman, S., and Hills, A. G. Albright's hereditary osteodystrophy comprising pseudohypoparathyroidism and pseudo-pseudohypoparathyroidism. *Ann. Intern. Med.* 56:315, 1962.
183. Marble, A. Renal glycosuria. *Amer. J. Med. Sci.* 183:811, 1932.
184. Marcet, A. Cited by Renander, A. [217].
185. Marshall, V. F., and Horwith, M. Oxalosis. *J. Urol.* 83:278, 1959.
186. Matthews, W. B. Familial calcification of the basal ganglia with response to parathormone. *J. Neurol. Neurosurg. Psychiat.* 20: 172, 1957.
187. Matthews, W. B., Milne, M. D., and Bell, M. The metabolic disorder in hepatolenticular degeneration. *Quart. J. Med.* 21: 425, 1952.
188. Menkes, J. H. Idiopathic hyperglycinemia: Isolation and identification of three previously undescribed urinary ketones. *J. Pediat.* 69:413, 1966.
189. Menkes, J. H., Hurst, P. L., and Craig, J. M. New syndrome: Progressive familial infantile cerebral dysfunction associated with unusual urinary substance. *Pediatrics* 14:462, 1954.
190. Milkman, L. A. Pseudofractures (hunger osteopathy, late rickets, osteomalacia); report of case. *Amer. J. Roentgen.* 24:29, 1930.
191. Mills, J. N., Thomas, S., and Williamson, K. S. The acute effect of hydrocortisone, deoxycorticosterone and aldosterone upon the excretion of sodium, potassium and acid by the human kidney. *J. Physiol.* (London) 151:312, 1960.
192. Milne, M. D. Unpublished observations.
193. Milne, M. D. Renal control of acid-base balance. *Lect. Sci. Basis Med.* 5:404, 1955.
194. Milne, M. D., Asatoor, A. M., Edwards, K. D., and Loughridge, L. W. The intestinal absorption defect in cystinuria. *Gut* 2:323, 1961.
195. Milne, M. D., Crawford, M. A., Girao, C. B., and Loughridge, L. W. The metabolic disorder in Hartnup disease. *Quart. J. Med.* 29 407, 1960.
196. Milne, M. D., Crawford, M. A., Girao, C. B., and Loughridge, L. W. The excretion of indolylacetic acid and related indolic acids in man and the rat. *Clin. Sci.* 19:165, 1960.
197. Milne, M. D., Scribner, B. H., and Crawford, M. A. Non-ionic diffusion and the excretion of weak acids and bases. *Amer. J. Med.* 24:709, 1958.

198. Milne, M. D., Stanbury, S. W., and Thomson, A. E. Observations on the Fanconi syndrome and renal hyperchloraemic acidosis in the adult. *Quart. J. Med.* 21:61, 1952.
199. Mitoma, C., Auld, R. M., and Udenfriend, S. On the nature of enzymatic defect in phenylpyruvic oligophrenia. *Proc. Soc. Exp. Biol. Med.* 94:634, 1957.
200. Moreigne, H. Étude sur la cystinurie. *Arch. Med. Exp. Anat. Path.* 11:254, 1899.
201. Morikawa, T., Tada, K., Ando, T., Yoshida, T., Yokoyama, Y., and Arikava, T. Prolinuria: Defect of intestinal absorption of imino acids and glycine. *Tohoku J. Exp. Med.* 90:105, 1966.
202. Morris, R. C., Jr., and Fudenberg, H. H. Impaired renal acidification in patients with hypergammaglobulinemia. *Medicine* (Balt.) 46:57, 1967.
203. Mudd, S. H., Finkelstein, J. D., Irreverre, F., and Laster, L. Homocystinuria: An enzymatic defect. *Science* 143:1443, 1964.
204. Mudge, G. H. Clinical patterns of tubular dysfunction. *Amer. J. Med.* 24:785, 1958.
205. Newton, M. A. A distinctive fraction of alkaline phosphatase in health and disease. *J. Clin. Path.* 19:491, 1966.
206. Nordmann, J., Nordmann, R., du Ruisseau, J. P., and Gauchery, O. Études sur le cycle tricarboxylique chez l'homme au moyen de la chromatographie sur papier des acides organiques. *Rev. Franc. Etud. Clin. Biol.* 1:67, 1956.
207. Oliver, J. Microcystic renal disease and its relation to "infantile nephrosis." *Amer. J. Dis. Child.* 100:312, 1960.
208. Orloff, J., and Berliner, R. W. The mechanism of the excretion of ammonia in the dog. *J. Clin. Invest.* 35:223, 1956.
209. Page, E. W., Glendening, M. B., Dignam, W., and Harper, H. A. The causes of histidinuria in normal pregnancy. *Amer. J. Obstet. Gynec.* 68:110, 1954.
210. Palmer, W. W. The titration of organic acids in urine. *J. Biol. Chem.* 68:245, 1926.
211. Perry, T. L., Hardnick, D. F., Dixon, G. H., Dolnan, C. L., and Hansen, S. Hypermethioninemia: A metabolic disorder associated with cirrhosis, islet cell hyperplasia and renal tubular degeneration. *Pediatrics* 36: 236, 1965.
212. Pitts, R. F., and Alexander, R. S. Renal reabsorptive mechanism for inorganic phosphate in normal and acidotic dogs. *Amer. J. Physiol.* 142:648, 1944.
213. Platt, R. Structural and functional adaptation in renal failure. *Brit. Med. J.* 1:1313, 1372, 1952.
214. Prout, W. Cited by Renander, A. [217].
215. Rathbun, J. C. "Hypophosphatasia," new developmental anomaly. *Amer. J. Dis. Child.* 75:822, 1948.
216. Read, A. E., Sherlock, S., and Harrison, C. V. Active "juvenile" cirrhosis considered as part of a systemic disease and the effect of corticosteroid therapy. *Gut* 4:378, 1963.
217. Renander, A. The roentgen density of the cystine calculus; a roentgenographic and experimental study including a comparison with more common uroliths. *Acta Radiol.* [Diagn.] (Stockholm) Suppl. 41, 1941.
218. Reubi, F. C. Glucose titration in renal glycosuria. In Lewis, A. A. G., and Wolstenholme, G. E. W. (Eds.), *Ciba Foundation Symposium on the Kidney.* London: Churchill, 1954. P. 96.
219. Robson, E. B., and Rose, G. A. The effect of intravenous lysine on the renal clearances of cystine, arginine and ornithine in normal subjects, in patients with cystinuria and Fanconi syndrome and in their relatives. *Clin. Sci.* 16:75, 1957.
220. Rosenberg, L. E., Downing, S., Durant, J. L., and Segal, S. Cystinuria: Biochemical evidence for three genetically distinct diseases. *J. Clin. Invest.* 45:365, 1966.
220a. Rosenberg, L. E., Downing, S. J., and Segal, S. Competitive inhibition of dibasic amino acid transport in rat kidney. *J. Biol. Chem.* 237:2265, 1962.
221. Rosenberg, L. E., Durant, J. L., and Albrecht, I. Genetic heterogeneity in cystinuria: Evidence for allelism. *Trans. Ass. Amer. Physicians* 79:284, 1966.
222. Rothstein, A., and Berke, H. Amino aciduria in uranium poisoning; the use of the amino-acid nitrogen to creatinine ratio in "spot" samples of urine. *J. Pharmacol. Exp. Ther.* 96:179, 1949.

223. Royer, P., and Prader, A. Les insuffisances congénitales du tubule rénale chez l'enfant. Clinique et thérapeutique. 16e Congrès des Pédiatres de Langue Française. Extrait du tome 1:263, 1957. L'expansion scientifique française, Paris.
224. Russell, R. G. G. Excretion of inorganic pyrophosphate in hypophosphatasia. *Lancet* 2:461, 1965.
225. Sandler, M., and Pare, C. M. B. Starvation amino-aciduria. *Lancet* 1:494, 1954.
226. Sass-Kortsak, A., Cherniak, M., Geiger, D. W., and Slater, R. J. Observations on ceruloplasmin in Wilson's disease. *J. Clin. Invest.* 38:1672, 1959.
227. Saunders, S. J., Irvine, R. O. H., Crawford, M. A., and Milne, M. D. Intracellular pH of potassium-deficient voluntary muscle. *Lancet* 1:468, 1960.
228. Scaglioni, P. R., and Lucey, J. F. Further observations on hypophosphatasia. *A.M.A. Amer. J. Dis. Child.* 92:493, 1956.
229. Schafer, I. A., Scriver, C. R., and Efron, M. L. Familial hyperprolinemia, cerebral dysfunction and renal anomalies occurring in a family with hereditary nephropathy and deafness. *New Eng. J. Med.* 267:51, 1962.
230. Scheinberg, H., and Gitlin, D. Deficiency of ceruloplasmin in patients with hepatolenticular degeneration (Wilson's disease). *Science* 116:484, 1952.
231. Schiess, W. A., Ayer, J. L., Lotspeich, W. D., and Pitts, R. F. The renal regulation of acid-base balance in man; factors affecting the excretion of titratable acid by the normal human subject. *J. Clin. Invest.* 27:57, 1948.
232. Schinke, R. N., McKusick, V. A., Huan, G. T., and Pollack, A. D. Homocystinuria: Studies of 20 families with 38 affected members. *J. Amer. Med. Ass.* 193:711, 1965.
233. Schneider, J. A., Bradley, K., and Seegmiller, J. E. Increased cystine in leucocytes from individuals homozygous and heterozygous for cystinosis. *Science* 157:1321, 1967.
234. Schwarz, V., Golberg, L., Komrower, G. M., and Holzel, A. Some disturbances of erythrocyte metabolism in galactosaemia. *Biochem. J.* 62:34, 1956.
235. Schwartz, W. B., Jenson, R. L., and Relman, A. S. Acidification of the urine and increased ammonium excretion without change in acid-base equilibrium: Sodium reabsorption as a stimulus to the acidifying process. *J. Clin. Invest.* 34:673, 1955.
236. Scowen, E. F., Stansfeld, A. G., and Watts, R. W. E. Oxalosis and primary hyperoxaluria. *J. Path. Bact.* 77:195, 1959.
237. Scriver, C. R. Hartnup disease: A genetic modification of intestinal and renal transport of certain neutral alpha-amino acids. *New Eng. J. Med.* 273:530, 1965.
238. Scriver, C. R. Renal tubular transport of proline, hydroxy-proline and glycine: III. Genetic basis for more than one mode of transport in human kidney. *J. Clin. Invest.* 47:823, 1968.
239. Scriver, C. R., Clow, C. L., and Silverberg, M. Hypermethioninaemia in acute tyrosinosis. *Lancet* 1:153, 1966.
240. Scriver, C. R., Pueschel, S., and Davies, E. Hyper-beta-alaninemia associated with beta-aminoaciduria and gamma-aminobutyric-acidemia, somnolence and seizures. *New Eng. J. Med.* 274:635, 1966.
241. Scriver, C. R., Schafer, I. A., and Efron, M. L. New renal tubular amino-acid transport system and a new hereditary disorder of amino-acid metabolism. *Nature* (London) 192:672, 1961.
242. Sealock, R. R., and Silberstein, H. E. Excretion of homogentisic acid and other tyrosine metabolites by vitamin C-deficient guinea pig. *J. Biol. Chem.* 135:251, 1940.
243. Seegmiller, J. E., Friedmann, T., Harrison, H. E., Wong, V., and Schneider, J. A. Cystinosis. *Ann. Intern. Med.* 68:883, 1968.
244. Seldin, D. W., and Wilson, J. D. Renal Tubular Acidosis. In Stanbury, J. B., Wyngaarden, J. B., and Fredrickson, D. M. (Eds.), *The Metabolic Basis of Inherited Disease* (2d ed.). New York: McGraw-Hill, 1966.
245. Sherlock, S. Pathogenesis and management of hepatic coma. *Amer. J. Med.* 24:805, 1958.
246. Shohl, A. T., and Butler, A. M. Citrates in treatment of infantile rickets. *New Eng. J. Med.* 220:515, 1939.

247. Sidbury, J. B., Jr. The enzymatic lesions in galactosemia. *J. Clin. Invest.* 36:929, 1957.

248. Sirota, J. H., and Hamerman, D. Renal function studies in an adult subject with the Fanconi syndrome. *Amer. J. Med.* 16:138, 1954.

249. Sjoerdsma, A., Weissbach, H., and Udenfriend, S. A clinical, physiologic and biochemical study of patients with malignant carcinoid (argentaffinoma). *Amer. J. Med.* 20:520, 1956.

250. Spencer, A. G., and Franglen, G. T. Gross amino-aciduria following a Lysol burn. *Lancet* 1:190, 1952.

251. Spencer, R. P., Brody, K. R., and Mautner, H. G. Intestinal transport of cystine analogues. *Nature* (London) 207:418, 1965.

252. Stanbury, S. W. Azotaemic renal osteodystrophy. *Brit. Med. Bull.* 13:57, 1957.

253. Stanbury, S. W., and Mahler, R. F. Salt-wasting renal disease; metabolic observations on a patient with "salt-losing nephritis." *Quart. J. Med.* 28:425, 1959.

254. Stein, W. H. Excretion of amino acids in cystinuria. *Proc. Soc. Exp. Biol. Med.* 78:705, 1951.

255. Stokes, G. S., Potts, J. T., Jr., Lotz, M., and Bartter, F. C. New agent in the treatment of cystinuria: N-acetyl-D-penicillamine. *Brit. Med. J.* 1:284, 1968.

256. Stowers, J. M., and Dent, C. E. Studies on the mechanism of the Fanconi syndrome. *Quart. J. Med.* 16:275, 1947.

257. Tada, K., Itu, H., Wada, Y., and Arakawa, T. Congenital tryptophanuria with dwarfism ("H" disease-like clinical features, without indicanuria and generalised aminoaciduria): A probably new inborn error of tryptophan metabolism. *Tohoku J. Exp. Med.* 80:118, 1963.

258. Tada, K., Marikawa, T., Ando, T., Yoshida, T., and Minagawa, A. Prolinuria: A new renal tubular defect in transport of proline and glycine. *Tohoku J. Exp. Med.* 87:133, 1965.

259. Taniguchi, K., and Gjessing, D. R. Studies on tyrosinosis: II. Activity of the transaminase, p-hydroxyphenylpyruvate oxidase, and homogentisic acid oxidase. *Brit. Med. J.* 1:968, 1965.

260. Thiele, F. H. Concerning cystinuria and diamines. *J. Physiol.* (London) 36:68, 1907.

261. Thier, S. O., Fox, M., Segal, S., and Rosenberg, L. E. Cystinuria: In vitro demonstration of an intestinal transport defect. *Science* 143:482, 1964.

262. Thorn, G. W., Koepf, G. F., and Clinton, M., Jr. Renal failure simulating adrenocortical insufficiency. *New Eng. J. Med.* 231:76, 1944.

263. Uzman, L. L. On the relationship of urinary copper excretion to the aminoaciduria in Wilson's disease (hepatolenticular degeneration). *Amer. J. Med. Sci.* 226:645, 1953.

264. Uzman, L. L., Iber, F. L., Chalmers, T. C., and Knowlton, M. The mechanism of copper deposition in the liver in hepatolenticular degeneration (Wilson's disease). *Amer. J. Med. Sci.* 231:511, 1956.

265. Van Slyke, D. D., and Palmer, W. W. Studies of acidosis; the titration of organic acids in urine. *J. Biol. Chem.* 41:567, 1920.

266. von Udransky, L., and Baumann, E. Ueber das Vorkommen von Diaminen, sogenannten Ptomainen, bei Cystinurie. *Z. Physiol. Chem.* 13:562, 1889.

267. Wada, Y., Tada, K., Minagawa, A., Yoshida, T., Norikawa, T., and Okamura, T. Hypervalinemia. Probably a new entity of inborn error of valine metabolism. *Tohoku J. Exp. Med.* 81:46, 1963.

268. Wallace, H. W., Moldave, K., and Meister, A. Studies on conversion of phenylalanine to tyrosine in phenylpyruvic oligophrenia. *Proc. Soc. Exp. Biol. Med.* 94:632, 1957.

269. Wallis, L. A., and Engle, R. L., Jr. The adult Fanconi syndrome: Review of eighteen cases. *Amer. J. Med.* 22:13, 1957.

270. Wallraff, E. B., Brodie, E. C., and Borden, A. L. Urinary excretion of amino acids in pregnancy. *J. Clin. Invest.* 29:1542, 1950.

271. Webber, W. A. Characteristics of acidic amino acid transport in mammalian kidney. *Canad. J. Biochem.* 41:131, 1963.

272. Webster, G. D., Jr., Huth, E. J., Elkinton, J. R., and McCance, R. A. The renal excretion of hydrogen ion in renal tubular acidosis; quantitative response to the car-

bonic anhydrase inhibitor, acetazolamide. *Amer. J. Med.* 29:576, 1960.

273. Welt, L. G., Hollander, W., Jr., and Blythe, W. B. The consequences of potassium depletion. *J. Chronic Dis.* 11:213, 1960.
274. Westall, R. G. Argininosuccinic aciduria: Identification and reactions of the abnormal metabolite in a newly described form of mental disease, with some preliminary metabolic studies. *Biochem. J.* 77:135, 1960.
275. Williams, H. E., and Smith, L. H., Jr. L-glyceric aciduria: New genetic variant of primary hyperoxaluria. *New Eng. J. Med.* 278:233, 1968.
276. Wilson, V. K., Thomson, M. L., and Dent, C. E. Amino-aciduria in lead poisoning; a case in childhood. *Lancet* 2:66, 1953.
277. Winters, R. W., Graham, J. B., Williams, T. F., McFalls, V. W., and Burnett, C. H. A genetic study of familial hypophosphatemia and vitamin D resistant rickets with a review of the literature. *Medicine* (Balt.) 37:97, 1958.
278. Wollaston, W. H. On cystic oxide, a new species of urinary calculus. *Phil. Trans. Roy. Soc. London* 100:223, 1810.
279. Wong, V. G., Lietman, P. S., and Seegmiller, J. E. Alterations of pigment epithelium in cystinosis. *Arch. Ophthal.* (Chicago) 77:361, 1967.
280. Wood, M. M. Central nervous system complications during I.N.H. treatment of pulmonary tuberculosis. *Brit. J. Tuberc.* 49:20, 1955.
281. Worthen, H. G., Vernier, R. L., and Good, R. A. Infantile nephrosis; clinical, biochemical, and morphologic studies of the syndrome. *A.M.A. Amer. J. Dis. Child.* 98:731, 1959.
282. Wrong, O., and Davies, H. E. F. The excretion of acid in renal disease. *Quart. J. Med.* 28:259, 1959.
283. Yeh, H. L., Frankl, W., Dunn, M. S., Parker, P., Hughes, B., and György, P. The urinary excretion of amino acids by a cystinuric subject. *Amer. J. Med. Sci.* 214:507, 1947.

31

The Kidney in Liver Disease

Solomon Papper and Carlos A. Vaamonde

There are many experimental and clinical observations indicating that disorders of the liver may be associated with renal abnormalities. It is known that liver damage due to choline deficiency may be associated with severe cortical and medullary necrosis and hemorrhage in the cortex and subcapsular areas of the kidney [45]. Numerous experiments have been undertaken to test the hypothesis that a damaged liver may liberate a substance which either directly or indirectly produces damage to the kidney [10, 83, 84]. The excellent work of Shorr and his associates [83, 84] is an example. These investigators demonstrated that in the animal with an experimentally damaged liver (as well as in patients with cirrhosis) the serum contains a relatively large amount of a vasodepressor material which has the property of decreasing the vasoconstrictor response to epinephrine. Under the same circumstances the serum concentration of a vasoexcitor material, which is believed to be of renal origin, is relatively reduced. Studies of this kind are of great interest, but it is clear that they do not prove a direct relationship between renal damage and a "toxic" material liberated by, or produced in, the abnormal liver.

Of special interest because of clinical observations to be described below, are some of the experimental studies concerned with changes in renal circulation in liver disease. Fajers [21, 22] has performed in rabbits extensive studies of the effects of experimental hepatic necrosis and of biliary tract obstruction on renal function and morphology. These studies indicate that hepatic necrosis and biliary tract obstruction alone generally result in only slight, if any, change in renal morphology and function. However, when either insult is combined with renal ischemia, there are alterations in the reabsorption of sodium and water and the kidney undergoes tubular degenerative changes. These effects are probably greater than those observed with ischemia alone. Fajers has interpreted his data as indicating that hepatic necrosis alone does not cause sufficient renal abnormality to produce renal failure; some additional factor such as ischemia must also be present.

Recent studies of experimental hypotension in jaundiced dogs [90] and of induced renal ischemia in jaundiced rats [18] or in rats infused with bile acids [2] give further support to Fajers hypothesis. Although many in vitro experiments have shown that bile components may be toxic to a variety of cell functions, most of the recently accumulated evidence indicates that bile, bilirubin, or bile acids per se are not toxic to the kidney [2], with the exception of the nephropathy recently described by Odell et al. [63] in the Gunn strain of rat.

Among the first precise references to the role of the kidney in clinical liver disease are those of Austin Flint [27], in 1863, and Gilbert and Lereboullet [29], in 1901, who reported oliguria in patients with cirrhosis. Since that time there have been many studies concerned with the role of the kidney in the development of ascites and edema [64]. It has been clear that certain clinical circumstances result in simultaneous injury to both the liver and the kidney — carbon tetrachloride poisoning, Weil's disease, yellow fever, Waterhouse-Friderichsen syndrome, generalized infection, toxemia of pregnancy, and circulatory collapse [73]. In addition, it is now known that patients with liver disease may develop renal failure of unknown cause in the course of their illness [3, 36, 64, 65, 82]. These clinical situations as well as the less well-defined observation that renal failure may follow surgery of the biliary tract have sometimes been included in the broad term *hepatorenal syndrome* [10, 38, 87]. This term has little advantage and perhaps bears the disadvantage of implying common pathogenesis which does not appear to be applicable. For this reason, we prefer to consider each of the above circumstances separately and for example specifically refer to the situation in cirrhosis as "renal failure of cirrhosis."

Acute Infectious Hepatitis

Conrad et al. [17], in a study of 25 servicemen with viral hepatitis, observed proteinuria, microscopic hematuria, or pyuria in a significant number of patients. These abnormalities were present only in the first 10 days of observation. The blood urea nitrogen and concentrating ability were reported to be normal. The same investigators performed percutaneous renal biopsy in 20 patients during the acute stage of the illness. While no pathognomonic lesion was found, they noted hyaline granular tubular changes and interstitial edema. The glomeruli were swollen and exhibited focal areas of hypercellularity with no evidence of inflammation. Repeat biopsy in five patients showed no histologic abnormality one year later.

Many studies suggest some impairment of renal function in acute hepatic disease, but the evidence for it is contradictory. Several studies report impaired concentrating ability as well as reduced urea and creatinine clearance indicating decreased glomerular filtration rate (GFR) [24, 37, 85]. Other studies have been concerned primarily with impairment in water diuresis, generally without measurement of renal hemodynamics. Thus Von Noorden [94] noted increased urine formation during the convalescent phase of "catarrhal" jaundice. This observation was extended by Jones and Eaton [41], who reviewed the intake and output records of their patients with hepatitis and reported that diuresis occurred early in the recovery period and might herald a favorable course. Impaired water diuresis has also been reported during acute hepatitis [1, 51].

Findings contrary to the foregoing were obtained by Papper et al. [69] in a study of the diuretic response to administered water in 10 patients with acute infectious hepatitis. In all instances the endogenous creatinine clearance was within normal limits, as was the magnitude of the diuretic response to administered water. All patients demonstrated a capacity to dilute the urine that was well within the normal range.

From the available data it is obvious that the matter of renal function in infectious hepatitis is not entirely resolved. It is clear, however, that extensive acute hepatic functional impairment may exist without adverse effect on glomerular filtration rate or water diuresis.

Laennec's Cirrhosis Without Ascites or Edema ("Compensated")

In three studies, a total of 11 patients without edema or ascites were observed to have a normal GFR as determined by the measurement of inulin or endogenous creatinine clearance [32, 57, 66]. In another study, two of five patients had normal inulin and para-aminohippurate (PAH) clearances, whereas in three, inulin clearance was definitely reduced [12]. McCloy et al. [60] have observed normal GFR and renal plasma flow (RPF) in six of seven patients with compensated cirrhosis. Klingler et al. [46] found normal GFR in 10 of 13 patients with cirrhosis without ascites.

Goodyer et al. [32] have demonstrated a normal natriuretic response to the administration of hypertonic saline in two nonedematous patients. Ralli et al. [75] described a normal peak flow of urine after a single water load, followed by a sharper decline than normal after maximal flow. Papper and Rosenbaum [66] observed a modest but definite reduction in diuretic response to administered water. This was associated with a lower rate of sodium excretion than was found in normal subjects when both groups were provided diets with an equal and large sodium content. In addition, these authors noted definite modification of the normal diurnal rhythm of sodium excretion, with relatively more sodium excreted at night than was observed in normal individuals. In recent studies Klingler et al. [46] have found normal water diuresis in 11 patients with compensated cirrhosis. Vaamonde et al. [91] found normal concentrating ability as determined by maximal urine osmolality ($U_{osm\ max}$) and tubular reabsorption of water $T^{c}_{H_2O}$) in most patients with compensated cirrhosis.

Thus while patients with compensated cirrhosis often have normal renal function defined in terms of hemodynamics, diluting ability, concentrating capacity, and sodium excretion, in others one may detect modest reduction in these functions.

Laennec's Cirrhosis with Ascites or Edema ("Decompensated")

Most investigative efforts in this field have been concerned with the patient with frankly decompensated cirrhosis. Many observations indicate anatomic and functional abnormalities in the kidney, although the precise relationship of structural and physiologic changes is not clear in most instances [64]. While knowledge of the functional changes has advanced, much remains to be done.

PATHOLOGY

Considerable controversy surrounds the matter of precise anatomic description of the kidney in patients with cirrhosis. For many years pathologists emphasized "bile" or "cholemic" nephrosis — that is, the presence of swollen tubular cells and bile casts. That this finding has any functional significance may be seriously questioned since azotemia may exist without bile nephrosis and the latter may be observed without any impairment in renal function [65, 73]. Other tubular changes varying from minimal degeneration to necrosis have been described in cirrhosis [7, 13, 73]. Glomerular alterations have also been described. Barr and Sommers [6] and Bloodworth and Sommers [9] have described a diffuse glomerular sclerosis which frequently accompanies cirrhosis of the liver. In an advanced state, this renal lesion consists of striking thickening of the glomerular stroma and increase in glomerular cellularity. The cause of the lesion is not known, and it has been observed in postnecrotic cirrhosis and biliary cirrhosis as well as in patients with Laennec's cirrhosis. Jones et al. [43] found some similar glomerular lesions, but in fewer patients, and furthermore he observed the same changes in 10 per cent of a control group without liver disease. Fisher and Hellstrom [26] reported similar glomerular lesions in 25 per cent of patients with cirrhosis and regarded the findings as nonspecific. According to Kimmelstiel [44], it is sometimes difficult to distinguish this lesion from mild diabetic glomerulosclerosis or from the aging process. Of interest is the older report of Patek et al. [72] in which lesions of chronic glomerulonephritis are recorded in 14 of 200 patients with Laennec's cirrhosis.

More recently Sakaguchi and Salomon and their associates [77, 78] have performed electron microscopic studies of renal biopsies from patients with cirrhosis of different severity. This group of investigators found some renal changes in all their patients, including those with early liver disease. They observed deposition of osmophilic granules, proteinaceous material, and irregular black particles mainly in the mesangial matrix. They also noted thickening of the glomerular basement membrane and mesangial matrix with some fusion and focal destruction of foot processes. Slight tubular changes consisting of hyaline droplets in proximal cells were also observed. Similar findings were observed by Fischer and Perez-Stable [26a].

The clinical significance of these anatomic observations is far from clear. Thus the lesion of glomerulosclerosis does not correlate with the presence or absence of proteinuria or azotemia. Furthermore, histologically the kidney in cirrhosis may show variations ranging from a normal appearance to one exhibiting a number of glomerular and tubular abnormalities. The nature and pathogenesis of the observed abnormalities are not clear. The functional and clinical significance of most of the observed morphologic changes must remain in doubt until more detailed studies correlating anatomic change with function are available.

RENAL HEMODYNAMICS

In patients with decompensated cirrhosis, GFR and RPF vary over a very broad spectrum ranging at the extremes from supernormal values to severe renal failure, and in many instances the GFR is perfectly normal [8, 19, 32, 42, 46, 56, 57, 60, 64, 67, 68, 71, 80, 86, 91]. While it is noted that the lowest values of GFR and RPF tend to be observed in the sickest patients, such an association is by no means invariable, and there is great variation in renal hemodynamics in all phases of the liver disease [46, 67]. The mechanisms responsible for the abnormal values are not readily apparent. Supernormal values have received relatively little investigative attention and are not explained [46, 64]. The mechanism responsible for reduction in renal hemodynamics is not known. It may in part be secondary to circulatory changes elsewhere in the body. The role of effective intravascular volume has recently received considerable attention [60, 70, 76, 88]. While total plasma volume may be increased in cirrhosis, it is known that, perhaps by virtue of its distribution, the physiologic circumstances may mimic a reduction in plasma volume in this disease. There are studies [76, 88] demonstrating that expansion of plasma volume may result in increased renal hemodynamics in some patients. However, this response is not uniform [88]. It is also possible that the reduced GFR may be related to intrarenal circulatory abnormalities of unknown cause.

Of interest are the studies of Gornel et al. [35], who observed that certain patients with impaired GFR as well as other cirrhotic patients with normal GFR respond to the administration of the pressor amine, metaraminol, with an increase in the clearance of inulin or creatinine. While this study does not localize the reasons for the reduction in GFR, it demonstrates that the GFR can be readily changed by a vasoactive drug that does not have a comparable action in patients without cirrhosis. The administration of angiotensin to patients with cirrhosis also results in natriuresis and diuresis [55].

Some patients with decompensated cirrhosis have reduced extraction of PAH [5, 80]. This observation is consistent either with altered intrarenal distribution of blood or with a defect in the tubular transport of PAH [80]. Circulatory features are also considered below in relation to the mechanism of renal failure in patients with cirrhosis.

The effect on renal function of increased abdominal pressure secondary to ascites formation has been the subject of some study. It is known that an increase in intraabdominal pressure in animals and in human subjects without cirrhosis may be followed by a decrease in glomerular filtration rate and renal plasma flow [11]. Leslie et al. [57] measured renal hemodynamics before and after abdominal paracentesis in two patients with cirrhosis. In neither instance was renal function significantly altered after the removal of the ascitic fluid. Lauler and Wesson [56] observed no significant change in inulin clearance after paracentesis in two patients studied.

Gordon [33] has studied this subject with continuous measurement of clearance following rapid paracentesis. His data indicate that abdominal paracentesis is generally followed by a definite rise in GFR and effective RPF, occurring within one hour after the paracentesis is performed. This increment is transient, however, and generally lasts no more than a few hours. Assumption of the prone position (while the patient was lying on a Stryker frame), allowing the abdominal contents to lie without support, resulted in transient improvement in the glomerular filtration rate. Although abdominal paracentesis and change in position may result in improved GFR and RPF, we doubt for two reasons that ascites per se is a fundamental factor in the observed decrease in GFR and RPF: First, the effects of abdominal paracentesis are short-lived; and second, many patients with extensive ascites have normal GFR and RPF.

IMPAIRED SODIUM EXCRETION

Since the work of Farnsworth and Krakusin [23] in 1948, there have been many reports which demonstrate that patients with decompensated Laennec's cirrhosis have a remarkable capacity for sodium retention; in fact, such patients frequently excrete urine which is almost free of sodium. When challenged with an acute sodium load, patients actively forming ascites or edema have definite limitation in their natriuretic response [32]. In addition, patients with decompensated cirrhosis may have ablation or gross reversal of the normal diurnal pattern of increased sodium excretion in the day compared with the night [30, 42].

The quantity of sodium excreted in the urine is the resultant of two operations, glomerular filtration and tubular reabsorption. As has been indicated, patients with normal GFR may have extensive ascites and edema and marked limitation in the renal excretion of sodium. This indicates that a reduction in GFR is not requisite for the accumulation of ascites and diminished sodium excretion. (However, in patients who have a reduction in GFR, it may play some role in limiting excretion.) When there is impaired sodium excretion in the presence of a normal filtered load of sodium, an increased tubular reabsorption of sodium must be the cause.

Although there is good evidence for increased proximal tubular reabsorption of sodium in cirrhosis [79], the mechanism whereby this occurs is not known. In dogs, acute partial thoracic inferior vena caval obstruction results in prevention and reversal of the decreased proximal tubular reabsorption of sodium that follows sodium loading [14]. The relevance of this model to the genesis of increased sodium reabsorption in man with cirrhosis is not known. Possible explanations for increased sodium reabsorption include primarily extrarenal as well as intrarenal mechanisms. Thus, a decrease in effective extracellular fluid volume, no matter how mediated, has been proposed [64]. More recent experimental work raises the theoretical possibility of decreased activity of a factor that inhibits reabsorption of sodium by the proximal nephron [50]. However, confirmation of the existence of such a factor is lacking. Intrarenal mechanisms may include: a decrease in GFR per nephron, when a reduction in GFR is present; and some as yet undefined alteration in intrarenal blood flow. The latter may result in redistribution of filtrate from cortical superficial nephrons (relative salt losers) to cortical juxtamedullary nephrons (relative salt retainers), as suggested for other edematous states [5a].

While aldosterone activity is increased during the formation of ascites, in our opinion this is only of secondary and quantitative relevance and does not constitute a prime mover.

IMPAIRED WATER EXCRETION

It has been known for a number of years that patients with decompensated cirrhosis may have some impairment in their capacity to have a normal water diuresis [75]. However, several studies have demonstrated that marked impairment of water diuresis is not as common or consistent an observation as is a decreased ability to excrete sodium [8, 62, 67, 95]. Although modest impairment of water diuresis occurs in a significant number of patients with cirrhosis, it is apparent, particularly in the study by Papper and Saxon [67], that inability to elaborate a urine more dilute than plasma is unusual, and is observed primarily in patients who are seriously ill and whose prognosis is relatively poor. These authors reported that 22 of 48 patients with decompensated cirrhosis had a peak urine flow greater than 9 ml. per minute after water loading. An additional 18 subjects had a maximal flow of 4 to 9 ml. per minute. In both these groups, in all instances studied, the urine concentration was less than 100 mOsm per kilogram of water. Eight subjects had a urine flow of less than 4 ml. per minute, and in only half of these was there failure to elaborate a dilute urine.

It is difficult to correlate the capacity for water diuresis with specific clinical features. The poorest diuretic response tends to occur in the sickest patients, but some patients who are equally sick in terms of their general appearance may have reasonably good water diuresis. In addition, maximal water diuresis does not correlate precisely with the degree of ascites or the level of jaundice.

The mechanism for the impairment in water diuresis is not fully known [64]. It is well recognized that the major determinant of diluting ability is the availability of sodium for reabsorption in the loop of Henle and distal tubule. In cirrhotic patients who have increased proximal tubular reabsorption of sodium, this factor limits the elaboration of free water [79]. Although a reduced GFR may play a role in some patients as previously indicated, diluting ability may be normal in patients with low GFR. Although increased antidiuretic hormone (ADH) activity may limit water excretion in some cirrhotic patients, it seems unlikely that it is an important or major determinant of abnormal water excretion under most circumstances. Whatever its pathogenesis, inability to elaborate a dilute urine may have serious prognostic significance.

Vaamonde et al. [91] have observed a reversible defect in concentrating ability in patients with decompensated cirrhosis. The data suggest that the distal nephron appears to respond normally to vasopressin [92] and that decreased availability of urea is a major factor in limiting urine maximal osmolality [93]. $T^{c}_{H_2O}$ formation was also decreased and could not be attributed to diminished distal delivery of sodium [74, 91].

Other tubular functions in cirrhosis have received relatively little attention [56]. Of interest is the recent observation by Shear et al. [81] concerning renal tubular acidosis in patients with cirrhosis. Nine of 15 patients had a defect in urinary acidification following acid loading. Total urinary hydrogen excretion after acidification was normal in most patients. However, urinary titratable acidity was reduced and ammonia excretion increased. Impaired renal potassium conservation was observed in six patients in conjunction with the acidification defect. There were no abnormalities in the phosphate and uric acid clearances and urinary amino acid excretion.

RENAL FUNCTION AND THE CLINICAL COURSE OF CIRRHOSIS

Most reported observations relate to groups of patients at various stages of cirrhosis. There are relatively few sequential observations of renal function in individual patients as their clinical course unfolds. Leslie et al. [57] reported an increase in renal hemodynamics with clinical improvement. Baldus et al. [4] found only minimal change in water diuresis after resolution of ascites. Vaamonde et al. [91] demonstrated improvement in concentrating ability as decompensated patients became compensated and conversely deterioration in concentrating ability when ascites formed in patients previously free of ascites. More recently Klingler et al. [46] have approached in prospective fashion the problem of changes in GFR, diluting ability, and sodium excretion in individual patients as their clinical course changed. They found that when compensated, GFR and diluting ability were generally within the normal range. Although there was a general tendency for an increase in urine flow, free water clearance, and sodium excretion with clinical improvement, particularly in patients with severe liver disease, some decompensated patients had a normal diuretic response to administered water which did not increase with compensation. There was no clear correlation of GFR or RPF with maximal urine flow or the clinical status.

The data suggest that in decompensated cirrhosis the spectrum of renal function is broad. A very general relationship of renal function to the severity of the liver disease exists although a lack of a uniformly consistent relationship between renal function and clinical course is apparent.

Renal Failure in Laennec's Cirrhosis

When oliguria occurs in Laennec's cirrhosis, it is generally attributable to a reduction in the rate of solute excretion, in particular sodium, rather than to kidney damage. The oliguria is seldom associated with any evidence of significant impairment of renal function as measured by reduction in glomerular filtration rate or by azotemia. However, there *are* instances in which oliguria in patients with cirrhosis is associated with the development of azotemia. Since its earliest descriptions, much controversy has developed about the existence of renal failure which cannot be explained on the basis of factors known to result in renal insufficiency (e.g., shock and overwhelming infection). In the past 15 years especially, this subject has been reinvestigated by many groups, and it is now clear that in patients with Laennec's cirrhosis renal failure may develop without apparent cause. In 1959 Papper et al. [65] reported in detail on 22 patients with otherwise unexplained renal failure. This series now has been extended to include 75 patients and, in conjunction with the studies of others [3, 36, 82], comprises the basis for the following observations.

CLINICAL FEATURES

Some of the clinical features of renal failure in Laennec's cirrhosis may be summarized as follows:

1. Although progressive and severe oliguria is the hallmark of the syndrome, we have now observed several patients with progressive renal failure in the absence of oliguria.

2. Renal failure may develop in the course of the disease without any apparent precipitating event. It may also occur following abdominal paracentesis, even when as little as 2 or 3 liters are removed, and sometimes is noted as liver failure progresses. We have also seen renal failure in patients with guaiac-positive stool in the absence of gross gastrointestinal hemorrhage, decrease in hematocrit, or shock.

3. Renal failure may develop with great rapidity. Because many of our patients had been studied previously for other reasons, we were able to determine that normal blood urea nitrogen or creatinine concentrations, normal glomerular filtration rate, and good urinary concentrating ability existed as recently as a few months, weeks, or even days before the development of renal failure. As will be discussed later, this has certain implications regarding the underlying mechanisms of the development of renal failure in patients with Laennec's cirrhosis.

4. In our series, ascites was generally present, but it varied considerably in degree from minimal to quite marked. Jaundice was extremely variable, ranging from minimal elevation of the serum bilirubin concentration to severe and progressive jaundice. Although in many instances renal failure occurred while jaundice deepened, it is noteworthy that in several patients jaundice was actually decreasing when renal failure developed.

5. In all but a few instances we observed a definite modest reduction in blood pressure from previous values.

6. Hepatic coma was present in more than half our patients.

7. The development of renal failure in the course of Laennec's cirrhosis is of grave prognostic significance. Only one patient in our entire group has had a spontaneous recovery. (We cannot exclude the possibility of unrelated acute renal disease in this exceptional case.) On the other hand, a few patients with recovery have been observed by others [3, 28, 31, 79a].

However, it is difficult to attribute death directly to renal failure in a patient whose serum creatinine concentration is 2.2 mg. per 100 ml., and whose blood urea nitrogen concentration is 40 mg. per 100 ml. While it is possible that patients with severe functional hepatic impairment may be more sensitive to unexcreted metabolic waste products than patients without liver disease, this explanation is entirely conjectural. It seems more likely that renal failure may be a reflection or a part of a broader lethal event, and that in general it is not, in itself, the most important determinant as to how long the patient will survive.

LABORATORY FEATURES

The following are the more significant laboratory features of our patients with renal failure in Laennec's cirrhosis.

1. The urine was generally acid and frequently contained small amounts of protein. Hyaline and granular casts as well as microscopic hematuria were commonly observed.

2. There was a striking decrease in glomerular filtration rate and renal plasma flow.

3. Urinary concentration was variable. In many instances the urine was scanty and quite concentrated (2 to 3.5 times plasma) early in the course of renal failure. In several patients death occurred while the urine was still concentrated. Most patients were observed to have a gradual decrease in urinary concentration toward that of plasma while they remained oliguric. Still other patients had urine concentrations only slightly above that of plasma at the time they were first seen.

Diluting ability is difficult to study and interpret in such patients. Many of them are so uncomfortable that ADH secretion may be stimulated for reasons unrelated to liver disease. A number of observations have been made under carefully controlled conditions, and with only rare exception these patients cannot elaborate a dilute urine [46, 53].

4. With the exception of an occasional patient with a urinary sodium concentration (U_{Na}) of 30 mEq. per liter, the U_{Na} was less than 10 mEq. per liter, including patients without oliguria. Indeed, it was usually only 1 to 2 mEq. per liter. This is in striking contradistinction to the usual situation in acute tubular necrosis, in which urinary sodium concentration is generally greater than 50 mEq. per liter.

5. In general, the levels of serum creatinine did not reach those seen in the terminal stages of primary renal disease, although one patient had a serum creatinine concentration of 14.3 mg. per 100 ml. An important fact, however, is that death occurred in patients whose serum creatinine concentration was as low as 2.2 mg. per 100 ml.

6. Serum sodium concentration is usually but not always reduced. It has been clearly shown that in early renal failure the serum sodium concentration is normal, and it appears to decline as the course evolves, perhaps as a consequence of administered water in excess of that excreted [3, 65, 82].

7. Autopsy did not reveal evidence of primary renal disease in any instance in our series. In some, no abnormalities were noted. The glomeruli often demonstrated the glomerulosclerosis described by Barr and Sommers [6] and by Bloodworth and Sommers [9]. Several patients, but not all, with severe jaundice had the findings described as "bile nephrosis" or "cholemic nephrosis." In addition, a number of tubular changes, varying from minimal dilatation and cell flattening to degenerative changes, were observed in our series. Acute tubular necrosis has on occasion been observed by others [34, 82]. As has been discussed above, the functional significance of these findings is not clear. The histologic appearance of the liver varied greatly.

PATHOGENESIS OF RENAL FAILURE

The etiology of the observed renal failure of cirrhosis is still not known. Its relationship to the modest reduction in GFR and RPF sometimes observed in other patients with Laennec's cirrhosis, whose course is entirely dissimilar, is not at all clear. It seems apparent, however, from the rapidity with which renal failure may occur, that one must search for the mechanism of its development among more acute and subacute varieties of renal dysfunction. Some of these possibilities warrant further consideration.

Hyponatremia is not likely to be related to the development of renal failure in cirrhosis, because the decrease in serum sodium concentration often follows the onset of renal failure and the early correction of hyponatremia does not result in improvement. Potassium deficiency, an additional possible explanation for the development of renal failure in cirrhosis, is not likely to be an important factor because many of our patients had a concentrated urine while they had azotemia, and because none of the characteristic histologic changes associated with potassium depletion were observed.

While the histologic lesion of acute tubular necrosis has been described in some patients with cirrhosis and renal failure [34, 82], it is unlikely that it accounts for the renal failure in any appreciable number of patients. While we recognize that one may have a course consistent with acute tubular necrosis at a time when examination of the kidney with light microscopy fails to reveal any abnormality, it seems unlikely that we should have as large a series as ours and not find a single instance of a typical lesion of tubular necrosis. Furthermore, the functional changes, especially maintained concentrating ability in some, the very low urinary sodium concentration, and the high creatinine U/P ratios constitute strong evidence against such a mechanism.

It is possible that certain metabolic disturbances associated with Laennec's cirrhosis may be involved in the pathogenesis of renal failure. We have mentioned the possibility that substances either produced by or inadequately detoxified by the diseased liver may affect renal function. However, at the present time, there is insufficient evidence to constitute proof. While the possibility that bilirubin itself may have an adverse effect on the kidney has not been completely excluded, several factors militate against this explanation: (1) renal failure may develop while jaundice is decreasing; (2) renal failure may be present in the absence of "bile nephrosis"; and (3) "bile nephrosis" may be observed in the absence of significant impairment in renal function.

The following evidence in man supports the view that circulatory disturbances involving the kidney account for the renal failure:

1. Renal failure may develop with great rapidity.

2. The capacity to elaborate a concentrated urine may be present despite marked reduction in GFR. In most instances urinary concentration may be observed to decrease with time and approach the osmolality of serum. These observations of a reduced GFR, an initially concentrated urine in many instances, and a striking reduction in the urine concentration of sodium are all consistent with some diminution in effective renal perfusion.

3. Although we excluded all patients with gross clinical shock from our series, a modest decrease in blood pressure was the rule.

4. The onset of renal failure following mild gastrointestinal bleeding (defined in our series as asymptomatic guaiac-positive stools without decrease in hematocrit or marked hypotension) or paracentesis may also lend support to the importance of circulatory derangements, since a reduction in "effective" fluid volume results under both circumstances.

5. The administration of isotonic saline, ascitic fluid, plasma, dextran, or whole blood have been shown to result in a transient increase in GFR, and sometimes in increased flow of a more dilute urine.

6. Administration of the pressor amine, metaraminol, is sometimes followed by increased inulin or creatinine clearance, and usually by some increase in urine flow and the rate of excretion of sodium, potassium, and total solutes.

7. The histologic appearance of the kidney, which is variously described as normal or as demonstrating some minimal abnormalities of the tubules, is consistent with decreased renal perfusion.

8. The recent observation that six of seven kidneys from six patients dying with this syndrome functioned promptly when used as the donor kidney in renal transplantation, is consistent with some readily reversible disturbance in the kidney such as one of a circulatory nature [48].

If the pathogenesis of the renal failure in Laennec's cirrhosis lies in a disturbance in renal circulation, one cannot offer a precise mechanism based on unequivocal experimental evidence. It is conceivable that the apparent renal afferent vasoconstriction may be entirely due to alterations in the extrarenal distribution of blood. Thus, it is known that many patients with cirrhosis including many with renal failure, have increased cardiac output generally assumed to be due to peripheral vasodilatation (of unknown cause), functioning in effect as an arteriovenous shunt mechanism [15, 47, 49, 61]. Of interest is the observation that patients with cirrhosis have decreased vascular sensitivity to administered angiotensin [40, 55]. It is also known that patients with advanced liver failure who may or may not have azotemia may have a reduction in cerebral [25] and hepatic blood flow [36] as well. Thus, one can think of a patient with cirrhosis with a high cardiac output and blood going preferentially to the "shunted areas," depriving the kidney (and perhaps other viscera) of blood [39, 52]. While this relatively simple mechanism cannot be dismissed entirely, there are some bits of evidence that question it as the sole explanation. Some patients with cirrhosis and renal failure have normal or even reduced cardiac output [15, 80, 88, 89]. With all the many determinants of cardiac output, aside from the presence of a shunt, perhaps the presence of normal or reduced cardiac output does not necessarily exclude such a mechanism. In any case, there may be other explanations for an altered extrarenal distribution of blood still making the kidney passively deprived. Although the nature of the functional changes are consistent with such a hypothesis, the severity of renal failure in some patients seems excessive, as compared, for example, to renal function in dehydration or congestive heart failure. In addition, in the latter instance the filtration fraction is generally increased, whereas in renal failure in cirrhosis, the filtration fraction is often reduced [80]. Finally, the response to expansion of the intravascular volume results in inconsistent and only transient improvement in renal function [35, 67, 76, 88].

Although one cannot exclude an extrarenal diversion of blood from the kidney as operative, at least in some patients with renal failure, the possibility of some basic alteration in intrarenal circulation continues to deserve serious consideration [54, 80]. Indeed, Epstein and his co-workers [20], utilizing the technics of xenon washout and selective renal arteriography in patients with cirrhosis and renal failure, have derived data consistent with preferential renal cortical ischemia. In addition, the changing nature of the xenon curves as well as normal filling of the entire arterial tree during postmortem angiography constitute further confirmation of the functional nature of the renal failure in cirrhosis. It is conceivable that a single substance, inadequately destroyed by the diseased liver or generated by it, is capable of producing both peripheral vasodilatation and, independently, vasoconstriction in other circulatory beds such as the kidney. However appealing such a formulation may be, it is *entirely* conjectural at this time.

In summary, the data suggest that renal failure in cirrhosis is due to a circulatory mechanism with afferent renal vasoconstriction. While the precise nature of the circulatory disturbance is not clear, one must consider (1) reduced renal perfusion secondary to altered systemic distribution of blood, and (2) abnormalities in intrarenal circulation. It is conceivable that both may be relevant.

TREATMENT

It is distressing to realize that we have nothing to add to our unsuccessful therapeutic efforts reported in 1959. While improvement in GFR may occur following infusion of whole blood, plasma, saline, dextran, ascitic fluid, metaraminol, and dopamine ([5b], these measures have only temporary effect. In no instance in our experience was the outcome altered. Even frequent attempts to expand plasma volume have been futile [16, 59]. Dialysis has also been used without success.

A major point, however, is to recognize that decreased urine volume and azotemia occurring in cirrhosis, may be due to a coincidental, unrecognized, and more remediable variety of renal disease. Therefore, the physician should consider dehydration, pyelonephritis, nephrotoxins, etc., in such instances and institute appropriate therapy.

It is difficult to be certain of what measures can be taken to prevent the development of renal failure in cirrhosis. However, it seems reasonable to believe that any factors resulting in decreased intravascular volume may be hazardous. Thus, for example, paracentesis should be undertaken with care and for the specific indications of pulmonary distress and abdominal pain.

The presence of renal failure may complicate the management of cirrhotic patients from other points of view [58]. Thus the rate of ammonia formation in the gastrointestinal tract may be increased, and with it the likelihood of hepatic coma. In addition, the choice and dosage of antibiotics for the prevention and treatment of hepatic coma and of incidental infection depend, at least in part, on knowledge of the renal capacity for excretion of individual drugs.

Summary

Renal failure without apparent cause may develop in the course of Laennec's cirrhosis. While the development of azotemia under these circumstances bears with it a very poor prognosis, the data suggest that the patients die *in* renal failure rather than *of* renal failure. The latter seems to be only a part of a broader, more fundamental disturbance. The pathogenesis of renal failure is not known, but the evidence supports an impairment in effective renal perfusion.

Acknowledgment

These studies were supported by National Institute of Health Grant No. 07665 from the U.S. Public Health Service.

References

1. Adlersberg, D., and Fox, C. L., Jr. Changes of the water tolerance test in hepatic disease. *Ann. Intern. Med.* 19:642, 1943.
2. Aoyagi, T., and Lowenstein, L. M. The effect of bile acids and renal ischemia on renal function. *J. Lab. Clin. Med.* 71:686, 1968.
3. Baldus, W. P., Feichter, R. N., and Summerskill, W. H. J. The kidney in cirrhosis: I. Clinical and biochemical features of azotemia in hepatic failure. *Ann. Intern. Med.* 60:353, 1964.
4. Baldus, W. P., Feichter, R. N., Summerskill, W. H. J., Hunt, J. C., and Wakim, K. E. The kidney in cirrhosis: II. Disorders of renal function. *Ann. Intern. Med.* 60:366, 1964.
5. Baldus, W. P., Summerskill, W. H. J., Hunt, J. C., and Maher, F. T. Renal circulation in cirrhosis: Observations based on catheterization of the renal vein. *J. Clin. Invest.* 43:1090, 1964.

5a. Barger, A. C. Renal hemodynamic factors in congestive heart failure. *Ann. N.Y. Acad. Sci.* 139:276, 1966.

5b. Barnabo, D. E., Baldus, W. P., and Maher, F. T. Effects of dopamine on renal function in patients with cirrhosis. *Gastroenterology* 58:524, 1970.

6. Barr, R. W., and Sommers, S. C. Endocrine abnormalities accompanying hepatic cirrhosis and hepatoma. *J. Clin. Endocr.* 17:1017, 1957.
7. Baxter, J. H., and Ashworth, C. T. Renal lesions in portal cirrhosis. *Arch. Path.* 41:476, 1946.
8. Bernstein, S. H., Weston, R. E., Ross, G., Grossman, J., Hanenson, I. B., and Leiter, L. Studies on intravenous water diuresis and nicotine and Pitressin antidiuresis in normal subjects and patients with liver disease. *J. Clin. Invest.* 32:422, 1953.
9. Bloodworth, J. M. B., Jr., and Sommers, S. C. "Cirrhotic glomerulosclerosis," a renal lesion associated with hepatic cirrhosis. *Lab. Invest* 8:962, 1959.
10. Boyce, F. F. *The Role of the Liver in Surgery*. Springfield, Ill.: Thomas, 1941.
11. Bradley, S. E., and Bradley, G. P. The effect of increased intra-abdominal pressure on renal function in man. *J. Clin. Invest.* 26: 1010, 1947.

12. Brandt, J. L., and Caccese, A. The effects of modified human globin on renal function in cirrhosis of the liver. *J. Lab. Clin. Med.* 39: 57, 1952.
13. Cachera, R., Darnis, F., and Lubetzki, J. Le rein des cirrhotiques. *Rev. Int. Hepat.* 3:603, 1953.
14. Cirksena, W. J., Dirks, J. H., and Berliner, R. W. Effect of thoracic cava obstruction on response of proximal tubule sodium reabsorption to saline infusion. *J. Clin. Invest.* 45:179, 1966.
15. Claypool, J. G., Delp, M., and Lin, T. K. Hemodynamic studies in patients with Laennec's cirrhosis. *Amer. J. Med. Sci.* 234:48, 1957.
16. Clermont, R. J., Vlahcevic, Z. R., Chalmers, T. C., Adham, N. F., Curtis, G. W., and Morrison, R. S. Intravenous therapy of massive ascites in patients with cirrhosis: II. Long term effects on survival and frequency of renal failure. *Gastroenterology* 53:220, 1967.
17. Conrad, M. E., Schwartz, F. D., and Young, A. A. Infectious hepatitis — A generalized disease. A study of renal, gastrointestinal, and hematologic abnormalities. *Amer. J. Med.* 37:789, 1964.
18. Dawson, J. L. Jaundice and anoxic renal damage: Protective effect of mannitol. *Brit. Med. J.* 1:810, 1964.
19. Epstein, F. H., Lesser, G. T., and Berger, E. Y. Renal function in decompensated cirrhosis of the liver. *Proc. Soc. Exp. Biol. Med.* 75:822, 1950.
20. Epstein, M., Berk, D. P., Hollenberg, N. K., Adams, D. F., Chalmers, T. C., Abrams, H. L., and Merrill, J. P. Renal failure in the patient with cirrhosis. *Amer. J. Med.* 49:175, 1970.
21. Fajers, C. Experimental studies in cholemic nephrosis. *Acta Path. Microbiol. Scand.* 41: 44, 1957.
22. Fajers, C. Experimental studies in the so-called hepato-renal syndrome. *Acta Path. Microbiol. Scand.* 44:5, 1958.
23. Farnsworth, E. B., and Krakusin, J. S. Electrolyte partition in patients with edema of various origins: Qualitative and quantitative definition of cations and anions in hepatic cirrhosis. *J. Lab. Clin. Med.* 33:1545, 1948.
24. Farquhar, J. C. Renal studies in acute infections (epidemic) hepatitis. *Amer. J. Med. Sci.* 218:291, 1949.
25. Fazekas, J. F., Tictin, H. E., Ehrmantrant, W. R., and Alman, R. W. Cerebral metabolism in hepatic insufficiency. *Amer. J. Med.* 21:843, 1956.
26. Fisher, E. R., and Hellstrom, H. R. The membranous and proliferative glomerulonephritis of hepatic cirrhosis. *Amer. J. Clin. Path.* 32:48, 1959.
26a. Fisher, E. R., and Perez-Stable, E. Cirrhotic (hepatic) lobular glomerulonephritis: Correlation of ultrastructural and clinical features. *Amer. J. Path.* 52:869, 1968.
27. Flint, A. Clinical report on hydroperitoneum, based on an analysis of forty-six cases. *Amer. J. Med. Sci.* 45:306, 1863.
28. Galambos, J. T., and Wilkinson, H. A., III. Reversible hyponatremia and azotemia in a patient with cirrhosis and ascites. *Amer. J. Dig. Dis.* 7:642, 1962.
29. Gilbert, A., and Lereboullet, P. Des urines rétardées (opsiurie) dans les cirrhoses. *Compt. Rend. Soc. Biol.* (Paris) 53:276, 1901.
30. Goldman, R. Studies in diurnal variation of water and electrolyte excretion: Nocturnal diuresis of water and sodium in congestive cardiac failure and cirrhosis of the liver. *J. Clin. Invest.* 30:1191, 1951.
31. Goldstein, H., and Boyle, J. D. Spontaneous recovery from the hepatorenal syndrome: Report of four cases. *New Eng. J. Med.* 272:895, 1965.
32. Goodyer, A. V. N., Relman, A. S., Lawrason, F. D., and Epstein, F. H. Salt retention in cirrhosis of the liver. *J. Clin. Invest.* 29:973, 1950.
33. Gordon, M. E. The acute effects of abdominal paracentesis in Laennec's cirrhosis upon exchanges of electrolytes and water, renal function and hemodynamics. *Amer. J. Gastroent.* 33:15, 1960.
34. Goresky, C. A., and Kumar, G. Renal failure in cirrhosis of the liver. *Canad. Med. Ass. J.* 90:353, 1964.
35. Gornel, D. L., Lancestremere, R. G., Papper, S., and Lowenstein, L. M. Acute changes in renal excretion of water and solute in patients with Laennec's cirrhosis, induced by the ad-

ministration of the pressor amine, metaraminol. *J. Clin. Invest.* 41:594, 1962.

36. Hecker, R., and Sherlock, S. Electrolyte and circulatory changes in terminal liver failure. *Lancet* 2:1121, 1956.
37. Heintzelmann, F. Nierenfunktionsundersøgelser hos patienter med hepatitis epidemica med henblik paa det hepato-renale syndrome. *Nord. Med.* 33:240, 1947.
38. Helwig, F. C., and Schutz, C. B. A liver kidney syndrome: Clinical, pathological and experimental studies. *Surg. Gynec. Obstet.* 55:570, 1932.
39. Hilton, J. G., Kanter, D. M., Hays, D. R., Bowen, E. H., Golub, J. R., Keating, J. H., and Wégria, R. The effect of acute arteriovenous fistula on renal functions. *J. Clin. Invest.* 34:732, 1955.
40. Johnston, C. I., and Jose, A. D. Reduced vascular response to angiotensin II in secondary hyperaldosteronism. *J. Clin. Invest.* 42:1411, 1963.
41. Jones, C. M., and Eaton, F. B. The prognostic significance of a spontaneous diuresis in acute or subacute disease of the liver. *New Eng. J. Med.* 213:907, 1935.
42. Jones, R. A., McDonald, G. O., and Last, J. H. Reversal of diurnal variation in renal function in cases of cirrhosis with ascites. *J. Clin. Invest.* 31:326, 1952.
43. Jones, W. A., Rao, D. R. G., and Braunstein, H. The renal glomerulus in cirrhosis of the liver. *Amer. J. Path.* 39:393, 1961.
44. Kimmelstiel, P. Diabetic Nephropathy. In Becker, E. L. (Ed.), *Structural Basis of Renal Disease.* New York: Hoeber Med. Div., Harper & Row, 1968. P. 462.
45. Klatskin, G., and Krehl, W. A. The effect of alcohol on the choline requirement: II. Incidence of renal necrosis in weanling rats following short term ingestion of alcohol. *J. Exp. Med.* 100:615, 1954.
46. Klingler, E. L., Jr., Vaamonde, C. A., Vaamonde, L. S., Lancestremere, R. G., Morosi, H. J., Frisch, E., and Papper, S. Renal function changes in cirrhosis of the liver: A Prospective study. *Arch. Intern. Med.* (Chicago) 125:1010, 1970.
47. Kontos, H. A., Shapiro, W., Mauck, H. P., and Patterson, J. L., Jr. General and regional circulatory alterations in cirrhosis of the liver. *Amer. J. Med.* 37:526, 1964.
48. Koppel, M. H., Coburn, J. W., Mims, M. M., Goldstein, H., Boyle, J. D., and Rubini, M. E. Transplantation of cadaveric kidneys from patients with hepatorenal syndrome: Evidence for the functional nature of renal failure in advanced liver disease. *New Eng. J. Med.* 280:1367, 1969.
49. Kowalski, H. J., and Abelmann, W. H. The cardiac output at rest in Laennec's cirrhosis. *J. Clin. Invest.* 32:1025, 1953.
50. Kurtzman, N. A., Hull, A. R., Martinez-Maldonado, M., Rector, F. C., Jr., and Seldin, D. W. Significance of natriuretic hormone in edematous states. *Amer. Soc. Nephrol. Abstracts* p. 36, 1967.
51. Labby, D. H., and Hoagland, C. L. Water storage and the movements of body fluids and chlorides during acute liver disease. *J. Clin. Invest.* 26:343, 1947.
52. Lancestremere, R. G., Davidson, P. L., Earley, L. E., O'Brien, F. J., and Papper, S. Renal failure in Laennec's cirrhosis: II. Simultaneous determination of cardiac output and renal hemodynamics. *J. Clin. Invest.* 41:1922, 1962.
53. Lancestremere, R. G., Davidson, P. L., Earley, L. E., O'Brien, F. J., and Papper, S. Renal failure in Laennec's cirrhosis: III. Diuretic response to administered water. *J. Lab. Clin. Med.* 60:967, 1962.
54.. Lancestremere, R. G., Klingler, E. L., Jr., Frisch, E., and Papper, S. Simultaneous determination of cardiac output and renal function in patients with Laennec's cirrhosis during the administration of the pressor amine, metaraminol. *J. Lab. Clin. Med.* 61:820, 1963.
55. Laragh, J. H., Cannon, P. J., Bentzel, C. J., Sicinski, A. M., and Meltzer, J. I. Angiotensin II, norepinephrine, and renal transport of electrolytes and water in normal man and in cirrhosis with ascites. *J. Clin. Invest.* 42:1179, 1963.
56. Lauler, D. P., and Wesson, L. G., Jr. Renal function in cirrhosis. *Clin. Res.* 8:382, 1960.
57. Leslie, S. H., Johnston, B., and Ralli, E. P. Renal function as a factor in fluid retention in patients with cirrhosis of the liver. *J. Clin. Invest.* 30:1200, 1951.

58. Lieber, C. S., and Davidson, C. S. Complications resulting from renal failure in patients with liver disease. *Arch. Intern. Med.* (Chicago) 106:749, 1960.
59. McCloy, R. M., Baldus, W. P., Maher, F. T., and Summerskill, W. H. J. Effects of changing plasma volume, serum albumin concentration, and plasma osmolality on renal function in cirrhosis. *Gastroenterology* 53: 229, 1967.
60. McCloy, R. M., Baldus, W. P., Tauxe, W. N., and Summerskill, W. H. J. Plasma volume and renal circulatory function in cirrhosis. *Ann. Intern. Med.* 66:307, 1967.
61. Murray, J. F., Dawson, A. M., and Sherlock, S. Circulatory changes in chronic liver disease. *Amer. J. Med.* 24:358, 1958.
62. Nelson, W. P., III, and Welt, L. G. The effects of Pitressin on the metabolism and excretion of water and electrolytes in normal subjects and patients with ascites. *J. Clin. Invest.* 31:392, 1952.
63. Odell, G. B., Natzschka, J. C., and Storey, G. N. B. Bilirubin nephropathy in the Gunn strain of rat. *Amer. J. Physiol.* 212:931, 1967.
64. Papper, S. The role of the kidney in Laennec's cirrhosis of the liver. *Medicine* (Balt.) 37:299, 1958.
65. Papper, S., Belsky, J. L., and Bleifer, K. H. Renal failure in Laennec's cirrhosis of the liver: I. Description of clinical and laboratory features. *Ann. Intern. Med.* 51:759, 1959.
66. Papper, S., and Rosenbaum, J. D. Abnormalities in the excretion of water and sodium in "compensated" cirrhosis of the liver. *J. Lab. Clin. Med.* 40:523, 1952.
67. Papper, S., and Saxon, L. The diuretic response to administered water in patients with liver disease: II. Laennec's cirrhosis of the liver. *A.M.A. Arch. Intern. Med.* 103:750, 1959.
68. Papper, S., and Saxon, L. The influence of intravenous infusion of sodium chloride solutions on the renal excretion of sodium in patients with cirrhosis of the liver. *J. Clin. Invest.* 35:728, 1956.
69. Papper, S., Seifer, H. W., and Saxon, L. The diuretic response to administered water in patients with liver disease: I. Acute infectious hepatitis. *A.M.A. Arch. Intern. Med.* 103:746, 1959.
70. Papper, S., and Vaamonde, C. A. Renal failure in cirrhosis — Role of plasma volume. *Ann. Intern. Med.* 68:958, 1968.
71. Paris, J. L'exploration du functionnement rénal au cours des affections hépatobiliares. *Rev. Int. Hepat.* 3:37, 1953.
72. Patek, A. J., Jr., Seegal, D., and Bevans, M. The coexistence of cirrhosis of the liver and glomerulonephritis: Report of 14 cases. *Amer. J. Med. Sci.* 221:77, 1951.
73. Popper, H., and Schaffner, F. *Liver: Structure and Function.* New York: Blakiston Div., McGraw-Hill, 1957.
74. Presser, J. I., Vaamonde, L. S., Vaamonde, C. A., and Papper, S. Renal concentrating ability in cirrhosis of the liver: IV. Failure of hypertonic saline to improve the $T^{c}_{H_2O}$ defect. *J. Clin. Invest.* 46:1106, 1967.
75. Ralli, E. P., Leslie, S. H., Stueck, G. H., Jr., and Laken, B. Studies of the serum and urine constituents in patients with cirrhosis of the liver during water tolerance tests. *Amer. J. Med.* 11:157, 1951.
76. Reynolds, T. B., Lieberman, F. L., and Redeker, A. G. Functional renal failure with cirrhosis: The effect of plasma expansion therapy. *Medicine* (Balt.) 46:191, 1967.
77. Sakaguchi, H., Dachs, S., Grishman, E., Paronetto, F., Salomon, M., and Churg, J. Hepatic glomerulosclerosis: An electron microscopy study of renal biopsies in liver diseases. *Lab. Invest.* 14:533, 1965.
78. Salomon, M. I., Sakaguchi, H., Churg, J., Dachs, S., Grishman, E., Mautner, W., Paronetto, F., and Rosenthal, W. S. Renal lesions in hepatic disease. *Arch. Intern. Med.* (Chicago) 115:704, 1965.
79. Schedl, H. P., and Bartter, F. C. An explanation for and experimental correction of the abnormal water diuresis in cirrhosis. *J. Clin. Invest.* 39:248, 1960.
79a. Schroeder, E. T., Numann, P. J., and Chamberlain, B. E. Functional renal failure in cirrhosis. Recovery after portocaval shunt. *Ann. Intern. Med.* 72:923, 1970.
80. Schroeder, E. T., Shear, L., Sancetta, S. M., and Gabuzda, G. J. Renal failure in patients

with cirrhosis of the liver: III. Evaluation of intrarenal blood flow by para-aminohippurate extraction and response to angiotensin. *Amer. J. Med.* 43:887, 1967.

81. Shear, L., Bonkowsky, H. L., and Gabuzda, G. L. Renal tubular acidosis in cirrhosis: A determinant of susceptibility to recurrent hepatic precoma. *New Eng. J. Med.* 280:1, 1969.
82. Shear, L., Kleinerman, J., and Gabuzda, G. J. Renal failure in patients with cirrhosis of the liver: I. Clinical and pathologic characteristics. *Amer. J. Med.* 39:184, 1965.
83. Shorr, E. Hepatorenal Vasotropic Factors in Experimental Cirrhosis. In Hoffbauer, F. W. (Ed.), *Liver Injury*. Transactions of the Sixth Conference. New York: Josiah Macy, Jr. Foundation, 1947.
84. Shorr, E., Zweifach, B. W., and Furchgott, R. F. Hepatorenal factors in circulatory hemostasis; influence of humoral factors of hepatorenal origin on vascular reactions to hemorrhage. *Ann. N.Y. Acad. Sci.* 49:571, 1948.
85. Siegler, P., and Faludi, G. Nierenfunktionsprüfungen bei Leberkranken. *Z. Ges. Inn. Med.* 8:607, 1953.
86. Strauss, M. B., Birchard, W. H., and Saxon, L. Correction of impaired water excretion in cirrhosis of the liver by alcohol ingestion or expansion of extracellular fluid volume: The role of the antidiuretic hormone. *Trans. Ass. Amer. Physicians* 69:222, 1956.
87. Thompson, L. L., Jr., Frazier, W. D., and Ravdin, I. S. The renal lesion in obstructive jaundice. *Amer. J. Med. Sci.* 199:305, 1940.
88. Tristani, F. E., and Cohn, J. N. Systemic and renal hemodynamics in oliguric hepatic failure: Effect of volume expansion. *J. Clin. Invest.* 46:1894, 1967.
89. Tyler, J. M., Jeffries, J. L., and Wilder, C. E. A study of the renal blood flow by nitrous oxide technique in normal and oliguric patients with cirrhosis of the liver. *Clin. Res.* 10:194, 1962.
90. Uchiyama, T. Experimental studies of hepatorenal relationship from the surgical point of view. *Arch. Jap. Chir.* 33:53, 1964.
91. Vaamonde, C. A., Vaamonde, L. S., Morosi, H. J., Klingler, E. L., Jr., and Papper, S. Renal concentrating ability in cirrhosis: I. Changes associated with the clinical status and course of the disease. *J. Lab. Clin. Med.* 70:179, 1967.
92. Vaamonde, C. A., Vaamonde, L. S., Morosi, H. J., Klingler, E. L., Jr., and Papper, S. Renal concentrating ability in cirrhosis: II. Role of vasopressin and urea, and comparison with diluting ability. Submitted for publication.
93. Vaamonde, C. A., Vaamonde, L. S., Presser, J. I., Morosi, H. J., Klingler, E. L., Jr., and Papper, S. Role of urea in the renal concentrating defect of cirrhosis. *Clin. Res.* 17: 451, 1969.
94. Von Noorden, C. *Metabolism and Practical Medicine. Vol. 2: Pathology*. Chicago: W. T. Keener, 1907. P. 267.
95. White, A. G., Rubin, G., and Leiter, L. Studies in edema: III. The effect of Pitressin on the renal excretion of water and electrolytes in patients with and without liver disease. *J. Clin. Invest.* 30:1287, 1951.

32

The Kidney in Pregnancy

Ethan A. H. Sims

In the course of pregnancy a previously healthy woman may be transformed into a patient with fluid retention, increased reactivity of the vascular and central nervous systems, and disturbance of the normal mechanisms for coagulation of the blood. Thus she becomes edematous and hypertensive, she may convulse, and infarction may develop in various vital organs. If a woman enters pregnancy with underlying kidney disease, she may react in a similarly adverse manner. The major objectives of this chapter are, first, to outline the physiologic changes in normal pregnancy, with attention to those factors that make a pregnant woman susceptible to such a physiologic upheaval, and second, to consider the various diseases of the kidney in the setting of pregnancy, with attention to the multiple factors that may lead to a common clinical state of preeclampsia.

Anatomic Changes of the Urinary Tract

The calyceal, pelvic, and ureteral dilatation, more marked on the right, which is seen in normal pregnancy has been reviewed by Crabtree [44] and by Fainstat [59]. There is good evidence from the work of Van Wagenen and Jenkins [224] that the dilatation results from endocrine effects, predominantly progesterone, but mechanical effects cannot be completely excluded. In the monkey the physiological dilatation of the ureter is dependent upon an intact placenta, but not upon the presence of the fetus [224]. The dilatation also occurs in the rat, in which no mechanical factor can be demonstrated [58].

Functional change accompanies the ureteral dilatation in human pregnancy. Traut and McLane [222] have shown that there is a decrease in the amplitude of the normal peristaltic pressure waves of the ureter. This starts at the third month and is maximal by the seventh or eighth month. During the last month of pregnancy, the normal rhythmic peristalsis returns. The physiologic dilatation of the urinary tract clears within two weeks after delivery in 60 per cent of patients, within six weeks in 94 per cent, and within 12 weeks in essentially all patients without underlying pathology [44].

Renal Function in Normal Pregnancy

As Homer Smith [205] stated two decades ago, "To a renal physiologist, a pregnant woman is a very interesting phenomenon. I do not know any other way to increase the filtration rate by 50 per cent or better for prolonged periods."

There are two main reasons why the physiologic increase of renal function in normal pregnancy has eluded many investigators until relatively recently. First, measurement of renal function in pregnancy presents special technical problems, and second, function varies with the particular stage of pregnancy, so that serial studies may be necessary to detect significant changes.

MEASUREMENT OF RENAL FUNCTION

The technical difficulties peculiar to pregnancy have been summarized by Chesley [30] and others [200]. To obtain satisfactory measurements, certain conditions must be met.

1. Adequate drainage of the bladder requires suprapubic pressure, occasional elevation of the fetal head, or shifting of the position of the patient to ensure complete collection and adequate irrigation. Catheterization is necessary for short-term clearance studies, but the risks of provoking urinary infection must be weighed against the possible benefits from the studies. The risk is minimal in women with normal urinary tracts and adequate flow. When there is increased susceptibility, prophylactic antibiotic therapy may be given following the studies, and in any event a subsequent culture of sterile-voided urine should be made.

2. The dead space of the urinary tract in pregnancy is doubled in size [116], with peak values between the twentieth and thirty-fifth weeks, and this doubling has important consequences. Levinsky and Berliner [108] have shown that with low rates of urine flow, and particularly with an enlarged dead space, the diffusion of water and solutes through the mucous membranes of the urinary tract is increased. Owing to the greater back diffusion of para-aminohippurate (PAH), the calculated renal plasma flow (RPF) is reduced by slow urine flow, and hence the filtration fraction (FF) is disproportionately increased. Thus adequate flows of urine are essential during measurement of renal clearances in pregnant subjects.

3. When there is glucosuria, special precautions must be taken to avoid conjugation of glucose with para-aminohippurate in measuring renal plasma flow [198].

4. Supine posture may sharply alter various measurements of renal function, especially in the second and third trimesters [35]. At these stages, patients must be kept in the lateral positions during clearance studies to obtain maximal values.

RENAL CLEARANCES IN NORMAL PREGNANCY

In 1951 Bucht [24], in Stockholm, published an extensive study which established clearly that from the second through the eighth month of pregnancy, clearances of inulin, PAH, and exogenous creatinine are increased. Independently and simultaneously, Bonsnes and Lange [17] reported similar findings. Earlier studies had supported the widely accepted conclusion that renal function did not differ from that in the nonpregnant subject. This misinterpretation occurred because measurements were made shortly before term and not serially.

Since 1951 a number of serial studies have been published in which patients served as their own controls. In 1956 Levitt [109] demonstrated a sustained rise in filtration rate in serial studies in 18 pregnant subjects comparable to that observed in earlier studies; RPF rose proportionately, but declined after the twentieth week, giving a rise in FF. At the same time Sims and Krantz [200] reported serial studies of 12 pregnant subjects with es-

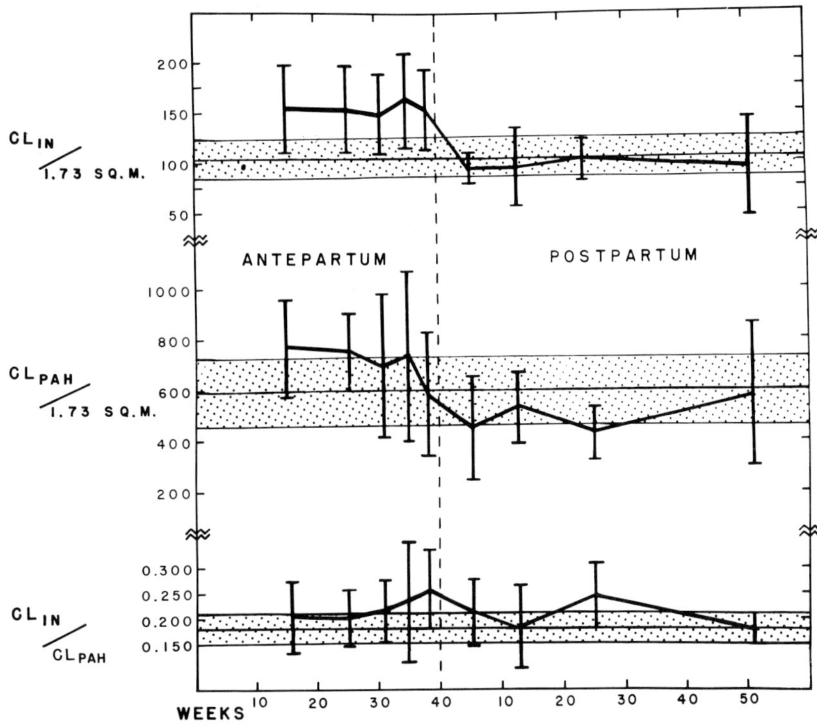

Figure 32-1. The mean values of clearance of insulin (CL_{IN}) and of PAH (CL_{PAH}) and of filtration fractions (CL_{IN}/CL_{PAH}) in 12 pregnant women studied during pregnancy and for a year following delivery. The vertical bars represent two standard deviations above and below the mean. The horizontal line and shaded area represent the corresponding values for nine nonpregnant control subjects. The decline in clearances prior to delivery is at least in part produced by supine posture. (From Sims and Krantz [200].)

sentially the same findings. Figure 32-1 shows the data in graphic form. The RPF and renal blood flow were approximately 25 per cent higher than control values throughout early and mid-pregnancy. The values declined to the range of the control subjects during the last trimester. As Chesley and Sloan [35] have suggested, a portion if not all of the decline may be the result of postural effects, as discussed below. They have shown that when measurements are made exclusively in the right lateral position RPF and GFR do not decline near term. Dignam et al. [52] also noted no reduction in RPF as the patient approached term. However, a glance at patients on an obstetric ward will show that pregnant women do not appreciate the dividend in function which is obtained by lying on their side. Therefore, supine measurements may represent their function state for much of the time. Further effects of posture are discussed below.

In Sims and Krantz's study [200] the glomerular filtration rate was increased approximately 50 per cent throughout pregnancy, returning early in the puerperium to the range seen in nonpregnant subjects (Fig. 32-1). The filtration fraction was significantly elevated throughout pregnancy, rising to approximately 40 per cent above control values as term was approached, and remaining inconstantly elevated during the early puerperium. The RPF was decreased significantly below that of control subjects for many months during the puerperium.

ENDOGENOUS CREATININE CLEARANCE

Measurement of endogenous creatinine clearance provides a more practical method of estimating glomerular filtration rate than use of inulin. Since longer collection periods may be employed, the exact urine volume is less critical and the hazards of catheterization may be avoided. The clearance closely parallels that of inulin in normal pregnancy [200]. Again, it is important that urine flow be ample and that the collection period be sufficiently prolonged so that dead-space error is minimized. To detect gross errors in collection, one should confirm that the actual quantity of creatinine excreted corresponds to the quantity excreted by a woman of average physique, or approximately 1 gm. per day. When renal function is impaired, serum creatinine rises and tubular secretion of creatinine is increased, so that the test is less representative of the true filtration rate.

EFFECT OF INCREASED FILTRATION RATE ON NORMAL CONCENTRATION OF SERUM CREATININE AND UREA

There is a correlation between an increase in GFR and a decrease in blood urea nitrogen and creatinine. More than thirty years ago Peters [153] emphasized that the concentration of the blood nonprotein nitrogen and urea falls in the later months of pregnancy. These observations have been confirmed and extended by measurement of creatinine, which during pregnancy is reduced to 0.46 ± 0.06 mg. (standard deviation) per 100 ml., from 0.67 ± 0.07 mg. per 100 ml. in nonpregnant subjects [200]. Plasma urea is similarly reduced to 8.7 ± 1.5 mg. per 100 ml. from 13.0 ± 3.0 mg. per 100 ml. [200].

Effect of Posture on Renal Function. The pregnant woman has marked circulatory changes that cannot be completely correlated with the increase in blood volume. These have been reviewed by Bader et al. [8] and more recently by Kerr [94]. When standing upright, the pregnant woman is subject to large translocations of fluid, as well as to the exaggerated mechanical effect of the pressure of the gravid uterus on the common iliac vein. Adaptation to these changes is imperfect since in the course of evolution man has only recently assumed an upright posture. In normal man a variety of maneuvers that reduce renal blood flow or produce venous congestion diminish renal function and sodium excretion. It is therefore not surprising that Pritchard et al. [164] found in near-term pregnant subjects that supine posture reduced the rate of excretion of sodium and urine flow. Chesley and Sloan [35] found that in the supine position GFR and effective RPF were reduced 20 per cent, and urine flow and sodium excretion 56 per cent in comparison with values for pregnant patients measured in the lateral position. Others [237] have found excretion of urate is similarly reduced by 43 per cent. The diminution in function in the supine position has usually been attributed to ureteral compression or particularly to venous compression by the gravid uterus, but Bieniarz et al. [14] have presented evidence that aortic compression is also important. Baird et al. [9] have studied postural changes in renal function in pregnancy by means of ^{131}I-renography. Their striking tracings have shown a marked reduction of excretion from the right kidney only when the patient was supine. At 37 weeks there was severe delay in excretion from both kidneys and slight impairment of excretory function, which was only partially relieved by change to lateral position. The important finding was that the delay in excretion was consistent with obstruction and stasis due to mechanical compression, which was at times complete. In the last trimester the postural changes in hemodynamics probably contribute to the impaired secretion and delayed excretion. Potential obstruction of this degree further complicates studies of renal function in pregnancy.

Assali et al. [6] have demonstrated that the pregnant woman is more susceptible than the nonpregnant subject to the effects of quiet standing, responding with a sharp drop in urine flow and in filtration. These postural decrements of function may in turn provoke compensatory increase in blood volume in the ambulatory woman.

CIRCADIAN RHYTHMS OF RENAL FUNCTION

Kalousek et al. [88] have shown that when pregnant women are studied during continuous recumbency in the lateral position, their circadian rhythms of urine flow, creatinine excretion, and electrolyte excretion are similar to those of nonpregnant subjects, with peaks in excretion of all of these parameters during the daytime. However, when normally active during the day, the response of pregnant subjects was variable, and there frequently were peaks of excretion of sodium during the night. It was concluded that posture played a major role in their production.

CAUSES OF THE INCREASED GLOMERULAR FILTRATION RATE AND PLASMA FLOW

Anatomic Factors. It appears that a true anatomic hypertrophy of the kidney does not take place during pregnancy. In guinea pigs the kidneys increase in weight only during the puerperium [203]. In a series of 20 rats no change in the weight of the kidneys in late pregnancy in rats was found when compared with their littermates; in fact, the renal weight per 100 gm. of rat had decreased from 0.71 to 0.60 gm. Since the rat kidney is capable of intermittency of glomerular flow, the number of active glomeruli was estimated by injecting a fluorescent dye and found to be identical in the pregnant and nonpregnant groups.

Circulatory Factors. The increase in renal plasma flow represents an increase in total renal blood flow, in spite of the lowered hematocrit of pregnancy [200]. The plasma, red cell, and total blood volumes increase in pregnancy [13]. It is not possible completely to correlate changes in blood volume and cardiac function with those in renal function, since we still do not know how early kidney function is augmented in pregnancy. During the latter part of pregnancy there is close correlation of renal function with the changes in cardiac output, as measured by Bader et al. [8]. However, as Kerr points out [94], the observed drop in cardiac output prior to delivery may also be an effect of supine posture.

It is of interest that at least one other species has supernormal renal function in pregnancy in common with man. In our laboratory, rats in the latter third of pregnancy were found to have a 28 per cent increase ($p < 0.05$) in endogenous creatinine clearance over that of nonpregnant littermates.

Endocrine Factors. There is much to suggest that endocrine factors mediate the increase in renal function in pregnancy and the regression of renal function in the postpartum period.

Although thyroid hormone is capable of augmenting renal function, there is no evidence that its activity is increased in pregnancy. On the other hand, there is increasing evidence [55, 145] that free plasma cortisol as well as that bound to corticosteroid-binding protein is increased in pregnancy, and this may augment renal function, either directly or indirectly, through retention of sodium.

It appears likely, however, that a major factor may be the growth-hormone-like action of placental lactogen, which is markedly increased in pregnancy [180]. Growth hormone enhances renal function in animals [240] and in man [68]. Since placental lactogen has many metabolic effects in common with growth hormone [11], it is likely, but as yet unproved, that it is also renotrophic. While less physiologically active than growth hormone, its effects may be considerable, since large quantities are in circulation.

EXCRETION OF HISTIDINE AND OTHER AMINO ACIDS IN NORMAL PREGNANCY

The observation that histidine is excreted in excess in pregnancy formed the basis 40 years ago of a test for pregnancy.

Page et al. [150] demonstrated that three factors were responsible for the increased excretion of histidine: (1) the increase in filtration rate during pregnancy accounted for about half of the excess excretion; (2) a reduced rate of entry of administered histidine into the intracellular compartment during pregnancy caused an elevation of plasma histidine and a further increase in the filtered load; and (3) although no sharp tubular Tm could be demonstrated for histidine, the percentage of the filtered histidine which was absorbed by the renal tubules was decreased during pregnancy, and this reduction accounted for one-fourth of the excess histidine excreted. Peterson and Frank [155] have attributed histidinuria to reduced tubular reabsorption, although the data, as was pointed out by Chesley [30], also indicated an increase in the filtered load.

It is now evident that the kidney is also prodigal of other amino acids. Wallraff [229] measured the excretion of 14 amino acids during pregnancy and found increased excretion in seven. Similarly Christensen et al. [39] found that the excretion of 12 of 19 to be increased, with corresponding reductions in plasma concentration. The total loss to the pregnant woman, however, is only moderate; in Wallraff's series [229] this amounted to 0.7 gm. per day of amino nitrogen.

Since creatine shares a common reabsorptive mechanism with several of the amino acids concerned [159], it is not surprising that creatinuria is a relatively constant finding in pregnancy, amounting to 0.15 gm. per day in early pregnancy, 0.33 gm. by the seventh month, and 0.77 gm. preceding delivery. Likewise, since creatine and guanidoacetic acid share a common reabsorptive mechanism [201] in which creatine is more actively reabsorbed, guanidoacetic aciduria would be expected in pregnancy. Zinneman, Seal, and Doe [246] have advanced indirect evidence that the increase in free plasma cortisol in pregnancy may be the cause of the increase in excretion of amino acids. They found that estrogen, progesterone, or a combination of the two had little effect on the pattern of excretion of amino acids, but that administration of cortisol produced aminoaciduria of a pattern strikingly similar to that seen in the last trimester of pregnancy.

RENAL CLEARANCE OF URIC ACID IN NORMAL PREGNANCY

Studies by Chesley [29] and Christensen and Steenstrup [40] have indicated an increased clearance of uric acid in pregnancy during all but the last weeks. Hayashi [76] found clearance of 18.4 $\pm$ S.D. 4.9 ml. per minute prior to the thirty-second week of gestation and 13.0 $\pm$ 4.0 ml. during later pregnancy. Serum uric acid concentrations were 3.2 $\pm$ 0.8 ml. and 3.0 $\pm$ 1.7 ml. in the two periods, respectively. These values are somewhat lower than the 3.57 $\pm$ 0.69 ml. reported by Pollak and Nettles [161] during the third trimester. Uric acid was analyzed in these studies by direct methods not employing uricase. Since uric acid has been shown to be actively secreted by the renal tubules, the lowering of the concentration in pregnancy may reflect increased secretion as well as increased filtration. The decline in late pregnancy may be a postural effect, since Weston and Lindheimer [237] have shown that the supine position not only blunts natriuresis but also decreases clearance of urate out of proportion to reduction of clearance of inulin.

The hyperuricemia noted in preeclampsia

and its relation to the increase in the concentration of lactate in the serum is discussed later in the section on *Preeclampsia.*

GLUCOSE EXCRETION AND RENAL GLUCOSURIA

Glucosuria of pregnancy has been recognized for over a century [154], and the reported incidence, variously estimated to be from 5 to 40 per cent, seems to vary with the diligence with which it is sought. Donato and Turchetti [56], in 1955, measured maximal tubular reabsorption of glucose (Tm_G), calculated from thiosulfate clearances, in two groups of glucosuric pregnant women and in control subjects. In one group there was a reduction of both GFR and Tm_G, which they attributed to chronic renal disease. In the other there was a disproportionate rise in GFR over Tm_G, and the glucosuria was attributed to increase in the filtered load of glucose. Friedberg [65] measured GFR by means of inulin and calculated the Tm_G in pregnant subjects with and without glucosuria and in control subjects, and in contrast found neither a rise in mean GFR in the glucosuric subjects nor a significant difference in Tm_G.

In similar studies Christensen [38] found the renal threshold for glucose in pregnancy to be reduced to 155 ± 17 mg. per 100 ml., as opposed to 194 ± 6.5 mg. per 100 ml. in the nonpregnant state. The Tm_G was essentially the same in pregnant and control subjects and therefore he concluded that increase in filtration rate was the major factor in production of glucosuria.

Welsh and Sims [235] have measured inulin clearances and maximal tubular reabsorption of glucose in 29 pregnant women, 16 without glucosuria and 13 with glucosuria, and in 15 nonpregnant controls. The mean GFR was the same for the two groups of pregnant women. The mean Tm_G was significantly lower in the pregnant women with glucosuria (310 ± 18 mg. per minute) than in those without glucosuria (378 ± 18 mg. per minute) or in the controls (366 ± 16 mg. per minute). Since the glucosuric patients were not studied before or after pregnancy as well, it is not possible to say whether the Tm_G was actually lowered during the pregnancy, or whether glucosuria merely developed as a result of the increase in the filtered load in patients who initially had a lower Tm_G.

The data are plotted in Figure 32-2, in which regression lines of Tm_G on GFR corrected to standard body surface area for the three groups are drawn. It should be noted that there is a normal variation of Tm_G with GFR, as the slope of the regression lines of Tm_G on GFR is essentially the same in all groups. This relationship was noted originally by Smith [204] in his initial studies of Tm_G. The Tm_G in some glucosuric women

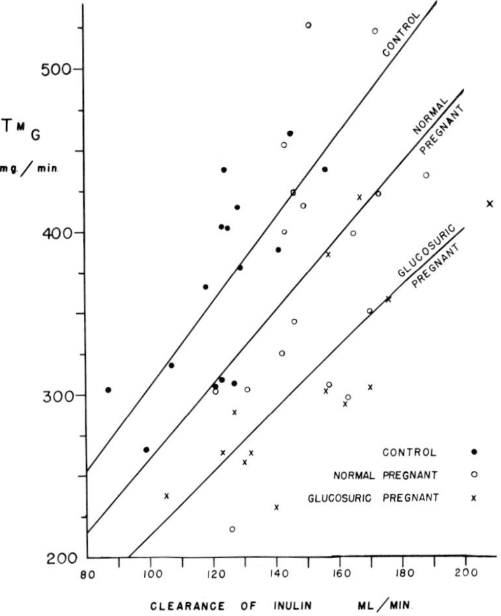

Figure 32-2. Regression lines of tubular maximum glucose reabsorption (Tm_G) on inulin clearance in normal women, normal pregnant women, and in glucosuric pregnant women, corrected to standard body surface area. (From Welsh and Sims [235].)

deceptively appears normal unless it is considered in relation to the GFR. The increased GFR without corresponding increase in Tm_G of the normal pregnant group is shown by the displacement to the right without significant change in the slope of the regression line of the normal pregnant group. The further displacement of the regression line of the glucosuric pregnant group reflects the lower Tm_G of this group when it is related to GFR. The data suggest that pregnancy increases the filtered load of glucose without producing an appreciable increase in the tubular capacity to reabsorb glucose, thus making all pregnant women more liable to develop glucosuria.

Reubi [170] made titration studies in patients with renal glucosuria in which the filtered load of glucose was progressively increased, and found that the disorder may be associated with both heterogeneous and homogeneous populations of nephrons, as indicated by the degree of splay of the curve as Tm_G is approached. Christensen's data [38] indicate no difference in the curves for pregnant and nonpregnant subjects, but recently Renschler and von Baeyer [169] have found a widening of the splay of the titration curve in 15 subjects, a high proportion of whom were glucosuric, and have concluded that reduced tubular reabsorption is the more important factor in producing the glucosuria. Serial studies starting prior to pregnancy, however, are needed to determine whether Tm_G is actually lowered during pregnancy.

The question is often raised as to whether glucosuria is not so ubiquitous in pregnancy as to be useless or misleading as a guide to detection of diabetes in pregnancy. Fine [63] has emphasized the frequency of glucosuria in pregnancy which he finds can be demonstrated by sensitive means in 70 per cent of pregnant women studied "around the clock." The Clinistix test, employing glucose oxidase, is unduly sensitive for use in pregnancy, detecting 10 to 100 mg. per 100 ml. of glucose, but has the advantage of specificity. The Clinitest, employing reduction of copper, is sensitive only to 150 mg. per 100 ml. In place of relying solely upon random checking for glucosuria, the stronger case can be made for testing with an abbreviated tolerance test all women at several intervals during pregnancy. If only a selected group are to be tested, the highest yield of diabetics will be from those with a positive family history of diabetes, or history of having delivered babies of large birth weight, or unexplained stillbirth. However, approximately one-fifth of patients with random glycosuria alone may be found to have gestational diabetes. Thus, Wright et al. [245] found latent diabetes in 13 per cent and asymptomatic diabetes in 6 per cent of 203 women who were glucosuric to Clinistix and Clinitest testing.

WATER AND SODIUM BALANCE IN NORMAL PREGNANCY

This subject has recently been reviewed by Hytten et al. [84], by Little [113], and by Chesley et al. [32].

During pregnancy there is an increase in blood volume of from 30 to 50 per cent, gradually reaching a peak by the twenty-eighth to thirty-fourth weeks, with a gradual decline as term is approached [94], and the pH of plasma increased, consistent with a respiratory alkalosis [113]. Plentl and Gray [160] have estimated by means of isotope dilution that the normal pregnant woman retains only the amount of sodium required by the conceptus and by the increased blood volume. The mean retention was 520 mEq. They also demonstrated retention of water in excess of sodium. In an extensive study by Hytten and his co-workers [84], it was shown that until the thirtieth week of pregnancy there is no water retention in excess of that required by the products of conception, the increased blood volume, and the reproductive organs. Later, however, a surplus of water, amounting at term to 1 to 2 liters, or as much as 5 liters in those with edema, is accumulated. Essentially the same changes have been described in total-body analyses of pregnant rats by Lichton [110, 111].

Whether some degree of edema in pregnancy is normal and physiologic has been a matter of debate for many years. In an extensive study by Thomson et al. [219] edema was found in 35 per cent of patients who remained normotensive, and the authors concluded that edema is physiologic and not of itself an ominous sign.

There has been much controversy over the question of whether restriction of intake of sodium is beneficial or harmful in pregnancy. The effects of variations in intake in normal and abnormal pregnancy are discussed in the section below on *Preeclampsia*. In this place it may be useful to review the factors in pregnancy which normally tend to retain sodium and those which promote natriuresis.

Factors Promoting Retention of Sodium. ESTROGENS. The role of estrogens in sodium and aldosterone metabolism is not entirely clear. Estradiol has been shown by Dignam et al. [53] to cause retention of sodium, and Little [113] has shown that this is more marked when hepatic inactivation is decreased in cirrhosis and in cardiac failure. On the other hand, Katz and Kappas [93] have suggested that an initial brief natriuresis in certain subjects may contribute to the increase in aldosterone secretion when estriol or estradiol is administered. The production of estrogen is increased in pregnancy, but not to a degree sufficient to increase aldosterone binding to plasma proteins; its possible effect upon reduction of hepatic metabolism of aldosterone is discussed by Tait and Little [216].

CORTISOL. Cortisol produces a net increase in the renal tubular reabsorption of sodium, with increased exchange of sodium for potassium. As noted above, there is evidence that free cortisol is increased in the plasma in pregnancy [145], but it is not certain whether other steroids compete for binding sites and blunt its physiologic action.

THE RENIN-ANGIOTENSIN SYSTEM AND ALDOSTERONE IN NORMAL PREGNANCY. It is well known that angiotensin II, formed from renin substrate (angiotensinogen) by the action of renin derived from the juxtaglomerular apparatus of the kidney, is a major factor controlling secretion of aldosterone. Plasma renin concentration has been found by Brown et al. [22] to be consistently elevated throughout pregnancy and for 24 hours or more following delivery. Helmer and Judson [77], however, have found values for renin activity in the normal range late in pregnancy. The same authors have found an increase in renin substrate (alpha-2 globulin) in normal pregnancy. Since the quantity of substrate in pregnancy is as high as in any known condition, approximately 30 per cent of the amount required to saturate the amount of enzyme normally present in plasma [202], this increase is consistent with the increased amount of angiotensin formed and may account for at least part of the increased renin activity. As Skinner et al. [202] have recently pointed out, it may be necessary to assay renin activity in the presence of added excess of substrate in order to measure accurately the quantity of enzyme present. It is probable that in pregnancy a portion of the increase in renin activity in the plasma is of extrarenal origin. An enzyme similar in activity to renin has been detected in human placenta by Hodari et al. [82] and others. It has been shown by Gross [74] that the pregnant and nonpregnant uterus of the rabbit contains a substance with renin-like activity. Talledo et al. [217] have found that in normal pregnancy, as in other conditions in which high renin activity is found, there is marked blunting of the pressor and renal effect of infusions of angiotensin II. They found that the same refractoriness to the renal, but not to the pressor response could be reproduced by administration of progesterone to normal nonpregnant women.

Aldosterone is secreted in very large amounts in normal pregnancy [231]. The concentration of free aldosterone in plasma is increased, since the hepatic blood flow and metabolic clearance rate (MCR) of aldosterone are unaltered in pregnancy [216] and since the MCR = secretion rate/plasma concentration. This increase is apparently provoked by the various natriuretic factors of pregnancy which are detailed below, particularly the spironolactone-like action of progesterone in competing with aldosterone at a renal tubular site. It is clear that aldosterone, in spite of this antagonism, continues to play a dynamic role in regulating sodium balance, since its secretion is responsive to variations in the intake of sodium [231]. Aldosterone is normally metabolized to two major metabolites, the 18-glucuronide and tetrahydroaldosterone (THA), which are physiologically inert. In pregnancy an alteration in aldosterone metabolism has been demonstrated by Tait and Little [215]. The splanchnic extraction of aldosterone is reduced, although the protein-binding of aldosterone in pregnancy is not increased. A larger proportion is excreted in pregnancy as the 18-glucuronide, and the increased formation appears to be in the splanchnic bed. THA is produced in the liver in nonpregnant subjects, but in pregnancy there may be an appreciable fetoplacental contribution.

ERECT POSTURE. As described above, the pregnant woman has considerable translocation of fluid to the lower part of the body when standing, even though increased capillary permeability cannot be demonstrated [87]. Assali et al. [6] have shown that quiet standing by pregnant women produced a greater fall in glomerular filtration rate and a greater increase in excretion of aldosterone than in nonpregnant subjects.

Factors Promoting Loss of Sodium. GLOMERULAR FILTRATION RATE. With the increase in the glomerular filtration rate in pregnancy, there is an increase of as much as 40 to 50 per cent in the amount of sodium presented to the renal tubules for reabsorption. An amount equal to five times the total body sodium is filtered per day. If tubular reabsorption of sodium were not proportionately increased, depletion of body sodium would lead to hypovolemia and increase in secretion of aldosterone.

PROGESTERONE. The secretion of progesterone by the placenta during the latter months of pregnancy is approximately 10 times that of the ovary during the luteal phase of the menstrual cycle, and the concentration of free progesterone in the plasma is increased [178]. It was suggested by Martin and Mills [122] that the spironolactone-like action of progesterone in antagonizing the renal tubular action of aldosterone may explain the increased secretion of aldosterone. Landau and Lugigihl [103] have shown progesterone to be natriuretic in nonpregnant subjects.

NATRIURETIC FACTOR. The evidence for a natriuretic factor or "third factor" which affects proximal tubular reabsorption of sodium in response to expansion of plasma volume has been discussed elsewhere in this book (pages 60, 249). To date conclusive demonstration of an assayable circulating factor has not been accomplished. However, some mechanism other than that involving change in filtration rate or aldosterone secretion apparently must be involved in the "escape" from the sodium-retaining effect of excess desoxycorticosterone or aldosterone in normal subjects. In the pregnant woman a third natriuretic mechanism or factor may be of considerable importance. Chesley and his associates [36] have shown that the normal pregnant woman is capable of excreting an average of 20 per cent of 400 mEq. of infused sodium within 20 minutes. Lindheimer and

Weston [112] have attempted to clarify the mechanism of natriuresis in pregnancy by capitalizing on the fact that the assumption of the supine position by a pregnant woman reduces the glomerular filtration rate. In pregnant subjects who were pretreated with mineralocorticoid and liberally infused with hypotonic saline solution, assumption of the supine position blunted natriuresis despite volume expansion and independent of changes in the amount of sodium filtered. Under conditions of maximal water diuresis, however, they found that there was a decrease in fractional reabsorption of filtrate at proximal tubular sites, suggesting a tubular readjustment independent of mineralocorticoid activity. There was also decrease in the fractional reabsorption of sodium at proximal nephron sites during volume expansion both before and after assumption of the supine position.

In summary, there are many factors, some of which are either strikingly increased in or are peculiar to pregnancy, which affect either the retention of or excretion of sodium. If any element in this precarious balance is abruptly altered, severe disturbance in electrolyte balance may result.

The Kidney in Pregnancy Complicated by Preeclampsia, Eclampsia, Hypertensive, or Renal Disease

In the following discussion a classification based upon that of the Chicago Lying-In Hospital [124] will be used. The categories have been extended, and additional categories added to include the disorders that must be considered in the differential diagnosis of the conditions which may simulate preeclampsia or which may lead to renal insufficiency in pregnancy. The use of the term *toxemia* has been avoided, and the term *preeclampsia* used whenever the specific entity with its characteristic renal pathology is indicated. We stand in need of a better term than "hypertensive disorders of pregnancy" to replace the by now archaic term toxemia, to cover the general group of hypertensive disorders. Preeclampsia is predominantly a disease of previously well primigravida in which hypertension and proteinuria, and usually edema, develop after the twentieth week of pregnancy. It is most commonly seen in those women between the ages of 15 and 29 and in those with twin pregnancies. It may appear before the twentieth week in those with hydatidiform mole. For detailed clinical description of the disorder, the reader is referred to current obstetric texts. A syndrome with the clinical features of preeclampsia and with its histologic renal lesion may be superimposed on or be a consequence of many of the conditions listed under the headings of hypertensive, renal, and genitourinary disorders. McCartney [125] has reviewed the dilemma presented by attempting to classify these disorders on clinical grounds. Rippmann [172] has entered a plea for a symptomatic classification which will permit grading of the gestoses of pregnancy in terms of severity.

- I. Hypertensive diseases peculiar to pregnancy (onset after 24 weeks and usually after 30 weeks)
  - A. Preeclampsia
    - 1. Mild
    - 2. Severe
  - B. Eclampsia
- II. Cardiac, vascular, renal diseases not peculiar to pregnancy (onset usually but not always before 24 weeks)
  - A. Hypertensive disease
    - 1. Essential hypertension
      - a. Mild
      - b. Severe
      - c. Malignant
      - d. With superimposed preeclampsia
    - 2. Coarctation of the aorta

   3. Unilateral renal arterial disease
   4. Primary hyperaldosteronism
   5. Pheochromocytoma
- B. Renal and genitourinary tract disease (any one of which may be associated with superimposed preeclampsia)
   1. Glomerulonephritis
      a. Acute
      b. Chronic
      c. Nephrotic syndrome
   2. Pyelonephritis
      a. Acute
      b. Chronic
   3. Asymptomatic bacteriuria
   4. Lupus erythematosus
      a. With glomerulitis
      b. With glomerulonephritis
   5. Scleroderma with renal involvement
   6. Periarteritis with renal involvement
   7. Acute renal failure
      a. Acute renal insufficiency
      b. Cortical necrosis
   8. Polycystic disease
- C. Diseases frequently associated with preeclampsia
   1. Diabetes mellitus (prediabetes, latent chemical, chemical, or overt diabetes)
      a. Without nephropathy
      b. With nephropathy
   2. Erythroblastosis fetalis

In the first edition of this book emphasis was placed in this chapter upon separating "true preeclampsia" from other disorders. As emphasized below, it appears that many diverse disorders may set in motion the chain of reactions producing the syndrome of preeclampsia, and that its features may be superimposed on a variety of diseases. It has been asked by Homer Smith with reference to hypertension whether the kidney is the culprit in the disease or its victim. During the past five years a mass of evidence has accumulated that in pregnancy the kidney is primarily the victim of a maternal disturbance that may be triggered in a variety of ways. Once victimized and injured, the kidney in turn contributes to the maternal disturbance, and a vicious cycle, which may culminate in the physiologic upheaval of eclampsia, is set in motion. Thus, to place the renal disorder in its true perspective, one must first consider the ways in which the maternal physiology may be disturbed. It is recognized in addition that there are both environmental and hereditary factors predisposing to the development of preeclampsia in pregnancy. In a study of daughters of patients with preeclampsia, using daughters-in-law as controls, Chesley et al. [33] have shown the importance of the latter, although dietary or environmental factors could not be excluded.

ROLE OF THE PLACENTA, UTERUS, AND FETUS IN THE ETIOLOGY OF PREECLAMPSIA

There is obstetric evidence that a viable placenta is essential to the development and perpetuation of preeclampsia, but that the fetus is not essential. There are several ways in which the placenta may be involved.

Ischemia. For many years attempts have been made with varying success to produce preeclampsia experimentally by compromising the uterine blood supply. Hodari [81] has reported that placing constricting Teflon bands about the uterine arteries of the dog before pregnancy leads predictably to a reversible syndrome of hypertension and proteinuria. This differs from human preeclampsia in that a striking hypernatremia develops and hypertension and proteinuria appear relatively earlier in pregnancy. It has not been shown that the renal lesion has the same characteristics as that of the human disorder. To my knowledge this important observation has not yet been confirmed in other laboratories. In later studies Hodari et al. [82] suggest that renin was produced either by the fetal kidney or by the placenta; in fact, in these studies, they showed that the placenta may indeed produce renin. Such a pressor mechanism, discussed in more detail below, would have obvious benefits to the mother by ensuring adequate uterine blood supply, in much the same way that the response to renal ischemia tends to restore renal blood flow. It has often been suggested that polyhydramnios, the primagravid state, or underlying arterial disease secondary to hypertension or diabetes predispose to preeclampsia by compromising uterine blood flow.

Robertson et al. [174] have contributed important studies of the basal arteries of the placental bed. In preeclampsia they find a distinctive vascular lesion consisting of fibrinoid necrosis and infiltration with foam and round cells. In essential hypertension there is hyperplastic arteriosclerosis more severe than would be expected in other organs in the nonpregnant patient with the same degree of hypertension. Purely on a morphologic basis they suggest in addition that there may be an immunologic component to the uterine lesions of preeclampsia.

Sophian [209] has long maintained that a uretero-renal vascular reflex provoked by distention of the uterus or placental ischemia leads to renal cortical ischemia and preeclampsia. This possibility has been given some support by the finding of Franklin and Winstone [64] that distention of the pregnant uterus of the rabbit leads to renal cortical ischemia and by that of Berger and Boucek [12] that experimental placental ischemia in the rabbit produced a syndrome resembling eclampsia. A pressor humoral factor was also demonstrated. In view of evidence cited below this factor may well be renin.

Maternal Rejection of the Placenta. In this era of organ transplantation, it still remains a remarkable and poorly understood, as well as fortunate, fact that the placenta and fetus are not more often rejected by the mother. There is accumulating evidence that the balance is a delicate and not always successful one. Simmons and Russell [197] have shown in mice that the trophoblast serves as both an anatomic and an immunologic barrier between mother and fetus. The fact that the placenta is accepted as a homograft is the more remarkable since it has been demonstrated by Dancis et al. [46], using production of runt disease in mice as an experimental model, that the placenta itself contains immunologically competent cells. A strain of guinea pigs which is susceptible to a spontaneous syndrome resembling preeclampsia has been shown by Rogers et al. [177] to have increased placental permeability to trypan blue. Langford et al. [106, 207] have produced hypertension and decreased renal renin content in pregnant, but not in nonpregnant, rats by injection of antiplacental serum; antikidney serum produced hypertension in both.

Using a passive hemagglutination reaction and Ouchterlony gel double diffusion technic, Wilner et al. [242] demonstrated antibodies against placenta in 40 per cent of 406 normal pregnant women, and against liver and kidney antigen in 24 per cent, but no increase in titer with successive pregnancies. They found a significant increase in patients with either primary or superimposed preeclampsia, but Riccioni and Turchetti [171] failed to confirm a significant increase. Using a more specific complement-fixing technic, however, Tomasi and Deftos [220] were unable to demonstrate antibodies against a variety of tissues in six normal pregnant women one month postpartum at a time when maximum titers against placenta might be expected. Serum complement (C′) titers are unchanged during the third trimester of pregnancy and in patients with clinical preeclampsia [163]. In diabetes mellitus and in erythroblastosis fetalis, both of which are associated with increased incidence of preeclampsia, Burstein et al. [26] have described proliferative vascular lesions of the placenta that bind fluorescent anti-insulin antibodies in diabetes and anti-Rh serum in erythroblastosis. The binding is specific, since it can be blocked by nonfluorescent antigen, and they suggest that in diabetes tissue-fixed antibodies react with exogenous or endogenous insulin. Aladjem [1] has described syncytial and stromal lesions of the placenta in gestational diabetes, the severity of which correlate with the fetal outcome. Such placental lesions may in turn affect its ability to inactivate pressor substances or may affect its production of steroids, with resulting effect upon maternal blood pressure and electrolyte balance. *In summary,* mechanisms are available for rejection of the placenta; whether they may play a role in initiating preeclampsia is discussed below.

RENIN-ANGIOTENSIN SYSTEM IN PREECLAMPSIA

The renin-angiotensin system and its effect upon aldosterone secretion in normal pregnancy has been discussed above. In 52 women with hypertensive pregnancy, Brown et al. [23] found renin activity within the range normal for pregnancy, except in one instance of hydatidiform mole and one of erythroblastosis. Helmer and Judson [77] found the concentration of renin substrate to be lower in preeclampsia, and this may reduce apparent renin activity, as emphasized by Skinner [202]. However, the sensitivity to infusion of angiotensin is greatly increased in hypertensive pregnancies [217], so the net physiologic effect may be greatly increased. Although renin may be of uterine or placental origin, Hodari et al. [82] found no increase in the amount of renin in placentas from hypertensive patients.

ROLE OF SEROTONIN AND CATECHOLAMINES AND OTHER PRESSOR AGENTS IN PREECLAMPSIA

Chesley [31] has recently reviewed the subject of vascular reactivity in normal and abnormal pregnancy. Senior et al. [190] have reported increased plasma concentrations of 5-hydroxytryptamine (serotonin) in pregnant women. The concentration was not further increased in hypertensive pregnancies, but significantly increased amounts were found in the placentas by biologic assay. This has been related by Sandler and Baldock [181] to monoamide oxidase (MAO) deficiency, and they have shown a reduced metabolism of 5-hydroxytryptamine, but not of tryptamine in preeclampsia. They suggest that placental ischemia resulting from the pressor agent further reduces the activity of the enzyme, establishing a vicious cycle. However, available evidence from the studies in Assali's laboratory [5] in ewes near term suggest that pressor agents do not cause uterine ischemia, since the uterine vasculature appears to respond like a passive conduit in which the flow of blood varies with the arterial perfusion pressure. In man, Dixon et al. [54a] have found that in preeclampsia the rate of clearance of radioactive sodium (^{24}Na) from the maternal placental blood lake is not enhanced when blood pressure is reduced by means of hydralazine. Injection of serotonin in laboratory animals produces renal lesions somewhat resembling those of preeclampsia, but what relevance, if any, this has to the disease in humans is uncertain.

Talledo et al. [217] have shown increased sensitivity to norepinephrine of preeclamptic women, but not of pregnant patients with essential hypertension. Raab et al. [166a] have shown an increased sensitivity to the pressor effect of epinephrine in pregnant women with edema or proteinuria during the current pregnancy or in those who subsequently develop hypertension. Three of 11 with marked pressor responses later developed eclampsia. There has been a long and so far fruitless search for a "toxic" or pressor substance released from the uterus in preeclampsia. The search has been punctuated by positive reports which have lacked confirmation, and later studies have failed to demonstrate such a substance [70]. Barnes and Kumar [10] have suggested that instead of producing such a substance, ischemia of the uterus and placenta may diminish their ability to detoxify pressor agents already in circulation. Support is given to this concept by DeMaria and See's observation [48] as well as that of Sandler and Baldock [181] that there is less MAO assayable in the placentas from preeclamptic pregnancies, and that the content of norepinephrine and of dihydroxyphenylalanine (DOPA) is increased. The MAO is concentrated in the syncytial layers of the placenta, and since it is the syncytiotrophoblast layer that disintegrates in preeclampsia, a vicious cycle may be set up.

DISTURBANCE OF THE COAGULATORY MECHANISM IN PREECLAMPSIA

Perhaps the most significant development in the field of hypertensive disorders of pregnancy in the past decade has been the realization of the widespread nature of disorders of the coagulation mechanism in abnormal pregnancy. The demonstration of fibrin deposits in even the early renal lesions of preeclampsia, as described below when the pathology of preeclampsia is considered, gives this added importance.

The normal mechanism of fibrinolysis and fibrinolytic activity has been reviewed by Sherry et al. [192]. Through the action of activated fibrinolysin or plasmin, split products of lower molecular weight may be formed from fibrin. Fibrinogen concentration normally increases throughout pregnancy and there is a decrease in fibrinolytic activity [15].

Since 1953 McKay and his associates [130] have been accumulating evidence that the more catastrophic forms of renal damage and damage to other organs, as in acute tubular necrosis, acute cortical necrosis, and severe eclampsia, are the result of the following sequence, which is similar to the generalized Shwartzman reaction in laboratory animals: There is initial degeneration of the labyrynthine and giant cell trophoblasts of the placenta. Focal deposits of fibrin form in the maternal spaces, and there is extension of parauterine thrombosis. A clot-promoting agent escapes into the circulation and produces intravascular thrombosis, with microemboli disseminating to lungs and other organs. Thrombocytopenia is a common finding, and McKay et al. [131] have found the adhesiveness of platelets to be increased in preeclampsia and attribute this to slow disseminated intravascular coagulation. There may be fibrin accumulation and extension of thrombosis in glomerular and other renal vessels, and essentially all organs of the body may be affected. As early as 1956 Magara and his group [120] noted that injection of a placental extract with pressor activity also provoked a Shwartzman reaction in pregnant rabbits and produced lesions resembling those of preeclampsia. In man the syndrome is most commonly associated with septicemia from infection with gram-negative organisms. Premature placental separation, with release of thromboplastin into the general circulation may produce a similar clinical situation. Jaameri et al. [84a] have demonstrated that there is 20 times as much trophoblastic tissue in uterine venous blood from preeclamptic as from normal pregnant subjects. This material is presumably trapped in the lungs, where it undergoes lysis, releasing thromboplastin and other substances into the systemic circulation. Such a mechanism, as originally suggested by Schmorl [185] could well initiate intravascular coagulation. Tissue damage and escape of trophoblasts into the circulation have also been mentioned as possible triggering mechanisms for intravascular coagulation. In pregnant animals the reaction may be provoked by injection of bacterial endotoxin [244], by infusion of thrombin [121], or by a diet low in tocopherol and containing distillates of oxidized cod liver oil [132].

There are also suggestions that an antigen-antibody reaction may predispose to hypercoagulability. Robbins and Stetson [173] have shown that either injection of antigen into an immunized animal or injection of antigen-antibody complex shortens coagulation time in the rabbit. Coagulation time of separated plasma is not affected, suggesting that the alteration may be in the platelets. Immune complexes formed in the circulation accelerate fibrin formation with deposition of fibrin in the glomeruli, and in vitro such complexes accelerate clotting, probably again through an effect upon platelets [225]. Some years ago Seegal and Loeb [186] suggested that antiplacental antigens might be a cause of preeclampsia. The evidence for and against placental rejection in pregnancy is reviewed above. Later, Steblay [212] demonstrated that antihuman placenta antibodies react with the same portion of the glomerulus as antihuman-basement-membrane antibody. Both react in an identical way with placenta. The immunofluorescent studies described below in relation to the pathology of the kidney in preeclampsia essentially exclude the possibility that antirenal-placental antibodies directly cause the renal damage in preeclampsia. It is more likely that such a mechanism may be involved in nephritis complicating pregnancy, or particularly in recurrent nephrotic syndrome of pregnancy. The work of Burstein et al. [26], also detailed below, suggests that in erythroblastosis and in diabetes an immune reaction may be associated with placental vascular damage.

ROLE OF WATER AND ELECTROLYTE RETENTION IN PREECLAMPSIA

The factors affecting sodium and water metabolism in normal pregnancy have been reviewed in a previous section. Again the reader is referred to the reviews of Hytten and Thomson [83], Little [113], and Chesley [32], and to that of Pirani and Pollak [157].

Evidence has accumulated that restriction of sodium may be deleterious in pregnancy, and that tolerance for high intake of sodium is high. Several studies have shown that a normal pregnant woman can excrete infused loads of sodium in excess of 400 mEq. as rapidly as the nonpregnant [36], but that the natriuresis is blunted in the supine position [112]. In a study of 28 women in a controlled environment, Gray et al. [73] were able only with difficulty to increase the intake of sodium during the third trimester. Those taking diets higher in sodium gained slightly more weight and retained more water, but their increase in aldosterone secretory rates was less than expected for the stage of pregnancy, and the net retention of exchangeable sodium was also less. That restriction of sodium may be deleterious is suggested by the findings of Wardlaw and Pike [230] in pregnant rats given varying amounts of sodium in their diet. Despite an increase in the percentage of sodium retained, those given a diet low in sodium had a reduction of muscle sodium and hyponatremia, and apparently did not have the expected increase in blood volume. Both pregnancy and decreasing intake of sodium were associated with increase in the width of the zona glomerulosa of the adrenal gland, and in all but the pregnant animals given the lowest intake of sodium, there was increased granulation of the juxtaglomerular apparatus. In this latter group renin secretion exceeding the rate of production was suspected.

It is well established that sodium is retained in greater amounts in preeclampsia than in normal pregnancy [113]. Water is retained in excess of sodium in preeclampsia [113] as in the latter weeks of normal pregnancy [84]. Paradoxically, it appears that in early preeclampsia there may be tolerance of a high intake of sodium. Dieckmann [50] found that 84 to 100 mEq. of sodium added to the usual diet of 100 women under suspicion of preeclampsia gave only slight increase in weight; in fact, 20 per cent lost weight. Robinson [175] carried out a field study of 1039 pregnant patients instructed to maintain a high sodium intake and of an equal number of controls. There was an apparent reduction in complications of pregnancy in the experimental group. However, any significant reduction in the frequency of preeclampsia should be sought among the primiparas; these were limited in number to 290 experimental subjects and controls, and the difference was not statistically significant. The experiments of Pike et al. [156], cited above, give support to the idea that ample sodium is not damaging and possibly may be beneficial in pregnancy and that restriction may be harmful. Giving a diet moderately low in sodium to pregnant rats reduced plasma and tissue sodium and produced small fetuses and small litters. The depleted dams exhibited renal sodium wasting under conditions in which conservation would be expected. On the other hand, very high intake had no adverse effect.

Over a relatively short period of 8 to 10 days, Bower [20] found no correlation between the clinical course or outcome in patients with mild preeclampsia and variations in intake of sodium from 2 to 25 gm. per day. In a similarly short study Mengert and Tacchi [134] found no different effect in preeclampsia of 10 gm. as opposed to 1 gm. of salt per day. However, Redd et al. [168] have reported that, when ambulatory, women with preeclampsia have a greater retention of sodium than do normal women, which may explain in part the benefit of bed rest in this condition. The above cases, as well as Robinson's, were mainly mild preeclampsia. In studying the response to salt loading of women with graded degrees of preeclampsia, Zuspan and Bell [248] found that women with moderate as opposed to mild degrees of preeclampsia tolerated additional sodium poorly. This is to be expected, particularly in patients with definitely impaired renal function. In patients who have been nephrectomized and are treated by hemodialysis, maintaining sodium balance is critical to prevention of hypertension, and the same must apply to pregnant women with definitely impaired renal function.

Previous studies have indicated that patients with essential hypertension in pregnancy also retain sodium abnormally. This is in contrast to the finding of an exaggerated natriuresis seen in nonpregnant hypertensive subjects similarly challenged with infusions of sodium. Sarles et al. [183] have pointed out that in these earlier studies the patients were not in positive sodium balance prior to the infusions and also that diagnoses were not firmly established. They have studied the response to infusion of 430 mEq. of sodium chloride to patients in whom the diagnoses were established by means of renal biopsy and adequate follow-up studies and who were maintained in positive sodium balance for at least seven days prior to testing. Those with preeclampsia reached a lower maximum rate of secretion of sodium following the infusion than did normal pregnant subjects, while the patients with essential hypertension had a striking natriuresis (Fig. 32-3). The patients in the two categories could be clearly separated. Patients with glomerulonephritis without severe impairment of renal function responded normally. Subsequent studies of patients with preeclampsia, which was superimposed on essential hypertension in two patients, on proliferative glomerulonephritis in one, and diabetic glomerulosclerosis in another, demonstrated the diminished natriuresis seen in pure preeclampsia. There were no complications from the relatively large intravenous infusions of sodium, perhaps because patients with GFR's below 60 ml. per minute were excluded. It seems likely that patients with nephritis and severely reduced filtration rates would respond as did those with preeclampsia.

ROLE OF ADRENAL STEROIDS IN PREECLAMPSIA

Administration of mineralocorticoid and excess sodium to animals may produce a syndrome somewhat resembling preeclampsia in man [4, 100]. There is no significant difference between the secretion rate of aldosterone in early preeclampsia and the elevated values seen in normal pregnancy [223, 232]. In severe preeclampsia there is a reduction in secretion to the range seen in nonpregnant women [232]. The physiologic effect may well be increased,

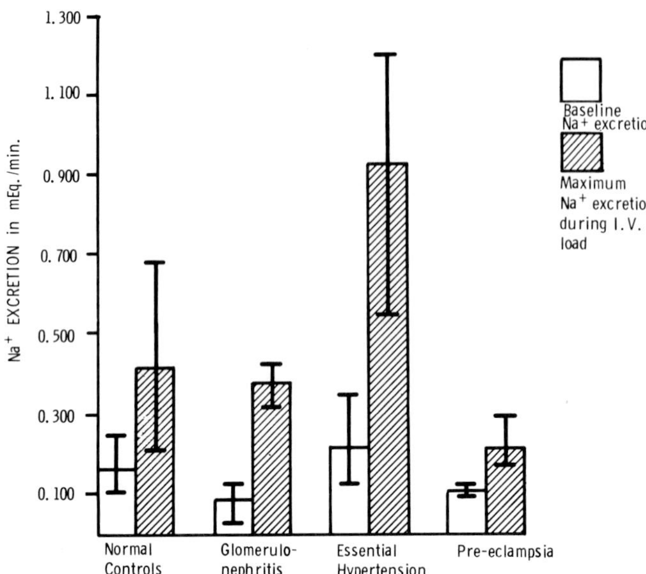

Figure 32-3. Baseline and maximal urinary sodium excretion during the intravenous infusion of 1000 ml. of 2.5 per cent sodium chloride over a one-hour period during the last trimester of pregnancy in five normal pregnant control subjects, four patients with chronic smoldering proliferative glomerulonephritis, eight patients with essential hypertension, and nine with preeclampsia established by renal biopsy. The height of the bars represents the mean and the vertical lines the observed range. (From Sarles et al. [183].)

however, as a result of diminished hepatic inactivation of the steroid, or other change in the formation of the metabolites of aldosterone. A decrease in the production of progesterone would diminish its spironolactone-like antagonism to the renal action of aldosterone. Kumar [99], however, found no measurable reduction of the content of progesterone in placentas of patients with preeclampsia. There is much to suggest that aldosterone plays only a facilitative role in preeclampsia. An aldosterone-producing adenoma has been tolerated during pregnancy without production of preeclampsia. In one instance the adenoma produced hypertension, but not preeclampsia [19] and in another instance [45] the symptoms were ameliorated during pregnancy. At the other extreme, preeclampsia has been reported in a patient with bilateral adrenalectomy [138].

ROLE OF ANTIDIURETIC HORMONE IN PREECLAMPSIA

The activity of antidiuretic hormone, as measured by bioassay in rats, in serum [66] and in urine [247] from normal pregnant patients, is not increased. The activity is not increased in mild preeclampsia, although increase in antidiuretic substances has been reported in severe preeclampsia. There is, however, no evidence to date that this is a primary factor in the production of the edema. In fact, several cases of preeclampsia have been reported in patients with diabetes insipidus [16].

ROLE OF THE KIDNEY IN PREECLAMPSIA

With the above background one may then consider whether the kidney is the culprit or the victim in preeclampsia.

Renal Function. The many studies of renal function in preeclampsia and eclampsia over the past 30 years have been reviewed by Smith [205], Pollak and Nettles [161], and Chesley [32]. Because of the formidable technical difficulties, no study is entirely satisfactory. Some investigators have resorted to induction of osmotic diuresis to maintain adequate urine flow [7a]. All studies have presumably been made with the patient in the supine position, which may have lowered the renal blood flow. In only two studies have diagnoses been established by renal biopsy, that of McCartney et al. [127] and that of Sarles et al. [183]. The results of selected major studies are summarized in Table 32-1.

Table 32-1. Glomerular Filtration Rate and Renal Plasma Flow in Eclampsia and Preeclampsia

Authors	Number of Cases	Filtration Rate (ml./min.)	Renal Plasma Flow (ml./min.)	Method and Remarks
Studies without biopsy-confirmed diagnoses:				
Corcoran & Page, 1941 [43a]	28	100 (60–145)	—	Inulin, Diodrast, & phenol red
Wellen et al., 1942 [233a]	13	105 (50–155)	612 (250–825)	Inulin & Diodrast
Bucht & Werkö, 1953 [25]	10 early[a] 18 late[a]	105 ± 7[b] 65 ± 7	498 ± 69 320 ± 69	Inulin & PAH 22 normals[c] Early C_{IN} 170 & C_{PAH} 800[a] Late C_{IN} 156 & C_{PAH} 571[a]
Assali et al., 1953 [7b]	9	77	577	Mannitol & PAH 9 normals C_M 109 and C_{PAH} 699
Chesley et al., 1958 [36]	13	103 ± 27.2	—	Inulin 11 normals: C_{IN} 145 ± 22.6 12 hypertensive: C_{IN} 136 ± 26.7
Studies with diagnoses confirmed by renal biopsy:				
McCartney et al., 1964 [127]	6	90 ± 29	—	Inulin at 36–40 weeks 7 normals: 133 ± 20
Sarles et al., 1968 [183]	9	120 (92–140)	560 (460–620)	Inulin & PAH last trimester

[a] Early = early pregnancy; late = late pregnancy.
[b] Standard error of the mean.
[c] Normal pregnant women (controls) by same authors.

Glomerular Filtration Rate. In comparison with values normal for the particular stage of pregnancy, the glomerular filtration rate (Table 32-1) is reduced in preeclampsia, including those cases in which the diagnoses were established by renal biopsy. In the small series of Sarles [183] there is no overlap of values with those of the control pregnant subjects, and in that of McCartney there is little overlap, although a few subjects have relatively normal filtration.

Effective Renal Plasma Flow. The most definitive of the earliest studies is that of Bucht and Werkö [25] in which comparison was made with normal pregnant women in a comparable stage of pregnancy. In many of the reported studies, however, the urine flows of less than 0.5 ml. per minute suggest that the clearances of PAH may have been spuriously lowered. In the study by Sarles et al. [183] of nine subjects with preeclampsia the range of plasma flow was below that of five normal pregnant subjects (Table 32-1).

Filtration Fraction. In only a small number of studies is it possible to calculate the filtration fraction (or the ratio of inulin to PAH clearance, representing the proportion of the plasma which forms the glomerular filtrate). Assali et al. [7a] and others [205] found a lower filtration fraction in their patients with apparent preeclampsia as opposed to those with a history of antecedent hypertension. In Sarles's study [183], in which patients with milder preeclampsia may have been selected, no such differential was noted.

Renal Concentrating Ability. In the study by McCartney et al. [127] of 22 patients with acute hypertension in pregnancy, in whom the etiology was determined by renal biopsy, the patients with the preeclamptic renal lesion were sharply differentiated with respect to one parameter. The mean value for the quantity of free water extracted per unit of glomerular filtration rate, $\frac{T^c_m H_2O}{C_{IN}} \times 100$, was 5.3 ± 1.1 S.D. ml. per minute in normal pregnant subjects and those with simple excessive gain in weight. It was reduced to 2.7 ± 0.9 ml. per minute in gravidas with nephrosclerosis, and to 2.7 ± 0.3 ml. per minute in those with chronic glomerulonephritis, but was increased to 7.5 ± 1.3 ml. per minute in those with preeclampsia. Thus, within the group of hypertensive patients there were no values within the range of those found in the preeclamptic patients. Unfortunately, the more readily measured parameters of concentrating power failed to show this sharp differential, and the technic of measurement is cumbersome, so that the procedure cannot be readily applied to clinical problems.

Proteinuria. It seems possible that delineating the pattern of proteinuria in the acute hypertensive disorders of pregnancy may ultimately aid in their differentiation, as has been the case in differentiating the nephrotic syndromes. A study of urine proteins by paper electrophoresis [27] and the study by McEwan [129] by immunoelectrophoresis are difficult to evaluate since the diagnoses are based only on clinical impressions.

Renal Pathology and Pathogenesis of Preeclampsia. The subject has been reviewed by Pirani [158]. Attention was first drawn by Löhlein [115], in 1918, to the glomerulus as the site of the major lesion in preeclampsia. A host of studies by light microscopy since then have given the erroneous impression that the characteristic lesion involved thickening of the basement membrane, although studies by modern light microscopy show that this is not so (Figs. 32-4, 32-5). It was not until percutaneous renal biopsy and electron microscopy were applied to the problem that the nature of the lesion and its specificity were clarified. One of the first such studies was that of Spargo, McCartney, and Winemiller in 1959 [210]. They noted a narrowing of the capillary lumen due to an increase in the cytoplasm of the endothelial cells, and such intracellular changes as droplet formation, vacuolization, formation of cytoplasmic strands, and an increase in particulate structures. This finding they termed *glomerular endotheliosis,* an entity different from other known lesions associated with the nephrotic syndrome. There was no thickening of the basement membrane and essentially no changes in epithelial cells or their foot processes. The typical renal lesion is seen in Figure 32-6. Pollak and Nettles [161] confirmed these findings and noted in addition enlargement and increase in granularity of the juxtaglomerular cells. Pirani [158] and Mautner [123] and their co-workers have further clarified the ultrastructure of the lesion. The extensive and serial studies of Altchek et al. [3] have shown an increase in mesangial cells and their matrix and the presence of deposits of several types between the endothelial cells and the basement membrane. They have quantitated the increase in granularity in the juxtaglomerular cells originally noted by Pollak and Nettles [161]. Altchek [2] has demonstrated that the typical glomerular lesions may appear with minimal, if any, clinical symptoms and may persist during pregnancy even though the clinical signs are ameliorated by vigorous therapy. Contrary to the suggestion of Dieckmann et al. [51], he found that the lesions believed to be pathog-

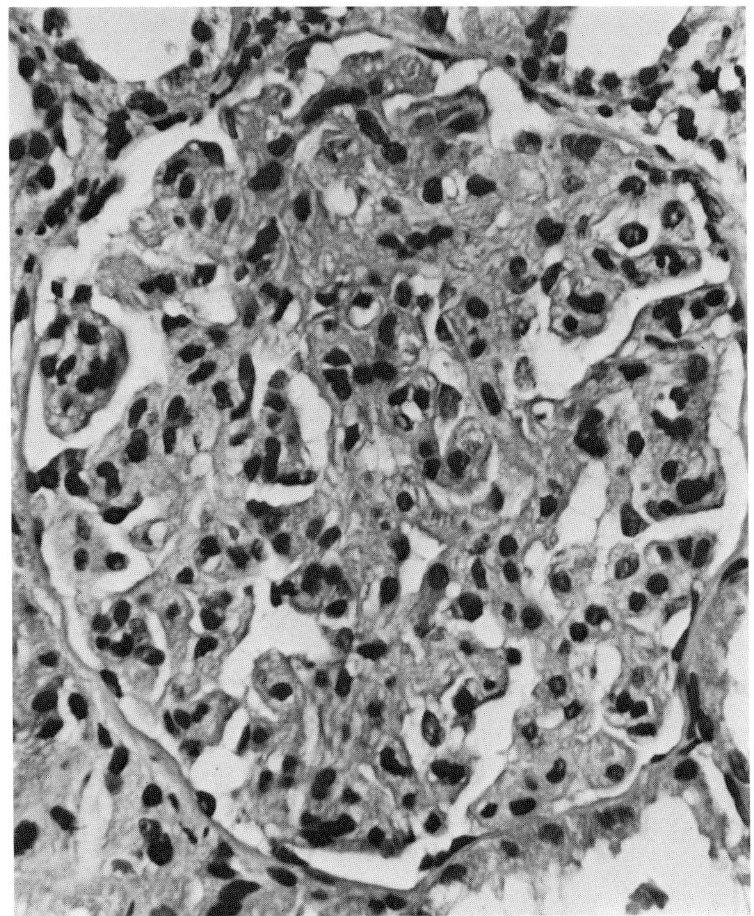

Figure 32-4. In preeclampsia the glomeruli are enlarged and bloodless due to swelling of intracapillary cells (endothelial and mesangial) which results in complete narrowing of capillary lumina. Hematoxylin and eosin. ×500, before 12% reduction. (Provided by Dr. C. L. Pirani and Dr. S. Madrigal.)

nomonic for preeclampsia developed in those patients with essential hypertension who developed the classic triad of symptoms of preeclampsia. Faith and Trump [60] have presented evidence that the glomerular endothelium apparently has phagocytic properties and that mesangial cells may migrate to form part of the capillary wall. Renal tubular cells and small arteries and arterioles show minor changes [158].

In fulminating eclampsia deposits of fibrin have been noted in the capillary loops, but their deposition has been regarded as a terminal event. Of great importance is the demonstration by Vassalli [226] and Morris [137] and their associates, using an immunofluorescent technic, that fibrin aggregates are present within the glomerular capillary endothelial cells and occasionally along the basement membrane in mild and moderate preeclampsia. Complement and immunoglobulins, on the other hand, were not demonstrable, whereas they may be readily demonstrated in lupus erythematosus and usually in glomerulonephritis. This does not, however, rule out other unrecognized immune reaction remote from the kidney as a prime or contributory cause. Such strong localization of fibrin in endothelial cells in the absence of deposition of immunoglobulins and complement along the basement membrane has been seen only in preeclampsia [128, 225], and the deposition may be

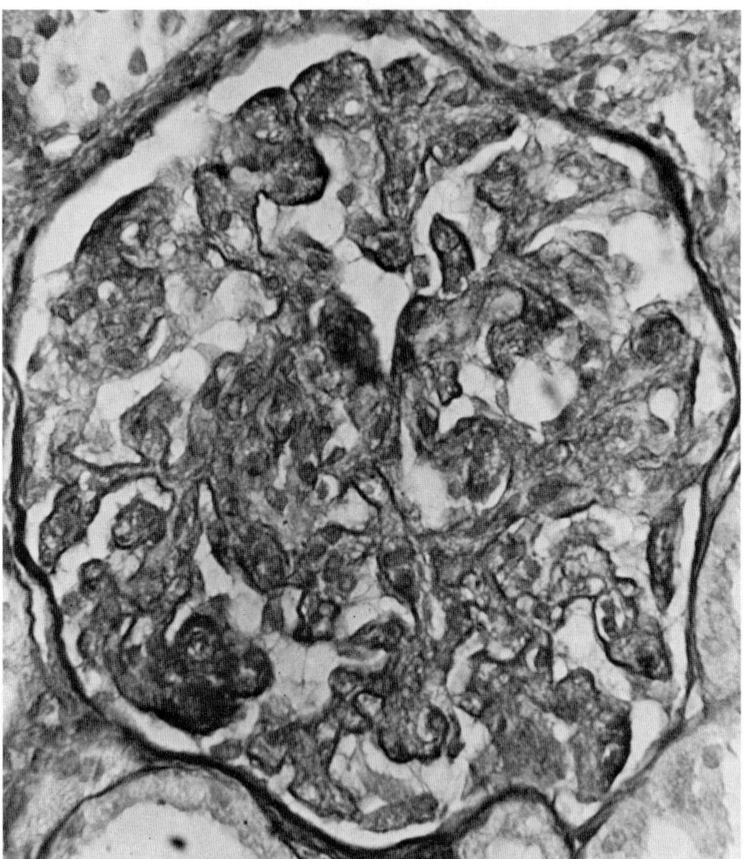

Figure 32-5. Glomerulus in preeclampsia. The Alcian blue–PAS stain reveals a moderate, diffuse increase in mesangial matrix with a fibrillar pattern. The peripheral basement membrane is not thickened. ×500, before 12% reduction. (Provided by Dr. V. E. Pollak.)

found before symptoms appear. Such fibrin deposition, demonstrated by fluorescent antifibrinogen serum, is shown in Figure 32-7, which is reprinted from the studies by Morris et al. [137]. They have found that infusion of thromboplastin in rabbits produced renal lesions similar to those in preeclampsia [227]. They suggest that the renal lesions are initiated by the formation in the circulation of fibrinogen derivatives by slow intravascular coagulation. Fibrin removed from the circulation by cells of the reticuloendothelial system is readily degraded, but while renal endothelial cells may be capable of phagocytosis, as suggested by Faith and Trump [60], they are more susceptible to damage. Morris et al. [137] found no gross evidence of a defect in coagulation in their patients, but cite the reduction in the number of circulating platelets in preeclampsia that has been noted by others as evidence of such a disturbance.

Ferris et al. [62a] have recently completed a clinical, biochemical, and histologic study of the preeclampsia-like syndrome that develops when pregnant sheep near term given a diet low in protein are exercised vigorously. By electron microscopy the renal lesion closely resembles that of preeclampsia in women. It will be of great value to know whether this lesion is associated with intracellular deposition of fibrin. Likewise it will be important to know whether similar deposition occurs in the preeclampsia-like syndrome resulting from uterine ischemia produced by the technic of Hodari [81].

Altered Reaction of the Kidney to Immune

column of Table 32-2 are listed a number of changes or derangements seen in normal pregnancy, which are normally balanced by other derangements but which, operating singly, could lead to a disease state. If any one of a variety of factors, as listed in the second column of Table 32-2, disturbs the equilibrium, disorders in three major areas may follow: (1) the mechanisms for coagulation of the blood, leading to formation of circulating fibrin aggregates which in turn result in glomerular capillary endothelial swelling; (2) decreased inactivation of pressor amines; and (3) retention of electrolytes and water secondary to the renal damage, to decreased inactivation of aldosterone, and possibly to decrease in the plasma progesterone, which normally opposes its action. Disproportionate increase in plasma volume in excess of that seen in normal pregnancy then increases the reactivity of the vascular tree to pressor agents, in much the same way that administration of mineralocorticoids with sodium increases responsiveness to catecholamines [166]. Like an atomic pile which has become "critical" and produces a self-sustaining reaction, each one of these three factors can aggravate the others, so that a truly explosive physiologic situation may develop. The resulting disorders are listed in the third column of Table 32-2.

DIAGNOSIS OF PREECLAMPSIA

The accuracy of the diagnosis of preeclampsia on the basis of clinical signs and routine laboratory aids is notoriously poor. Pollak and Nettles [161] found that the clinical diagnosis was correct in only 26 out of 35 patients studied by renal biopsy. In a series of patients studied by McCartney [125], all of whom met the criteria for diagnosis of "toxemia of pregnancy" of the American Committee for Maternal Welfare, 43 per cent of the primigravida fulfilling the criteria for preeclampsia had underlying chronic renal disease on biopsy. Similarly, 21 per cent of multigravida fulfilling the clinical criteria for hypertensive vascular disease with superimposed toxemia had chronic renal disease. Such a diagnostic score admittedly provides an uncertain basis for clinical management and an inadequate basis for clinical investigation. If a disorder of the coagulation mechanism ultimately proves to be a consistent finding in preeclampsia, whether primary or secondary, its early detection would be of value. Progressively simpler technics for measuring fibrin split products in the serum are being developed (135, 212a). A rapid method for measuring fibrinogen split-products in the serum has recently been described [135]; it remains to be learned whether increase in such split products may serve to indicate the development of glomerular capillary endotheliosis and preeclampsia.

Measurement of serum uric acid as a valuable aid in the diagnosis of preeclampsia is discussed in the following section. A further aid in the detection of preeclampsia or impaired renal function is the serum creatinine or blood urea. As emphasized above in considering the kidney in normal pregnancy, the normal range of these excretory products in the plasma is markedly reduced due to the increase in filtration rate. At the present time the only certain means of diagnosis is by means of renal biopsy. But in any given case the possible benefits of biopsy must be weighed against the increased hazard of this procedure in pregnancy. Schewitz et al. [184] have emphasized the relatively high frequency of serious bleeding following biopsy, either percutaneous or open.

A valuable clinical sign is spasm of the retinal arterioles, which Pollak and Nettles [161] found in 30 of 35 patients with histologically proved preeclampsia, and in only 2 of 10 with hypertension and arteriolar sclerosis.

The concentration of *uric acid* in the serum has long been considered an aid in the diagnosis and the evaluation of the prognosis in preeclampsia, for reasons which now appear to be well founded. Since the original observation by Stander and Cadden [211], many

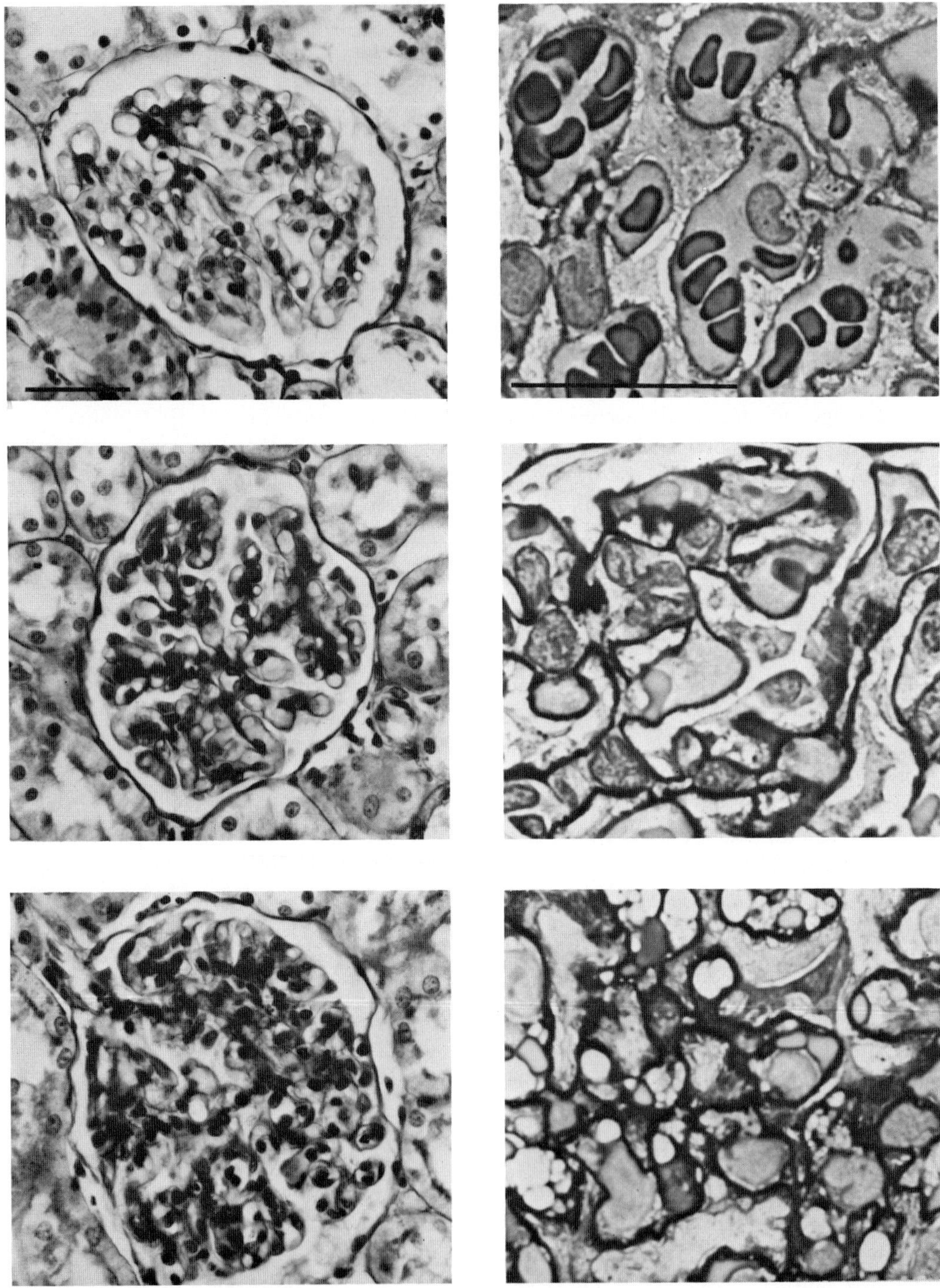

Figure 32-8. The glomerular reaction to antikidney gamma globulin and its modification in pregnancy. Glomeruli embedded in paraffin and stained with periodic acid–Schiff (PAS) stain are shown on the left, and

Table 32-2. Factors Which May Contribute to the Syndrome of Preeclampsia

Initial Equilibrium	Intercurrent Factors	Result
Uterus and placenta increasing blood flow ↗ placental MAO ↗ placental progesterone	Compromise of uterine & placental blood supply due to: Mechanical effects Vascular disease Possible immunologic rejection of placenta	Uterine ischemia degeneration of trophoblasts ↘ MAO & ↘ inactivation of pressor amines ↗ placental & fetal renin (not proved) ↘ progesterone
Cardiovascular ↗ blood volume Renin-angiotensin-adrenal ↗ renin and renin substrate Increased angiotensin II & angiotensinase ↗ aldosterone secretory rate	Immune reaction associated with: Erythroblastosis fetalis Diabetes mellitus Collagen disease	↘ Renin substrate normal but possible inappropriate renin activity ↗ Sensitivity to angiotensin II & pressor agents
Coagulatory mechanisms ↘ fibrinolytic activity ↗ platelet agglutination ↗ coagulability	Intercurrent infection Antecedent hypertensive vascular disease	Intravascular coagulation Fibrin aggregates giving disseminated circulatory damage
Orthostatic effects ↗ translocation of fluid when upright		
Kidney ↗ renal blood flow ↗ glomerular filtration	Antecedent primary renal disease Urinary tract infection	Glomerular capillary endotheliosis ↘ RBF and ↘ GFR ↗ JGA hypertrophy *Proteinuria*
Net Balance Decreased vascular reactivity	—	Sodium retention & hypervolemia. *Edema* ↗ vascular reactivity & *hypertension*

thin sections fixed in osmium tetroxide and embedded in araldite and stained with methenamine–silver nitrate on the right. Scale = 104. The *upper* photographs are of the glomeruli of a pregnant rat given rabbit gamma globulin on the tenth day of pregnancy and killed on the eighteenth day as a control. The *middle* photographs are of the glomerulus of a nonpregnant rat eight days after injection of antikidney rabbit gamma globulin (AKRGG). The findings are typical of the Masugi type of immune nephrosis in the rat with slight increase of PAS-positive material in the mesangial region, increase in mesangial cells, and thickening of the basement membrane. The *lower* photographs are of the glomeruli of a pregnant rat given AKRGG in similar manner on the tenth day of pregnancy and killed on the eighteenth day. Almost all the capillary loops are occluded by vacuoles in the endothelial cells and by increase in the endothelial cells. The basement membrane is also slightly thickened. Electron microscopic studies were confirmatory of the predominantly endothelial reaction of the pregnant animal to antikidney gamma globulin. (From Shirai et al. [193].)

studies have demonstrated a close correlation between the severity of preeclampsia and the increase in serum uric acid. Values ranging from 5.0 mg. per 100 ml. in mild preeclampsia to 7.5 mg. in eclampsia have been reported by Lancet and Fisher [102]. Seitchik et al. [189] have shown by measuring the turnover rate of ^{15}N-labeled urate that the rate of production of urate is not increased under these conditions. Seitchik studies [188] and those of Chesley and Williams [37] suggested that net tubular reabsorption of urate was increased. Since urate may be actively secreted, and there is much to suggest that, the defect may lie in decreased secretion.

It has long been known that lactic acid is increased in the serum in eclampsia. In 1935 Quick [165] suggested that the increased circulating lactate competes with urate for excretion. Handler [75] has demonstrated that in normal pregnancy infusions of lactate depress uric acid secretion. In 14 patients with mild preeclampsia he found that there was an insignificant increase in blood lactate and a slight decrease from that of control subjects in the ratio of clearance of urate to that of creatinine, but an insignificant increase in serum uric acid. In eclampsia there was insignificant negative correlation between the degree of hyperuricemia and the ratio of uric acid clearance to that of endogenous creatinine. It appears that increased lactate may be one factor, but not necessarily the only factor, affecting tubular secretion of urate in pregnancy.

The role of lactic acid is of particular importance since there is considerable evidence [75] that in preeclampsia and eclampsia the uterus, placenta, and fetus are major sources of lactic acid. This in turn may be a consequence of the reduction in uterine blood flow which Assali et al. [7] had observed in toxemic prognancies. Consistent with this, Kuhlbäck and Widholm [98] have found the serum uric acid to be an aid in evaluating fetal prognosis following preeclampsia.

The first study in which exact histologic diagnosis by percutaneous renal biopsy was correlated with the degree of hyperuricemia was that of Pollak and Nettles [161]. Patients with uncomplicated vascular disease did not have hyperuricemia. Thirty-three patients with preeclampsia had a rise in serum urate from a mean of 3.57 ± 0.69 (S.D.) to 6.43 ± 1.74 mg. per 100 ml. When the cases were grouped on

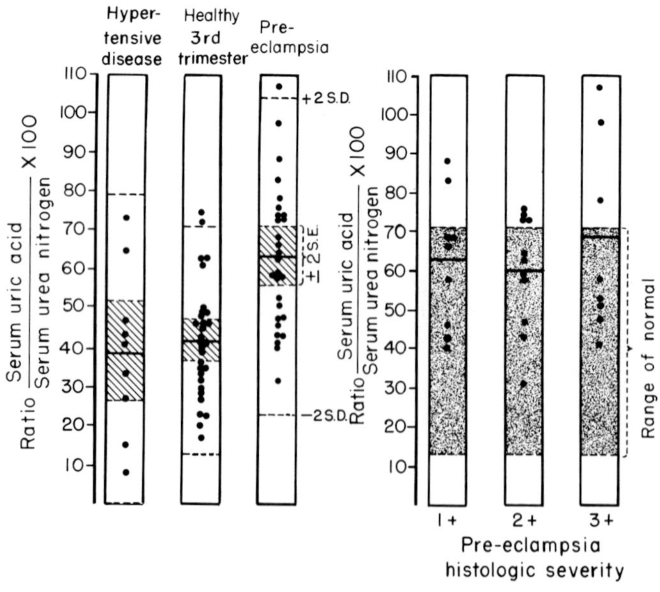

Figure 32-9. Serum ratios of uric acid to urea nitrogen in (*left*) hypertensive women, healthy women, and women with preeclampsia (all in the last trimester of pregnancy), and (*right*) in cases of preeclampsia graded according to the severity of the lesions in renal biopsy specimens. (From Pollak and Nettles [161].)

the basis of the histologic findings into three categories of increasing severity, the means were 5.53 ± 1.74 mg., 6.33 ± 1.37 mg., and 7.76 ± 1.54 mg. per 100 ml., respectively. The mean value even in those patients with slight histologic changes is significantly different from the normal pregnant mean. Even when allowance is made for the lowered range of normal values in pregnancy, the correlation between blood urea or nonprotein nitrogen and the presence or severity of preeclampsia is not as good. The ratio of uric acid to urea nitrogen also showed a poor correlation (Fig. 32-9). This provides further evidence that serum uric acid is a sensitive diagnostic, and possibly prognostic, clinical index of preeclampsia.

It should be borne in mind that metabolites of salicylates may interfere with the chemical determination of uric acid when uricase is not used for specificity. Also, the ubiquitous thiazide diuretics may produce hyperuricemia.

PREVENTION AND TREATMENT OF PREECLAMPSIA

For reasons that are not well understood, the frequency of preeclampsia is decreasing. Restriction of dietary sodium in the early stages of pregnancy appears not to be a critical factor, for the reasons discussed above. Gray [72] has also recently pointed out the futility and possible hazards of the use of thiazide diuretics as a prophylaxis against preeclampsia. The renal lesions may progress in spite of depletion of sodium [2], and sodium or potassium depletion may add a prerenal factor to renal and circulatory insufficiency. In some areas of the country severe electrolyte depletion with hypovolemia as a result of overzealous use of potent diuretics has represented a more frequent threat to pregnant patients than severe preeclampsia. This may be increasingly true if even more potent diuretics such as ethacrynic acid or furosemide are accepted for use in pregnancy. However, later in the course of the disease excessive intake of sodium may exaggerate the hypertension, as emphasized above.

If intravascular formation of fibrin aggregates plays an important role in the development of the renal lesion in preeclampsia and in the pathology of eclampsia, could treatment be directed specifically against this process? The anticoagulant warfarin in high dosage has been shown by McCluskey et al. [128] to prevent the fibrin accumulation, swelling, and proliferation of intracapillary cells in experimental nephritis. Also Müller-Berghaus and McKay [140] have shown that alpha-adrenergic blockade prevents the Shwartzman reaction and localization of renal thrombi following injection of endotoxin in pregnant rats. Some very preliminary studies reporting the use of heparin with favorable effects in severe preeclampsia were reported by Page [149] and Maeck and Zilliacus [119]. In certain cases recently reviewed by Brain et al. [21] in which intravascular hemolysis and thrombocytopenia have been evident, treatment with heparin has been successful. With the evidence at hand it is not possible to say whether treatment with anticoagulants would be effective in altering the underlying pathology in early preeclampsia, and whether the benefits would justify the evident risks. Carefully controlled studies in an adequate number of histologically diagnosed patients are needed to answer this question. Such studies would have to include serial renal functional and histologic studies with demonstration of glomerular fibrin deposition by the fluorescent-antibody technic. If a sensitive method were available to detect excessive intravascular coagulation early in the course of pregnancy, particularly in those patients with high frequency of toxemia, it is possible that prophylactic treatment might be justified.

Man is one of the few species developing preeclampsia, and is also one of the few that habitually walks erect on his hind legs. In view of the marked effects of posture on renal function and sodium balance in pregnant women, it is logical to give a trial of complete bed rest as a means of mobilizing edema fluid.

It is often more effective than the use of diuretics. While a pregnant patient remains ambulatory, postural translocation of fluid may stimulate the mechanisms for retention of sodium. There may be edema, but also a functional hypovolemia, and use of diuretics may aggravate this hypovolemia and produce relative sodium depletion. On the other hand, because of mechanical factors it is important that the pregnant woman avoid a supine position, particularly if there is polyhydramnios. Finally, it should be mentioned that the most effective and permanent treatment is delivery of the fetus and placenta.

LATE SEQUELAE OF PREECLAMPSIA AND ECLAMPSIA

It has been difficult to evaluate the immediate and remote consequences of preeclampsia or eclampsia because of uncertainty as to whether there may have been antecedent renal disease, and because control groups have not been comparable with respect to racial and economic background. These difficulties have been considered by Pollak and Nettles [161], Pirani and Pollak [157], and Epstein [57].

Many studies have emphasized that there is a familial frequency of eclampsia. Perhaps the best controlled study is that of Chesley and his co-workers [33], already referred to, in which it was found that the frequency of preeclamptic episodes in daughters of mothers who had had eclampsia in their first pregnancy was significantly greater than that in their daughters-in-law.

It now appears that the renal lesion of preeclampsia may not be as reversible as was once thought [157, 161]. Altchek et al. [3] state that five months after the acute episode patches of increased mesangial matrix can be detected histologically. In an important prospective study Dennis et al. [49] found in 118 serial biopsies in 61 patients with preeclampsia persistent glomerular changes in 37 per cent six months postpartum and in 13 per cent one to four years postpartum. Arteriolar lesions were found in 47 and 20 per cent, respectively. Forty-eight per cent of the preeclamptic patients and 62 per cent of eclamptic patients had recurrence of hypertension, and fixed hypertension developed in 18 to 19 per cent. In the same series of patients Dennis et al. [49] state that there are two types of renal lesion in preeclampsia, one predominately glomerular, which tends to revert to normal, and the other involving arteriolar changes, which persist and are correlated with an increased frequency of recurrent and permanent hypertension. Since the incidence of hypertensive sequelae is higher than in other reported series, one wonders, however, whether there was a higher proportion of Negroes among the patients, since they are known to be more prone to hypertensive disease, and whether there were any unique dietary factors. These findings are in sharp contrast to the findings in the fifth periodic review of the series of eclamptic patients at the Margaret Hague Maternity Hospital from 1931 to 1951 by Chesley et al. [34]. White primiparous eclamptic women had no increase in remote over predicted deaths and no increase in observed over expected frequency of hypertension. Only 25 per cent of the deaths were cardiovascular in origin, but multiparous patients with eclampsia had 2.6 times the expected mortality. In approximately one-third of the pregnancies following eclampsia the women were hypertensive, but this tended to be mild. The prognosis was again worse for multipara than for primipara. The striking 10-fold increase over the expected frequency of diabetes in this series of patients who had eclampsia as multipara is discussed below.

Epstein [57] has made a carefully controlled retrospective study of the frequency of hypertension following preeclampsia, diagnosed on clinical grounds. The results are at variance with those of Chesley et al. [34]. The incidence of hypertension after an average of 15 years in those with a history of preeclampsia was 40 per cent, or three to five times greater than in the control subjects. Obesity was excluded as a variable. Since there was no increase in late hypertension in siblings of the patients with hypertensive pregnancies, it was concluded that the episodes of "toxemia" were etiologic. However, since patients with hypertension, edema, and proteinuria were considered as a single group and since half were multipara at the time of their hypertensive pregnancies, it is unlikely on the basis of clinical evaluation alone that all represented uncomplicated preeclampsia. Also, since the control subjects were parous women who had escaped hypertension during their pregnancies, it is possible that some then-latent hypertensive patients were excluded from the control series. Final definitive answers will have to await the completion of prospective studies with precise initial diagnosis of preeclampsia.

Diseases Not Peculiar to Pregnancy

HYPERTENSIVE DISEASE

Essential Hypertension. Classically, essential hypertension in pregnancy is noted before the twenty-fourth week and is less associated with edema and proteinuria, retinal sheen, and retinal vasospasm. There is no hyperuricemia as in advanced preeclampsia. The hypertension may persist between pregnancies, and there may be a family history of hypertension. At best, however, the diagnosis is one of exclusion. Earlier studies [205] have indicated that the filtration fraction is increased and that the glomerular filtration rate is higher in patients with clinical diagnosis of hypertensive vascular disease as opposed to those with preeclampsia.

As described above in relation to retention of sodium in preeclampsia, the patient with essential hypertension in pregnancy is set apart from the one with preeclampsia in the ability to respond with striking natriuresis to intravenous administration of sodium. Sarles et al. [183] have shown that to demonstrate this difference, patients must be maintained with a positive balance of sodium prior to testing.

When pregnancy occurs with a background of antecedent hypertension, the kidney either may appear normal histologically or may have varying degrees of arteriolar change [161]. It was the original conclusion of Dieckmann et al. [51] that when hypertension, proteinuria, and edema developed during the last 14 weeks of pregnancy in a patient with renal vascular disease, it represented an exacerbation of the disease rather than that of superimposed preeclampsia. As noted above, however, Altchek [2] has found in such cases the renal lesions which are believed to be specific for preeclampsia, and McCartney [126] has reported in multigravida fulfilling clinical criteria for essential hypertension with superimposed preeclampsia normal renal histology in 55 per cent, chronic renal disease in 25 per cent, and the lesions characteristic of preeclampsia in 20 per cent.

Coarctation and Hypoplasia of the Aorta. One might expect in the light of Hodari's experiments [81], in which a preeclampsia-like syndrome was produced in animals by placing Teflon bands about the uterine vessels prior to pregnancy, that coarctation of the aorta would predispose to preeclampsia. As in other forms of hypertension, however, there may be a lowering of blood pressure during pregnancy, and, as pointed out by Shanahan et al. [191] preeclampsia has not been reported. In reviewing the numerous later reports of pregnancy associated with coarctation of the aorta, the authors found cases with various complications, but none in which a definite diagnosis of preeclampsia was established [117]. Apparently adequate hypertrophy of the collateral circulation is possible.

This is not true, however, in the case of hypoplasia of the aorta. Clemetson [41] has reported 10 obstetric cases with early and severe preeclampsia and early intrauterine fetal death in whom the findings on aortography suggested hypoplasia. Gordon and McKay [71] report a similar case with hypoplasia of the aorta found at operation. The possible benefit of presacral neurectomy, carried out on this patient and five of Clemetson's patients, is difficult to evaluate. Pregnancy in association with aortic hypoplasia provides a natural and confirmatory counterpart to Hodari's experiments described above with reference to the role of ischemia in preeclampsia.

Unilateral Renal Arterial Disease. Under appropriate conditions constriction of the renal artery may produce a syndrome of severe hypertension somewhat resembling preeclampsia in pregnant dogs and rabbits [54]. Under other conditions, however, such constriction in animals may have no effect or may even lower blood pressure in early pregnancy [43, 151]. Palmer [151a] reports one illuminating instance of a woman with calcified hydronephrotic kidney who had two hypertensive pregnancies with partial subsidence of hypertension between pregnancies. Nephrectomy early in a third pregnancy was followed by complete remission of hypertension. Landesman et al. [104] have reported constricting renal arterial lesions in nine women with antecedent hypertensive pregnancies, and estimate the frequency of such lesions as occurring in between 5 and 10 per cent of all severely hypertensive pregnancies. Diagnosis can be made with safety by percutaneous transfemoral aortography by the technic of Seldinger in the immediate postpartum period. This procedure should be a part of the postpartum study of patients with recurrent hypertension in pregnancy, rapidly progressive hypertension, hypertension with superimposed preeclampsia, or disparity in the size of the two kidneys.

Hyperaldosteronism. Hyperaldosteronism is a rare cause of hypertensive pregnancy. Boucher and Mason [19] have reported the case of a woman with severe hypertension during a fourth pregnancy which was associated with polyuria and weakness aggravated by thiazide diuretics. A left adrenal adenoma was found on surgical exploration.

Pheochromocytoma. Pheochromocytoma in pregnancy is rare, but when it occurs there is a mortality of approximately 50 per cent. Only about half the patients have been correctly diagnosed [28, 47].

RENAL DISEASE

Acute Glomerulonephritis. There is no evidence for an increased frequency of complications of pregnancy in patients with healed acute nephritis [89]. Patients with a clinical history and findings suggesting acute nephritis during pregnancy have been reported [218]. In Wilson's [243] three cases there was early fetal loss. There is some suggestion in the series of Rauramo et al. [167] that there is an increased frequency of complications of pregnancy and prematurity in patients pregnant within three years following acute glomerulonephritis, although the intervals following apparent complete healing are not specified. It seems reasonable to postpone pregnancy for at least a year after complete healing has been demonstrated.

Chronic Glomerulonephritis. The studies of Wellen et al. [234] and of Werkö and Bucht [236] suggest that the trophic factors of pregnancy may actually increase renal function in damaged kidneys. The available studies have been critically reviewed by Oken [147] and MacKay [118], and in general it can be said that if the only symptom of renal disease is proteinuria, the pregnancy may have no adverse effect on mother or child. On the other hand, if there is hypertension as well, an exacerbation of the renal insufficiency or development of superimposed preeclampsia may be expected. If, in addition, the concentration of blood urea nitrogen is increased, particularly if it is above 28 mg. per 100 ml., the likelihood of fetal loss or of serious progression of disease in the mother is very great and pregnancy may be contraindicated. It should be borne in mind that the BUN is normally reduced in pregnancy and at best is a poor index of early impairment of renal function. A complete study of such a patient should include serial measurement of endogenous creatinine clearance, quantitation of the excretion of protein in the urine, careful microscopic examination of the urine, assessment of anemia, and pyelography when feasible.

Severe azotemia does not absolutely preclude successful completion of pregnancy. Herwig et al. [78] have reported a case in which such a patient was treated by hemodialysis throughout pregnancy and was delivered of a viable infant. As emphasized below in the section on bacteriuria, it is important that superinfection be excluded in patients with glomerulonephritis.

Nephrotic Syndrome in Pregnancy. The nephrotic syndrome constitutes a constellation of symptoms and signs — namely, hypoproteinemia, proteinuria, edema, with or without hypertension, or hypercholesterolemia.

The specific causes such as lupus erythematosus, diabetes mellitus, and renal amyloidosis must be excluded, as well as the more rare causes of the syndrome. It is apparent that any renal disease may occur coincidentally with pregnancy. In the patients in whom a specific etiology can be excluded, the findings on renal biopsy are usually typical of membranous glomerulonephritis. A rare form of nephrosis is the nephrotic syndrome of pregnancy, described in more detail by Schreiner elsewhere in this volume (page 570.) In this syndrome proteinuria and edema recur with each pregnancy, only to remit without sequelae in the intervals between. It is suggested, but not proved, that this may represent a reaction to some antigen associated with the products of conception.

Oken [147], who has summarized the findings in the many cases of nephrosis reported in the literature to 1966, points out that relative infertility and advice against pregnancy eliminates from pregnancy many of the patients who might represent poor risks. In general, both mother and child have weathered pregnancy well in all series that have been reported [86, 146, 187], since renal function is usually little impaired and may even be above normal. In one instance improvement in symptoms was noted during pregnancy [152]. As in chronic nephritis, when hypertension or azotemia are present, there is less likelihood of successful outcome. Particularly in an adult, the nephrotic syndrome may carry a poor long-term prognosis, and this outlook is not altered by pregnancy. Again, superimposed urinary infection should be watched for and appropriately treated. Treatment with hydroxycorticoids in the dosage usual for this condition has been well tolerated during pregnancy.

Pyelonephritis, Acute and Chronic. In 1937 Peters [153] wrote "Attention might well be diverted from preconceived notions of the nature of toxemias to a more exact descriptive analysis of these conditions and their relation to analogous diseases in the nonpregnant. . . . it is distinctly worthwhile to pay more attention in history and examination to infectious processes." This comment was prompted by a retrospective study of 320 patients with toxemia of pregnancy, in 41 of whom evidence of pyelonephritis was found. Many factors may predispose the pregnant patient to pyelonephritis, although studies are not available which show an unusual prevalence over comparable nonpregnant subjects. These include the physiologic dilatation of the uterus and renal pelvis with both hypertrophy and hypotonia. The volume of bladder urine, however, is unaltered [92]. There may be an endocrine factor predisposing to infection in early pregnancy, since, as Kass has noted [92], significant bacteriuria may develop before the anatomic changes are established. The renal glucosuria of pregnancy or glucosuria in the diabetic patients may also predispose to infection. Finally, potassium deficiency from hyperemesis or from kaluretic diuretics may contribute to development of pyelonephritis, as

Muehrcke [139] has emphasized. Pyelonephritis in pregnancy may be silent and yet significant and should be suspected when proteinuria is found without hypertension or retinal changes of preeclampsia.

The exact relationship of pyelonephritis and bacteriuria to hypertensive disease of pregnancy remains uncertain. Stuart et al. [213] and Norden and Kilpatrick [143] have found a significant correlation between bacteriuria and hypertensive disease, but the results of other studies are conflicting [238]. Kincaid-Smith [95] could not demonstrate that eradication of bacteriuria affected the frequency of hypertensive disease in their series of bacteriuric patients. She attributes this to the underlying renal disease, since she has demonstrated a much higher incidence of radiologic abnormalities among her Australian patients with bacteriuria [96].

The diagnosis of pyelonephritis in pregnancy is usually based upon recognition of characteristic symptoms and examination and culture of the urine. However, as Kincaid-Smith has emphasized [96], if there are more than two recurrences of bacteriuria after courses of treatment, pyelography with appropriate shielding should be carried out, since calculi or obstructive lesions amenable to correction may be detected. Otherwise pyelography should be postponed until six to eight weeks after delivery when the physiologic changes of the urinary tract have returned to normal.

Treatment of pyelonephritis in pregnancy follows the principles outlined in Chapter 18, with the important additional consideration that antibiotic agents must be selected so as to avoid toxicity to the fetus or hepatic toxicity to the mother. These limitations are discussed at the end of the following section.

Bacteriuria. The opportunities in obstetrics for effective preventive medicine have been greatly increased by the recognition that bacteriuria is an infection which may have important consequences. Kass [91] emphasized the relationship between asymptomatic bacteriuria and subsequent pyelonephritis and showed that treatment was effective in its prevention. Critical evaluations of the many studies of the relationship between bacteriuria and complications of pregnancy have been published by Norden and Kass [142], by Whalley [238], and by Kincaid-Smith [96]. The reported frequency of bacteriuria in pregnancy in the most reliable studies ranges between 4 and 7 per cent [142]. The incidence is affected by age, parity, and socioeconomic status. The sickle cell trait increases the incidence in Negro women [239]. Norden and Kass [142] estimate that in populations with low income the rates of bacteriuria increase from about 2 per cent in primigravida under age 21 to 8 to 10 per cent in multipara over 35 years of age. As noted below, the incidence in patients with diabetes is considerably higher than in nondiabetic women. The detection of significant bacteriuria and the probable site of infection have been described in Chapter 18.

BACTERIURIA IN ASSOCIATION WITH KNOWN RENAL DISEASE. It is doubly important to exclude bacteriuria in patients with known renal disease, such as chronic nephritis and diabetic intercapillary glomerulosclerosis, since such patients may be more vulnerable to ascending infection than normal subjects. In experimental nephrosis in rats Shirai et al. [193] have shown that such increased susceptibility can be demonstrated. Schreiner (Chapter 16) has pointed out the same susceptibility in man, and the series of Pollack and Nettles [161] includes a pregnant patient with glomerulonephritis and superimposed pyelonephritis. Superinfection should be suspected when the course of the disease accelerates.

Unfortunately, while spontaneous cure of bacteriuria certainly does occur, it is not possible to predict which patients will be cured and which will undergo crippling illness. Kincaid-Smith [96], in her series in Australia, found that at least 25 per cent had infection persisting for 0.5 to 12 months following pregnancy, 20 to 30 per cent had bacteriuria persisting for years following intermittent treatment, and about one-third had persistent symptomatic or recurrent urinary tract infection.

RELATION OF BACTERIURIA TO PYELONEPHRITIS. While the incidence of pyelonephritis developing in the course of pregnancy in untreated bacteriuric women is difficult to estimate [142], it is undeniable that detection of bacteriuria delineates the patients at risk. The evidence is equally strong that adequate treatment of bacteriuric patients discovered at the first prenatal visit will prevent 75 to 85 per cent of all prenatal pyelonephritis [142]. An average of about 1 per cent of women who do not have bacteriuria on the initial examination will develop overt disease.

A relationship between bacteriuria and prematurity was emphasized by Kass [92]. This is a matter of great potential importance, since prematurity accounts for 60 per cent of fetal deaths. A host of subsequent studies, some employing inadequate technics or too few patients for statistical significance, have given discordant results. However, Kincaid-Smith [96] has taken nine of the larger studies and analyzed the results statistically as a single group. The increase in frequency of prematurity was found to be highly significant ($p < 0.001$). In the large Australian series, a high incidence of radiologic abnormalities was found, and Kincaid-Smith [96] suggests that the underlying renal disease rather than the bacteriuria itself may be responsible for the high frequency of prematurity. So far, it has not been statistically proved that treatment of the bacteriuria per se reduces the rate of prematurity, nor is it clear which women among the bacteriurics are at greatest risk or for what reason. In Little's series in England [114], prematurity was more frequent in those with infection difficult to eradicate.

TREATMENT OF PYELONEPHRITIS AND BACTERIURIA IN PREGNANCY. There are special hazards in the treatment of urinary infection in pregnancy involving a risk of injury to the patient or the fetus. These have been reviewed recently by Weinstein and Dalton [233]. Thus, streptomycin may lead to eighth nerve damage in the fetus. Long-acting sulfonamides used near term may contribute to kernicterus in the infant. Pregnant women are peculiarly susceptible to severe hepatic toxicity from tetracyclines, particularly when there is renal insufficiency. In general, the sulfonamides are the drugs of choice for initial treatment, and later, if necessary, nitrofurantoin or ampicillin are recommended. Kincaid-Smith [96] has emphasized that ampicillin should be given in dosage of at least 2 gm. per day. In view of the risks of antibiotic treatment in pregnancy and also the risk of masking underlying renal disease, it appears preferable, as Williams et al. [241] and Kincaid-Smith [96] have suggested, to give short courses of treatment in conjunction with clinical and bacteriologic follow-up studies. If there is more than one recurrence, intravenous pyelography should be carried out.

In summary, there are areas of conflicting evidence regarding the exact relationship of bacteriuria to complications of pregnancy, and further large well-controlled studies are required to answer the important questions that have been raised. However, it is already clear that detection of bacteriuria indicates the patients at the greatest risk. The association between bacteriuria and later development of pyelonephritis is well established, and treatment is effective in largely preventing this important complication. There is a higher prevalence of patients with underlying renal disease of urologic abnormalities in the group with bacteriuria, particularly with infections that are resistant to treatment. There may be a direct or indirect relationship to development of preeclampsia, hypertensive disease, and prematurity. Thus, it is fair to say that the detection and appropriate treatment of bacteriuria in pregnancy is a mandatory component of good obstetric practice.

Lupus Nephritis. Lupus erythematosus should be suspected particularly in women with a history of frequent spontaneous abortions, unexplained proteinuria, nephrotic syndrome, or falsely positive serology. Approximately two-thirds of the patients with disseminated lupus have renal involvement. Its occurrence in pregnancy has been reviewed by Murray [141] and by Oken [147]. Pollak et al. [162] have demonstrated that there are two histologic forms of lupus nephritis: (1) glomerulitis, in which the pathology is mild and limited to the glomerulus; and (2) glomerulonephritis, in which involvement is more severe, and there are tubular and interstitial lesions as well. In contrast to the glomerular capillary endotheliosis of preeclampsia, in which fibrin aggregates but not gamma globulin or complement can be demonstrated, DNA antigen-antibody complexes can be demonstrated in glomerular deposits, together with immunoglobulins and complement and also with fibrinogen in variable amounts [97]. Since the condition is both potentially serious and may be amenable to treatment, renal biopsy to establish the diagnosis and the histologic severity is clearly indicated. Garstein et al. [67] have studied 33 pregnancies in 21 patients with lupus nephritis, and in 17, renal biopsies were performed. Four patients with histologically proved severe glomerulonephritis died during pregnancy. There was a threefold increase in the statistical risk of exacerbation during the first half of pregnancy over that prior to pregnancy, but during the latter half the risk was not statistically greater. During the 8 weeks of the postpartum period the risk was increased eightfold over that in subsequent weeks. The fetal loss was approximately 30 per cent, and this appeared to be independent of the effect of therapy on the mother. As in the case of chronic nephritis, normotensive patients may tolerate pregnancy well provided renal function is adequate and they are adequately treated. The pregnant patients tolerated corticosteroids in the dosage usually given to nonpregnant patients. In periods of greatest risk, such as the immediate postpartum period, increased amounts of steroid may be required. In view of the high fetal risk, however, the possibility of fetal damage from high dosage of steroid, and the increased risk of exacerbation of a potentially fatal illness, therapeutic abortion is to be considered in all but mild cases readily controlled.

Scleroderma. Scleroderma with renal involvement has been reported by Fear [62] as a rare cause of the syndrome of preeclampsia.

Periarteritis Nodosum. Periarteritis nodosum may closely simulate severe preeclampsia or eclampsia. Five instances of this rare and to date uniformly fatal complication of pregnancy have been reported by Siegler and Spain [196].

Acute Renal Failure. ACUTE RENAL INSUFFICIENCY. Acute renal insufficiency, often associated with acute tubular necrosis, is one of the most unfortunate lesions associated with pregnancy and is one to which the pregnant woman is peculiarly susceptible. This subject has been reviewed in detail by Ober et al. [144], and by Smith et al. [206]. The causes which are peculiar to pregnancy form an impressive list:

1. *Circulatory collapse* in some form underlies and is an essential component of most episodes of acute renal insufficiency. Early in pregnancy this may be caused by severe electrolyte depletion resulting from hyperemesis gravidarum. In such patients Ober et al. [144] have noted the distal renal tubular lesions characteristic of potassium depletion. Circulatory collapse and shock may of course follow hemorrhage from a variety of obstetric complications or disasters, as well as from amniotic fluid embolism.

Depletion of sodium with hypovolemia resulting from misguided use of diuretic agents may contribute to acute renal insufficiency by increasing susceptibility to damage from other insults, such as intravascular hemolysis. Whereas severe preeclampsia was once the more common medical emergency in pregnancy, it now appears that sodium depletion from strenuous diuresis with increasingly potent agents resulting in circulatory insufficiency and prerenal insufficiency is seen more frequently. In dogs a sizable infusion of hemolyzed cells may be given with impunity provided hydration is adequate [69]. However, with antecedent dehydration the same insult results in renal damage.

2. *Hemolytic episodes.* In addition to the factors seen in nonpregnant subjects, abortifacients and pelvic infection with *Clostridium welchii* may contribute to hemolysis in pregnancy.

3. *Infection.* Severe septicemias of endometrial or renal origin may lead to acute renal failure, particularly when associated with circulatory collapse.

4. *Severe preeclampsia or eclampsia,* particularly when complicated by any of the above, may lead to acute renal insufficiency. Not infrequently the cumulative action of a combination of sedative and hypotensive agents leads to severe circulatory collapse and renal ischemia. In this case the resulting tubular necrosis may be a product as much of the therpay as of the underlying renal lesion or preeclampsia.

5. *Disturbance of coagulation mechanisms* in preeclampsia has been discussed above. It is apparent that the various factors that may trigger such a disturbance are operative to varying degrees in the circumstances which lead to development of acute renal insufficiency. These may be formation of intravascular thrombi which further compromise the circulation of the kidney and other organs. When consumptive coagulopathy can be demonstrated, heparinization is indicated.

6. *Unexplained irreversible postpartum renal failure* associated with cardiomyopathy developing two to five weeks after delivery in four patients has recently been described by Robson et al. [176]. All were multipara, delivered at home, and had had pregnancies normal except for borderline hypertension in three and minimal proteinuria in one. A unique and uniform renal lesion included focal glomerular necrosis and arteriolar vascular changes and, on electron microscopy, a thick and irregular rarefied layer between basement membrane and capillary endothelial cells. An adverse reaction to oxytocic drugs could not be excluded.

ACUTE CORTICAL NECROSIS. A majority of the foregoing causes result in acute renal insufficiency which is potentially reversible [144]. A more ominous variant of acute renal failure, however, is acute cortical necrosis. This is most frequently associated with circulatory collapse following the hemorrhage of abruptio placentae. Here there is strong evidence that intravascular coagulation and the Shwartzman reaction play a major role [130]. Lee [107] has produced the lesion experimentally in rabbits by immunologic means combined with blockade of the reticuloendothelial system, and suggests that there may be an immunologic basis to production of cortical necrosis by bacterial endotoxin. The striking cortical distribution of the necrosis suggests local impairment or redistribution of renal circulation, although the evidence for this in man has been controversial. Kupic and Abrams [101] have recently reviewed this evidence, and have shown by renal angiography that in dogs subjected to hemorrhagic shock there is reduced cortical perfusion and sustained medullary perfusion.

The *diagnosis* of acute tubular necrosis in obstetric oliguria or anuria is made on clinical evidence. Renal biopsy is not indicated, since the findings could not be expected to modify initial treatment. If severe oliguria persists and cortical necrosis is suspected, biopsy may be justified for establishing prognosis and planning subsequent management. Even so, the lesions may be patchy and the findings may be misleading.

The *prophylaxis and clinical management* of acute renal failure with few exceptions differs little from that in nonpregnant patients. When there is evidence of acute or chronic disseminated intravascular coagulation in association with an obstetric catastrophe, the underlying disorder should be treated when possible. The therapeutic considerations in this difficult situation, which may involve both increased coagulation and increased bleeding, have recently been reviewed by Verstraete and Vermylen [228]. As Scott [185a] has pointed out, "giving fibrinogen in the consumptive phase of a disorder of coagulation is akin to attempting to rebuild a house on fire rather than summon the fire-brigade." One might add that it is tossing lumber into the flames as well. Verstraete and Vermylen [228] have reported good success in treating 18 women with the acute defibrination syndrome with simultaneous administration of fibrinogen (4 to 6 gm.), whole blood, and heparin (25 mg. — 2500 units) intravenously, usually followed by an infusion of 125 mg. of heparin over 8 to 12 hours. There were no instances of acute renal failure, and they recommend that fibrinogen never be given without antecedent heparinization.

In borderline situations in which acute renal failure may be expected, intravenous mannitol may be preventive. When renal failure is established, peritoneal or hemodialysis should not be withheld as a last resort. Particularly since many of the patients may have become edematous or overhydrated in an attempt to "open up the kidneys," dialysis under conditions adjusted to remove salt and water may be extremely beneficial.

Polycystic Disease. Polycystic disease is a progressive renal dysplasia inherited as an autosomal dominant. Fortunately the usual age at which symptoms appear is in the early forties, and hypertension, proteinuria, or azotemia due to this condition is rare in pregnancy. The general rule that applies to other forms of chronic renal disease also applies to polycystic disease. The likelihood of an uncomplicated pregnancy diminishes as hypertension becomes apparent, and with increasing azotemia the prognosis for the fetus in particular becomes increasingly poor.

In the retrospective study of Landesman and Scherr [105] 23 patients with undetected polycystic disease had 48 uncomplicated pregnancies. Four with known disease had aggravation of hypertension and a course resembling superimposed preeclampsia. Higgins [79] has reported a more benign course in patients with less-advanced disease. On the other hand, the report of Millar [136] documents the fact that those with hypertension, proteinuria, and azotemia have an unsuccessful outcome.

There is an increased susceptibility to pyelonephritis in patients with polycystic disease [79]. Thus, the possibility of cystic disease should be kept in mind in those with pyelonephritis, as well as in those with albuminuria early in pregnancy. It goes without saying that if a patient with polycystic disease is determined to have children, she should have them before the age at which the disease presents a problem.

DISEASES FREQUENTLY ASSOCIATED WITH PREECLAMPSIA

Diabetes Mellitus, Without Nephropathy. The increased incidence of abortion and of the clinical syndrome of preeclampsia in overt diabetes mellitus is well known, but it is less well established that the patient with latent diabetes or even prediabetes in the strict sense of the term has an increased susceptibility to development of preeclampsia. At the time of the fifth periodic review of the 206 eclamptic patients of Chesley et al. [34] the frequency of diabetes was found to be five times that expected in women who had had eclampsia as primiparas and 10 times that expected in those who had had eclampsia as multiparas. It is probable that a portion of the patients who had died of cardiovascular disease before follow-up examination may have had undetected diabetes, perhaps masked by an elevated renal threshold for glucose. The diabetes was detected from 3 to 35 years after the eclamptic episode, with an average age in the early fifties. Many of these women had infants with excessively large birth weights. These striking statistics underscore the importance of excluding diabetes as a concomitant of preeclampsia, and also of excluding latent diabetes in studies of preeclampsia. Since the frequency of bacteriuria in pregnant diabetic patients is as high or higher than in nondiabetic persons [199], there may also be an increased incidence of urinary infection predisposing to preeclampsia. Much evidence is accumulating that early recognition and treatment of the pregnant woman with latent diabetes is beneficial to both mother and child.

Diabetes Mellitus with Nephropathy. It may not be justified to attempt to classify diabetic patients according to presence or absence of nephropathy, since early in the course of diabetes in patients with grossly normal renal function ultramicroscopic thickening of the basement membranes may be found [179]. There is no reason, however, to believe that such early lesions affect the clinical course of pregnancy. On the other hand, many juvenile diabetic persons of long standing are now surviving to the childbearing age and enter pregnancy with significant renal disease, together with great determination to have a normal child. Burstein et al. [26] have described proliferative vascular lesions of the placenta in diabetic patients. Since fluorescent anti-insulin antibody localized in these lesions, and since the binding was blocked by excess of antigen, they suggest that the binding is specific and that the lesions may be produced by a reaction of tissue-fixed antibody with endogenous or exogenous insulin.

Studies in our laboratory [198] have indicated that a pregnant diabetic patient with significant renal disease may still have enhancement of renal function during pregnancy. Serial measurements of renal function were made in eight patients with diabetes of 8 to 13 years' duration. Four had retinopathy, three early intercapillary glomerulosclerosis proved by renal biopsy, and four pyelonephritis on clinical evidence. The increase in all measurements of renal function in all patients except one was comparable to that of nondiabetic pregnant subjects, except that the filtration fraction was somewhat lower.

The experience with a group of 41 patients with more severely compromised renal function is summarized by Oppé et al. [148]. Such patients, falling into class F of White's classification, comprise only about 4 per cent of pregnancies in a diabetic population. All had azotemia, hypertension, and proteinuria. The fetal wastage was 55 per cent. Therapeutic abortion was induced in 8 because of decreasing renal function or increasing retinitis. Birth weights were small. The net impact of pregnancy upon the renal disease was not determined.

It will be of value to know whether, when the pregnant diabetic patient develops apparent superimposed preeclampsia, there is deposition of fibrin in the glomerular capillary endothelium. In two of the patients of Morris et al. [137] with diabetes and suspected preeclampsia such deposition was not found.

Erythroblastosis Fetalis. Although an association was not apparent in earlier studies, erythroblastosis fetalis with hydrops fetalis may cause a syndrome resembling, if not identical with, preeclampsia [80]. John and Duncan [85] have reported 30 such instances out of a series of 34 cases. The onset of edema is apt to be earlier in pregnancy than in preeclampsia without Rh incompatibility. Burstein et al. [26] have reported proliferative vascular lesions of the placenta which bind fluorescent anti-Rh serum similar to those which they have reported in diabetes. Whether there is a disturbance of the coagulation mechanism as well and whether fibrin deposits can be demonstrated in the glomeruli in this condition is not yet known.

Summary

The kidney in pregnancy undergoes an hypertrophy of function so that normal values of substances cleared by filtration must be revised downward. The ability to reabsorb glucose is not increased in proportion to the filtration rate, so that there is an increased frequency of glucosuria.

There is a precarious balance between those factors contributing to retention of sodium and of water and those making for loss, and the pregnant woman is more susceptible to postural effects on water and electrolyte balance. There are many ways in which this balance may be disturbed, and an important one of these appears to be disturbance of the coagulation mechanism with formation of fibrin aggregates which on contact with the glomerular endothelial cells may produce the capillary endotheliosis typical of preeclampsia. Such a disturbance may be triggered by a variety of stimuli, including infection and uterine ischemia with release of thromboplastic substance from the placental trophoblast. Another is a diminution in the uterine and placental inactivation of pressor substances. Thus the kidney may well be the victim rather than the culprit in a disorder which becomes self-perpetuating.

There is increasing evidence that there is a close interrelationship between asymptomatic bacteriuria and certain complications of pregnancy, particularly pyelonephritis, and that the incidence of these may be favorably influenced by treatment.

Acknowledgments

The author's investigations have been supported by grants from the U.S. Public Health Service: RG-3745 (later, HD-00460) and 5 T01 AM-5086, and from the Vermont Heart Association.

References

1. Aladjem, S. Morphologic aspects of the placenta in gestational diabetes seen by phase-contrast microscopy: An anatomico-clinical correlation. *Amer. J. Obstet. Gynec.* 99:341, 1967.
2. Altchek, A. Electron microscopy of renal biopsies in toxemia of pregnancy. *J.A.M.A.* 175:791, 1961.
3. Altchek, A., Albright, N. L., and Somers, S. C. The renal pathology of toxemia of pregnancy. *Obstet. Gynec.* 31:595, 1968.
4. Arhelger, R. B., Douglas, B. H., and Langford, H. G. Experimental toxemia of pregnancy: Fine structure of renal lesions. *Arch. Path.* (Chicago) 84:393, 1967.
5. Assali, N. S. (Ed.). *Biology of Gestation.* Vol. 1: *The Maternal Organism.* New York: Academic, 1968. P. 185.
6. Assali, N. S., Dignam, W. J., and Dasgupta, K. Renal function in human pregnancy: II. Effects of venous pooling on renal hemodynamics and water electrolyte, and aldosterone excretion during normal gestation. *J. Lab. Clin. Med.* 54:394, 1959.
7. Assali, N. S., Douglass, R. A., Baird, W. W., and Nicholson, D. B. Measurement of uterine blood flow and uterine metabolism with the N_2O method in normotensive and toxemic pregnancy. *Clin. Res. Proc.* 2:102, 1954.

7a. Assali, N. S., Kaplan, S. A., Fomon, S. J., and Douglass, R. A., Jr. Renal function studies in toxemia of pregnancy: Excretion of solutes and renal hemodynamics during osmotic diuresis in hydropenia. *J. Clin. Invest.* 32:44, 1953.

8. Bader, R. A., Bader, M. E., Rose, D. J., and Braunwald, E. Hemodynamics at rest and

during exercise in normal pregnancy as studied by cardiac catheterization. *J. Clin. Invest.* 34:1524, 1955.

9. Baird, D. T., Gasson, P. W., and Doig, A. The renogram in pregnancy, with particular reference to the changes produced by alternation in posture. *Amer. J. Obstet. Gynec.* 95:597, 1966.
10. Barnes, A. C., and Kumar, D. Significance of cardiovascular alterations in pre-eclampsia-eclampsia: A review. *Mod. Conc. Cardiovasc. Dis.* 33:841, 1964.
11. Beck, P., and Daughaday, W. H. Human placental lactogen: Studies of its acute metabolic effects and disposition in normal man. *J. Clin. Invest.* 46:103, 1967.
12. Berger, M., and Boucek, R. J. Irreversible uterine and renal changes induced by placental ischemia. *Amer. J. Obstet. Gynec.* 89:230, 1964.
13. Berlin, N. I., Goetsch, C., Hyde, G. M., and Parsons, R. J. The blood volume in pregnancy as determined by P^{32}-labeled red blood cells. *Surg. Gynec. Obstet.* 97: 173, 1953.
14. Bieniarz, J., Maqueda, E., and Caldeyro-Barcia, R. Compression of aorta by the uterus in late human pregnancy: I. Variations between femoral and brachial artery pressure with changes from hypertension to hypotension. *Amer. J. Obstet. Gynec.* 95:795, 1966.
15. Biezenski, J. J., and Moore, H. C. Fibrinolysis in normal pregnancy. *J. Clin. Path.* 11:306, 1958.
16. Bloemers, D. Diabetes insipidus and toxaemia of pregnancy. *J. Obstet. Gynaec. Brit. Comm.* 68:322, 1961.
17. Bonsnes, R. W., and Lange, W. A. Inulin clearance during pregnancy. (Abstract.) *Fed. Proc.* 9:154, 1950.
18. Boonshaft, B., O'Connell, J. M. B., Hayes, J. M., and Schreiner, G. E. Serum renin activity during normal pregnancy: Effect of alterations of posture and sodium intake. *J. Clin. Endocr.* 28:1641, 1968.
19. Boucher, B. J., and Mason, A. S. Conn's syndrome with associated pregnancy. *Proc. Roy. Soc. Med.* 58:575, 1965.
20. Bower, D. The influence of dietary salt intake on pre-eclampsia. *J. Obstet. Gynaec. Brit. Comm.* 71:123, 1964.
21. Brain, M. C., Kuah, K-B, and Dixon, H. G. Heparin treatment of haemolysis and thrombocytopenia in pre-eclampsia. *J. Obstet. Gynaec. Brit. Comm.* 74:702, 1967.
22. Brown, J. J., Davies, D. L., Doak, P. B., Lever, A. F., and Robertson, J. I. S. Serial estimation of plasma renin concentration during pregnancy and after parturition. *J. Endocr.* 35:373, 1966.
23. Brown, J. J., Davies, D. L., Doak, P. B., Lever, A. F., Robertson, J. I. S., and Trust, P. Plasma renin concentration in the hypertensive diseases of pregnancy. *J. Obstet. Gynaec. Brit. Comm.* 73:410, 1966.
24. Bucht, H. Studies on renal function in man: With special reference to glomerular filtration and renal plasma flow in pregnancy. *Scand. J. Clin. Lab. Invest.* 3 (Suppl. 3):1, 1951.
25. Bucht, H., and Werkö, L. Glomerular filtration rate and renal blood flood in hypertensive toxaemia of pregnancy. *J. Obstet. Gynaec. Brit. Emp.* 60:157, 1953.
26. Burstein, R., Berns, A. W., Hirata, Y., and Blumenthal, H. T. A comparative histo- and immunopathological study of the placenta in diabetes mellitus and in erythroblastosis fetalis. *Amer. J. Obstet. Gynec.* 86: 66, 1963.
27. Buzanowski, Z., Chojnowska, I., Myszkowski, L., and Sadowski, J. The electrophoretic pattern of proteinuria in cases of normal labor and in the course of toxemia of pregnancy. *Pol. Med. J.* 5:217, 1966.
28. Cannon, J. F. Pregnancy and pheochromocytoma. *Obstet. Gynec.* 11:43, 1958.
29. Chesley, L. C. Simultaneous renal clearances of urea and uric acid in the differential diagnosis of the late toxemias. *Amer. J. Obstet. Gynec.* 59:960, 1950.
30. Chesley, L. C. Renal functional changes in normal pregnancy. *Clin. Obstet. Gynec.* 3: 349, 1960.
31. Chesley, L. C. Vascular reactivity in normal and toxemic pregnancy. *Clin. Obstet. Gynec.* 9:871, 1966.

32. Chesley, L. C. Kidney Fluid and Electrolytes. In Assali, N. C. (Ed.), *Pathophysiology of Gestational Disorders*. New York: Academic Press. In press.
33. Chesley, L. C., Annitto, J. E., and Cosgrove, R. A. The familial factor in toxemia of pregnancy. *Obstet. Gynec.* 32:303, 1968.
34. Chesley, L. C., Annitto, J. E., and Cosgrove, R. A. Long-term follow-up study of eclamptic women: Fifth periodic report. *Amer. J. Obstet. Gynec.* 101:886, 1968.
35. Chesley, L. C., and Sloan, D. M. The effect of posture on renal function in late pregnancy. *Amer. J. Obstet. Gynec.* 89:754, 1964.
36. Chesley, L. C., Valenti, C., and Rein, H. Excretion of sodium loads by nonpregnant and pregnant normal, hypertensive, and pre-eclamptic women. *Metabolism* 7:575, 1958.
37. Chesley, L. C., and Williams, L. O. Renal glomerular and tubular function in relation to hyperuricemia of pre-eclampsia and eclampsia. *Amer. J. Obstet. Gynec.* 50:367, 1945.
38. Christensen, P. J. Tubular reabsorption of glucose during pregnancy. *Scand. J. Clin. Lab. Invest.* 10:364, 1958.
39. Christensen, P. J., Date, J. W., Schønheyder, F., and Volqvartz, K. Amino acids in blood plasma and urine during pregnancy. *Scand. J. Clin. Lab. Invest.* 9:54, 1957.
40. Christensen, P. J., and Steenstrup, O. R. Uric acid excretion with increasing plasma glucose concentration (pregnant and nonpregnant cases). *Scand. J. Clin. Lab. Invest.* 10:182, 1958.
41. Clemetson, C. A. B. Aortic hypoplasia and its significance in the aetiology of pre-eclamptic toxaemia. *J. Obstet. Gynaec. Brit. Emp.* 67:90, 1960.
42. Cobbs, C. G., Strickler, J. C., McGovern, J. H., and Kaye, D. The postpartum renal status of women with untreated asymptomatic bacteriuria during pregnancy. *Amer. J. Obstet. Gynec.* 99:221, 1967.
43. Corbit, J. D. The effect of pregnancy upon experimental hypertension in the rabbit. *Amer. J. Med. Sci.* 201:876, 1941.
43a. Corcoran, A. C., and Page, I. H. Renal function in late toxemia of pregnancy. *Amer. J. Med. Sci.* 201:385, 1941.
44. Crabtree, E. G. *Urological Diseases of Pregnancy*. Boston: Little, Brown, 1942. P. 61.
45. Crane, M. G., Andes, J. P., Harris, J. J., and Slate, W. G. Primary aldosteronism in pregnancy. *Obstet. Gynec.* 23:200, 1964.
46. Dancis, J., Samuels, B. D., and Douglas, G. W. Immunological competence of placenta. *Science* 136:382, 1962.
47. Dean, R. E. Pheochromocytoma and pregnancy. *Obstet. Gynec.* 11:35, 1958.
48. DeMaria, F. J., and See, H. Y. C. Role of the placenta in pre-eclampsia. *Amer. J. Obstet. Gynec.* 94:471, 1966.
49. Dennis, E. J., McIver, F. A., and Smythe, C. M. Renal biopsy in pregnancy. *Clin. Obstet. Gynec.* 11:473, 1968.
50. Dieckmann, W. J. *The Toxemias of Pregnancy* (2d ed.). St. Louis: Mosby, 1952.
51. Dieckmann, W. J., McCartney, C. P., and Harrod, J. P. Kidney biopsies in multiparous patients with vascular renal disease in pregnancy. *Amer. J. Obstet. Gynec.* 75: 634, 1958.
52. Dignam, W. S., Titus, P., and Assali, N. S. Renal function in human pregnancy: I. Changes in glomerular filtration rate and renal plasma flow. *Proc. Soc. Exp. Biol. Med.* 97:512, 1958.
53. Dignam, W. S., Voskian, J., and Assali, N. S. Effects of estrogens on renal hemodynamics and excretion of electrolytes in human subjects. *J. Clin. Endocr.* 16:1032, 1956.
54. Dill, L. V., and Erickson, C. C. Eclampsia-like syndrome occurring in pregnant dogs and rabbits following renal artery constriction. *Proc. Soc. Exp. Biol. Med.* 39:362, 1938.
54a. Dixon, H. G., Browne, J. C. McC., and Davey, D. A. Choriodecidual and myometrial blood-flow. *Lancet* 2:369, 1963.
55. Doe, R. P., Dickinson, P. B., Swaim, W. R., Zinneman, H. H., and Seal, U. S. Nonprotein-bound 17-OHCS at 9 AM and 9 PM in normals, pregnancy, estrogen-treated females, and males with cancer of the pros-

tate. (Abstract #80.) *Pgm, The Endocrine Society,* 1967. P. 68.

56. Donato, L., and Turchetti, G. Renal glycosuria in pregnancy. *Acta Med. Scand.* 152:223, 1955.
57. Epstein, F. H. Late vascular effects of toxemia of pregnancy. *New Eng. J. Med.* 271:391, 1964.
58. Fainstat, F. "Physiological hydroureter" of pregnancy in a four-legged animal. *Amer. J. Obstet. Gynec.* 87:486, 1963.
59. Fainstat., T. Ureteral dilatation in pregnancy: A review. *Obstet. Gynec. Survey* 18:845, 1963.
60. Faith, G. C., and Trump, B. F. The glomerular capillary wall in human kidney disease: Acute glomerulonephritis, systemic lupus erythematosus, and preeclampsia-eclampsia. Comparative electron microscopic observations and a review. *Lab. Invest.* 15:1682, 1966.
61. Farquhar, M. G. Review of Normal and Pathologic Glomerular Ultrastructure. In Metcoff, J. (Ed.), *Proceedings of the Tenth Annual Conference on the Nephrotic Syndrome.* Washington, D.C.: National Kidney Disease Foundation, Inc., 1959. Vol. 22, pp. 2–30.
62. Fear, R. E. Eclampsia superimposed on renal scleroderma: A rare cause of maternal and fetal mortality. *Obstet. Gynec.* 31: 69, 1968.

62a. Ferris, T. F., Herdson, P. B., Dunnill, M. S., and Lee, M. R. Toxemia of pregnancy in sheep: A clinical, physiological, and pathological study. *J. Clin. Invest.* 48: 1643, 1969.

63. Fine, J. Glycosuria of pregnancy. *Brit. Med. J.* 1:205, 1967.
64. Franklin, K. J., and Winstone, N. E. A review of some experimental findings of obstetrical interest. *J. Obstet. Gynaec. Brit. Emp.* 62:29, 1955.
65. Friedberg, V. Über die Entstehung der Glykosurie in der Schwangerschaft. *Gynaecologia* (Basel) 146:431, 1958.
66. Friedberg, V., Vorherr, H., and Schulte, G. Adiuretinuntersuchungen während der normalen Schwangerschaft und bei Gestosen. *Arch. Gynaek.* 192:483, 1960.
67. Garstein, M., Pollak, V. E., and Kark, R. M. Systemic lupus erythematosus and pregnancy. *New Eng. J. Med.* 267:165, 1962.
68. Gershberg, H. Metabolic and renotropic effects of human growth hormone in disease. *J. Clin. Endocr.* 20:1107, 1960.
69. Goldberg, M. Studies of the acute renal effects of hemolyzed red blood cells in dogs including estimations of renal blood flow with krypton. *J. Clin. Invest.* 41:2112, 1962.
70. Gomel, V., and Hardwick, D. F. Search for a pressor substance in toxemia of pregnancy. *Amer. J. Obstet. Gynec.* 94:308, 1966.
71. Gordon, G., and McKay, R. T. Preeclampsia associated with hypoplasia of the aorta. *J. Obstet. Gynaec. Brit. Comm.* 71:785, 1964.
72. Gray, M. J. Use and abuse of thiazides in pregnancy. *Clin. Obstet. Gynec.* 11:568, 1968.
73. Gray, M. J., Munro, A. B., Sims, E. A. H., Meeker, C. I., Solomon, S., and Watanabe, M. Regulation of sodium and total body water metabolism in pregnancy. *Amer. J. Obstet. Gynec.* 89:760, 1964.
74. Gross, F. Renin-like substance in placenta and uterus of the rabbit. *Lancet* 2:590, 1964.
75. Handler, J. S. The role of lactic acid in the reduced excretion of uric acid in toxemia of pregnancy. *J. Clin. Invest.* 39:1526, 1960.
76. Hayashi, T. Uric acid and endogenous creatinine clearance studies in normal pregnancy and toxemias of pregnancy. *Amer. J. Obstet. Gynec.* 71:859, 1956.
77. Helmer, O. M., and Judson, W. E. Influence of high renin substrate levels on renin-angiotensin system in pregnancy. *Amer. J. Obstet. Gynec.* 99:9, 1967.
78. Herwig, K. R., Merrill, J. P., Jackson, R. L., and Oken, D. E. Chronic renal disease and pregnancy: Case report of azotemia, hemodialysis, and delivery of a viable infant. *Amer. J. Obstet. Gynec.* 92: 1117, 1965.
79. Higgins, C. C. Bilateral polycystic kidney

disease: A review of ninety-four cases. *A.M.A. Arch. Surg.* 65:318, 1952.

80. Hirsch, M. R., and Mark, M. S. Pseudotoxemia and erythroblastosis. Report of a case. *Obstet. Gynec.* 24:47, 1964.
81. Hodari, A. A. Chronic uterine ischemia and reversible experimental "toxemia of pregnancy." *Amer. J. Obstet. Gynec.* 97:597, 1967.
82. Hodari, A. A., Smeby, R., and Bumpus, F. M. A renin-like substance in the human placenta. *Obstet. Gynec.* 29:313, 1967.
83. Hytten, F. E., and Thomson, A. M. Maternal Physiological Adjustments. In Assali, N. S. (Ed.), *Biology of Gestation. The Maternal Organism.* New York: Academic, 1968. Vol. I, Chap. 8, p. 449.
84. Hytten, F. E., Thomson, A. M., and Taggart, N. Total body water in normal pregnancy. *J. Obstet. Gynaec. Brit. Comm.* 73:553, 1966.

84a. Jäämeri, K. E. U., Koivuniemi, A. P., and Carpen, E. O. Occurrence of trophoblasts in the blood of toxaemic patients. *Gynaecologia* 160:315, 1965.

85. John A. H., and Duncan, A. S. The maternal syndrome associated with hydrops foetalis. *J. Obstet. Gynaec. Brit. Comm.* 71:61, 1964.
86. Johnston, C. I., Johnson, J. R., and Reader, R. The nephrotic syndrome in pregnancy. *Aust. Ann. Med.* 12:342, 1963.
87. Jones, E. M. Capillary permeability to plasma proteins during pregnancy. *J. Obstet. Gynaec. Brit. Comm.* 75:295, 1968.
88. Kalousek, G., Hlavacek, C., Nedoss, B., and Pollak, V. E. Circadian rhythms of creatinine and electrolyte excretion in healthy pregnant women. *Amer. J. Obstet. Gynec.* In press.
89. Kaplan, A. L., Smith, J. P., and Tillman, A. J. B. Healed acute and chronic nephritis in pregnancy. *Amer. J. Obstet. Gynec.* 83:1519, 1962.
90. Kaplan, S. L., and Grumbach, M. M. Studies of a human and simian placental hormone with growth hormone-like and prolactin-like activities. *J. Clin. Endocr.* 24:80, 1964.
91. Kass, E. H. Asymptomatic infections of the urinary tract. *Trans. Ass. Amer. Physicians* 69:56, 1956.
92. Kass, E. H. The Role of Asymptomatic Bacteriuria in the Pathogenesis of Pyelonephritis. In Quinn, E. L., and Kass, E. H. (Eds.), *Biology of Pyelonephritis.* (Henry Ford Hospital International Symposium.) Boston: Little, Brown, 1960. Chap. 28.
93. Katz, F. H., and Kappas, A. The effects of estradiol and estriol on plasma levels of cortisol and thyroid hormone-binding globulins and on aldosterone and cortisol secretion rates in man. *J. Clin. Invest.* 46:1768, 1967.
94. Kerr, M. G. Cardiovascular dynamics in pregnancy and labour. *Brit. Med. Bull.* 24:19, 1968.
95. Kincaid-Smith, P. Bacteriuria in Pregnancy. In Kass, E. H. (Ed.), *Progress in Pyelonephritis.* Philadelphia: Davis, 1965. P. 11.
96. Kincaid-Smith, P. Bacteriuria and urinary infection in pregnancy. *Clin. Obstet. Gynec.* 11:533, 1968.
97. Koffler, D., and Kunkel, H. G. Mechanisms of renal injury in systemic lupus erythematosus. (Editorial.) *Amer. J. Med.* 45:165, 1968.
98. Kuhlbäck, B., and Widholm, O. Serum uric acid in toxaemia of pregnancy with special reference to the prognosis of the foetus. *Acta Obstet. Gynec. Scand.* 43:330, 1964.
99. Kumar, D. Tissue progesterone concentrations of placentas in pre-eclamptic patients. *Amer. J. Obstet. Gynec.* 95:594, 1966.
100. Kumar, D., and Barnes, A. C. Aldosterone in normal and abnormal pregnancy. *Obstet. Gynec. Survey* 15:625, 1960.
101. Kupic, E. A., and Abrams, H. L. Renal vascular alterations induced by hemorrhagic hypotension; preliminary observations. *Invest. Radiol.* 3:345, 1968.
102. Lancet, M., and Fisher, I. L. The value of blood uric acid levels in toxaemia of pregnancy. *J. Obstet. Gynaec. Brit. Emp.* 63:116, 1956.
103. Landau, R. L., and Lubigihl, K. Inhibition of the sodium-retaining influence of

aldosterone by progesterone. *J. Clin. Endocr.* 18:1237, 1958.

104. Landesman, R., Halpern, M., and Knapp, R. C. Renal artery lesions associated with the toxemias of pregnancy. *Obstet. Gynec.* 18:645, 1961.
105. Landesman, R., and Scherr, L. Congenital polycystic kidney disease in pregnancy. *Obstet. Gynec.* 8:673, 1956.
106. Langford, H. G., Douglas, B. H., and Arhelger, R. B. A model of pre-eclampsia: I. Blood pressure changes produced by anti-placenta serum. *Johns Hopkins Med. J.* 120:213, 1967.
107. Lee, L. Antigen-antibody reaction in the pathogenesis of bilateral renal cortical necrosis. *J. Exp. Med.* 117:365, 1963.
108. Levinsky, N. G., and Berliner, R. W. Changes in composition of the urine in ureter and bladder at low urine flow. *Amer. J. Physiol.* 196:549, 1959.
109. Levitt, M. F. Clinical conference on medical hazards of pregnancy. (Discussion.) *J. Mount Sinai Hosp. N.Y.* 24:472, 1957.
110. Lichton, I. J. Salt saving in the pregnant rat. *Amer. J. Physiol.* 201:765, 1961.
111. Lichton, I. J. Urinary excretion of water, sodium and total solutes by the pregnant rat. *Amer. J. Physiol.* 204:563, 1963.
112. Lindheimer, M., and Weston, P. The effect of hypotonic expansion on sodium, water and urea excretion in late pregnancy: The influence of posture on these results. *J. Clin. Invest.* 48:947, 1969.
113. Little, B. Water and electrolyte balance during pregnancy. *Anesthesiology* 26:400, 1965.
114. Little, P. J. The incidence of urinary infection in 5000 pregnant women. *Lancet* 2:925, 1966.
115. Löhlein, M. Zur Pathogenese der Nierenkrankheiten: II. Nephritis und Nephrose mit besonderer Berücksichtigung der Nephropathia gravidarum. *Deutsch. Med. Wschr.* 44:1187, 1918.
116. Longo, L. D., and Assali, N. S. Renal function in human pregnancy: IV. The urinary tract "dead space" during normal gestation. *Amer. J. Obstet. Gynec.* 80:495, 1960.
117. MacDonald, D. Coarctation of the aorta in pregnancy. *J. Irish. Med. Ass.* 54:168, 1964.
118. MacKay, E. V. Pregnancy and renal disease: A ten-year survey. *Aust. New Zeal. J. Obstet. Gynaec.* 3:21, 1963.
119. Maeck, J. V. S., and Zilliacus, H. Heparin in the treatment of toxemia of pregnancy. *Amer. J. Obstet. Gynec.* 55:326, 1948.
120. Magara, M. A Study on the intrinsic factors of the toxaemia of pregnancy. *Acta Path. Microbiol. Scand.* 24:670, 1961.
121. Margaretten, W., Zunker, H. O., and McKay, D. G. Production of the generalized Shwartzman reaction in pregnant rats by intravenous infusion of thrombin. *Lab. Invest.* 13:552, 1964.
122. Martin, J. D., and Mills, I. H. Aldosterone excretion in normal and toxaemic pregnancies. *Brit. Med. J.* 2:571, 1956.
123. Mautner, W., Churg, J., Grishman, E., and Dachs, S. Preeclamptic nephropathy. *Lab. Invest.* 11:518, 1962.
124. McCartney, C. P. Toxemias of Pregnancy. In Greenhill, J. P., *Obstetrics* (12th ed.). Philadelphia: Saunders, 1960. P. 381.
125. McCartney, C. P. Toxemia of pregnancy — classification. *Clin. Obstet. Gynec.* 9:864, 1966.
126. McCartney, C. P. Renal morphology and function among patients with preeclampsia and gravidas with essential hypertension. *Clin. Obstet. Gynec.* 11:506, 1968.
127. McCartney, C. P., Spargo, B., Lorincz, A. B., Lefebvre, Y., and Newton, R. E. Renal structure and function in pregnant patients with acute hypertension; osmolar concentration. *Amer. J. Obstet. Gynec.* 90: 579, 1964.
128. McCluskey, R. T., Vassalli, P., Gallo, G., and Baldwin, D. S. An immunofluorescent study of pathogenic mechanisms in glomerular disease. *New Eng. J. Med.* 274:695, 1966.
129. McEwan, H. P. Investigation of proteinuria in pregnancy by immuno-electrophoresis. *J. Obstet. Gynaec. Brit. Comm.* 75:289, 1968.
130. McKay, D. G. *Disseminated Intravascular Coagulation: An Intermediary Mechanism*

of Disease. New York: Hoeber Med. Div., Harper & Row, 1965.

131. McKay, D. G., DeBacalao, E. B., and Sedlis, A. Platelet adhesiveness in toxemia of pregnancy. *Amer. J. Obstet. Gynec.* 90:1315, 1964.

132. McKay, D. G., Goldenberg, V., Kaunitz, H., and Csavossy, I. Experimental eclampsia: An electron microscope study and review. *Arch. Path.* (Chicago) 84:557, 1967.

133. McKay, D. G., Merrill, S. J., Weiner, A. E., Hertig, A. T., and Reid, D. E. Pathologic anatomy of eclampsia, bilateral renal cortical necrosis, pituitary necrosis, and other acute fatal complications of pregnancy, and its possible relationship to generalized Shwartzman phenomenon. *Amer. J. Obstet. Gynec.* 66:507, 1953.

134. Mengert, W. F., and Tacchi, D. A. Pregnancy toxemia and sodium chloride: A preliminary report. *Amer. J. Obstet. Gynec.* 81: 601, 1961.

135. Mertens, B. F., McDuffie, F. C., Bowie, E. J. W., and Owen, C. A. Rapid sensitive method for measuring fibrinogen split-products in human serum. *Mayo Clin. Proc.* 44: 114, 1969.

136. Millar, W. G. Pregnancy and polycystic disease of the kidneys. *J. Obstet. Gynaec. Brit. Emp.* 60:868, 1953.

137. Morris, R. H., Vassalli, P., Beller, F. K., and McCluskey, R. T. Immunofluorescent studies of renal biopsies in the diagnosis of toxemia of pregnancy. *Obstet. Gynec.* 24:32, 1964.

138. Moses, A. M., Lobotsky, J., and Lloyd, C. W. The occurrence of pre-eclampsia in a bilaterally adrenalectomized woman. *J. Clin. Endocr.* 19:987, 1959.

139. Muehrcke, R. C. Prolonged potassium deficiency and chronic pyelonephritis in man and animals. In Quinn, E. L., and Kass, E. H. (Eds.), *Biology of Pyelonephritis.* (Henry Ford Hospital International Symposium.) Boston: Little, Brown, 1959. Chap. 40.

140. Müller-Berghaus, G., and McKay, D. G. Prevention of the generalized Shwartzman reaction in pregnant rats by alpha-adrenergic blocking agents. *Lab. Invest.* 17:276, 1967.

141. Murray, F. A. Lupus erythematosus in pregnancy. *J. Obstet. Gynaec. Brit. Emp.* 65:401, 1958.

142. Norden, C. W., and Kass, E. H. Bacteriuria of pregnancy: A critical appraisal. *Ann. Rev. Med.* 19:431, 1968.

143. Norden, C. W., and Kilpatrick, W. H. Bacteriuria in Pregnancy. In Kass, E. H. (Ed.), *Progress in Pyelonephritis.* Philadelphia: Davis, 1965.

144. Ober, W. B., Reid, D. E., Romney, S. L., and Merrill, J. P. Renal lesions and acute renal failure in pregnancy. *Amer. J. Med.* 21:781, 1956.

145. O'Connell, M., and Welsh, G. W., 3rd. Unbound plasma cortisol in pregnant and Enovid-E treated women as determined by ultrafiltration. *J. Clin. Endocr.* 29:563, 1969.

146. Ojo, O. A., and Akinkugbe, O. O. The nephrotic syndrome in pregnancy. *J. Obstet. Gynaec. Brit. Comm.* 74:919, 1967.

147. Oken, D. E. Chronic renal diseases and pregnancy: A review. *Amer. J. Obstet. Gynec.* 94:1023, 1966.

148. Oppé, T. E., Hsia, D. Y., and Gellis, S. S. Pregnancy in the diabetic mother with nephritis. *Lancet* 1:353, 1957.

149. Page, E. W. Use of heparin in pre-eclampsia. (Abstract.) *Amer. J. Med.* 4:784, 1948.

150. Page, E. W., Glendening, M. B., Dignam, W., and Harper, H. A. The causes of histidinuria in normal pregnancy. *Amer. J. Obstet. Gynec.* 68:110, 1954.

151. Page, E. W., Patton, H. S., and Ogden, E. The effect of pregnancy on experimental hypertension. *Amer. J. Obstet. Gynec.* 41: 53, 1941.

151a. Palmer, J. K. Hypertension and unilateral renal disease. *Amer. Surg.* 20:744, 1954.

152. Peters, A. Nephrosis during pregnancy: Report of a case. *Obstet. Gynec.* 17:202, 1961.

153. Peters, J. P. Toxemia of pregnancy. *Yale J. Biol. Med.* 9:311, 1937.

154. Peters, J. P., and Van Slyke, D. D. *Quan-*

G. F. Diabetes and latent diabetes in pregnancy. *Brit. Med. Bull.* 24:25, 1968.

246. Zinneman, H. H., Seal, U. S., and Doe, R. P. Urinary amino acids in pregnancy, following progesterone, and estrogen-progesterone. *J. Clin. Endocr.* 27:397, 1967.
247. Zuspan, F. P., Barnes, A. C., and Dillhoefer, J. R. The urinary excretion of antidiuretic substances by the obstetric and gynecologic patient. *Amer. J. Obstet. Gynec.* 76:619, 1958.
248. Zuspan, F. P., and Bell, J. D. Variable salt-loading during pregnancy with preeclampsia. *Obstet. Gynec.* 18:530, 1961.

33

The Kidney in Sickle Cell Anemia

Louis G. Welt and Carl B. Lyle, Jr.

Sickle cell disease is an inherited molecular disorder in which the basic alteration consists in the substitution of one amino acid for another: valine for glutamic acid in the globin portion of hemoglobin [15, 28]. As a consequence, the red cells containing this altered molecule develop unusual shapes, which are described in the title of the first report of this entity by Herrick [14] in 1910: "Peculiar elongated and sickle-shaped red blood corpuscles in a case of severe anemia."

The assumption of these bizarre shapes is said to be conducive to an increase in the viscosity of the blood, which promotes a slowed circulation with congestion and stagnation in the minute vessels. This, in turn, may lead to improper blood supply to visceral tissues with morphologic and functional changes which are reflected in signs and symptoms involving many organs [43]. Patients with sickle cell disease grow improperly and reproduce poorly. They are anemic, and they complain of pains in joints, bones, muscles, and the abdomen. They have lesions which could be manifestations of infarctions in the skin, bone, spleen, lungs, heart, kidneys, and in the central nervous system. However, actual thrombotic lesions are unusual. The anemia is due to the shortened life span of these erythrocytes and may be severe; in conjunction with morphologic alterations in the myocardium, it leads to cardiac enlargement and frequently to heart failure.

It is estimated that 8 per cent of American Negroes have red cells that sickle, and that one in 40 with such cells has sickle cell disease [29]. The distinction between sickle cell trait and sickle cell disease was clarified by the demonstration by Pauling et al. [30] of the different electrophoretic mobility of sickle (S) hemoglobin compared with that of normal (A) hemoglobin, and by Neel's studies [29] of the genetic aspects. The latter investigator predicted that patients with sickle cell trait would be heterozygous (SA) with respect to the abnormal hemoglobin and hence only approximately half their hemoglobin would be abnormal, whereas those with the disease would be homozygous (SS) and have essentially all of the hemoglobin as the altered molecule. Electrophoretic technics have provided support for this hypothesis, and this is the current interpretation. These technics have made it possible to discriminate not only between SS and SA hemoglobinopathies but also among other sickle cell variants, such as the combination of S with C or D hemoglobin or with the trait for thalassemia.

Despite the multisystemic character of the disorder, this chapter will concern itself solely with the renal manifestations, which consist of gross hematuria, inability to concentrate the urine appropriately, rare instances of the nephrotic syndrome, and, uncommonly, significant renal insufficiency leading to uremia. Both gross hematuria and the urine-concentrating defect are observed in patients with sickle cell trait (SA) as well as sickle cell disease (SS).

Renal Pathology

The pathology of the kidney in sickle cell disorders has received attention, but the descriptions offer difficulties in interpretation, for several reasons. The first concerns the discrimination between the disease (SS) and the trait (SA); since this was often difficult before the development of electrophoretic technics, there is uncertainty as to which features of the renal pathology might characterize each one. Another hazard arises from the fact that pathologic material has been obtained from individuals of different ages, which makes it difficult to decide which alterations may be of a primary nature and which may arise from secondary consequences. The more primary lesions are probably seen only in very young children, and particular emphasis must be placed on the alterations seen in this age group. Finally, since the functional defect characterized by an inability to concentrate the urine is noted in patients with the trait as well as the disease, it is most important to discover, if possible, what morphologic changes might be common to both.

GROSS PATHOLOGY

In descriptions of the gross pathology [4, 8, 18, 25, 27, 33, 38, 44, 45] the usual comments include references to the fact that, in general, the kidneys are normal or even somewhat increased in size, rather than atrophic. Nevertheless, the external surface is often finely and irregularly scarred and, on occasion, mottled with numerous yellow-gray, sharply demarcated foci, which are rhomboid or wedge-shaped. Shrunken areas are observed beneath this surface manifestation of disease, and these have the configuration of old, small infarcts.

MICROSCOPIC PATHOLOGY

One of the outstanding features of the kidney is the appearance of the small vessels. These are dilated and filled with sickled erythrocytes. However, this clumping and marked sickling of the red cells could be an artifact of fixation of the tissue.

The glomeruli are enlarged and the enlargement appears disproportionately great when compared with the increase in size in other anemic states. Bernstein and Whitten [4] confined their study to the younger age group with anemia to avoid the influence of time and secondary change. They noted not only that the glomeruli appeared large but also that, in particular, when the size was systematically estimated and compared with the size of the glomeruli in normal subjects, there was a distinct difference between patients with sickle cell disease and normal persons with respect to the juxtamedullary glomeruli. In addition to enlarged and engorged glomeruli, there is some glomerulosclerosis, which later progresses to complete obliteration of the tufts.

The tubules are both dilated and atrophic; some are plugged with necrotic debris; there are evidences of active necrosis and regeneration of tubular epithelium simultaneously. There is considerable deposition of hemosiderin pigment in the tubular cells. In some areas there are scars where the population of tubules and collecting ducts has diminished in numbers and where there is fibrous tissue replacement, an occasional tubular retention cyst, and stromal edema.

Mostofi et al. [27] reported a study in which the observations were limited to the appearance of the kidneys removed because of unilateral hematuria. They noted vascular congestion in both the cortex and the medulla, and, in addition, congestion and hemorrhage in the renal pelves and ureters and, occasionally, papillary necrosis. The most prominent alteration was the severe stasis in the peritubular capillaries of both the cortex and the medulla, but most marked in the capillaries of the medulla, with extravasation of blood into the peritubular areas.

In lesions that appeared to be older, there was partial or complete loss of epithelium in the segments involved. In addition, there were small empty spaces partially lined by remnants of tubular epithelial cells or entirely lined with fibrous tissue. The edematous connective tissue was infiltrated with lymphocytes, monocytes, and hemosiderin-laden macrophages.

Renal Hemodynamics

Most observers [5, 9, 10, 21] have found that the glomerular filtration rate (GFR) tends to be elevated in young patients with sickle cell disease and that this function begins to diminish to depressed levels in early adulthood, between the ages of 20 and 30 years. After the third decade, GFR, estimated renal plasma flow, and tubular maximum for para-aminohippurate (Tm_{PAH}) all diminish.

Renal Concentrating Ability

Many early reports of isolated instances of sickle cell disease contain comments concerning the apparent inability of these patients to elaborate a concentrated urine. This inability has now been documented many times and appears to be clearly established as a common and early manifestation of sickle cell disease *and* trait [20, 26, 34, 40, 46, 47]. Certain characteristics and features of this inability warrant comment. First of all, it is not simply a reflection of the anemia per se. This is attested by the fact that such a defect is not a usual accompaniment of other states of anemia [35, 46] and also by the fact that it is seen in patients with the trait who are not anemic.

Despite these observations, it is important to point out that the concentrating defect is partially reversed after blood transfusion in children. Keitel et al. [17] reported that multiple transfusions in seven patients were accompanied by an increase from 533–682 mOsm to 942–1042 mOsm in the maximal ability to concentrate the urine. In older patients the reversibility was either less marked or not observed at all. Keitel's patients were able to dilute the urine in a normal fashion [16]. This reversibility of the concentrating defect with transfusions with group A blood has been confirmed [36]. Another interesting feature of this defect is that children who are unable to concentrate the urine maximally when provoked with water deprivation and Pitressin may nevertheless have normal values for negative free-water clearance ($T^{C}_{H_2O}$) when undergoing a solute diuresis [13, 22, 41, 42].

The reader should refer to Chapter 2 for a thorough consideration of the urine-concentrating mechanisms. For our purposes we may ascribe inability to concentrate the urine to one or more of the following alterations:

1. A constant solute diuresis involving some or all nephrons.
2. An inability to elaborate a hyperosmotic

interstitium, owing to some intrinsic defect in the countercurrent multiplier mechanism.

3. An increased blood flow in the vasa recta, such that the high interstitial osmolality is more readily dissipated.

4. An alteration in the trapping characteristics of the circulation [22].

5. A failure to achieve osmotic equilibration across the distal convolution, so that hypotonic fluid is brought to the beginning of the collecting tubule.

6. A failure to achieve osmotic equilibration across the collecting tubular epithelium, so that the final urine is less concentrated than the papillary interstitium.

Although in general the GFR is normal or increased, there is no evidence that these patients undergo a solute diuresis that involves *all* the nephrons. The fact that the concentrating defect is reversible argues against the probability that there is a permanent primary defect in the countercurrent multiplier mechanism. This is suggested also by the fact that these patients can dilute the urine properly [16]. There may conceivably be an increase in medullary blood flow in the vasa recta, but no technic is available to determine this. Levitt et al. [22] suggest that the trapping mechanism of the circulation becomes inefficient owing to alterations in the vessels such that diffusion of solutes from the efferent capillary loop diminishes, whereas that from the afferent loop continues in normal fashion. This is a remote possibility and is as yet untestable. These patients do not excrete hypotonic urine under a solute diuresis with mannitol, which argues against a failure to achieve osmotic equilibrium across the distal convolutional tubular epithelium; and finally, the fact that they may have *normal* values for $T^{C}_{H_2O}$ argues against a failure of osmotic equilibration across the collecting tubular epithelium as well.

Perillie and Epstein [31] have referred to the fact that a hypertonic environment promotes sickling and argued that slowing of blood flow in the vasa recta as sickle cells pass through the hypertonic environment might minimize the effectiveness of the countercurrent multiplier system by imposing some limitation on the reabsorption of sodium in this region. This argument suggests that a diminished rate of medullary blood flow imposes a significant restriction on the delivery of oxygen and substrates to the loops of Henle. This, in turn, might impair the ability to transport sodium efficiently and minimize the intensity of the osmotic gradient and in this fashion result in a less concentrated urine. This hypothesis seems quite reasonable and is supported by the improvement in urine concentration that may be achieved in young patients when their sickle hemoglobin red cells are replaced with erythrocytes containing normal hemoglobin by the use of multiple transfusions. Alternative explanations include modifications in the medullary circulation and rates of medullary blood flow [12].

The fact that the concentrating defect becomes more intense with time and is less readily reversible with transfusions in the older age groups could merely be a reflection of the consequences of the more obvious structural damage that obtains with time. Since the major portion of these pathologic alterations is in the medulla, it is clear that a permanent concentrating defect might easily emerge.

Hematuria

In 1948 Abel and Brown [1] described the case of a 24-year-old Negro soldier who underwent a left nephrectomy for gross hematuria. Examination of the removed kidney revealed numerous sickled cells in the vasculature; there were a few submucosal hemorrhages, but no other alterations to account for the hematuria. The disorder was attributed to sickle cell disease, although no supporting hematologic evidence was available. Since that time, 120 instances of gross hematuria have been reported in individuals with laboratory evidence of one of the sickle hemoglobinopathies.

These cases have been reviewed by Lucas and Bullock [23]. The earlier reports did not provide sufficient data to establish exactly what form of hemoglobinopathy was present. Approximately 64 of the reported cases had electrophoretic patterns to confirm the diagnosis. Of these, 7 had the homozygous (SS) pattern; but only 4 in this group had the classic picture of *gross* painless hematuria. In 39 instances the hemoglobin pattern was SA, and in 17 it was SC. Although the entire group is probably too small to reflect the frequency of hematuria in each variant of sickling, it is of interest that this distribution conforms reasonably well with the relative frequency of SS, SA, and SC [7, 29].

It is difficult to determine the frequency of hematuria in sickle hemoglobinopathies, but one report [23] suggests that over 20 per cent of hospitalized patients with electrophoretic patterns of SS, SA, or SC had manifest hematuria at some time. Another study suggests that approximately one-third of Negroes with gross hematuria have an accompanying abnormal hemoglobin [6]. The majority of the reported instances have occurred in males, but this may well be a nonrepresentative preponderance, since most of the early series were from Veterans Administration hospitals.

The bleeding was noted to be from the left ureteral orifice in 62 of the 75 instances in which unilateral hematuria was documented. Of the 95 instances in which roentgenographic evidence was recorded, pyelography, either intravenous or retrograde, revealed abnormalities in 37. These changes usually suggested a filling defect [26].

The pathologic alterations have already been alluded to. The changes that seem most likely to be contributory to hematuria are the rather common findings of papillary congestion, submucosal hemorrhage, and occasional frank papillary necrosis. The precise reason why these alterations occur is unknown, except insofar as they can be attributed to the increased viscosity of blood containing sickled erythrocytes, with consequent stasis, congestion, and hypoxia. Knochel [19] has discussed the influences that tend to increase the degree of sickling in the renal medulla and papilla as alluded to earlier [31]. He has advanced some notions concerning therapy which include the infusion of distilled water and the implementation of diureses with solute loads and diuretic agents which should diminish the degree of sickling and may reduce the intensity of hematuria. In addition, it is possible that these changes are responsible for hematuria through defects regarded as characteristic of so-called essential hematuria [24, 37].

Nephrotic Syndrome

Three reports have appeared of the association of sickle cell disease and the nephrotic syndrome [2, 3, 37]. The association of the two disorders may simply be a coincidence. Biopsies in four patients revealed areas of normal tissue interspersed with areas of far-advanced pyelonephritis or parenchymatous scarring. Glomeruli varied from those that were normal to those with membranous thickening, to those that were partially or completely hyalinized (see Chapter 16).

Renal Insufficiency

Although patients exhibit functional defects (alluded to earlier in this chapter) which tend to become more intense with time, significant renal insufficiency with uremia is rare as the cause of death in sickle cell disease [11, 39].

References

1. Abel, M. S., and Brown, C. R. Sickle cell disease with severe hematuria simulating renal neoplasm. *J.A.M.A.* 136:624, 1948.
2. Berman, L. B., and Schreiner, G. E. Clinical and histologic spectrum of the nephrotic syndrome. *Amer. J. Med.* 24:249, 1958.
3. Berman, L. B., and Tublin, I. The nephropathies of sickle cell disease. *A.M.A. Arch. Intern. Med.* 103:602, 1959.
4. Bernstein, J., and Whitten, C. F. A histologic appraisal of the kidney in sickle cell anemia. *Arch. Path.* (Chicago) 70:407, 1960.
5. Calcagno, P. L., McLavy, J., and Kelley, T. Glomerular filtration rate in children with sickle cell disease. *J. Pediat.* 5:127, 1950.
6. Chapman, A. Z., Reeder, P. S., Friedman, I. A., and Baker, L. A. Gross hematuria in sickle cell trait and sickle cell hemoglobin-C disease. *Amer. J. Med.* 19:733, 1955.
7. Chernoff, A. I. The human hemoglobin in health and disease. *Amer. J. Hum. Genet.* 13:151, 1961.
8. Diggs, L. W., and Ching, R. E. Pathology of sickle cell anemia. *Southern Med. J.* 27:839, 1934.
9. Etteldorf, J. N., Smith, J. D., Tuttle, A. H., and Diggs, L. W. Renal hemodynamic studies in adults with sickle cell anemia. *Amer. J. Med.* 18:243, 1955.
10. Etteldorf, J. N., Tuttle, A. H., and Clayton, G. W. Renal hemodynamics in children with sickle cell anemia. *A.M.A. Amer. J. Dis. Child.* 83:185, 1952.
11. Evans, P. V., and Symmes, A. T. Bone marrow infarction with fat embolism and nephrosis in sickle cell disease. *J. Indiana Med. Ass.* 50:1101, 1957.
12. Hatch, F. E., Culbertson, J. W., and Diggs, L. W. Nature of the renal concentrating defect in sickle cell disease. *J. Clin. Invest.* 46:336, 1967.
13. Heinemann, H. O., and Cheung, M. W. Renal concentrating mechanism in sickle-cell anemia. *J. Lab. Clin. Med.* 49:923, 1957.
14. Herrick, J. B. Peculiar elongated and sickle-shaped red blood corpuscles in a case of severe anemia. *Arch. Intern. Med.* 6:517, 1910.
15. Ingram, V. M. Gene mutations in human haemoglobin: The chemical differences between normal and sickle cell haemoglobin. *Nature* (London) 180:326, 1957.
16. Keitel, H. G. Water metabolism in sickle cell anemia. *A.M.A. Amer. J. Dis. Child.* 94:549, 1957.
17. Keitel, H. G., Thompson, D., and Itano, H. A. Hyposthenuria in sickle cell anemia: A reversible renal defect. *J. Clin. Invest.* 35:998, 1956.
18. Kimmelstiel, P. Vascular occlusion and ischemic infarction in sickle cell disease. *Amer. J. Med. Sci.* 216:11, 1948.
19. Knochel, J. P. Hematuria in sickle cell trait. *Arch. Intern. Med.* (Chicago) 123:160, 1969.
20. Kunz, H. W., Mellin, G. W., Cheung, M. W., and Pratt, E. L. Impairment of urinary concentration in sickle cell anemia. *A.M.A. Amer. J. Dis. Child.* 86:512, 1953.
21. Levin, W. C., Gregory, R., and Bennett, A. The effect of chronic anemia on renal function as measured by inulin and Diodrast clearances. *J. Lab. Clin. Med.* 32:1433, 1947.
22. Levitt, M. F., Hauser, A. D., Levy, M. S., and Polimeros, D. The renal concentrating defect in sickle cell disease. *Amer. J. Med.* 29:611, 1960.
23. Lucas, W. M., and Bullock, W. H. Hematuria in sickle cell disease. *J. Urol.* 83:733, 1960.
24. MacMahon, H. E., and Latorracia, R. Essential renal hematuria. *J. Urol.* 71:667, 1954.
25. Margolies, M. P. Sickle cell anemia. *Medicine* (Balt.) 30:357, 1951.
26. McCrory, W. M., Goren, N., and Gornfeld, D. Demonstration of impairment of urinary concentration ability, or "Pitressin resistance" in children with sickle anemia. *A.M.A. Amer. J. Dis. Child.* 86:512, 1953.
27. Mostofi, F. K., Vorder Bruegge, C. F., and Diggs, L. W. Lesions in kidneys removed for unilateral hematuria in sickle-cell disease. *A.M.A. Arch. Path.* 63:336, 1957.

28. Murayama, M. Structure of sickle cell hemoglobin and molecular mechanism of the sickling phenomenon. *Clin. Chem.* 13:578, 1967.

29. Neel, J. V. The inheritance of sickle cell anemia. *Science* 110:64, 1949.

30. Pauling, L., Itano, H. A., Singer, S. J., and Wells, I. C. Sickle cell anemia, a molecular disease. *Science* 110:543, 1949.

31. Perillie, P. E., and Epstein, F. H. Sickling phenomenon produced by hypertonic solutions: A possible explanation for the hyposthenuria of sicklemia. *J. Clin. Invest.* 42:570, 1963.

32. Pytel, A. Renal fornical hemorrhages: Their pathogenesis and treatment. *J. Urol.* 83:783, 1960.

33. Schlitt, L. E., and Keitel, H. G. Renal manifestations of sickle cell disease: A review. *Amer. J. Med. Sci.* 239:773, 1960.

34. Schlitt, L. E., and Keitel, H. G. Pathogenesis of hyposthenuria in persons with sickle cell anemia or the sickle cell trait. *Pediatrics* 26:249, 1960.

35. Smith, H. W. *The Kidney: Structure and Function in Health and Disease.* New York: Oxford University Press, 1951.

36. Statius Van Eps, L. W., Schouten, H., laPorte-Wijsman, L. W., and Struyker Boudier, A. M. The influence of red blood cell transfusions on the hyposthenuria and renal hemodynamics of sickle cell anemia. *Clin. Chim. Acta* 17:449, 1967.

37. Sweeney, M. J., Dobbins, W. T., and Etteldorf, J. N. Renal disease with elements of the nephrotic syndrome associated with sickle cell anemia. *J. Pediat.* 60:42, 1962.

38. Sydenstricker, V. P. Sickle cell anemia. *Southern Med. J.* 17:177, 1924.

39. Tellem, M., Rubenstone, A. I., and Frumin, A. M. Renal failure and other unusual manifestations in sickle cell trait. *A.M.A. Arch. Path.* 63:508, 1957.

40. Vandepitte, J. Some Remarks on the Pathology of Haemoglobin S. In Jonxis, J. H. P., and Delafresnaye, J. F. (Eds.), *Abnormal Haemoglobins.* (A symposium.) Springfield, Ill.: Thomas, 1959. P. 123.

41. Whitten, C. F., and Younces, A. A. An evaluation of Tm^C H_2O in children with sickle-cell anemia. *A.M.A. Amer. J. Dis. Child.* 96:446, 1958.

42. Whitten, C. F., and Younces, A. A. A comparative study of renal concentrating ability in children with sickle cell anemia and in normal children. *J. Lab. Clin. Med.* 55:400, 1960.

43. Wintrobe, M. *Clinical Hematology* (5th ed.). Philadelphia: Lea & Febiger, 1961. Chap. 13.

44. Wollstein, M., and Kreidel, K. V. Case report: Sickle cell anemia. *Amer. J. Dis. Child.* 36:998, 1928.

45. Yater, W. M., and Hansmann, G. H. Sickle-cell anemia: A new cause of cor pulmonale. *Amer. J. Med. Sci.* 191:474, 1936.

46. Zarafonetis, C. J. D., McMaster, J. D., Molthau, L., and Steiger, W. A. Apparent renal defect in sicklemic individuals. *Amer. J. Med. Sci.* 232:76, 1956.

47. Zarafonetis, C. J. D., Steiger, W. A., Molthau, L., McMaster, J., and Colville, V. F. Renal defect associated with sickle cell trait and sickle cell disease. *J. Lab. Clin. Med.* 44:959, 1954.

34

Genetics in Renal Disease

Gerald T. Perkoff and William S. Sly

That renal disease may be hereditary has been known since the nineteenth century, and several case reports were made then describing patients who were said to have hereditary hematuria, nephritis, or Bright's disease [2, 4–6, 8, 12, 16, 23, 26, 29]. Polycystic disease was described clearly in 1888 [17], and in 1902 Guthrie made the classic report of what we now know as hereditary nephritis [10]. Guthrie's family was restudied by several groups of workers, including Kendall and Hertz [15], who first applied the term "nephritis" to involved members of this family, and by Alport [1], who first recognized the association of nerve deafness with this illness. That functional abnormalities of the kidney could be hereditary was pointed out by Garrod [7], who included cystinuria in the initial group of "inborn errors of metabolism" he described. As late as 1934, however, Osman [22] stated: "It is fortunate that heredity is not a conspicuous feature of those forms of renal disease which occur with any frequency. Indeed, for practical purposes, only two need be considered in this connection — nephritis and polycystic disease of the kidneys."

From this small beginning, the past two decades have seen rapid growth of knowledge. Clinical and biochemical genetics have expanded, and the mechanisms by which genetically determined diseases occur are better understood. It is not surprising, therefore, that the number of diverse renal diseases now known to be hereditary has increased from a few to 30 or more [24]. A classification of the hereditary renal diseases, modified from that presented earlier, follows:

Diffuse Nephropathies in Which Renal Disease Is a Major If Not the Sole Abnormality

Noncystic renal diseases:
- Hereditary chronic nephritis:
  - With nerve deafness and ocular defects
  - Without nerve deafness and ocular defects
  - With polyneuropathy
- Familial hyperprolinemia with renal anomalies
- Familial Mediterranean fever with renal amyloidosis
- Urticaria, deafness, and amyloidosis

Cystic diseases of the kidney
- Polycystic disease
  - In adults
  - In infants
- Cystic disease of the liver and kidneys
- Medullary cystic disease (familial juvenile nephronophthisis)
- Infantile nephrosis

Hereditary functional abnormalities of the kidney
- Abnormalities of the proximal segment of the tubule:
  - Cystinuria
  - Hartnup disease
  - Glycinuria
  - Fanconi syndrome
  - Hypophosphatemia and vitamin D-resistant rickets
  - Renal glycosuria
  - Pseudohypoparathyroidism
  - Cerebrooculorenal dystrophy
- Abnormalities of the distal segment of the tubule:
  - Renal tubular acidosis
  - Nephrogenic diabetes insipidus
- Unspecified renal tubular abnormalities
  - Idiopathic hereditary urolithiasis

Hereditary congenital anomalies and tumors of the genitourinary tract
- Unilateral hydronephrosis
- Congenital megaloureter
- Congenital renal and ear anomalies
- Renal agenesis
- Hypernephroma
- Sarcoma

Review of Current Concepts of Genetics

If the growth in the body of information on hereditary renal diseases has been rapid and impressive, the increase in interest and knowledge in the whole field of genetics has been spectacular. So great have been the recent advances in our understanding of what genes are and how they act that we believe it important to review some aspects of this progress briefly in this chapter to serve as a framework for understanding genetic mechanisms in renal diseases. A suitable source for additional general reading on medical genetics is the recent text of Thompson and Thompson [28] which was written for use by medical students and physicians.

PRESENTLY ACCEPTED PRECEPTS

The current concepts of molecular genetics can best be reviewed by considering a series of presently accepted precepts:

1. *The genetic information resides in the nucleus coded in the deoxyribonucleic acid (DNA).* The earliest evidence for this concept came from experiments of Griffith [9] who reported, in 1928, that mice given rough form, unencapsulated benign pneumococci would die if they also were given heat-killed smooth form, encapsulated organisms. Only smooth virulent forms could be recovered from the dead mice, indicating that the rough forms had been "transformed" to the smooth by something associated with the heat-killed smooth forms given earlier. The change was permanent; recovered smooth forms gave rise to further smooth forms and never to rough. In 1944 Avery et al. [3] demonstrated that the active principle which induced transformation from rough to smooth pneumococci was DNA. Destruction of the DNA in an extract from heat-killed, smooth pneumococci destroyed the transforming capacity of the extract, clearly implicating the DNA as the agent leading to genetic transformation. In 1952 Hershey and Chase [13] reported an ingenious experiment which showed that bacteriophage DNA is all that is injected when a phage infects *Escherichia coli* and that it is this component which carries the information for self-propagation.

2. *The three-dimensional structure of DNA is that of a helical double-stranded molecule composed of two complementary polynucleotide chains.* Chemical analysis of DNA showed

it to be made of purines, pyrimidines, deoxyribose, and phosphate. Two purines, adenine and guanine (A and G), and two pyrimidines, thymine and cytosine (T and C), form the nitrogen bases of DNA. Each base is joined to a deoxyribose group and a phosphate group to form a nucleotide unit. A polynucleotide chain is formed from a series of nucleotides by means of bonds from the sugar of one nucleotide to the phosphate group of another, and so on. Chemical analysis reveals a specific quantitative relationship among the nucleotides. For each nucleotide of adenine, there is one of thymine. For each nucleotide of guanine, there is one of cytosine. Wilkins and Franklin [32] deduced from x-ray diffraction patterns that the DNA structure was helical. Integrating the chemical and x-ray data, Watson and Crick [30], in 1953, proposed the three-dimensional model of DNA structure which did so much to launch the recent era of molecular biology. The double helical model proposed resembles a twisted ladder. Each vertical segment of the ladder is formed by a backbone of alternating phosphate and sugar (deoxyribose) molecules. Forming the rungs of the ladder are the complementary base pairs A=T and G=C. The members of each base pair are attached to one strand of the phosphate-sugar backbone through the deoxyribose by covalent bonds and to their complementary base through weaker hydrogen bonds. Watson and Crick proposed that the two complementary strands could separate and that each strand could serve as template for synthesis of a new complementary strand. The limitations of hydrogen bonding are such that only an A can bond with a T, and only a G with a C. Thus, fidelity of replication is guaranteed by the base sequence of the template on which the complementary strand is assembled. An important prediction of this model for DNA duplication is that one round of replication should produce from one parent molecule two progeny molecules, each identical to the parent molecule, and each having one intact parental strand and one newly synthesized complementary strand. Meselson and Stahl's elegant physical experiments [20] confirmed this prediction for *E. coli* DNA in 1958. Thus, DNA duplication explains one important aspect of transmission of genetic information. In human cells there is an additional well-developed mechanism which aligns the newly doubled chromosomes symmetrically on the mitotic spindle apparatus and guides their division and distribution into daughter cells so that each of the two daughter cells receives an identical complement of 46 chromosomes.

3. *The gene (DNA) directs synthesis of a protein.* The genetic information resides in the nucleus. Yet the ultimate gene products are proteins which are assembled on the ribosomes outside the nucleus. Although some details of the mechanism by which DNA directs protein synthesis still remain to be elucidated, a number of important observations have been made. First, it was found that in vitro protein synthesis appeared to require a special or complementary RNA which resembled DNA in its base sequence. Soon afterward an enzyme which could use the DNA template to produce a complementary RNA was found and purified. Then synthetic polymers of ribopolynucleotides were shown to stimulate amino acid incorporation into polypeptide by cell-free extracts from bacteria or from mammalian tissues, and these synthetic RNA's could satisfy the requirement for a complementary RNA. Furthermore, polyuridylic acid directed only the incorporation of phenylalanine, the product being a peptide chain composed only of phenylalanine. These experiments provided the approach for a systematic and now nearly complete elucidation of the genetic code [21].

Thus, the picture emerged that DNA serves as the template for synthesis of a complementary "messenger" RNA. The messenger RNA molecule leaves the nucleus and binds to the ribosome in the cytoplasm. The ribosome is the structure on which the protein is assembled from "activated" amino acids. The messenger RNA on the ribosome specifies which amino acid can join the growing polypeptide chain by providing a recognition code word to which a "transfer RNA" carrying a specific amino acid can bind and thereby add the amino acid it carries to the growing polypeptide chain.

4. *The genetic code is a nonoverlapping, triplet code, and is universal.* The in vitro studies of Nirenberg and others [21] provided evidence that the genetic code is a nonoverlapping triplet code in which one gene is a double-stranded sequence of nucleotide triplets. The DNA specifies a sequence of nucleotides in messenger RNA that is complementary to one of the two DNA strands. Only one of the two strands in DNA codes for protein synthesis. The sequence of messenger RNA triplets in turn specifies the primary sequence of the protein which is assembled on the ribosome. One triplet code word in the gene is composed of three DNA bases and corresponds to the code word for one specific amino acid. It appears that the same DNA code words are used by all organisms for the same amino acids. Thus, if the average protein is 150 amino acids long, it corresponds to a messenger RNA molecule 150 triplets long (450 nucleotides) and in turn to a gene in the twisted-ladder image that is 450 rungs long. If the genetic information which specifies a protein is a unique sequence of nucleotide triplets in DNA, genetic misinformation produced by mutation represents an alteration in this unique sequence of DNA code words. This change alters either the amount or the structure of the protein specified by that gene. Because most mutations affect one or very few genes, they produce no visible alteration in the chromosome.

5. *Regulation of gene action controls cell differentiation.* It was clear from studies of microorganisms that not all genes are continuously active. Some enzymes (called inducible) are made only in response to the presence of a given substrate. For example, the several linked genes specifying enzymes involved in lactose utilization are simultaneously induced by lactose; the dozen or more closely linked genes involved in histidine biosynthesis are coordinately repressed (turned off) by histidine. These observations led to the formulation of the "operon theory" of gene action which states that blocks of functionally and anatomically linked genes form an operon which is turned on or off as a unit by interaction with a repressor at a key structural site within the operon [14]. From these bacterial studies come precedents for regulatory gene mutations which produce alterations in the rate of synthesis of the gene product, not through an alteration in the structural gene, but through an alteration in a control gene.

The mechanisms of gene regulation governing differentiation of human cell lines are not yet clear, but regulation of gene activity is very important. The DNA in the nucleus of dividing cells is dynamic. During various stages of the cell cycle it varies from being very disperse (interphase), when it is most active in terms of directing protein synthesis, to being tightly folded or coiled, when it is not active in directing protein synthesis. In addition to varying degrees of gene activity during the cell cycle, there is variation in gene expression from cell to cell which leads to cell differentiation. All human somatic cells contain the same amount of genetic material. Thus, the renal tubule cell and the liver cell have the same total genetic information. What determines appearance of specialized function (differentiation) is the selective expression of some genes in one cell type and of other genes in another cell type. Although some genes which are expressed in renal tubular cells probably are also expressed in other cells (e.g., genes for enzymes involved in energy metabolism), expression of certain other genes is probably unique to renal tubular cells (e.g., genes for certain transport proteins). On the other hand, some genes are not expressed at all in renal tubular cells (e.g., hemoglobin genes). In fact the kidney itself is composed of cells of many different cell types, and each cell type probably reflects the expression of a small but very specific group of the total genes present.

Differentiation is related to genetic diseases in several ways. First, certain genes may produce malformations by adversely affecting the delicate process of organ differentiation. Second, failure to activate a given gene may produce a functional loss of the gene product even though the structural gene for the protein is normal. Third, differentiation may partly explain the organ selectivity of certain genetic diseases. The more differentiated a cell line or organ becomes, the more unique its function. A cell line in which a unique genetically determined function is expressed is potentially a target for a genetic disease limited to that organ. A gene expressed in only two or three organs might produce clinical effects, if defective, in only those two or three organs. However, it is also possible for a defective gene which is expressed primarily in one organ to have widespread secondary affects on many organs. Until the basic defect in a genetic disease is established, it is usually difficult to decide whether a "pleiotrophic" gene affects many organs because of loss of one function expressed in all of these organs, or because of loss of a more localized function which produces indirect effects on other more generally distributed biochemical processes.

6. *Patterns of inheritance provide at least a rough clue to genetic mechanisms.* Ultimately the cause of any hereditary disease is the defective gene. Generally speaking it can be assumed that the defective gene normally specifies the primary sequence of a protein or else alters the rate of synthesis of the protein. The protein specified by the defective gene might be a structural protein (e.g., collagen) or an enzyme (e.g., catalase). The normal functional role of the protein in question will determine the biochemical and clinical manifestations of a deficiency or a structural abnormality of that protein.

The biochemical mechanisms by which defective genes produce clinical abnormalities are very diverse. There are storage diseases, transport defects, hemoglobinopathies, and blocks in both biosynthetic and degradative pathways, to mention a few. Even the same clinical finding (e.g., aminoaciduria) can be produced by a variety of different altered genes. One clear example of such genetic heterogeneity is found in the group of diseases called the mucopolysaccharidoses. Although originally thought to be one syndrome (Hurler's), it is now clear that at least six distinct genetic mucopolysaccharidoses can be distinguished on clinical, biochemical, or genetic grounds [19].

In some ways the pattern of inheritance can give a rough clue to the genetic mechanism of an inherited disease. Recessively inherited disorders often are the result of enzyme deficiencies. Thus, one functional gene usually provides sufficient enzyme for the organism to carry out most of its essential biochemical reactions, but loss of both produces disease. Usually no abnormality is seen in the person heterozygous for an enzyme deficiency. However, by direct enzyme assay or by certain indirect provocative tests one can often identify the unaffected carrier of such an enzyme defect. Dominantly inherited conditions less often involve enzymatic proteins. Presumably they more often involve genes specifying structural proteins. In such disorders there often are variable degrees of abnormality despite the presence of one normal gene for the structural protein. Yet, these generalizations have their exceptions. Transport proteins, for example, have properties of both structural proteins and enzymes. In some of the diseases to be discussed, both the mode of inheritance and the biochemical mechanisms are reasonably well understood. In many, however, the mechanism by which the defective gene produces the clinical illness has yet to be established.

7. *Recognizable chromosome aberrations are NOT involved in most hereditary renal diseases.* It is important to remember that most inherited diseases result from alterations involving a small segment of the DNA of a single gene. Thus, no visible chromosome aberration is to be expected. On the other hand, a morphologically abnormal chromosome with either a deficiency (deletion) or excess of chromosome material that is large enough to detect microscopically implies an imbalance of a sizable number of genes. Such chromosome abnormalities often produce birth defects involving many organs, one of which may be the kidney. Thus, although chromosome studies are usually not informative in the recognized simply-inherited renal diseases, they may be helpful in patients with a renal lesion associated with multiple birth defects, whether or not the multiple birth defects appear to be inherited.

Several abnormalities of chromosome number with an extra chromosome are compatible with life. These are not hereditary in the usual sense but result from accidents in germ cell formation and can be considered chromosome packaging errors. A gamete with an extra chromosome can unite with a normal gamete to produce a zygote with 47 chromosomes. Such an individual may be viable if the extra chromosome is a chromosome number 21, 18, 13–15, a Y, or an X. Although an additional chromosome 21 causes mongolism and may produce up to 50 congenital malformations, the kidney is not often involved. In contrast, trisomy E_1 (trisomy 18) and trisomy D_1 (trisomy 13–15) each produces a characteristic clinical syndrome with multiple birth defects and with a high incidence of renal anomalies [25, 27]. A monosomy (a missing member of a pair of chromosomes) appears to be compatible with life only if the missing member is a sex chromosome. Patients with only one sex chromosome (45, XO) have Turner's syndrome. Although they have a female phenotype, they have short stature, ovarian dysgenesis, and a variable number of other abnormalities including web-neck, sexual infantilism, and cubitus valgus. Two-thirds of 25 children with proved XO karyotype were found to have genitourinary anomalies [18].

Comments

It is hoped that this brief chapter will serve as an introduction to this complex, interesting, and rapidly changing subject and that it will provide a framework of orientation for the reader in relation to the specific disease descriptions which follow. Much more is known now than at the time of the earlier edition of this book. It is particularly encouraging to note that study of the hereditary functional abnormalities of the kidney has increased our understanding of the mechanisms of renal function and that new technics applied to such disorders as cystic diseases of the kidney have provided much information about renal development. Further study of this group of renal diseases no doubt will be of great value.

References

1. Alport, A. C. Hereditary familial congenital haemorrhagic nephritis. *Brit. Med. J.* 1: 504, 1927.
2. Attlee, W. H. W. Three cases of recurrent haematuria occurring in one family. *St. Bart. Hosp. Journal* 9:41, 1901.
3. Avery, O. T., Macleod, C. M., and McCarty, M. Studies on chemical nature of substance inducing transformation by desoxyribonucleic acid fraction isolated from Pneumococcus Type III. *J. Exp. Med.* 79: 137, 1944.
4. Brill, N. E., and Libman, E. A contribution to the subject of chronic interstitial

nephritis and arteritis in the young, and family nephritis, with a note on calcification in the liver. *J. Exp. Med.* 4:541, 1899.

5. Eichhorst, H. In Senator H. (Ed.), *Erkrankungen der Nieren. Spezielle Pathologie und Therapie.* Vienna: Nothnagel, 1899. Vol. 19, p. 249.
6. Forster, R. Über Schrumpfniere im Kindesalter. *Jb. Kinderheilk.* 26:38, 1887.
7. Garrod, A. E. Inborn errors of metabolism. *Lancet* 2:1908 (Lecture I, p. 1; Lecture II, p. 73; Lecture III, p. 142; Lecture IV, p. 214).
8. Goodheart, J. F. In Keating, J. M. (Ed.), *Acute and Chronic Bright's Disease.* Vol. 3. *Cyclopedia of Diseases of Children.* Philadelphia: Lippincott, 1890. P. 532.
9. Griffith, F. The significance of pneumococcal types. *J. Hyg.* (Camb.) 27:113, 1928.
10. Guthrie, L. G. "Idiopathic" or congenital hereditary and family haematuria. *Lancet* 1:1243, 1902.
11. Hartman, P. E., and Suskind, S. R. *Gene Action.* Englewood Cliffs, N.J.: Prentice Hall, 1965.
12. Hellendall, H. Hereditare Schrumpfnieren im frehen Kindewaiter. *Arch. Kinderheilk.* 22:61, 1882.
13. Hershey, A. D., and Chase, M. Independent functions of viral protein and nucleic acid in growth of bacteriophage. *J. Gen. Physiol.* 36:39, 1952.
14. Jacob, F., and Monod, J. Genetic regulatory mechanisms in the synthesis of proteins. *J. Molec. Biol.* 3:318, 1961.
15. Kendall, G., and Hertz, A. C. Hereditary familial congenital haemorrhagic nephritis. *Guy. Hosp. Rep.* 66:137, 1962.
16. Kidd, J. The inheritance of Bright's disease of the kidney. *Practitioner* 29:104, 1882.
17. Lejars, F. *Du Gros Rein Polykystique de l'Adulte.* Paris: Steinhill, 1888.
18. Lemli, L., and Smith, D. W. The XO syndrome: A study of the differentiated phenotype in 25 patients. *J. Pediat.* 63:577, 1963.
19. Mellman, W. J. The genetic basis for the variability of genetic diseases. *J. Pediat.* 72:727, 1968.
20. Meselson, M., and Stahl, F. W. The replication of DNA in *Escherichia coli. Proc. Nat. Acad. Sci. U.S.A.* 44:671, 1958.
21. Nirenberg, M., Casky, T., Marshall, R., Brimacombe, R., Kellog, D., Doctor, B., Hatfield, D., Levin, J., Rottman, F., Pestaka, S., Wilcox, M., and Anderson, F. The RNA code and protein synthesis. *Cold Spring Harbor Sympos. Quant. Biol.* 31:11, 1966.
22. Osman, A. A. Hereditary Renal Diseases. In Blacker, C. P. (Ed.), *The Chances of Morbid Inheritance.* Baltimore: Wood, 1934. P. 449.
23. Pel, P. K. Die Erblichkeit der chronischen Nephritis. *Z. Klin. Med.* 38:127, 1899.
24. Perkoff, G. T. The hereditary renal diseases. *New Eng. J. Med.* 277:79, 129, 1967.
25. Rohde, R. A., Hodgman, J. E., Cleland, R. S. Multiple congenital anomalies in the E_1 trisomy (Group 16–18) syndrome. *Pediatrics* 33:258, 1964.
26. Romme, R. L'heredite dans la nephrite chronique. *Presse Med.* 2:362, 1899.
27. Smith, D. W., Patau, K., Thermau, E., Inhorn, S., and DeMars, R. The D_1 syndrome. *J. Pediat.* 62:326, 1963.
28. Thompson, J. S., and Thompson, M. W. *Genetics in Medicine.* Philadelphia: Saunders, 1967.
29. Tyson, J. *A Treatise on Bright's Disease and Diabetes, with Special Reference to Pathology and Therapeutics, Including a Section on Retinitis and Bright's Disease.* Philadelphia: Lindsay & Blakiston, 1881. P. 166.
30. Watson, J. D., and Crick, F. H. C. Molecular structure of nucleic acids — a structure for deoxyribose nucleic acid. *Nature* (London) 171:737, 1953.
31. Whalen, R. E., and McIntosh, H. D. Spectrum of hereditary renal diseases. *Amer. J. Med.* 33:282, 1962.
32. Wilkins, M. H. F., and Franklin, N. Unpublished observations. Quoted by Watson, J., and Crick, F. H. C. [30].
33. Zubay, G. Molecular model of protein synthesis. *Science* 140:1092, 1963.

35

Polycystic Disease of the Kidneys

O. Z. Dalgaard

Bilateral polycystic kidneys, by far the most important developmental disturbance in the architecture of the renal parenchyma, are found in two forms, one in adults and the other in infants and children. Since the two forms have different modes of inheritance and different clinical manifestations, these aspects will be discussed independently.

This remarkable malformation has attracted the attention of so many investigators since the first French description that the literature is voluminous. The classic monograph of Lejars [62] in 1888 deserves mention. Case reports and clinical studies have appeared with increasing frequency since that date, among the most illuminating of which has been a series of outstanding works from the Mayo Clinic: Braasch [14] on clinical data, Schacht [97] on hypertension, Braasch and Schacht [15] on pathology and clinical findings, Walthers and Braasch [108] on surgical treatment, Braasch and Hendrick [16] on classification of cysts, Rall and Odel [89] on clinical findings, Comfort et al. [28] on polycystic liver, and Simon and Thompson [99] on clinical manifestations. To avoid a laborious chronological exposition, the most important observations of the various authors are referred to in the clinical analysis of the individual problems and in the discussion of my series of 350 cases of bilateral polycystic disease of the kidney in adults.

Definition and Classification

A polycystic kidney is a kidney the tissue of which is displaced by a large number of tightly packed cysts so that the cystic volume predominates over the solid parts to a considerable degree. In outward appearance it can best be compared to a bunch of grapes [65]. Macroscopically, or often only microscopically, small islands of normal, secreting kidney parenchyma are seen between the individual cysts. In most cases a considerable increase in kidney size results from the cyst formation. The size of the cysts is in no way dependent on the age of the patient. Very large polycystic kidneys may be found in infants, and hypoplastic kidneys with cyst formation in older children and adults. Not infrequently polycystic kidneys attain an enormous size and weight. Nonetheless they retain normal kidney shape and fibrous capsule, although the surface is irregular and knobby as a result of the cysts, which can vary in size from the microscopic to that of a closed fist, and may project above the level of the kidney tissue. On the cut surface the cysts are often so closely packed that there are only narrow partitions between them. In some polycystic kidneys the cut surface has a honeycomb appearance (see Fig. 35-1).

The cyst wall is usually covered with flat epithelial cells, but in the case of large cysts only by the remains of epithelium. On the inner walls there are often bulges from projecting ridges containing ground substance resembling connective tissue, in which glomeruli and renal tubules are found, often partly atrophic or incompletely developed, but in many cases quite normal.

Lambert's studies [60, 61] are of great interest. On the basis of careful serial sections of cystic nephrons in four adult cases of polycystic kidneys, he described three groups of cysts, according to their anatomic localization: glomerular, tubular, and excretory cysts. The glomerular cysts are always closed units, whereas both the tubular and the excretory cysts may communicate with tubules which presumably drain into the kidney pelvis. In the infantile form of polycystic kidneys, only closed cysts are found. Osathanondh and Potter [78a] suggest that there are four types of polycystic kidneys on the basis of microdissection of the kidneys of 30 patients: type 1, caused by hyperplasia of interstitial portions of collecting tubules (this condition is always bilateral and is fatal soon after birth); type 2, caused by inhibition of ampullary activity; type 3, owing to multiple abnormalities of development; and type 4, caused by urethral obstruction.

The content of the cysts varies in color from clear light yellow, resembling urine, to dark brown or yellowish-red after hemorrhage and after changes in the blood pigment. It may be thick as a result of inflammation; it may contain protein, be shiny from cholesterol deposits, or be cloudy from calcium precipitates. Urine constituents can often be demonstrated.

Cystic nephrons [60] in adults retain their function and take part in the formation of

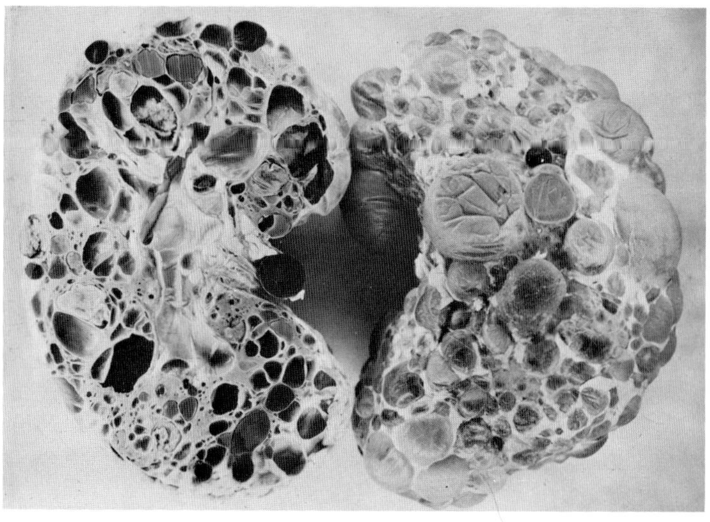

Figure 35-1. Bilateral polycystic disease of the kidneys in a 49-year-old woman.

urine. Bricker and Patton [17] carried out studies involving, among others, inulin, para-aminohippurate, and endogenous creatinine determinations at the time of surgical operation on six adults with polycystic kidneys, on a 21-month-old child, and on five patients with simple cysts of the kidney. Many of the cysts in the polycystic kidneys of the adults, and some of the cysts in the child's kidneys, were in functional connection with open nephrons. Simple cysts, on the other hand, did not seem to have this connection.

The significance of the participation of the cystic nephrons in the maintenance of the renal function is unknown. The polycystic conversion of the kidneys ultimately leads to death of the patient in uremia.

Other Types of Renal Cysts

The existence of the unilateral polycystic kidney is doubted by some authors, but it is a fact that it is found both in adults and in children. Several cases have been reported in which an apparently normal kidney became large and polycystic many years after its polycystic mate was removed [8, 73a]. Bell [8] notes that the unilateral polycystic kidney is very much smaller than the bilateral type, but that the destruction of the parenchyma is just as complete. He therefore prefers to classify these kidneys as hypoplastic kidneys, since hypoplasia is their most outstanding characteristic. He found a frequency of approximately 8 per cent.

Braasch and Hendrick [16] classify the various other forms of kidney cysts as follows: (1) retention or inflammatory cysts (usually of little or no significance); (2) simple cysts (single, multiple, multilocular, and hemorrhagic); (3) peripelvic (pyelogenic) cysts; (4) parapelvic cysts; (5) cysts secondary to pathologic changes in the kidney (calculus, hypernephroma, tuberculosis, pyelonephritis, hematoma, and echinococcus).

Careful examination of adult kidneys at autopsy reveals that over 50 per cent contain one or more small macroscopic cysts. These cysts seldom cause complications. (The best studies concerning such cysts are those by Bell [8], Braasch and Hendrick [16], Glaser [38], and Hepler [50].) Although there may be 8 to 10 large simple cysts in a kidney, such multiple cysts do not represent a hereditary disease [16]. If there are many small simple cysts, it may be difficult to distinguish the disease from an early and mild stage of polycystic kidneys which has not progressed enough to cause renal insufficiency.

The term *multilocular cysts* designates large cysts split into multiple minor compartments. They must not be confused with unilateral polycystic kidneys. Excellent reports on this subject have been made [37, 87]. Occasionally a hypernephroma contains cysts, and can be confused with simple cysts [16, 20].

Peripelvic cysts lie adjacent to the kidney pelvis and communicate with it directly, usually through a calyx, whereas parapelvic cysts are located adjacent to the kidney pelvis without being directly connected with it [16].

In their monograph on congenital multicystic dysplasia, Parkkulainen et al. [80] discuss the differential diagnosis of this congenital disorder from true polycystic disease, in which the connective tissue is normal and does not contain any primitive dysplastic structures.

Microcystic disease of the renal medulla is described in Chapter 36.

Frequency of Bilateral Polycystic Kidneys in Adults

The frequency of polycystic kidneys in clinical material and the frequency of polycystic kidneys at autopsy are shown in Tables 35-1 and 35-2. The clinical figures are naturally not directly comparable with the figures from autopsies.

Table 35-1. Frequency of Polycystic Kidneys in Adults from Clinical Material

Year	Author	Clinic	Number of Polycystic Kidneys/Number of Admissions	Ratio
1925	Cairns	London Hospital	79:389,773	1:4933
1933	Braasch & Schacht	Mayo Clinic	193:680,000	1:3523
1934	Oppenheimer[a]	Mount Sinai Hospital, N.Y.	60:220,000	1:3666
1949	Fergusson[a]	Central Middlesex Hospital, England	29:c. 100,000	1:3500
1952	Higgins	Cleveland Clinic		1:4000
1954	Arrigoni et al.	Istituto di Urologia, Milano	24:8211	1:342
1955	Simon & Thompson	Mayo Clinic	366:?	1:2438

[a] A few cases of polycystic kidneys in infants and children are included.

The frequency of polycystic kidneys based on autopsy varies greatly in different reports, depending in part on whether kidneys have been included which (1) are full of cysts but still have enough parenchyma for normal functioning, (2) are involved unilaterally, or (3) are only partly replaced by cysts. The frequency likewise depends on the age distribution of the autopsy material, and on how many stillbirths and young infants are included [8].

The morbid risk (or disease expectancy) of developing polycystic kidneys by 80 years of age is estimated as being less than 1 per 1000 [29].

Etiology and Pathogenesis

The innumerable theories concerning the etiology of polycystic kidneys in adults and infants have been summarized very clearly and comprehensively by Berner [9] and Lambert [60]. Almost all investigators have adopted the point of view that the most important causal element is a hereditary factor, both in the congenital form of the disease and in the adult form. Steiner [103] was the first to conclude that an "outstandingly hereditary character" was the cause of polycystic kidneys.

On the question of pathogenesis, practically every author has his own theory. These can

Table 35-2. Frequency of Polycystic Kidneys in Adults at Autopsy

Year	Author	Place	Number of Polycystic Kidneys/Number of Autopsies	Ratio
1897	Naumann	Kiel	16:10,177	1:636
1928	Ssokoloff	Leningrad	192:50,198	1:261
1933	Braasch & Schacht	Mayo Clinic	9:9171	1:1019
1933	Roscher	Oslo	7:3995	1:571
1934	Oppenheimer[a]	Mount Sinai Hospital, N.Y.	14:6000	1:428
1935	Pabst[a]	Göttingen	38:8423	1:222
1949	Fergusson[a]	Central Middlesex Hospital, England	16:c. 6000	1:375
1950	Bell	Minnesota	70:54,552	1:779
1954	Dalgaard	Copenhagen	143:98,000	1:773
1955	Simon & Thompson	Mayo Clinic	35:?	1:323

[a] A few cases of polycystic kidneys in infants and children are included.

be put into the following groups: retention theories, malformation theories, tumor theories, and "combination" theories. It would be unreasonable to go further into all these more or less fantastic ideas here, as they are pure speculation. Lambert's classic work [60] may be consulted for summaries. In short, nothing certain is known about the pathogenesis.

Inheritance

Polycystic kidneys in adults show a regular autosomal dominant heredity [4, 24, 34, 109], while polycystic kidneys in infants appear to be due to an autosomal recessive, at least in some families [19, 22, 72, 100, 110, 112] (see Fig. 35-2).

The dominant gene has an extraordinarily high penetrance (in the pathologic-anatomic sense), being in the neighborhood of 100 per cent if the individual lives to the age of 80. When the clinical tracing of the genetic carriers becomes more refined, this high penetrance percentage will also be revealed clinically in an earlier age group, so that the risk curve will have a steeper form and approach more and more the theoretically expected [29].

On the basis of data showing concordance and discordance between the right and left sides of the body, the estimated penetrance appears to be extraordinarily high [29]. The use of studies of twins to appraise the intimate interplay between nature and nurture is unique, but it has not yet been possible to collect enough unbiased findings in twins to elucidate interplay between heredity and environment or determine the penetrance [29].

The genetically determined disease process is latent for many years and then becomes manifest in a kidney tissue that has apparently developed and functioned normally. Cyst formation usually occurs synchronously in the two kidneys and proceeds at more or less the same pace in each, although deviations occur, particularly in the early stages, resulting in asymmetry between the two sides. An intrafamily correlation is found, since there appears to be a similarity in the onset, clinical course, and picture of the disease [29] as it manifests itself in different members of the family. The reasons may lie partly in the genes themselves, partly in environmental influences; it has not been possible to analyze the extent to which each is responsible. The theory that has been advanced, without sound basis, that polycystic kidneys occur at an increasingly earlier age from generation to generation (anticipation) must be rejected [29].

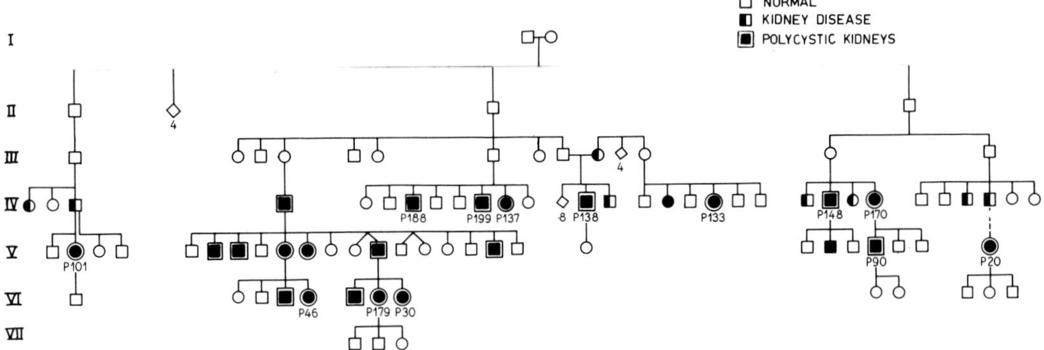

Figure 35-2. Polycystic kidneys in the direct line in three generations. Two families with polycystic kidneys have intermarried.

By Haldane's indirect method [45], based on determinations of the incidence of the malformation in the general population and the relative fitness,* the spontaneous mutation rate is calculated as being 6.5×10^{-5} to 12×10^{-5} mutations per gene per generation [29].

Liver cysts are found in one-third of individuals with polycystic kidneys. Because of the rarity of polycystic disease of the liver in the general population, it is evident that there must be an etiologic association between polycystic kidneys and polycystic liver. Many investigations suggest a significant association between polycystic kidneys and aneurysm of the basal arteries of the brain. It appears more likely that the malformations are caused by a single gene with multiple effects modified by environmental factors and by other genes than that they are caused by different closely linked genes. In the syndrome of malformations — polycystic kidneys, polycystic liver, and congenital aneurysm of the basal arteries of the brain — there is a wide variation in the frequency with which polycystic liver appears but congenital aneurysm appears only rarely [29]. The quantitative variations in the expression of the malformation (the expressivity) are discussed in detail in the clinical section. The cause of the qualitative variations in the genetic effect (the specificity) can lie partly in the genes themselves, partly in the influence of neighboring genes, and partly in environmental factors. The gene of polycystic kidneys in adults cannot be placed on the sex chromosome, as there is no sex linkage, complete or partial [29]. It either lies on another autosome than the genes for seven blood groups thus far investigated, or its distance from these is considerable if they do lie on the same autosome [46].

* The relative fitness is considered equal to the product of the "relative reproductive span" [91] and the reproductive capacity.

Gross Pathologic Findings

Autopsy was carried out in my series in 173 cases. In 157 it was reported that both kidneys were enlarged, and in three cases that one kidney only was enlarged.

Cysts of the liver were found in 43 per cent. There were occasional cysts in other organs — ovarian cysts in four cases, cysts of the uterus in one, an esophageal cyst in one, a cerebral cyst in one, and a cerebellar cyst in one.

In 50 per cent, the weight of the heart was greater than 1/200 of the body weight, or it was stated that the heart was enlarged. These data correspond closely to the finding of Rall and Odel [89] of hypertrophy of the heart in 52 per cent. Sieber [98] found 48 cases of hypertrophy of the heart in 140 autopsies, but observed rightly that the figure presumably would be greater still if a detailed autopsy report were available in every case.

Coronary thrombosis with acute myocardial infarction was found in only 3 per cent, although coronary arteriosclerosis was found in 40 per cent.

Cerebral hemorrhage was found in 11 per cent. This figure corresponds to that of Rall and Odel [89], who found cerebral hemorrhage in 9 per cent. (Raaschou [88] found the same frequency of cerebral hemorrhage in a series of autopsies on patients without polycystic disease.) Subarachnoid hemorrhage was found in a further 4 per cent. Renal calculus was found in 11 per cent. Renal cancer and horseshoe kidney were each found once.

Oppenheimer [78] divided inflammation into three main types. In the first type pyelitis, pyelonephritis, and infected hydronephrosis are present. In my series 20 cases of this type were found. The second type is characterized by purulent infection localized in the individual cysts; four such cases were encountered. In the third type, diffuse infection of the remaining parenchyma and of the cysts (pyonephrosis) is found, with occasional complicating perforation and perinephritic abscess. Five cases were found in my material.

Diagnosis

In the diagnosis of polycystic kidneys, the skill of the physician may be tested severely. It is not remarkable that the condition is often first demonstrated unexpectedly at operation or autopsy (in my series 134 of 350 cases were discovered at autopsy). In advanced cases, however, the diagnosis is usually not difficult, provided the disease is kept in mind. The most important desideratum is a thorough family history.

The palpation of both kidney regions must be carried out thoroughly. In the earlier stages, the disease is perhaps not considered, either because of lack of symptoms or because the kidneys cannot be palpated. At this stage the diagnosis can be made only by urography. If both kidneys are enlarged, the diagnosis usually presents little difficulty. When only one kidney is enlarged, diagnostic difficulties arise, and the disease is frequently confused with tumor and hydronephrosis. It is not unusual to find a pronounced difference of size even when both kidneys are enlarged. There may also be a pronounced difference in their function. When the disease is demonstrated in only one kidney, whether by palpation or urography, it does not follow that it is not bilateral. When neither of the kidneys is enlarged, the diagnosis is even more difficult. Urography may then provide the correct diagnosis, but the erroneous diagnosis of chronic glomerulonephritis or nephrosclerosis is common.

If a history is given of intermittent hematuria, lumbar pain, or pyuria, pointing to renal disease, the patient should undergo a complete urologic examination. A urologic examination is necessary also when hypertension is present, to eliminate not only the diagnosis of unilateral renal disease but also the diagnosis of polycystic kidneys [52]. Urine analysis, renal function tests, and blood examinations are of little diagnostic value early in the disease. If reduced renal function should be demonstrated, however, radiologic examination may provide the correct diagnosis.

RADIOLOGIC APPEARANCE

The cysts are localized in the kidney parenchyma, and in the majority of cases the size of the kidney is increased. This characteristic is the basis of diagnosis of polycystic kidneys by radiology. The methods of radiologic investigation available today and their use in the diagnosis of polycystic kidneys will be briefly mentioned.

The outer surface of the kidney has a characteristic appearance due to the cysts, which may sometimes be seen in a preliminary film of the abdomen, by tomography, possibly combined with intravenous urography or retrograde pyelography, and by retroperitoneal insufflation of carbon dioxide presacrally, possibly combined with urography or pyelography, although this is rarely required.

Furthermore, the cysts may deform the inner surface of the kidney parenchyma toward the kidney pelvis and calyces. These changes will be revealed by retrograde pyelography and intravenous urography, both possibly combined with tomography. If the kidney parenchyma becomes filled with cysts, the kidney blood vessels are deformed and partly atrophic, and these alterations may be seen by aortography. Finally, it is possible to visualize the kidney parenchyma itself by nephrography, by nephrotomography, and in the nephrographic phase of aortography.

Hickel and Cornet [51] have subdivided polycystic kidneys into three clinical-radiologic forms: (1) those which are easy to diagnose clinically and radiologically (the kidneys are palpable, enlarged, and knobby; the deformities of the kidney pelvis and calyces are clas-

Table 35-3. Frequency of Symptoms of Polycystic Kidneys from Case Histories of 350 Adults

Symptoms	Of 350 Persons		Of 254 Deceased Persons		Of 96 Living Persons		Of 193 Males		Of 157 Females	
	Number with Symptom	Per Cent with Symptom	Number with Symptom	Per Cent with Symptom	Number with Symptom	Per Cent with Symptom	Number with Symptom	Per Cent with Symptom	Number with Symptom	Per Cent with Symptom
Pain & indefinite abdominal symptoms	208	59	141	56	67	70	133	69	75	48
Renal colic & possible passage of stone	64	18	38	15	26	27	26	14	38	24
Hematuria	158	45	113	44	45	47	82	43	76	48
Cardiovascular symptoms, including hypertension	162	46	120	47	42	44	90	47	72	46
Uremia	154	44	148	58	6	6	99	51	55	35
Palpable tumor	213	61	152	60	61	64	141	73	72	46
Proteinuria	261	75	199	78	63	66	160	83	101	64
Pyuria & bacteriuria	160	46	119	47	41	43	120	62	40	26
Renal insufficiency	110	32	104	41	6	6	65	34	45	29

sic and bilateral; the clinical diagnosis is usually made before the radiologic diagnosis); (2) those which are difficult to diagnose (the kidneys are not palpable; the result of laboratory examination is not convincing; the radiologic anomalies are not pronounced and are liable to be overlooked; or the radiologic picture at first sight is only pathologic on one side); and (3) those in which it is impossible to make the diagnosis (the clinical and laboratory signs are unconvincing; the radiologic signs are without decisive value — small cysts).

Figures 35-3, 35-4, and 35-5 are roentgen pictures selected to show the greatest and most typical changes.

Enlargement of one or both kidneys, although frequently found [2], is not, however, diagnostic, since a kidney without cysts can be enlarged because of congenital anomalies, hydronephrosis, or unilateral hyperplasia due to a nonfunctioning or absent mate. The scalloped outline characteristic of a polycystic kidney may be seen in noncystic kidneys as a result of scars or persisting fetal lobulation.

Parenchymal thickening of over 3 cm., providing it is not caused by a locally expanding process, is stressed by Billing [11] as practically pathognomonic of polycystic kidney. He pointed out that the "worm-eaten" parenchyma seen in a nephrogram made by aortography is also pathognomonic. The calyces can be elongated [2]. The cysts press the calyces from their normal course, so that they become tortuous and run in unusual directions. The necks of the calyces become slender, elongated, and curved. The calyx can also show a club- or

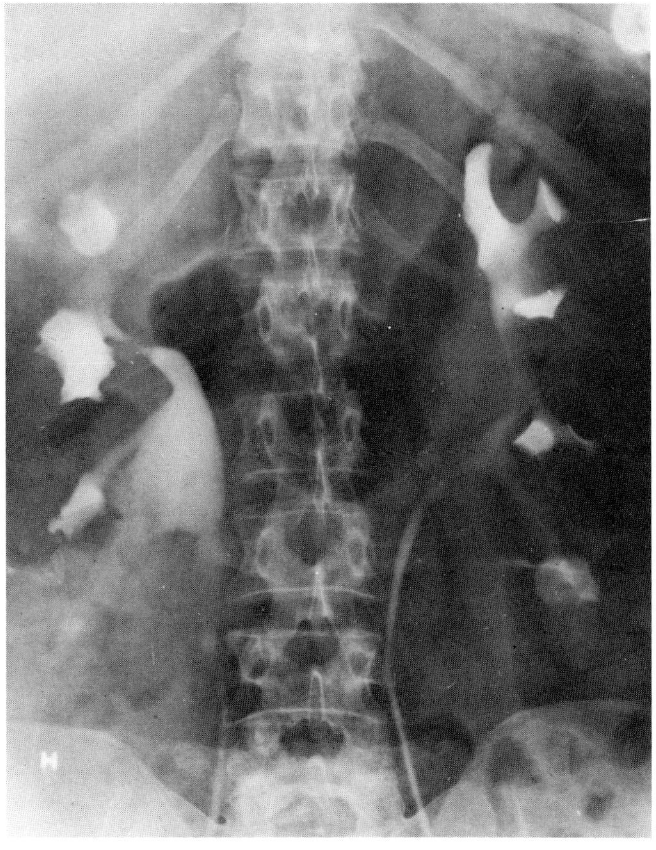

Figure 35-3. Both kidneys are enormously large in this pyelogram, the left one being 19 cm. long. The calyces are elongated and dislocated from each other. The longitudinal axes of the pelves are parallel to the vertebral column.

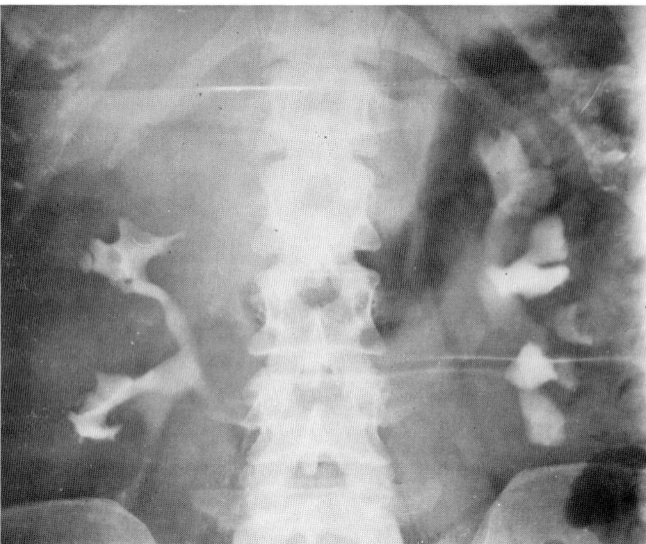

Figure 35-4. On the left side the calyces are plump and broadened, particularly above. On the right side an enlarged, coarsely humped kidney shadow is seen. The calyces here are elongated, slender, distorted, and dislocated from each other.

flask-shaped expansion [42]. A bowl-shaped deformation of the calyx develops when large cysts cause the papilla to arch forward into the calyx [47]. The lunate form occurs when smaller cysts project into the wall of the flask-shaped expanded calyx [109]. The fornices also undergo changes in configuration [14], becoming flattened and broadened when the cysts expand the papilla. Extension of the kidney pelvis itself can occur along with the enlargement of the kidney [2]. Multiple cyst impressions can be seen in the pelvis, and the pelvis can be horn-shaped [11]. The superior and inferior main calyx can lie at right angles to the kidney pelvis [49]. A lateral displacement of the kidney can arise, so that the kidney is axially rotated, with its longitudinal axis no longer parallel to the lateral border of the psoas muscle but more parallel to the spinal column.

As mentioned previously, it may be impossible to draw a sharp line between the variation in width seen in normal pyelograms and that which is characteristic for polycystic kidneys. Henninger and Weiss [49] stressed in this connection the significance of the personal experience and intuition of the investigator. A painstaking analysis of the pyelogram of the least modified kidney in cases of anatomically asymmetric development is the most important basis for a correct appreciation of the early radiologic stages.

If the pyelogram shows suspicious conditions only on one side, with the other side normal, or if the suspected abnormality on the one side is restricted to a portion of the pyelogram — for example, to only an extension of one calyceal neck — then other diagnoses must be considered. The aim of the roentgenologist should be to diagnose polycystic kidneys with such certainty that operation for suspected tumor will not be required [43].

Recent investigations [33] suggest that in the future it may be possible to make the diagnosis earlier than at present. By the method of Evans et al. [33], in which intravenous urography with large quantities of contrast medium is combined with tomography, exact delineation of the actual kidney morphology should be possible. This composite technic is termed nephrotomography, and when further developed will undoubtedly have great value

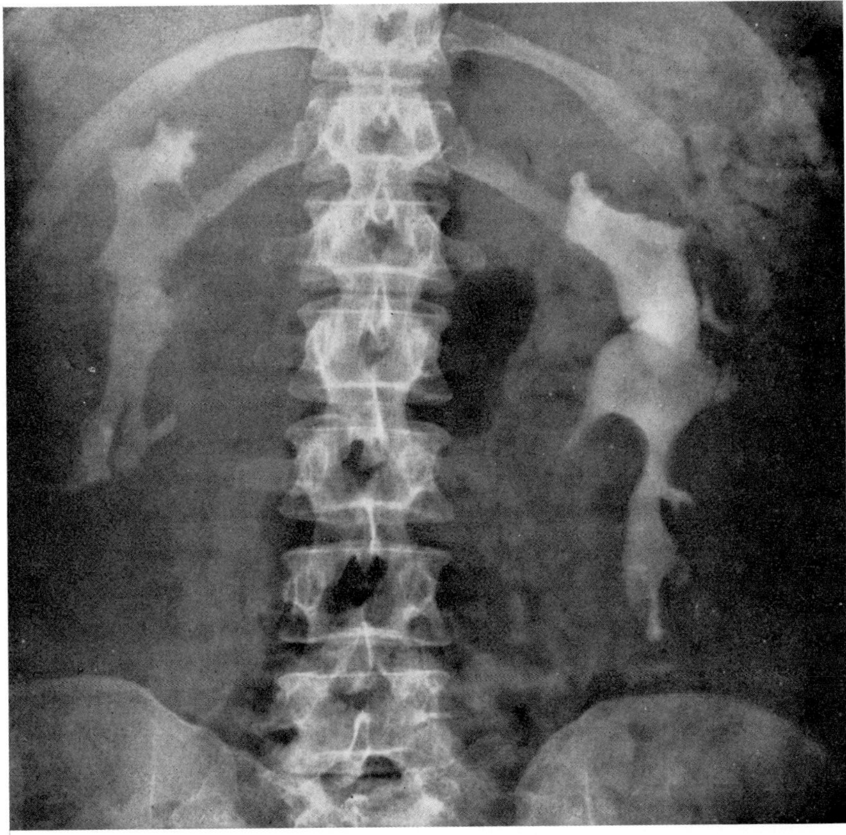

Figure 35-5. The kidneys in this pyelogram are considerably enlarged (the left one 16.5 cm. long). They are displaced laterally. There are multiple cyst impressions. The longitudinal axes are parallel to the vertebral column.

in the differential diagnosis between cysts and neoplasms. Isotope-scan will demonstrate the increased size of the kidney, and the cystic areas will be indicated by areas of diminished or absent radioactivity.

It is important to keep in mind that no matter how great the diagnostic value of a urogram may be, it cannot be used for prognosis, since the urogram shows only the gross anatomic changes, the development of which need not run parallel with the functional impairment. It is the latter which is of particular significance for the prognosis.

No doubt in the future renal biopsy will enable earlier diagnosis than any radiologic method permits.

DIFFERENTIAL DIAGNOSIS

The most important differential diagnosis by far is between neoplasms of the kidney and polycystic kidneys. As polycystic kidneys and neoplasms of the kidney can show precisely the same symptoms, and as the classic symptoms of polycystic disease are far from always present, diagnostic uncertainty is common. Since neoplasms of the kidney are very seldom bilateral, the presence of bilateral, palpable enlargement of the kidneys argues against tumor, as do bilateral pyelographic changes.

Patients with chronic pyelonephritis can show all the symptoms of patients with polycystic kidneys, but cases of primary chronic pyelonephritis with enlarged kidneys probably do not occur. The disease can also be confused with chronic glomerulonephritis. When hypertension is the major manifestation, the malformation can be erroneously diagnosed as nephrosclerosis.

The differential diagnosis between polycystic kidneys and pyonephrosis has been discussed exhaustively by Goldstein and Klotz [40]. If symptoms of pyonephrosis are found in both kidneys, a diagnosis of bilateral polycystic kidneys must primarily be considered, because this disease is much more frequent than bilateral pyonephrosis in otherwise normal kidneys. The diagnosis of polycystic kidneys should be made tentatively when there are reduced kidney function and typical changes in the pyelograms on both sides. If these are present together with pyuria from one or both kidneys, the diagnosis of pyonephrosis in polycystic kidneys is obvious. If there are symptoms of pyonephrosis on the one side and symptoms typical of uncomplicated polycystic kidney on the other side, the diagnosis of polycystic kidneys must be made, as this disease is almost always bilateral. Pyonephrosis without polycystic kidney should be suspected when the retrograde pyelogram does not show the typical signs of polycystic kidneys.

In the differential diagnosis from bilateral hydronephrosis, it must be remembered that there is usually no reason for dilated pelves in the case of polycystic kidneys unless there is accompanying bilateral obstruction of the ureters or obstruction of the bladder.

Innumerable other faulty diagnoses have been reported, some of them other kidney diseases, such as solitary cysts of the kidney, echinococcal cysts of the kidney, and nephroptosis, and occasionally tumors and cysts in other abdominal organs [5, 30, 98, 102, 105]

Clinical Aspects

FORMS OF THE DISEASE

Numerous authors have attempted to group the disease into various clinical forms. Albarran and Imbert [3] recognized three forms: (1) *forme urémique,* characterized by indefinite general symptoms and the sudden occurrence of symptoms of uremic intoxication, generally leading to death within eight days and at the latest after three weeks; (2) *forme Brightique,* the clinical picture developing as in Bright's disease and characterized by edema, hypertension, and hypertrophy of the heart, the course being very protracted and even extending over a period of 20 years; (3) *forme rénale chirurgicale,* characterized in most cases by unilateral, periodically recurring renal colic and leading within one to three years to death in uremia.

Maier [68] classified the disease into two forms, one with predominantly systemic manifestations, and a second with symptoms suggesting those forms of renal disease in which mechanical disturbances, hematuria, anuria, or uremic symptoms also appear. Braasch [14] distinguished three stages: (1) the latent stage, (2) the stage of kidney enlargement and hematuria, and (3) the stage with uremia.

Talman [105] found three main types: (1) cases in which the disease takes a symptom-free course; (2) cases with renal insufficiency, and (3) cases with secondary manifestations or complications (e.g., symptoms of pressure on neighboring organs, nephroptosis, and so on). Bell [8] found three types: (1) an early type, in which the disease can be diagnosed either by finding palpable kidneys before any symptoms have developed — although the kidneys are usually not palpable before the onset of symptoms — or, often, by an abnormal urogram in the absence of clinical symptoms; (2) the surgical type, in which there is a palpable kidney with localized pain, fever, leukocytosis, and sometimes hematuria with bleeding from one kidney only; (3) the medical type, in which the symptoms are those of renal insufficiency and the clinical picture is that found in chronic glomerulonephritis or pyelonephritis. The onset of uremia may be sudden, but more often it develops slowly over a period of years. Oppenheimer [78] subdivided the disease into no fewer than eight clinical forms.

In my own attempt at a classification of the disease into various clinical groups, it has been impossible to arrange a more specific grouping than a rough classification into three stages: a first stage, in which the patient shows no symptoms referable to the disease; a second stage, in which the patient shows a greater or lesser number of symptoms; and the final stage, in which the symptoms of uremia predominate. The individual clinical pictures either overlap or present intermediate forms. An analysis has shown that the various symptoms and complications can be freely combined with each other.

SEX AND AGE DISTRIBUTION

My material comprises 350 patients, 193 women and 157 men. There is no significant difference due to sex. The age at the time of diagnosis varied from 16 to 85 years (mean, 47.2 years). This age distribution corresponds to what other authors have found [4, 34, 39, 52, 75, 78, 89, 99]. The majority of the patients had symptoms for a long time before the diagnosis was made. The age at which the disease started varied between 8 years and 77 years. The mean age at onset was 40.7 years [29], which is comparable to the 41.5 years found by Oppenheimer [78] for the first symptoms (see Fig. 35-6).

PAIN

Pain is an important finding in polycystic kidneys and has a widely varying character. At times there is troublesome pressure in the lumbar region, at other times a persistent feeling of pain located in one or both loins and radiating to the back or chest, epigastrium, or groin. In other cases there is violent pain, either in intermittent attacks or continuously. At the same time there is often great tenderness on pressing on one or both lumbar regions. The pain arises or is increased by vigorous movements, on walking, or on sitting still for a long time, so that the patient is occasionally forced to remain in bed for most of the day. It is possible that the pain is caused by the mechanical effect of pressure on adjacent organs and traction on the kidney pedicle, etc. Pain and vague abdominal symptoms are found very often (in 59 per cent of cases) and

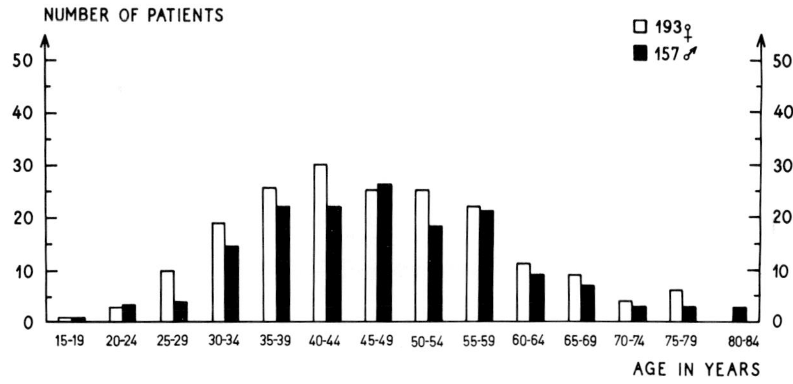

Figure 35-6. Age and sex distribution of 350 adult patients with polycystic kidneys at the time of diagnosis.

are significantly more frequent in women than in men. The pain begins early in the course of the disease. Rall and Odel [89] found lumbar and abdominal pain in 28 per cent of cases, Higgins [52] in 33 per cent.

RENAL COLIC AND THE PASSAGE OF A RENAL CALCULUS

These are among the noninflammatory complications accompanying polycystic kidneys. It is difficult to delimit the symptoms, as colicky pain often occurs on the passage of blood clots; further, the pain of polycystic kidneys can itself be of a colicky character. These two last-named forms of colic have as far as possible not been included. Colic or the passage of a calculus (or both) occurred in 18 per cent of my series, and was significantly more frequent in men than in women. There was a more or less uniform distribution for the first appearance of the symptom throughout the period of the disease. Rall and Odel [89] found associated nephrolithiasis in 14 per cent of their cases. Oppenheimer [78] found colic in 9 cases out of 60, and 14 cases of kidney or ureter stone from case history, roentgenogram, operation, or autopsy. The occurrence of stone in polycystic kidneys is, however, unusual.

HEMATURIA

Hematuria is an important and frequent complication, which very often causes the patient to seek medical advice. It may be of short or long duration, unilateral or bilateral, insignificant or violent, even a danger to life. It often occurs periodically at intervals of years. Persistent hematuria can result in severe anemia. Frequently the hematuria occurs quite unexpectedly; in other cases after trauma, lifting heavy loads, etc. At times the hematuria is accompanied by pain and even by true renal colic. The urine may consist solely of blood, resemble coffee grains, or be faintly red. This manifestation mostly appears in the middle of the course of the disease.

Braasch [14] found hematuria in 40 per cent of cases. Braasch and Schacht [15] found macroscopic hematuria in 34 per cent and microscopic hematuria in 44 per cent. Rall and Odel [89] reported painless hematuria in 13 per cent and hematuria accompanied by kidney pain in 10 per cent. Laboratory tests further showed grade 1–2 hematuria in 16 per cent and grade 3–4 hematuria in 9 per cent. Simon and Thompson [99] found that about half the patients developed macroscopic hematuria in the course of the disease.

Anuria is usually due to some mechanical impediment to urinary flow except when it occurs in the terminal stage of the disease. Gross enlargement of a functioning kidney may compress the ureter, and therefore ureteral catheterization is indicated.

Reversible acute renal failure was observed in 27 of 154 patients by Funck-Brentano et al. [37a]. In 21 of the 27 cases the cause was a water and electrolyte imbalance often due to sodium depletion from excessive restriction of dietary sodium associated with electrolyte loss from vomiting. Correction of the functional disorder restored the patient to his previous condition.

CARDIOVASCULAR SYMPTOMS

Cardiovascular symptoms, including hypertension, appeared frequently (46 per cent of my cases), and equally in both sexes, generally quite late in the course of disease. There are no data as to whether they are more common than in the corresponding age group in the general population. Edema occurred only rarely (8 per cent).

Sieber [98] found hypertrophy of the left ventricle among only 48 patients out of 212, either by examination during life or at autopsy. He found atheromatous changes in 20 per cent of these cases. Other investigators have reported a much greater proportion of cases with vascular lesions. Newman [75], for example, found changes in 60 per cent.

UREMIA

Uremia is frequent in the terminal stage of polycystic kidneys. In many cases it develops slowly and insidiously, and the time of its onset may be difficult to establish. It is often stressed as an important clinical experience that patients are surprisingly little troubled by uremia — for example, by Lejars [62] as early as 1888. Uremia occurred often, in 44 per cent, in my cases, and with a significantly greater frequency in women than in men.

According to Bell's experience [8], extensive impairment of renal function was found in two-thirds of cases on the first occasion when the patients consulted their physician. The majority of symptoms were due to renal insufficiency and were reminiscent of those occurring in chronic glomerulonephritis and pyelonephritis. Braasch and Schacht [15] found nausea and vomiting in 50 out of 193 cases, usually caused by renal insufficiency. Loss of weight was noted in 115 cases (76 per cent), and weakness, usually pronounced, was present in 40 cases. Both symptoms were presumably the result of renal insufficiency. On the other hand Rall and Odel [89], in their material from the Mayo Clinic, found uremia in only 2 cases (1 per cent) at the time of the diagnosis, and Newman [75] found uremia in only 5 out of 57 patients. The diagnoses in these two series must have been made exceedingly early in the disease.

PALPABLE RENAL MASSES

Palpable renal masses in polycystic disease are of great clinical significance. One or both kidneys may be enlarged to such a degree that upward arching of the abdominal wall is visible on inspection, and the abdominal circumference may be increased, possibly asymmetrically. Palpation is frequently difficult because of muscular tension, adiposity, and tenderness.

In my series, when masses could be felt both kidneys could be palpated in 64 per cent of cases, while only one kidney was felt in 36 per cent. Such masses were present very frequently, and significantly more often in women than in men, possibly because palpation is often easier in women. The sign first appears halfway through the course of the disease.

Braasch and Schacht [15] found bilateral palpable tumors in 78 per cent of cases, unilateral palpable tumors in 16 per cent, and no palpable enlargement in 6 per cent; and although both kidneys usually were enlarged, there was often a pronounced difference in their size. These authors expressed surprise that even greatly enlarged kidneys had escaped discovery during routine abdominal examination. Rall and Odel [89] found palpably enlarged kidneys or kidney in 72 per cent of their cases. Higgins [52] found bilateral kidney tumors in 55 per cent of cases, unilateral enlargement of the kidneys in 25 per cent, and no enlargement in 15 per cent; he was unable to decide the matter in 3 per cent. In all, one or both kidneys were palpably enlarged in 80 per cent of cases. Simon and Thompson [99] found bilateral enlargement of the kidneys in 51 per cent of cases, and unilateral enlargement in 27 per cent.

PROTEINURIA

Proteinuria was the most frequent finding on routine examination of the urine in my series. It varied from a slight trace to considerable amounts, and was observed very frequently (75 per cent of my cases), more often in women than in men. No proteinuria was found at any time in 20 per cent. It appears temporarily in some cases. A slight degree of proteinuria is thus the most frequent finding.

Braasch and Schacht [15] found proteinuria in 95 per cent of cases, usually in slight amounts. Oppenheimer [78] demonstrated proteinuria in 71 per cent. Newman [75] found that it was present in 88 per cent of cases, from slight traces to large amounts. He stressed that those patients who only had a slight trace of proteinuria often did not undergo urologic examination, as only slight importance was attached to this single finding. Rall and Odel [89] found proteinuria in 78 per cent of cases.

PYURIA AND BACTERIURIA

Cases with typical symptoms of urinary tract infection, such as pain, fever, chills, dysuria, and pollakiuria, and cases in which only microscopic examination or culture of urine indicated infection were included in my study of pyuria and bacteriuria.

These manifestations were very frequent, 46 per cent of cases, with a significant preponderance in women. The reason for this is presumed to be anatomic. Pyuria and bacteriuria commenced generally halfway through the course of the disease.

Oppenheimer [78] found signs of mild infection in 50 per cent of cases and severe infection in 32 per cent. Rall and Odel [89] found pyuria in 69 per cent of cases. Higgins [52] found an abnormal number of pus cells in 60 per cent and positive urine cultures in 50 per cent of cases. Simon and Thompson [99] found that at one time or another approximately one-third of their patients had had infection of the urinary tract. Goldstein and Klotz [40] stressed that the urinary findings do not necessarily correspond to the pathologic extent of the infection. The high frequency of infection in polycystic kidneys might indicate that these kidneys are particularly susceptible to infection.

RENAL FUNCTION

Renal function is frequently reduced in polycystic disease. Several renal function tests are required to evaluate the magnitude of change. The stage of the disease is an important determinant of the result.

At the time of follow-up examination, reduced renal function was found in 77 per cent of my patients (mostly raised blood urea or nonprotein nitrogen).

Determination of the hemoglobin value gives a simple but nonspecific evaluation of the kidney function. Seventy per cent of the patients in my series had a reduced hemoglobin value.

Cylindruria (particularly granular) was found on urine microscopy in only 8.5 per cent. This sign of degeneration of the tubular epithelium is thus infrequent in polycystic kidneys.

Spontaneous urinary concentration to 1.022 or above was found in 33 patients. Thus it could be considered that tubular function was either normal or only moderately reduced. The concentration test (Addis-Shevky and/or Strauss test) was carried out in 71 patients. In 8 the specific gravity was normal (greater than or equal to 1.022); 52 had hyposthenuria (between 1.010 and 1.022); and 11 had isosthenuria (less than or equal to 1.010). It was astonishing to find how frequently patients reported having suffered from thirst, polydipsia, and polyuria at an early stage of the disease.

Braasch [14] found the following distribution among 41 patients: 17 had a specific gravity of urine between 1.015 and 1.031, 14 between 1.010 and 1.015, and 9 less than 1.010. Braasch and Schacht [15] found the specific gravity less than 1.010 in 40.4 per cent of cases. Higgins [52] found the specific gravity less than 1.015 in 58 per cent and less than 1.010 in 30 per cent of cases.

Glomerular filtration rate as determined by urea clearance values was normal in eight of my patients on whom it was measured at the time the diagnosis was made by urography. There was thus no correlation in these cases between the destructive effect of the cysts on the kidney tissue and the deforming action of the cysts as indicated in the pyelogram.

Examination of discrete renal functions based on the modern renal function tests has been made in only a few cases — notably by Bricker and Patton [17, 81] (see page 1225).

Renal insufficiency demonstrated by renal function tests was seen in 32 per cent of my cases. It had a late onset and no sex differential.

Braasch and Schacht [15] found blood urea values of 40 mg. per 100 ml. or more in 67 per cent of their cases. In 10 per cent the values were greater than 200 mg. per 100 ml. They found the degree to which the patients could develop a tolerance to renal insufficiency with a blood urea concentration of more than 100 mg. per 100 ml. worthy of note. They observed a number of cases in which the blood urea value lay between 130 and 200 mg. per 100 ml., yet these patients remained in good health over a period of years. This was also the case where the creatinine value was between 3 and 10 mg. per 100 ml. I have had the same experience. Rall and Odel [89] found increased blood urea (more than 40 mg. per 100 ml.) in 36 per cent of cases at the time of diagnosis. In Higgins' material [52] the blood urea values were above 40 mg. per 100 ml. in 70 per cent of cases, over 60 mg. per 100 ml. in 35 per cent of cases, and over 80 mg. per 100 ml. in 15 per cent.

ARTERIAL HYPERTENSION

Hypertension (an arterial blood pressure of 160/100 mm. Hg or more, or a systolic blood pressure of 180 mm. Hg or more) was found in 42 per cent of women and 39 per cent of men. Thirty-two per cent of women and 23 per cent of men had an arterial blood pressure which exceeded the normal limits as defined by Master et al. [70].

Schacht [97], employing a systolic blood pressure of 145 mm. Hg as the upper limit for normal blood pressure, found hypertension in 75 per cent of 74 patients. In order to eliminate such factors as age, sex, and renal infection, he selected a group of 72 patients of the same age and sex distribution who were suffering from chronic bilateral pyelonephritis, and found that blood pressure was increased in only 26 per cent.

Rall and Odel [89] found a blood pressure greater than 140/90 mm. Hg in 73 per cent of cases. Higgins [52] found the blood pressure greater than 145/90 in 73 per cent of cases.

The best material on ophthalmoscopy is that of Rall and Odel [89]. In 71.5 per cent of their patients, the fundi had changes typical of hypertension, and though attempts were made to correlate these findings with the degree of severity of the hypertension and the degree of renal insufficiency, no clear relationship could be established. Schacht [97] found sclerosis of the retinal arterioles in 68 per cent of cases, and Braasch and Schacht [15] found abnormalities in the eye grounds in 57 per cent of cases.

RISK OF PATIENTS HAVING VARIOUS SYMPTOMS

The magnitude of risk of patients showing various symptoms by a certain age will always be higher than the frequency found empirically, shown in Table 35-4.

The mutual course of the risk curves (Figs. 35-7, 35-8) is significant. The risk that the polycystic kidneys are so enlarged that they can be palpated by the age of 35 is 11 per cent, while the risk of uremia is only 2 per cent. By the age of 50 the corresponding percentages are 55 and 41, and by the age of 65 they are 74 and 61.

The increase in kidney size takes place before there is functional destruction. In my opinion, this is a central point in the character of the disease, and a characteristic that facilitates both the clinical and the roentgenologic diagnosis.

When symptoms first arise, or at least within six months of the first occurrence of a symptom, pain is experienced by 46 per cent of the patients, the kidneys can be felt in 26 per cent, and uremia is present in 12 per cent. Within 10 years of the first symptom, 66 per cent have

Table 35-4. Age at Onset of Pain, Palpable Kidneys, and Uremia

Age Period	Pain: Observations[a]	Pain: Onset[b]	Pain: Risk[c] (per cent)	Palpable Kidneys: Observations	Palpable Kidneys: Onset	Palpable Kidneys: Risk (per cent)	Uremia: Observations	Uremia: Onset	Uremia: Risk (per cent)
5– 9	346	1	0	—	—	—	—	—	—
10–14	346	0	0	—	—	—	—	—	—
15–19	346	6	2	338	2	1	—	—	—
20–24	344	12	6	333	5	2	—	—	—
25–29	337	14	10	323	11	5	337	2	1
30–34	320	23	17	304	18	11	320	4	2
35–39	289	31	28	269	35	22	289	14	7
40–44	250	32	40	221	40	35	250	20	14
45–49	200	25	53	168	29	45	200	30	26
50–54	143	24	70	119	25	55	143	32	41
55–59	89	10	81	77	18	65	89	21	53
60–64	51	6	93	45	14	74	51	9	61
65–69	29	1	96	25	6	80	29	11	73

[a] Total number of patients observed in the age period.
[b] Number of patients with the onset of the manifestation during the age period.
[c] Risk, in per cent, of developing the manifestation during or before the end of the specified age period.

pain, the kidneys can be felt in 59 per cent, and there is uremia in 38 per cent of the cases.

COMPLICATIONS

Complications can be divided into two main groups, inflammatory and noninflammatory [5, 27]. Inflammation can be due either to ascending or to hematogenous infection, and may appear as pyelitis, pyelonephritis, inflammation of individual cysts or, with spread of infection, as pyonephrosis, perinephritis, or paranephritis, possibly with generalized sepsis. Tuberculous infection in polycystic kidneys is rare.

Noninflammatory changes comprise rupture of cysts, hemorrhage into cysts, and angulation of the ureter by cystic compression or displacement of the kidney, with consequent hydronephrosis together with calculus formation. Furthermore, very large cystic kidneys can

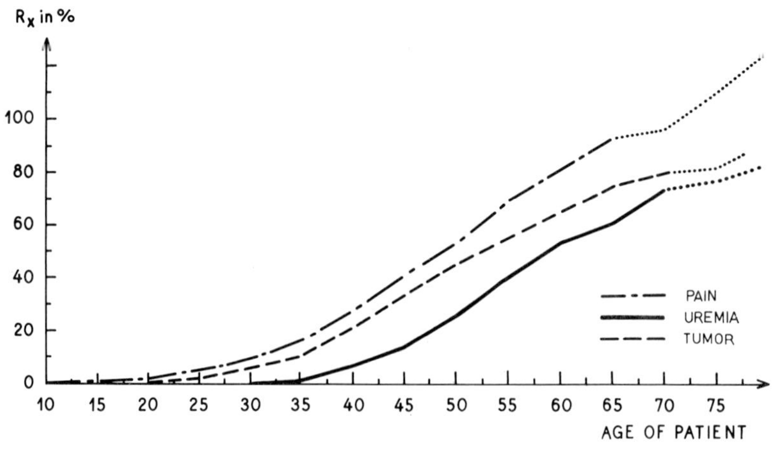

Figure 35-7. Risk (R_x in %) of onset of pain, uremia, and palpable kidneys within the ages indicated.

Figure 35-8. Risk (R_x in %) of onset of pain, uremia, and palpable kidneys in relation to the duration of disease.

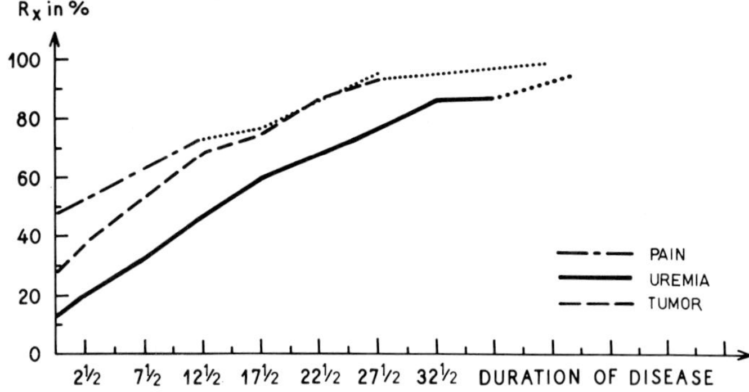

produce symptoms of compression and displacement in the abdomen. Malignant tumors are rare.

EFFECT OF PREGNANCY

The effect of pregnancy on the progress of polycystic kidneys is unknown. Of the 193 women with polycystic kidneys in my series, 65 per cent had been pregnant one or more times, and 61 per cent had one or more live births. Pregnancy followed by live births is thus very frequent. Perhaps this desirable outcome is due to the fact that the births occur early in the course of polycystic kidney disease. It would be of great interest if we could describe for the entire period of pregnancy the nature and frequency of the complications it introduces in polycystic kidneys, but opportunities are very rare. To judge whether pregnancy and birth have any influence on the spontaneous course of polycystic kidney disease it is necessary to provide a comparative control material of nonpregnant women. As the great majority of the women with polycystic kidneys in my series were pregnant during the study, and as the preponderance of the most serious cases was in the group of nonpregnant women, it was impossible to resolve this question.

Bell [8] is of the opinion that pregnancy increases the load on the kidneys, and not only intensifies all symptoms already present but also evokes symptoms in a latent stage of the disease.

Among Higgins' [52] patients there were 51 women, of whom 42 had had from one to nine pregnancies. Renal complications were no more numerous than in normal women. Higgins is of the opinion, however, that repeated pregnancies should be advised against, because of both the increased burden on the already affected kidneys and the likelihood of transmitting the disease to the child. Like my own material, the literature gives many examples of multiparity without complications.

Prognosis

In the majority of cases the cystic conversion of the kidneys progresses relentlessly, and uremia gradually develops in the majority of patients. However, there are wide variations in the course of the disease. In some rare patients the malformation does not appear to produce any symptoms whatever; in others it appears to remain almost unchanged for many years; but in many patients the disease is acute and fulminant in its manifestations, with death ensuing shortly after the onset of symptoms. It is impossible, in my study, to determine with certainty those cases in which a more benign course of the disease might be anticipated, although a certain familial uniformity in the course of the disease and in its characteristics was demonstrated [29].

SURVIVAL IN RELATION TO THE ONSET OF THE DISEASE

As the symptoms in polycystic kidneys usually develop gradually, it may be difficult for the patient to determine the precise time when the disease began. The dependence of the length of survival on the age at onset is emphasized by dividing the patients into two groups, one group above the age of 50 years at onset and the other group below the age of 50 years. In my group of patients in whom the disease started before the fiftieth year, 44 per cent of the women and 33 per cent of the men were alive after 12½ years, while in the general population 94 per cent of the women and 95 per cent of the men were alive after this time. In the group of patients in whom the disease first appeared after the fiftieth year, 54 per cent of the women, but only 14 per cent of the men, were alive 2½ years after the commencement of the disease, in contrast to 98 per cent and 97 per cent in the general population. The number of cases in this group, however, is small.

In Braasch and Schacht's patients [15], 22 among 74 deceased patients, or 36 per cent, died within 2 years after the onset of the first symptom, while 11, or 15 per cent, died between 2 and 4 years after the first symptoms had appeared. Thus, in these two groups 45 per cent of the patients were alive at least 4 years after the onset of the first symptoms.

Rall and Odel [89] were able to establish the time of onset of symptoms for 43 patients with some precision, and to observe them till death. The average time interval was 9.3 years.

SURVIVAL AFTER FIRST PALPATION OF POLYCYSTIC KIDNEYS

Table 35-5 illustrates the survival times of patients with polycystic kidneys from the time the kidneys were first palpable. It appears certain that very often polycystic kid-

Table 35-5. Survival in Per Cent at Given Times After the Onset of Certain Symptoms of Polycystic Kidneys, by Sex and Age at Onset

		Under 50 Years of Age (time in years)								Over 50 Years of Age (time in years)				
		0	2.5	7.5	12.5	17.5	22.5	27.5		0	2.5	7.5	12.5	17.5
Normal population[a]														
Women		100	99	97	94	91	87	81		100	98	91	82	69
Men		100	99	97	95	92	88	81		100	97	90	80	67
	No.								No.					
First symptom														
Women	41	100	91	64	44	29	19	4	11	100	54	18	9	—
Men	27	100	70	55	33	18	11	7	7	100	14	—	—	—
Kidney palpated														
Women	37	100	58	39	28	17	6	—	16	100	31	19	13	—
Men	15	100	53	7	7	7	—	—	6	100	33	17	17	—
Uremia														
Women	44	100	7	—	—	—	—	—	50	100	—	—	—	—
Men	29	100	3	—	—	—	—	—	30	100	—	—	—	—

		(time in years)							(time in years)			
	No.	0	0.5	1.5	2.5	3.5	4.5	No.	0	0.5	1.5	2.5
Uremia												
Women	44	100	27	18	7	2	—	50	100	24	4	—
Men	29	100	34	14	3	—	—	30	100	17	3	—

[a] Figures are for the Danish population for 1926–1930.

Table 35-6. Clinical Aspects in Relation to Prognosis in Polycystic Renal Disease

	Patients		Lived 5 or More Years	
Clinical Data	Total	Traced	Number	Survival Rate[a] (per cent)
Symptoms				
Asymptomatic[b]	89	72	43	59.7
Pain	163	128	82	64.1
Hematuria[c]	154	114	54	47.4
Infections[d]	170	130	69	53.1
Gastrointestinal	28	18	0	—
Blood pressure				
Normal	152	129	88	68.2
Moderately elevated	118	88	46	52.3
Severely elevated	84	62	24	38.7
Not recorded	12	—	—	—
Renal function				
Normal	187	156	133	85.3
Impaired	164	118	25	21.2
Not recorded	15	—	—	—
Hemoglobin				
Normal	253	196	136	69.4
Moderately decreased	73	57	19	33.3
Severely decreased	29	27	4	14.8
Not recorded	11	—	—	—
Total patients	366	288	160	55.6

[a] Based on traced patients. Inquiry as of January 1, 1954.
[b] Patients with microhematuria and pyuria are excluded.
[c] Includes 39 patients with microhematuria only and 115 with gross hematuria.
[d] Includes 93 patients with asymptomatic pyuria and 77 with symptoms of urinary infection.
SOURCE: From Simon, H. B., and Thompson, G. J. [99].

neys were first palpated long after the actual time at which they could have been palpated; thus, the survival times after this sign was first noticed are too short. For the same reason, the figures in the table are safe minimum figures.

Table 35-6 relates the length of survival in Simon and Thompson's cases [99] to some of the clinical manifestations of polycystic disease of the kidneys. An asymptomatic patient or one complaining only of lumbar pain tends to have a better prognosis than the patient with urinary infection. Since symptoms were multiple in most cases, these figures include patients with other manifestations. Hematuria is definitely an unfavorable symptom, and with hypertension of any marked degree the prognosis is poor. Anemia also indicates a serious outlook. Gastrointestinal disturbances due to advanced renal insufficiency are most ominous.

SURVIVAL AFTER DEVELOPMENT OF UREMIA

Uremia is a frequent terminal event in the clinical course of polycystic kidneys. In many cases it develops slowly and insidiously, so that the time of onset becomes manifest only because of other factors, such as the onset of infection of the urinary tract. All patients died within four years after the onset of uremia in my series. Simon and Thompson [99] found that all patients died within three years after the onset of the uremia.

Rall and Odel [89] were able to determine the time of onset of uremia in 17 patients more or less precisely, as indicated by a concentration of blood urea of more than 40 mg. per 100 ml. These patients survived, on the average, 2.2 years, and one patient survived 5.5 years. Rall and Odel's findings [89] give a rather more optimistic picture than is otherwise found in the literature, but their criterion for uremia is rather low.

It is often stressed that patients with polycystic kidneys characteristically have a uremic stage of long duration, and may have azotemia for a long time before the onset of the more severe "clinical uremia." This situation is perhaps due to the slowly progressive nature of the impairment in renal function, and to the fact that such patients often do not have hypertension. The best estimate of their chance of survival presumably would be obtained by examining urea or creatinine clearance.

For comparison, patients suffering from hypertension with nephrosclerosis may be in such bad condition (among other reasons, because of heart damage) that they have uremia for only a few weeks, while patients with chronic glomerulonephritis usually have a longer uremic stage, and patients with chronic pyelonephritis may have as long a uremic stage as patients with polycystic kidneys [88].

Compared with the normal population, patients with polycystic kidneys have a considerably increased mortality, particularly the older ones. The men are likely to die before the women. (This can perhaps be explained by the fact that the disease is observed later in men.)

AGE AT DEATH AND CAUSES OF DEATH

The mean age at death in my entire series was 51.5 years. The mean age at death as given by Oppenheimer [78] was 50 years, by Rall and Odel [89] 49.3 years, and by Higgins [52] 50 years (see Fig. 35-9).

Since there could be several concurrent causes, it was often difficult to establish the actual cause of death in my series, but three main causes predominated: uremia, cerebral hemorrhage, and cardiac disease. Out of 254 patients, 59 per cent died from uremia, 13 per cent died from cerebral hemorrhage, and only 6 per cent died from cardiac disease; 22 per cent died from other causes.

Sieber's findings [98] in 98 patients who were not operated on agree with mine. In his group, 50 patients died of uremia, 7 of apoplexy, 1 of rupture of the heart, 2 of cardiac insufficiency, and the remainder of various other diseases. Acute and chronic affections of the lungs, accounting for 16 deaths, were the second most frequent causes of death in the entire group.

Newman [75] found 13 deaths from ure-

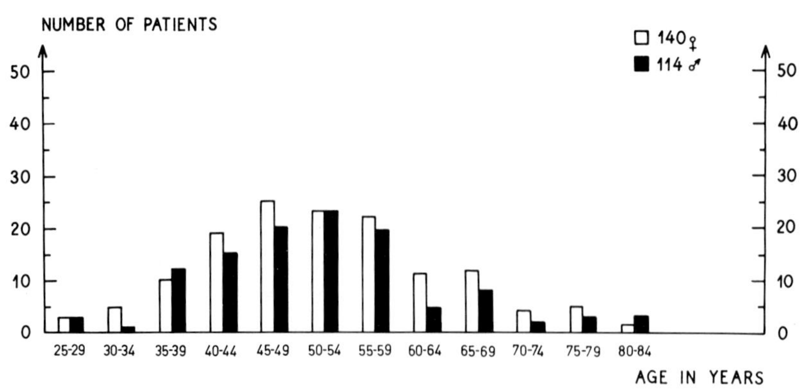

Figure 35-9. Age and sex distribution of 254 adult patients with polycystic kidneys at the time of death.

mia among 19 patients, whereas Rall and Odel [89] give renal insufficiency with uremia as the cause of death in only 9 cases among 46 patients.

Surgical Treatment in Adults

The most important question is whether operative treatment helps the basic disease — the gradual polycystic conversion of the kidney parenchyma, resulting sooner or later in the complete functional destruction of both kidneys.

In 1911 Rovsing [94] published his classic work on the treatment of polycystic kidneys by multiple puncture. On the basis of his experience in three cases, he was of the opinion that an unmistakable improvement in kidney function occurred, and that it was explicable on the assumption that much potentially functional but actually nonfunctioning kidney tissue had been squeezed between the cysts and again became functioning as a result of emptying the cysts. This theory could also explain the apparent improvement in the general condition of the patients and the apparent increase in their life span. Rovsing stressed that there was, of course, no question of curing the disease or of averting its fatal termination, but the fact that the patients had been freed of pain encouraged him to carry out the operation in all his cases of polycystic kidneys.

Since then, many reports of investigations have appeared, discussing the value of the operation. Lund [67] and Braasch [14] advised Rovsing's operation in mild cases. Payr [82] modified the operation slightly, using ignipuncture to avoid bleeding when the cysts are punctured. Gottlieb [41], Rovsing [95, 96], and Henninger and Weiss [49] were all much in favor of ignipuncture of the cysts.

In 1929 Meltzer [73] sent out a questionnaire to members of the American Urological Association and collected 111 cases of polycystic kidneys in which there had been surgical intervention. In 59 cases nephrectomy was carried out and in 31 cases Rovsing's puncture of the cysts. Meltzer analyzed the postoperative risk for the patients and concluded that the prognosis is more hopeful than is commonly believed.

In 1934 Walthers and Braasch [108] analyzed the operative results for 85 patients operated on at the Mayo Clinic. They concluded that the value of the Rovsing operation, carried out with the object of removing pressure on remaining renal parenchyma, still remained undetermined. Theoretically, there was much to be said in favor of the operation but, unfortunately, secondary infection or a persistent urinary fistula sometimes developed after it, requiring nephrectomy. They felt that if such complications could be avoided, the operation deserved wider use.

In the Scandinavian literature there is Köhler's investigation [58]. He held that there was everything to gain and nothing to lose by surgical intervention, and operated conservatively by opening the cysts and applying "varicocide." Mayers [71] applied quinine hydrochloride and quinine dihydrochloride; Nielsen [76] used dextrose (50 per cent).

Yates-Bell [113] recommends Rovsing's operation. Eighteen patients were so treated. Two patients died soon after operation; the 16 others benefited in one way or another. Relief from pain and hematuria and temporary relief of hypertension were common. Length of life may have been increased when the operation was performed early. Renal function was always lowered for a short time. After recovery renal function is unlikely to improve but deterioration may be delayed, particularly when a considerable portion of the kidney can be preserved. This may be possible in patients treated early, who are the ones most likely to benefit, and is an important feature to consider in determining treatment. Since Yates-Bell has not compared the course of the disease following operation with its natural course, his conclusions remain unproved.

Other authors are very much against operation. Lowsley [66] believed that "the less one does in the way of a surgical traumatic nature for these patients the better off they are," and Keys [56] has stated that "the patient may be more comfortable after Rovsing's operation of multiple puncture of the cysts, but the improvement is doubtless psychic, and surgery is a clumsy instrument for psychotherapy."

Goldstein [39] was the first to attempt a comparison of the results achieved by operation with the results in an equal number of cases in which only conservative treatment had been employed. His material consisted of 18 patients treated conservatively and 18 patients operated on. Of the former, seven were too great a risk for operation and the other 11 refused operation. Of the 18 who were operated on, two had nephrectomy and 16 had Goldstein's operation. This is a modification of Rovsing's operation: extraperitoneal exposure of the kidney, decapsulation, incision and excision of the cysts, nephrostomy, nephropexy, and formation of a temporary nephrocutaneous, nonurinary fistula, with, finally, the subsequent percutaneous puncture of re-formed or large cysts.

The operative results were very promising. The pain disappeared postoperatively in practically all cases, but there were no changes in blood pressure or in proteinuria after the operation. The blood urea nitrogen and excretory function tests showed pronounced postoperative improvement. Goldstein concluded that there was no hope of cure at the moment, but that no effort should be spared to relieve the patients by making an early diagnosis. The mean duration of life after the diagnosis had been made was twice as long with surgical intervention as without it. The ages of the 18 patients operated on ranged from 24 to 48 years, with a mean of 35 years, while the ages of the controls ranged from 3½ months to 60 years, with a mean of 33 years. Unfortunately, the ages of the individual patients are not given in Goldstein's report, but the control material includes children, who always die very soon after birth if they have polycystic kidneys, and older people, in whom one would expect the spontaneous course of the disease to be adverse. Because the age distributions in the experimental group and in the control group differ, they cannot be profitably compared. Furthermore, the fall in the blood urea nitrogen cannot be taken without question as a sign of improvement in the postoperative renal function, for the level of the blood urea depends both on the nitrogen turnover and on renal function. If the patients receive less protein, the nitrogen turnover and blood urea both fall. In a more recent paper Goldstein [40a] advised the same treatment.

A considerably superior and much more critical investigation is that of Simon and Thompson [99]. They carried out a comparison of the survival time for 230 patients nonsurgically treated, 28 patients treated by nephrectomy, and 26 patients treated by puncture of the cysts. Their results conform very closely to those obtained in my investigation.

On the whole, the condition of the surgical group was better than that of the nonsurgical. In the surgical group the average age was 42.7 years; 23 per cent of the patients had anemia, 35 per cent hypertension, and 24 per cent renal insufficiency. In the nonsurgical group the average age was 44.2 years, 29 per cent of the patients had anemia, 61 per cent hypertension, and 51 per cent renal insufficiency. As a result it might have been anticipated that the overall survival in the surgical group would be better, and indeed it was.

Table 35-7 compares the five-year survival rates after the two principal surgical procedures with the five-year survival rate in nonsurgical cases after these forms of treatment and also gives the various clinical manifestations of the disease. Surgical treatment was

Table 35-7. Comparison of Survival Rates after Nephrectomy and Cyst Puncture with Survival Rates in Nonsurgical Cases: Relationship of Clinical Signs[a]

Type of Therapy	Total Patients in Series	Renal Function		Blood Pressure			Hemoglobin		
		Normal	Impaired	Normal	Moderately Elevated	Severely Elevated	Normal	Moderately Decreased	Severely Decreased
Nonsurgical (average age, 44 yr.)									
Traced patients	230	111	105	91	76	56	151	48	24
5-year survival rate (%)	50.0	82.9	20.0	57.1	53.7	39.3	64.9	29.2	12.5
Nephrectomy alone (average age, 40 yr.)									
Traced patients	28	21	7	19	5	2	21	4	2
5-year survival rate (%)	82.1	95.2	42.9	94.7	40.0	50.0	90.5	50.0	50.0
Cyst puncture alone (average age, 45 yr.)									
Traced patients	26	20	6	15	7	4	20	5	1
5-year survival rate (%)	69.2	85.0	16.7	93.3	42.9	25.0	75.0	60.0	—

[a] Four patients treated with multiple surgical procedures are excluded from this analysis.
SOURCE: From Simon, H. B., and Thompson, G. J. [99].

carried out on a total of 119 patients among the 350 patients with bilateral polycystic kidneys in my series. In 90 patients the operation was unilateral, in 29 patients it was bilateral. Thirteen patients were operated on by several methods. Three of these died immediately following operation. Thirty-two had nephrectomy and 7 died immediately following the operation. Fifty-four had Rovsing's operation; 7 died immediately. Finally, of 20 patients who underwent exploratory operation, 4 died immediately after operation, either with or without an accompanying operation on another abdominal organ. The indications for operation in my series are shown in Table 35-8.

Table 35-8. Indications for Operation in Polycystic Kidneys in 119 Patients

Operations	Suspected Neoplasm	Therapy	Pain	Hematuria	Calculus	Pyonephrosis or Abscess	Tuberculosis	Various
Various (exploration, puncture, nephrolithotomy, nephrectomy, and decapsulation)	9	1	10	1	3	2	—	—
Nephrectomy	16	—	2	2	—	5	1	6
Rovsing's operation	17	25	19	3	—	1	—	1
Explorative for kidney disease	17	—	2	—	—	—	—	2
Totals	59	26	33	6	3	8	1	9

To be able to judge whether operation on patients with polycystic kidneys has any effect, it is necessary to have a control series of unoperated patients with the disease. The stage of their disease at the commencement of the period of observation should be identical with that of the operated patients at the time of the operation. Then it must be demonstrated in a statistically significant number of cases that the course of the disease following operation is more favorable than the natural course of the disease under conservative treatment. Unfortunately, such data are not available in the literature nor from my series, since cases were selected for operation partly on the basis of the stage and severity of the disease and because nephrectomy was largely limited to asymmetrically involved cases. It is also obvious that the result of an operation will always be much better earlier in the course of the disease than later, irrespective of whether or not the operation has actually had any effect on the prolongation of life.

Observations [81] made before and after surgical decompression of both kidneys in one case and of one kidney in another case gave no evidence of improved renal function; on the contrary, clearance values decreased after each operative procedure. Moreover there was no tendency for function to improve appreciably with time, and final follow-up observations in both subjects demonstrated values for all measurements of function well below control levels. The recent evidence that cystic nephrons in polycystic kidneys retain functional activity makes it mandatory to establish beyond doubt that the decompressive procedure is not detrimental [17a]. Although the contribution of the cystic units to the overall functional capacity of polycystic kidneys has not yet been assessed, it is conceivable that destruction of large numbers of functioning cystic nephrons in a kidney with diminished functional reserve will further compromise its functional ability.

Special Indications for Operative Intervention

The treatment of polycystic kidneys is first and foremost medical, but surgical intervention may be necessary. No type of treatment cures the basic disease, which is generalized and bilateral, but treatment may prevent or relieve the complications which sooner or later threaten life.

Removal of a polycystic kidney because it is riddled with cysts is a procedure to be advised against, since functional tissue may still be present. As the disease must always be considered bilateral, a person with one kidney is always in a worse position than a person with two.

If pyonephrosis supervenes and antibiotic treatment fails, it may be necessary to carry out nephrectomy, but a very conservative attitude should be adopted in patients with polycystic kidneys, and if nephrectomy seems indicated, adequate function in the other kidney must be demonstrated.

Surgical intervention may be necessary in patients suffering from unbearable persistent and incapacitating pain, and in such a case Rovsing's operation is advised.

Profuse steady bleeding, which cannot be treated conservatively by rest in bed and blood transfusions, but necessitates operation, possibly nephrectomy, is rare.

Other conditions which might indicate operation are perinephritic abscess, calculus, and tuberculosis. When a calculus is without symptoms, conservative treatment is indicated. It is possible that the continually improved control of infection will reduce the risk of calculus formation, which up to now has been 24 per cent by the age of 65.

General Measures of Treatment

The risk of developing infection in the form of pyelonephritis, intracystic infection, or perinephritis is 59 per cent by the age of 65, but the majority of patients can now be treated with effective chemotherapeutic and antibiotic agents. Catheterization or endoscopy must be avoided as far as possible, as the danger of infection is great. It is of major importance that all cases of acute inflammation be treated, so as to reduce damage to the parenchyma and the danger that the infection may become chronic. The need for surgical intervention, with drainage of renal and perirenal abscesses, will undoubtedly be lessened by treatment with chemotherapeutic and antibiotic agents, and there should be fewer deaths from uncontrollable infections.

In a significant number of 55 patients with marked renal failure [4a] there was an obligatory urinary loss of electrolytes unaffected by dietary restriction; this is why some patients on a strict low-salt diet are the victims of severe salt loss which in turn depresses renal excretory function and aggravates considerably the degree of nitrogen retention. For this reason, salt should not be restricted too severely in patients with polycystic disease. This rule may at times be difficult to apply in cases complicated by severe hypertension, and it is advisable to check the sodium balance and blood pressure at frequent intervals since it may be necessary to alter the sodium intake from time to time. Treatment of hypertension, if it is of minor degree, may be indicated. However, if hypertension is of major severity, even if renal function is little or not at all impaired, treatment is very important since significant persistent elevation of the blood pressure has a deleterious influence on the course of the disorder.

Uremia, which occurs so commonly in patients with polycystic kidneys, often responds well to treatment, in comparison with its response in the majority of other chronic kidney diseases. Dietary protein restriction in the presence of renal failure and treatment of the other manifestations of renal insufficiency such as hyperchloremic acidosis and hypocalcemia are outlined in other chapters and need not be repeated here. Anuria calls for ureteral catheterization which often will be sufficient to restore urinary flow.

Regular follow-up examination once every 3 months is essential in the management of these patients, to ensure the early recognition of water and electrolyte disturbances and hypertension. With effective treatment prolonged survival is possible. Treatment by hemodialysis may be indicated when there has been an acute worsening of the patient's condition in an early stage [73a]. When the stage of terminal uremia is reached, maintenance dialysis and kidney transplantation may be indicated.

Associated Anomalies

POLYCYSTIC LIVER

Cysts of the liver, like cysts of the kidneys, can be single or multiple. Single cysts can be simple or multilocular; multiple cysts can vary in number from a few to so many that the liver sometimes fills most of the abdomen and appears to be completely replaced by the cysts. The size of the cysts can likewise vary; some are microscopic and others large enough to contain one or more liters of fluid.

The similarity in the pathologic anatomy, and possibly also in the pathogenesis, has caused some authors to group all cases together, irrespective of the size and number of the cysts [28]. Others [1, 7] have been more inclined to ascribe a different etiology to the two diseases, among other reasons because polycystic liver is frequently associated with cyst formations in other organs, while this is not observed in the case of the large solitary cystadenoma.

Poinso et al. [84], in an outstanding monograph, have thrown light on the etiology, pathogenesis, pathologic anatomy, clinical features, diagnosis, prognosis, and treatment. Their study, based almost entirely on case histories drawn from the literature, comprises 224 polycystic livers. Polycystic kidneys were associated in 120 cases (53 per cent). Oppenheimer [78] found polycystic liver present in 4 of 14 autopsies of patients with polycystic kidneys, Rall and Odel [89] in 15 of 46 autopsies, and Küster [59] in 41 of 249 autopsies of patients with polycystic kidneys.

In my material of 173 autopsies, cysts of the liver were found in 75 cases. From one to several cysts were found in 19 per cent of the cases, and in 21 per cent of the cases the liver was riddled with cysts. There are no reports on the frequency of polycystic liver found at autopsy in general, but it is a rare condition. Data from families in which cysts of the liver were found in addition to several cases of polycystic kidneys have been collected by numerous writers [24, 53, 90, 103, 106, 109]. In my material there were 14 families in which one or more individuals were found with both polycystic kidneys and polycystic liver (Fig. 35-10).

In view of the frequency of polycystic livers in patients with polycystic kidneys, the possibility of a chance coincidence between the two malformations can be excluded. I have found a regular transition from polycystic liver degeneration to the solitary liver cyst.

ANEURYSMS OF THE BASAL ARTERIES OF THE BRAIN

The first case of simultaneous occurrence of polycystic kidneys and basilar aneurysm in a patient was reported, in 1901, from Scandinavia by Borelius [12]. Since then, about 50 cases have been published in the world literature [10, 18, 86].

Dunger [32] left unanswered the question whether these vascular dilatations arise as a result of increased blood pressure, special toxic action perhaps playing a part, or whether they might be due to a congenital lack of resistance in the wall of the vessel, an assumption which Dunger found in general agreement with the character of the malformation in polycystic kidneys.

Whether there is a causal relation between polycystic kidneys and aneurysm of the basal arteries of the brain is a matter that can be determined only by statistical analysis of the autopsy material [10, 18, 29, 104]. This shows a significant association for the two malformations. However, the central question—whether the connection found between the two malformations is really due to a common cause and pathogenesis or whether other factors, such as hypertension in patients with polycystic kidneys, are responsible—is undecided. It is my opinion that the theory of a common cause has not been demonstrated, but is likely enough.

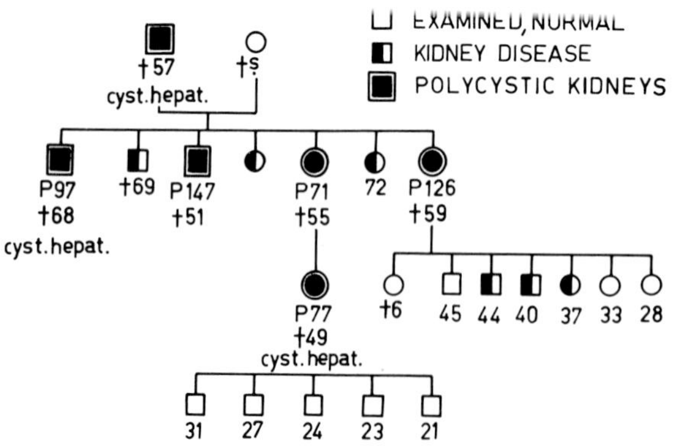

Figure 35-10. Polycystic kidneys in the direct line in three generations, without skipping. Cysts of the liver.

Patients known to have polycystic kidneys who manifest migraine headache or symptoms of cerebrovascular accident should be promptly examined if intracranial aneurysms are to be discovered in time to permit proper treatment. This is especially true in those who have a favorable life expectancy in terms of renal reserve [86] (Fig. 35-11).

CYSTS IN OTHER ORGANS

The occurrence of cysts in other organs in association with renal cysts is much less frequent than is their occurrence in the liver. Nonetheless, on occasion, cyst formation, in association with renal cysts, has been described in the pancreas, lungs, spleen, ovaries, testes, epididymis, thyroid gland, uterus, bladder, and other organs [10, 89, 98]. In my material, there were eight cases in which cysts were found in other organs than the kidneys and the liver. Whether the cyst formation in these organs is purely coincidental cannot be determined.

In the world literature, only two cases are mentioned in which polycystic disease of the kidneys and von Hippel-Lindau's disease have occurred simultaneously [31, 36].

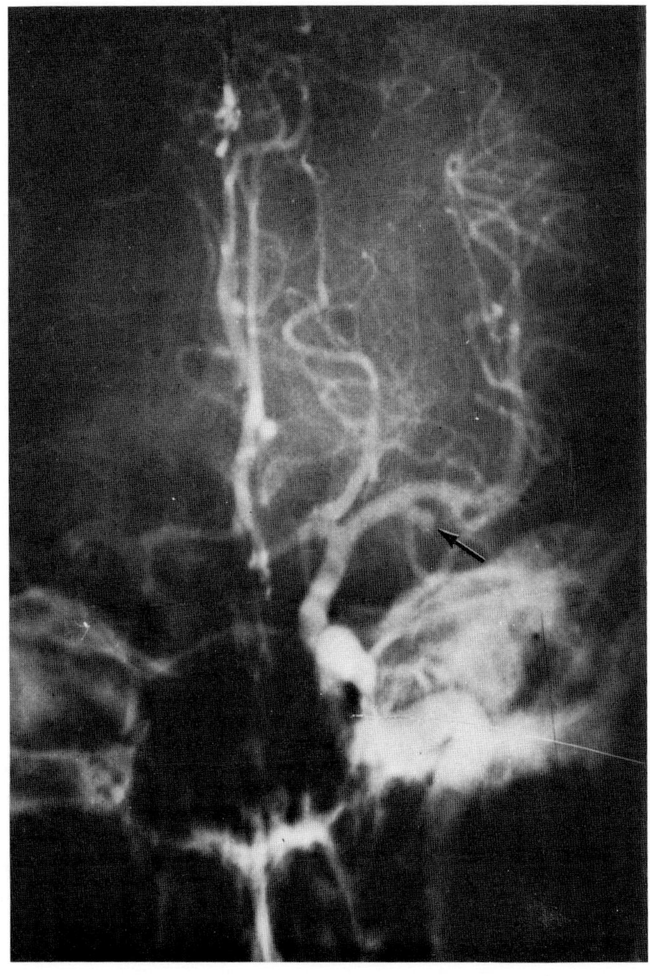

Figure 35-11. A 31-year-old man with familial polycystic kidneys was admitted with subarachnoid hemorrhage. (The 24-hour creatinine clearance showed 50 per cent of normal function.) Arteriography showed a saccular aneurysm, 5 mm. in diameter, of the left medial cerebral artery. Surgical correction with a silver clip placed across the base of the aneurysm was successful. The patient recovered.

Bilateral Polycystic Kidneys in Infants and Children

In the congenital form of polycystic kidneys the defect, already present at birth, must be considered as the final stage of a developmental process which has been going on during fetal life. The main question is whether the malformation is an etiologic entity. In the 26 cases reported in the world literature [29] in which congenital polycystic kidneys arose in two or more siblings and in which the kidneys were described, the kidneys were always enlarged except in one family.

Potter's autopsy material [85] of 50 cases could be divided on the basis of the histologic picture into two main groups: 44 cases in which the amount of connective tissue was increased, and 6 in which it was normal. Thus the former type was by far the more common. However, it is interesting that the latter type included a pair of siblings who had enlarged kidneys. It is natural, therefore, to imagine that two forms of polycystic kidneys occur: one in which the kidneys often assume enormous proportions, have a spongy appearance, and show familial incidence (recessive inheritance), and another in which the most characteristic feature is that the kidneys are hypoplastic.

The frequency of congenital polycystic kidneys at autopsy is shown in Table 35-9. Of 42 children [29], 15 were stillborn or died immediately after birth, 14 died during the first 24 hours of life, four died during the first month, and six died during the first year. One child survived for 13 months, one was alive at the age of five years, and one died at the age of 11 years.

Treatment is fundamentally the same as in adults. Following nephrectomy, in congenital polycystic disease, half of the patients die during the immediate postoperative period, and a third die of renal failure within the first postoperative month [25].

The reported frequency of congenital polycystic kidney varies from 1 case in 6000 births [29] to 1 in 14,000 [23]. The malformation appears so infrequently in children that it must be considered a curiosity. Albarran and Imbert [3] collected 22 cases from the literature for the ages between eight weeks and 19 years, Sieber [98] added 10 cases from the literature, and Olesen [77] added a further nine cases from the literature. The clinical manifestations of the disease do not differ essentially from those in adults. Palpation of a large nodular mass in the renal region must necessarily suggest polycystic disease, particularly when found bilaterally. Complete urologic investigation is necessary and pyelography is usually confirmatory. At times the kidneys are so enormously enlarged that they obstruct delivery [111]. Urinalysis commonly leads to the diagnosis of chronic interstitial nephritis, and elevated blood urea nitrogen is

Table 35-9. Frequency of Cogenital Polycystic Kidneys in Infants at Autopsy

Year	Author	Place	Number of Polycystic Kidneys/Number of Autopsies	Ratio
1930	Bardram	Copenhagen	12:4435	1:370
1933	Roscher	Oslo	7:1532	1:219
1950	Bell	Minnesota, U.S.A.	14:4512	1:322
1951	Campbell	U.S.A.	70:15,919	1:227
1952	Potter	U.S.A.	50:16,000	1:320
1957	Dalgaard	Copenhagen	24:10,734 (from 147,046 births)	1:448

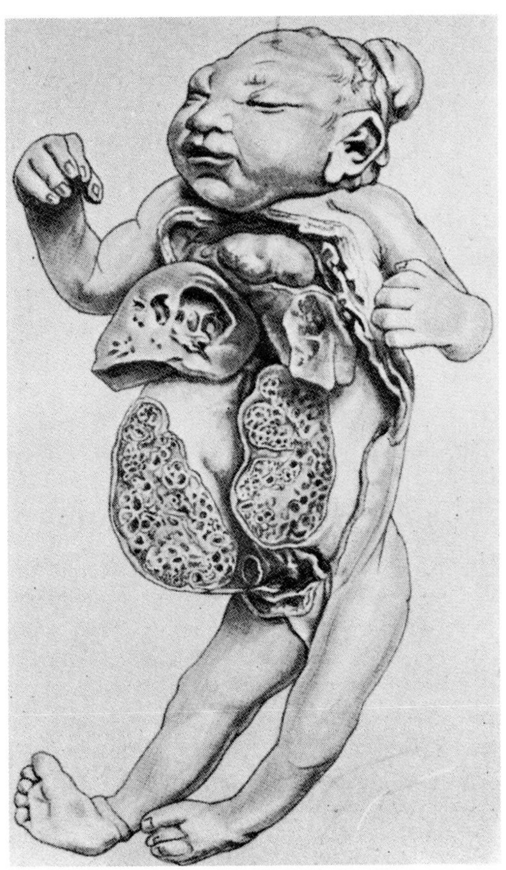

Figure 35-12. Dysencephalia splanchnocystica. (From Gruber, G. B. [44].)

the rule. The blood pressure may or may not be elevated. When anuria is present the diagnosis of polycystic kidneys must always be suspected. Renal rickets has developed in some children with polycystic disease [57]. In the differential diagnosis the possibility of Wilms's tumor must be considered.

The malformations related to congenital polycystic kidneys are usually divided into two groups: those caused by changes in a single portion of the embryonic disc, and those caused by an abnormal duplication of the embryonic area, with the result that individuals are produced with partially but not completely duplicated body structures.

Four sibling pairs with polycystic kidneys and polycystic liver have been reported in the literature [21, 26, 64, 69]. In addition, one of Bunting's and both of Marquardt's cases had polycystic pancreas. Cysts of the liver, pancreas, spleen, or other organs have also been described in numerous single cases. In my material, one case with cysts of the liver was found. In Campbell's autopsy material [25] of 50 cases, associated urogenital malformations were found in 39. Urologic malformations were found in 7 cases in my material, malformations in the alimentary canal in 3 cases, in the cardiovascular system in 3 cases, in the musculoskeletal system in 6 cases, and in the central nervous system in 8 cases.

Gruber [44] set up a complex of malformations, acrocephalosyndactyly and dysencephalia splanchnocystica, and collected 16 cases with polycystic kidneys, dysencephaly and possibly dysphalangia and malformations of the eye. The material has been supplemented by four cases [83] in which one or more of the above-mentioned malformations were present in addition to polycystic kidneys.

Familial observations have also been made. Polydactylism has been found among other malformations in two sibships, in addition to polycystic kidneys [19, 72]. Meningocele or encephalocele has occurred in three sibs in addition to polycystic kidneys. Families have been reported in which, besides the individual with polycystic kidneys, there are individuals with other malformations. There are no reports of bilateral polycystic kidneys with double malformations, but one case has been reported [96] of a hypoplastic unilateral polycystic kidney in an ileothoracopagus.

Thus, the literature mentions almost all possible disturbances of development among simultaneously occurring malformations. It is quite impossible to decide whether the malformations are determined by a pleiotropic gene, occur together on account of gene linkage, or are determined by external factors.

References

1. Adler, H. Beitrag zur operativen Behandlung der Cystadenome der Leber. *Zbl. Chir.* 63:987, 1936.
2. Adrian, C., and von Lichtenberg, A. Die klinische Bedeutung der Missbildungen der Niere, des Nierenbeckens und der Harnleiters. *Z. Urol. Chir.* 1:139, 1913.
3. Albarran, J., and Imbert, L. *Tumeur de Rein.* Paris: Masson et Cie, 1903. Pp. 34, 537, 570.
4. Arrigoni, G., Cresseri, A., and Lovati, G. *Ricerche Genetiche sul Rene Policistico.* Rome: Ium Sumposium Internationale Geneticate Medicae, 1954. P. 242.

4a. Assa, S., and Vantelon, J. La maladie polykystique des reins (étude de 150 cas). *Path. Biol.* (Paris) 10:237, 1962.

5. Backofen, O. *Das Krankheitsbild der polycystischen Nierendegeneration (Genese und klinischer Verlauf).* Taucha b. Leipzig, 1930. Pp. 5, 24, 60, 64.
6. Bardram, E. Congenital kidney malformations and oligohydramnios. *Acta Obstet. Gynec. Scand.* 10:134, 1930.
7. Beattie, D. A., and Robertson, H. D. Case of simple cyst of liver, with analysis of 62 other cases. *Lancet* 1:674, 1932.
8. Bell, E. T. *Renal Diseases.* London: Kimpton, 1950. P. 87.
9. Berner, O. *Die Cystenniere. Studien über ihre pathologische Anatomie.* Jena: Fischer, 1913. Pp. 6, 69.
10. Bigelow, N. H. The association of polycystic kidneys with intracranial aneurysms and other dilated disorders. *Amer. J. Med. Sci.* 225:485, 1953.
11. Billing, L. The roentgen diagnosis of polycystic kidneys. *Acta Radiol.* [Diag.] Stockholm 41:305, 1954.
12. Borelius, J. Zur Genese und klinischen Diagnose der polyzystischen Degeneration der Nieren. *Nord. Med. Ark.* 34:1, 1901.
13. Borst, J. R. Disturbances in water- and salt metabolism in the final stage of chronic renal insufficiency. *Acta Med. Scand.* 136:1, 1949.
14. Braasch, W. F. Clinical data of polycystic kidney. *Surg. Gynec. Obstet.* 23:697, 1916.
15. Braasch, W. F., and Schacht, F. W. Pathological and clinical data concerning polycystic kidney. *Surg. Gynec. Obstet.* 57:467, 1933.
16. Braasch, W. F., and Hendrick, J. A. Renal cysts, simple and otherwise. *J. Urol.* 51:1, 1944.
17. Bricker, N. S., and Patton, J. F. Cystic disease of the kidneys: A study of dynamics and chemical composition of cyst fluid. *Amer. J. Med.* 18:207, 1955.

17a. Bricker, N. S., and Patton, J. F. Renal function studies in polycystic disease of the kidneys — with observations on the effects of surgical decompression. *New Eng. J. Med.* 256:212, 1957.

18. Brown, R. A. P. Polycystic disease of the kidneys and intracranial aneurisms. The aetiology and interrelationship of the conditions: Review of recent literature and report of seven cases in which both conditions coexisted. *Glasgow Med. J.* 32:333, 1951.
19. Brückner, C. Zweimalige Entbindung derselben Frau von Missgeburten mit vergrösserten Nieren. *Arch. Path. Anat.* 46:503, 1869.
20. Bugbee, H. G., and Wollstein, M. Surgical pathology of the urinary tract in infants. *J.A.M.A.* 83:1887, 1924.
21. Bunting, C. H. Congenital cystic kidney and liver with family tendency. *J. Exp. Med.* 8:271, 1906.
22. Burger, C. *Über cystoide Degeneration der Niere bei Neugeborenen.* Bonn: Carthaus, 1867. P. 25.
23. Böök, J. A. The incidence of congenital diseases and defects in a South Swedish population. *Acta Genet.* (Basel) 2:289, 1951.
24. Cairns, H. W. B. Heredity in polycystic disease of the kidneys. *Quart. J. Med.* 18: 359, 1925.
25. Campbell, G. S., Bick, H. D., Paulsen, E. P., Lober, P. H., Watson, C. J., and Varco, R. L. Bleeding esophageal varices with polycystic liver; report of three cases. *New Eng. J. Med.* 259:904, 1958.
26. Campbell, M. *Clinical Pediatric Urology.* Philadelphia: Saunders, 1951. P. 181.

27. Cantus, H. *Über Cystennieren und ihre Diagnose*. Bonn: Trapp, 1931. Pp. 27, 32.
28. Comfort, M. W., Gray, H. K., Dahlin, D. C., and Whitesell, F. B. Polycystic disease of the liver: A study of 24 cases. *Gastroenterology* 20:60, 1952.
29. Dalgaard, O. Z. *Bilateral Polycystic Disease of the Kidneys. A Follow-up of Two Hundred and Eighty-four Patients and Their Families*. University of Copenhagen, M.D. Thesis. Copenhagen: Munksgaard, 1957. Supplement 328, 1957. *Acta Med. Scand*. Opera ex Domo Biologiae Hereditariae Humanae Universitatis Hafniensis, vol. 38.
30. Davis, J. E. Surgical pathology of malformations in kidneys and urethra. *J. Urol.* 20: 1, 155, 283, 1928.
31. Donat, R. *Ein Beitrag zu dominant vererbbaren vielfachen Geschwulstbildungen*. Kiel: Ehlers, 1935. P. 3.
32. Dunger, R. Zur Lehre von der Cystenniere, mit besonderer Berücksichtigung ihrer Heredität. *Beitr. Path. Anat.* 35:445, 1904.
33. Evans, J. A., Dubilier, W., and Monteith, J. C. Nephrotomography: A preliminary report. *Amer. J. Roentgenol.* 71:213, 1954.
34. Fergusson, J. D. Observations on familial polycystic disease of the kidney. *Proc. Roy. Soc. Med.* 42:806, 1949.
35. Fiessinger, N. Cited by Poinso et al. [84]. P. 80.
36. Fraenkel. *Virchow. Arch.* 230, 1921. Cited by Donat [31].
37. Frazier, T. H. Multilocular cysts of the kidney. *J. Urol.* 65:351, 1951.
37a. Funck-Brentano, J. L., Vantelon, J., and Lopez-Alvarez, R. Les accidents évolitifs de la maladie polykystique des reins: 154 observations personelles. *Presse Med.* 72: 1583, 1964.
38. Glaser, S. Simple renal cysts. *Brit. J. Surg.* 40:74, 1952.
39. Goldstein, A. E. Polycystic renal diseases with particular reference to author's surgical procedure. *J. Urol.* 66:163, 1951.
40. Goldstein, A. E., and Klotz, B. Pyonephrosis in congenital polycystic kidneys. *Surgery* 6:730, 1939.
40a. Goldstein, A. E., and Goldstein, R. B. Polycystic renal disease; and analysis of operative and nonoperative cases. *J. Urol.* 84:268, 1960.
41. Gottlieb, J. G. Über die cystische Entartung der Nieren. *Z. Urol. Chir.* 17:256, 1925.
42. Grauhan, M. Die Klinik der Missbildungen der Niere und des Harnleiters. *Verh. Deutsch. Ges. Urol.* Sonderband 180, 1929.
43. Grauhan, M. Gehört die Cysterniere zu den mit Sicherheit diagnostizierbaren Erkrankungen? *Deutsch. Z. Chir.* 197:205, 1926.
44. Gruber, G. B. Beiträge zur Frage "Gekoppelter" Missbildungen. (Akrocephalo-Syndactylie und Dysencephalia splanchnocystica). *Beitr. Path. Anat.* 93:459, 1934.
45. Haldane, J. B. S. *The Causes of Evolution*. London: Longmans, Green, 1932. P. 171.
46. Hauge, M. Om blodtypernes anvendelse i den humane genetik. Thesis. Copenhagen, 1962.
47. Hennig, O. Über den Wert der röntgenologischen Darstellung von Cystennieren. *Z. Urol. Chir.* 27:106, 1929.
48. Henninger, H. Die Anzeigestellung zur Operation der angeborenen Zystenniere. *Wien. Klin. Wchnschr.* 51:525, 1938.
49. Henninger, H., and Weiss, K. Zuk Klinik der kongenitalen Cystennieren. *Z. Urol. Chir.* 44:221, 1938.
50. Hepler, A. B. Solitary cyst of the kidney. *Surg. Gynec. Obstet.* 50:668, 1930.
51. Hickel, R., and Cornet, P. Les signes radiologiques de la maladie polykystique des reins. *J. Radiol. Electr.* 30:113, 1949.
52. Higgins, C. C. Bilateral polycystic kidney disease: Review of 94 cases. *A.M.A. Arch. Surg.* 65:318, 1952.
53. Höhne, E. Ein Beitrag zur polycystischen Nierenentartung. *Deutsch. Med. Wschr.* 22: 757, 1896.
54. Kemp, T. Om svangerskabsafbrydelse på eugenisk indikation. *Ugeskr. Laeg.* 102: 373, 1940.
55. Kemp, T. *Genetics and Disease*. Copenhagen: Munksgaard, 1951. Pp. 59, 193.

56. Keys. Cited by Milliken, L. F. *Clinics* 3:90, 1944.
57. Kretschmer, H. L. Renal rickets and polycystic disease of the kidney. *J. Urol.* 59:773, 1948.
58. Köhler, B. Surgical treatment of polycystic kidney. *Acta Chir. Scand.* 96:283, 1947.
59. Küster, E. Die Chirurgie der Nieren, der Harnleiter und der Nebennieren. Cystenniere und Nierencysten. In *Deutsche Chirurgie,* 52C. Stuttgart: F. Enke, 1896–1902. Pp. 511, 561.
60. Lambert, P. *Le Rein Polykystique. Etude Morphologique, Clinique et Physiopathologique.* Paris: Masson, 1943. Pp. 14, 34, 84, 130.
61. Lambert, P. Polycystic disease of the kidney: A review. *Arch. Path.* 44:34, 1947.
62. Lejars, F. *Du Gros Rein Polykystique de l'Adulte.* Paris: Steinheill, 1888. Pp. 5, 55.
63. Lelievre, A., and Walther, P. Cinque cas des reins polycystiques à l'appui de la théorie dysembryoplastique. *Bull. Soc. Anat. Paris.* 94:34, 1924.
64. Lightwood, R., and Loots, G. H. Three cases of familial congenital cystic disease of kidney and liver. *Proc. Roy. Soc. Med.* 25: 1230, 1932.
65. Littre, M. Observations sur les reins d'un faetus humain de neuf mois. *Bibliothèque Choisie de Médicine par Planque* 22:8, 1763.
66. Lowsley, 1929. Cited by Meltzer [73].
67. Lund, F. B. Rovsing's operation for congenital cystic kidney. *J.A.M.A.* 63:1083, 1914.
68. Maier, O. Die echte polycystische Niere, ihre Aetiologie und chirurgische Behandlung. *Arch. Klin. Chir.* 132:226, 1924.
69. Marquardt, W. *Cystenniere, Cystenleber und Cystenpankreas bei zwei Geschwistern mit Besonderer Berücksichtigung der Vererbung der cystischen Missbildung parenchymatösen* Organe. Tübingen, 1934. Pp. 3, 14.
70. Master, A. M., Garfield, C. I., and Walters, M. B. *Normal Blood Pressure and Hypertension.* Philadelphia: Lea & Febiger, 1952. Pp. 37, 86, 87.
71. Mayers, M. M. Polycystic kidney disease. *J. Urol.* 59:471, 1948.
72. Meckel, J. F. Beschreibung zweier, durch sehr ähnliche Bildungs Abweichungen entstellter Geschwister. *Deutsch. Arch. Physiol.* 7:99, 1822.
73. Meltzer, M. Surgical polycystic kidney. *Amer. J. Surg.* 7:420, 1929.
73a. Menasche, V., and Smith, D. R. Apparently unilateral polycystic kidney. *Amer. J. Dis. Child.* 94:313, 1957.
73b. Nakamoto, S., and Kolff, W. J. Chronic uremia due to polycystic renal disease treated with the artificial kidney. *A.M.A. Arch. Intern. Med.* 101:921, 1958.
74. Naumann, H. *Über die Häufigkeit der Bildungsanomalien der Niere.* Kiel, 1897. Cited by Backofen [5].
75. Newman, H. R. Congenital polycystic kidney disease. *Amer. J. Surg.* 80:410, 1950.
76. Nielsen, S. S. Infisert cystenyre. *Nord. Med.* 44:1145, 1950.
77. Olesen, I. Congenit cystenyre hos et barn. Et tilfaelde. *Ugeskr. Laeg.* 116:399, 1950.
78. Oppenheimer, G. D. Polycystic disease of the kidney. *Ann. Surg.* 100:1136, 1934.
78a. Osathanondh, V., and Patter, E. L. Pathogenesis of polycystic kidneys. *Arch. Path.* (Chicago) 77:466, 1964.
79. Pabst, E. *Nierencysten und Cystennieren im Leichenöffnungsgut des Göttingener Pathologischen Institutes 1907–33.* Göttingen, 1935. P. 1.
80. Parkkulainen, K. V., Hjelt, L. v., and Sirola, K. Congenital multicystic dysplasia of the kidney: Report of nineteen cases with discussion on the etiology, nomenclature and classification of the cystic dysplasias of the kidney. *Acta Chir. Scand.* Suppl. 244, 1959.
81. Patton, J. F., and Bricker, N. S. Renal function studies in polycystic disease of the kidney: A preliminary report. *J. Urol.* 72:285, 1954.
82. Payr, E. Die operative Behandlung- Ignipunktur- mancher Fälle polycystischer Nierendegeneration. Bemerkungen zur Pathologie und Klinik. *Z. Urol. Chir.* 12:254, 1923.
83. Pohlmann, F. *Über das Vorkommen hinterer Hirnbruchbildung mit vielcystischen Formfehler von Eingeweidedrüsten und mit*

Vielfingerigkeit. Göttingen: Pieper, 1935. P. 3.

84. Poinso, R., Monges, H., and Payan, H. *La Maladie Kystique du Foie*. Expansion scientifique française, 1954. Pp. 17, 39.
85. Potter, E. L. *Pathology of the Fetus and the Newborn*. Chicago: Year Book, 1952. P. 368.
86. Poutasse, E. F., Gardner, W. J., and McCormack, L. J. Polycystic kidney disease and intracranial aneurysm. *J.A.M.A.* 154:741, 1954.
87. Powell, T., Shackman, R., and Johnson, H. D. Multilocular cysts of the kidney. *Brit. J. Urol.* 23:142, 1951.
88. Raaschou, F. Does urine stasis have any influence on the development of arterial hypertension? *Acta Med. Scand.* 133:31, 1949.
89. Rall, J. E., and Odel, H. M. Congenital polycystic disease of the kidney: Review of the literature and data on 207 cases. *Amer. J. Med. Sci.* 218:399, 1949.
90. Reason, C. H. Heredity and polycystic disease of the kidneys. *Canad. Med. Ass. J.* 29:612, 1933.
91. Reed, T. E., and Neel, J. V. Genetic study of multiple polyposis of colon (with appendix deriving method of estimating relative fitness). *Amer. J. Hum. Genet.* 7:236, 1955.
92. Roscher, F. Über die Häufigkeit, die Art und die pathogenische Bedeutung von Missbildungen der Niere und der Harnwege. Eine Übersicht über das Material des Pathologisch-Anatomischen Instituts der norwegischen Universitätsklinik betreffend Missbildungen der Nieren und der Harnwege in den Jahren 1914–1930. *Acta Chir. Scand.* 70:493, 1933.
93. Röver, O. *Betrachtungen zur Frage des Ileothoracopagus*. Göttingen, 1936. P. 91.
94. Rovsing, T. Behandling af de multiloculaere nyrekystom med multiple punkturer. *Hospitalstid.* 4:105, 1911.
95. Rovsing, T. Det multiloculaere nyrekystoms behandling med bemaerkninger om sygdommens natur. *Bibl. Laeg.* 118:275, 1926.
96. Rovsing, T. Die Behandlung der multilokulären Nierencysten nebst Bemerkungen über die Art dieses Leidens. *Deutsch. Med. Wschr.* 52:614, 1926.
97. Schacht, F. W. Hypertension in cases of congenital polycystic kidney. *Arch. Intern. Med.* 47:500, 1931.
98. Sieber, F. Über Cystennieren bei Erwachsenen. *Deutsch. Z. Chir.* 79:406, 1905.
99. Simon, H. B., and Thompson, G. J. Congenital renal polycystic disease: A clinical and therapeutic study of three hundred sixty-six cases. *J.A.M.A.* 159:657, 1955.
100. Singer, F. *Ein Fall von Hydrops Renum Cystique Congenius*. Greifswald, 1894. P. 5.
101. Ssokoloff, N. *Vestnik. Khir. Grekoo.* 40:135, 1928. Cited by Talman [105].
102. Steglich, W. *Cystennieren und Solitärcysten der Niere*. Leipzig, 1935. Pp. 5, 20, 29, 34.
103. Steiner. Über grosscystiche Degeneration der Nieren und der Leber. *Deutsch. Med. Wschr.* 25:677, 1899.
104. Suter, W. Congenital aneurism of basal cerebral arteries and cystic kidneys. *Schweiz. Med. Wschr.* 79:471, 1949.
105. Talman, I. M. Cystennieren. *Z. Urol. Chir.* 28:180, 1929.
106. Thompson, T. *The Pathology and Clinical Features of Generalized Cystic Disease of the kidneys in Adults*. M.B. Thesis. Cambridge, 1903.
107. Virchow, R. *Verh. Physiol. Med. Ges. Würzburg* 5:447, 1855.
108. Walters, W., and Braasch, W. F. Surgical aspects of polycystic kidneys. Report of 85 surgical cases. *Surg. Gynec. Obstet.* 58:647, 1934.
109. Ward-Steward. Cited by Henninger and Weiss [49].
110. Werner, M. Erbbiologie und Erbpathologie des Harnapparates. In Just, G. (Ed.), *Handbuch der Erbbiologie des Menschen*. Berlin: Springer, 1940. Vol. 4, p. 828.
111. Wobus, R. E. Congenital polycystic kidney with a report of four cases, occurring in children of the same mother. *Surg. Gynec. Obstet.* 27:423, 1918.

112. Wolff, W. Geburtsbehinderung durch vergrösserte Nieren. *Klin. Wschr.* 4:480, 1867.
113. Yates-Bell, J. G. Rovsing's operation for polycystic kidney. *Lancet* 1:126, 1957.
114. Zemitsch, W. Hochdruck und Nierenfunktion bei Cystennieren. *Zbl. Inn. Med.* 60:272, 1939.

36

Microcystic Disease of the Renal Medulla

Maurice B. Strauss

Multiple cysts in the renal medulla are encountered in two widely divergent clinical syndromes. One, designated medullary cystic disease, usually manifests itself by the insidious onset of anemia and leads to death in uremia, frequently in the second or third decade of life. The other, termed medullary sponge kidney, is devoid of symptomatic manifestations in the absence of complications, is discovered on urographic examination, and hence has been reported largely in the radiologic literature.

Cysts of the medullary portions of the kidney are not uncommon apart from these two syndromes and may occur in the course of bacterial pyelonephritis, in association with congenital polycystic disease (see Chapter 35), as a concomitant or result of a variety of congenital and acquired renal disorders, and in the absence of any ascertainable cause. Since cases in these categories present no clearly recognizable clinical syndromes, they are not considered in this chapter.

Medullary Cystic Disease

The clinical and pathologic features of this disorder were first clearly delineated in a single case report by Smith and Graham in 1945 [31]. Although a few writers had described medullary renal cysts earlier, insufficient details were reported to classify these cases. Warfield T. Longcope may well have been the first to correlate the clinical and pathologic aspects, as noted by Smith and Graham, but the report of his patient, who died in 1941, was not published until 1954 when Hogness and Burnell included it with their description of three cases taken from files of the Presbyterian Hospital [13].

In 1951 Fanconi and his colleagues reported seven cases of renal disease in two sibships under the designation "familial juvenile nephronophthisis" [10]. The clinical features were similar in all and to those encountered in medullary cystic disease. Although cysts were not specifically described, several may be seen in the published photograph of the bisected kidney of one of their cases.

In the ensuing decades, many more cases have been described from both sides of the Atlantic, almost invariably as "medullary cystic disease" in the United States and as "familial juvenile nephronophthisis" in Europe. It has become clear that macroscopic cysts are not invariably found in all cases, although microscopic cysts or cystic dilatation of tubules are almost always present. In the autumn of 1967, Herdman et al. [12] and Mongeau and Worthen [23], working independently, published papers indicating that the two conditions were clinically indistinguishable, except genetically, and they suggested that published descriptions and photographs of pathologic material were also identical. At the same time, Strauss and Sommers [34], having had the opportunity of comparing, side by side, histologic sections of cases diagnosed as nephronophthisis in Norway or Sweden with similar sections from published cases of medullary cystic disease of their own, were unable to detect distinguishing features between the two conditions.

In the earlier reports of medullary cystic disease the cases were of sporadic occurrence, and although many of the patients were young, the average age at death being 27 years, at least one patient survived until the sixth decade [33]. Obviously, cases were not reported as instances of familial juvenile nephronophthisis if they were sporadic or the patient had reached adult life. However, in view of the fact that otherwise the clinical and pathologic features are identical, these aspects can be described together regardless of the nosologic designation under which the cases were reported.

CLINICAL ASPECTS

As mentioned above, the disorder is predominantly one of youth, with no predilection for either sex. The most common manifestations which lead to the seeking of medical attention are ascribable to anemia, from which virtually all patients suffer except the asymptomatic cases detected in family surveys. The anemia has an insidious onset, is normocytic and normochromic in type, varies considerably in severity, and can be ascribed to chronic renal insufficiency (see Chapter 7). Often the azotemia is discovered during a search for the cause of anemia, since routine urinalysis generally reveals no or minimal proteinuria and only rarely a few red or white blood cells or casts. However, a history of polyuria and nycturia can generally be elicited, usually of such long duration that neither is often a complaint.

Physical examination is generally unremarkable except for pallor. The blood pressure is usually normal, occasionally becoming moderately elevated later in the course of the disease. Bone changes are rarely clinically manifest, and then only in children, who may also suffer from retarded growth.

Laboratory data are those expected in chronic renal insufficiency. There is an inability to concentrate, but not to dilute, the urine. The hyposthenuria, so generally present, accounts in part for the minimal or absent proteinuria on qualitative testing of random urine specimens and the sparsity of formed elements in the urinary sediment. Blood urea nitrogen concentration may be as low as 50 mg. or exceed 350 mg. per 100 ml. terminally. Serum creatinine concentration has varied greatly, often being in the range of 10 to 20 mg. per 100 ml. when the patient is first seen, and rising to 30 mg. or more per 100 ml. later in the course. The anemia at first is usually of moderate degree (hemoglobin, approximately 10 gm. per 100 ml.), but it often becomes quite severe. Serum phosphorus is generally elevated and is usually accompanied by a depressed level of serum calcium. The bicarbonate is almost always reduced, although symptoms of acidosis are unusual. Serum alkaline phosphatase is generally elevated in the young.

Urinary salt-wasting is frequently observed. In fact, severe salt-wasting, requiring an intake of several hundred milliequivalents of sodium daily to maintain balance, was the dominant manifestation in a patient reported by Thorn et al. [35] under the title "Renal Failure Simulating Adrenocortical Insufficiency" in 1944, the year preceding Smith and Graham's publication. The published description of the kidneys is typical of medullary cystic disease of the kidney, as were the actual sections I examined more than 15 years after the patient's death.

As suggested by the long history of polyuria before the occurrence of other manifestations of renal disease, an inability to concentrate the urine has been noted in a number of patients in the pre-azotemic phase of the disorder. In several cases a reduction in the ability to acidify the urine has been noted [10b, 12], and in one case an inability to dilute the urine normally, increased excretion of amino acids, and a "tubular" type of proteinuria [10b]. These findings and the anatomic evidence speak for the primacy of tubular disease with glomerular insufficiency secondary.

RADIOGRAPHY

Intravenous urography has seldom been rewarding in view of the markedly diminished renal function of most patients. Retrograde pyelography may be normal or indicative of reduced kidney size. In one case renal arteriography [23] showed small kidneys with very thin cortices, distended medullary vessels, poor delineation between cortex and medulla, and radiolucencies suggesting the presence of cysts. This has not been found in other cases [2a, 10a].

COURSE AND TREATMENT

The course has been quite variable, depending on how advanced the renal insufficiency was when the patients were first seen. Inexorable progression appears to be the rule, but a number of patients have survived for some years.

Treatment is that employed for renal insufficiency as outlined in earlier chapters, including dialysis and transplantation in suitable cases. Particular attention must be paid to an adequate intake of sodium, both as the chloride and the bicarbonate, in the severe salt-wasting form of the disorder, especially in the later stages when too little salt rapidly leads to hypovolemia and a small excess to salt retention, edema, and a rise in blood pressure.

PATHOLOGIC ANATOMY

The kidneys at autopsy are generally equally reduced in size. The capsule may or may not strip easily, revealing a smooth or slightly nodular surface. The calyceal and pelvic mucosa is smooth and not thickened. The cortex is thin and differentiated with difficulty from the medulla. Cysts varying in size from less than a millimeter to more than a centimeter in diameter are located for the most part just beneath the cortex (Fig. 36-1).

Microscopic examination confirms the gross impression of a thin and poorly demarcated cortex and shows a majority of the glomeruli to be partially or completely hyalinized. Some glomeruli are abnormally small (about half the usual size), suggesting a process that began in the perinatal period. The remaining glomeruli show no abnormality other than hypertrophy in some. Periglomerular fibrosis may be seen. Practically all the cortical tubules except for a few proximal convolutions have an atrophic or unspecialized epithelium and are engulfed in fibrous tissue. Many tubules have evidently disappeared. The cortical collecting ducts are tortuous and irregularly dilated, and some have either a hyperplastic or an immature type of epithelium.

The medulla is enlarged by multiple cysts varying in size from 100 microns to 1 cm. or more in diameter. The medullary cysts are restricted to, or predominantly near, the corticomedullary junction, although an occasional cyst may be found in the cortex or pyramids. The cysts are lined with low cuboidal or flattened epithelium, sometimes containing scanty amorphous eosinophilic material (Fig. 36-2),

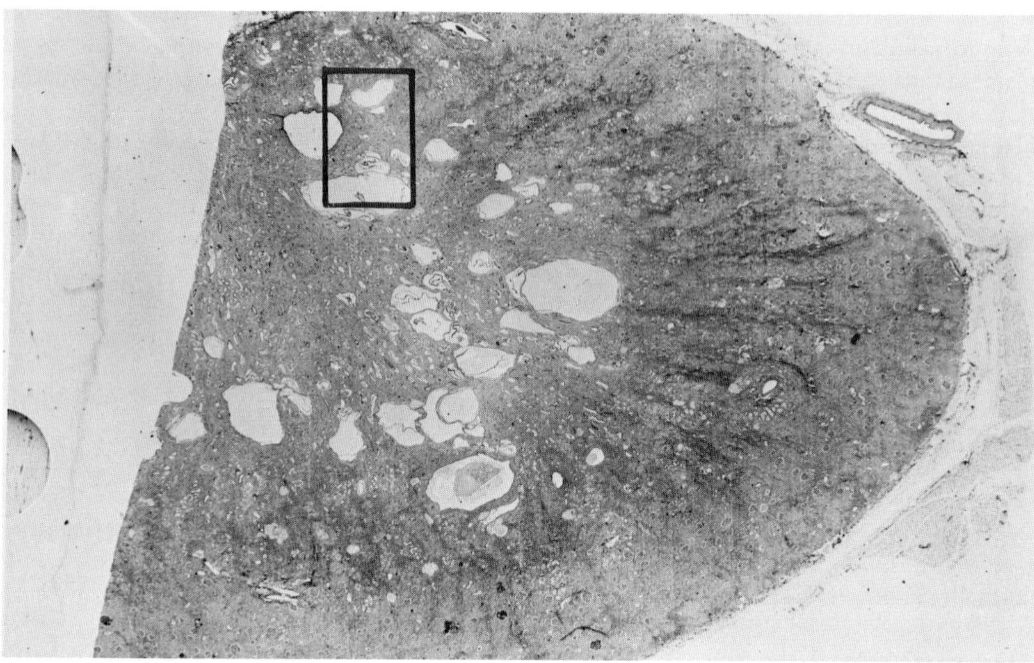

Figure 36-1. Section of the kidney of a 10-year-old boy showing multiple thin-walled cysts occupying the medulla. The cortex is thin (2 mm.), and many of the glomeruli are hyalinized. The remaining glomeruli are intact, often hypertrophied. ×10, before 15% reduction.

and sometimes causing compression and distortion of adjacent tubules.

The uninvolved collecting ducts are distorted, and near the papilla are sometimes extremely narrowed or obliterated, with concentrically thickened PAS-positive basement membranes (Fig. 36-3). The renal pelvic epithelium is usually partly or entirely of the immature metanephric type.

The renal arteries, arterioles, and veins may or may not show intrinsic fibromuscular thickening. The interstitial tissue, aside from extensive diffuse fibrosis and localized lymphangiectasis, contains many lymphocytes, some macrophages and occasionally plasma cells, phagocytized pigment, and calcific foci (Fig. 36-4). Focal dense scars, colloid casts, and interstitial leukocytic infiltrates (including plasma cells) may be encountered, giving the appearance (often misnamed) of chronic pyelonephritis.

Electron microscopic examination [12] has revealed that the most extensive alteration is interstitial fibrosis consisting of wide bands of collagen fibrils mixed with amorphous and fibrillar membrane-like material and cellular processes and nuclei. The basement membranes of tubules are greatly thickened, with either lamination or irregular scalloped extensions projecting into the cytoplasm of the tubule cells. It is thought that dilated segments of tubules derive from proximal and distal tubules as well as from collecting ducts. Cysts are associated with attenuated tubular cytoplasm and extreme basement-membrane thickening. In one asymptomatic sibling of a patient with advanced disease, cysts appeared to be derived from distal tubules or collecting ducts. Microdissection in the advanced case led to a similar conclusion [12].

The parathyroid glands are often markedly enlarged and extremely hyperplastic. In asso-

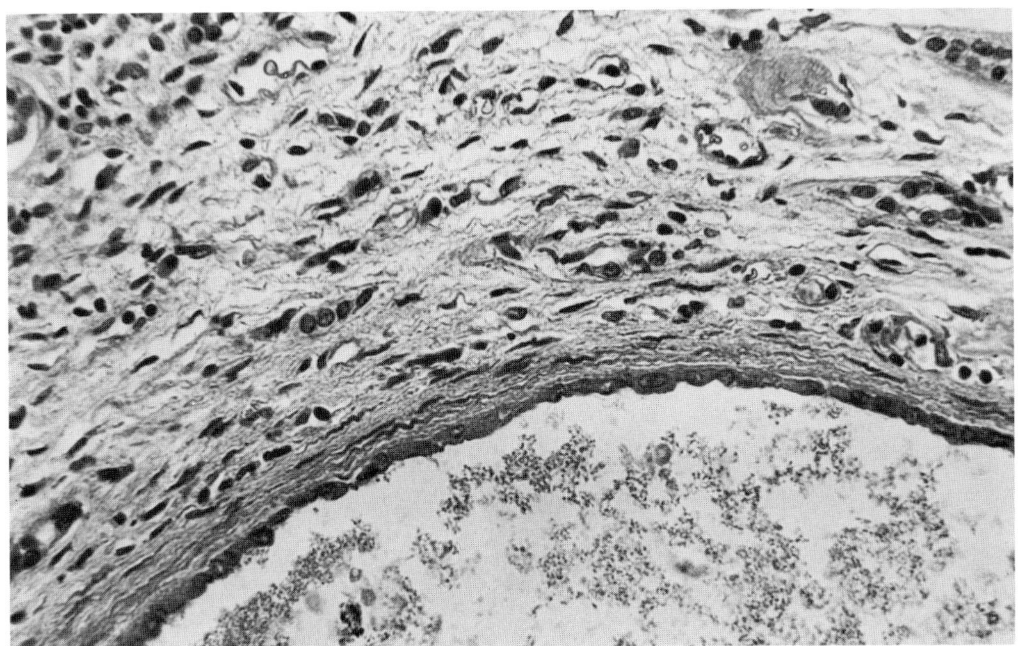

Figure 36-2. Section of cyst wall from a 15-year-old girl, showing the single layer of flattened epithelium lining the cyst and surrounded by connective tissue. ×200, before 15% reduction.

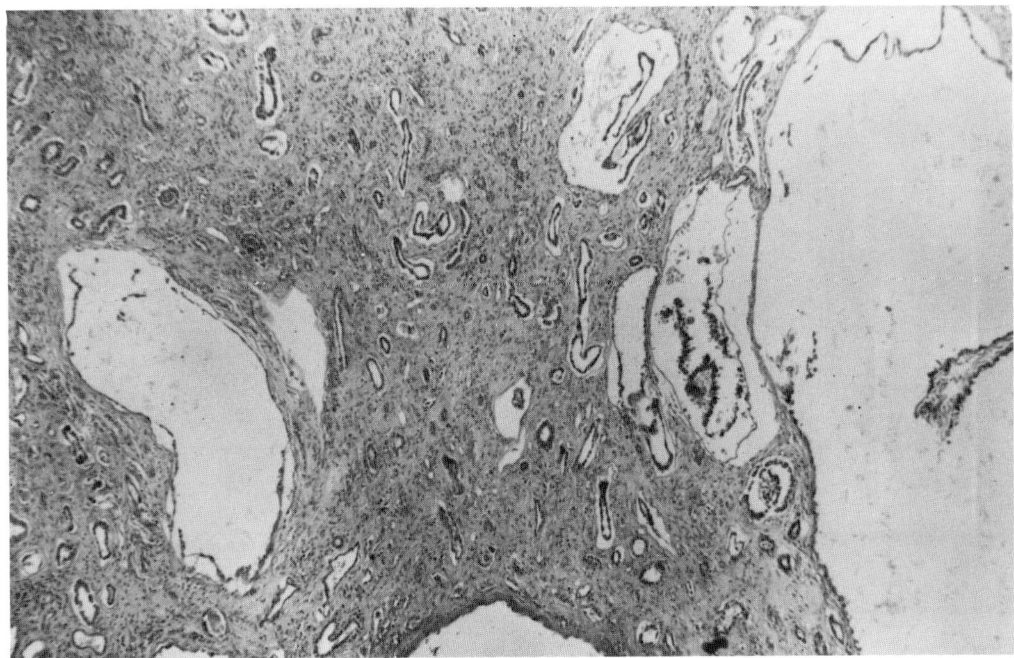

Figure 36-3. Higher magnification of the area outlined by the rectangle in Figure 36-1, showing the atrophic and dilated tubules and cysts surrounded by relatively acellular connective tissue. ×80, before 15% reduction.

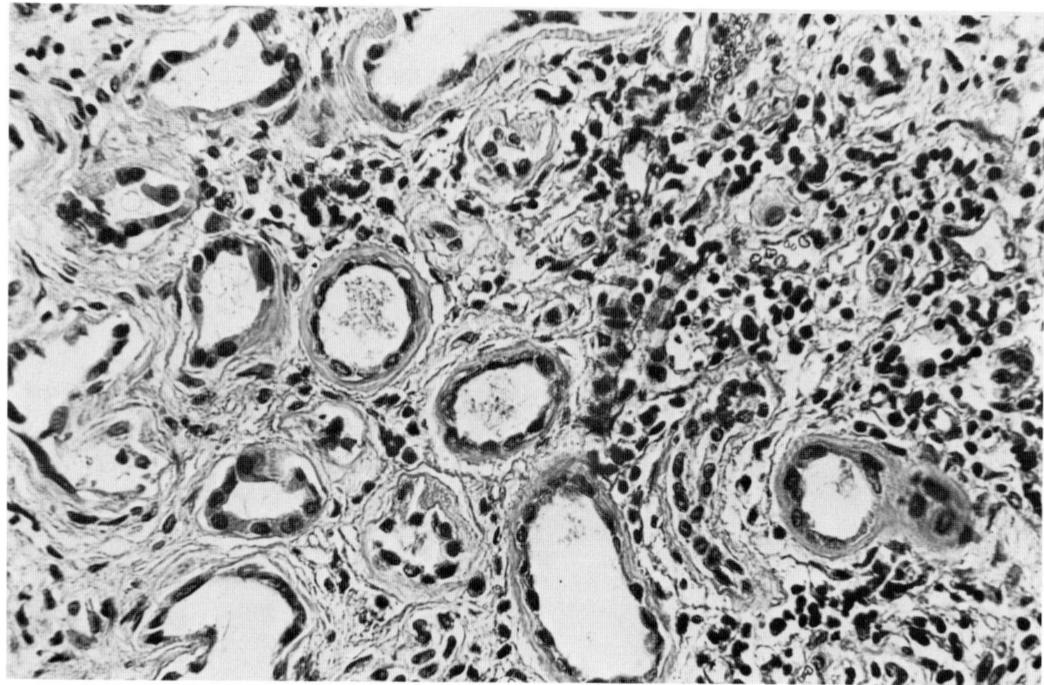

Figure 36-4. Section from the same case as Figure 36-2, showing collars of hyaline material surrounding tubules. ×200, before 15% reduction.

ciation with this finding are bone changes both of renal rickets and of osteitis fibrosa cystica. The bone marrow is hypoplastic and may have areas of fibrosis. The adrenal glands are enlarged, with the zona glomerulosa moderately prominent, in the cases with marked salt-wasting.

OCULAR DEFECTS

Retinal dysplasia (retinitis pigmentosa, tapetoretinal degeneration) has been reported in association with medullary cystic disease in families in which cases occurred in siblings only — that is, in those in whom recessive inheritance is suggested [17, 19a, 21, 30]. It was not observed in the 18 sporadic cases reported in 1962 [33] nor in the 30 cases in which dominant inheritance occurred [11].

In one of the sibships [21] eye disease alone occurred once as did renal disease without eye involvement. Three siblings had both and one neither. The parents, aged 60 and 61, had neither renal nor eye disease. In another family [30], seven siblings were normal, four had both renal and eye disease, and two had definite retinal dysplasia and probable nephropathy. The father, aged 48, was normal, and the mother, aged 40, had the eye disorder only. In a third sibship there was no knowledge of familial abnormalities, but both children were blind from infancy and died at 8 and 9 years of age from renal failure [17].

A most astounding Australian family has been reported on by Fairley et al. [8]. Two generations were free of renal or ocular abnormalities, including both parents. Three of 5 children were blind from birth, the older two because of central cataracts, the youngest from retinal dystrophy. The oldest boy died at 22 years of age from uremia secondary to what appeared at autopsy to be typical enlarged polycystic kidneys of the familial variety.

(However, not a single one of Dalgaard's 254 patients with this disorder died so young, and none had ocular defects — see Chapter 35.) A daughter, the second child, died at age 18 years with typical findings of medullary cystic disease. The next two siblings both had proteinuria but no other renal abnormality; one, an 18-year-old girl, had severe myopia; the other, a 16-year-old boy, had no ocular defect. The fifth child, a 14-year-old girl, who had retinal dystrophy and proteinuria without evidence of renal functional impairment, showed on intravenous urography the typical pattern of medullary sponge kidney (see below). Fairley et al. concluded that several alternative explanations were possible, which seems warranted. For the other three families recessive inheritance of both ocular and renal defects, with linkage or variable penetrance, seems likely but not proved.

PATHOPHYSIOLOGY

The earliest manifestations observed by patients are polyuria and nycturia, reflected in asymptomatic siblings who subsequently develop the disease by an inability to concentrate the urine. There may also be defective urinary acidification. Both are consistent with a distal tubular or collecting duct defect. It is of interest that the cystic disease that develops after several months of feeding diphenylamine to rats is limited to the collecting duct. Early, when anatomic changes are minimal and glomerular filtration rate and proximal tubular function are normal, marked reduction in concentrating ability is noted [14]. No gross evidence of disordered proximal tubular function (glucosuria or marked aminoaciduria) has been reported.

The mechanism of the marked salt-wasting in many cases of medullary cystic disease, and occasionally in other types of kidney disorder, is not yet clear. Although consistent with the osmotic effect of a normal urea load imposed upon a greatly diminished number of nephrons [32], it must be noted how rarely it is encountered in other types of renal failure of equal or greater severity. Furthermore, reduction of blood urea levels by dialysis in those with severe salt-wasting has been found to have little or no effect on urinary salt excretion. In contrast, lowering the urea load in patients without a salt-losing disorder decreases the urine volume [22].

The apparent normality or even hypertrophy of the remaining glomeruli in this disorder, together with the dilation and atrophy of many of the remaining tubules, suggests the possibility that the filtered load of sodium exceeds the reabsorptive capacity of the tubules. An inability to establish the usual large gradient between urine and serum appears to be one mechanism for the modest salt-conserving disability of the usual patient with renal failure [4]. Data in one case of medullary cystic disease revealed a maximal gradient between urine and serum sodium concentrations of 42 mEq. per liter [33], a value consistent with this hypothesis.

GENETICS

A few general comments seem in order preliminary to discussion of medullary cystic disease. Similar phenotypes may be produced by different genetic mechanisms. For example, retinitis pigmentosa [9] and familial spastic paraplegia [19] may show autosomal dominant, autosomal recessive, or sex-linked recessive inheritance. Glycogen storage disease and cystinuria are further examples. In addition, environmental factors may lead to disorders which cannot be distinguished from those genetically determined. The best example of such a phenocopy is the deaf-mutism resulting from maternal rubella early in pregnancy, which is identical to the inherited form controlled by a recessive gene. Finally, the occurrence of multiple cases of a disorder not only in siblings but also in more than one generation of a family does not necessarily indicate an inherited defect. Balkan nephropathy, for example, is almost certainly not a genetic defect although the possibility of a genetic defect permitting it to develop as a result of environmental toxic or infectious factors cannot be excluded [3]. Kuru, a slow virus disease, is another example [20].

Of the 18 cases of medullary cystic disease which I collected in 1962 [33] a family history of renal disease was absent in 16. In one family traced for three generations, no members had kidney disease. Twenty-nine individuals survived for 60 to 90 years, two died of cancer in their mid-forties, and the parents of the affected patient, who were in their mid-sixties, were free of renal disease and had normal ability to concentrate the urine [6]. None of this, however, excludes recessive inheritance.

In the cases described under the term familial juvenile nephronophthisis there obviously was more than one individual per family affected. In all verified instances, parents were not affected and the siblings were randomly distributed as to age and sex, consistent with autosomal recessive inheritance, but so few data are available that definite conclusions cannot be reached [28]. In some of the North American families a similar pattern existed [12] as well as in the South African family of Senior et al. [30]. One of the two families of Mongeau and Worthen [23] is suggestive of autosomal recessive inheritance with involvement of one individual in each of three generations. In their other family, in a large family studied by Nelsen [25], and in the very impressive family of Goldman et al. [11] autosomal dominant transmission is probable. However, over 50 per cent of the family members at risk (in four generations) were affected, abnormal females outnumbered abnormal males and no male-to-male transmission was observed, leading Perkoff [28] to raise the question of either sex-linkage or preferential segregation of an abnormal autosome which was more likely to remain with the oocyte than to migrate randomly to the polar body. Gardner [10a] has also reported a large family in which autosomal dominant inheritance appears likely, and has added further data on the family of Goldman et al. [11].

PATHOGENESIS

The pathogenesis of cystic disease of the renal medulla remains as obscure as that of the more common familial polycystic disease (Chapter 35). A decade ago the disorder was considered an unusual result of bacterial pyelonephritis. A developmental defect, genetically determined in several ways or acquired in utero or subsequently, remains probable. Herdman et al. [12] have suggested that an inborn error of metabolism first causes functional, then secondarily, structural changes in the kidney. Since a kidney transplanted into one of their patients showed no evidence of involvement after two years, they deduced that the metabolic abnormality resided in the patient's kidneys rather than in a systemic defect such as hyperoxaluria. Gardner [10a] has reported survival of normal renal function in 3 transplanted kidneys for three or more years.

Medullary Sponge Kidney

Beitzke [1], in 1908, reported that in four autopsies performed on unrelated individuals dying of nonrenal disorders he had found cysts lined with cuboidal epithelium, often several layers thick, largely limited to the medulla and papilla. Calcium deposits were found in some cysts and a "black stone" in one.

Thirty years later the Italian radiologist Lenarduzzi [15] demonstrated x-ray films which showed small punctate calcifications in areas of both kidneys corresponding to the pyramids of Malpighi. At retrograde pyelography the contrast medium was seen to pass up through normal pelvocalyceal systems into dilated collecting ducts. Ten years later Cacchi and Ricci [2] gave the condition the name sponge kidney (*rene a spugna*) in describing 5 cases, one of which was the original case of Lenarduzzi. Unilateral nephrectomy on one of the patients afforded them anatomic material similar in gross and microscopic appearance to that of Beitzke. Since then several hundred cases have been reported, mostly in radiologic and urologic journals, often as single case reports and rarely illustrated with histologic sections. In 1959 Ekström and his co-workers [7] published their splendid monograph based on 44 patients, the majority of whom had been under observation for from 2 to 20 or more years. Histologic examination was made on 15 specimens obtained from partial or total nephrectomies. This most complete study can be recommended most highly and has been drawn on heavily for this section.

As far as can be ascertained, sponge kidney is entirely asymptomatic unless accompanied by the passage of stones, obstruction, or infection. Whether or not hematuria occurs in the absence of stones remains unknown. If, as is generally held, the disorder is a developmental defect, it is clear that there must be a long asymptomatic period since the majority of patients do not have symptoms until after the age of 40. Indeed, it is probable that many cases never become symptomatic.

The prevalence of sponge kidney is unknown. Why it has not been recognized at autopsy more often in the 60 years since Beitzke's report is unclear. Possibly it was classified in the wastebasket of "chronic pyelonephritis." Palubinskas [26] found 14 cases in 2465 consecutive urograms, an incidence of 0.5 per cent. However, since urography is most often performed for the investigation of urinary complaints, this figure probably is much greater than the true prevalence in asymptomatic individuals. Since the injection of contrast material and exposure to x-irradiation of normal subjects cannot be justified, it can only be hoped that autopsy data concerning this condition will be forthcoming in the future.

Although males outnumber females by 2:1 when all reported cases are considered, Ekström et al. [7], MacDougall and Prout [18] and others have found an almost equal sex distribution. There is no apparent racial or familial* preponderance although most cases have been reported by Italian, Scandinavian, and French physicians. This is presumably because of the neglect of the subject in Anglo-Saxon literature until the last decade. The age of the patient when the diagnosis was first made has varied from the first to the eighth decade, with about two-thirds of reported cases in the 30- to 60-year range and about one-third in the fifth decade. This is in contrast to the uremic form of medullary cystic disease (see above) as well as to the familial type of polycystic kidney disease (Chapter 35).

UROGRAPHIC APPEARANCE

Since the diagnosis of sponge kidney is essentially dependent on radiologic examination, it may be well to commence with a description of the characteristic appearance seen on x-ray films. Moderate enlargement of one or both kidneys occurs in about one-third of the cases. Radiopaque calculi, varying in size from being barely visible to 5 mm. or more, and varying in number from a solitary stone to hundreds, are seen on plain films of the kidneys in most cases.

On intravenous urography the density of the contrast material is invariably normal in the absence of complicating obstructive hydronephrosis or secondary infectious pyelonephritis. A typical feature is that the cavities are the first structures to be filled with contrast medium, that they appear more distinct on applying pressure to the ureter, and that they remain filled temporarily after pressure has been removed and the pelvis emptied of contrast medium. Many of the cavities contain calculi, slightly smaller than the cavity itself.

* Although it is stated that 6 members of one family had sponge kidney, no radiologic or pathologic confirmation was given [29]. In another article on sponge kidney with a familial incidence [5], the author himself questions whether the condition described was not familial renal tubular acidosis with secondary nephrocalcinosis.

The cavities vary from barely discernible to about 7 mm. in size. They may appear simply as greatly dilated collecting tubules, as round or oval cavities, or as triangular-shaped or irregularly shaped spaces. They are invariably confined to the pyramids and mainly in the papillary portion, practically never extending to the corticomedullary junction. There may be only a few cavities in a single pyramid of one kidney, or every pyramid of both kidneys may have multiple cavities. Enlargement of the involved pyramids and of the corresponding calyces is common. Cavities may all be of one configuration, or two or three shapes may be seen in a single pyramid. In general, over long periods of repeated urography the visible lesions remain unaltered although the number and the size of calculi increase [7].

Palubinskas [27] has put together a series of photographs of renal pyramids observed upon urography in various individuals in which normal and affected blend imperceptibly from the normally observed "pyramidal blush" to the full-blown diagnostic picture of medullary sponge kidney. In addition, he has depicted six pyramids from a single patient with sponge kidney showing similar gradations.

Retrograde pyelography seldom reveals as many cavities as urography (Fig. 36-5). This has been assumed to be due to "sphincters" at

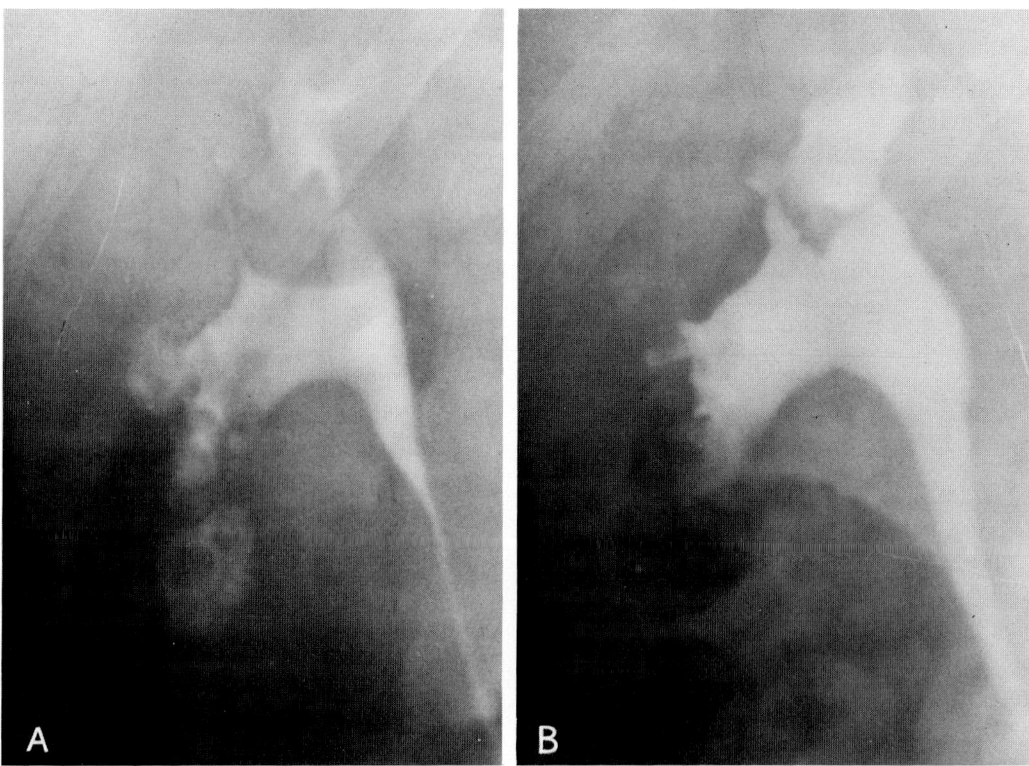

Figure 36-5. A. Appearance of sponge kidney on roentgenologic examination following intravenous injection of contrast material. Note the many spaces of various shape and size lying adjacent to the calcyces. Plain films revealed a number of small opaque calculi in these areas. B. Appearance of the same kidney as in A on retrograde pyelography. Most of the spaces filled with contrast material after intravenous urography are not filled by the retrograde injection.

the papillary orifices of the collecting ducts which do not permit reflux. However, when calculi have eroded through, this mechanism presumably is destroyed. Conversely, cavities not visible on urography may be seen on retrograde study, suggesting that they open on the calyx but are no longer connected to functioning nephrons.

CLINICAL MANIFESTATIONS

As mentioned above, it is doubtful whether medullary sponge kidney produces any symptoms at all in the absence of complications. This view is shared by Ekström et al. [7], who point out that although "silent" gross or microscopic hematuria occurred in eight of their patients who at the time had no visible concretions in the pyramids, the stones may have been so tiny as to be invisible on radiographs or the hematuria may have been unrelated to the sponge kidney which was found incidental to urography performed in search of a cause of bleeding. Of their remaining 36 cases, acute renal colic was the first manifestation in 25, of whom the passage of a stone was verified in 19; seven had urinary tract infection; and four were asymptomatic, urologic investigation being incidental to other problems.

Major symptoms during the follow-up period included recurrent renal colic in 19, macroscopic hematuria in 29, and recurrent acute or chronic infection in 12. How the calculi escape from the cysts has not been determined, but they are probably extruded as a result of their eroding through the pyramid. Although passage down the ureter often produces colic, many calculi are so small as to be passed painlessly. The high frequency of urinary tract infection has been ascribed to the fact that any anatomic abnormality in the kidney appears to favor bacterial localization. To what extent instrumentation leads to retrograde infection is unknown.

Renal function in uncomplicated cases is generally normal. Blood urea nitrogen is not elevated, and creatinine clearance is normal. PAH clearance in the few cases examined was normal. Slight reduction in maximal urinary concentration may be encountered in patients with extensive bilateral involvement. In cases complicated by infection, an impaired urine-concentrating ability is more common. Inability to acidify the urine maximally has been reported [24] as has defective ammonium excretion [16] and hypercalciuria [7].

Few of the cases have been confirmed pathologically, and as noted below, other conditions may present a somewhat similar radiologic appearance. Many writers have assumed that the uremic form of medullary cystic disease is a late stage of sponge kidney, further confusing the issue.

PATHOLOGIC FINDINGS

Although anatomic examination has been carried out in only about 10 per cent of cases, the gross and microscopic appearance of the uncomplicated case is characteristic. The kidneys generally are of normal size or moderately enlarged in the more extensively involved cases. The lesions are limited to the pyramids which are paler than normal and irregularly demarcated. Neither the cortex nor its extension in the columns of Bertin is involved. The pyramids, when extensively involved, are often enlarged and bulge into the calyces. In such cases the cortex and columns of Bertin appear narrower than usual. The papillary region shows varying numbers of cavities, ranging in size from the barely visible up to 7 to 8 mm., and containing clear to opaque, liquid, jelly-like, or grumous material, and frequently smooth-surfaced calculi, pale yellow to black in color. In the absence of secondary infection, pelvic and calyceal mucosa is normal.

Microscopically both dilatation of collecting ducts and rounded or irregularly shaped cysts are seen (Fig. 36-6). Connection with tubules or renal pelvis is obvious in some but not all cases. In others the cysts appear to be isolated.

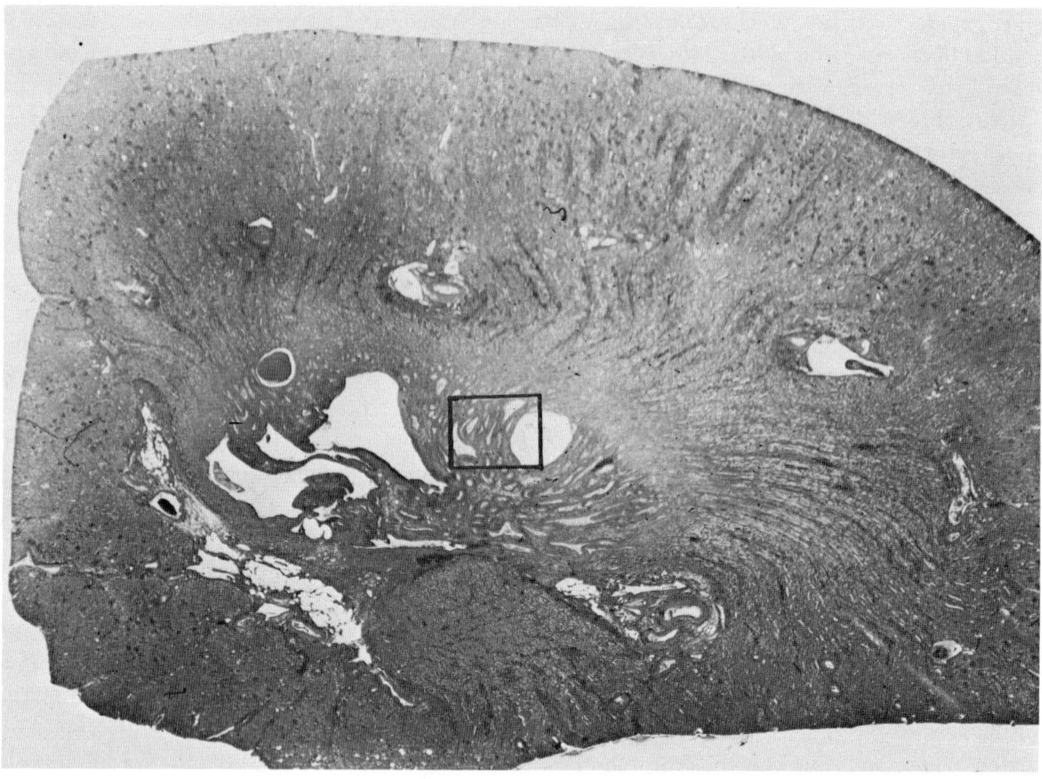

Figure 36-6. Section of lower pole of sponge kidney removed surgically in the case shown in Figure 36-5. Note the normal cortex and glomeruli. The medulla shows numerous cysts and cleft-like dilatations of the tubules. Calculi occupy several of the cysts. ×6, before 15% reduction.

The cysts may contain desquamated cells, precipitated calcium salts, or solid calculi (Fig. 36-6). The dilated tubules may be lined with either more or less normal-appearing cells or several layers of cuboidal or columnar cells of transitional type (Fig. 36-7). The larger cysts are usually lined with a single layer of cuboidal or flattened epithelial cells (Fig. 36-8), or in cavities containing calculi, the epithelium may have been shed. Many cysts communicate with the calyces. Collecting tubules appear to open into others. The cortex ordinarily shows no abnormalities unless there has been concomitant infection. Even in the absence of any evidence of prior infection, the connective tissue in the affected areas is infiltrated with round cells and an occasional eosinophil. Ekström et al. [7] determined that the concretions are most often pure apatite or apatite with more or less calcium oxalate or ammonium magnesium sulfate.

As can be seen from the photomicrographs, the histologic appearance is entirely different from that seen in the uremic form of medullary cystic disease. Except for the fact that cystic areas occur in the same general region of the kidney, there are no similarities clinically or pathologically.

DIFFERENTIAL DIAGNOSIS

A number of conditions may present a roentgenologic appearance similar to that of medullary sponge kidney. In some of these, differentiation is unimportant; in others, such

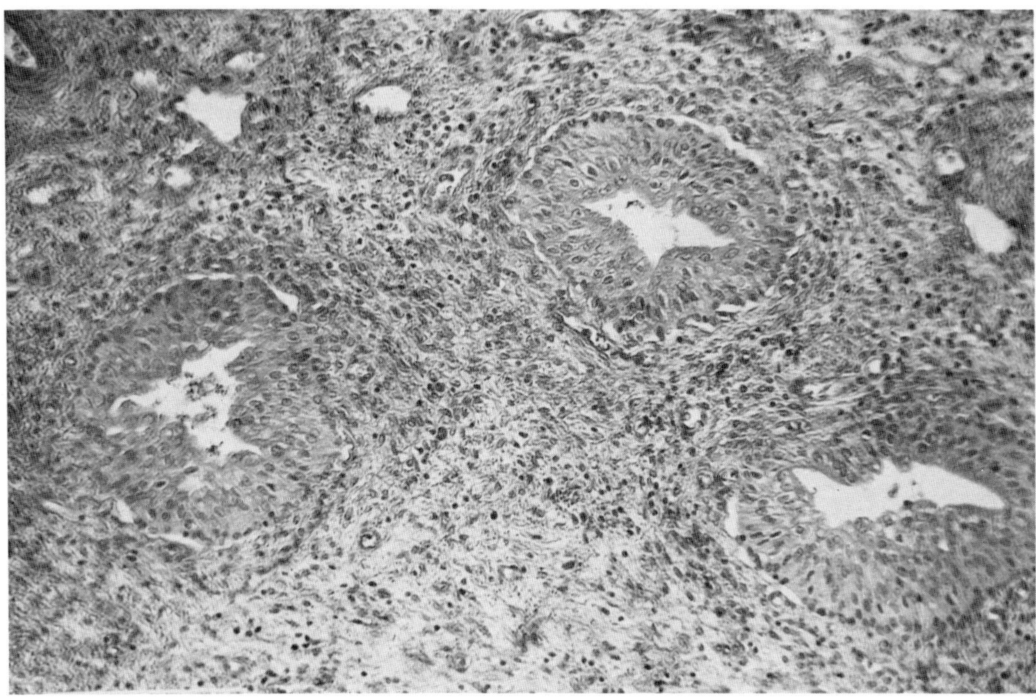

Figure 36-7. Collecting tubules from the same case as Figure 36-6, showing columnar epithelium three and more cells in depth lining the tubules and surrounded by proliferation of interstitial tissue. ×120, before 15% reduction.

as renal tuberculosis, appropriate treatment is of vital import. Thus, it was the fear that the condition was tuberculous which led to the generous biopsy in the case from which the photomicrographs shown above were obtained a decade ago. In nephrocalcinosis due to hyperparathyroidism or in renal tubular acidosis, appropriate management is, of course, of great importance.

Calyceal diverticula and cysts, pyelonephritis cysts, those secondary to papillary necrosis, and other urinary tract abnormalities may be difficult to differentiate at times but seldom present a problem in management. "Tubular stasis" may resemble the form of sponge kidney in which only collecting-duct ectasia exists. However, it is said that these ducts empty more promptly upon relief of abdominal compression.

TREATMENT

Since uncomplicated cases are asymptomatic, no therapy is required. There is no known way to prevent calculus formation in the cavities. The treatment of impacted stones and of urinary tract infection does not differ from the therapy of these conditions in the absence of sponge kidney. However, the knowledge that the disorder is so frequently bilateral must temper the surgeon's hand. Although partial or complete nephrectomy has been performed for the relief of recurrent stone formation accompanied by bacterial pyelonephritis that was otherwise uncontrollable, such procedures should not be entered upon lightly. In the case of recurrent stone passage with the disorder limited to one pole or to one kidney, surgical excision has also been employed. Massive hematuria may re-

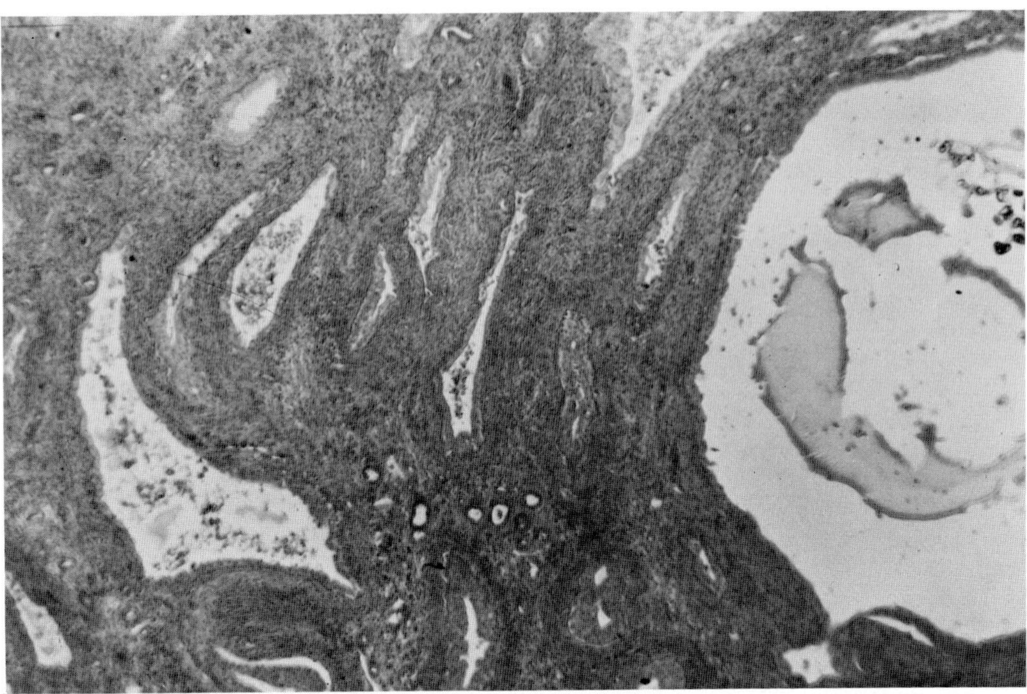

Figure 36-8. Higher magnification of the area outlined by the rectangle in Figure 35-6. The epithelial lining of the dilated tubules is several layers thick. The cyst, containing bluish-staining material (calcium?), is lined by a single layer of cuboidal epithelium. ×80, before 15% reduction.

quire blood transfusion, but I know of no instance in which nephrectomy was indicated.

PROGNOSIS

Twenty-one of the 44 patients of Ekström et al. [7] have been followed for from 5 to more than 15 years with one death from bronchogenic carcinoma at 12 years. Recurring stone passage, hydronephrosis (which occurred from obstruction in almost half the patients), and recurring pyelonephritis have led to renal functional impairment in five. Four patients subjected to unilateral nephrectomy developed serious disorder in the remaining kidney. It appears that conservatism and the avoidance of unnecessary instrumentation are in order.

PATHOGENESIS

A considerable number of writers on sponge kidney have engaged in speculation concerning its pathogenesis which has been as sterile as speculation concerning the pathogenesis of the common form of polycystic kidneys. Furthermore, they have frequently confused this disorder with the uremic form of medullary cystic disease. That the latter is not the end result or late stage of sponge kidney is indicated not only by the dissimilar histologic appearance of the kidneys but also by the fact that the latter is a disorder of middle to late adult life while medullary cystic disease is prone to kill in adolescence and early adulthood.

References

1. Beitzke, H. Ueber Zysten im Nierenmark. *Charité-Ann.* 32:285, 1908.
2. Cacchi, R., and Ricci, V. Sur une rare maladie kystique multiple des pyramides rénales, le "rein en éponge." *J. Urol. Nephrol.* (Paris) 55:497, 1949.

2a. Case records of the Massachusetts General Hospital. *New Eng. J. Med.* 282:799, 1970.

3. Ciba Foundation Study Group No. 30. *The Balkan Nephropathy.* Boston: Little, Brown, 1967.
4. Coleman, A. J., Arias, M., Carter, N. W., Rector, F. C., Jr., and Seldin, D. W. The mechanism of salt wastage in chronic renal disease. *J. Clin. Invest.* 45:1116, 1966.
5. Deck, M. D. F. Medullary sponge kidney with renal tubular acidosis: A report of 3 cases. *J. Urol.* 94:330, 1965.
6. Editorial. Cystic diseases of kidney. *New Eng. J. Med.* 274:1029, 1966.
7. Ekström, T., Engfeldt, B., Lagergren, C., and Lindvall, N. *Medullary Sponge Kidney.* Stockholm: Almqvist & Wiksell, 1959.
8. Fairley, K. F., Leighton, P. W., and Kincaid-Smith, P. Familial visual defects associated with polycystic kidney and medullary sponge kidney. *British Med. J.* 1:1060, 1963.
9. Falls, H. F., and Cotterman, C. W. Choroidoretinal degeneration: A sex-linked form in which heterozygous women exhibit a tapeto-like retinal reflex. *Arch. Ophthal.* 40:685, 1948.
10. Fanconi, G., Hanhart, E., v. Albertini, A., Ühlinger, E., Dolivo, G., and Prader, A. Die familiäre juvenile Nephronophthise (die idiopathische parenchymatöse Schrumpfniere). *Helv. Paediat. Acta* 6:1, 1951.

10a. Gardner, K. D., Jr. Evolution of clinical signs in adult-onset cystic disease of the renal medulla. *Ann. Intern. Med.* 74:47, 1971.

10b. Giselson, N., Heinegard, D., Holmberg, C-G., Lindberg, L-G., Lindstedt, E., Lindstedt, G., and Schersten, B. Renal medullary cystic disease or familial juvenile nephronophthisis: A renal tubular disease. Biochemical findings in two siblings. *Amer. J. Med.* 48:174, 1970.

11. Goldman, S. H., Walker, S. R., Merigan, T. C., Jr., Gardner, K. D., Jr., and Ball, J. M. C. Hereditary occurrence of cystic disease of renal medulla. *New Eng. J. Med.* 274:984, 1966.
12. Herdman, R. C., Good, R. A., and Vernier, R. L. Medullary cystic disease in two siblings. *Amer. J. Med.* 43:335, 1967.
13. Hogness, J. R., and Burnell, J. M. Medullary cysts of kidneys. *A.M.A. Arch. Intern. Med.* 93:355, 1954.
14. Kime, S. W., Jr., McNamara, J. J., Luse, S., Farmer, S., Silbert, C., and Bricker, N. S. Experimental polycystic renal disease in rats: Electron microscopy, function, and susceptibility to pyelonephritis. *J. Lab. Clin. Med.* 60:64, 1962.
15. Lenarduzzi, G. Reperto pielografico poco commune (dilatazione delle vie urinarie intrarenali). *Radiol. Med.* (Torino) 26:346, 1939.
16. Levin, N. W., Rosenberg, B., Zwi, S., and Reid, F. P. Medullary cystic disease of the kidney, with some observations on ammonium excretion. *Amer. J. Med.* 30:807, 1961.
17. Løken, A. G., Hanssen, O., Halvorsen, S., and Jølster, N. J. Hereditary renal dysplasia and blindness. *Acta Paediat. Scand.* 50:177, 1961.
18. MacDougall, J. A., and Prout, W. G. Medullary sponge kidney: Clinical appraisal and report of twelve cases. *Brit. J. Surg.* 55:130, 1968.
19. Mahloudji, M., and Chuke, P. O. Familial spastic paraplegia with retinal degeneration. *Johns Hopkins Med. J.* 123:142, 1968.

19a. Mainzer, F., Saldino, R. M., Ozonoff, M. B., and Minagi, H. Familial nephropathy associated with retinitis pigmentosa, cerebellar ataxia and skeletal abnormalities. *Amer. J. Med.* 49:556, 1970.

20. Mathews, J. D., Glasse, R., and Lindenbaum, S. Kuru and cannibalism. *Lancet* 2:449, 1968.
21. Meier, D. A., and Hess, J. W. Familial nephropathy with retinitis pigmentosa: New oculorenal syndrome in adults. *Amer. J. Med.* 39:58, 1965.

22. Merrill, J. P. Quoted in Strauss, M. B., and Welt, L. G. (Eds.), *Diseases of the Kidney* (1st ed.). Boston: Little, Brown, 1963. P. 946.
23. Mongeau, J. G., and Worthen, H. G. Nephronophthisis and medullary cystic disease. *Amer. J. Med.* 43:345, 1967.
24. Morris, R. C., Yamauchi, H., Palubinskas, A. J., and Howenstine, J. Medullary sponge kidney. *Amer. J. Med.* 38:883, 1965.
25. Nelsen, C. E. Personal communication.
26. Palubinskas, A. J. Medullary sponge kidney. *Radiology* 76:911, 1961.
27. Palubinskas, A. J. Renal pyramidal structure opacification in excretory urography and its relation to medullary sponge kidney. *Radiology* 81:963, 1963.
28. Perkoff, G. T. The hereditary renal diseases. *New Eng. J. Med.* 277:79, 1967.
29. Pyrah, L. N. Medullary sponge kidney. *J. Urol.* 95:274, 1966.
30. Senior, B., Friedmann, A. I., and Braudo, J. L. Juvenile familial nephropathy with tapetoretinal degeneration. *Amer. J. Ophthal.* 52:625, 1963.
31. Smith, C. H., and Graham, J. B. Congenital medullary cysts of kidneys with severe refractory anemia. *Amer. J. Dis. Child.* 69:369, 1945.
32. Stanbury, S. W., and Mahler, R. F. Salt-wasting renal disease: Metabolic observations on a patient with "salt-losing nephritis." *Quart. J. Med.* 28:425, 1959.
33. Strauss, M. B. Clinical and pathological aspects of cystic disease of renal medulla: Analysis of eighteen cases. *Ann. Intern. Med.* 57:373, 1962.
34. Strauss, M. B., and Sommers, S. C. Medullary cystic disease and familial juvenile nephronophthisis: Clinical and pathological identity. *New Eng. J. Med.* 277:863, 1967.
35. Thorn, G. W., Koepf, G. F., and Clinton, M., Jr. Renal failure simulating adrenocortical insufficiency. *New Eng. J. Med.* 231:76, 1944.

37

Hereditary Chronic Nephritis

Gerald T. Perkoff

The early history of hereditary chronic nephritis, *hereditary nephritis,* or *Alport's syndrome* is characterized by intermittent reports of case and family studies beginning in 1881 and ending with those of Alport in 1927 [1, 2, 4, 10, 13, 16, 19, 20, 22, 24, 30, 37]. Then, from 1927 to 1951, little was added concerning this disease. But beginning in 1951 [34], the numbers of families in which hereditary chronic nephritis was recognized grew apace, so that by 1968 over 50 families were known throughout the world. A detailed review of this literature has been presented [32]. The disease is being diagnosed everywhere with increasing frequency.

Clinical Manifestations and Course of the Disease

The clinical features of the illness were described best by Guthrie [20], Kendall and Hertz [23], and Alport [1] in successive studies of the same family. Thus, hematuria, nerve deafness, and chronic renal insufficiency more severe in males than in females have been recognized hallmarks of the disease for four decades.

Early in hereditary chronic nephritis the patient usually has no symptoms, even though the urinary sediment may have been grossly abnormal since infancy. *Episodic hematuria* frequently begins in childhood, and rarely may be massive enough to lead to *renal colic.* Such episodes sometimes are preceded by a few days by an upper-respiratory-tract infection, but this is not always so. In a small number of patients characteristic urinary tract infection occurs intermittently, with the usual symptoms of fever, backache, dysuria, and urinary frequency as the presenting complaints instead of hematuria. When this occurs, organisms customarily associated with urinary tract infections usually can be cultured from the urine, and the patient's signs and symptoms respond to appropriate antibiotic or chemotherapy.

A marked sex difference in the severity of the disease is the most striking clinical feature of hereditary chronic nephritis. As a rule, involved females remain well throughout their lives, and very few are thought to have died of their disease. Most of the affected males die before the age of 40 years. In these patients, chronic renal insufficiency begins between the ages of 20 and 30 years. Initially the only symptom may be mild weakness. Later, easy fatigability, lassitude, and weight loss develop. Pallor, tetany, and the complex electrolyte abnormalities of uremia appear late in the course of the disease. Hypertension is not a prominent feature of hereditary chronic nephritis; when present, it usually is a moderate and late manifestation of the renal insufficiency.

ASSOCIATED CLINICAL FEATURES

Several extrarenal abnormalities occur in patients with hereditary chronic nephritis [21]; some (e.g., iliac horns, skin changes) may indicate a subtype of the disease. Nerve deafness is regularly associated with hereditary chronic nephritis [33], and frequently ocular abnormalities are present [5–7, 17, 41]. Although clinically evident deafness occurs primarily only in uremic males, this abnormality may occur as an isolated feature of the disease. Such patients can transmit the renal disease to their children. With few exceptions — the most notable one is Alport's family — deafness is recognized in women only by audiometry. In my group of patients, 10 men who died in uremia had had obvious nerve deafness. By audiometry of 86 other family members, nine other men were found to have nerve deafness, but only one female had deafness despite the fact that more women than men were tested. That woman had renal disease as well as nerve deafness. Although very few studies have been made, thus far no specific histopathologic changes have been found in the inner ear at autopsy in such patients [33, 49].

The ocular abnormalities are varied [5–7, 17, 41]. Thus congenital cataracts, congenital nystagmus, myopia, spherophakia, and anterior lenticonus all have been reported in patients with hereditary chronic nephritis — usually but not always in those patients with both renal disease and nerve deafness.

LABORATORY FINDINGS

The only consistent abnormalities are in the urinary sediment. Marked changes may be found even in infants, and consist, then as later, of pyuria, hematuria, and cylindruria. Proteinuria is less common and rarely is of major proportions; the nephrotic syndrome is found only rarely.

From a diagnostic point of view, biochemical laboratory studies are unrewarding. Occasionally hypercholesterolemia and hyperlipidemia in the absence of the nephrotic syndrome [9], or aminoaciduria of a variable and nonspecific type has been found [28, 48]. Generally, however, such measurements give normal results.

Pathologic Anatomy

The anatomic changes in the kidney in hereditary chronic nephritis vary greatly, depending on the stage of the disease. Early in the course of the disease, percutaneous renal biopsy shows only minor, nonspecific changes. A few red blood cells may be found in the renal tubules [36]; an occasional glomerulus sometimes is found to be hyalinized, and tiny interstitial foci of mononuclear cells are noted [33]. Perhaps of greater importance is that careful search sometimes reveals foci of lipid-filled foam cells (Fig. 37-1) scattered throughout the biopsy specimen. Most commonly these are seen in the interstitium near the corticomedullary junction, but they may be located anywhere in the specimen. The possible significance of these cells and the controversy which has arisen concerning them is discussed in a later paragraph.

In biopsy specimens taken later, when the disease has progressed, or in autopsy specimens, the changes are more striking. Grossly,

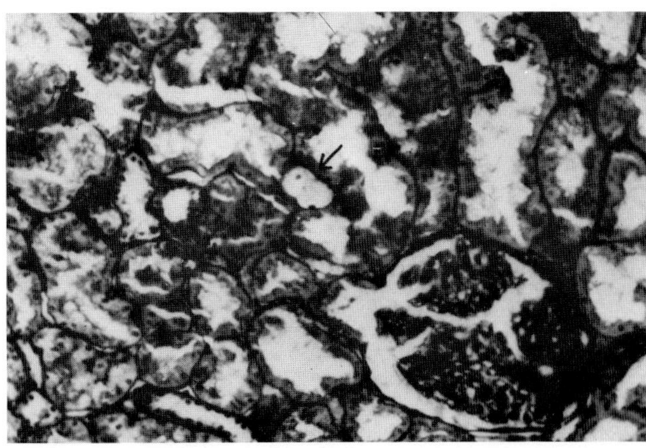

Figure 37-1. Low power photomicrograph of a renal biopsy specimen. The glomerulus shows thickening of the fibrous material of the stalk and focal thickening of Bowman's capsule. In addition, two foam cells (*arrow*) are seen to the right of the glomerulus. Periodic acid–Schiff stain. (From Perkoff, G. T., Nugent, C. A., Jr., Dolowitz, D. A., Stephens, F. E., Carnes, W. H., and Tyler, F. H. [33].)

the kidneys are small and on sagittal section both the cortex and the medulla are thinned. Diffuse linear streaks of lipid may be seen throughout the organ (Fig. 37-2). On microscopic examination, typical interstitial pyelonephritis has been found in some instances, whereas glomerulonephritis was described in others. In some cases both types of change were present. A prominent feature of the late cases is the presence of rows of lipid-filled foam cells throughout the cortex but most numerous near the corticomedullary junction. These correspond to the lipid streaking areas seen in the gross specimen (Figs. 37-3 and 37-4). In addition, foam cells may be found in the glomeruli and in the tubular epithelium per se.

The nature, significance, and specificity of the renal foam cells are uncertain. Whalen et al. [49], Rosen et al. [38], and Sanerkin [39] have shown that such cells may occur in chronic glomerulonephritis, lipoid nephrosis, and membranous glomerulonephritis, even though there is no positive family history for renal disease, nerve deafness, or ocular abnormalities. However, such cells are found more frequently in patients with hereditary nephritis than in patients with any other disease. Krickstein et al. [25] studied tissue from 9 autopsies, 7 renal biopsies, and 2 nephrectomy specimens representing material from members of 13 unrelated families. Interstitial foam cells were found in 6 of the 9 autopsy specimens, both nephrectomy specimens, and 3 of

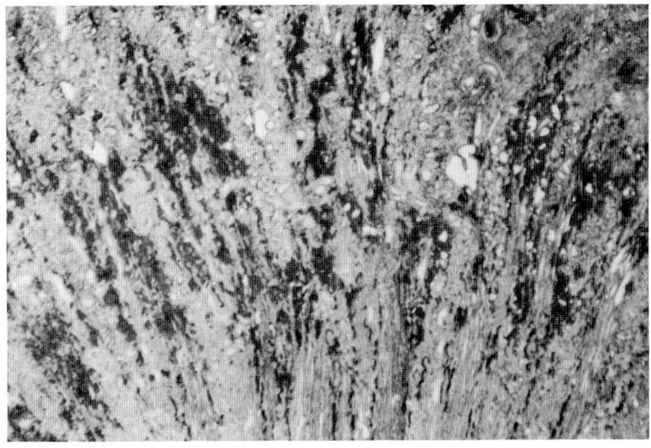

Figure 37-2. Lipid-filled foam cells in lower cortex correspond to yellow streaks seen grossly (Oil red 0 stain × 8, before 25% reduction). (From Krickstein, H. I., Gloor, F. J., and Blagk, K. [25].)

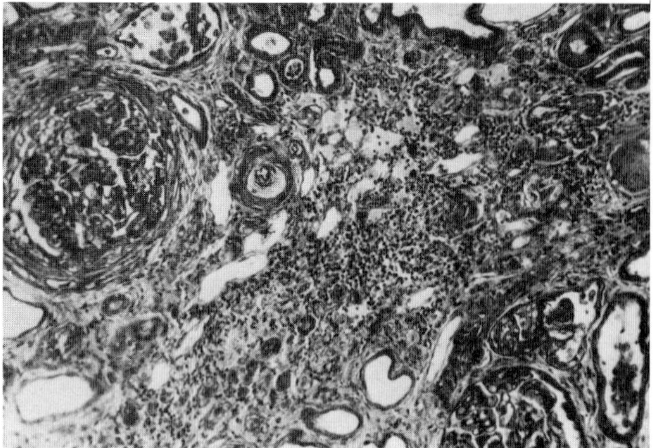

Figure 37-3. Autopsy kidney specimen. Numerous foam cells are seen scattered through the interstitial tissue. The glomerulus shows a characteristic crescent. Moderate interstitial lymphocytic infiltrate is present. (From Perkoff, G. T., Nugent, C. A., Jr., Dolowitz, D. A., Stephens, F. E., Carnes, W. H., and Tyler, F. H. [33].)

the 7 biopsy specimens. In addition, lipid was observed in glomerular podocytes, capsular epithelial cells, and some renal arteriolar endothelial cells. These authors suggested that most of the foam cells are of tubular rather than of interstitial origin, and emphasized their usefulness in the anatomic diagnosis of the disease. They also described clearly the "mixed" nephritis characteristic of the disorder. Many but not all of the glomeruli were abnormal, some showing changes like those in classic glomerulonephritis. But some normal glomeruli also were present, and the cortical stroma showed diffuse fibrosis and moderate infiltration with inflammatory cells (Fig. 37-3). Nephrocalcinosis was common in areas of the densest collections of foam cells. Histochemical studies showed that the lipid in these cells was cholesterol and neutral and phospholipids, but direct biochemical studies have not been done.

Microdissection studies of kidneys from a few patients with hereditary nephritis now have been reported, and interesting changes were found [47]. The collecting tubules had fewer arborizations than normal and showed small diverticulae. The distal segments of the renal tubules were unusually thin; only minimal abnormalities were noted in the proximal segments. These changes suggest that hereditary nephritis might be secondary to developmental abnormalities of the tubules, but how

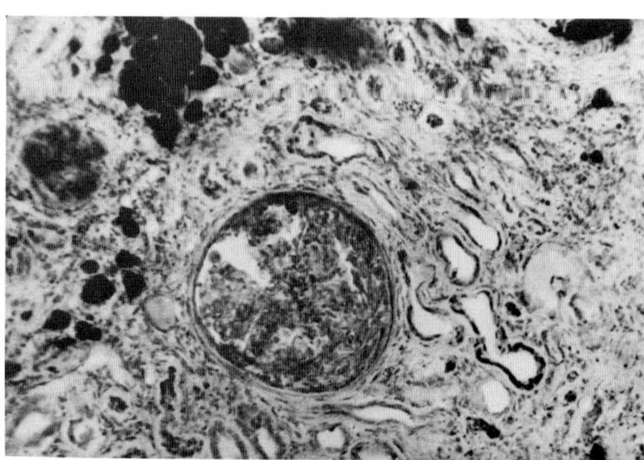

Figure 37-4. Sudan stain of kidney shown in Figure 37-3. (From Perkoff, G. T., Nugent, C. A., Jr., Dolowitz, D. A., Stephens, F. E., Carnes, W. H., and Tyler, F. H. [33].)

the latter could result in glomerular lesions and foam cells is unclear; increased susceptibility to renal infection might well result from tubular anomalies.

Treatment

There is no definitive therapy for hereditary chronic nephritis. Since it seems possible that part of the renal damage is due to the periodic episodes of renal infection that sometimes occur in this disease, the urine should be cultured periodically and appropriate therapy instituted if significant bacteriuria is found. Similarly, episodes of clinically apparent pyelonephritis should be treated vigorously. The management of uremia secondary to hereditary chronic nephritis is the same as that necessary in other chronic renal diseases.

Subtypes of Hereditary Chronic Nephritis

HEREDITARY CHRONIC NEPHRITIS WITHOUT NERVE DEAFNESS OR OCULAR DEFECTS

A number of families now have been reported in which exactly the same kind of renal disease as that discussed so far appears to occur, but without the major associated clinical findings of nerve deafness or ocular defects [18]. In some where the information is reasonably adequate, the mechanism of inheritance may be different, suggesting that in those instances a truly separate type of disease is occurring. The data are sparse, however, and these variations may represent nothing more than variable expression of the disease. At times, all the abnormalities known to occur singly in separate families have been found together in one family, suggesting that the variability may be extreme. In this regard, the report of Dubach et al. [9] is of special interest. These workers studied a family in which hereditary chronic nephritis, deafness, hyperlipidemia, renal foam cells, hyperprolinemia, and hyperprolinuria all occurred. As discussed below, hyperprolinemia may be associated with renal anomalies, or diffuse renal fibrosis, but in the patients of Dubach et al. the renal disease clearly was hereditary chronic nephritis.

Hereditary chronic nephritis has been reported with polyneuropathy [27], but this association is known for nonhereditary chronic renal disease as well. Also, two families were reported in which peroneal muscular atrophy (Charcot-Marie-Tooth disease) occurred together with hereditary chronic nephritis in a manner suggesting that one trait might be responsible for both clinical syndromes [26]. Whether or not this truly is the case is unknown.

FAMILIAL HYPERPROLINEMIA WITH RENAL DISEASE

Another variety of hereditary diffuse nephropathy thought to be separate from hereditary chronic nephritis is that associated with hyperprolinemia, prolinuria, hydroxyprolinuria, and glycinuria. In the first such family described [40], four siblings had renal "hypoplasia" and ectasias of the urinary tract, with superimposed pyelonephritis demonstrated at autopsy in one case. The presenting manifestation was hematuria; two patients had nerve deafness. Seizures and an abnormal electroencephalogram were found in five patients, and mental deficiency was present in one in the family of the propositus. However, renal disease and deafness were frequent in the mother's relatives and were unassociated with either the amino acid abnormality or the seizure disorder. The renal disease and deafness were inherited in a manner consistent with autosomal dominant inheritance. Since the hyperprolinemia and seizure disorder occurred in only one sibship in this family, the relation between the biochemical changes and the renal disease and deafness remained uncertain. Later studies of this family showed that tubular transport of L-proline was a saturable process, and that as proline approached the saturation limit for its own transport, it inhibited the transport of hydroxyproline and glycine. These data explain the unusual pattern of aminoaciduria found in familial hyperprolinemia.

The discovery of a second family with renal disease and hyperprolinemia provided an additional opportunity for study of this interesting disorder [11]. Efron and her associates described a man with renal disease who had mild mental retardation, renal insufficiency associated with signs of renal infection, unilateral hydronephrosis, aplasia of the opposite kidney, and hyperprolinemia. Hereditary renal disease again was found throughout the maternal side of the kindred. Neither deafness nor seizures were present in any family member, and, as in the first family, definite hyperprolinemia was present only in the sibship of the propositus. Extensive study revealed that the patient had markedly decreased activity of hepatic proline oxidase, but that the ability to metabolize hydroxyproline was normal. Thus, the enzyme defect in this syndrome appears to be proline oxidase deficiency, but the role of the enzyme defect in the renal disease is uncertain. In both families renal disease was present in several generations on the maternal side of the kindred, but hyperprolinemia occurred only in the sibship of the propositus. It was postulated, therefore, that the renal disease might be due to a single gene, in each instance found in the mother's family, and the proline oxidase deficiency to inheritance of a separate gene from both parents. The association with renal disease in two unrelated families would then be explained by proximity of the abnormal genes on the same chromosome. An alternative hypothesis was proposed that also could explain the observations — that is, the renal disease is associated with some "silent factor" that, when it exists together with a single gene for proline oxidase deficiency, in some way results in manifest aminoaciduria. How the family studied by Dubach et al. fits with the two just described is unknown, and the reason why renal anomalies or fibrosis (or both) occur in some families with hyperprolinemia, and hereditary chronic nephritis, foam cells, and hyperlipidemia occur in another is unexplained.

It is worthy of note that a second type of hyperprolinemia, related to deficiency of the enzyme Δ1-proline-5-carboxylic acid dehydrogenase, is unassociated with renal disease. One family now is known in which hydroxyprolinemia was associated with hematuria, pyuria, and mental deficiency; in this family, deficiency of hydroxyproline oxidase apparently was at fault [12].

Mechanism of Inheritance

The mechanism of inheritance of hereditary chronic nephritis has been debated. Autosomal dominant inheritance was assumed to be operative in earlier families, but the data were too sparse to be clear. Later, although large families occasionally were found in which the disease occurred with a typical autosomal dominant pattern of inheritance [31], in most reported large families peculiar sex ratios were observed [33]. In particular, in kindreds at risk, there were more abnormal females than males, and the vast majority of offspring of involved males were involved females. Male-to-male transmission of the disease is unusual but has been observed. Two major hypotheses have been advanced to explain these findings:

1. The disease is transmitted by partially sex-linked dominant inheritance [43]. A pedigree chart from such a family is shown in Figure 37-5. According to this hypothesis, the gene for hereditary nephritis is located on the portion of the X chromosome that might be homologous with the Y chromosome. Since most abnormal males could transmit the disease only to daughters, and involved females could transmit it to daughters and sons alike,

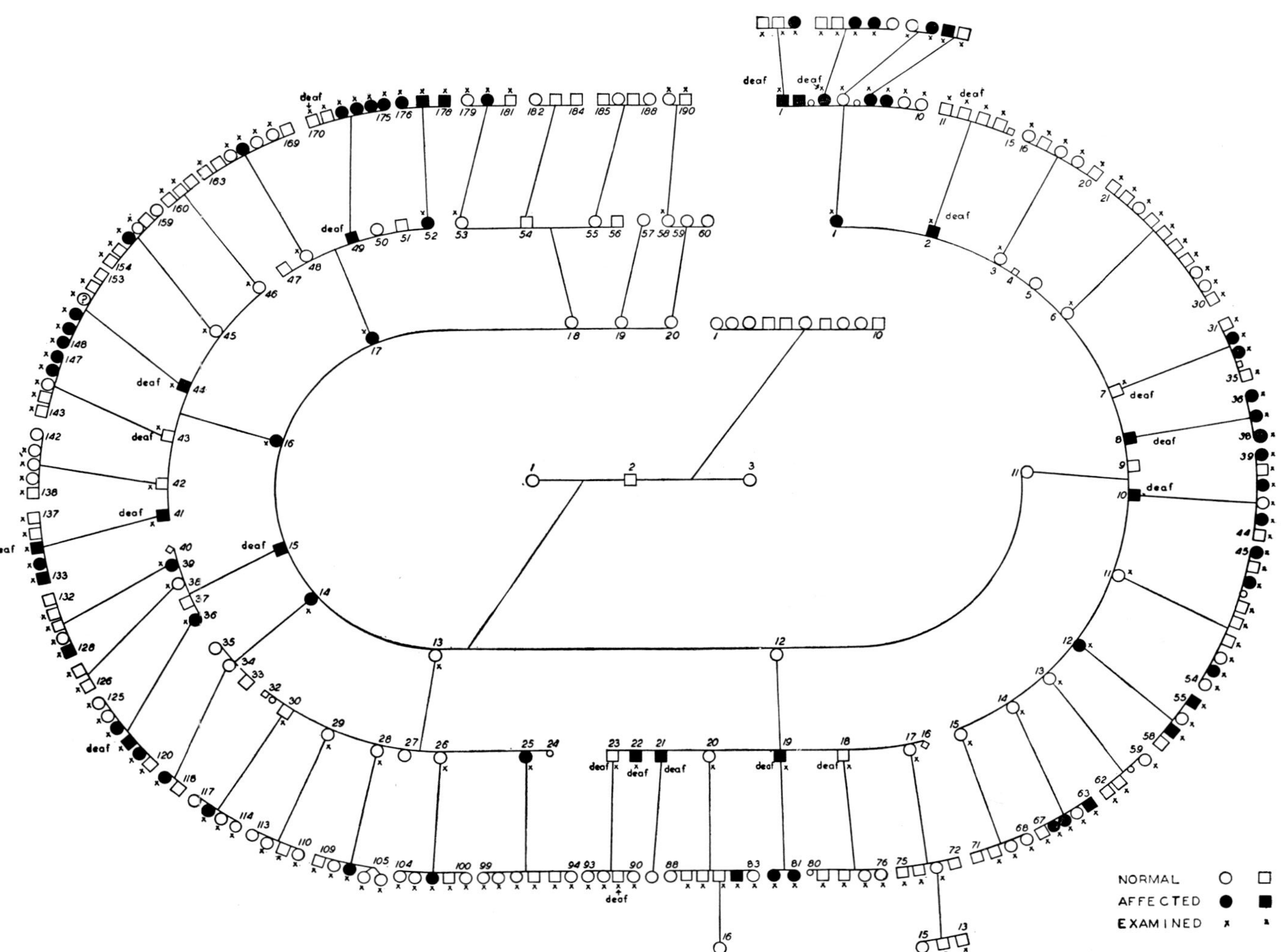

Figure 37-5. Pedigree chart from a large family with hereditary chronic nephritis. Unusual sex ratios, as shown here, led to the hypothesis that the mechanism of inheritance was that of a partially sex-linked dominant trait.

this would account for the unusual sex ratios. The occasional male-to-male transmission could be explained by the rare occurrence of crossing over between the homologous portions of X and Y. However, it is now uncertain that X and Y can be homologous, and if not, crossing over could not occur. For this reason, the hypothesis has been questioned.

2. Another mechanism postulated is that of preferential segregation and chromosomal association [8]. According to this hypothesis the gene for hereditary nephritis is located on an abnormal autosome that is thought to be more likely to remain with the oocyte than to migrate randomly to the polar body. If that were the case, an excessive number of abnormal offspring of heterozygous females should be found. Although that is true for the female children, it is not true for males. This disparity could be explained by excessive fetal loss of involved males, but such a loss has not been shown. Cohen et al. [8] did not find a deficiency of affected males and believed that the hypothesis of preferential segregation and chromosomal association explained all the genetic data in this disorder. Dr. ten Bokkel Huinink originally considered his data compatible with complete sex-linkage; later he proposed that autosomal dominant inheritance with incomplete penetrance of a pathologic pleiotropic gene was the best explanation in his families [45]. In at least some families (Fig. 37-6), straightforward dominant inheritance appears to be operative. The matter remains unsettled.

Glycolipid Lipidosis (Fabry's Disease)

Although it is a generalized disorder rather than a specific hereditary nephritis, a discussion of glycolipid lipidosis (Fabry's disease) is included in this chapter because of its major renal involvement and because the enzyme defect now is known.

Originally described as a disease of the skin [14], and not reported in this country until 1955 [15], glycolipid lipidosis now has been reported in more than 100 patients. It is known to involve many organs, the renal abnormality being particularly severe and, rather than being a benign vascular disease as originally thought, it is a serious disorder of lipid storage.

CLINICAL MANIFESTATIONS

The clinical features are evident mainly in affected males [50] and in general can be divided into three stages [35]. In childhood and adolescence, crises characterized by fever, burning or lightning pains of the extremities, abdominal pain, and paresthesia occur. Vascular lesions appear on the skin, particularly on the buttocks, scrotum, penis, and lower back; they may also be found around the umbilicus, on the conjunctivae, and on the lips, but to a lesser extent. Proteinuria is noted at this stage, and persists later as the other symptoms subside. In some but not all patients hypohidrosis develops. The skin lesions increase in number and renal function slowly deteriorates. The late phase is one of hypertension, progressive uremia, and death by the fifth decade. Additional frequent clinical features are signs of central nervous system involvement [50], including seizures, hemiplegia, hemianesthesia, aphasia, and cerebral hemorrhage, as well as pulmonary signs, varicose veins and hemorrhoids, and muscle and joint pain. Also characteristic, and particularly useful in genetic studies as indicators of involvement, are eye signs, especially corneal haziness and opacities [29, 42].

HISTOLOGIC FINDINGS

The microscopical anatomy [44] is characterized by foamy macrophages and reticuloendothelial cells located in the bone marrow, spleen, and liver, by lipid deposits in the smooth muscles of blood vessels, of the vermiform appendix, and occasionally of the skin, and by striking deposition of foamy lipid in the renal glomeruli and distal tubular seg-

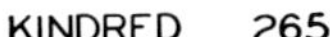

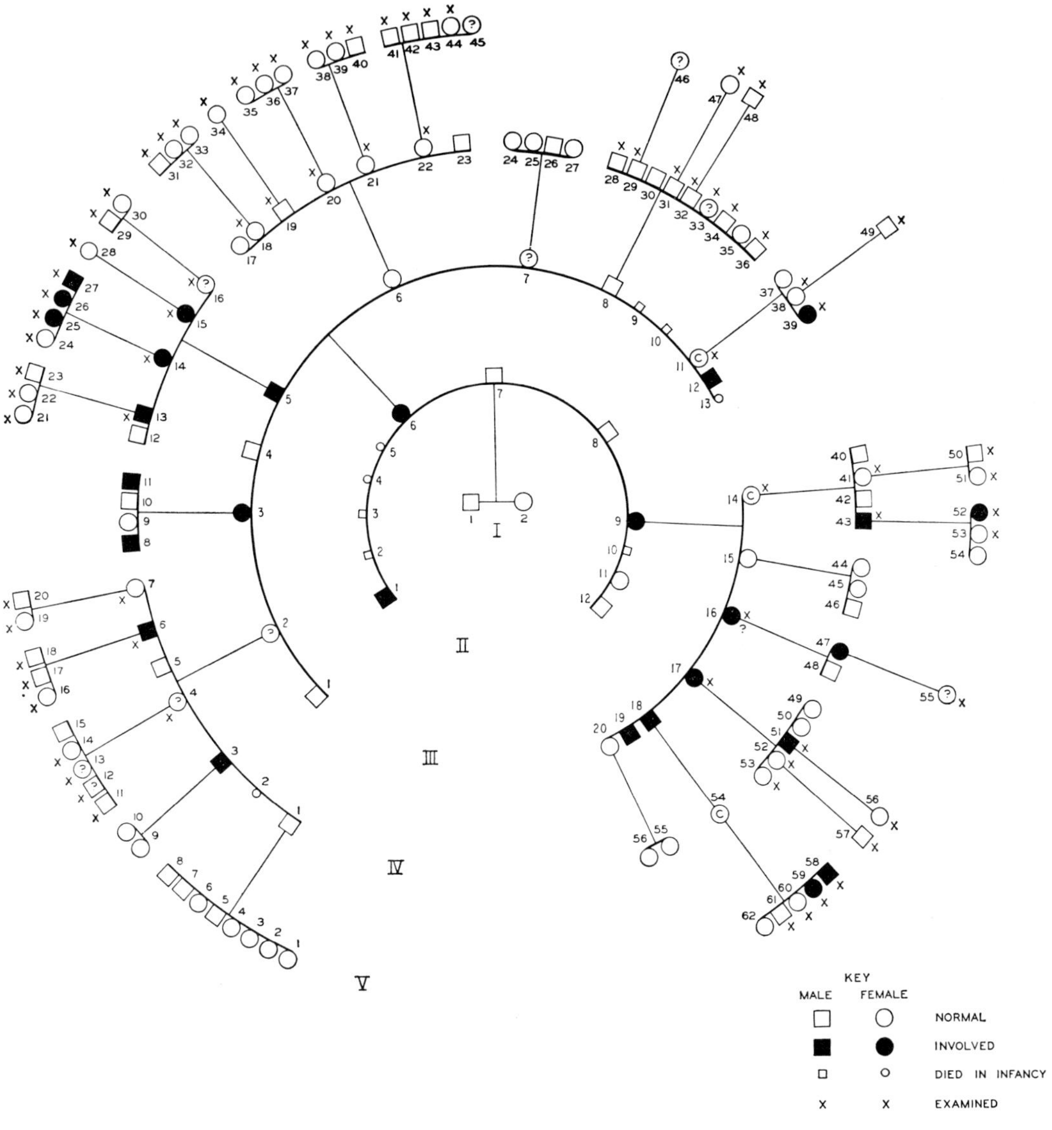

Figure 37-6. Pedigree of hereditary chronic nephritis compatible with dominant inheritance.

ments. Foamy macrophages may be found in the urine, and have diagnostic significance. Electron microscopy shows osmophilic material in lamellar structures in the kidneys and elsewhere.

The composition of the lipid deposits and the nature of the enzyme defect have been worked out [43a, 44]. Analysis of the renal tissue from one patient led to the isolation and characterization of an unusual glycolipid, ceramide trihexoside, with the molar ratios for long-chain base, fatty acid, glucose, and galactose of 1:1:1:2. Neither sialic acid nor hexosamine was present. The ceramide portion of the molecule could be shown to be attached to the glucose portion of glucopyranosyl-(4-1)-galactopyranosyl-(4-1)-galactopyranoside. The fatty acid composition closely resembled the distribution found in ceramide trihexoside of normal kidney. An additional glycolipid found in smaller concentrations was shown to be a dihexoside with an oligosaccharide portion consisting of galactopyranosyl-(4-1)-galactopyranoside. Similar glycolipid is assumed to be distributed widely outside the kidney, so that the term glycolipid lipidosis, indicating that the disease is a lipid-storage disorder, is appropriate. The major glycolipid accumulation almost certainly results from deficiency of the enzyme ceramidetrihexosidase. Brady et al. [3], in studies of biopsy specimens of intestinal mucosa, found no activity of this enzyme in two involved homozygous males, and intermediate activity in samples from a heterozygous female.

GENETICS

The genetics of glycolipid lipidosis appears to be that of an incompletely recessive or "intermediate" X-linked trait with evidence of linkage to the Xga blood group [29]. Originally it was thought that classic sex-linked recessive inheritance offered an explanation, but the recognition of the corneal abnormalities and the fact that their occurrence in females with minimal signs of disease could be used as a reliable discriminant in genetic studies [29] showed that both males and females were involved, but that full expression of the disorder rarely occurred in women. Thus, homozygous males have severe disease, and heterozygous females transmit the disease but, with rare exceptions, show only minor changes themselves. These observations fit well with the results of the enzyme assays for ceramidetrihexosidase in representative subjects.

References

1. Alport, A. C. Hereditary familial congenital haemorrhagic nephritis. *Brit. Med. J.* 1:504, 1927.
2. Attlee, W. H. W. Three cases of recurrent haematuria occurring in one family. *St. Bart. Hosp. J.* 9:41, 1901.
3. Brady, R. O., Gal, A. E., Bradley, R. M., Martensson, E., Warshaw, A. L., and Laster, L. Enzymatic defect in Fabry's disease: Ceramidetrihexosidase deficiency. *New Eng. J. Med.* 276:1163, 1967.
4. Brill, N. E., and Libman, E. A contribution to the subject of chronic interstitial nephritis and arteritis in the young, and family nephritis, with a note on calcification in the liver. *J. Exp. Med.* 4:541, 1899.
5. Brownell, R. D., and Wolter, J. R. Anterior lenticonus in familial haemorrhagic nephritis: Demonstration of lens pathology. *Arch. Ophthal.* (Chicago) 74:481, 1964.
6. Cassady, G., Brown, K., Cohen, M., and DeMaria, W. Hereditary renal dysfunction and deafness. *Pediatrics* 35:967, 1965.
7. Chappell, A., and Kelsey, W. M. Hereditary nephritis. *Amer. J. Dis. Child.* 99:401, 1960.
8. Cohen, M. M., Cassady, G., and Hanna, B. L. Genetic study of hereditary renal dysfunction with associated nerve deafness. *Amer. J. Hum. Genet.* 13:379, 1961.
9. Dubach, U. C., Minder, F. C., and Antener, I. Familial nephropathy and deafness. First observation of family and close relatives in Switzerland. *Helv. Med. Acta* 33:36, 1966.
10. Eason, J., Smith, G. L. M., and Buchanan, G. Hereditary and familial nephritis. *Lancet* 2:639, 1924.
11. Efron, M. L. Familial hyperprolinemia: Report of second case, associated with renal malformations, hereditary hematuria and mild mental retardation, with demonstration of enzyme defect. *New Eng. J. Med.* 272:1243, 1965.

12. Efron, M. L., Bixby, E. M., Palatto, L. G., and Pryles, C. V. Hydroxyprolinemia associated with mental deficiency. *New Eng. J. Med.* 267:1193, 1962.
13. Eichhorst, H. In Senator H. (Ed.), *Erkrankungen der Nieren. Spezielle Pathologie und Therapie.* Vienna: Nothnagel, 1899. Vol. 19, p. 249.
14. Fabry, J. Ein Beitrag zur Kenntis der Purpura haemorrhagica Nodularis (Purpura papulosa hemorrhagica Hebrae). *Arch. Derm. Syph.* 43:187, 1898.
15. Fessas, P., Wintrobe, M. M., and Cartwright, G. E. Angiokeratoma corporis diffusum universale (Fabry): First American report of rare disorder. *A.M.A. Arch. Intern. Med.* 95:469, 1955.
16. Forster, R. Über Schrumpfniere im Kindesalter. *Jahrb. Kinderheilk.* 26:38, 1887.
17. Goldbloom, R. B., Fraser, F. C., Waugh, D., Arnovitch, M., and Wiglesworth, F. W. Hereditary renal disease associated with nerve deafness and ocular lesions. *Pediatrics* 20:241, 1957.
18. Goldman, R., and Haberfelde, G. C. Hereditary nephritis: Report of kindred. *New Eng. J. Med.* 261:734, 1959.
19. Goodheart, J. F. In Keating, J. M. (Ed.), *Acute and Chronic Bright's Disease. Cyclopedia of Diseases of Children.* Philadelphia: Lippincott, 1890. Vol. 3, pp. 532–558.
20. Guthrie, L. G. "Idiopathic" or congenital hereditary and family haematuria. *Lancet* 1:1243, 1902.
21. Hawkins, C. F., and Smith, O. E. Renal dysplasia in family with multiple hereditary abnormalities including iliac horns. *Lancet* 1:803, 1950.
22. Hellendall, H. Hereditare Schrumpfnieren im frehen Kindewaiter. *Arch. Kinderheilk.* 22:61, 1882.
23. Kendall, G., and Hertz, A. C. Hereditary familial congenital haemorrhagic nephritis. *Guy. Hosp. Rep.* 66:137, 1962.
24. Kidd, J. The inheritance of Bright's disease of the kidney. *Practitioner* 29:104, 1882.
25. Krickstein, H. I., Gloor, F. J., and Blagk, K. Renal pathology in hereditary nephritis with nerve deafness. *Arch. Path.* (Chicago) 82:506, 1966.
26. Lemieux, G., and Neemek, J. A. Charcot-Marie-Tooth disease and nephritis. *Canad. Med. Ass. J.* 97:1193, 1967.
27. Marin, O. S. M., and Tyler, H. R. Hereditary interstitial nephritis associated with polyneuropathy. *Neurology* (Minneap.) 11: 999, 1961.
28. Ohlsson, L. Congenital renal disease, deafness and myopia in one family. *Acta Med. Scand.* 174:77, 1963.
29. Opitz, J. M., Stiles, F. C., Wise, D., Race, R. R., Sauger, R., von Gemmingen, G. R., Kierlund, R. R., Cross, E. G., and De Groot, W. P. Genetics of angiokeratoma corporis diffusum (Fabry's disease) and its linkage relations with Xg locus. *Amer. J. Hum. Genet.* 17:325, 1965.
30. Pel, P. K. Die Erblichkeit der chronischen Nephritis. *Z. Klin. Med.* 38:127, 1899.
31. Perkoff, G. T. Familial aspects of diffuse renal diseases. *Ann. Rev. Med.* 15:115, 1964.
32. Perkoff, G. T. The hereditary renal diseases. *New Eng. J. Med.* 277:79, 129, 1967.
33. Perkoff, G. T., Nugent, C. A., Jr., Dolowitz, D. A., Stephens, F. E., Carnes, W. H., and Tyler, F. H. A follow-up study of hereditary chronic nephritis. *A.M.A. Arch. Intern. Med.* 102:733, 1958.
34. Perkoff, G. T., Stephens, F. E., Dolowitz, D. A., and Tyler, F. H. Clinical study of hereditary interstitial pyelonephritis. *A.M.A. Arch. Intern. Med.* 88:191, 1951.
35. Rahman, A. N., Simeone, F. A., Hackel, D. B., Hall, P. W., III, Hirsch, E. Z., and Harris, J. W. Angiokeratoma corporis diffusum universale (hereditary dystopic lipidosis). *Trans. Ass. Amer. Physicians* 74:366, 1961.
36. Reyersbach, G. C., and Butler, A. M. Congenital hereditary hematuria. *New Eng. J. Med.* 251:377, 1954.
37. Romme, R. L'hérédité dans la nephrite chronique. *Presse Med.* 2:362, 1899.
38. Rosen, S., Pirani, C. L., and Muehrcke, R. C. Renal interstitial foam cells. *Amer. J. Clin. Path.* 45:32, 1966.
39. Sanerkin, S. G. On the nature of "interstitial foam cells" in chronic glomerulonephritis. *J. Path. Bact.* 86:135, 1963.

40. Schafer, I. A., Scriver, C. R., and Efron, M. L. Familial hyperprolinemia, cerebral dysfunction and renal anomalies occurring in family with hereditary nephropathy and deafness. *New Eng. J. Med.* 267:51, 1962.
41. Sohar, E. Renal disease, inner ear deafness, and ocular changes: New heredofamilial syndrome. *A.M.A. Arch. Intern. Med.* 97: 627, 1956.
42. Spaeth, G. L., and Frost, P. Fabry's disease: Its ocular manifestations. *Arch. Ophthal.* (Chicago) 74:760, 1965.
43. Stephens, F. E., Perkoff, G. T., Dolowitz, D. A., and Tyler, F. H. Partially sex-linked dominant inheritance of interstitial pyelonephritis. *Amer. J. Hum. Genet.* 3:303, 1951.
43a. Sweeley, C. C., and Klionsky, B. Fabry's disease: Classification as sphingolipidosis and partial characterization of novel glycolipid. *J. Biol. Chem.* 238:3148, 1963.
44. Sweeley, C. C., and Klionsky, B. Glycolipid Lipidosis: Fabry's Disease. In Stanbury, J. B., Wyngaarden, J. B., and Fredrickson, D. S. (Eds.), *The Metabolic Basis of Inherited Disease.* New York: McGraw-Hill, 1966. Chap. 29, p. 618.
45. ten Bokkel Huinink, J. A. Hereditaire Nefritis met Perceptive Slechthorendheid (Alport-Syndroom) en Een Familie met Hereditaire Idiopathische Schromplenieren. Thoben Offset Nijmegen, 1967.
46. Tyson, J. *A Treatise on Bright's Disease and Diabetes with Special Reference to Pathology and Therapeutics Including a Section on Retinitis and Bright's Disease.* Philadelphia: Lindsay & Blakiston, 1881. P. 166.
47. Van Buchem, F. S. P., and Beetstra, A. Hereditary renal disease associated with deafness — Alport's syndrome. *Acta Med. Scand.* 179:319, 1966.
48. Wallace, I. R., and Jones, J. H. Familial glomerulonephritis and aminoaciduria. *Lancet* 1:941, 1960.
49. Whalen, R. E., Huang, S., Peschel, E., and McIntosh, H. D. Hereditary nephropathy, deafness and renal foam cells. *Amer. J. Med.* 31:171, 1961.
50. Wise, D., Wallace, H. J., and Jellinek, E. H. Angiokeratoma corporis diffusum: Clinical study of eight affected families. *Quart. J. Med.* 31:177, 1961.

38

Vasopressin-Resistant Diabetes Insipidus

Jack Orloff and Maurice B. Burg

Vasopressin-resistant diabetes insipidus is a rare hereditary disorder characterized by insensitivity of the renal tubule to vasopressin. The disease was first described by Forssman [33] and Waring et al. [71]. It occurs with greatest frequency in male subjects. The essential features of the syndrome — namely, polyuria, polydipsia, and excretion of persistently hypotonic urine — resemble those of diabetes insipidus due to posterior pituitary insufficiency. It is distinguished from the latter by the inability of vasopressin to correct the disturbance in water conservation. The name nephrogenic diabetes insipidus was introduced by Williams and Henry [73] to emphasize the renal basis of the disorder.

Physiologic Considerations

The role of vasopressin in the mechanism of urinary dilution and concentration has been described in detail elsewhere (see pages 48–59). The hormone reduces urine flow by increasing the permeability of the distal convolution and collecting system to water, thereby facilitating osmotic flow of water out of the tubule lumen into the surrounding interstitium. The elaboration of urine more concentrated than plasma is accomplished by osmotic equilibration of collecting duct fluid with the hypertonic medullary tissue. It is sufficient to state that all the clinical manifestations of vasopressin-resistant diabetes insipidus may be ascribed to deficient reabsorption of water from the distal nephron. The unremitting water diuresis resembles in all respects the response of normal man to water ingestion and suppression of antidiuretic hormone release. It results from persistent impermeability of the distal convolution and collecting duct to water, owing to inability of the luminal membrane to respond to antidiuretic hormone. Despite inability to concentrate the urine, the diluting process is not impaired, as is indicated by the normal relationship between urine concentration and solute excretion during forced osmotic diuresis [59].

The only other abnormalities in renal function observed are those secondary either to dehydration, a frequent occurrence in the improperly managed or unrecognized case, or to hydronephrosis, a common complication of the syndrome. In the absence of these conditions, renal blood flow, glomerular filtration rate, glucose reabsorption, phosphate and amino acid transport, and other discrete tubular processes are unaffected [47, 55, 59, 66, 71, 73]. Acid-base balance and electrolyte metabolism are also generally unaltered, as evidenced by normal plasma electrolyte patterns in properly hydrated subjects. It has been reported that the sodium chloride concentration of sweat from infants affected with this disorder may be elevated [53].

Pathogenesis

There is little question that the disease is of renal origin. The neurohypophyseal system is apparently intact, as is evidenced by absence of anatomic changes and the presence of antidiuretic substance in both blood and urine under appropriate circumstances [1, 20, 52, 54, 55, 72]. Although chemical characterization of the antidiuretic substance elaborated in these subjects has not been accomplished, it is unlikely that an abnormal hormone is produced to which the kidney does not respond [24, 42]. The physiologic abnormalities are not corrected by administration of commercial vasopressin (Pitressin), lysine or arginine vasopressin, or oxytocin [56]. Abnormally rapid degradation of circulating hormones is unlikely in view of the observation that massive doses of vasopressin, though incapable of reducing urine flow, do produce abdominal pain and blanching, known side effects of the hormone [20, 44, 55, 56].

The precise defect responsible for the insensitivity of the renal tubule to vasopressin is unknown. No structural changes in the kidney have been observed using conventional technics [47, 55, 71, 72]. However, on the basis of microdissection studies, abnormal shortening of the proximal tubule has been reported [21, 55]. Darmady et al. [21] ascribe the clinical abnormalities to the shortened tubule rather than to unresponsiveness of the distal nephron to antidiuretic hormone. They reasoned that the shortened proximal segment permits escape of a larger fraction of glomerular filtrate than normal and that increased flow of dilute urine from the loop results in the excretion of hypotonic urine despite normal permeability to water of the distal nephron. This is reminiscent of the explanation for the development of isosthenuria in osmotic diuresis. The hypothesis does not account for the absence of an effect of vasopressin in patients with the fully expressed disorder, for the characteristic excretion of persistently dilute urine of low osmolality, and for the normal diluting capacity observed during variations in solute excretion [59]. Furthermore, although patients with cystinosis are also reported to have shortened proximal tubules [21], any defect in concentrating ability which they may have is considerably less than that in patients with vasopressin-resistant diabetes insipidus.

By analogy with other inherited metabolic disorders it is reasonable to ascribe the lack of response to the hormone to the formation of an abnormal protein which results in an altered enzyme system or receptor site within the tubule membrane.

As indicated earlier, vasopressin had been shown to increase the permeability of certain epithelial membranes (toad bladder and frog skin) to water by enlarging aqueous channels or pores in the membrane [2, 49]. Similar changes in the tubule membrane undoubtedly facilitate osmotic flow of water out of the lumen into the surrounding interstitium. This is supported by the observation that vasopressin increases the osmotic permeability to water of the distal tubule [74] and collecting system [36]. According to Fong et al. [32], vasopressin must first attach to the membrane by linkage involving the S-S bridge of the vasopressin molecule and the sulfhydryl groups of the membrane. If the membrane were incapable of binding vasopressin, as a consequence of a structural abnormality in the protein matrix, its effect would be blocked. The proposal of Ginetzinsky [35] that vasopressin causes the renal tubule to secrete hyaluronidase which then hydrolyzes hyaluronic acid in the tubule, rendering it more permeable to water, has been adopted by Dicker and Eggleton [24]. These authors have stated that vasopressin increases hyaluronidase excretion in normal man undergoing water diuresis but does not in vasopressin-resistant diabetes insipidus [25, 26]. Although this hypothesis may serve to implicate the hyaluronidase system in the pathogenesis of the syndrome, the observations in normal man have not been confirmed by others [5]. Furthermore, bovine testicular hyaluronidase does not accelerate water movement across the toad and frog bladder, whereas vasopressin does [25, 51].

Orloff and Handler [57, 58] have observed that adenosine-3′,5′-phosphate (cyclic AMP), as well as an inhibitor of its degradation, theophylline, produces effects similar to those of vasopressin in the toad bladder. Thus both agents increase the osmotic flow of water across the membrane as does vasopressin. The authors have proposed, by analogy with other hormonal effects [70], that vasopressin exerts its effect on permeability by stimulating the production and accumulation of cyclic AMP in the renal tubule cells. They have also suggested by analogy with the other hormonal effects [70] that vasopressin increases the activity of adenyl cyclase (the enzyme which accelerates the conversion of ATP to cyclic AMP) in kidney [58]. Cyclic AMP mimics vasopressin in the collecting tubule [36] as in toad bladder, and the neurohypophyseal hormone increases cyclic AMP concentration [8] and enhances adenyl cyclase activity in renal tissue [12]. It is apparent that if the renal enzyme systems necessary for either the production, accumulation, or subsequent channeling of cyclic AMP into other metabolic pools were absent or inactive in this disorder, vasopressin would be ineffective.

Genetics

Vasopressin-resistant diabetes insipidus is an inherited disease which occurs with greatest frequency in male members of affected families. The mode of inheritance has not yet been definitively established, and it is possible that more than one mechanism is involved. However, the original contention that the defect was limited to males and transmitted as a sex-linked recessive [33, 73] is erroneous. A number of females have been reported in whom the disease was fully as severe as that uniformly observed in the male [9, 17, 20, 59]. Furthermore, female siblings and relatives of affected males not only may transmit the defect but also may exhibit a subclinical form of the disorder [11]. In such heterozygous females, although polyuria is absent and hypertonic urine may be elaborated, the response to both dehydration and exogenous vasopressin is considerably depressed. The occurrence of this form of the disease in male subjects has not as yet been documented; however, no systematic study has excluded it. The overwhelming preponderance of males among patients with the disease and the absence of incomplete forms of the disorder in this sex may indicate a high degree of expressivity in males and a low degree of expressivity in females.

Although conceding that vasopressin-resistant diabetes insipidus is most reasonably viewed as a dominant sex-linked disorder with variable expressivity in heterozygous female carriers, a number of investigators have suggested that autosomal dominance with some degree of sex limitation may account for some of the cases [9, 13, 63]. Supporting evidence is derived largely from a pedigree described by

Cannon [9] in which six examples of male-to-male transmission were noted. If one excludes these as uncertain, then the pedigree conforms closely to sex-linked inheritance. This has been emphasized to us by Allen [56]. Autosomal inheritance requires that one-half the male offspring of affected males should be affected and one-half the female offspring should be carriers. In Cannon's pedigree, 6 of the 44 children were affected and virtually all the females who had children either were diseased or had affected children. These discrepancies make autosomal inheritance an unlikely possibility and support the view that the disease is sex-linked, with variable expressivity in females.

Clinical Aspects

Although the disease is undoubtedly present at birth, it is frequently unrecognized in infancy except in families with previously diagnosed cases. The characteristic syndrome of polyuria, polydipsia, and the excretion of persistently hypotonic urine is observed only when hydration is adequate. For obvious reasons these signs in the newborn child rarely engender suspicion. Most often no abnormality is suspected until signs of severe dehydration, fever, vomiting, hyperosmolality, and convulsions develop. Even under these circumstances the urine is generally less concentrated than plasma, and this finding readily establishes the diagnosis. Unrecognized or inadequately treated dehydration undoubtedly accounts for the high infant mortality in the disease.

As was indicated earlier, neither the copious urine flow nor the hypotonic urine is altered by administration of large doses of vasopressin. The response to hypertonic saline and to water restriction, on the other hand, is qualitatively similar to that observed in patients with posterior pituitary insufficiency. It is significant that although urine osmolality may rise following severe dehydration, elaboration of hypertonic urine has not been observed in patients in whom the defect was complete [19, 59]. In contrast, hypertonic urine may be elaborated in severely dehydrated subjects with posterior pituitary diabetes insipidus and in those cases of vasopressin-resistant diabetes insipidus in which the abnormality is not fully expressed. This last has been reported by Carter and Simpkiss [11], who noted partial responsiveness to vasopressin in female siblings and relatives of patients with the fully expressed disorder. Childs and Sidbury [13] have reported similar observations in two mothers of patients with the disease. It is notable that whereas the fully expressed disease occurs in both males and females, incomplete expressivity has thus far been observed only in female subjects.

Many authors have emphasized the relatively high frequency of both mental and physical retardation in children with vasopressin-resistant diabetes insipidus [30, 34, 41, 47, 55, 65, 72, 73]. These are not generally caused by associated genetic defects but are related to the uncontrolled polyuria. Structural brain damage when present is apparently occasioned by the repeated episodes of severe dehydration. Even when hydration is adequate, malnutrition and resultant altered growth patterns may develop. They are thought to be caused by the exhausting influence of the persistent polydipsia. Excessive drinking interferes with food intake, and limits the time available for play and rest. Hillman et al. [41] were able to improve both the mental performance and the nutritional status of an infant with the disease by reducing solute intake and thereby minimizing obligatory water loss and thirst.

Bladder distention and hydronephrosis are other common complications of vasopressin-resistant diabetes insipidus [14, 68]. These are of mechanical origin and are a consequence of voluntary retention of large volumes of fluid. It is probable that some degree of hydronephrosis and bladder distention is present in most, if not all, patients with the disorder.

Diagnosis

The disease is readily diagnosed in hydrated polyuric individuals in whom vasopressin is ineffective, particularly if a family history of the disease is obtained. However, as was noted earlier, the polyuric infant, particularly if a member of an otherwise unaffected family, is rarely suspected of having the disorder. Repeated episodes of fever, dehydration, constipation, and obvious failure to thrive should occasion suspicion.

It is important to note that persistent hypotonicity of urine is the only specific laboratory finding in the disease. Other abnormalities in urine and plasma composition when observed are a consequence of severe dehydration. The lack of response to vasopressin is characteristic, but should be viewed in the context of present concepts concerning concentration and dilution (see pages 48–59). It must be stressed that even in the absence of vasopressin an increase in urine osmolality may be provided by a diminution in glomerular filtration rate and renal blood flow, as well as by a rise in solute excretion [4, 59]. Dehydration insofar as it reduces volume flow through the nephron (and perhaps medullary blood flow) may result in a rise in urine osmolality in these individuals. The effects are generally minimal and if viewed in the correct perspective should not lead to erroneous diagnosis of vasopressin responsiveness. Infusion of hypertonic saline (the Carter-Robbins test) [10] will uniformly augment urine flow in patients with this disorder as in posterior pituitary insufficiency.

Differential Diagnosis

The distinction between vasopressin-resistant diabetes insipidus and neurohypophyseal forms of diabetes insipidus is generally made with ease. However, a hereditary form of the pituitary disease exists which also may manifest itself in childhood [33]. Furthermore, de Wardener and others [22, 48] have observed that diminished responsiveness to vasopressin may develop in patients with posterior pituitary insufficiency and in those with psychogenic polydipsia. The limitation in concentrating ability is reversible and should not occasion a mistaken diagnosis of the incompletely expressed form of vasopressin-resistant diabetes insipidus if a prolonged period of limited water intake precedes final evaluation. It is of interest that relative vasopressin insensitivity has been produced in animals and in normal man by forced and protracted water ingestion [23]. Hays and Leaf [39] contend that membrane permeability is temporarily diminished consequent to chronic depression of the osmolality of the fluid bathing the border of the tubule cell. Harrington and Valtin [37], on the other hand, contend that membrane permeability is normal but that a persistently subnormal osmolality of the renal papilla is responsible for the concentrating defect.

A variety of conditions resemble the mild forms of vasopressin-resistant diabetes insipidus superficially in that either isosthenuria or a marked limitation in maximal concentrating ability is present [31]. These include azotemia [60], cystinosis [6, 43], obstructive uropathy [27, 43], hypokalemic nephropathy [62], hypercalcemia [15], sickle cell disease [45], renal tubular acidosis [16], medullary cystic disease [43], cystic disease of the kidney [43], and amyloid disease of the kidney [64]. Each of these has characteristic findings that should permit ready differentiation.

As was indicated earlier, mild, incomplete forms of the disease exist in female siblings and relatives of affected males. These patients are frequently asymptomatic but when examined reveal variable degrees of reduction in maximal concentrating ability. The diagnosis is made with certainty only if a family history of the disease is present.

Therapy

Although as yet there is no specific means of increasing vasopressin responsiveness in this disaese, polyuria may be minimized by limiting solute intake [34, 41, 55, 72] or by administering chlorothiazide-like derivatives over prolonged periods of time [17]. These manipulations are rarely necessary in the adult, since dehydration is readily prevented by permitting free access to water. Plasma osmolality, an index of the state of bodily hydration, is maintained relatively constant in all but the smallest infant, despite absence of the hypothalamico-hypophyseal renal regulatory system. Clearly thirst rather than vasopressin-dependent variable reabsorption of water in the distal nephron assumes a primary regulatory role in this disorder. Parenteral therapy, on the other hand, may be a life-saving measure in severely dehydrated subjects, particularly infants. Five per cent dextrose in water is not the fluid of choice in dehydrated individuals with vasopressin-resistant diabetes insipidus, as it may be in other causes of dehydration [56]. Since urine osmolality cannot exceed that of plasma, the obligatory water loss which may be associated with glycosuria induced by the intravenous injection of 5% dextrose in water may aggravate, rather than alleviate, the hyperosmolality. Successful correction of dehydration has been achieved by administering 2.5 to 3.0% dextrose in water [56]. Under these circumstances it is possible to administer adequate solute-free water and to limit the extent of obligatory water and solute loss in the urine.

Chlorothiazide and certain of its derivatives have proved to be of considerable therapeutic importance in this disease. Crawford and Kennedy [17] were the first to note that chronic administration of these derivatives to patients with diabetes insipidus led to a marked reduction in urine flow and an increase in urine concentration. The effect of the thiazides is considerably greater if patients are also maintained on a low-sodium diet. The increase in urine osmolality is in accord with its effect in normal animals and man during water diuresis [28, 40]. In these, the drug interferes with sodium chloride reabsorption in the diluting segment of the nephron. However, this effect alone cannot account for the reduction in urine volume. The latter is probably attributable to a decrease in the fraction of glomerular filtrate escaping reabsorption in the proximal segment. The diminution in volume flow to the distal nephron provides the basis for the reduction in urine volume observed and also contributes to the rise in urine osmolality. Earley and Orloff [29] have presented evidence consistent with the view that enhanced proximal reabsorption is related to the induction of a mild degree of sodium depletion by the drug. They have also shown that once a sodium deficit is achieved, relative antidiuresis is maintained without further drug administration so long as the sodium deficit is maintained by rigid salt restriction. Their findings are in accord with those of Havard and Wood [38], who considered the antidiuresis to be due to urinary salt loss, and of Cutler et al. [18], who were unable to elicit an antidiuretic response to chlorothiazide when sufficient sodium was administered to prevent the development of a negative salt balance. Also, other diuretic drugs have an effect similar to chlorothiazide provided their use is accompanied by salt depletion [7, 29, 50, 61, 69]. The proposal that the diuretic agent interferes with aldosterone activity [46] is not supported by the data of other investigators [29].

Although chlorothiazide may prove a useful therapeutic agent in this disorder, particularly insofar as it limits nocturia in children, it is essential to note that administration is not without hazard. It must be given in association with a low-sodium diet in order to exert its maximal antidiuretic effect, and potassium must be added to the diet to prevent the development of hypokalemia. Adverse hematologic effects of chlorothiazide have also been observed [67].

References

1. Baratz, R. A., Doig, A., and Adatto, I. J. Plasma antidiuretic activity and free water clearance following osmoreceptor and neurohypophyseal stimulation in human subjects. *J. Clin. Invest.* 39:1539, 1960.
2. Bentley, P. J. The effects of neurohypophysial extracts on water transfer across the wall of the isolated urinary bladder of the toad *Bufo marinus. J. Endocr.* 17:201, 1958.
3. Bentley, P. J. Hyaluronidase, corticosteroids, and the action of neurohypophysial hormone on the urinary bladder of the frog. *J. Endocr.* 24:407, 1962.
4. Berliner, R. W., and Davidson, D. G. Production of hypertonic urine in the absence of pituitary antidiuretic hormone. *J. Clin. Invest.* 36:1416, 1957.
5. Berlyne, G. M. Urinary hyaluronidase: A method of assay and investigation of its relationship to the urine concentrating mechanism. *Clin. Sci.* 19:619, 1960.
6. Bickel, H., Baar, H. S., Astley, R., Douglas, A. A., Finch, E., Harris, H., Harvey, C. C., Hickmans, E. M., Philpott, M. G., Smallwood, W. C., Smelli, J. M., and Teall, C. G. Cystine storage disease with aminoaciduria and dwarfism (Lignac-Fanconi disease). *Acta Paediat.* 42 (Suppl. 90):1, 1952.
7. Brown, D., Reynolds, J., Michael, A., and Ulstrom, R. The use and mode of action of ethacrynic acid in nephrogenic diabetes insipidus. *Pediatrics* 37:447, 1966.
8. Brown, E., Clarke, D. L., Roux, V., and Sherman, G. H. The stimulation of adenosine 3′,5′-monophosphate production by antidiuretic factors. *J. Biol. Chem.* 238:852, 1963.
9. Cannon, J. F. Diabetes insipidus: Clinical and experimental studies with consideration of genetic relationships. *A.M.A. Arch. Intern. Med.* 96:215, 1955.
10. Carter, A. C., and Robbins, J. The use of hypertonic saline infusions in the differential diagnosis of diabetes insipidus and psychogenic polydipsia. *J. Clin. Endocr.* 7:753, 1947.
11. Carter, C., and Simpkiss, M. The "carrier" state in nephrogenic diabetes insipidus. *Lancet* 2:1069, 1956.
12. Chase, L., and Aurbach, G. Renal adenyl cyclase: Anatomically separate site for parathyroid hormone and vasopressin. *Science* 159:545, 1968.
13. Childs, B., and Sidbury, J. B. A survey of genetics as it applies to problems in medicine. *Pediatrics* 20:177, 1957.
14. Chung, R. C. H., and Mantell, L. K. Urographic changes in diabetes insipidus. *J.A.M.A.* 150:1307, 1952.
15. Cohen, S. I., Fitzgerald, M. G., Fourman, P., Griffeths, W. J., and de Wardener, H. E. Polyuria in hyperparathyroidism. *Quart. J. Med.* 26:423, 1957.
16. Cooke, R. E., and Kleeman, C. R. Distal tubular dysfunction with renal calcification. *Yale J. Biol. Med.* 23:199, 1950.
17. Crawford, J. D., and Kennedy, G. C. Chlorothiazide in diabetes insipidus. *Nature* (London) 183:891, 1959.
18. Cutler, R., Kleeman, C. R., Kowling, J. T., and Maxwell, M. H. Physiological studies in a family with nephrogenic (vasopressin-resistant) diabetes insipidus (N.D.I.) *J. Clin. Invest.* 39:980, 1960.
19. Cutler, R. E., Kleeman, C., Maxwell, M., and Dowling, J. Physiological studies in nephrogenic diabetes insipidus. *J. Clin. Endocr.* 22:827, 1962.
20. Dancis, J., Birmingham, J. R., and Leslie, S. H. Congenital diabetes insipidus resistant to treatment with Pitressin. *Amer. J. Dis. Child.* 75:316, 1948.
21. Darmady, E., Prince, J., and Stranack, F.

The proximal convoluted tubule in the renal handling of water. *Lancet* 2:1254, 1964.

22. de Wardener, H. E. *The Kidney*. Boston: Little, Brown, 1958.
23. de Wardener, H. E., and Herxheimer, A. The effect of a high water intake on the kidney's ability to concentrate the urine in man. *J. Physiol.* (London) 139:42, 1957.
24. Dicker, S. E., and Eggleton, M. G. Hyaluronidase and antidiuretic activity in urine of man. *J. Physiol.* (London) 154:378, 1960.
25. Dicker, S. E., and Eggleton, M. G. Nephrogenic diabetes insipidus. *Clin. Sci.* 24:81, 1963.
26. Dicker, S. E., and Franklin, C. S. The isolation of hyaluronic acid and chondroitin sulfate from kidneys and their reaction with urinary hyaluronidase. *J. Physiol.* (London) 186:110, 1966.
27. Earley, L. E. Extreme polyuria in obstructive uropathy: Report of a case of "water-losing nephritis" in an infant, with a discussion of polyuria. *New Eng. J. Med.* 255: 600, 1956.
28. Earley, L. E., Kahn, M., and Orloff, J. The effects of infusions of chlorothiazide on urinary dilution and concentration in the dog. *J. Clin. Invest.* 40:857, 1961.
29. Earley, L. E., and Orloff, J. The mechanism of antidiuresis associated with the administration of hydrochlorothiazide to patients with vasopressin-resistant diabetes insipidus. *J. Clin. Invest.* 41:1988, 1962.
30. Ellborg, A., and Forssman, H. Nephrogenic diabetes insipidus in children. *Acta Paediat.* 44:209, 1955.
31. Epstein, F. Disorders of renal concentrating ability. *Yale J. Biol. Med.* 39:186, 1966.
32. Fong, C. T. O., Silver, L., Christman, D. R., and Schwartz, I. L. On the mechanism of action of the antidiuretic hormone (vasopressin). *Proc. Nat. Acad. Sci. U.S.A.* 46: 1273, 1960.
33. Forssman, H. On hereditary diabetes insipidus: With special reference to a sex-linked form. *Acta Med. Scand.* 121 (Suppl. 159):1, 1956.
34. Gaitier, E., and Simpkiss, M. The management of nephrogenic diabetes insipidus in early life. *Acta Paediat.* 46:354, 1957.
35. Ginetzinsky, A. G. Role of hyaluronidase in the re-absorption of water in renal tubules: The mechanism of action of the antidiuretic hormone. *Nature* (London) 182:1218, 1958.
36. Grantham, J., and Burg, M. Effect of vasopressin and cyclic AMP on permeability of isolated collecting tubules. *Amer. J. Physiol.* 211:255, 1966.
37. Harrington, A., and Valtin, H. Impaired urinary concentration after vasopressin and its gradual correction in hypothalamic diabetes insipidus. *J. Clin. Invest.* 47:502, 1968.
38. Havard, C. W. H., and Wood, P. H. N. Antidiuretic properties of hydrochlorothiazide in diabetes insipidus. *Brit. Med. J.* 1: 1306, 1960.
39. Hays, R. M., and Leaf, A. The problem of clinical vasopressin resistance: In vitro studies. *Ann. Intern. Med.* 54:700, 1961.
40. Heinemann, H. O., Demartini, F. E., and Laragh, J. H. The effect of chlorothiazide on renal excretion of electrolytes and free water. *Amer. J. Med.* 26:853, 1959.
41. Hillman, D. A., Olcay, N., Porter, P., Cushman, A., and Talbot, N. B. Renal (vasopressin-resistant) diabetes insipidus: Definition of the effects of a homeostatic limitation in capacity to conserve water on the physical, intellectual, and emotional development of a child. *Pediatrics* 21:430, 1958.
42. Holliday, M., Burstin, C., and Hurrah, J. Evidence that the antidiuretic substance in the plasma of children with nephrogenic diabetes insipidus is antidiuretic hormone. *Pediatrics* 32:384, 1963.
43. Holliday, M., Eagan, T., Morris, C., Janah, A., and Hurrah, J. Pitressin-resistant hyposthenuria in chronic renal disease. *Amer. J. Med.* 42:378, 1967.
44. Kao, M. Y. C., and Steiner, M. M. Diabetes insipidus in infancy resistant to Pitressin. *Pediatrics* 12:400, 1953.
45. Keitel, H. G., Thompson, D., and Itano, H. A. Hyposthenuria in sickle cell anemia: A reversible renal defect. *J. Clin. Invest.* 35:998, 1956.
46. Kennedy, G. C., and Crawford, J. D. A comparison of the effects of adrenalectomy

and of chlorothiazide in experimental diabetes insipidus. *J. Endocr.* 22:77, 1961.
47. Kirman, B. H., Black, J. A., Wilkinson, R. H., and Evans, P. R. Familial Pitressin-resistant diabetes insipidus with mental defect. *Arch. Dis. Child.* 31:59, 1956.
48. Kleeman, C. R., Maxwell, M. H., and Witkin, S. Functional isosthenuria: An isolated reversible renal tubular defect. *A.M.A. Arch. Intern. Med.* 101:1023, 1958.
49. Koefoed-Johnson, V., and Ussing, H. H. The contributions of diffusion and flow to the passage of H_2O through living membranes: Effect of neurohypophyseal hormone on isolated Anuran skin. *Acta Physiol. Scand.* 28:60, 1953.
50. Kowarski, A., Berant, M., Grossman, M., and Migeon, C. Antidiuretic properties of aldactone (spironolactone) in diabetes insipidus. Studies on the mechanism of antidiuresis. *Bull. Johns Hopkins Hosp.* 119: 413, 1966.
51. Leaf, A. Some actions of neurohypophyseal hormones on a living membrane. *J. Gen. Physiol.* 43:175, 1960.
52. Linneweh, F., Buchborn, E., and Dellbrüch, B. Familiärer renaler diabetes insipidus. *Klin. Wschr.* 35:22, 1957.
53. Lobeck, C., Barta, R., and Mangos, J. Study of sweat in Pitressin-resistant diabetes insipidus. *J. Pediat.* 62:868, 1963.
54. Luder, J., and Burnett, D. A congenital renal tubular defect. *Arch. Dis. Child.* 29: 44, 1954.
55. MacDonald, W. B. Congenital Pitressin-resistant diabetes insipidus of renal origin. *Pediatrics* 15:298, 1955.
56. Orloff, J., and Burg, M. Vasopressin-Resistant Diabetes Insipidus. In Stanbury, J. B., Wyngaarden, J. B., and Fredrickson, D. S. (Eds.), *The Metabolic Basis of Inherited Disease.* New York: McGraw-Hill, 1960. Chap. 40.
57. Orloff, J., and Handler, J. S. The similarity of effects of vasopressin, adenosine-3′, 5′-phosphate (cyclic AMP) and theophylline on the toad bladder. *J. Clin. Invest.* 41:702, 1962.
58. Orloff, J., and Handler, J. S. The role of adenosine 3′, 5′-phosphate in the action of antidiuretic hormone. *Amer. J. Med.* 42:757, 1967.
59. Orloff, J., and Walser, M. Water and solute excretion in Pitressin-resistant diabetes insipidus. *Clin. Res. Proc.* 4:136, 1956.
60. Platt, R. Renal failure. *Lancet* 1:1239, 1951.
61. Ramos, G., Rivera, A., Pena, J., and Dies, F. Mechanism of the antidiuretic effect of saluretic drugs. *Clin. Pharmacol. Ther.* 8:557, 1967.
62. Relman, A. S., and Schwartz, W. B. The kidney in potassium depletion. *Amer. J. Med.* 24:764, 1958.
63. Robinson, M. G., and Kaplan, S. A. Inheritance of vasopressin-resistant ("nephrogenic") diabetes insipidus. *Amer. J. Dis. Child.* 99:164, 1960.
64. Roussak, N. J., and Oleesky, S. Water losing nephritis: A syndrome simulating diabetes insipidus. *Quart. J. Med.* 23:147, 1954.
65. Ruess, A., and Rosenthal, I. Intelligence in nephrogenic diabetes insipidus. *Amer. J. Dis. Child.* 105:358, 1963.
66. Schoen, E. J. Renal diabetes insipidus. *Pediatrics* 26:808, 1960.
67. Schotland, M., Grumbach, M., and Strauss, J. The effects of chlorothiazides on nephrogenic diabetes insipidus. *Pediatrics* 31:741, 1963.
68. Silverstein, E., and Tobian, L. Pitressin-resistant diabetes insipidus with massive hydronephritis. *Amer. J. Med.* 30:819, 1961.
69. Skadhauge, E. Studies of the antidiuresis induced by natrichloriuretic drugs in rats with diabetes insipidus. *Quart. J. Exp. Physiol.* 51:297, 1966.
70. Sutherland, E. W., and Rall, T. W. The relation of adenosine-3′, 5′-phosphate and phosphorylase to the actions of catecholamines and other hormones. *Pharmacol. Rev.* 12:265, 1960.
71. Waring, A. J., Laslo, K., and Tappan, V. A congenital defect of water metabolism. *Amer. J. Dis. Child.* 69:323, 1945.
72. Wattiez, R., Loeb, H., Bellens, R., and van Geffel, R. Diabète insipide pitressino-résistant. *Helv. Paediat. Acta* 12:643, 1957.
73. Williams, R. H., and Henry, C. Nephro-

genic diabetes insipidus: Transmitted by females and appearing during infancy in males. *Ann. Intern. Med.* 27:84, 1947.

74. Wirz, H. Der osmotische druck in den corticalen tubule der rattenniere. *Helv. Physiol. Pharmacol. Acta* 14:353, 1956.

39

Congenital Malformations of the Kidney

Joseph M. Hayman, Jr.

With increasing progress in reconstructive and plastic surgery has come an increased interest in congenital anomalies [60], since it is realized that in some cases early recognition may permit surgical correction. Polycystic kidney disease and cystic disease of the renal medulla have been discussed extensively in Chapters 35 and 36 and accordingly are omitted from this chapter.

Some anomalies are evident at birth; others give rise to no symptoms until late childhood or even middle age. These are usually complicated by infection and secondary changes. Some anomalies, such as fused kidney or simple double ureter, are harmless, but if they are discovered on a routine examination, the patient's symptoms and pain are apt to be erroneously attributed to them.

The most serious anomalies are those in which there is an insufficient amount of functioning kidney tissue, either because of a primary renal defect, or because of destruction of parenchyma resulting from obstruction in the lower urinary tract. Such parenchymal destruction from back pressure may occur in utero in spite of placental function. Hypoplastic kidneys and atrophic pyelonephritis with ureteral abnormalities are occasionally responsible for uremia in infancy, but usually not for a number of years. In these cases there are few symptoms of kidney disease, but the child does not grow and develops osteodystrophy (renal rickets). Many anomalies, particularly those associated with obstruction, predispose to infection and prevent cure of the infection until the obstruction is removed. In Smith and Orkin's analysis [52] of 471 congenital anomalies of the kidneys and ureters, only 20 per cent were without secondary associated pathology, especially infection. Renal anomalies are rarely the cause of enuresis, which in the majority of cases is simply the persistence of the infantile habit of bladder function on a psychogenic basis.

The great majority of the congenital malformations of the kidney are explainable in terms of deviations or defects in normal development. It therefore seems appropriate to begin this chapter with a brief review of normal embryologic development of the permanent kidney [40, 44].

Embryology of the Kidney

In the course of development of the adult mammal, three distinct excretory organs are formed. The first of these is the *pronephros,* remnants of which rarely may persist to produce cysts in the adult human. The second excretory organ is the *mesonephros,* parts of which normally persist to form parts of the genital system. In the male, some of the mesonephric tubules form the epididymis, and the mesonephric duct, the vas deferens. In the female, the only remnants of the mesonephros are the minute appendages of the ovary, the epoophoron and paroophoron.

The permanent kidney, or *metanephros,* is derived from two sources. The first is a bud or diverticulum which appears in the mesonephric duct just cephalad to the point where it opens into the cloaca. This anlage is destined to form the ureter, pelvis of the kidney, and the collecting ducts. As this bud grows cephalad, it is invested about its distal end with mesoderm from the nephrogenic cord, from which the permanent renal tubules develop. The pelvic end of the diverticulum divides to form the major and minor calyces within the surrounding mass of nephrogenic mesoderm. From the tip of each minor calyx a number of straight collecting tubules develop. The group of straight collecting tubules arising from a minor calyx, together with the nephrons which eventually drain into it, constitute a renal unit. The convoluted tubules, loops of Henle, and arched collecting tubules are all derived from the nephrogenic mesoderm. The glomerular portion of the nephron develops most rapidly and becomes a large, well-formed, and apparently functioning structure before the tubular portion shows any appreciable degree of differentiation [42]. Contrary to the older view, it seems that the glomerular capillaries develop in situ in the endothelial cell mass, and that branches of the afferent arteriole from the renal artery do not connect with the primitive glomerulus until a few capillary spaces are formed [57]. The glomeruli of the oldest nephrons lie closest to the medulla, their loops of Henle are the longest, and their convoluted tubules the most complex. The first-formed glomeruli are nearest the corticomedullary junction, those formed later lying progressively further out in the cortex. By the end of the fifth fetal month some 10 to 20 generations of straight tubules have been formed, and about 30 per cent of the glomeruli are mature. As later generations of collecting tubules develop, and as the pelvis and calyces expand, some of the first orders of straight tubules are incorporated and disappear.

At birth there are approximately a million to a million and a quarter nephrons in each kidney. Some are incompletely developed at birth, but there is no formation of new nephrons after birth, and no regeneration of a nephron whose glomerulus has been destroyed. The blood supply of the kidney is usually derived from a single renal artery which does not divide until it has entered the substance of the kidney at the hilus. Division of the renal artery into two or more branches before reaching the kidney and accessory renal arteries are common abnormalities.

When the kidneys are first formed, they lie approximately opposite the fourth lumbar segment; in their final position they are at the level of the twelfth thoracic or first lumbar vertebra. This "ascent" of the kidney is due in part to the rapid growth of the caudal part of the body, and in part to the cephalic movement of the kidneys out of the pelvic part of the body below the bifurcation of the aorta [27]. In this ascent they are rotated a quarter turn, so that their convex borders, instead of being directed dorsally, become directed laterally. Also during this movement they are squeezed together as they pass out of the pelvis, and may even fuse and remain fused during the remainder of their ascent. Abnormalities in the position and rotation of the kidneys are attributable to aberrations during this movement in the course of embryonic life.

Classification

The classification of congenital abnormalities of the kidney is usually based on that proposed by Papin and Eisendrath [43] or as modified by Gutierrez [29] or Kissane [33]. Papen and Eisendrath's classification, somewhat condensed and slightly modified, is as follows:

1. Anomalies of number (e.g., solitary, supernumerary)
2. Anomalies of volume (e.g., hypoplasia, hypertrophy, supplementary lobe)
3. Anomalies of differentiation (e.g., renal dysplasia)
4. Anomalies of location (e.g., simple unilateral or bilateral ectopia, crossed ectopia with or without fusion)
5. Median line fusion (e.g., horseshoe, L-shaped, cake, sigmoid kidney)
6. Anomalies of rotation
7. Anomalies of vessels
8. Anomalies of pelvis and ureter
9. Renal cysts

ANOMALIES OF NUMBER

Bilateral Renal Agenesis. This lesion of course is incompatible with survival for more than a few days [25]. In true agenesis, as distinguished from aplasia, the ureter is also absent. The failure of the ureteric bud to develop from the lower end of the mesonephric duct accounts for the failure of the metanephros to develop. The nephrogenic blastema develops metanephric tubules only when it is stimulated by the growth of the ureter into it [28]. Ashley and Mostofi [4], on the other hand, believe that the formation of the definitive kidney depends both on the presence of the ureteric bud and on the existence of an adequate nephrogenic blastoderm, and that the ureteric bud develops in response to induction from the developing metanephros. Besides a genetic defect, Fraser and Fainstat [24] believe that an environmental or toxic agent may at times be responsible. Such an agent would be most damaging if present at the time the pronephros is developing, at about the fourth week of pregnancy. In one of their cases the mother had taken quinine and castor oil six weeks after her last menstrual period. With bilateral agenesis, the perinephric fascia cannot be identified in the retroperitoneal space; in unilateral absence of the kidney, the fascia does not develop on the affected side. If the ureter is partially represented, the fascia is poorly developed and ends with the cephalad tip of the ureter [9].

The incidence of renal agenesis is greater than is commonly supposed. Davidson and Ross [19], in 1954, were able to collect 232 acceptable cases, including five of their own. As these authors point out, the frequency depends on whether the lesion is related to total autopsies (0.01 to 0.04 per cent), to postmortem examinations on stillbirths and infants dying within six weeks (0.3 per cent), or to deliveries (0.04 per cent). The longest recorded survival of an infant without kidneys is 39 days: the great majority either are stillborn or live less than 24 hours. Death is usually due to prematurity or to other deformities; it is due to uremia only in the few who survive for one or more days. Males are affected more frequently than females (ratio of 2.5:1). Perhaps, as suggested by Davidson and Ross, there is some obscure connection with the fact that the mesonephric duct normally undergoes involution in the female. There are at least two reports of the defect in siblings [49]. Six affected infants were accompanied by a normal twin.

Although bilateral renal agenesis has usually

been recognized only at postmortem examination, antemortem recognition has been made possible by Potter's observations, particularly of the face. Potter's description [46] is worth quoting: "The most striking feature consists of an increase in width between the eyes and the presence of an unusually prominent fold at the inner canthus of each eye. The fold sweeps downward and laterally to form a wide semicircle under the inferior medial aspect of each orbital space. Other changes which, when combined with the appearance of the eyes, give the face of the infant a resemblance to that of a person of very advanced age — an extreme premature senility as it were — are a flattening and slight broadening of the nose, an unusually receding chin, and large, low set ears which have proportionately little cartilage." Bilateral agenesis is usually associated with oligohydramnios [7], and this association has been put forward as an argument for the theory that urine has an important part in the formation of the amniotic fluid [58]. Other congenital defects are common. Bilateral pulmonary hypoplasia is almost constant, and major deformities of the legs or sirenomelia occur in 20 to 30 per cent [6].

Unilateral Agenesis. This anomaly is compatible with normal life and development. The incidence is about 1:1000 autopsies and 1:1500 urologic studies [27]. The ureter is absent in the majority of cases. The single kidney usually shows considerable hypertrophy [20]. The pathogenesis is the same as in bilateral agenesis: failure of the ureteric bud to develop from the mesonephric duct on the affected side. Potter [38] called attention to the absence of the fallopian tube as well as the lower müllerian derivative on the same side in cases of unilateral renal agenesis in females, a unicornuate uterus developing from a single müllerian duct. The possibility of a solitary kidney should be considered in any case of malformation of the uterus. Normal pregnancy is possible with a solitary kidney although the total fetal loss is high [22]. Recognition of a single kidney is obviously important if infection, calculus, or renal tumor develops, and particularly when surgery is contemplated [3]. Most authorities regard it as an absolute contraindication to percutaneous renal biopsy. Nondescent of the ipsolateral testis may be a useful sign in some cases. The most common reason for medical consultation is urinary tract infection. The diagnosis may be suspected from a flat plate of the abdomen by the absence of one renal outline, asymmetry of the psoas shadows, and an enlarged renal shadow on the opposite side. Conroy and Walker [18] believe that a single kidney with normal function is not a contraindication to military or combat service.

Supernumerary Kidney. This is probably the rarest of renal abnormalities. The first case is said to have been described by Martins in 1656. Carlson [16] was able to collect 51 cases in 1950, in only four of which was the diagnosis made preoperatively. Begg [8] reported the case of a 42-year-old woman who by pyelograms had six functioning kidneys, three on each side. Tölle [55] described two patients with two complete kidneys on each side, and four ureters. It is probable that with the increasingly common use of intravenous pyelography more cases will be reported.

The diagnosis of supernumerary kidney should include only cases in which the structure resembles the normal kidney in every particular, has a separate blood supply and excretory duct, and is completely separated from the other kidney on the same side. The so-called fused supernumerary kidney does not have a separate blood supply, and should be classed with supernumerary renal buds.

The development of a supernumerary kidney depends upon the presence of an additional ureteral bud. As this grows cephalad, either there has to be a splitting of the nephrogenic blastema or two separate metanephric blastemas must be present, which partially or completely reduplicated ureteral stalks enter. The supernumerary kidney is usually smaller and lower than the normal kidney and has reduced function.

Symptoms may be absent in supernumerary kidney. When present, they are due to such complicating lesions as infection, stone, obstruction, hydronephrosis, tumor, or, with ureteral ectopy, urinary leakage. Treatment is directed at the diseased supernumerary organ, and generally requires nephrectomy providing that adequate renal tissue will remain.

ANOMALIES OF VOLUME

Renal Hypoplasia. In renal hypoplasia the organ is small or infantile, but has essentially normal parenchyma and a patent ureter. There may be the normal division of medullary and cortical substance, or the pyramidal structure may be absent. While glomerular and tubular development may be rudimentary, and the glomeruli may even show hyaline degeneration, the majority of hypoplastic kidneys are simply diminutive organs with cells smaller than normal and with a greately reduced number of nephrons and calyces [11]. The hypoplastic kidney usually lies closer than normal to the spine. The blood supply is reduced, and the vessels often show sclerotic changes. This inadequate blood supply may be responsible for the inability of the hypoplastic kidney to hypertrophy when the other kidney is removed.

The frequency of renal hypoplasia is approximately 1:50, somewhat higher than agenesis. It may be unilateral or bilateral. When unilateral, the other kidney shows compensatory hypertrophy and is usually adequate to maintain life and normal renal function. Associated congenital abnormalities, such as situs inversus, ectopic position of the normal kidney, double ureters, and cardiovascular defects, are common. When renal hypoplasia is bilateral, there is usually insufficient tissue to maintain life for more than a few years; growth is retarded, "renal rickets" develops, and death occurs in uremia in childhood or early adolescence. Fleisher [23] believes lateral displacement of the nipples should lead to a suspicion of bilateral renal hypoplasia.

The hypoplastic kidney is very prone to infection, and this tendency frequently makes the differential diagnosis from atrophic pyelonephritis very difficult. In fact, Emmett et al. [21] do not believe that the differentiation can be made clinically, urographically, or pathologically. They believe that the number of calyces is an unreliable criterion. Certainly such a case as that reported by Slungaard and Jaeck [51] in which the total renal weight at 10 years was only 18 gm., and in which the left kidney showed six calyces and the right four, may be assumed to represent congenital hypoplasia even though histologically the picture was that of glomerulonephritis. Failure to grow has been noted after the first year.

Some cases of both unilateral renal hypoplasia and atrophic pyelonephritis are associated with hypertension [10]. Nephrectomy has resulted in a return of blood pressure to normal in about the same proportion of cases (30 to 40 per cent) whether the final diagnosis was congenital hypoplasia or atrophic pyelonephritis. It is essential, of course, to determine the function of the other kidney before surgery, as a number of tragedies have resulted from the removal of one of two hypoplastic organs.

The Ask-Upmark kidney is a rare form of true hypoplasia in which nephrogenesis has been arrested in one or a few adjacent renal lobules after formation of the juxtomedullary nephrons. It is characterized by a deep transverse groove on its cortical surface and ectasia of the corresponding calyx [5].

Congenital Renal Hypertrophy. This is a congenital compensatory mechanism associated with contralateral hypoplasia or agenesis. The kidney is considerably increased not only in size but also in functional capacity. The renal pelvis is also unusually large. While a congenital hypertrophic kidney may enable its bearer to reach advanced age, infection or acute injury is more likely to jeopardize life than when two kidneys are present. It is of surgical diagnostic concern since it may be mistaken for a tumor and removed without establishment of adequate function from the other kidney.

Supplementary Lobe. Supplementary lobe or redundancy of renal parenchyma is characterized by a double row of pyramids. It is an extremely rare anomaly, and is only a postmortem finding. The occasional distinct bulge found in one kidney, composed of apparently normal nephrons, and supernumerary renal buds attached to a more or less normal kidney should be included in the same grouping. These two anomalies are of no clinical significance.

Fetal Lobulation. The fetal and infantile kidney normally has a lobular surface, corresponding to the embryologic development of the renal parenchyma as lobules around the divisions of the ureter and its calyceal branches. As the kidney grows, these surface markings gradually disappear, and cannot be recognized after a child is 4 or 5 years old. Fetal lobulation, however, persists in 3 to 4 per cent of individuals into adult life. It has no clinical significance. It was described in Malpighi's paper in 1666 [37].

Unusually short, long, club, or dumbbell kidneys are not uncommon, but are of no significance. However, surgical exploration of a renal pelvis that is entirely intrarenal may be difficult.

ANOMALIES OF DIFFERENTIATION

Renal Dysplasia or Dysgenesis. This condition differs from agenesis or absence of a kidney in that some tissue is present which can be recognized as related to renal structure, but there is no true kidney. It represents a disturbed differentiation of nephrogenic tissue with persistence of structure inappropriate to the gestational age of the patient. Grossly, a dysplastic kidney consists of a disorderly mass of cysts, ranging in size from barely visible to several centimeters in diameter. The mass is not reniform but resembles a bunch of grapes. The ureter is usually absent. Associated defects in other organs are common. A few abnormal undeveloped structures resembling glomeruli may be present; Emmett et al. [21] and Campbell [15] believe that if glomeruli are present, the condition should be classified as hypoplasia rather than dysplasia. Occasionally a dysplasic organ may cause pain by sclerotic compression of nerve endings, and relief may follow its removal. Unilateral renal dysplasia is the most common abdominal abnormal mass palpable in the newborn infant, exceeding both Wilms's tumor and neuroblastoma [34].

Renal dysplasia has the same clinical significance as renal agenesis; bilateral dysplasia is incompatible with life. In unilateral dysplasia the prognosis is excellent if other malformations are absent. Late symptoms, such as hypertension, do not develop.

ANOMALIES OF LOCATION

Congenital Renal Ectopia. This anomaly may involve one or both kidneys. The ectopic organ may be located anywhere from the pelvis to the thorax. Although one or both kidneys, with or without the corresponding adrenal gland, may be found in the thorax or posterior mediastinum, this is due to congenital or acquired defects in the diaphragm. Thus a thoracic kidney, even though present at birth, does not represent true renal ectopia. Congenital ectopic kidneys are held in their abnormal position chiefly by anomalous vascular attachments, representing persistence of the renal blood supply of earlier fetal life. Ectopic kidneys are usually abnormal in shape, and are smaller and more lobulated than normal kidneys. The length of the ureter corresponds to the location of the kidney, in contrast to acquired ectopia or ptosis in which the ureter is of normal length and the vascular supply of normal origin. The origin of the vascular supply distinguishes congenital from acquired ectopia.

The kidney may be ectopic on its own side or on the opposite side, where it may be either fused or unfused with its mate (crossed ectopia). In a number of cases a solitary kidney has been in an ectopic location [2, 14, 38]. Rarely the ureter from a solitary kidney empties into the bladder on the opposite side. There is no satisfactory embryologic explanation. Thoracic kidneys are rare, and must be differentiated from other low intrathoracic masses [32]. The diagnosis has often been made only at thoracotomy.

The frequency of simple unilateral ectopia is about 1:800. The condition is more common in males, and on the left side. The ectopic kidney is most often in the pelvis, with the sacroiliac region the second most common site, but it may be between the bladder and rectum, behind the rectum, in a scrotal hernia, or in the thorax.

Ectopic kidneys commonly show malrotation, the renal pelves usually facing forward. An ectopic kidney may displace or compress the bowel, leading to severe constipation. A pelvic kidney may interfere with normal childbirth. Renal ectopia is clinically important because the abnormally placed kidney is particularly prone to infection, may cause lower abdominal pain by pressure on nerves, blood vessels, or neighboring organs, and, if palpable, may be mistaken for a neoplasm or another organ. Palpation of an ectopic kidney may be followed by albuminuria and hematuria.

Crossed Ectopia. In crossed ectopia bilateral embryologic development begins normally, but early in the ascent of the kidneys one organ crosses to the opposite side, where it may remain distinct or become fused with its mate. The reason or mechanism for this migration is unknown. The ureter of the crossed kidney crosses the midline and opens into the bladder in the normal position [2]. The blood supply of the ectopic kidney is always anomalous, and its source depends upon whether the ectopia developed early or later in the ascent of the kidney. If the dystopia occurs late, the blood supply will be from the original site of the kidney. The vascular supply may arise from the aorta or the iliac or hypogastric arteries. Crossed renal ectopia is said to occur about once in 2000 cases, but there were only four instances in Campbell's 51,880 cases [15], an incidence of about one case in 13,000. Abeshouse [1] was able to collect 337 cases from the literature in 1947. The symptoms in crossed ectopia are the same as those caused by disease in a normally placed organ, but the pain is at the site of the ectopic organ. Diagnosis is made by pyelography. Crossed renal ectopia of a solitary kidney is a rare lesion [47, 59].

Crossed ectopia with fusion may be considered a transition from the horseshoe kidney. The ectopic organ is below the normal one and is abnormal in form and size. The kidneys may be fused end to end, side to side, or in an S or I shape. Fused ectopia makes any indicated surgery difficult and often impossible.

MEDIAN LINE FUSION

Horseshoe Kidney. Little has been added to our knowledge of the horseshoe kidney since the publication of Gutierrez's monograph [30] in 1934. The best explanation for the formation of the horseshoe kidney is fusion of the two nephrogenic blastemas as they are squeezed together by the umbilical arteries during the ascent of the kidneys from the pelvis at about 30 days (9 mm. embryo). However, the position of the ureters suggests that fusion may take place at a later period. If fusion precedes rotation, the ureters leave anteriorly; if it occurs after rotation, they leave medially.

In the horseshoe kidney the two organs are fused across the midline by an isthmus which may be a solid mass of renal tissue or only a dense band of fibrous tissue. Fusion is at the lower pole in 90 per cent of cases. The horseshoe kidney usually lies anterior to the aorta and vena cava, but it has been found behind and even between them. The horseshoe kidney is rarely in the normal position; it usually overlies the lower lumbar vertebrae, and may be in the pelvis, where it is held by an early establishment of an abnormally low vascular supply from the aorta or iliac vessels.

The frequency of horseshoe kidney has been variously reported as from 1:300 to 1:1800. The anomaly is about twice as frequent in males as in females. While horseshoe kidney is not incompatible with normal duration of life, it is not an innocent congenital anomaly. Only 18 of 31 cases followed for 10 years by Glenn [26] remained asymptomatic. It is susceptible to contusion or rupture from trauma to the abdomen, and the angulation of the ureters predisposes to obstruction and pyelonephritis. Patients with horseshoe kidneys may suffer episodes of abdominal pain and vasomotor disturbances that can be relieved by anteflexion of the trunk. Many cases are associated not only with other abnormalities of the urogenital tract but also with defects in the cardiovascular and gastrointestinal systems.

Lump, Shield, and Cake Kidneys. These anomalies are extremely rare, only 11 cases having been collected by Miller et al. [39] in 1956. Both kidneys are fused into a solid, irregular organ located over the sacral area or in the pelvis. The renal pelves are usually anterior, while the blood supply enters the posterior aspect. Symptoms are due to complications, as in the horseshoe kidney, or there may be pain due to pull of the mass on the vascular pedicle. The renal mass may be palpable, and be mistaken for a tumor.

ANOMALIES OF ROTATION

At the end of the first month of fetal life, the renal hilus and pelvis face ventrally. During its ascent, the kidney undergoes rotation on its long axis so that the pelvis comes to face mesially, i.e., toward the spine. If this fails to occur, all degrees of faulty rotation (renal torsion) are encountered. In underrotation the pelvis faces anteriorly, and in overrotation laterally or, in rare cases, even posteriorly. Excessive rotation is rare, but may occur with or without crossed ectopia. Faulty rotation in itself is of no clinical significance, but if kept in mind, the interpretation of many puzzling pyelograms is made far easier.

ANOMALIES OF VESSELS

During their migration the kidneys are constantly supplied by the neighboring blood vessels. Thus they make new connections, while the old ones are obliterated and disappear. However, some of these older vessels may remain as anomalous vessels, usually accessory. Anomalous renal arteries may arise as branches of the middle sacral, iliac, or lumbar arteries [13]. These enter the lower pole of the kidney and may cross ventral to the ureter, and cause intermittent or constant obstruction. The kidney may receive vessels from the phrenic or suprarenal arteries which enter the upper pole. These anomalous vessels are often called polar arteries. "In many mammals, one of the mesonephric branches becomes the permanent renal artery, but in man by the time the kidney has reached its permanent position, the mesonephric tubules and arteries are degenerating, and at about eight weeks an appropriately placed member of the periaortic capillary plexus on each side suddenly enlarges and assumes arterial characteristics to become the definite renal artery" [12]. Normally there is one renal artery to each kidney, which divides into two or three branches on entering the hilus, or not until it has entered the substance of the kidney.

Anomalous renal arteries are usually symptomless unless they cause ureteral obstruction. They are believed to cause pain occasionally by traction, which has been relieved by division of the artery [41]. It is not clear whether the pain is due to pull on the artery itself or on periarterial nerves.

Congenital arteriovenous anastomosis is a rare lesion, only 24 cases having been reported [36]. Symptoms are directly proportional to the size of the fistula, and are usually those of hypertension or high output heart failure. Diagnosis is made by angiography, and nephrectomy is usually necessary.

ANOMALIES OF THE PELVIS AND URETER

Normally the ureteral stalk expands into a single ampullary pelvis which divides into two or three major calyces. An early division may occur, just external to the hilus. The kidney then has two pelves, an upper and a lower. The ureter may divide anywhere from the hilus to the bladder, each branch leading to a distinct pelvis. If the division is in the bladder wall, there are two ureteral meati, and the condition is called double ureter. With two ureters, there are two pelves. The renal mass may be single, indented, or so separated as to be called a double kidney. With two ureters, that from the upper pelvis always enters the bladder more mesially and lower than that from the lower pelvis.

There are a large number of congenital anomalies of the ureter — in number, termination, caliber, and structure. These are chiefly of interest to the urologist [15, 48]. They are of concern to the physician only because they predispose to infection and obstruction. The clinical examination of any patient with persistent infection should include urologic study, particularly intravenous pyelography. Unrecognized ureteral obstruction, whether from a congenital stenosis or valve, or a megaloureter from absence of normal parasympathetic innervation [51], frequently results in progressive destruction of the renal mass by back pressure. Early recognition and surgical correction is the only method of treatment. In many instances a case of full-blown "renal rickets" goes unrecognized and neglected for too long. Pyuria, with or without positive urine culture, or persistent loin pain demands the most careful and thorough urologic study.

CONGENITAL CYSTS

Congenital cysts include polycystic disease and medullary cystic disease (see Chapters 35 and 36). In addition, congenital cysts include solitary cysts, multilocular cystic disease, and several other rare forms.

Congenital solitary cysts are rare. In Campbell's series [15] of 19,046 autopsies on infants and children, the incidence was 1:1731. Small solitary cysts are not unusual and have no significance. The cause of the solitary cyst is obscure. In the adult it is difficult to determine whether a solitary cyst is congenital or the result of inflammation and tubular destruction. Solitary cysts are more common in the lower pole. As the cyst enlarges, it destroys the surrounding renal parenchyma by compression. The cysts vary from 1 to 10 cm. or more in diameter, and are thin-walled and serosa-lined, and contain a fluid which resembles a transudate of plasma [17]. Occasionally a solitary cyst gives rise to hematuria or is responsible for hypertension. Solitary cyst is frequently mistaken for tumor on urologic study; the differentiation is made by angiography. Treatment is by nephrectomy or excision of the cyst, depending on the amount of renal parenchyma remaining.

Congenital multilocular cystic disease is rare, only 40 cases having been reported up to 1963 [56]. These cysts are unilateral, solitary, multilocular, do not communicate with the pelvis, have a definite epithelial lining, and contain no renal elements within the cyst. The etiology is obscure. Theories of persistence of fetal tubules or failure of union cannot explain the multilocular nature of the cysts or the absence of renal tissue between them. About half these cysts are discovered in childhood because of hematuria or a palpable mass in the loin. However, they may produce no symptoms until old age. They are usually mistaken for a tumor.

Another rare form of congenital cyst has been described under the name *congenital unilateral multicystic disease,* which is believed to be distinct from polycystic disease and multilocular cysts [53]. The lesion consists of replacement of the normal kidney by a conglomeration of various-sized cysts, with either no discernible renal tissue or only a few remnants with fibrotic atrophy and dilated tubular structures.

There are other congenital cysts and diverticula of the calyces and ureter. These are described in Campbell's monograph [15], and are of significance only when they become infected or contain stones.

References

1. Abeshouse, B. S. Crossed ectopia with fusion: Review of the literature and report of four cases. *Amer. J. Surg.* 73:658, 1947.
2. Alexander, J. D., King, K. B., and Fromm, C. S. Congenital solitary kidney with crossed ureter. *J. Urol.* 64:230, 1950.
3. Anderson, E. E., and Harrison, J. H. The surgical importance of the solitary kidney. *New Eng. J. Med.* 273:683, 1965.
4. Ashley, D. B. J., and Mostofi, F. K. Renal agenesis and dysgenesis. *J. Urol.* 83:211, 1960.
5. Ask-Upmark, E. Über juvenile maligne Nephrosklerose und ihr Verhaltnis zu Storung in der Nierent wichlung. *Acta Path. Microbiol. Scand.* 6:383, 1929.
6. Bain, A. D., Beath, M. M., and Flint, W. F. Sirenomelia and monomelia with renal agenesis and amnion nodosum. *Arch. Dis. Child.* 35:250, 1960.
7. Bain, A. D., Smith, I. I., and Gould, I. K. Newborn after prolonged leakage of liquor amnii. *Brit. Med. J.* 2:598, 1964.
8. Begg, R. C. Sextuplicitas renum: A case of six functioning kidneys and ureters in an adult female. *J. Urol.* 70:686, 1953.
9. Benjamin, J. A., and Tobin, C. E. Abnormalities of the kidneys, ureters, and perinephric fascia: Anatomic and clinical study. *J. Urol.* 65:715, 1951.
10. Boeminghaus, H. Nierenhypoplasie und Hochdruck. *Z. Urol.* 51:323, 1938.
11. Boissonnat, P. What to call the hypoplastic kidney? *Arch. Dis. Child.* 37:142, 1962.
12. Bremer, J. L. The origin of the renal arteries in mammals and its anomalies. *Amer. J. Anat.* 18:179, 1915.
13. Bremer, J. L. *Congenital Anomalies of the Viscera.* Cambridge, Mass.: Harvard University Press, 1957.
14. Butler, T. J. Solitary ectopic pelvic kidneys: Fifty-three cases. *Brit. J. Surg.* 38:522, 1951.
15. Campbell, M. *Urology.* Philadelphia: Saunders, 1954.
16. Carlson, H. E. Supernumerary kidney: A summary of fifty-one reported cases. *J. Urol.* 64:224, 1950.
17. Clarke, B. G., Hurwitz, I. S., and Dubinsky, E. Solitary serous cysts of the kidney: Biochemical, cytological, and histological studies. *J. Urol.* 75:772, 1956.
18. Conroy, T. F., and Walker, J. H. Congenital solitary kidney: Case reports and consideration of military significance. *J. Urol.* 53:4, 1945.
19. Davidson, W. M., and Ross, I. G. M. Bilateral absence of the kidneys and related congenital disorders. *J. Path. Bact.* 68:459, 1954.
20. Doroshow, L. D., and Abeshouse, B. S. Congenital unilateral solitary kidney: Report of 37 cases and a review of the literature. *Urol. Survey* 11:219, 1961.
21. Emmett, J. L., Alvarez-Irena, J. J., and McDonald, J. R. Atrophic pyelonephritis versus congenital renal hypoplasia. *J.A.M.A.* 148:1470, 1952.
22. Felding, C. Obstetric studies in women with congenital solitary kidneys. *Acta Obstet. Gynec. Scand.* 44:555, 1966.
23. Fleisher, D. S. Lateral displacement of the nipple, a sign of bilateral renal hypoplasia. *J. Pediat.* 69:806, 1966.
24. Fraser, F. C., and Fainstat, T. D. Causes of congenital defects. *A.M.A. Amer. J. Dis. Child.* 82:593, 1951.
25. Frumkin, J., and Marz, R. Bilateral renal agenesis. *J. Urol.* 71:268, 1954.
26. Glenn, J. F. Analysis of 51 patients with horseshoe kidney. *New Eng. J. Med.* 261:684, 1959.

27. Gruenwald, P. The normal changes in the position of the embryonic kidney. *Anat. Rec.* 85:163, 1943.
28. Gruenwald, P. Mechanisms of abnormal development. *Arch. Path.* 46:495, 1947.
29. Gutierrez, R. Surgical aspects of renal agenesis. *Arch. Surg.* 27:686, 1933.
30. Gutierrez, R. *The Clinical Management of Horseshoe Kidney*. New York: Hoeber, 1934.
31. Helper, A. B. Solitary cysts of kidney: Report of seven cases and observations on pathogenesis of these cysts. *Surg. Gynec. Obstet.* 50:668, 1930.
32. Hill, J. E., and Bunts, R. C. Thoracic kidney: Case reports. *J. Urol.* 84:460, 1960.
33. Kissane, J. M. Congenital Malformations. In Heptinstall, R. H., *Pathology of the Kidney*. Boston: Little, Brown, 1966.
34. Longino, L. A., and Martin, L. W. Abdominal masses in the newborn infant. *Pediatrics* 21:596, 1958.
35. Longo, V. J., and Thompson, G. J. Congenital solitary kidney. *J. Urol.* 68:63, 1952.
36. Malloy, T. R., Leberman, P. R., and Murphy, J. J. Renal arteriovenous fistula. *J. Urol.* 98:40, 1967.
37. Malpighi, M. *De Vicerum Structura Excercitio Anatomica*. Bononiae: Montii, 1666.
38. McCrea, L. E. Congenital solitary pelvic kidney. *J. Urol.* 48:58, 1942.
39. Miller, A. L., Jr., Brown, A. W., and Tomskey, G. C. Pelvic fused kidney. *J. Urol.* 75:17, 1956.
40. Nicholson, G. W. The kidneys and development. *Guy. Hosp. Rep.* 77:362, 1927.
41. Ockerbald, N. F. Aberrant renal arteries. *J. Urol.* 67:810, 1927.
42. Osathanondh, V., and Potter, E. L. Development of the human kidney as shown by microdissection: II. Renal pelvis, calyces, and papillae. III. Formation and interrelationship of collecting tubules and nephrons. *Arch. Path.* (Chicago) 76:277, 290, 1963.
43. Papin, E., and Eisendrath, D. N. Classification of renal and ureteral anomalies. *Ann. Surg.* 85:735, 1927.
44. Patten, B. M. *Human Embryology* (2d ed.). New York: McGraw-Hill, 1953.
45. Potter, E. L. *Pathology of the Foetus and Newborn*. Chicago: Year Book Publishers, 1952.
46. Potter, E. L. Facial characteristics of infants with bilateral renal agenesis. *Amer. J. Obstet. Gynec.* 51:845, 1946.
47. Purpon, I. Crossed renal ectopy with solitary kidney: A review of the literature. *J. Urol.* 90:13, 1963.
48. Rolnick, H. C. *Practice of Urology*. Philadelphia: Lippincott, 1949.
49. Schmidt, E. C. H., Hartley, A. A., and Bower, R. Renal aplasia in sisters. *A.M.A. Arch. Path.* 54:403, 1952.
50. Shiller, W. R., and Wiswell, O. B. A fused pelvic (cake) kidney. *J. Urol.* 78:9, 1957.
51. Slungaard, R. K., and Jaeck, J. L. Bilateral dwarfed kidneys. *A.M.A. Amer. J. Dis. Child.* 97:575, 1959.
52. Smith, E. C., and Orkin, L. A. A clinical and statistical study of 471 congenital anomalies of the kidneys and ureters. *J. Urol.* 53:11, 1945.
53. Spence, H. M. Congenital unilateral multicystic kidney: An entity to be distinguished from polycystic kidney disease and other cystic disorders. *J. Urol.* 74:693, 1955.
54. Swenson, O., MacMahon, H. E., Jaques, W. E., and Campbell, J. S. New concepts of the etiology of megalo-ureters. *New Eng. J. Med.* 246:41, 1952.
55. Tölle, R. Zur Kasuistik der Doppelniere. *Z. Urol.* 49:501, 1956.
56. Uson, A. C., and Melicow, M. M. Multilocular cysts of the kidney with intrapelvic herniation of a "daughter" cyst: Report of four cases. *J. Urol.* 89:341, 1963.
57. Vernier, R. L., and Birch-Anderson, A. Studies of the human fetal kidney. *J. Pediat.* 60:754, 1962.
58. Weber, L. L., and Israel, S. L. Renal agenesis and oligohydramnios. *Obstet. Gynec.* 12:575, 1958.
59. Weiss, R. M., Maloney, P. K., Jr., and Beland, G. A. Crossed ectopia of a solitary kidney. *J. Urol.* 94:320, 1965.
60. Williams, D. I. Congenital anomalies of the genito-urinary tract. *Practitioner* 186:467, 1961.

40

Renal Tuberculosis

Herman Wechsler

Tuberculosis of the kidney is no longer the dread disease it was only two generations ago. The usual course of this disease was progressive parenchymatous destruction of one or both kidneys, with death usually resulting from uremia in three to five years. Surgical removal of the kidney first obviously involved was undertaken with the hope that it would halt the spread of the process to the other kidney.

Frequency

The frequency of renal tuberculosis has shown no decline in recent decades. In spite of newer and more efficient drugs and greater experience with the chemotherapy of tuberculosis, the number of new patients, as reported by a nationwide Veterans Administration survey, remains constant. It is likely that the reservoir of infection will continue to produce patients 2 to 20 years after the primary infection. Most cases occur in young adults, between the ages of 20 and 40 years. Cases in early childhood are reported, and also, with increased longevity, a greater number in persons over age 60. In fact, the second highest incidence of renal tuberculosis is in elderly persons. Unless the diagnosis is suspected early, many persons are doomed to ineffective treatment for many years, with varying degrees of morbidity, or to premature death. Renal tuberculosis in children under 10 years of age is not common. Even in hospitals with large pediatric services, no case of renal tuberculosis may be found.

Pathologic Changes

Tuberculosis of the kidney must be considered a disease which arises from infection of the lungs or hilar lymph nodes. The infection is blood-borne equally to both kidneys, and seeding occurs simultaneously in both organs (Fig. 40-1). Medlar's careful work [6] has now been widely accepted and is the basis for this hemic dissemination theory. Serial secions of kidneys show miliary tubercles in both kidneys. These may be dormant for many years, then begin to spread and develop caseation and eventual cavitation. The factor that precipitates this change re-

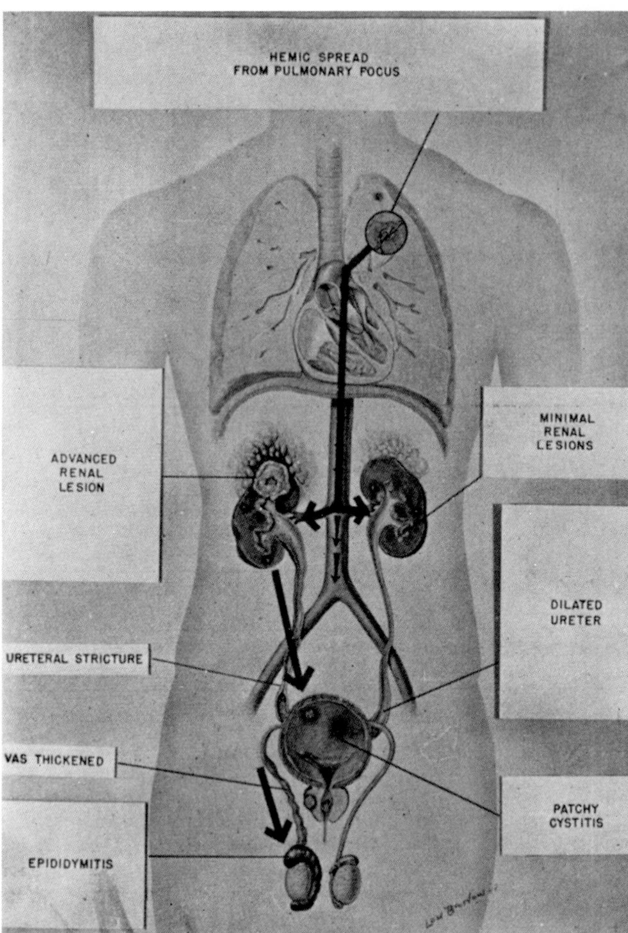

Figure 40-1. Pathogenesis of tuberculosis of the genitourinary tract.

mains obscure. One may speculate that it is host and tissue immunity, decreased resistance with age, or perhaps a reinfection.

The early lesion is a tubercle in the glomerulus. If healing occurs, organisms are contained and do not spill into the tubule. However, when healing does not occur and a sloughing renal lesion, however small, follows, then spillage occurs and *Mycobacterium tuberculosis* can be recovered in the urine. At this stage of the disease, there are no x-ray findings pathognomonic of the infection, and the urine may show only a few white blood cells (Fig. 40-2). It is not generally understood that patients with minimal renal tuberculosis do not have either a characteristic x-ray finding or, in fact, any x-ray evidence of disease. In this stage, the minimal, noncavitary lesion tends to heal spontaneously, but a few of these tiny lesions are likely to progress. It has been estimated that 25 per cent of a group of 5000 patients who died in Bellevue Hospital of pulmonary tuberculosis had these small tubercles in their kidneys [5].

About 4 per cent of the initial tubercles develop destructive tuberculosis. In the narrow loop of Henle, several tubercles coalesce, finally caseate and slough into a calyx. This now open cavity in the medullary area can be outlined by x-ray. It steadily enlarges, and the entire lobule or pyramid may be destroyed. The lesion may be compared with the open

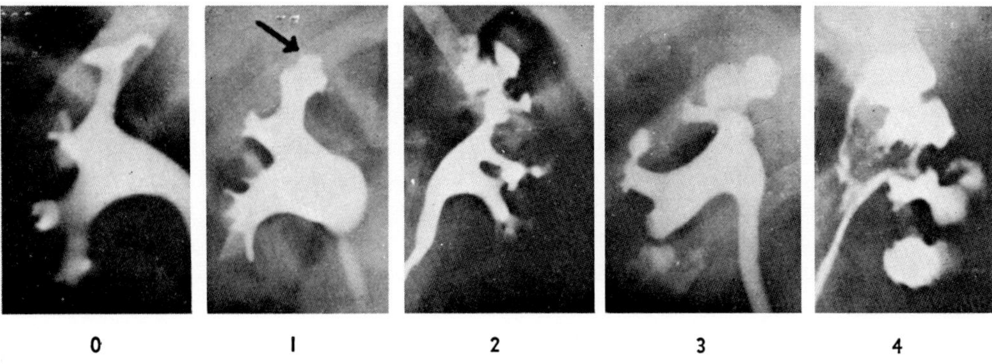

0	NO ROENTGEN ABNORMALITY VISIBLE BUT URETERAL URINE POSITIVE FOR TUBERCLE BACILLI	SMALL RENAL LESIONS	0
1	DEFINITE SLIGHT ROENTGEN ABNORMALITY, BUT NOT DIAGNOSTIC FOR TUBERCULOSIS, INCLUDES DOUBTFUL CALYCEAL DISTORTIONS, AND SLIGHT BUT DEFINITE IRREGULARITIES OF THE PELVIS OR UPPER URETER. URETERAL URINE POSITIVE FOR TUBERCLE BACILLI.	MEDIUM-SIZED RENAL LESIONS	1
2	ONE CALYX ONLY, WITH DEFINITE ROENTGEN CHANGES CHARACTERISTIC OF TUBERCULOSIS. URETERAL OR VOIDED URINE CULTURE POSITIVE.		2
3	TWO CALYCES SHOWING THE DISTORTIONS OF TUBERCULOSIS. URETERAL OR VOIDED URINE CULTURE POSITIVE.	LARGE RENAL LESIONS	3
4	THREE OR MORE CALYCES OBVIOUSLY TUBERCULOUS BY X-RAY. URETERAL OR VOIDED URINE CULTURE POSITIVE. MASSIVE PUTTY TYPE LESIONS IN THIS CATEGORY.		4

Figure 40-2. A roentgen classification of tuberculous kidney lesions. Group 0, without x-ray abnormality, represents a minimal lesion. Groups 1 and 2, with one cavity, are moderately advanced; and Groups 3 and 4, with two or more cavities, are far advanced.

cavity of pulmonary tuberculosis. Spontaneous healing of such a cavity is rare compared with the healing of the tubercles. The urine at this stage contains many white and red blood cells, in addition to *M. tuberculosis.* This lesion is termed the moderately advanced renal lesion.

When caseation is progressive, the disease may spread to involve the entire renal pelvis, and tuberculous granulations may cover all the calyces. If the caseous material is contained, a large mass forms which causes bulging against the renal capsule. If it calcifies, it will give a characteristic x-ray finding. If the caseous contents slough out, a large ragged cavity remains, and this too can be diagnostic on x-ray. When the walls of the cavity contract, indentations occur on the outer surfaces of the kidney, marking the site of the diseased pyramids. This indentation serves as a guidepost to the surgeon seeking to resect part of a kidney. When, roentgenologically, two or more cavities can be seen, advanced, destructive renal tuberculosis is present.

Diagnosis

The diagnosis is made by finding *M. tuberculosis* in the urine. This examination has undergone a change in the past decade. Most laboratories prefer to process the first morning specimen. Two reasons have been used to support this method: (1) the chance of contamination is less with a single morning specimen, as compared with the 24-hour urine; and (2) the belief of some microbiologists that the first voided urine yields higher positive cultures for *M. tuberculosis* than does the 24-hour urine. The latter is not necessarily valid, since the shower of organisms is intermittent and may occur at any hour of the day.

What is important is that a single negative finding is inconclusive. Specimens should be obtained for three days in succession, then repeated. Ideally twelve specimens should be secured. The guinea pig inoculation is also difficult to secure due to laboratory problems. I reserve this method now for use with the patient in whom the diagnosis is clinically suggestive but bacteriologically negative. Often this will be positive and help to clear a baffling case.

Symptoms

The earliest symptom in the child may be dysuria [3]. This is accompanied by mild, dull pain in the kidney region. Painless, gross hematuria is another important and fairly common occurrence. In adulthood [8] the symptoms of bladder distress and hematuria rank second to epididymitis, at least in the male. Thirty-six per cent of 127 male patients in whom renal tuberculosis was diagnosed presented themselves because of epididymitis. Twenty per cent suffered from bladder symptoms such as frequency, burning, and dysuria, while another 20 per cent first sought medical attention because of painless hematuria. Sixteen per cent of patients were investigated because pyuria had been found. In 10 per cent of the patients, no symptoms were present that required the patient to seek the aid of a doctor.

Treatment

SURGERY

Formerly it was believed and hoped that removal of a badly infected and destroyed kidney would prevent subsequent infection of the remaining kidney. With the knowledge that the infection is bilateral, removal of a kidney is no longer the treatment of choice. I have not found it necessary to remove a kidney in more than 17 years. Partial resection of the kidney [2] has also been used in the treatment of renal tuberculosis. When one pole of the kidney was found to be the only apparent source of involvement, partial resection of the kidney was offered, often with spectacular success (see Fig. 40-3). Renal tissue was preserved, and that basically is the best treatment for renal tuberculosis.

With the advent of chemotherapy, it is no

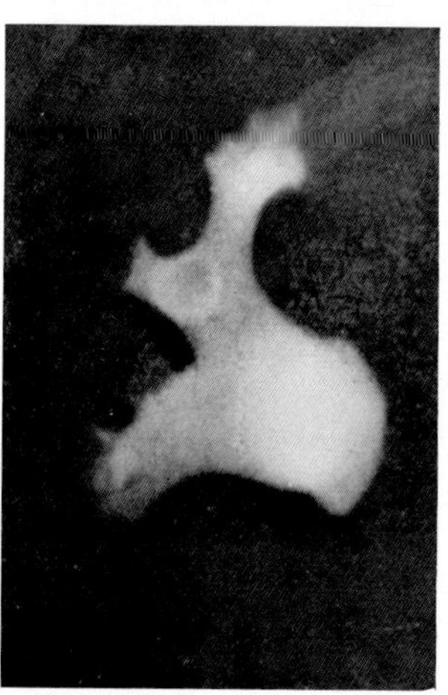

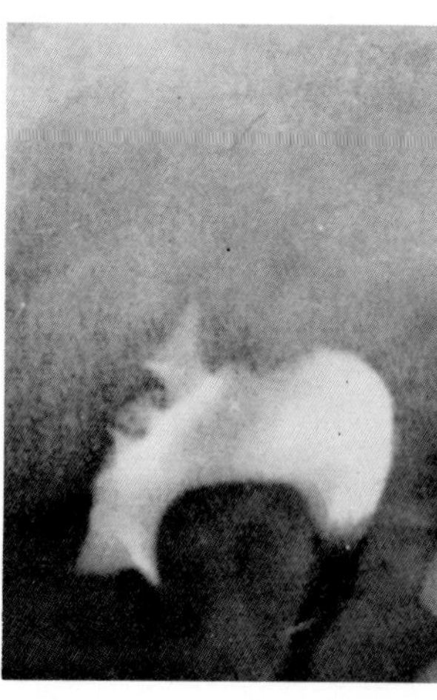

Figure 40-3. Tuberculous involvement of the upper pole of the kidney (left) treated by partial nephrectomy (right).

longer necessary to remove either part or all of a kidney. Results have been excellent and the preservation of renal tissue has been greater than with excisional surgery. Even in patients with an apparently destroyed kidney, I have deferred surgery. These patients can be observed at regular intervals, and if the infected kidney commences to produce systemic toxicity, it can be easily removed. My patients with one kidney so damaged that it possesses only a few functioning nephrons, have done well thus far for as long as 15 years. They have been spared a major surgical operation, have not developed hypertension, and have not shown any spread of the tuberculous infection [1].

It should be borne in mind that whenever the diagnosis of pyelonephritis is made, tuberculosis must be considered as a possible cause.

CHEMOTHERAPY

The pyelographic evidence in Figure 40-4 shows the destructive changes in untreated renal tuberculosis. Neither the surgeon nor the physician could offer the patient more than a faint hope of controlling the disease. In less than 20 years, chemotherapy changed a virtually hopeless situation to one compatible with a normal, productive life.

Streptomycin. Streptomycin was successfully used in the treatment of renal tuberculosis in 1947. When given in a daily dose of 1 gm. for 60 to 120 days, it halted the ravages of the infection and converted the urine to negative in a short time. This happy condition, however, did not persist. Within three to five years, almost 80 per cent of the patients had positive urines again. A serious complication was injury to the eighth nerve; fortunately it was often reversible. The vestibular impairment has been more common and more persistent than the auditory component. Dihydrostreptomycin was used in an attempt to avoid this damage, but not successfully, since the auditory loss with this drug was more frequent, sudden, and too often permanent. Combinations of the two drugs were no better. An audiogram should always be done be-

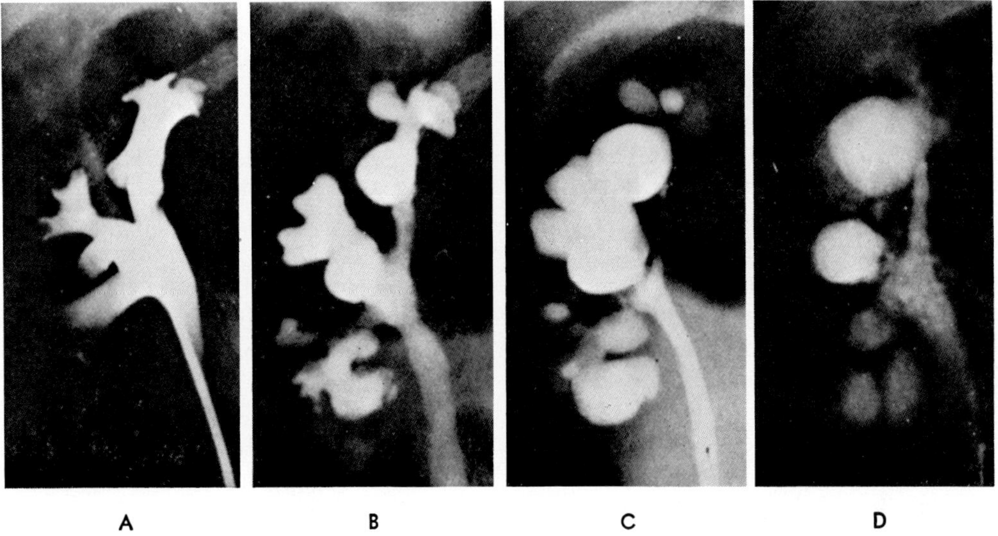

Figure 40-4. Progression of untreated renal tuberculosis. A. At time of diagnosis. Urine positive for tubercle bacilli. B. One and one-half years later. C. Three years after diagnosis. D. Three and one-half years after initial examination.

fore treatment with either drug is started, and at regular intervals thereafter.

Para-aminosalicylic Acid (PAS). It was soon noted that para-aminosalicylic acid was effective in the treatment of tuberculosis. When used alone, it is comparatively ineffective, but in combination with streptomycin or isoniazid, PAS enhances the antimicrobial effect of these drugs. Of greater importance is the additional finding that the likelihood of bacteria developing resistance to the drugs is diminished. PAS itself, like streptomycin, is a bacteriostatic agent. The major obstacle to its use is the gastrointestinal side effects, including nausea, vomiting, anorexia, diarrhea, and vague abdominal distress. The usual dose is 5 gm. of the sodium or potassium salt three times a day, preferably after meals. I have noted that when PAS is given to groups on a hospital ward, there seems to be less gastrointestinal disturbance than when it is taken alone at home. Group psychotherapy thus appears to play an important role in patient acceptance of PAS.

Isoniazid (INH). In 1952 isoniazid, although known for about 40 years, was introduced in the treatment of tuberculosis. It was soon found to be very effective, although bacteriostatic rather than bacteriocidal. Bacterial resistance often develops in two to four months. However, when INH is used in combination with other drugs, the development of resistance is markedly diminished and in renal tuberculosis is minimal. Little toxicity is seen with INH, and is usually limited to the central or peripheral nervous system, more often the latter. To forestall neuritis, a daily dose of pyridoxine, vitamin B_6, 50 to 100 mg., is added to the regimen and has proved very effective. The usual dose of INH is 100 mg. three times a day. I have seen no increased effectiveness from higher doses such as has been reported with pulmonary tuberculosis. Weekly urine examinations and blood urea determination at least once each month are helpful in guiding the physician as to dosage. INH is excreted in the urine, and if renal function is or becomes impaired, blood levels may become elevated to dangerous heights.

Cycloserine. In 1954 cycloserine (Seromycin) was found useful in the treatment of tuberculosis. It was first used in a daily dose of 1 gm., but many patients had toxic reactions referable to the central nervous system. Convulsive seizures, varying from petit mal to grand mal, and drowsiness and mental confusion were observed in at least 8 per cent of the patients. With reduction of the daily dose to 0.5 gm., these toxic manifestations were practically eliminated, and the therapeutic effect remained satisfactory. Excretion is through the kidney, and the drug is beneficial in the treatment of renal tuberculosis as a substitute for streptomycin. If blood levels are kept below 30 micrograms per 100 ml., patients do not exhibit alarming symptoms. A distinct advantage is that oral medication replaces an injection and therefore it is likely that treatment will be more faithfully followed.

Thiocarbanidin. Thiocarbanidin (Thioban) was introduced as another effective drug, given orally in a daily dose of 1 gm. Its use in renal tuberculosis has been discontinued because absorption from the intestinal tract is minimal. Until this drug can be better absorbed and excreted through the kidneys, its use in renal tuberculosis is of little value.

Kanamycin. Kanamycin (Kantrex) was added to the armamentarium when it was found to be useful against *M. tuberculosis.* The development of bacterial resistance has not been very great, but, as with streptomycin, eighth nerve disturbance has been a serious complication. When 1 gm. was injected daily, as at first, the frequency of deafness, usually irreversible, was high. It was soon noted that the high tones were lost first and later the low tones. When the dosage was changed to 1 gm. twice a week, the frequency of deafness dropped to a marked degree. As with other such drugs, audiometric studies should be done before, and regularly during treatment.

Fortunately, the high-tone loss, which occurs first and is not as disabling as the loss of low tones, serves as a warning. As with INH, urine examination and estimation of the blood urea nitrogen level are important guideposts in the use of this drug.

Ethionamide. Ethionamide, a derivative of nicotinic acid, has been found to be of value in the treatment of tuberculous patients. The dosage has varied from 0.5 to 1.0 gm. daily. This agent has not caused any serious effects to the present time, but some patients have reported gastrointestinal intolerance, which has not required special treatment, nor has therapy had to be discontinued.

Ethambutol. I have been using ethambutol (Myambutol) and am satisfied that it is useful in the treatment of genitourinary tuberculosis [4]. Its adverse effect on visual acuity must be considered. All patients should have a complete eye examination before treatment; this should include color perception and visual fields. During treatment, monthly eye tests with the Snellen chart will serve to delineate a loss in acuity in either eye. Further loss should be considered sufficient reason for discontinuing ethambutol. Loss of visual acuity has not occurred in a small series of patients. No other symptoms have been noted, and patient acceptance has been good.

Bed Rest. In general, treatment for renal tuberculosis [7] is best initiated in the hospital. Bed rest is not as essential as was once thought. However, patients do better at the height of their illness by preserving their strength. Perhaps, too, bed rest increases renal blood flow which promotes healing. The patients are allowed to get up for their meals, to use the bathroom, and to walk about for an hour twice a day. At the end of six months, if improvement has been satisfactory as evidenced by the general condition of the patient in addition to the normal temperature, pulse, sedimentation rate, and urinary findings, further freedom can be given. Treatment should then be continued at home for another six months so that the patient will receive a year's treatment with a maximum of rest. Actually the indigent person often receives the better treatment, since he is likely to be cared for in the hospital for a full year and frequently for the full course of two years.

Usually after one year of treatment the patient is well enough to return to work. If possible, there should not be an immediate change to full-time work from the hospital regimen. It is desirable at first to secure a half day's work, which can be lengthened in a few months to full time as rehabilitation appears secure. Treatment is continued during this second year, so that the patient receives two years of continuous therapy. If there is doubt that full recovery has been obtained, treatment may be given for another year and even for five years.

Drug Regimens. As noted previously, the use of a single drug in therapy was effective only temporarily, and patients relapsed in high numbers within three years. The use of two drugs has been more satisfactory, but the use of three drugs in the treatment of renal tuberculosis has been tested by time and found to give the best results, as will be seen from Figure 40-5. When the period is extended from one year to two years, results seem to be even better, but sufficient time has not elapsed

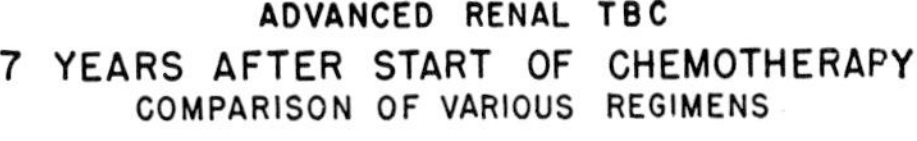

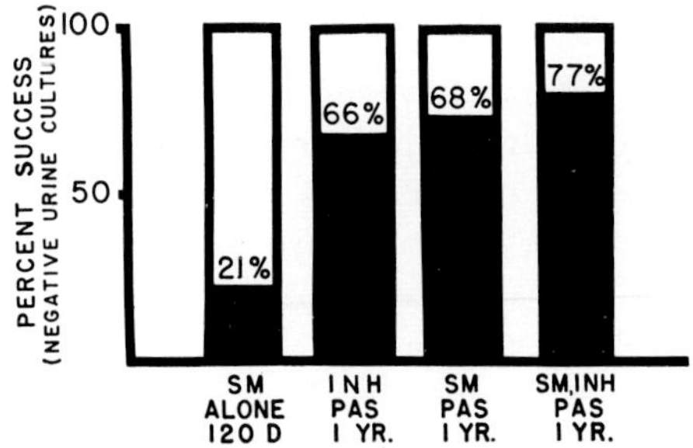

Figure 40-5. Results of various treatment regimens in renal tuberculosis. SM, streptomycin; INH, isoniazid; PAS, para-aminosalicylic acid.

for a proper evaluation. My clinical impression is that the increase in treatment time has been most salutary. The following regimen can be used safely and with assurance of good results:

INH: 100 mg. three times a day
PAS: 5 gm. three times a day
Streptomycin: 1 gm. injected twice a week
Pyridoxine: 50 mg. twice a day

If preferred, kanamycin can be substituted for the streptomycin. It should be injected deeply; otherwise some pain is noted.

Another regimen which has been found to be satisfactory, although not tested as long, is:

INH: 100 mg. three times a day
PAS: 5 gm. three times a day
Cycloserine: 250 mg. twice a day
Pyridoxine: 50 mg. twice a day

An advantage of this combination is that no injections are given; hence, the patient's acceptance is at its fullest and he can be trusted to take the medication at home. Appearance at the doctor's office can become a chore in time, and this regimen reduces the need for it.

Another regimen which has been tested for about ten years appears to be satisfactory with the follow-up studies. Only time will permit it to be properly evaluated. It consists of:

INH: 100 mg. three times a day
Cycloserine: 250 mg. twice a day
Ethionamide: 250 mg. three times a day
Pyridoxine: 50 mg. twice a day

With this regimen, no longer the latest in a continuing study of chemotherapy for renal tuberculosis, the conversion to a negative urine has been good. Patients have tolerated the treatment well, and toxicity has been low and thus far of no significance.

The newest regimen has been found to be satisfactory, with urine conversion and patient acceptance. I have no follow-up studies available. Treatment is entirely oral, all the medication being given at one time in the morning to obtain a high serum level. The dosage of ethambutol is given as 25 mg. per kilogram of body weight for two months and is then lowered to 15 mg. per kilogram for the balance of the two years. The tablet is supplied in 100 mg. and 400 mg. sizes which limits the number of tablets given to the patient.

INH: 300 mg. daily
Cycloserine: 0.5 gm. daily
Ethambutol: Dosage based on weight of patient, 25 mg. per kilogram for 60 days, then 15 mg. per kilogram to completion of therapy
Pyridoxine: 100 mg. daily

Treatment of renal tuberculosis can be carried out by any physician sympathetic with the care of a long-term patient. If he prefers, the physician can have the oral medication taken in one dose during the day. It may be shown soon that antituberculosis drugs may be at least as effective in a single high dose as in the time-honored regimen of divided dosage. During the course of chemotherapy, complete blood and urine studies as well as x-ray examinations should be made at four-month intervals for the first two years and yearly thereafter for another eight years. Since the course of tuberculosis is not known, the patient should be examined completely every two years after the tenth year, probably for the rest of his life. While this may appear to be exacting, it is better to find a lesion or reconversion of urine early than to have the patient report with a set of serious symptoms. Although the disappearance of tuberculosis has been forecast time and again, the eradication of this disease requires that one rid the patient of active disease and make follow-up examination a continuing process.

References

1. Bloom, S., Wechsler, H., and Lattimer, J. K. Results of long-term study of non-functioning tuberculous kidneys. *J. Urol.* 104:654, 1970.
2. Lattimer, J. K. Partial nephrectomy for tuberculosis. *Amer. Rev. Tuberc.* 66:744, 1952.
3. Lattimer, J. K., and Boyes, T. Renal tuberculosis in children. *Pediatrics* 22:1193, 1958.
4. Lattimer, J. K., and Wechsler, H. Current Trends in Renal Tuberculosis. Transactions of the 25th Research Conference in Pulmonary Disease, Jan. 23–27, 1966. Pp. 2–3.
5. Medlar, E. M. Cases of renal infection in pulmonary tuberculosis. Evidence of healed tuberculous lesions. *Amer. J. Path.* 2:401, 1926.
6. Medlar, E. M. The pathogenesis of minimal pulmonary tuberculosis. *Amer. Rev. Tuberc.* 58:583, 1948.
7. Wechsler, H., Lattimer, J. K., Garcia, M. A., and Kavookjian, H. Chemotherapy of renal tuberculosis. *New York J. Med.* 59:49, 1959.
8. Wechsler, H., Westfall, M., and Lattimer, J. K. The earliest signs and symptoms in 127 male patients with genitourinary tuberculosis. *J. Urol.* 83:801, 1960.

41

Tumors of the Kidney

J. Hartwell Harrison and Edward M. Mahoney

Renal tumors constitute a group of neoplasms that are difficult to detect and treat because of their anatomic location and their biologic characteristics. They imitate many trivial and serious illnesses and have justifiably been referred to as "the great imitator." The inaccessible location of the kidney, surrounded by a fibrous-fatty perinephric cushion, beneath the diaphragm, behind the peritoneum and its contained viscera, results in late recognition of this tumor. The growth of the tumor usually is slow as it expands in the renal parenchyma; often encapsulated, it characteristically metastasizes into the venous channels of the kidney, one of the most highly vascularized organs of the body [50]. Because of these characteristics, tumors of the kidney are late in producing symptoms, and signs are late in developing (Fig. 41-1). Until more specific diagnostic and screening tests become available, one must rely on detailed scrutiny of abnormal elements in the urine and upon careful evaluation of symptoms, physical examination, clinical pathology, and the several more refined radiographic technics available today.

Frequency

Cancer of the kidney comprises 2.8 per cent of all malignancies and ranks thirteenth in frequency of all carcinomas [9]. Renal cell carcinoma makes up 83 per cent of all renal cancers for all age groups [44]. The peak incidence occurs in the sixth decade [8]. In children malignant renal tumors may represent as high as 20 per cent of all malignancies, and are predominantly nephroblastomas [19]. In both children and adults, renal malignancies are consistently twice as common in males as in females. Race incidence is statistically significant only in that Negro males have a lower incidence than Caucasian males (Table 41-1). During the last 10 years there has been no significant statistical change in the death rate from carcinoma of the prostate, kidney, and bladder, in contrast to the lower frequency

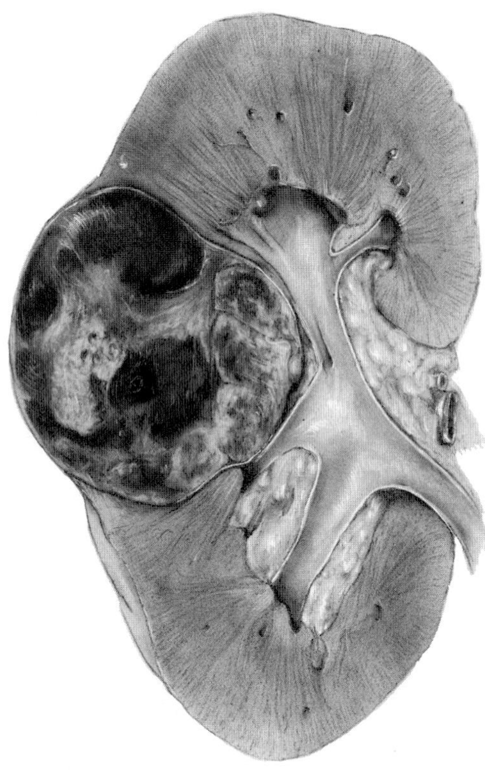

Figure 41-1. Sagittal section of right kidney bearing encapsulated renal cell carcinoma that shows early encroachment on the renal pelvis and expanding growth beyond the greater convexity of the kidney. This drawing by Barbara Clark of the specimen removed by W. C. Quinby in 1939 clearly shows why symptoms and signs are late in developing. Microscopic hematuria was the earliest local symptom in this case.

of each as recorded for 1940. Geography is not a factor in overall statistics, but might become so if information regarding type of renal tumor were available.

Etiologic factors in man remain obscure despite extensive animal studies. Heredity does not play a significant role except in Lindau-von Hippel disease. Viruses have not been implicated in man. No correlation with toxic agents is known with reference to parenchymatous tumors in contradistinction to transitional cell tumors which may be produced with certain hydrocarbons. Irradiation is implicated only in those few instances of patients with renal cell cancer where Thorotrast (a weak alpha-particle emitter) has been used for excretory urography years earlier. Except by animal implication, cigarette smoking is not correlated with renal cell cancer. There has been no direct evidence of cigarette smoking causing renal tumors in man; however, such tumors have occurred in rats after exposure to by-products of tobacco smoke such as the nitrosamine compounds [47, 84].

Pathology and Pathophysiology

BENIGN RENAL TUMORS

The frequency of benign renal tumors far exceeds that of malignant renal tumors in large randomly selected autopsy series [20]. Most of these benign neoplasms are small, subcapsular incidental findings of no clinical significance. Nonepithelial tumors of mesenchymal origin, the most common of which are fibromas, leiomyomas, and lipomas, have an incidence of 5 per cent or less and rarely are of clinical significance. Hemangiomas are small, cause intermittent hematuria, are difficult to diagnose, and often are found deep in the mucous membrane of the renal pelvis or parenchyma (Fig. 41-2).

Benign epithelial tumors occur more frequently than the neoplasms of mesenchymal origin. Small cortical adenomas, arising less often in small cysts and occurring more often in the older age groups, make up the majority of the benign epithelial tumors.

The nearly indistinguishable histologic pattern of a renal adenoma and well-differentiated renal cell carcinoma has led to the arbitrary classification of lesions measuring 3 cm. or less as benign adenomas. While lesions less than 3 cm. in diameter rarely produce metastases, Bell [8] has reported metastases from a tumor 1.5 cm. in diameter and the Peter Bent Brigham series includes two lesions 2.0 and 2.5 cm. with metastases.

Table 41-1. Death Rates from Genitourinary Malignant Neoplasms, Per 100,000 Population, by Age, Race, and Sex — United States, 1965[a]

Neoplasms	Ages: Under 25	25–44	45–64	65–84	85+	Total 1965	Total 1940
Prostate							
White	0	0.1	9.6	148.8	500.0	16.5	14.1
Nonwhite	0	0.3	26.8	241.7	382.9	18.7	8.2
Kidney							
White Male	0.3	0.8	8.1	22.4	17.8	3.9	2.4
Female	0.3	0.5	3.4	11.6	18.3	2.3	1.5
Nonwhite Male	0.3	1.2	5.6	15.3	4.9	2.2	1.0
Female	0.4	0.5	2.7	7.1	3.7	1.2	0.7
Bladder and other							
White Male	0	0.3	7.5	49.7	110.8	6.2	5.5
Female	0	0.1	2.4	17.7	58.7	2.8	2.8
Nonwhite Male	0	0.3	10.2	32.3	31.7	3.6	2.4
Female	0	0.3	6.0	20.3	25.9	2.4	1.5

[a] Provided by Dr. Jane Worcester, Professor of Biostatistics and Epidemiology, Harvard School of Public Health.

MALIGNANT TUMORS

Renal Cell Carcinoma. Renal cell carcinoma comprises 90 per cent of renal malignant tumors in the adult. This percentage in the literature corresponds with that in the Peter Bent Brigham Hospital [34a] series of 104 malignant renal tumors removed surgically or identified at autopsy, of which 84 were typical renal cell carcinomas. The term renal cell carcinoma is preferable to hypernephroma, Grawitz's tumor, or hypernephroid carcinoma, since the origin is of renal tubular epithelium rather than from aberrant adrenal tissue within the kidney. Electron microscopic studies demonstrate convincing similarities between tumor cells and those of the normal proximal convoluted tubule. Other clinical and pathologic observations supporting the renal tubular origin are: (1) the infrequency of aberrant adrenal tissue within the kidney in comparison with the incidence of renal cell carcinoma; (2) the fact that tumors of the adrenal cortex are often benign; (3) neoplastic changes in adrenal rests are extremely rare; and (4) adrenal neoplasms produce hormonal disturbances that are not seen in patients with renal cell carcinoma.

The small renal adenoma found incidentally at autopsy without metastases is ordinarily indistinguishable microscopically from a well-differentiated renal cell carcinoma. The arbitrary classification of lesions measuring 3 cm. or less in diameter as benign adenoma can be hazardous, as previously referred to in Bell's report and as observed in the Peter Bent Brigham series. The rare demonstration of metastatic spread from a small renal cell carcinoma has led to the concept that the so-called "adenoma" is a small renal carcinoma, which may metastasize upon attaining a larger size. The relatively slow rate of growth of most renal cell carcinomas is recognized, and does influence the clinical management of patients suffering from this cancer. One such patient with a 10 cm., slowly enlarging, nonmetastasizing renal lesion was observed for 10 years before her systemic disease allowed operation and removal of a typical renal cell carcinoma. The

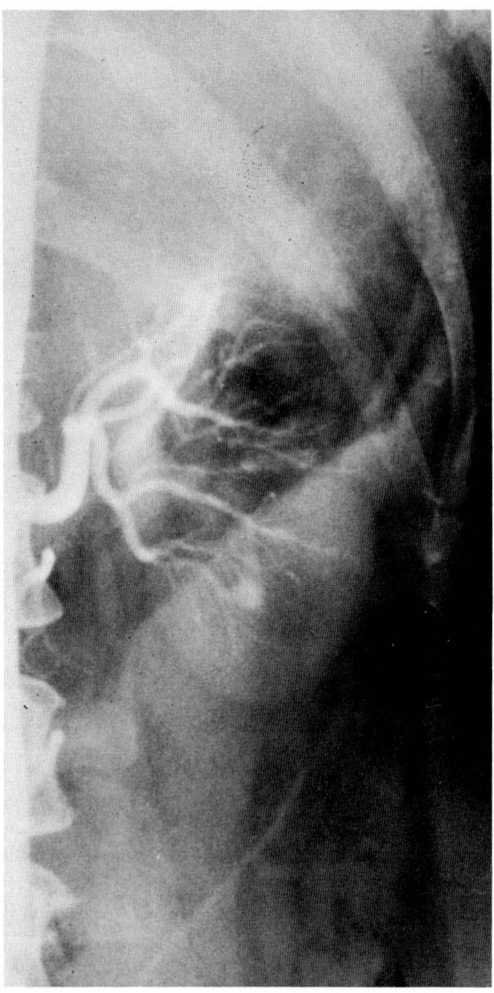

Figure 41-2. Selective renal angiogram with epinephrine added to the contrast media reveals a cluster of noncontracting arteriovenous shunts beneath the mucous membrane of a calyx in the lower pole of the kidney. Resection by partial nephrectomy cured this 43-year-old woman of recurrent gross hematuria of 4 years' duration. (Courtesy of Dr. Richard Basch.)

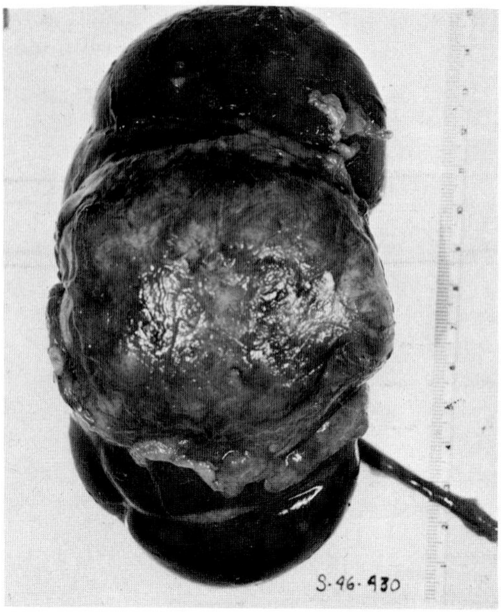

Figure 41-3. Renal cell carcinoma arising in the midportion of the renal parenchyma. It has grown through its own capsule and that of the kidney.

great majority of these neoplasms are basically encapsulated, adenomatous in nature, and on cut surface are bright yellow or orange and show areas of necrosis. In the Peter Bent Brigham series [20], the right and left kidneys were involved with equal frequency. In some series, as high as 50 per cent were found to have a microscopically perforated but grossly intact capsule (Fig. 41-3). They tend to grow around and into venous channels. Renal vein involvement is a common feature of larger tumors, affording direct access to the bloodstream for hematogenous spread and embolization. Centrifugal growth results in direct invasion of the perinephrium and surrounding viscera, particularly the colon. The lymphogenous spread is of clinical significance and is chiefly to the regional nodes. Proximity of the lateral aortic nodes to the cisterna chyli allows malignant cells access to the thoracic duct, superior vena cava, and lungs.

The predominant cell types in renal cell carcinoma are the clear cell, containing lipid and glycogen, and the granular cell. They are arranged in cords or clusters forming tubular or papillary patterns. The typical lesion has inconspicuous fibrous stroma but is richly vascular. In the Peter Bent Brigham series, 80 per cent of the tumors were composed of clear cells, or combinations of clear and granular cells. Only 19 neoplasms were of the pure granular cell type. While Dick and Flint [22] found histologic grading of no help in assessing prognosis, Riches [65] considers grading to be of major significance. It is our conviction that it is important to observe and describe the degree of histologic differentiation in trying to anticipate the prognosis.

Most of the tumors for which the patient seeks medical care are over 5 cm. in diameter. At operation more than 55 per cent [50] have already invaded veins. This does not mean, however, that distant metastases have already occurred. Metastases have been documented by Bennington and Kradjian [9] in 523 cases, thus: lung, 55 per cent; lymph nodes, 33 per cent; liver, 33 per cent; bone, 32 per cent; adrenal, 19 per cent; opposite kidney, 11 per cent; brain, 5 per cent; and heart, 5 per cent. Infrequently, a tumor reaches 10 to 20 cm. in breadth without invading or metastasizing.

Nephroblastoma or Wilms's Tumor. The nephroblastoma (Wilms's tumor) is the most common tumor of the urinary tract in children, and occurs in both the fetus and the newborn infant. While primarily a neoplasm of childhood, nephroblastoma has been reported in every decade, including one octagenarian [39]. It occurs equally often in either sex. There is no predilection to either right or left kidney, and it is bilateral in 2 to 5 per cent of cases. Of 189 cases reviewed by Riches [64], 50 per cent occurred between two and four years of age. In a collected series of 856 cases, Abeshouse [2] found the average age of onset to be 3.2 years.

Nephroblastoma is considered to originate from embryonic nephrogenic tissue (the metanephrogenic blastema) and develops during fetal life. A genetic etiologic influence is implicated by reports of occurrence in a family and in identical twins [29, 48].

Although the nephroblastoma when small is encapsulated, its invasive biologic potential is such that it may break through the capsule with minor trauma or injudicious palpation and spread directly to contiguous structures. These tumors are usually large, weighing from 200 to 4000 gm., grayish-white in color grossly, and usually feel solid to palpation unless hemorrhage or cystic degenerative changes have taken place. On section, nephroblastomas have a solid white, pinkish-white, or grayish-yellow surface. Histologic examination reveals both epithelial and mesodermal elements. The epithelial elements may be undifferentiated or, on occasion, acinar or tubular in structure. Mesodermal structures may include smooth and striated muscle, connective tissue, bone, and cartilage, but calcification in this tumor is rare. The prognosis cannot be correlated with the histologic type or character of the tumor. However, local recurrence may be anticipated if the capsule has been broken before or during surgery.

While most of the patients, 50 to 60 per cent, present with an incidentally discovered abdominal mass without symptoms, a remaining 30 per cent have variable pain, presumably due to capsular invasion or traction on the renal pedicle. Lattimer et al. [43], in a review of 285 children with abdominal masses, found half of these to be of renal origin and 30 per cent resulted from Wilms's tumor. Hematuria occurs in 5 to 10 per cent of cases and suggests invasion of the renal pelvis or major renal vein thrombosis; in Riches' [64] series hematuria constituted a bad prognostic sign.

The differential diagnosis lies most commonly between neuroblastoma, hydronephrosis, and renal cyst. The diagnosis of neuroblastoma is facilitated by its characteristic calcification demonstrated by x-ray study and an increased urinary excretion of vanillylmandelic acid and homovanillylmandelic acid. Radiologic examination will demonstrate the neuroblastoma to be extrinsic to the kidney, while the Wilms's tumor will usually alter the internal architecture of the kidney, and more commonly shows nonvisualization by excretory urography. In the pediatric age group, enlargement of the kidney is most commonly due to hydronephrosis secondary to congenital obstruction. Duplication of the kidney with hydronephrosis of one segment may also cause enlargement without visualization by excretory urography. In the newborn infant, renal enlargement with failure to excrete dye is most frequently due to multicystic disease of the kidney.

Metastatic characteristics are helpful in differentiating Wilms's tumor from neuroblastoma. While both spread to liver, neuroblastoma metastases have a predilection for bone, and Wilms's tumor for lung. Osseous metastases are very rare with Wilms's tumor [38]. Pulmonary metastatic disease is the cause of death in nearly all children with Wilms's tumor.

Tumors of Renal Pelvis and Ureter. Malignant tumors of the renal pelvis and ureter comprise between 14 per cent [40] and 30 per cent [66] of all renal tumors. Most of these tumors are of epithelial origin and are divided into transitional cell papilloma, transitional cell carcinoma, squamous or epidermoid carcinoma, and adenocarcinoma. The transitional cell neoplasms tend to be papillary and make up 75 per cent of the tumors, while the squamous cell is solid, plaque-like, and often ulcerated. They may spread by direct extension as well as by lymphatic and hematogenous routes. They have a particular tendency to be associated with similar lesions elsewhere in the urothelium, giving the appearance of multicentric foci. Twenty-five per cent of patients with renal pelvic tumors were reported by Culp [21] to have also similar ureteral tumors. These characteristics have significant bearing on the management of these neoplasms. Perhaps the entire urinary tract epithelium has the potential of producing these tumors when exposed to urine-borne carcinogens such as the toxic aminophenols [41] found in urine of heavy cigarette smokers. Squamous cell carcinomas are associated with specific factors causing metaplasia and clinically, in several series, are found concurrently with renal calculi in 50 per cent of cases. These tumors tend to outgrow their blood supply, superficial necrosis, ulceration, and bleeding being the result. They may arise as simple papillomas which progress to papillary carcinomas and invasive transitional cell carcinomas. When they are primary in the ureter, obstruction may be the first pathologic event, but more frequently it is hematuria.

Mesothelial Tumors. The mesothelial tumors are sarcoma, leiomyosarcoma, and neuroblastoma; they are quite malignant. In a series of 100 consecutive neoplasms surgically treated at the Peter Bent Brigham Hospital one each of the following of mesothelial origin were found: embryonal carcinoma, fibrosarcoma, spindle cell sarcoma, leiomyoliposarcoma, carcinoma of the adrenal cortex, and carcinosarcoma. Eighty per cent of neuroblastomas occur in children under three years of age and carried a grave prognosis prior to the use of x-ray, surgery, and chemotherapy which resulted in marked improvement [83].

Diagnosis

SYMPTOMS

Renal neoplasms, particularly renal cell carcinoma, may present confusing systemic symptoms for long periods before the tumor is detected. The classic triad of hematuria, pain, and a palpable mass is absent in between 32 and 86 per cent of varying reported series of patients with proved renal carcinoma. Approximately 47 per cent of patients presenting with the triad will have metastases at that time. Thirty per cent will have nonurologic signs and symptoms only.

Hematuria. Hematuria, usually painless, is the most common and most important sign. It occurs in between 50 and 75 per cent of cases, and is unfortunately a late event suggesting invasion of the vascular or collecting

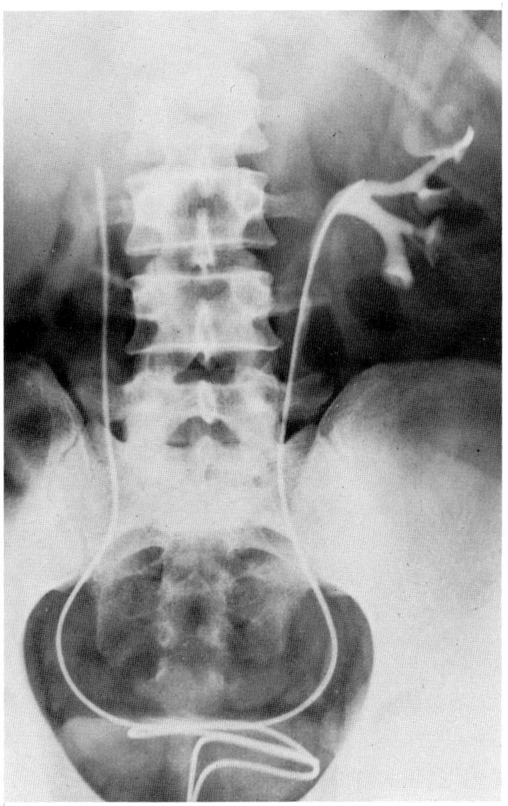

Figure 41-4. Left retrograde pyelogram showing an expansile lesion of the upper calyx which also enlarges the upper pole of the kidney. Painless hematuria was the initial event, and neoplastic cells were found in urine collected from the left renal pelvis by ureteral catheter.

system (Figs. 41-4, 41-5). In 80 patients with renal cell carcinoma reviewed by Crocker from the Peter Bent Brigham Hospital [20], 36 presented with gross hematuria, and of these pathologic examination of the renal tumor revealed 50 per cent of the tumors involved the renal pelvis, and all demonstrated microscopic or gross blood-vessel invasion. In an earlier series [45a] of 100 cases from the same hospital, hematuria occurred in 76 patients. This lower frequency of hematuria, a late sign, may suggest earlier detection of renal neoplasms in the more recent series. The neoplasms of the renal pelvis tend to bleed earlier, and consequently may be discovered in time for surgical cure even though there are multiple foci in pelvis, ureter, and bladder.

Hematuria was typically painless and transitory in an otherwise healthy person, and often preceded other symptoms by months or even years. At times it was accompanied by ureteral colic due to passage of clots and, for this reason, simulated a ureteral calculus. Occasionally hemorrhage was so severe as to cause total retention of urine owing to a blood clot in the bladder.

Pain. Flank pain occurred in 31 of 81 patients with renal cell carcinoma, and was the initial symptom in 14 [20]. The pain was more frequently continuous and of an aching character, but in some was severe and intermittent. Primary pain of renal neoplasm is produced by distention of the renal capsule, obstruction of the ureteropelvic junction with resulting hydronephrosis, and local extension to involve contiguous structures (Fig. 41-6). Capsular invasion was found by pathologic examination in 14 of 33 patients with symptoms of pain. Passage of blood clot through the ureter and obstruction of the vesical neck by blood clot in the bladder may result in renal colic and acute urinary retention.

Secondary pain is produced by metastases and may be completely disabling, particularly when located in the paravertebral areas encroaching on nerves, or when involving bone. The accompanying features of the metastatic lesions such as weight loss, fever, anemia, anorexia, constipation, nausea, vomiting, dehydration, indigestion, easy fatigability, malaise, and weakness are more common than pain.

Reflex Gastrointestinal Disturbances. Reflex disturbances of the gastrointestinal tract, particularly nausea and vomiting, were the chief complaint in 3 per cent, and occurred in 18 per cent leading to initial treatment on the Medical Service [20]. Two patients had undergone removal of a normal appendix some months before.

Palpable Mass. The presence of an ab-

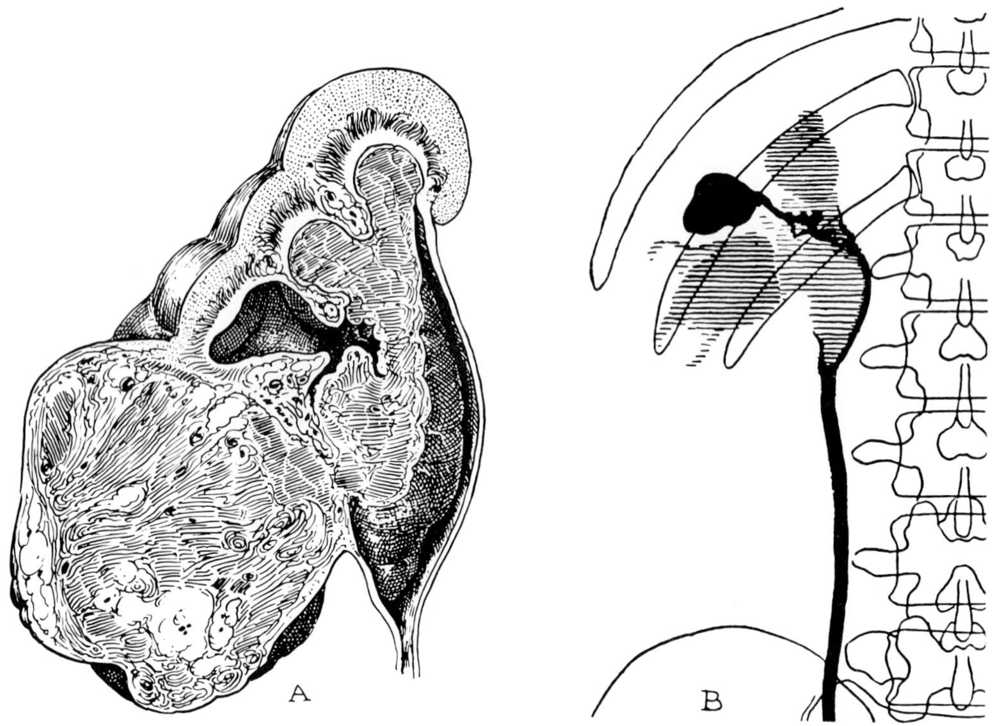

Figure 41-5. A. Drawing of renal cell carcinoma with direct invasion of vasculature and mucous membrane of the calyces and pelvis, demonstrating the mechanism of hematuria. B. Drawing of urogram demonstrating the corresponding radiologic findings in invasion of renal collecting system. (Courtesy of the late Dr. John Homans.)

dominal mass was discovered by the patient and constituted a primary complaint in 7 per cent of cases. In the two Peter Bent Brigham Hospital series [20, 34a] a renal mass was palpable in 60 per cent and 50 per cent of the patients, respectively. In addition to size per se of the neoplasm, other factors such as whether the patient is slender in which case a ptotic or lower renal pole is easily palpable or whether the patient is obese with increased anteroposterior diameter has considerable bearing on the incidence or discovery of this sign. Large lesions may be asymptomatic and difficult to palpate, but generally indicate an advanced lesion. In the second series [20] 14 patients with a palpable mass noted flank pain, while 25 did not. Tumors weighing 400 gm. or more were palpable in 21 of 27 cases, whereas of those weighing less than 400 gm. only 10 of 38 were noted on physical examination.

Fever. Fever of unknown origin occurs with a sufficient frequency to constitute an important symptom of renal cell carcinoma. Most series show an incidence of 10 to 20 per cent

Figure 41-6. A. Retrograde pyelogram performed because of left-sided flank pain, hematuria, and a palpable mass in the left side. B. Gross specimen of tumor of left kidney that is well encapsulated and growing in the lower half of the organ. C. The tumor on section shows extensive invasion of the remaining pelvis, parenchyma, and veins of the kidney as well as severe necrosis and hemorrhage produced by the growth of the tumor exceeding its blood supply.

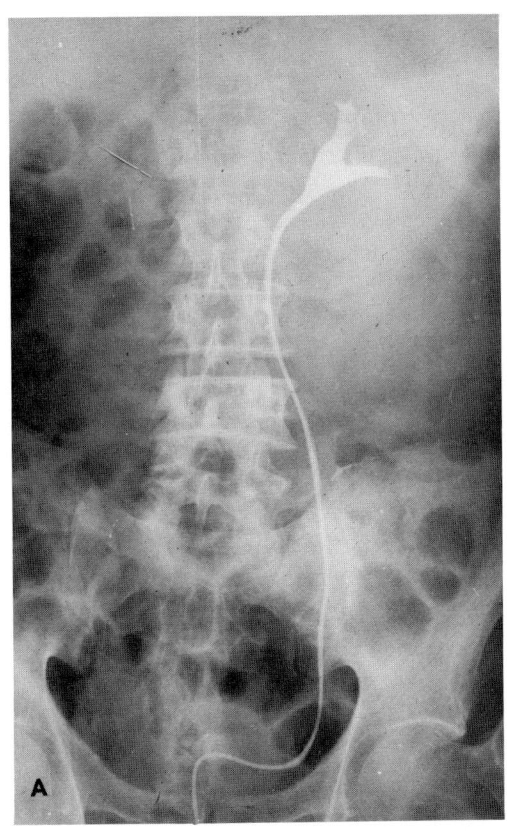
A

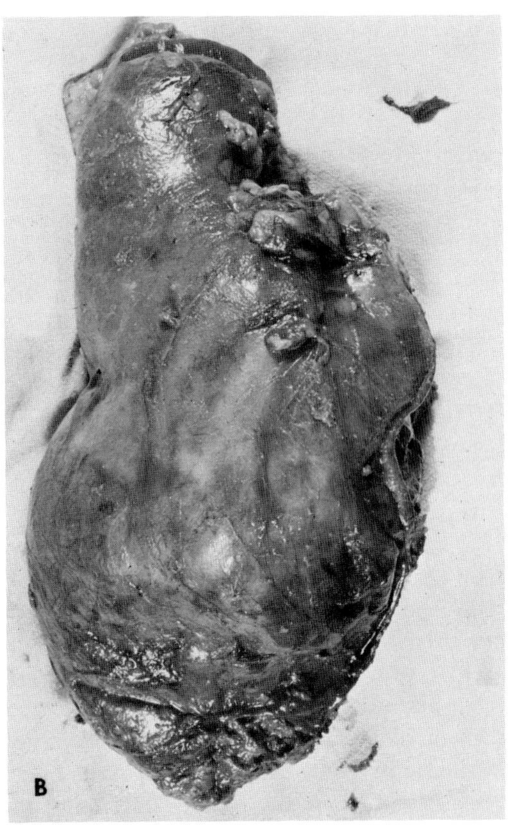
B

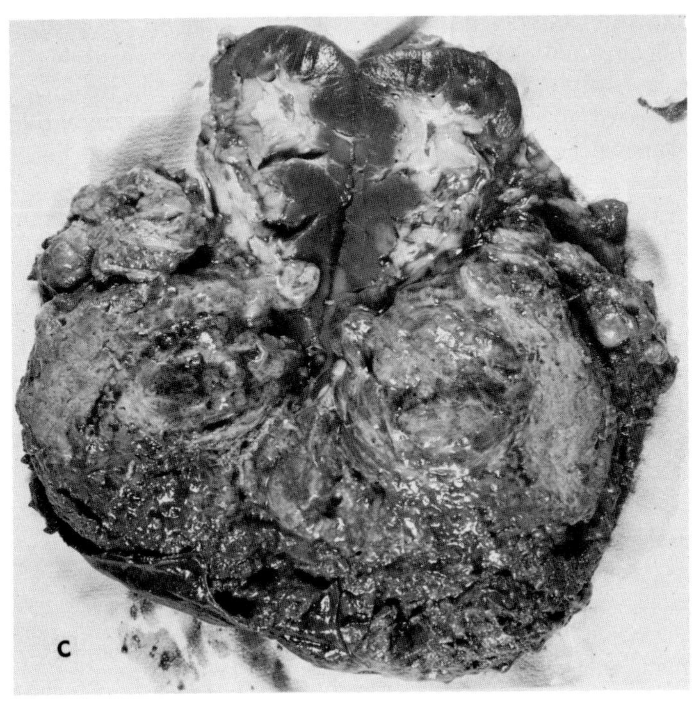
C

of cases. Of Bottiger's [12] 136 patients, 41 per cent had fever, and in 12 per cent, it was the presenting complaint. The fever is ordinarily low grade but has been reported as high as 105°F. It is usually accompanied by normocytic anemia, leukocytosis, and a rapid erythrocyte sedimentation rate. With removal of the offending kidney, the fever usually disappears.

PHYSICAL SIGNS

Hypertension of moderate to severe degree has been described in significant numbers of patients in several series. Morlock and Horton [52] noted hypertension in 144 of 335 patients with renal cell carcinoma; 18 became normotensive after removal of the neoplasm. Roberts [69], in 1961, and Luke et al. [45], in 1965, each reported a case of hypertension due to renal artery compression by tumor with return of blood pressure to normal following nephrectomy. Two exactly similar cases have been described in the Peter Bent Brigham Hospital series [20].

Hepatic vein obstruction, with physical findings of hepatomegaly and ascites, was caused by renal carcinoma in 9 of 49 patients reported by Parker et al. [60]. Vena caval obstruction may be suspected when an abdominal bruit, ascites, edema of the lower extremities and scrotum, and dilated abdominal veins are present. In such cases, it has been recommended that venography be used for assessment of neoplastic extension.

The appearance of a left varicocele of fairly acute onset which does not empty with recumbency may indicate the presence of a renal neoplasm. The frequency of occurrence with renal neoplasm in Graham's [33] series of 195 cases was 3 per cent.

Weight loss with characteristic findings is not uncommon. Graham has documented a frequency of 29 per cent in patients with renal cell carcinoma.

The neurologic findings of Lindau–von Hippel disease, hemangioblastoma of cerebellum or medulla oblongata, should suggest the presence of the frequently associated renal cell carcinoma. Another rare finding is priapism of which there have been 12 recorded instances, each due to metastasis to the spinal cord or penis.

The only characteristic physical sign of a renal tumor is a palpable mass that is movable but not tender. There is no muscle spasm unless perinephric hemorrhage has occurred. This is in contrast to the perinephric abscess, which is fixed and tender. The conditions to be considered in the differential diagnosis of a palpable mass in the retroperitoneum are tumor of the kidney, hydronephrosis, pyonephrosis, cortical or perinephric abscess, solitary or multiple cysts, neoplasm of the adrenal glands or tail of the pancreas, and neuroblastoma.

Cystadenoma or neoplasm of the tail of the pancreas have become involved with the upper pole or medial aspect of the left kidney in several instances, creating a problem in differential diagnosis. Various retroperitoneal tumors arising in the perinephrium, such as fibroma, lipoma, neurofibroma, retroperitoneal cysts, lymphosarcoma, paraganglioma, and tumors of the genital ridge, may displace both kidney and ureter (Fig. 41-7). They may cause ureteral obstruction and hydronephrosis, and metastases from small tumors of the testes to the retroperitoneum may present primarily as a lesion of the latter area. Tumors of the genital ridge may arise anywhere in the retroperitoneal space from the testis to the diaphragm. Adrenal cortical neoplasms and pheochromocytomas may present as large masses and be differentiated by clinical laboratory assessment of their hormonal secretion. However, large pheochromocytomas are on occasion nonsecreting. Nesbit [53] has emphasized that palpable tumors of the left kidney have frequently been described as having a notch and thus may be incorrectly interpreted as splenomegaly.

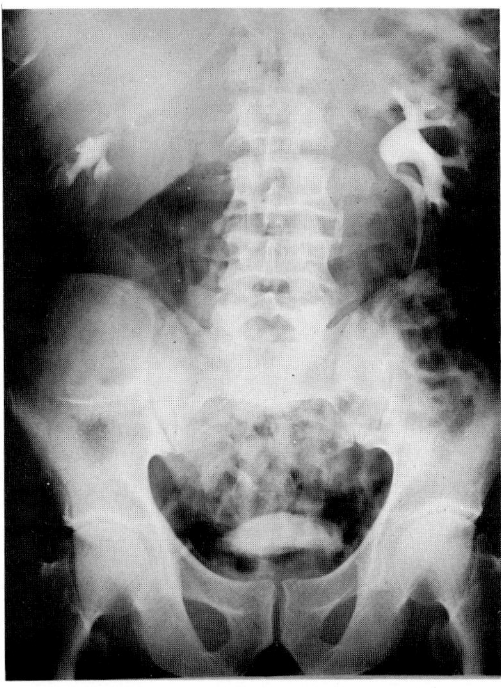

Figure 41-7. Excretory urogram showing displacement of the right kidney laterally by tumor of the kidney and metastasis in the left retroperitoneal area displacing the left ureter laterally in a manner similar to the displacement caused by genital ridge, testicular metastases, and retroperitoneal neoplasms.

LABORATORY FINDINGS

While no single laboratory test is sufficiently specific or accurate to establish, or to rule out, the diagnosis of renal tumor, taken together they are invaluable in developing a clinical impression. Hematuria, gross or microscopic, as already discussed, is the common presenting manifestation of a renal tumor. The urinary sediment, however, may demonstrate pyuria when concurrent infection is present.

Cytology. The urinary sediment, when stained with toluidine blue or polychrome methylene blue and eosin, affords easy and rapid identification of malignant tumor cells in the cystoscopic laboratory. The Papanicolaou technic [26, 27, 35] is nearly alway positive in patients with tumors of the renal pelvis. Less accuracy is found in renal cell carcinoma unless invasion of the renal collecting system has taken place, thus allowing shedding of neoplastic cells into the urine (see Fig. 41-5). Concurrent infection, hematuria, and degenerative changes present a diagnostic challenge to the cytologist. However, a positive cytologic examination demands explanation (Fig. 41-8), and in a recent case, recurring hematuria and positive cytology only, with negative pyelography and selective angiography, led to successful removal of a pelvic tumor by nephrectomy. Gross inspection and frozen sections of the removed kidney defied diagnosis, and only permanent microscopic studies demonstrated the grade 2 calyceal and pelvic neoplasm.

Erythrocytosis. Polycythemia, first described in 1929 [10, 28] in patients with renal cell carcinoma, has been calculated by various authors to have an incidence of between 1.8 and 6.0 per cent [9]. The absence of splenomegaly, thrombocytosis, and leukocytosis, and the presence of an elevated sedimentation rate distinguish this erythrocytosis from polycythemia vera. Elaboration of erythropoietin by tumor cells [80] has been well established, but venous stasis caused by a large tumor may be a contributory factor. Investigation of all patients with above-normal hematocrits has and will lead to earlier diagnosis.

Anemia. While polycythemia has captured medical interest, normochromic normocytic anemia is far more common, with an incidence demonstrated by Clarke and Goade [18] of 25 per cent in renal carcinoma. The anemia is not related to blood loss from the kidney in most instances. Pennington [61] believes that the anemia is caused by toxic depression of bone marrow and inadequate stimulation of bone marrow.

Leukocytosis. This is not a common finding but has been reported by Hensler [36] and Reiss [63] to exist on occasion to an extreme degree.

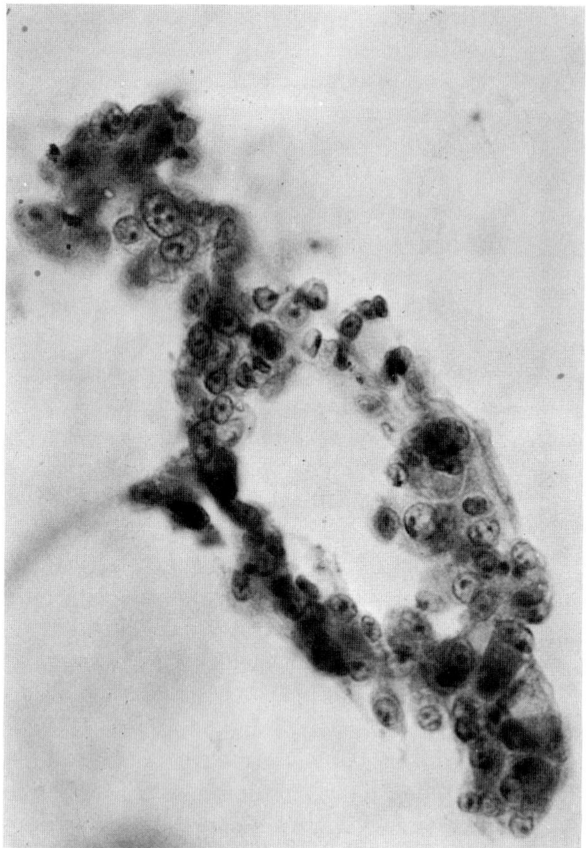

Figure 41-8. Papanicolaou stain showing mitotic figures from the urinary sediment of a patient with papillary carcinoma.

Hypercalcemia. In patients with renal cell carcinoma hypercalcemia occurs relatively frequently and on occasion has been rapidly progressive or fatal. The elevation of blood calcium in the absence of osseous lesions, coupled with a low serum phosphorus, and the demonstration by Goldberg et al. [31] of tumor antigen, similar to parathyroid hormone, have suggested tumor production of hormone as the probable mechanism. Both serum calcium and phosphorus have returned to normal after removal of the offending neoplasm.

Erythrocyte Sedimentation Rate. This simple laboratory test has been found elevated by Olovson [57] in two-thirds of a series of 109 patients with renal carcinoma and in 81 per cent of patients reported by Ochsner [55]. This often neglected simple determination is one of the most constant tests to be abnormal.

Serum Alkaline Phosphatase and C-reactive Protein. Elevation of the serum alkaline phosphatase may occur in the absence of liver disease, with return to normal levels after removal of the neoplasm. Determinations of the C-reactive protein are measurements of the reaction of the capsule of pneumococci to serum of patients with tumor. Their value as a means of differentiating cyst from tumor has been limited by a frequency of over 10 per cent false-negative results [51].

Urinary Lactic Dehydrogenase and Alkaline Phosphatase. Elevations of urinary LDH enzyme activity are found in patients with urinary tract malignancy of any type or location [81]. Urinary alkaline phosphatase is above normal in patients with malignancy of the kidney, but generally it is not elevated in patients with lower urinary tract neoplasm. Active glomerulonephritis, acute tubular necrosis, diabetic nephrosclerosis, systemic lupus erythematosus, pyuria of any origin, and renal infarction all cause the urinary LDH activity to rise. Use of these tests must therefore be for broad screening of renal disease and, in the case of the individual patient, adjunctive to the other criteria for diagnosis of renal neoplasm.

RADIOLOGIC EXAMINATION

Plain film of the abdomen, excretory urography, cystoscopic examination with ureteral catheterization, and retrograde pyelography are invaluable screening and diagnostic technics which lead to the accurate localization of pathologic lesions in the kidney in practically all cases. However, during the past 10 years new and modified radiologic technics, such as nephrotomography and selective renal angiography, have brought about an accuracy of identification of pathology of 95 to 100 per cent. This has been particularly true in differentiating renal cyst from renal neoplasm (Figs. 41-9, 41-10). In utilizing these technics one progresses logically from the simpler and less complicated to the more complex and delicate as is necessary according to the individual demands of each patient.

Plain Film. In a film of good technical quality the plain film of the abdomen will reveal location, size, contour, and whether or not there are two kidneys. Calcification in renal space-occupying lesions will be visible. Austen [4] demonstrated calcification in 16 per cent of renal carcinomas, while Phillips, Chin, and Palubinskas [62a] reported calcification in only 7 per cent. Other series, on the other hand, reported a 3 per cent incidence of calcification in benign cysts. Thus calcification in a space-occupying lesion increases the probability of neoplasm but does not exclude the possibility of a benign lesion. The pathologic physiology of this phenomenon was described by MacCallum [46] and attributed to a propensity to calcium deposition from healthy tissues in contact with the periphery of ischemic or necrotic areas.

Excretory Urography. This technic will ordinarily demonstrate a renal space-occupying lesion with considerable accuracy (Fig. 41-11). Correlation of such findings with the source of bleeding as demonstrated by cystoscopic observation and by sampling of urine from each renal pelvis by ureteral catheterization is of obvious importance. The usual contraindications of sensitivity to contrast media may be always circumvented by premedication with antihistaminics and cortisone, and by an anesthetist in attendance. Increased dosage of administered contrast media will often result in satisfactory urograms despite moderate degrees of azotemia, unless failure to excrete is caused by arterial occlusion, spasm, or interruption (Fig. 41-12).

Retrograde Pyelography. Retrograde pyelography provides detailed radiologic visualization of the architecture of the renal collecting system, particularly when accompanied by fluoroscopy and spot films. The problems of contrast-media sensitivity and failure to excrete in presence of azotemia found in excretory urography are easily solved by ureteral catheterization, function studies, and retrograde pyelography. Cystoscopic examination should be performed whenever necessary but only under ideal aseptic conditions such as are found in the operating room environment. Even the sickest patient can easily tolerate ureteral catheterization under local instillation anesthesia.

Nephrotomography. This technic is essentially high-dosage excretory urography combined with body-section roentgenography (tomography). During the nephrographic phase, characterized by parenchymatous opacification, cysts appear radiolucent and thin walled (Fig. 41-13). Southwood and Marshall [75] and Chynn and Evans [17]

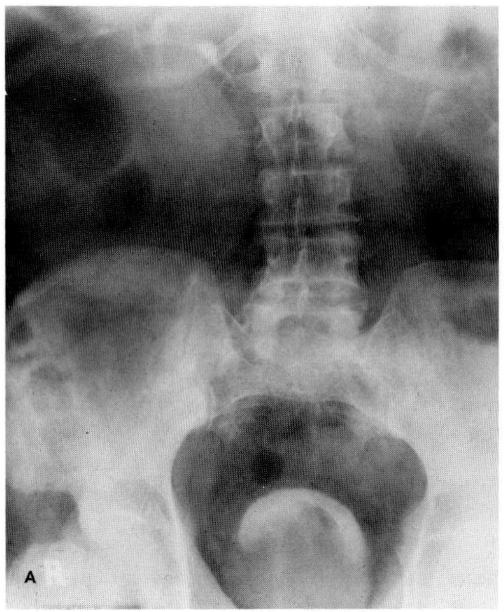

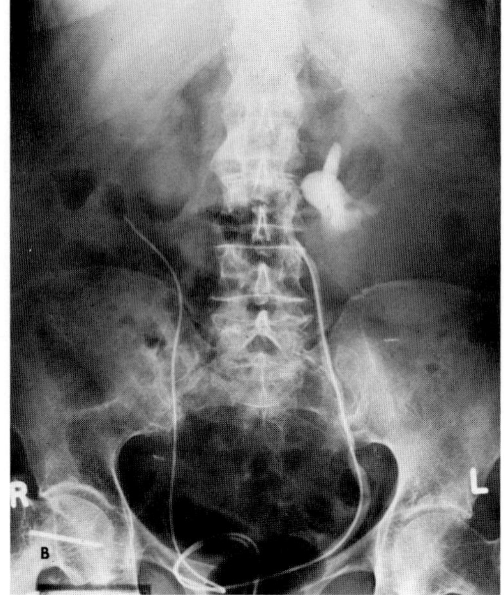

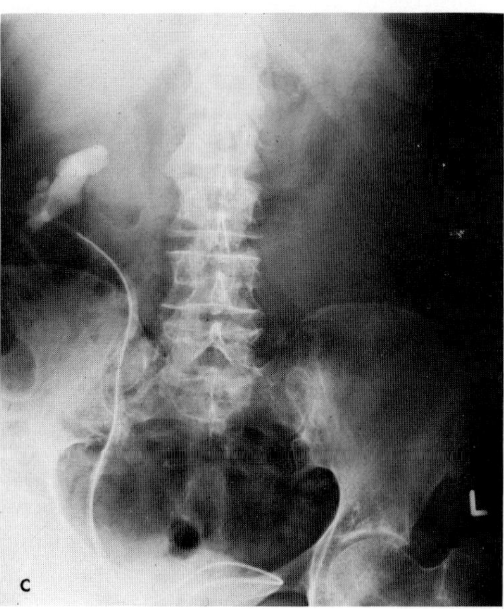

Figure 41-9. A. Excretory urogram in a 60-year-old man showing a large rounded shadow below the right kidney with spreading of the renal pelvis. The left renal pelvis is normal, and there is the filling defect of an intravesical enlargement of the prostate deforming the contour of the urinary bladder. A huge cyst of the right kidney was removed, followed by suprapubic transvesical prostatectomy. Both were benign. B. Retrograde pyelogram of the left kidney shows a huge rounded shadow in the region of the left kidney and a grossly distorted renal pelvis and calyces. The right renal shadow is also irregular and enlarged. C. Right pyelogram also shows an abnormal-appearing pelvis. Operation revealed that the mass in the left renal area was an encapsulated renal cell carcinoma. Left nephrectomy was performed, and partial nephrectomy on the right two years later was done for renal cell carcinoma involving this kidney and perinephrium. The x-ray similarity to cyst and bilateral renal involvement by primary carcinoma in the kidney is illustrated by this case.

demonstrated a 95 per cent diagnostic accuracy in a series of 580 consecutive cases. Extensive necrosis within a neoplasm may lead to difficulty in interpreting the x-ray findings.

Aortography and Selective Renal Angiography. These technics can be safely performed using a percutaneous femoral [73] or, less often, brachial catheter. The demonstration of tumor vessels within the space-occupying lesion is about 95 per cent accurate in the diagnosis of neoplasm (Fig. 41-14).

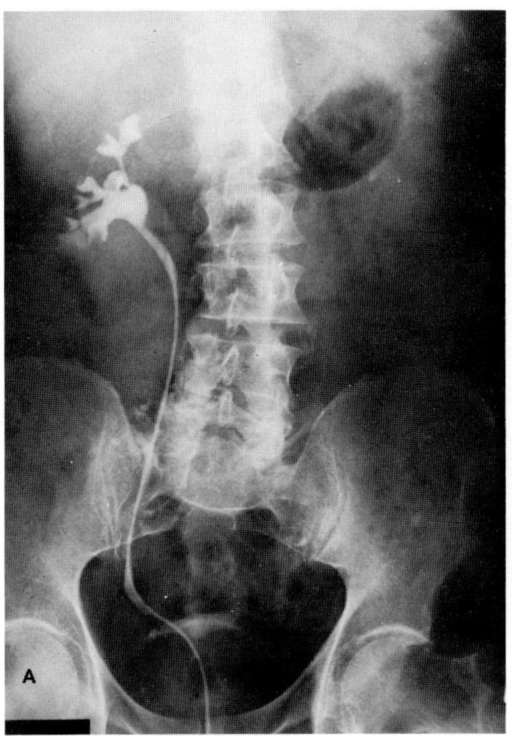

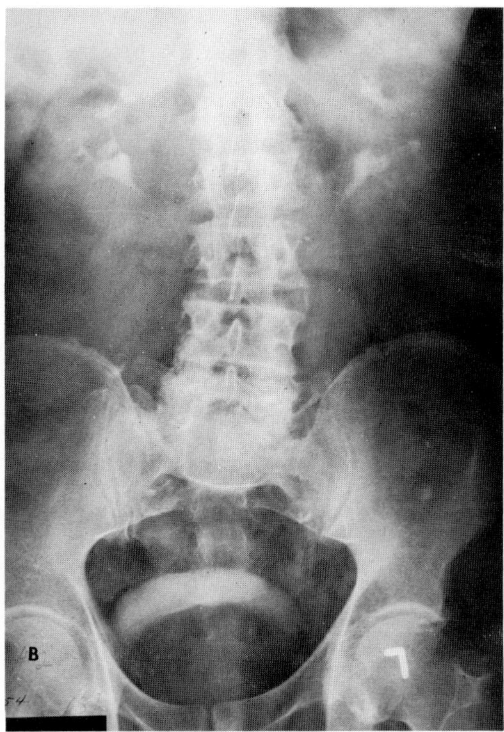

Figure 41-10. Excretory urogram (A) and retrograde pyelogram (B) showing a rounded shadow in the iliac fossa and lower portion of the right kidney with slight spreading of the lower calyces only. The preoperative diagnosis was cyst of lower pole of kidney. Needle aspiration yielded no fluid and at operation nephrectomy was done for a large encapsulated renal cell carcinoma. The patient survived for 10 years, when he died of rupture of an aortic aneurysm.

The addition of epinephrine to the contrast media, described by Abrams [3], is of great value and allows contrast of the normal contracting vasculature, with the unresponsive dilated vessels and arteriovenous shunting in the vasculature of neoplasms. In addition, the surgeon is afforded knowledge of any aberrant renal blood supply which may be invaluable at operation. The venous phase of angiography may delineate the presence of tumor within the renal vein. This information forewarns and guides the surgeon to a more successful cancer operation.

Other Radiologic Technics. Other radiologic methods are available, each with specific indications. *Abdominal venography* may delineate vena caval extension of the tumor. *Lymphangiography* is generally not performed, but it may be valuable in defining lymph node metastases in tumors of the renal pelvis. Retroperitoneal carbon dioxide insufflation adds little to tomography and is plagued by false-positive findings. Percutaneous biopsy or introduction of contrast media into the lesion introduces the unwarranted danger of local neoplastic spread, and is to be avoided in all suspected lesions. *Radioisotope scanning* shows renal tumors as "cold spots" and provides valuable information by a means that is safe and painless to the patient. *Pre-*

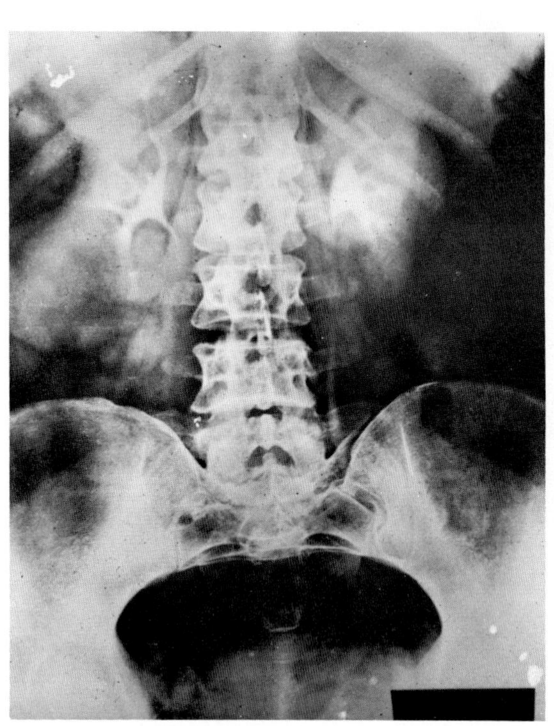

A

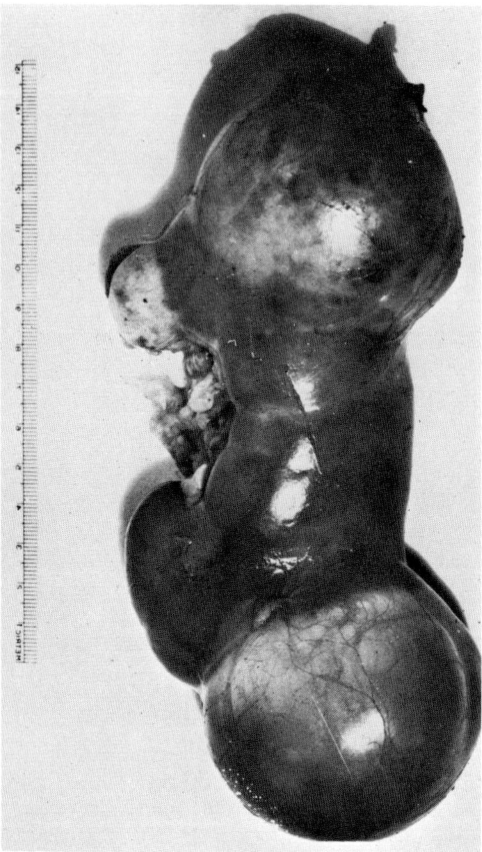

B

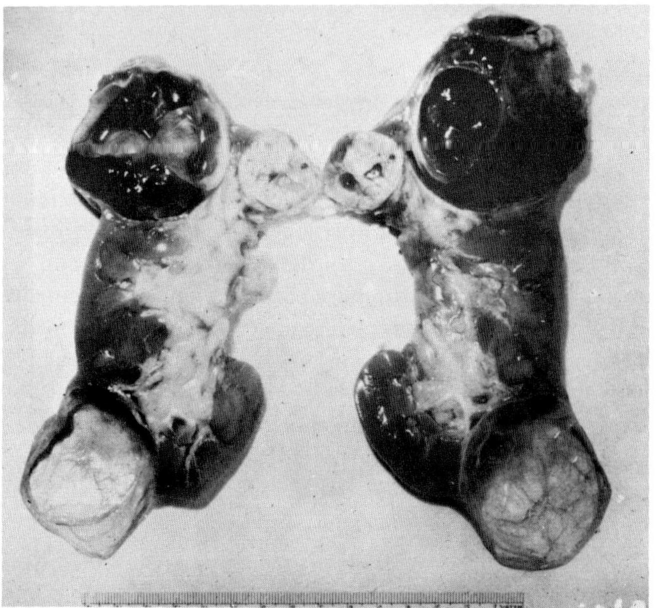

C

Figure 41-11. A. Excretory urogram demonstrating two radiologically indistinguishable space-occupying lesions in the upper and lower poles of the left kidney. (Film reversed.) B. Gross specimen of this kidney reveals a solitary cyst in the lower pole and a large encapsulated renal cell carcinoma in the upper pole of the organ as well as a smaller separate neoplasm mesial to the latter. C. Sagittal section of kidney showing the lower cyst and the two upper tumors each of which on section contains cysts. This is a very important illustration of the relationship of cyst and tumor and shows the importance of exploration of renal cysts.

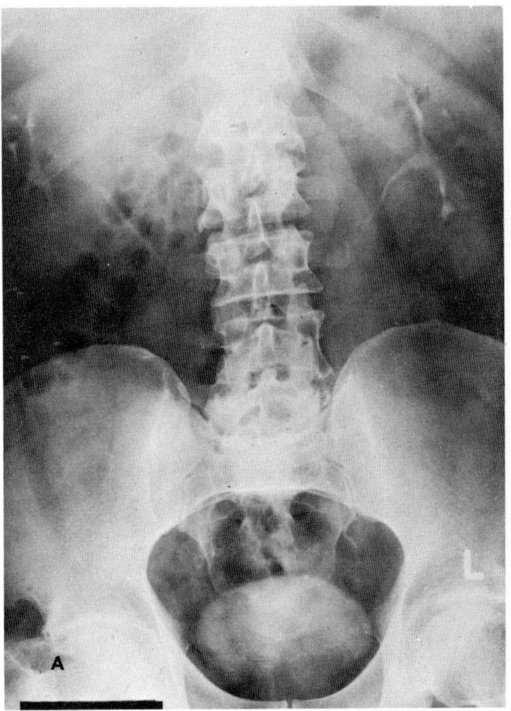

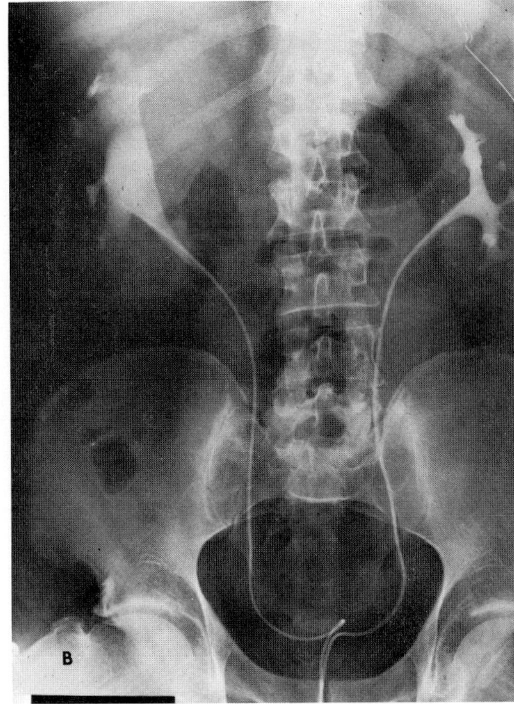

Figure 41-12. A. Excretory urogram showing incomplete outline of each renal pelvis — fairly normal on left but grossly abnormal on right with displacement of kidney, pelvis, and ureter laterally and superiorly. There is incomplete filling of calyces on each side but especially on the right superiorly. B. Bilateral retrograde pyelogram showing the shadow of a mass involving the upper pole of the right kidney, with dilatation of the pelvis and great spreading of the upper calyx. There is good filling of both renal pelves with the contrast medium. All details of the left pyelogram are clear and normal. A and B compare excretory and retrograde pyelography detail and show how each technic supplements the other. Right nephrectomy was carried out with the successful removal of a large renal cell carcinoma. The patient was well for 10 years and subsequently died of pulmonary metastases.

operative barium enema is essential to demonstrate displacement of the colon and to evaluate the possible invasion of this organ.

Treatment

RENAL CELL CARCINOMA

Nephrectomy. Radical excision of the renal tumor offers the only hope for cure. The surgeon benefiting by described diagnostic procedures may approach operation with knowledge concerning: (1) any aberrant blood supply of the kidney that might otherwise contribute to blood loss; (2) perinephric extension that would indicate wider excision for cure; (3) the probable status of renal vein or vena caval invasion by tumor thrombus as well as the state of peripheral venous collaterals; and (4) a 95 per cent certain preoperative diagnosis obviating unnecessary intraoperative maneuvers involving risk of bleeding and spreading of tumor.

Renal cell carcinoma treated by nephrectomy has in various series shown a five-year survival of from 30 to 65 per cent (Fig. 41-15). The higher per cent of cure occurred in patients undergoing concurrent lymphadenec-

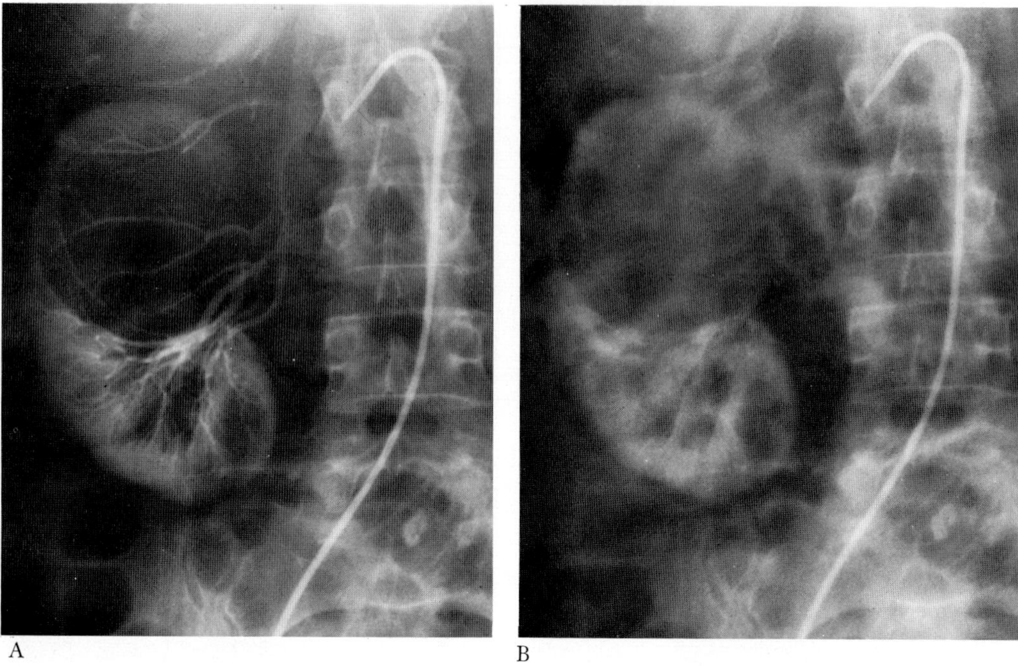

Figure 41-13. A. Selective arteriogram showing the vasculature of a kidney bearing a translucent cyst of the upper pole. Persistent pain demanded unroofing and excision. B. Nephrographic phase of a selective renal angiogram demonstrating the characteristic radiolucency and thin wall of a benign solitary cyst in the upper pole of the kidney. (Courtesy of Dr. Herbert Abrams.)

tomy. The overall 10-year survival is between 18 and 23 per cent. Renal vein involvement generally decreased five-year survival from 55 per cent to 29 per cent in McDonald and Priestly's series [49]. Invasion of the renal pelvis has a similar statistical influence. The presence of local lymph node metastases even with extensive lymphadenectomy reduced the five-year survival from 65 per cent to 42 per cent [70]. The figures of Kaufman and Mims [40] relating to survival are shown in Figure 41-16.

METASTATIC DISEASE. The presence of metastases does not contraindicate nephrectomy because a number of benefits accrue to the removal of the primary tumor, such as relief of pain, arrest of hemorrhage, relief of toxic absorption, improvement of anemia, and relief of pyrexia (Fig. 41-17). It is a sound principle to remove the primary tumor when feasible also because it can then produce no more metastases. In rare instances, the metastases of renal cell carcinoma have been documented to regress after removal of the primary. Everson and Cole [23], in 1966, carefully recorded regression in 31 cases, usually after excision of the renal neoplasm. Histologic evidence was reported in 2 of the 31, while the remainder were assessed radiologically. This fact may allow some doubt as to validity in some cases. It seems appropriate to mention the case of a patient whose apparent pulmonary metastasis proved to be a benign hamartoma and another whose femoral metastasis proved to be a benign cyst of the neck of the femur. The latter had a radiographic appearance similar to that in Figure 41-10. Each of these patients had had previous nephrectomy for renal cell carcinoma. Though rare, excision of a solitary metastasis after re-

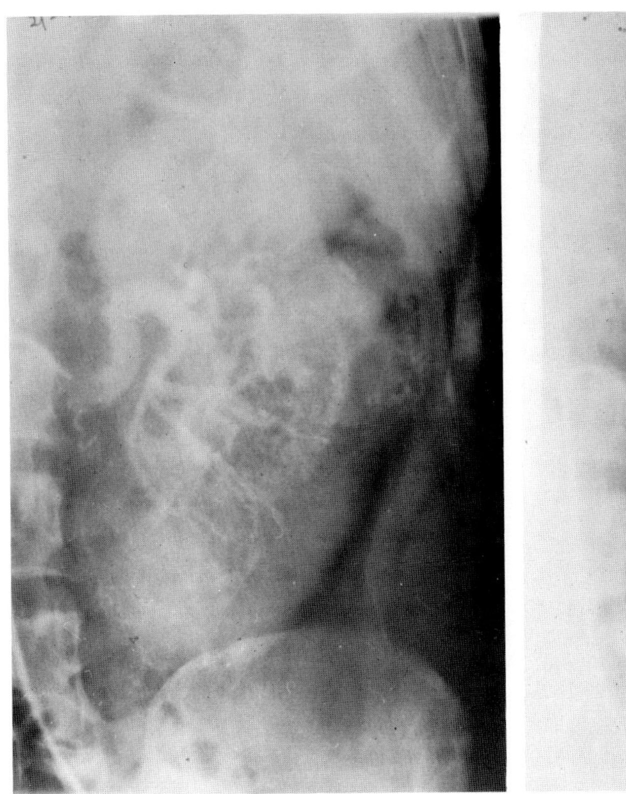

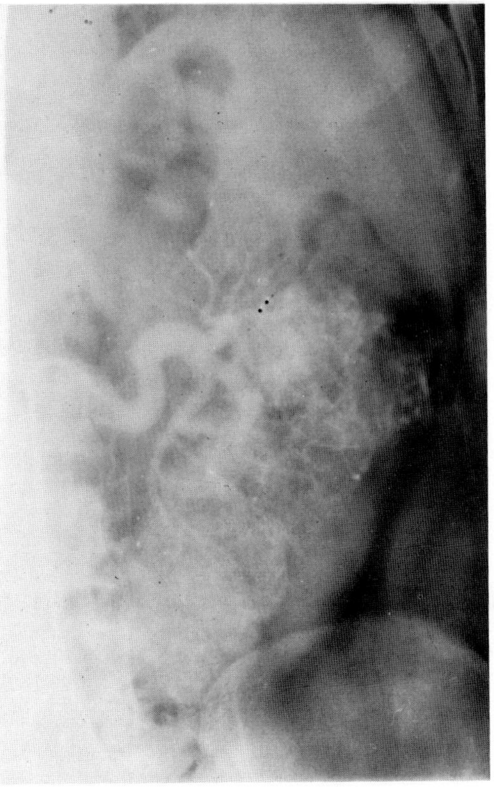

Figure 41-14. Arteriogram of left solitary remaining kidney shows the abnormal vascular pattern caused by renal cell carcinoma invading the perinephrium. Gross hematuria and pain of one month's duration were relieved by x-irradiation, testosterone proprionate, and four weeks' hospitalization. The patient is well and active at home four months later. (Courtesy of Dr. Herbert Abrams.)

moval of the primary has brought a five-year [15, 72, 76, 78] or 10-year survival [6, 71]. Smallwood and Kickham [74] reported a 10-year survival after extirpation of a lesion of the scalp, clavicle, and the primary, but recorded the appearance of other metastases in the eighth year. The variable biologic behavior of renal neoplasm is shown in Figure 41-18 which illustrates a pulmonary metastasis from renal carcinoma that became larger after nephrectomy and regressed with testosterone proprionate therapy. She was well for two years after lobectomy but now, in the third year, has multiple pulmonary metastases and is again receiving testosterone therapy.

Renal arteriography has demonstrated and located soft tissue as well as osseous painful metastatic lesions. This information has been valuable in allowing accurate irradiation of the lesion and has brought about nearly complete relief of pain. Osseous metastases particularly may respond to radiation and hormonal therapy, with regression and disappearance of pain.

Irradiation. Sir Eric Riches has demonstrated that renal cell carcinoma may respond to radiotherapy. In his series of 362 inoperable patients, the five-year survival without treatment was 0.5 per cent, in contrast to 6 per cent with radiotherapy alone. In a recent review [67], Riches points out that improvement beyond three years was related to lack of renal

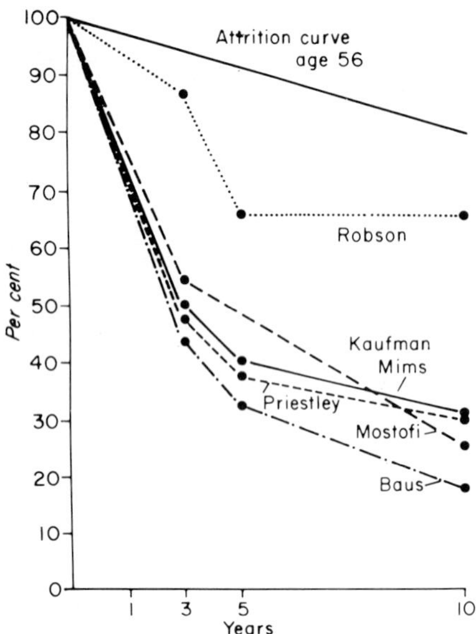

Figure 41-15. Crude survival curves of several large series of cases of renal cell carcinoma treated surgically and followed for 10 years. (From *Tumors of the Kidney* by Joseph J. Kaufman and Matlock M. Mims, in "Current Problems in Surgery." Copyright © 1966, Year Book Medical Publishers, Inc. Used by permission of Year Book Medical Publishers.)

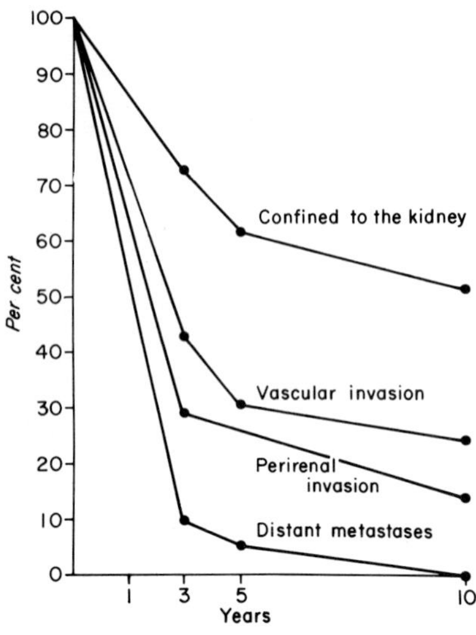

Figure 41-16. Survival curves according to degree of invasion and based on 100 cases reported by Kaufman and Mims. (From *Tumors of the Kidney* by Joseph J. Kaufman and Matlock M. Mims, in "Current Problems in Surgery." Copyright © 1966, Year Book Medical Publishers, Inc. Used by permission of Year Book Medical Publishers.)

vein involvement and to a well-differentiated tumor growth rather than to a postoperative irradiation. He now favors preoperative irradiation of 3000 rads for the purpose of decreasing the spread of tumor during operation, and to reduce the size of the tumor. Eleven cases considered inoperable because of the huge size of the tumor have been reported by Riches to have become easily operable after preoperative irradiation. While awaiting assessment of the value of x-ray treatment in a statistically significant number of patients, preoperative irradiation is rarely invoked in the treatment of these tumors today. The shrinkage of some huge tumors after irradiation is attributed to decrease in vascularity and lymphedema with perhaps some specific effect on the growth of the tumor itself (see Fig. 41-14).

Chemotherapy. Chemotherapy for treatment of renal neoplasms, with the exception of nephroblastoma, has been ineffectual in nearly all reports [30, 77] in the literature. Such treatment may occasionally be warranted in metastatic disease, but only after irradiation, surgery, and hormonal measures have been exhausted.

Hormonal Therapy. The variable growth and behavior of renal cell carcinoma have been thought by Bloom [11] to be related to a "host resistance" factor which may be hormonal. Kirkman [42] demonstrated a high incidence of renal cell carcinoma in hamsters receiving diethylstilbestrol. Tumors in most reports develop about seven months after beginning of estrogen administration. The carcinogenic effect is confined to males, or to females that have been oophorectomized. Tumor growth in hamsters is inhibited by simultaneous administration of testosterone or progesterone. Extrapolating the experimental observations to the clinical situation, Bloom

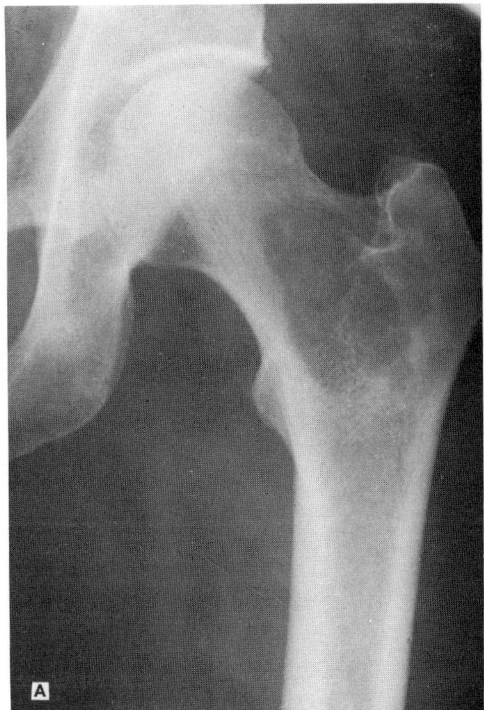

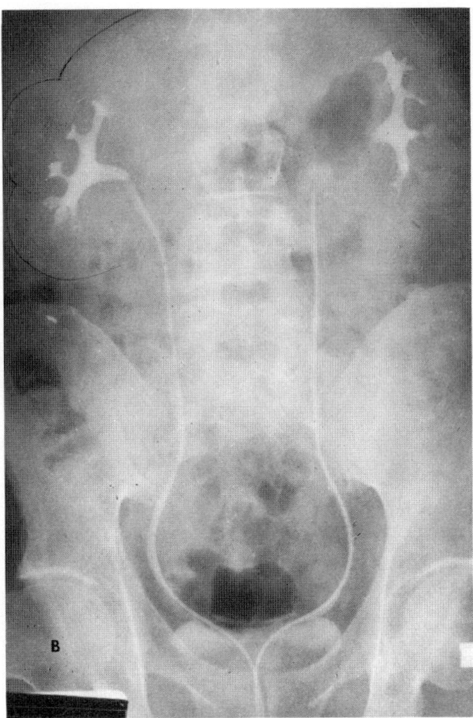

Figure 41-17. A. Roentgenogram of the left hip showing an osteoclastic lesion of the neck of the femur of a 42-year-old man which at biopsy proved to resemble renal cell carcinoma. B. Bilateral retrograde pyelograms which outline normal renal pelves; urine from the right kidney showed a few erythrocytes and epithelial cells that were definitely neoplastic. A convexity was present in the midportion of the lateral border of the right kidney which proved to be a renal cell carcinoma at exploration; right nephrectomy was performed.

[11] reported radiologic or clinical improvement in eight (21 per cent) of 38 patients receiving hormonal therapy within two to six weeks of commencing treatment. The agents used were medroxyprogesterone acetate and testosterone proprionate for seven and one patients, respectively. The response has been reported as complete or partial regression of two months' to three years' duration.

Endocrine treatment not only has been found more effective than chemotherapy with cytotoxic agents but also has the significant advantages of being anabolic and nontoxic systemically. The results in the management of renal cell carcinoma involving a remaining or solitary kidney have been recently reported [60] and suggest further the benefits of combined treatment with radiation and hormonal therapy.

WILMS'S TUMOR

The cure of any renal neoplasm is primarily accomplished by early surgical removal. During the past three decades the survival rate has steadily improved. William E. Ladd, M.D., of the Children's Medical Center in Boston, advocated the transperitoneal approach, early ligation of the pedicle, meticulous care not to rupture the tumor capsule, and excision of the neoplasm irrespective of size. In a series of patients treated between 1931 and 1939, Ladd, by operation alone, increased the cure rate to 32 per cent with a startling lack of operative mortality. Gross

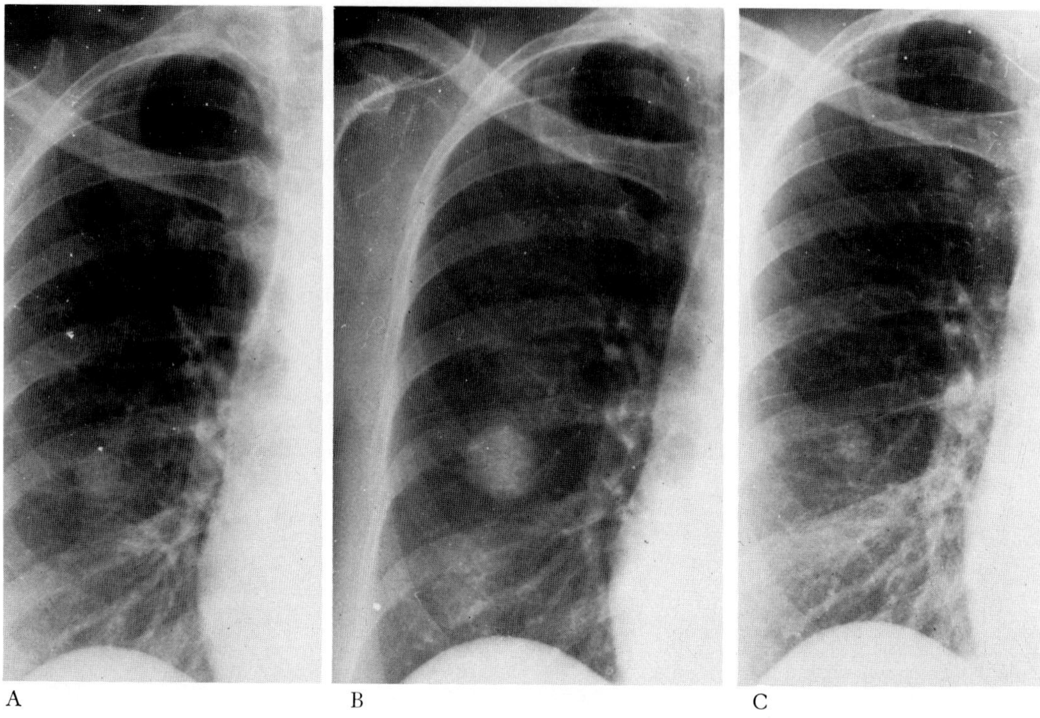

Figure 41-18. A small pulmonary metastasis (A) that became larger after nephrectomy (B) and regressed after testosterone proprionate therapy (C). Lobectomy was then carried out, and the patient was well for two years. Multiple pulmonary metastases are now evident in the third year.

adopted the thoracoabdominal approach and, utilizing postoperative irradiation, attained a 47 per cent [34] cure rate by 1956. The previous 20-year cure rate had been 40 per cent. Gross had tried preoperative radiotherapy and found the results discouraging. Several disadvantages of the preoperative irradiation were (1) delay of definitive surgery, (2) liquefaction of the neoplasm making intraoperative rupture more likely, and (3) more difficult definition of the margin of the tumor. Postoperative radiotherapy to the renal fossa has been used in nearly all patients since 1940. In infants under one year of age whose neoplasm has been removed without rupture, irradiation has been omitted both because of the improved prognosis in this group and to avoid skeletal abnormalities. An important feature of the biologic behavior of this tumor is that metastases and or recurrence usually become manifest within two years. Survival without recurrence or metastases for two years is usually commensurate with cure.

A search by Farber [25] and his associates for anticancer chemicals in the treatment of Wilms's tumor was rewarded after eight years by finding in 1954 that actinomycin D was effective in mouse tumors. After evaluation of its toxicity, a clinical trial demonstrated disappearance of pulmonary metastases both radiologically and by postmortem examination. Encouraged by such observations, Farber [24] was able in 1966 to report on 134 patients treated by combined surgery, postoperative irradiation, and actinomycin D. In 53 children without metastases, a two-year survival rate of 89 per cent was attained. This compared favorably with the 40 per cent survival rate found prior to the use of actinomycin D. A Wilms's tumor with a solitary pulmonary metastasis has been successfully treated by surgical excision with some long-term survivals [82]. Multiple pulmonary metastases have been treated by Farber with a combination of actinomycin D and radiotherapy in amounts not harmful to the lungs with an apparent two- to nine-year cure of 58 per cent in a series of 15 patients.

TUMORS OF THE RENAL PELVIS AND URETER

Papillary tumors of the renal pelvis must be all considered malignant. They are usually multiple, involving the ureter and often the bladder as well (Figs. 41-19, 41-20, 41-21). Because of the multiplicity of these tumors, a total nephroureterectomy including a cuff of bladder must be accomplished. A careful study of the patient's occupation and possible exposure to carcinogenic agents of a chemical nature should be made in all instances. Squamous cell carcinoma or epidermoid carcinoma of the renal pelvis is usually associated with chronic suppurative infection and calculous disease. It is quite malignant and tends to spread by lymphatics and by direct extension as well as hematogenously. Papillary tumors

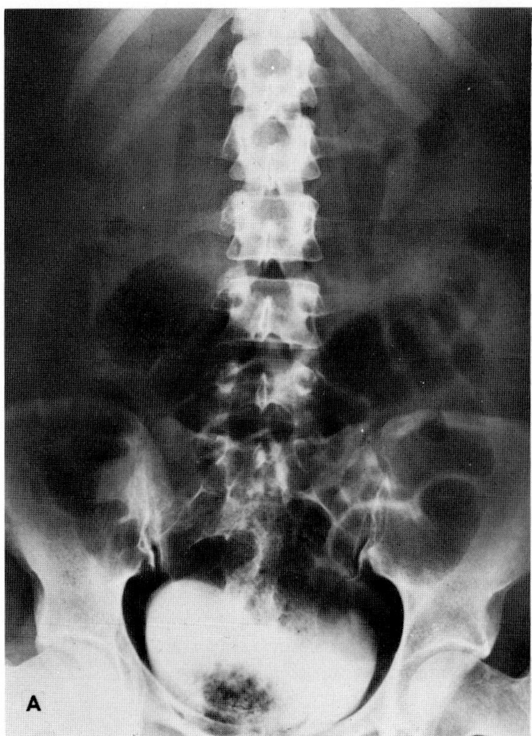

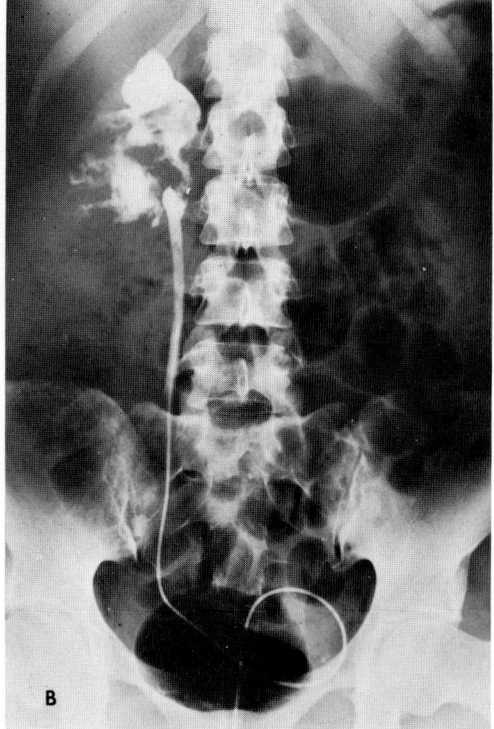

Figure 41-19. A. Cystogram showing a large filling defect caused by papillary transitional cell carcinoma in the urinary bladder of a 45-year-old woman. The patient was admitted to the hospital with pain in the right flank, where a palpable tender mass was present. The urine was both bloody and purulent; hematuria had been intermittent for six months. B. Retrograde pyelogram made on the right side shows a very irregular filling of the renal pelvis and upper ureter suggesting invasion of the renal parenchyma by primary tumor in the renal pelvis. Right nephroureterectomy and partial cystectomy were carried out for papillary transitional cell carcinoma of the right kidney, ureter, and right side of bladder. The patient died 18 months later of cerebral metastases.

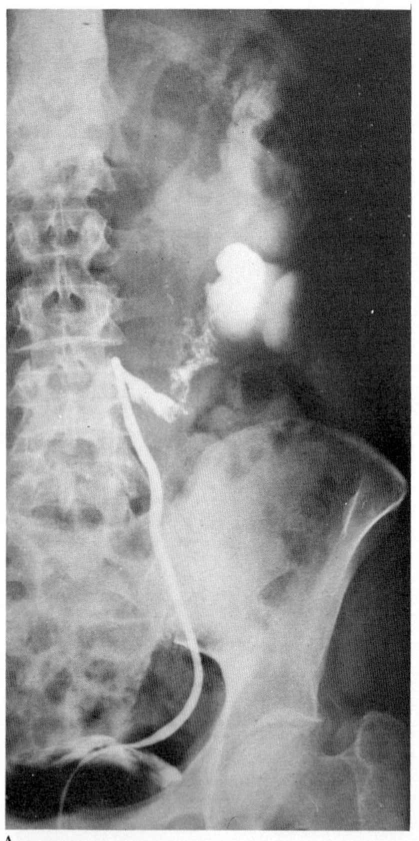
A

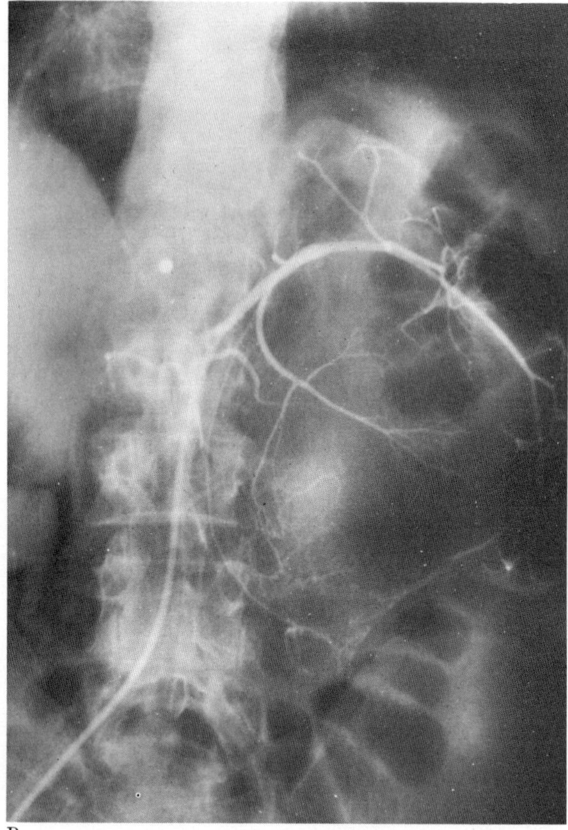
B

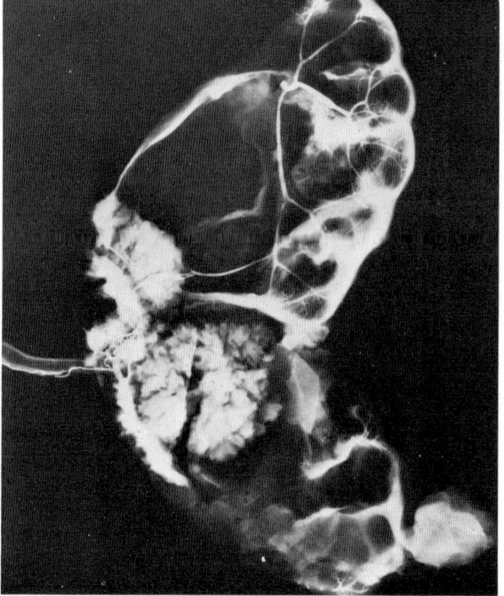
C

Figure 41-20. A. Papillary transitional cell carcinoma causing ureteropelvic obstruction and presenting an extreme irregularity in the ureterogram. B. Selective angiogram shows a widely spread renal vasculature caused by the large hydronephrosis and an abnormal pattern of vessels in the tumor itself. C. In vitro radiograph of the injected specimen shows this large congenital hydronephrosis bearing an extensive papillary carcinoma in the renal pelvis. This had caused no hematuria, but complete obstruction prevented positive urinary cytology.

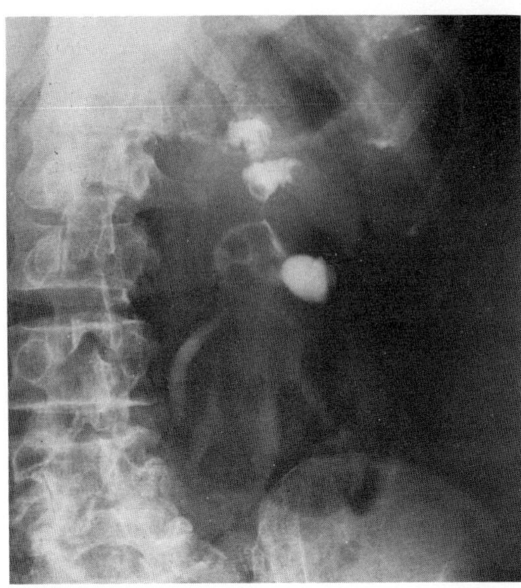

Figure 41-21. Left retrograde pyelogram showing a negative filling defect in the pelvis, dilatation and erosive irregularity of the only calyces not obliterated. Nephrectomy was carried out. Tuberculosis of the kidney complicated by epidermoid carcinoma of the renal pelvis was found.

have an equal potential for spread, but they tend to invade blood vessels even more than the squamous cell carcinoma. Squamous cell carcinoma has a poor prognosis. The diagnosis is made late; the tumor has usually been present for a long time before discovery. The papillary tumors of the renal pelvis are discovered usually as a result of hematuria, whereas those of epidermoid or squamous cell type are found in the course of the treatment of chronic suppurative infection and stone (Fig. 41-21). Hematuria was present in 80 per cent of 59 cases reported by Newman et al. [54] and in 92 per cent of 37 patients reported by Grace et al. [32]. Exfoliative cytology of the urine will usually be positive in cases of papillary tumor of the renal pelvis, and in most cases of epidermoid carcinoma (Fig. 41-22). These tests will be positive also in those cases in which renal carcinomas have invaded the renal pelvis.

The most important feature of the treatment of tumors of the renal pelvis following nephroureterectomy is cystoscopic examination repeated at intervals of two to three months for evidence of new tumors in the urinary bladder, so that they may be destroyed by electrocoagulation or irradiation. We prefer electrocoagulation for this purpose. Cytologic examination of the urine is helpful and will show neoplastic cells in more than 90 per cent of cases with recurrence. It is not uncommon for distant metastases to the brain, spinal cord, and lung to occur by hematogenous routes from these tumors.

The results of surgery for tumors of the renal pelvis and ureter are of interest. Riches [64] found a 40 per cent five-year survival (10 of 25 patients). All the tumors that were removed from the survivors were of low-grade malignancy. Recurrence or metastasis occurred in 33 per cent of the total group. Among the seven patients having solid or transitional cell lesions, the longest survival was nine months; metastases occurred in five cases.

A recent series, reported by Grace et al. [32] in 1967, shows a 36 per cent five-year survival, demonstrating that the survival rate remains unchanged and discouragingly low for surgical treatment alone of the tumors of the renal pelvis. The need for an improved treatment is apparent, but to date the effect of more radical surgery with lymph node dissection, or combinations of surgery with irradiation and or chemotherapy has not been determined. Papillary tumors have a much better prognosis than the undifferentiated sessile and infiltrating lesions.

The recurrence rate of neoplasm in the ureteral stump following nephrectomy and partial ureterectomy have been found to be 27 per cent by O'Conor [56] and 17 per cent by Riches et al. [68]. In patients with primary ureteral carcinoma treated by partial ureterectomy, a recurrence rate between 9 and 12 per cent in the ureteral stump has been reported [1, 37, 79]. The occurrence of bilateral neo-

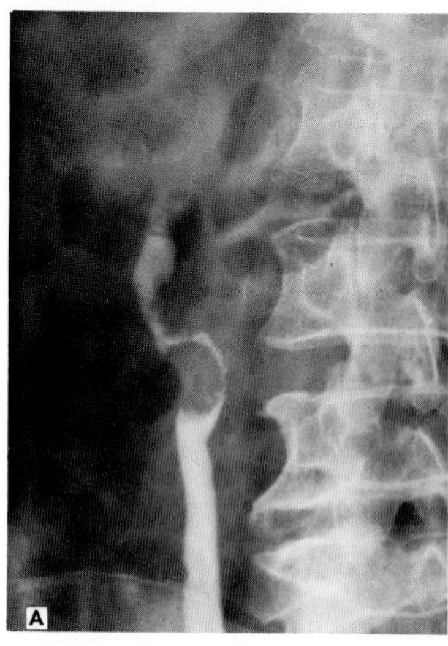

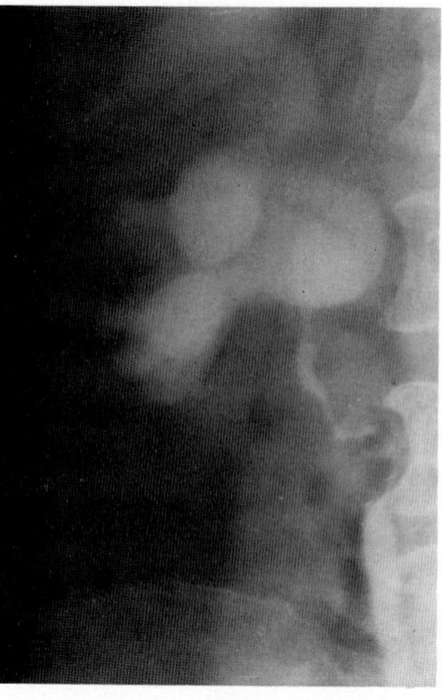

Figure 41-22. A. Retrograde and excretory ureterogram and pyelogram showing a filling defect of the ureter caused by intrinsic carcinoma of the upper ureter with hydronephrosis due to obstruction. B. Urinary sediment from right ureteral catheter shows pleomorphic bizarre mitotic figures characteristic of carcinoma. C. Papanicolaou stain of urinary sediment of another patient having carcinoma of the ureter showing mitotic figures characteristic of neoplasms.

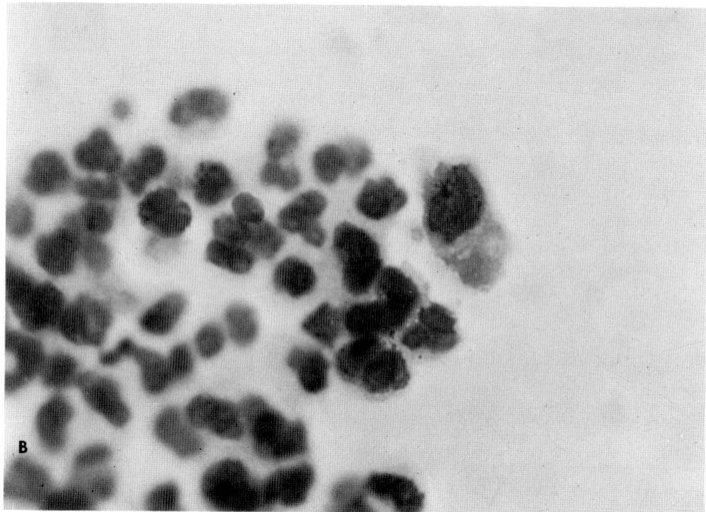

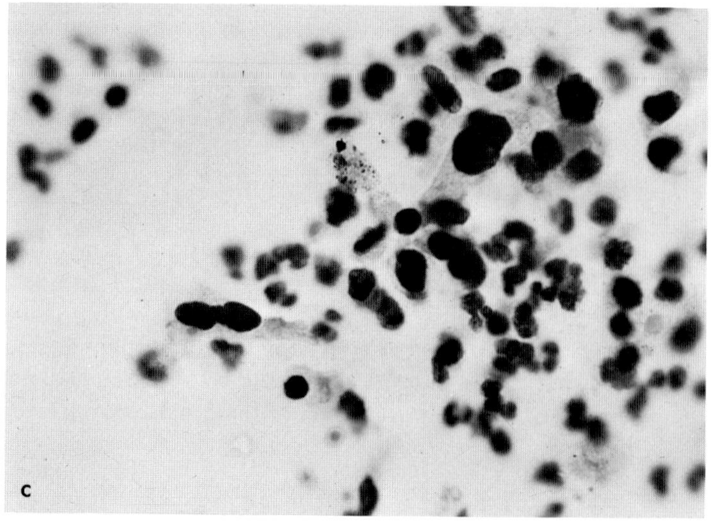

plasia of the upper urinary tract is rare, but 14 cases of simultaneous and 8 cases of asynchronous lesions have been described in the literature [62]. Papillary tumors have a much better prognosis than the undifferentiated sessile and infiltrating neoplasms.

Conclusions

In the last 25 years the death rate from tumors of the kidney has increased significantly (see Table 41-1). A vigorous search for more effective screening tests, such as enzymatic studies, and an increased utilization of cytologic examination of the urine and excretory urography should lead to a more frequent early discovery of this insidious lesion, with greater possibility for cure. That renal tumors may cause polycythemia, anemia, fever, weight loss, rapid sedimentation rate, leukocytosis, and malaise without local symptoms or signs needs further emphasis; in 75 per cent of cases hematuria leads to their discovery. A plain film of the abdomen will often detect changes in size and contour of the kidney, indicating the necessity for more definitive x-ray examinations.

Advances in the surgery of renal tumor in the last two decades include a less hesitant attitude toward removal of the primary tumor, excision of the neoplasm with lymphadenectomy and wider margin after division of the renal pedicle, removal of solitary metastases, and the combined use of chemotherapy and irradiation in selected cases. The thoracoabdominal approach of Chute has rendered safer the removal of large tumors, and Nagamatsu's osteoplastic flap has facilitated surgical exposure of renal tumors. Early removal of a renal neoplasm must be accomplished if the results of treatment are to be improved. Since symptoms appear late in the growth of these tumors, more widespread use of objective diagnostic facilities must be stimulated and a higher degree of suspicion cultivated regarding slight abnormalities of blood, urine, and temperature.

References

1. Abeshouse, B. S. Primary benign and malignant tumors of the ureter: Review of the literature and report of one benign and 12 malignant tumors. *Amer. J. Surg.* 91:237, 1956.
2. Abeshouse, B. S. Management of Wilms' tumor as determined by national survey and review of the literature. *J. Urol.* 77:792, 1957.
3. Abrams, H. L. The response of neoplastic renal vessels to epinephrine in man. *Radiology* 82:217, 1964.
4. Austen, G., Jr. Calcification of renal tumors. *Amer. J. Roentgen.* 49:580, 1943.
5. Bailey, O. T., and Harrison, J. H. Large benign renal neoplasms: Their pathology and clinical behavior with report of five cases. *J. Urol.* 38:509, 1937.
6. Barney, J. J. D. A twelve-year cure following nephrectomy for adenocarcinoma and lobectomy for solitary metastasis. *J. Urol.* 52:406, 1944.
7. Beare, J. B., and McDonald, J. R. Involvement of the renal capsule in surgically removed hypernephroma: A gross and histopathologic study. *J. Urol.* 61:857, 1949.
8. Bell, E. T. *Renal Diseases.* Philadelphia: Lea & Febiger, 1947. P. 420.
9. Bennington, J. L., and Kradjian, R. M. *Renal Carcinoma.* Philadelphia: Saunders, 1967.
10. Bliss, T. L. Basal metabolism in polycythemia vera. *Ann. Intern. Med.* 2:1155, 1929.
11. Bloom, H. J. B. Cancer of the urogenital tract: Kidney. The basis for hormonal therapy. *J.A.M.A.* 204:605, 1968.
12. Bottiger, L. E. Fever of unknown origin:

IV. Fever in carcinoma of the kidney. *Acta Med. Scand.* 156:477, 1957.

13. Cahill, G. F. Cancer of kidneys, adrenals and testes. *J.A.M.A.* 138:357, 1948.
14. Caplan, B., Halasz, N. A., and Bloomer, W. E. Resection and ligation of the suprarenal inferior vena cava. *J. Urol.* 92:25, 1964.
15. Chute, R., Ireland, E. F., and Houghton, J. D. Solitary distant metastases from unsuspected renal carcinoma. *J. Urol.* 80:420, 1958.
16. Chute, R. L., Soutter, L., and Kerr, W. J. Value of the thoracoabdominal incision in removal of the kidney. *New Eng. J. Med.* 241:951, 1949.
17. Chynn, K. Y., and Evans, J. A. Nephrotomography in the differentiation of renal cyst from neoplasm: A review of 500 cases. *J. Urol.* 83:21, 1960.
18. Clarke, B. G., and Goade, W. J., Jr. Fever and anemia in renal cancer. *New Eng. J. Med.* 254:107, 1956.
19. Cresson, S. L., and Pilling, G. P. Renal tumors. *Pediat. Clin. N. Amer.* 6:473, 1959.
20. Crocker, D. W. Renal Tumors. In S. C. Somers (Ed.), *Pathology Annual.* New York: Appleton-Century-Crofts, Division of Meredith, 1967. P. 243.
21. Culp, O. S. Treatment of tumors of the renal pelvis and ureter. *Trans. Amer. Ass. Genitourin. Surg.* 47:101, 1955.
22. Dick, V. S., and Flint, L. D. The prognosis of renal tumors. *Surg. Clin. N. Amer.* 31:633, 1951.
23. Everson, T. C., and Cole, W. E. *Spontaneous Regression of Cancer.* Philadelphia: Saunders, 1966. P. 11.
24. Farber, S. Chemotherapy in treatment of leukemia and Wilms' tumor. *J.A.M.A.* 198:826, 1966.
25. Farber, S., Maddock, C. L., and Swaffield, M. N. Studies on the carcinolytic and other biological activity of actinomycin D. *Proc. Amer. Ass. Cancer Res.* 2:104, 1956.
26. Foot, N. C., and Papanicolaou, G. N. Early renal carcinoma in situ detected by means of smears of fixed urinary sediment. *J.A.M.A.* 139:356, 1949.
27. Foot, N. C., Papanicolaou, G. N., Holmquist, N. D., and Seybolt, J. F. Exfoliative cytology of the urinary sediment; a review of 2829 cases. *Cancer* 11:127, 1958.
28. Forsell, J. Polycythemia in a patient with hypernephroma. *Nord. Med.* 30:1415, 1946.
29. Gaulin, E. Simultaneous Wilms' tumors in identical twins. *J. Urol.* 66:547, 1951.
30. Glenn, J. F., and Hunt, L. D. Chemotherapy of nephrocarcinoma: A report of two cases. *Cancer Chemother. Rep.* 27:63, 1963.
31. Goldberg, M. F., Tashjian, A. H., Jr., Order, S. E., and Dammin, G. J. Renal adenocarcinoma containing a parathyroid hormone-like substance and associated with marked hypercalcemia. *Amer. J. Med.* 36:805, 1964.
32. Grace, D. A., Taylor, W. N., and Winter, C. C. Carcinoma of the renal pelvis: A 15-year review. *J. Urol.* 98:566, 1967.
33. Graham, A. P. Malignancy of the kidney Survey of 195 cases. *J. Urol.* 58:10, 1947.
34. Gross, R. E., and Newhouser, E. B. D. Treatment of mixed tumors of the kidney in childhood. *Pediatrics* 6:843, 1950.

34a. Harrison, J. H. Tumors of the Kidney. In Strauss, M. B., and Welt, L. G. (Eds.), *Diseases of the Kidney.* Boston: Little, Brown 1963. Chap. 37.

35. Harrison, J. H., Botsford, T. W., and Tucker, M. R. The use of the smear of the urinary sediment in the diagnosis and management of neoplasm of the kidney and bladder. *Surg. Gynec. Obstet.* 92:129, 1951.
36. Hensler, L. Hohe Leukocytose durch Karzinom. *Schweiz. Med. Wschr.* 83:1032, 1953.
37. Holtz, F. Papillomas and primary carcinoma of the ureter: Report of 20 cases. *J. Urol.* 88:380, 1962.
38. Hope, J. W. Radiographic differential diagnosis. *J.A.M.A.* 204:983, 1968.
39. Jenkins, R. H. Embryonal adenomyosarcoma of the kidney in adults. *New Eng. J. Med.* 205:472, 1931.
40. Kaufman, J. J., and Mims, M. M. *Tumors of the Kidney.* Chicago: Year Book, 1966.
41. Kerr, W. K. Notes on cancer and smoking linked chemically. *Med. World News,* April 9, 1965. P. 30.
42. Kirkman, H. Estrogen-induced tumors of

the kidney in the Syrian hamster. *Nat. Cancer Inst. Monogr.* No. 1, 1959.

43. Lattimer, J. K., Melicow, M. M., and Uson, A. C. Wilms' tumor: A report of 71 cases. *J. Urol.* 80:401, 1958.
44. Lucke, B., and Schlumberger, H. G. Tumors of the Kidney, Renal Pelvis, and Ureter. In *Atlas of Tumor Pathology.* Washington, D.C.: Armed Forces Institute of Pathology, 1957. Section VIII, Fascicle 30.
45. Luke, R. G., Kennedy, A. C., Stirling, W. B., and McDonald, G. A. Renal artery stenosis, hypertension, and polycythaemia. *Brit. Med. J.* 1:164, 1965.
46. MacCallum, W. G. A. *Textbook of Pathology.* Philadelphia: Saunders, 1940.
47. Magee, P. N., and Barnes, J. M. Induction of kidney tumours in rat with dimethylnitrosamine (N-nitrosodimethylamine). *J. Path. Bact.* 84:19, 1962.
48. Maslow, L. A. Wilms' tumor: Report of three cases and possible fourth one in the same family. *J. Urol.* 43:43, 1940.
49. McDonald, J. T., and Priestley, J. R. Malignant tumors of the kidney: Surgical and prognostic significance of tumor thrombosis of the renal vein. *Surg. Gynec. Obstet.* 77:295, 1943.
50. Melicow, M. M. Classification of renal neoplasms: A clinical and pathological study based on 199 cases. *J. Urol.* 51:333, 1944.
51. Miller, H. C. Use of C-reactive protein in distinguishing renal cyst from tumor. *Invest. Urol.* 1:514, 1964.
52. Morlock, C. G., and Horton, B. T. Variations in systolic blood pressure in renal tumors: A study of 491 cases. *Amer. J. Med. Sci.* 191:647, 1936.
53. Nesbit, R. M. *Fundamentals of Urology.* Ann Arbor: University of Michigan Press, 1950.
54. Newman, D. M., Allen, L. E., Wishard, W. N., Jr., Nourse, M. H., and Mertz, J. H. O. Transitional cell carcinoma of the upper urinary tract. *J. Urol.* 98:322, 1967.
55. Ochsner, M. G. Renal cell carcinoma: Five-year follow-up study of 70 cases. *J. Urol.* 93:361, 1965.
56. O'Conor, V. J. The diagnosis of tumors of the renal pelvis and ureter. *J. Urol.* 75:416, 1956.
57. Olovson, T. Die Senkungreaktion beim Hypernephroma: Erfahrungen von 109 operierten Fallen. *Acta Chir. Scand.* 93:503, 1946.
58. Orr, L. M., Anderson, E. E., and Harrison, J. H. Carcinoma arising in the hypoplastic kidney. *J. Urol.* 96:203, 1966.
59. Parker, R. G. Occlusion of the hepatic veins in man. *Medicine* (Balt.) 38:369, 1959.
60. Parker, R. M., Timothy, R. P., Harrison, J. H. Carcinoma in the solitary kidney. *Trans. Amer. Ass. Genitourin. Surg.* In press.
61. Pennington, D. G. Anaemia and polycythaemia with renal diseases. *Postgrad. Med.* 38:497, 1962.
62. Perlmutter, A. D., Retik, A. B., and Harrison, J. H. Simultaneous bilateral carcinoma of the ureter present for five years before surgery. *J. Urol.* 93:582, 1965.

62a. Phillips, T. L., Chin, F. G., and Palubinskas, A. J. Calcification in renal masses: An 11-year survey. *Radiology* 80:786, 1963.

63. Reiss, O. Leukemoid reaction due to hypernephroma. *J.A.M.A.* 180:1126, 1962.
64. Riches, E. W. Malignant Disease of the Urinary Tract. Lettsomian Lectures. *Trans. Med. Soc. London* 74:77, 1957–58.
65. Riches, E. W. Factors in the prognosis of carcinoma of the kidney. *J. Urol.* 79:190, 1958.
66. Riches, E. W. *Tumors of the Kidney and Ureter.* Baltimore: Williams & Wilkins, 1964.
67. Riches, E. Cancer of the urogenital tract: The place of irradiation. *J.A.M.A.* 204:230, 1968.
68. Riches, E. W., Griffiths, I. H., and Thackeray, A. C. New growth of kidney and ureter. *Brit. J. Urol.* 23:296, 1951.
69. Roberts, L. Case report: Hypertension due to renal tumour. *Med. Serv. J. Canada* 17:179, 1961.
70. Robson, C. J. Radical nephrectomy for renal cell carcinoma. *J. Urol.* 89:37, 1963.
71. Sammellas, W. Adenocarcinoma of the kidney: A 10 year apparent cure following resection of a solitary pulmonary metastasis. *J. Urol.* 90:250, 1963.

72. Scudder, C. L. The bone metastases of hypernephroma: A completed record of a case with solitary bone metastasis. *Ann. Surg.* 52:533, 1910.
73. Seldinger, S. I. Catheter replacement of needle in percutaneous arteriography: New technique. *Acta Radiol.* 39:368, 1953.
74. Smallwood, C. T., and Kickham, C. J. E. Renal cell carcinoma with nephrectomy and excision of 2 lesions: 10 year survival. In press.
75. Southwood, W. F., and Marshall, V. F. A clinical evaluation of nephrotomography. *Brit. J. Urol.* 30:127, 1958.
76. Starr, A., and Miller, G. M. Solitary jejunal metastasis twenty years after removal of a renal cell carcinoma. *New Eng. J. Med.* 246:250, 1952.
77. Straffon, R. H. Cancer chemotherapy in the urologic patient. *J. Urol.* 86:259, 1961.
78. Straus, F. H., and Scanlon, E. F. Five-year survival after hepatic lobectomy for metastatic hypernephroma. *A.M.A. Arch. Surg.* 72:328, 1956.
79. Thomas, G. J., and Regnier, E. A. Tumors of the kidney pelvis and ureter. *J. Urol.* 11:205, 1924.
80. Thorling, E. B., and Ersbak, J. Erythrocytosis and hypernephroma. *Scand. J. Haemat.* 1:38, 1964.
81. Wacker, W. E. C., and Dorfman, L. E. Urinary lactic dehydrogenase activity: I. Screening method for detection of cancer of kidneys and bladder. *J.A.M.A.* 181:972, 1962.
82. White, J. G., and Krivit, W. Surgical excision of pulmonary metastases. *Pediatrics* 29:927, 1962.
83. Wittenborg, M. H. Roentgen therapy in neuroblastoma: A review of 73 cases. *Radiology* 54:679, 1950.
84. Zak, F. G., Holzner, J. H., Singer, E. J., and Popper, H. Renal and pulmonary tumors in rats fed dimethylnitrosamine. *Cancer Res.* 20:96, 1960.

42

Pediatric Nephrology

Chester M. Edelmann, Jr., and Henry L. Barnett

Management of the child with renal disease requires not only knowledge of those aspects of disease peculiar to the pediatric age group but also a thorough understanding of developmental aspects of renal physiology. In this chapter no attempt is made to present an exhaustive review of pediatric nephrology. Following a brief review of developmental renal physiology, clinical evaluation of the pediatric patient is presented and disorders of the kidney are discussed, with particular emphasis on those aspects in infants and children that differ from the disorders in adults, as discussed elsewhere in this volume.

Developmental Physiology

The role of the fetal kidney and its contribution to the maintenance of body homeostasis in the fetus remain speculative. The contribution of fetal urine to the formation of amniotic fluid is evidenced by the state of oligohydramnios that inevitably accompanies renal agenesis [20, 21, 37, 390]. However, body composition of the fetus does not appear to be affected by renal agenesis, showing that the placenta can, and under normal circumstances probably does, assume responsibility for excretory and regulatory functions in utero. Although it has been shown in a variety of mammals that the fetal kidney is capable of performing a number of functions, including urinary dilution, reabsorption of phosphate, acidification, and transport of organic materials [7–9, 54, 74, 333, 336, 339, 367, 445, 475, 506], it appears likely that these functions proceed incidentally to the welfare of the developing fetus and simply represent the prenatal expression of the renal functional capacity that increases rapidly from the moment of birth. The rapid onset of renal function postnatally in the youngest viable premature infant attests to the functional capacity of the fetus.

Renal blood flow and glomerular filtration rate in the fetus are maintained at low levels [7, 9, 54, 445]. In the first few days after birth, a striking increase in these functions is observed, followed by a progressive rise over the subsequent weeks and months, mature levels being achieved toward the end of the first year of life [7, 25, 29, 30, 105, 333, 341, 441, 487, 513, 525].

The similarity between the structure of the

fetal glomerulus and the alveolar wall was pointed out by Clara [91] in 1936. These observations were extended by Jäykkä [254], who suggested that in the fetus the turgid cells of the juxtaglomerular apparatus in the walls of the afferent arterioles may obstruct the flow of blood into the glomeruli. He observed that following birth these cells disappear, permitting the arterioles to open up, presumably allowing for an increased flow of blood through the kidney. These observations were extended in 1966 by Naeye [365], who measured arteriolar wall-to-lumen ratios and demonstrated that subsequent to birth a progressive vasodilatation of the renal vessels occurs.

Studies in piglets [204] have demonstrated that the marked increase in renal blood flow observed during the first six weeks of life results from an increase in both cardiac output and fractional blood flow to the kidney, providing further evidence for decreasing vascular resistance in the kidney during this period. However, cardiac index in the human neonate is virtually at adult levels [179], making it almost certain that changes in renal arteriolar resistance account for the large increases in renal blood flow and glomerular filtration rate during the transition from fetal to extrauterine life, and the subsequent progression to mature levels. It should be emphasized, however, that the control mechanism (or mechanisms) for these changes remains entirely unknown.

STRUCTURAL AND FUNCTIONAL GLOMERULOTUBULAR RELATIONSHIPS

Following the demonstration that glomerular filtration rates (GFR) in infants are well below those observed in adults [25], limitations in various tubular functions have been ascribed generally as secondary to the low rates of glomerular filtration. Many explanations have been offered for the low GFR in the infant, including inadequate systemic arterial pressure for filtration, an insufficient number or small size of glomeruli, and a poorly permeable glomerular epithelial lining [477]. Each of these possibilities may play some role, but together they are insufficient to account for the low filtration rates that are observed [138]. Changes in blood pressure during the first year of life are small compared to the large increase in filtration rate. In the human, formation of new glomeruli ceases when the fetus weighs between 2100 and 2500 gm. [392], and from their earliest formation, all glomeruli have functional afferent and efferent arterioles [391]. At term, the glomerular surface area available for filtration is more than adequate quantitatively to permit a higher filtration rate [138, 160]. The cuboidal epithelium of the glomerular membrane cannot be considered to limit filtration [14, 508], since, as pointed out by McCance [333], some time before the end of gestation higher filtration rates are observed, despite the presence of columnar epithelium covering the glomerular tufts [9, 54].

As early as 1948, West et al. [525] suggested that renal blood flow appeared to increase in proportion to the development of the renal tubules and that in early infancy there were functional imbalances between glomeruli and tubules in favor of the former. In a review of this subject in 1966, Edelmann [138] suggested that the rate of development of tubular functions sets the pace for overall renal maturation and that the low rates of glomerular filtration in early infancy are the consequence of tubular immaturity.

The human kidney at term contains approximately one million nephrons [392]. Since the glomerular filtration rate during the first few weeks of life is approximately 6 to 7 ml. per minute (uncorrected for body size) and by the end of the first year usually is no higher than 30 ml. per minute, it is apparent that the glomerular filtration rate per nephron is low during this entire period. Furthermore, glomerular filtration rate per gram of kidney is low in the newborn infant and reaches levels observed in the adult only after six to nine months [138, 441], indicating relative as well as absolute changes during this period. In considering the glomerular filtration rate per nephron, however, one must take into account the size of the nephron or the magnitude of tubular mass per nephron. Measurements of filtration rate and tubular size have not been made in the same subjects. However, the data of Fetterman et al. [160] indicate that proximal tubular volume in the term infant is one-tenth that of the adult, whereas the filtration rate is about one-twentieth that of the adult, confirming the presence of a filtration rate per nephron that is low even relative to the small size of the tubule.

Despite this low filtration rate per nephron, functional data in the infant indicate glomerular preponderance, suggesting, therefore, that there may be significant tubular immaturity out of proportion to tubular size. High ratios of glomerular filtration rate to Tm_G [501] and to Tm_{PAH} [31, 525] have been found in young infants, supporting the concept that the rate of filtration is excessive relative to tubular functional capacity.

Simultaneous measurements during infancy of glomerular filtration rate, based on the clearance of inulin or mannitol, and effective renal plasma flow (ERPF), based on the clearance of para-aminohippurate (PAH) or diodone, have revealed values of filtration fraction (GFR/ERPF) ranging from 0.32 to 0.34 [31, 71, 105, 441, 513, 525], as compared to the range of values from 0.19 to 0.20 in adult man. These data appear to provide additional evidence for glomerular preponderance during this period. However, in 1963 Calcagno and Rubin [71] found that the renal extraction of PAH during the first three months of life ranged from 0.5 to 0.8, on the average 30 per cent below the average adult value of 0.95. Recalculation of the ratio of glomerular filtration rate to renal plasma flow in these young infants resulted in a mean filtration fraction of 0.23, a value only slightly higher than that observed in adults. The authors presumed that the decreased extraction of PAH was due to a decrease in tubular mass or tubular function. However, examination of their data indicates that the extractions they measured were independent of the plasma concentrations of PAH, suggesting that the low values were not the result of tubular saturation but a consequence of a portion of the blood not perfusing the proximal tubules of the cortex. This interpretation is consistent with the observation that the medullary and juxtamedullary circulation develops at a more rapid rate than that of the outer cortical nephrons [310, 477]. Additional evidence in favor of this conclusion is the work of Barger [23] and his associates, who did silicone-rubber injection studies in young puppies. The earliest renal filling was in the juxtamedullary cortex and developing vasa recta; their findings were interpreted as evidence for increased vascular resistance in the outer cortex in early life. Since the clearance of inulin provides an estimate of combined cortical and juxtamedullary glomerular filtration and the clearance of PAH likely reflects cortical blood flow, it is not possible in the infant to use the ratio of these two clearances as an index of the balance between glomerular and tubular functions.

The available functional data suggest that immaturity of renal function is characterized by glomerulotubular imbalance, glomerular preponderance, and decreased fractional reabsorption in the proximal tubule. The renal threshold for bicarbonate is depressed in both premature and full-term infants [137, 502]. Although glucose reabsorption has not been studied extensively in the infant, the maximal rate of reabsorption is low [501]. Glucose titration curves have not been done in infants, but it might be anticipated that a low threshold and considerable splay of the titration curve would be demonstrable. Although there is a limited response to saline loading [106, 108, 333, 337, 339], owing to the low rates of glomerular filtration, it is not known whether infants have the capacity to conserve sodium during periods of severe deprivation. It has recently been shown that infants excrete a higher percentage of their filtered load of amino acids than do older children and adults [61]. Similarly, the rate of tubular reabsorption of phosphate is low [107, 347, 405].

These data indicating a high rate of glomerular filtration relative to tubular functional capacity are reminiscent of the findings in human and experimental renal disease, in which it has been shown that there is a high filtration rate per nephron and glomerular preponderance [58]. Although it may be distasteful to some developmentalists, it is tempting to consider the possibility that the functional pattern of the neonatal kidney may be determined, at least in part, by a similar state of glomerulotubular imbalance [57, 397, 405, 406, 418, 456, 463, 471].

Fetterman and his associates [160] have approached this problem morphologically in a study of the growth of glomeruli and proximal convolutions, using the technic of microdissection. They demonstrated that although neither glomerular nor tubular size approach that of the adult until several years of age, the ratio of glomerular surface area to proximal tubular volume, used as an index of anatomic balance, is extremely high at birth, falls rapidly during the first year of life, and then levels off or continues to decline slowly thereafter. These anatomic data suggest striking glomerular preponderance during the first year of life.

In addition, these workers [160] have shown that the anatomic structure of the kidney of the infant reveals a degree of heterogeneity that is far in excess of that observed in later life. Heterogeneity of structure has been considered to play a major role in the functional disturbances of the diseased kidney [376], and it may contribute to the functional pattern of the neonatal kidney as well [138].

RENAL CONTROL MECHANISMS

Osmolality of Extracellular Fluid: Concentration and Dilution of the Urine. Within a few days of birth, the diuretic response of the infant is prompt and comparable to the adult with respect to the degree of urinary dilution [11, 35, 72, 128, 334], indicating that even the very young infant is able to transport sodium adequately in the diluting segment of the nephron. In most instances, however, the rate of urine flow lags far behind that of older subjects [11, 35, 128]. Nevertheless, if one examines the response in terms of rate of urine flow or production of free water per 100 ml. of glomerular filtrate, values in the infant exceed those in the adult. This observation indicates that in the infant fractional reabsorption in the proximal tubule is less than that in the adult, at least under the conditions of volume expansion with water. It also fits well with the concept previously presented of a high glomerular filtration rate relative to proximal tubular functional capacity.

In view of the fact that in the infant juxtamedullary and medullary structures are more highly developed than those of the cortex, it is not surprising that despite a relatively high rate of delivery of fluid to the loop and distal tubule, diluting capacity is comparable to that observed in the adult. Nevertheless, the young animal ceases to excrete water at an accelerated rate before the entire load of water has been voided [11, 334, 338], suggesting a degree of immaturity of this control mechanism. In combination with the fact that the absolute rate of water excretion is low, this renders the infant more vulnerable than older subjects to the injudicious administration of water.

Following water deprivation, young infants generally fail to concentrate their urine to levels commonly observed in older children and adults [72, 122, 128, 130, 132, 215, 338, 473]. In view of their small nephrons and the importance of the length of the loop of Henle in the concentrating mechanism, this observation is not surprising [128]. It has been shown, however, that a major portion of the limitation in concentrating capacity in the infant results from the low rate of excretion of urea due to the strongly anabolic state that prevails during that period of life [122, 130, 132]. When the rate of excretion of urea is increased by feeding urea or high-protein diets, significant increases in concentrating capacity are observed [122, 130, 132].

The studies of Heller in newborn rats [223] and in humans [225] and those of Dickers and Tyler [114] in dogs and puppies suggested no limitation in availability of antidiuretic hormone in the neonate. Heller and Lederis [224] subsequently found less vasopressor and oxytocic activities in the pituitary glands of young rats, but they confirmed the previous findings in human infants. This question has been reopened by Janovský et al. [252], who were able to detect antidiuretic activity in the plasma following administration of hypertonic saline only in infants more than 3½ months of age.

Yunibhand and Held [539, 540] have shown that the pattern of change in urea, sodium, and water content in the renal medulla of 45-day-old albino rats during prolonged water deprivation is similar to maturational changes that occur in rats during the first few weeks of life. This suggests that continued exposure to the stimulus of antidiuretic hormone may play an important role in normal development. If so, the suggestion by Janovský and his associates [252] that antidiuretic hormone may be limited in infants before 3½ months of age takes on added significance.

The degree of permeability to water achieved by the nephron of the neonate in response to antidiuretic hormone (ADH) is unresolved. Edelmann and his associates [132] suggested that the response to the hormone was intact. However, Martínek et al. [329] concluded that resistance to ADH is demonstrable in young infants. During mannitol osmotic diuresis, urines hypotonic to plasma may be observed in young infants [127], suggesting incomplete equilibration of the tubular fluid with the interstitium, due either to a difference in the characteristics of the distal or collecting tubules, or both, or to an impaired response to ADH.

Thus, concentrating performance in the neonate and young infant is limited principally by the metabolically low rate of excretion of urea; concentrating capacity is limited moderately by the shortness of the loop of Henle, and possibly by a limitation in the availability of, or the responsiveness of the distal and collecting tubule to, antidiuretic hormone, or both. A further possibility, thus far not tested, is a limitation in the capacity of the cells to pump sodium against a gradient. The ability of the infant of only a few days of age to produce a urine of low osmolality in response to water loading, as discussed above, renders the latter possibility unlikely.

Volume of Extracellular Fluid: Renal Excretion and Conservation of Sodium. Infants and other young animals switched abruptly to a milk rich in sodium content have been shown to gain weight and become edematous [165, 190, 337]. However, when piglets are acutely volume-expanded by giving them a load of isotonic sodium chloride, fractional sodium excretion reaches levels similar to those observed in adult animals — that is, 15 per cent or more of the filtered load is excreted in the urine [135]. Thus, although the low glomerular filtration rates of this period limit the absolute rate at which sodium can be excreted, the renal response to a large degree of volume expansion is vigorous.

Recent data suggest that renal control of sodium excretion is influenced markedly by changes in vascular volume apparently mediated by hormonal or hemodynamic factors (or both) [57]. It is of interest in this regard that the extracellular volume of the newborn infant constitutes 45 per cent of body weight as compared to the value in adults of 18 per cent [168]. This may indicate that the renal control mechanisms for sodium in the infant reflect a state of immaturity in responding only to large changes in volume.

Infants fed diets providing a wide range of

intake of electrolytes do well, indicating considerable capacity for renal adjustment to variation in sodium intake. In a study by Staninсová and her associates [483], infants three to five months of age were fed human milk, providing 1 mEq. of sodium per kilogram of body weight, or a cow's milk formula, providing 3 mEq. of sodium per kilogram of body weight. The clearance of sodium in the group of infants receiving human milk was 0.098 ml. per minute. Infants receiving cow's milk had a clearance of sodium of 0.286 ml. per minute. These observations suggest that a control mechanism for sodium balance is functional in the infant and that an appropriate sodium balance is maintained by renal adjustment of the percentage of the filtered sodium that is reabsorbed.

Nevertheless, infants fed diets with a high sodium content appear to develop a significant expansion of their extracellular compartment, as compared with infants fed diets with lower sodium content [256]. This might mean that infants come into balance during periods of increased sodium intake only after a significant expansion of the extracellular volume has ensued. Janovský and his associates [253] did daily balance studies in six infants switched from a milk containing 7 mEq. of sodium per liter to a milk containing 137 mEq. of sodium per liter. Each infant demonstrated a marked increase in the rate of excretion and the clearance of sodium during the first 24 hours of high sodium intake, the clearance of sodium ranging from 0.51 to 2.62 ml. per minute in four infants two weeks of age and from 0.59 to 1.35 ml. per minute in two infants seven weeks of age. Even if the expansion of extracellular volume were accompanied by an increase in GFR, there must have been a significant increase in fractional excretion. If one assumes a filtration rate in the two-week-old infants of 8 ml. per minute, their fractional excretion of sodium during the first 24 hours of high salt intake ranged from 5 to 15 per cent, as compared with excretion of 0.5 to 1.0 per cent of the filtered sodium on the preceding control day. Although the change may not have been related entirely to the effects of volume expansion, since each infant had an increase in the concentration of sodium in serum, the data do suggest that the infant demonstrates little or no delay in his response to an increased intake of sodium. This does not imply, of course, that the same control mechanisms that are active in older children and adults are operative in infants. It should be noted that in infants, as in older patients with renal insufficiency, the low filtration rate imposes the requirement that in order to maintain sodium balance during intake of an increased amount of sodium, a high fractional excretion must be attained [471].

If it is true that the nephron in the immature kidney is overperfused, with decreased fractional reabsorption in the proximal tubule, as discussed above, one might anticipate a limited capacity to produce a urine low in sodium content in response to sodium deprivation. On the other hand, the relatively greater level of function of the juxtamedullary nephrons, with their long loops of Henle, might be expected to increase the capacity for tubular conservation of sodium. In support of this are studies demonstrating a relatively large capacity for production of free water [11, 35, 72, 135, 334]. No firm data are available concerning the response of infants or other young animals to severe restriction beyond the first few days of life, although preliminary data in our laboratory on young puppies suggests no limitation.

Hydrogen Ion Balance: Renal Reabsorption of Bicarbonate and Excretion of Hydrogen Ion. The observation that infants maintain a lower pH and concentration of bicarbonate in blood has focused attention on the capacity of the kidney to excrete hydrogen ion. During the first few days of life infants do not excrete strongly acid urines [339]. After the first week or two, however, their capacity to acidify the urine is comparable to that observed in older children and adults [138, 196].

Very young infants, puppies, and piglets excrete little phosphate in their urine and therefore are limited in their capacity to excrete titratable acid, despite imposition of an acid load [100, 164, 221, 339, 442]. If given additional phosphate, the excretion of titratable acid increases [229].

During the first few weeks of life, infants excrete significantly less ammonium in their urine in response to administration of ammonium chloride or calcium chloride than do older children, when compared on the basis of body surface area [196, 221]. When compared on the basis of glomerular filtration rate, however, no differences are found between young infants and older children. After one month of age, infants fed cow's milk formulas excrete hydrogen ion in response to ammonium chloride at a rate comparable to that observed in older children [137]. Due to their high rates of excretion of phosphate, their rate of excretion of titratable acid is greater than that in older children, whereas their rate of excretion of ammonium continues to be somewhat lower. These data, plus the recent demonstration that infants are in negative balance for hydrogen ion, render it unlikely that infants maintain a lower blood bicarbonate and pH due to a limitation in the capacity to excrete hydrogen ion.

Investigation of bicarbonate excretion in young infants has demonstrated a renal threshold for bicarbonate that is significantly lower than that found in adults [137, 502]. Thus it appears likely that the "physiologic acidosis" of infants is related to the level of the renal bicarbonate threshold. Presently there is no explanation for the low renal threshold during infancy, but it may be related to nephron heterogeneity, a difference in the kinetics of bicarbonate reabsorption during this period, or a low fractional reabsorption of sodium in the proximal tubule [137, 397]. The similarity to patients with renal disease has been discussed above.

MECHANISMS CONTROLLING RENAL GROWTH AND MATURATION

The concept of alteration in structure and function to meet the needs of the organism is not a new one [197]. In utero, when the kidney does not need to function as an excretory or regulatory organ, renal blood flow, glomerular filtration, and tubular functions all are at low levels. Immediately following birth the kidney must replace the placenta as the organ primarily responsible for maintenance of homeostasis. The abrupt increase in renal blood flow and filtration rate following birth is evidence of the kidney's assumption of this role. Barnett and his associates [29] concluded from a study of premature infants of different postgestational age but similar weight that the duration of extrauterine life may be a more important factor than body size in determining the level of renal function.

Noting that premature infants fed a high protein intake for four weeks were shown to have approximately twice the level of Tm_{PAH}, as compared with infants fed low-protein diets [68], Edelmann and Wolfish [139] postulated that the magnitude of the work load imposed upon the kidney by diet might be a major factor in determining the rate of renal maturation after birth. Infants fed high-protein, high-solute diets from birth were compared with infants fed low-protein, low-solute diets. After four weeks the clearances of inulin and PAH and the capacity to excrete hydrogen ion were approximately double in the first group [139].

What common features, if any, are shared by renal growth induced by maturational demands for increased function, on the one hand, and the hypertrophy that occurs in the contralateral kidney following unilateral nephrectomy or in the residual nephrons in the chronically diseased kidney, on the other hand, is not known. The degree of compensatory renal hypertrophy following unilateral nephrectomy in rats and puppies has been shown to become less and less with advancing age [250, 323], suggesting a dependence upon normal growth mechanisms. Similarly, renal hypertrophy in chickens induced by dietary loads of sodium chloride has been found to be most marked in animals undergoing rapid growth [275]. In this regard it is of interest that both the study of Calcagno and Lowe [68] and that of Edelmann and Wolfish [139] involved rapidly maturing premature infants. The effect of diet could not be reproduced in full-term infants [68].

COMMENTS

In infancy the low glomerular filtration rate and limitation in tubular functions limit the maximal response of the kidney under conditions of stress. For example, although the response to salt or water loading or to acidosis may be qualitatively normal, the quantitative response generally is less than that observed in older subjects, rendering the infant more vulnerable to the stresses imposed by disease or injudicious medical management, especially in the administration of electrolyte solutions and drugs [26].

It is of interest that in infancy the fact that the medullary region is more developed than the cortical permits the infant to withstand the stress of deprivation better than that of loading. Both anatomic and functional data are consistent with the existence of glomerulotubular imbalance and glomerular preponderance. This state renders it difficult for the infant to conserve substances such as glucose, amino acids, phosphate, and bicarbonate which are reabsorbed in the proximal tubule.

Nevertheless it is apparent from the sustained growth and well-being of the healthy infant, despite wide fluctuation in dietary intake, that control mechanisms responsible for maintenance of body homeostasis are operative. On the basis of studies in newborn rats, Oh and associates have commented on the "extraordinary capability of the neonatal kidneys for defense and regulation of body fluids," despite the limitations of immaturity [373]. Insufficient data are available to determine if these regulatory mechanisms are as finely tuned as in older children or adults or if the kidney requires greater stimuli to demonstrate a response.

McCance and his associates [330–333] emphasized the importance to the neonate of the process of growth in assisting the kidney in maintenance of homeostasis by reducing the excretory load imposed upon the kidney by the diet. In addition, the potential for growth and hypertrophy that is intrinsic to the kidney of the infant provides him, in defense of disease, with a reserve that is greater than that present at an older age.

Clinical Evaluation of Renal Function

Investigation of the pediatric patient for renal disease does not differ essentially from that of the adult, as described in Chapter 3. In this section some of the practical and technical problems in evaluating renal function in infants and small children are discussed and normal values for the pediatric age group are presented [32, 34, 242].

With sufficient patience and attention to technical details adequate urine specimens for chemical, microscopic, and bacteriologic examination can be obtained from even the smallest infant. Nurses experienced in working with children will be able to obtain midstream, clean-voided urine specimens from children as young as two to three years of age. In the child who is unable to void on request, a urine specimen is obtained by means of a plastic collector affixed after local cleansing of the perineum. Although results on specimens obtained by this technic are not as reliable as those from a midstream, clean-voided specimen, experience with thousands of infants and small children has proved this method to be entirely satisfactory, if meticulous care is given to the technic of cleansing. In subjects in whom it is not possible to obtain midstream, clean-voided urine specimens for bacteriologic examination, the technic of suprapubic aspiration of urine is useful. Application of this procedure to infants and children has been described by Pryles and his associates [396], Nelson and Peters [366], and Stamey and his co-workers [482].

Infants cannot be relied upon to empty their bladder completely with each voiding. Therefore, timed specimens obtained using this technic are open to serious question, except for the collection of 24-hour specimens in which, if the times of initial emptying and final voiding are accurately noted and recorded, the error becomes negligible.

Obtaining blood samples from infants and small children presents technical problems that are readily overcome with good instruction and experience. All clinical measurements of renal function utilizing classic clearance technics are applicable to infants and children. Important data should not be missed because of the difficulty in performing clearance measurements in small subjects. An indwelling needle secured in a superficial vein makes it possible to obtain multiple blood samples without repeated venipuncture. In infants and children too small to void voluntarily and frequently, the bladder is catheterized with a straight catheter of appropriate size. This is inserted so that the opening is just within the bladder. Bladder emptying is assured by suprapubic compression, both before and after installation of a few milliliters of air or saline. Since the rate of urine flow in infants is low, we have found it convenient to drain the catheter directly into chemically clean, sterile, graduated cylinders of appropriate size. Such short-term periods of catheterization have not induced infection *if meticulous aseptic technic is used*. The importance of a nurse to comfort and quiet an infant or toddler and the enormous distractive value of a television set for the older child cannot be overemphasized.

PROTEINURIA

Data concerning the rate of excretion of protein in healthy infants and children of various ages are not entirely adequate. It has been shown that the common finding in neonates of a positive reaction for protein may be due to the presence of urates and not protein [121]. Contamination with other substances, such as benzalkonium, also can cause falsely positive results [414]. In the examination of 500 newborn infants, we have found no proteinuria using a method adequate to detect 5 mg. of protein per 100 ml. Urine specimens collected from healthy children will, in the great majority of instances, have a negative or occasional trace reaction for protein, using either Albustix or 10% sulfosalicylic acid [167, 278, 398, 399). In most children with a positive result, a repeat examination will be negative. Subjects with persistently positive results must be considered abnormal. Since the rate of excretion of protein increases during ambulation, we have found it convenient to quantitate the rate of excretion on overnight timed collections. With this method we consider any value greater than 10 to 15 mg. per 12 hours as abnormal. This is in general agreement with the findings of Rigas and Heller [407], who examined 15 adults ranging in age from 24 to 30 years and found proteinuria ranging from 30.5 to 49.6 mg. per 24 hours. Lyttle [322] examined 161 12-hour urine specimens collected from 74 children aged 4 to 12 years; 106 specimens had 20 mg. or less of protein; only 13 specimens had greater than 35 mg. of protein per 12-hour urine sample.

URINARY SEDIMENT

In the healthy subject, routine examination of the sediment from 10 ml. of freshly voided urine, centrifuged for 5 to 10 minutes, usually reveals not more than 2 to 4 white blood cells per high power field and no red blood cells or casts. One or two red blood cells should be considered suspicious; more than that number is probably abnormal [533].

Houston [244] has shown that there is a poor concordance between the number of cells per high power field counted in the sediment of a centrifuged urine and the number of cells per cubic millimeter determined by use of a counting chamber. These results confirm the finding of previous investigators. Zero to ten white blood cells per cubic millimeter of urine is normal, 11 to 100 is probably abnormal, and more than 100 is definitely abnormal [243].

Although routine examination of a freshly voided urine specimen is adequate in most instances, the semiquantitative examination made possible by an Addis count is of considerable value in detecting minimal abnormalities. We see repeated instances of significantly abnormal Addis counts in children considered to have negative urines by routine examinations. Children excrete no more than 250,000 red blood cells per 12 hours, and usually less than half this number. The rate of excretion of white blood cells is approximately double that of red blood cells.

BACTERIURIA

Bacteriuria in infants and children can be evaluated by a variety of methods. The most immediate information can be obtained from examination of a freshly voided urine. Detection of bacteria in a gram-stain preparation of the uncentrifuged urine correlates with a bacterial count of over 10^5 organisms per milliliter. We have found it more useful to examine a gram-stained sediment from a centrifuged urine specimen. Urines containing in excess of 10^5 organisms per milliliter reveal either great numbers of organisms in every field or solid sheets of bacteria. Absent or occasional organisms indicate a count of less than 10^3. Scattered bacteria in every field examined indicates counts between 10^3 and 10^5. Cultural methods of quantitating bacteria, using calibrated loops or pipette dilutions of urine, are described in detail in Chapter 18.

It has been demonstrated by Kunin and his associates [277, 278] that bacteriuria is almost nonexistent in healthy school boys, but has a prevalence rate in school girls of 1.1 per cent. Randolph and Greenfield [398] reported bacteriuria in 4.5 per cent of female and 0.5 per cent of male infants from birth to 24 months of age. Although positive results were confirmed by repeated examination, urine collections were made using a sterile-bag technic and the details of cleansing were not given, raising the possibility of false-positive results. Nevertheless, urologic examination of 7 of the 10 infants found to have persistent bacteriuria revealed abnormalities in all but one.

Several studies have suggested a frequency of bacteriuria in the newborn infant ranging as high as 24 per cent [1, 51, 306, 307, 342]. In a recent survey of 836 newborn infants in our unit, repeated examinations revealed more than 10^5 organisms per milliliter of urine in less than 1 per cent, with an even distribution between males and females. The difference in this study from previous reports is attributed to the attention paid to cleansing of the perineum and genitalia prior to application of the collection bag and the confirmation of positive results by examination of urines obtained by suprapubic puncture. Recently, O'Brien and his associates [371] found only one infant with bacteriuria in 1000 neonates examined.

GLOMERULAR FILTRATION RATE

As estimated from the clearance of inulin, the rate of glomerular filtration in children aged 2 to 12 years is 127 ± 19* ml. per minute per 1.73 square meters of body surface area. In the first few days of life, GFR in full-term infants may be as low as 25 to 30 ml. per minute; it usually reaches values of 50 to 60 ml. per minute by several weeks of age, from

* Normal values are given as the mean (± standard deviation) calculated from data from this laboratory and from the literature.

which point it gradually increases to mature levels over the course of the subsequent months.*

Although each has its limitations, both urea and creatinine clearances provide reasonable estimates of GFR (see page 107). At rates of urine flow above 2 ml. per minute per 1.73 square meters, approximately 60 per cent of filtered urea is excreted. Since the portion excreted falls unpredictably when the rate of urine flow falls below 2 ml. per minute, it is essential to maintain rates above this level throughout the study. On the assumption that the clearance of urea represents 60 per cent of the GFR, normal values for subjects of various ages can be obtained from the values given for inulin clearance. The rate of urea clearance in children two years of age and older is 75 ml. per minute per 1.73 square meters of body surface area, with 55 to 60 ml. per minute usually taken as the lower limit of normal.

Creatinine clearance has the advantage of being much less dependent on the rate of urine flow. Clearances can be performed, therefore, on 12-hour or 24-hour urine specimens, minimizing collection and timing errors. Although the normal values given in the literature vary enormously, depending mainly upon the analytical methods employed, it may be assumed that creatinine clearance is equal to or somewhat greater than the true GFR (see page 37). In chronic renal disease, when the filtration rate has fallen to 25 ml. per minute or below, the marked increase in filtration rate per nephron results in the urea and creatinine clearances coming closer and closer to the inulin clearance.

We have confirmed in children the finding of Lubowitz and his associates in adults [318] that in subjects with advanced renal disease, one-half the sum of the urea and creatinine clearances provides an accurate estimate of the glomerular filtration rate, as determined by the clearance of inulin.

CONCENTRATING CAPACITY

If the Addis count specimen is collected during water deprivation, an estimate of concentrating capacity may be obtained. The child is instructed to have no fluids after 1 P.M. on the day the collection is begun, and to withhold fluids until the collection is completed. On very hot days, minimal fluids in the form of ice may be permitted. Starting in the evening, urine is collected as a single overnight specimen of 8 to 12 hours' duration. Under these conditions urinary osmolality in healthy children 2 to 16 years of age averages 1089 mOsm per kilogram of water with a lower limit of 870 mOsm [131]. Data in children under two years are limited, and it may be difficult and undesirable to withhold fluids completely in such subjects. Infants between three months and two years should be able to achieve a urine osmolality of 800 mOsm per kilogram. During the period one week to three months, an osmolality of 700 or more is expected [32, 34, 388, 531].

URINARY ACIDIFICATION AND EXCRETION OF HYDROGEN ION

The simplest way to assess renal acidifying mechanisms is with the short ammonium chloride loading test [133, 137]. A sufficient dose of ammonium chloride is given by mouth over the course of an hour to lower the plasma bicarbonate several millimoles per liter. Two 60-minute urine collections are made three to five hours after administration of the ammonium chloride, and a sample for blood pH, carbon dioxide tension, and total carbon dioxide content is obtained at the midpoint. Table 42-1 gives the normal values in healthy infants and children. If the urinary pH fails to fall to the expected level, the possibility of a low

* The following values, expressed as milliliters per minute per 1.73 square meters of body surface area, have been compiled: 2 to 8 days, 38 ± 11 ml. per minute; 4 to 28 days, 48 ± 10 ml. per minute; 37 to 95 days, 58 ± 14 ml. per minute; 1 to 5.9 months, 77 ± 18 ml. per minute; 6 to 11.9 months, 103 ± 27 ml. per minute; and 12 to 19 months, 127 ± 32 ml. per minute.

Table 42-1. Excretion of Hydrogen Ion in Response to Acute Administration of Ammonium Chloride

Subject	Urine pH	Titratable Acid (μEq./min./1.73 m^2)	Ammonium (μEq./min./1.73 m^2)
Infants during first year of life	≦5.0	62 (43–111)	57 (42–79)
Children 3 to 15 years old	≦5.5	52 (33–71)	73 (46–100)

bicarbonate threshold must be considered. An additional dose of ammonium chloride may be needed to rule out this possibility [133].

Similar data have been obtained with a three- to five-day ammonium chloride loading test by Gordon et al. [196], Fomon et al. [164], and Peonides [381]. Lestradet and his associates [296] studied hydrogen ion excretion following intravenous administration of arginine hydrochloride, and Rubin et al. [442] observed the effects of orally administered calcium chloride.

RENAL BIOPSY

The importance of histologic, histochemical, and immunochemical examinations of tissue obtained by biopsy is discussed in Chapter 5. The fact that performance of percutaneous needle biopsy in infants and children is technically more difficult than in adults should not be used as a reason for not performing a biopsy when indicated. We have been able to biopsy successfully even the smallest of infants, utilizing direct visualization of the kidney with an image-intensifier fluoroscope [136]. With this technic, success can be anticipated in 99 per cent of attempts.

Renal Failure

The pathophysiology, clinical problems, and principles of treatment of acute and chronic renal failure are basically similar in infants, children, and adults. For a detailed discussion of these conditions the reader is referred to Chapters 15–17. The emphasis here is on certain points of particular significance with regard to the pediatric patient.

ACUTE RENAL FAILURE

Acute renal failure is a relatively uncommon condition in the pediatric age group if one considers only true renal failure due to renal parenchymal disease. However, the categories of prerenal, renal, and postrenal failure apply to infants and children as well as to adults. Considered in this broader sense renal failure becomes much more common, due primarily to the frequency of prerenal failure in infants and small children with dehydration secondary to gastroenteritis and other diseases. Thus, in a sixteen-month period in Athens, Greece, Doxiadis [120] observed 47 infants who presented with blood urea levels between 50 and 500 mg. per 100 ml. Only four had true renal failure, which may have been prerenal at the onset.

Obstructive uropathy, a rare cause of acute renal failure in older infants and children, must be considered strongly in the anuric newborn infant.

The most frequent causes of true renal failure in children are diffuse parenchymal diseases such as acute glomerulonephritis (page 1366) and the hemolytic-uremic syndrome (page 1373). Acute cortical and tubular necroses, probably the most common causes of acute renal failure in adults, are observed in the pediatric age group, but not commonly [44, 56, 76, 78, 80, 147, 400, 413, 495]. Most cases have been reported in the newborn infant, and are attributed to obstetrical complications, asphyxia, erythroblastosis, sepsis, dehydration, and hemorrhage. Six infants with bilateral hemorrhagic necrosis of the renal pyramids, not associated with renal vein thrombosis, were reported by Thomas [495]. The lesion was attributed to prolonged labor and anoxia. Scattered reports of renal cortical and medullary necrosis in older infants and children have been attributed to the usual factors, including circulatory collapse, infection, nephrotoxins, vascular disease, burns, and transfusion reactions.

Treatment of acute renal failure in children is identical with that in adults [182, 239, 261]. The technical difficulty encountered in infants and small children in measuring intake and output makes the accurate recording of daily weight extremely important.

Water intake is limited to 200 to 300 ml. per square meter of body surface area per day, plus replacement of urinary output. A weight loss of 0.5 per cent per day indicates an appropriate water balance. Urinary sodium excretion is replaced with sodium bicarbonate. Serious hyperkaliuria usually can be avoided by eliminating the intake of potassium. If the serum potassium rises above 6 mEq. per liter or if the electrocardiogram shows changes indicating potassium excess, therapy with a cation-exchange resin (Kayexalate) is given in a dose of 1 gm. per kilogram of body weight per day.

Attempts should be made to maintain good nutrition, through the use of nonprotein, electrolyte-free foods, although this is almost an impossible task in the face of severe renal failure. If that state is prolonged, nutrition can be maintained only in association with dialysis.

Dialytic therapy can be done, when indicated, even in the smallest infant, in whom peritoneal dialysis is usually the method of choice. Further details concerning peritoneal and extracorporeal dialysis are given below.

The prognosis in acute renal failure depends in large part on the underlying etiology. It is our impression that the recovery rate from acute renal failure in general is better in children than in adults. For example, during the course of acute glomerulonephritis a period of severe oliguria of more than two or three days' duration is an ominous prognostic sign in the adult. In contrast, it is not uncommon for a child to have restoration of a significant level of renal function following severe oliguria of several days' duration.

CHRONIC RENAL FAILURE

Chronic renal failure is encountered in the pediatric age group as a consequence of congenital abnormalities, other forms of obstructive uropathy, neurologic disease interfering with normal bladder function, various forms of progressive glomerulonephritis, and pyelonephritis.

Therapy of infants and children with chronic renal insufficiency, based on a thorough understanding of the pathophysiology of uremia, is extremely gratifying. Regulation of diet is a primary means of treating chronic uremia [40, 185, 394]. However, it is particularly important in children to avoid arbitrary and unnecessary restrictions. Every effort must be given to provide a palatable, well-balanced, nutritionally adequate diet. In patients with severe renal insufficiency, dietary protein is restricted initially to 0.3 to 0.5 gm. per kilogram per day. This allowance is then increased empirically, as tolerated. Although milk is a poor source of protein in advanced renal insufficiency, due to its high solute content, infants with renal insufficiency often do very well on "humanized milk" formulas with low concentrations of both electrolyte and protein. Of great importance is restriction of biologically poor vegetable protein. Animal protein should be utilized exclusively in providing the day's allowance. Experience is beginning to accumulate in the treatment of patients with advanced renal insufficiency (rates of glomerular filtration as low as 1 to 2 ml. per minute) with synthetic diets designed to maintain adequate nutritional intake with proteins of high biologic value and virtually no electrolytes. It should be noted that several authors have emphasized the failure of adults to adhere to strict, unpalatable dietary regimens [394]. The feasibility of these technics in children, particularly in combination with intermittent dialysis, presently is unknown. However, the principles underlying this type of therapy have been applied with success to infants and small children with lesser degrees of renal failure, using naturally available foods and special food products such as Resource Baking Mix* and Controlyte* for preparation of low-protein, low-sodium, low-potassium bread, cookies, milk shakes, and so forth.

Arbitrary restriction of dietary sodium is one of the most common errors in treatment of patients with renal disease. A low sodium intake may result in a negative sodium balance, depletion of extracellular volume, and deterioration of renal function. Until the terminal stages a normal sodium intake is usually well tolerated.

In mild degrees of renal insufficiency gastrointestinal symptoms usually respond well to restriction of dietary protein. Anorexia, nausea, and vomiting may become severe in the later stages of disease. Prochlorperazine (0.4 mg. per kilogram per 24 hours) and chlorpromazine (2 mg. per kilogram per 24 hours) given by mouth in three or four doses, may be very effective.

Mild degrees of acidosis usually respond to restriction of dietary protein. Severer degrees of acidosis can usually be controlled by administration of sodium bicarbonate or citrate, which are well tolerated until renal insufficiency is far advanced. Initial dosages of 1 to 3 mEq. per kilogram per day may be given, adjusting the dosage according to the response of the patient. Aluminum and magnesium hydroxide, used primarily to correct hyperphosphatemia, may also serve to correct acidosis. A dosage of 50 to 150 mg. per kilogram per day can be given.

If dietary restriction of sodium proves insufficient in the patient with persistent edema, diuretic therapy can be employed. Hydrochlorothiazide, 2 to 4 mg. per kilogram per day, is given, and spironolactone can be added in a dosage of 10 to 20 mg. per kilogram per day. Recent experience with furosemide in children suggests that it is currently the most useful diuretic. We have used it in a dose of 1 to 2 mg. per kilogram given orally once or twice a day.

Hyperkalemia is usually not a problem except in patients with very advanced disease or during decompensation associated with intercurrent illness. The addition of Kayexalate, in a starting dosage of 0.5 to 1.5 gm. per kilogram per day, will induce a negative potassium balance and bring serum levels into the normal range. Hypokalemia may develop from injudicious use of diuretic agents or as a consequence of anorexia, diarrhea, or vomiting. Correction is achieved by addition of a potassium supplement in a dosage of 3 to 5 mEq. per kilogram per day.

Hypocalcemia and bone disease are frequently encountered in children with renal insufficiency. Therapy includes provision of dietary supplements of calcium and administration of vitamin D. Calcium, usually given as calcium lactate, is administered in an amount calculated to provide 10 to 20 mg. of calcium per kilogram per day. Vitamin D, given initially in a dose of 10,000 to 20,000 units per day, is increased as needed to levels as high as several hundred thousand units per day.

As in adults, certain children appear to develop severe degrees of secondary hyperparathyroidism and the bony lesions of osteitis fibrosa. Parathyroidectomy has been carried out in a number of these children, with excellent results.

Control of hypertension is an important part of the therapy of chronic renal failure.

* D. M. Doyle Pharmaceutical Co., Minneapolis, Minn.

Reserpine is the safest and simplest antihypertensive agent available, and is given in a dosage of 0.01 to 0.03 mg. per kilogram per day in one or two divided doses. If ineffective, hydralazine can be added to the regimen in a starting dose of 1 to 2 mg. per kilogram per day, in four divided doses, increasing over a period of time to levels as high as 20 mg. per kilogram. If blood pressure has not returned to normal levels with those agents, guanethidine or alpha-methyldopa can be given, in starting dosages of 0.2 mg. per kilogram per day and 10 mg. per kilogram per day, respectively. Guanethidine is given as a single daily dose, alpha-methyldopa is divided into two or three doses daily.

Specific therapy of the anemia of chronic renal insufficiency is not available. Unless extremely severe, it is usually asymptomatic, so that transfusions should be given as infrequently as possible; if transfusions are required, packed cells should be given. The transfusion must be given slowly and with extreme caution, since severe hypertension may be noted in a child after administration of only a small amount of blood. For this reason, the simultaneous administration of blood and a potent diuretic, such as furosemide, has been proposed.

It is important to realize that the irritative neuromuscular phenomena commonly seen in children with chronic uremia are rarely due to hypocalcemia. Treatment is limited to sedation, which is nonspecific and usually unsatisfactory. The severe generalized itching that is occasionally observed in advanced uremia has recently been attributed to secondary hyperparathyroidism. Treatment is nonspecific although in some patients this symptom has been relieved after parathyroidectomy.

DIALYSIS

Peritoneal dialysis has been used frequently in the treatment of infants and children with acute renal failure and, to a much lesser degree, in patients with chronic renal failure [148, 149, 150, 156, 157, 257, 312, 327, 401, 460]. The procedure, technically simpler than hemodialysis, is tolerated even by small infants. The 2-liter exchanges commonly employed in adults are too large for children. In older children a 1-liter exchange is used. In younger children and infants 50 to 100 ml. per kilogram per exchange has been recommended. Commercially available catheters are suitable for use in children and are inserted after distending the abdomen by instillation through a No. 18 needle of a volume of fluid equal to one exchange. This permits positioning the catheter within the peritoneal cavity so that free return of fluid is obtained. Commercial dialysis fluid, with 5 mg. per liter of heparin, is used with or without added potassium.

Usually 1.5% glucose dialysis fluid is employed. If it is desired to remove additional fluid from the patient, a mixture of equal parts of 1.5 and 7.0% glucose may be employed. We have avoided the use of 7.0% glucose dialysis fluid alone, to avoid excessively rapid transfer of fluid.

Peritoneal urea clearances relatively greater than those obtained in adults have been reported in children. It has been suggested that this is due to greater permeability of the peritoneal membrane, or that the peritoneal surface area is greater relative to body size in children than in adults.

Dialysis can be maintained continuously for periods up to 72 hours or more, as needed clinically, with the risk of peritonitis increasing as the duration of dialysis is prolonged. In one child, whom we maintained with a single catheter for a period of more than three months, peritonitis did occur but was controlled with antibiotic therapy.

A major disadvantage of peritoneal dialysis is the large loss of protein in the peritoneal fluid. This may be particularly troublesome in patients being maintained chronically.

Adults with terminal renal failure have been maintained with chronic hemodialysis for periods of several years. Attempts at such therapy in children have been very limited and, in general, discouraging [13, 55, 82, 90, 161, 247, 258, 294]. In addition to the technical difficulties encountered in carrying out hemodialysis in small subjects, children are prone to frequent problems with cannulas and medical complications, and they often adjust poorly psychologically. Furthermore, hemodialysis in children often fails to restore appetite, good health, and general well-being, despite apparently adequate biochemical control. Hutchings et al. [247] reported on a 14-year-old girl who was maintained on chronic hemodialysis for a period of 18 months. She failed to grow normally and did not mature sexually. Schribner [457] has stated that an absolute contraindication to chronic dialysis is the child who has not achieved full growth and sexual maturation. However, some of the patients reported by Fine et al. [161, 162] have shown excellent growth. Nevertheless, the major role of hemodialysis in children appears to be in the treatment of acute renal failure and the support and preparation of patients prior to renal hemotransplantation.

The technics of hemodialysis in children are essentialy the same as in adults. Descriptions of technics applicable to the pediatric age group have been presented by Lee and Sharpstone [294], Chamberlain and his associates [82], Kallen and his co-workers [258], and Fine and his associates [161]. Maintenance of cannulas may be a serious problem in young children with small blood vessels. Recently, the technic of Brescia and his associates [55] of creating an arteriovenous fistula has been applied with success in the pediatric age group.

TRANSPLANTATION

As survival figures following renal homotransplantation steadily improve, this procedure more and more becomes the one of choice in the management of terminal renal failure [408]. This is particularly true for children in whom chronic dialysis as definitive therapy generally has been unsuccessful. Recent experience indicates that remarkably good results can be anticipated when the donor is a living relative, matched for histocompatibility antigens. Since children are likely to have healthy, young parents who are ideal subjects to serve as donors, transplantation may turn out to have its greatest success in the pediatric age group. In addition, children appear to develop less toxicity during immunosuppressive therapy, and they are likely to be free from diseases of other body systems.

Relatively few renal transplants have been performed in children, and most of these have been in teen-agers. However, transplantation has been attempted in the young infant and success has been achieved in very small children.

Renal Diseases in Infants and Children

The focus of the discussion in this section is on differences between renal diseases in infants and children and renal diseases in adults. Theoretically, such differences could be due to either occurrence of unique diseases in different age groups, unique responses of individuals of different ages to the same disease, or a combination of the two. Special attention is given here also to renal diseases of adults which may have their origin during childhood.

The most obvious unique renal diseases of childhood are those congenital anomalies, such as renal agenesis, which are incompatible with survival. However, there are other diseases that occur with much greater frequency, if not exclusively, during childhood — for example, the hemolytic-uremic syndrome as the sole manifestation of thrombotic microangiopathy is far more frequent in children than in adults [386]. The same is true for the idiopathic form (or forms) of the nephrotic syndrome and also for poststreptococcal glomerulonephritis, the age distribution of the latter being related probably to that of streptococcal infections.

It is generally believed that the immature kidney may respond uniquely to a given stimulus, and there is some experimental evidence in support of this concept. However, there is little if any firm clinical evidence for such unique responses. The response of the fetal kidney to ureteral obstruction may be one example [43]. The congenital form of the nephrotic syndrome was considered as an example of a unique response, but until more is known about the cause of any type of idiopathic nephrotic syndrome, it cannot be determined whether the congenital form represents a unique response or, as seems more likely, a unique disease. Similarly, there are speculations, but no firm evidence, concerning whether differences in prognosis in diseases such as acute glomerulonephritis and the idiopathic nephrotic syndrome in children and adults are due to differences in responses or in disease. Finally, the reported increased severity of renal involvement in children with disseminated lupus erythematosus may represent a unique renal response [351].

The ultimate goal in the study of renal diseases is their prevention, which requires knowledge about their origins. There are many important examples of renal diseases of adults which have their origin in childhood. In some of these, early detection can lead either to therapeutic cures or to prevention of secondary renal damage. For example, there are few instances in all of clinical medicine where early diagnosis and proper treatment is more effective in preventing what may be a fatal disease than in the case of the child with correctable obstructive uropathy.

In several renal diseases of unknown origin in adults, it has been suspected that the disease may have begun during childhood. In many of these cases, however, including the controversial question of the origin of chronic glomerulonephritis [27], firm evidence for such a relationship is lacking.

In the following sections most of the renal diseases that occur in children are discussed. There are three important subjects — congenital malformations, urinary tract infections, and urolithiasis — which are covered thoroughly elsewhere in this volume and are therefore not included in this chapter.

ACUTE GLOMERULONEPHRITIS

Careful examination of epidemiologic and laboratory evidence and of clinical experience indicates that, except for an apparent quantitative difference in prognosis, acute glomerulonephritis in children does not differ importantly from the disease in adults [66, 104, 116, 117, 163, 170, 199, 228, 255, 301, 346, 383, 443, 484, 511].

Pathogenesis. There is no evidence that the pathogenesis and especially the relationship with nephritogenic strains of group A beta-hemolytic streptococci is different in children from that in adults. Although not documented to our knowledge, the frequency of streptococcal infections in sites other than the pharynx, and especially of the skin [49], may be higher in children than in adults, but, contrary to an earlier view, the site and type of streptococcal infection does not appear to influence the incidence or severity of acute glomerulonephritis.

It is not possible to state with any reliable supporting evidence whether glomerulonephritis following infections not of hemolytic streptococcal origin occurs more or less frequently in children than in adults. Inferences may be made, however, from data on the epidemiology of some of the other infections associated with acute glomerulonephritis. The diffuse type of glomerulonephritis found in patients with subacute bacterial endocarditis (page 439) is probably more common in adults than in children, whereas glomerulonephritis associated with viral infections, especially the common exanthematous diseases such as varicella, undoubtedly occur more frequently in children [299, 538].

Renal Pathology. The renal lesion of acute glomerulonephritis in children differs in no way from that observed in adults [116, 117, 199, 299, 511]. Examination of both biopsy and autopsy specimens from patients with glomerulonephritis by light and electron microscopy as well as with immunofluorescent technics have revealed no age-related features.

Clinical Aspects. The clinical aspects of acute glomerulonephritis in children are very similar to those in adults. In fact, most descriptions of the clinical aspects are based largely on observations made on patients having the disease during childhood and adolescence, since most of the cases occur during these periods.

Epidemiology. Systematic examination of the urine of children recovering from streptococcal infections has provided clinical evidence that many patients with acute glomerulonephritis are not diagnosed because they either are asymptomatic or have such mild symptoms that the disease is not suspected and the urine is not examined. The performance by Dodge and his co-workers [117] of percutaneous renal biopsies in family contacts of patients with acute glomerulonephritis has now confirmed the diagnosis in such children not suspected of having the disease. Although the proportion of patients whose disease may be undiagnosed cannot be estimated with any assurance, the figure is probably high enough that any epidemiologic studies must be interpreted with the knowledge that the population being described is the empirical one composed of recognized or manifest cases. Reports of patients with poststreptococcal glomerulonephritis with minimal or no urinary findings, which may be more frequent in children than adults, complicate epidemiologic analyses even further [5, 95, 246].

An analysis of the age of onset of clinically recognizable acute glomerulonephritis in 214 children during their first 12 years of life showed a peak incidence between 6 and 7 years, with about 60 per cent of cases occurring between 5 and 10 years and 95 per cent between 2 and 12 years of age [28]. Although it does occur, the disease is rare under one year of age, due probably to the low prevalence of streptococcal infections during this period. The high incidence during early school years may also be related to the high prevalence of streptococcal infections during that time.

Acute glomerulonephritis occurs more frequently in boys than in girls, the ratio being as high as 2:1 in some series. This difference in the frequency of the disease in the two sexes, which is unexplained, is also present in adults.

Clinical Features. With minor exceptions, the presenting features of acute glomerulonephritis in children are quite similar to those described for adults. The possibility of a child presenting with minimal urinary abnormalities should not be overlooked [5, 95, 246, 259]. Marked weakness, seen occasionally in adults as the outstanding symptom and persisting for several months after the acute attack, is rarely seen in children. On the other hand, acute abdominal pain is a rather frequent presenting symptom in children, although it is uncommon in adults. The occasional occurrence of mild hyperlipemia and hypoalbuminemia early and transiently in the course of acute glomerulonephritis in children has not, to our knowledge, been reported in adults.

Early recognition and prompt treatment of the early complications of acute glomerulonephritis — that is, hypertension, cardiac failure, and renal failure — are as imperative in children as in adults. In general the symptoms and general principles of treatment are similar in both age groups. A generalized convulsion as the presenting symptom of acute glomerulonephritis is not common at any age, but it is probably more frequent in children than in adults. Although hypertension may not be the sole cause for such convulsions, it is consistently present, and *detection of an elevated blood pressure may be the first evidence that an isolated convulsion in a child is due to acute glomerulonephritis.* In assessing the blood pressure it is important to appreciate the changing normal ranges in children of different ages.

The clinical manifestations of congestive cardiac failure and the pulmonary findings in children with acute glomerulonephritis are similar to those of adults [163]. The young child with acute renal failure has different metabolic requirements which, as discussed elsewhere, must be appreciated in assessing his clinical status.

Treatment. The principles both of the general treatment of children with acute glomerulonephritis and of the early complications are similar to those recommended for adults. Avoidance of prolonged restriction of dietary protein is especially important in the growing child; we recommend and urge no dietary alterations in children with acute glomerulonephritis after the early symptomatic period.

Because it is still recommended frequently, we are even more concerned with the avoidance of prolonged restriction of activity in asymptomatic children recovering from acute glomerulonephritis [255, 346]. Restricting activity until all laboratory findings have returned to normal involves, on the average, a period of three months if a normal sedimentation rate is required, and six months if disappearance of proteinuria and a normal urinary sediment as judged from Addis counts are used as criteria of recovery. At the upper range, use of these criteria for restricting activity may involve periods up to two or more years. Absence of evidence supporting the impression that prolonged bed rest has a favorable effect in asymptomatic patients with acute glomerulonephritis (page 447) and systematic observations revealing that early ambulation is beneficial are discussed elsewhere [255, 256]. In the developing child it is especially important to avoid unnecessary restriction of activity. We recommend that gradual resumption of full activity be permitted after the acute symptoms and signs have subsided. The great majority of our patients are back to full activity six to eight weeks after the onset of acute glomerulonephritis.

Prognosis. It is generally accepted that the overall prognosis of acute glomerulonephritis is better in children than in adults [104, 117, 135, 170, 199, 228, 255, 301, 346, 383], and possible explanations for this difference have been presented. Our own experience conforms with that of Herbert [228] that practically 100 per cent of those who survive the initial illness recover completely.

In the past the majority of deaths in both age groups, and especially in children, were due to extension of the preceding streptococcal infection, congestive heart failure, or hypertension with central nervous system complications. Death from these causes is now rare. In a prospective study of 362 children with acute glomerulonephritis [199], there were no deaths attributable to these complications. Early deaths are now caused almost exclusively by acute renal failure, which appears to be more frequent and more severe in adults than in children.

The proportion of patients who fail to heal following what appears clinically to be acute glomerulonephritis is generally estimated to range from 30 to 50 per cent in adults and from 0 to 10 per cent in children. These estimates, based previously on clinical data alone, must be reexamined to include the relationship between the clinical and the pathologic features of the disease [117, 135, 199, 411, 511]. Understanding the nature and course of the disease (or diseases) in these patients requires additional information on several important questions. The one that has been argued most extensively is whether acute glomerulonephritis in children is an antecedent of chronic nephritis in adults. Prospective studies have revealed complete healing in such a high proportion of children whose disease is recognized that a relationship with chronic nephritis in adults seems very unlikely. At least two possible situations could negate this suggestion. In the first place, acute glomerulonephritis in children whose clinical features are so mild that the disease is not recognized could, unlike the recognized form, lead to a latent disease first manifested as chronic nephritis of unknown cause in adults. Our experience and that of most [246], although not all [116], other pediatric nephrologists suggests that the severity of the clinical manifestations correlates with the severity of the pathologic change in the glomerulus and with the prognosis (see below). It seems unlikely, therefore, that complete healing would occur less frequently in children with the mildest clinical disease. In addition, in at least one investigation of the prevalence of abnormal Addis counts among apparently healthy adolescent boys, some of whom could be expected to have "latent" glomerulonephritis, the number with significant proteinuria or hematuria, or both, did not support the concept that unrecognized acute glomerulonephritis in children is a frequent antecedent of chronic nephritis in adults.

The preceding discussion does not exclude completely the second possibility — that is, what appears clinically to be complete healing may be associated histologically with pathologic processes which might lead to future disease after a long latent period. Persistent histologic alterations observed in renal biopsies of children who clinically have recovered completely provide tentative support for this concept [199]. Until much more evidence is at hand, however, it does not seem reasonable to assume that there is a relationship between acute glomerulonephritis in children and chronic nephritis of unknown cause in adults.

Another important unanswered question concerns the nature of the disease (or diseases) in children with apparent acute glomerulonephritis who *do* fail to heal [117, 135, 511]. Percutaneous renal biopsy has shown that some patients in these groups had preexisting glomerular disease, the proportion being lower in children than in adults. Such exacerbations of preexisting renal disease may follow streptococcal as well as other infections, which in itself does not establish the diagnosis of acute poststreptococcal glomerulonephritis.

Excluding these patients, there remains a very small number of patients with clinically typical acute glomerulonephritis who develop chronic renal disease. In our experience these children have had severe symptoms initially, with depressed renal function that, though it may improve, does not return to normal. They progress, therefore, from what appears to be acute glomerulonephritis directly to chronic renal insufficiency over a period of months or years. The nature of the disease (or diseases) in these children remains unclear. Renal biopsies in a large number of children with acute glomerulonephritis suggest that at least some of these children may have had so many glomeruli destroyed in the initial episode, that chronic renal insufficiency developed even though there was no continuing activity of the initial disease process [199, 246].

FOCAL GLOMERULONEPHRITIS

Focal glomerulonephritis (see Chapter 14) refers to conditions in which only some of the glomeruli reveal abnormalities in contrast to the diffuse involvement seen in most types of nephritis. This form of glomerular disease has been found in association with collagen diseases, may occur as a complication of bacteremia, and apparently may occur de novo [140, 227, 425, 523].

Focal glomerular lesions occur in patients during infection, particularly with bloodstream invasion by pathogenic organisms such as staphylococcus, gonococcus, and pneumococcus. These focal lesions result in urinary abnormalities, but they do not produce renal insufficiency. They are considered to be a manifestation of bacteremia and not a specific renal disease entity.

The lesions of periarteritis, systemic lupus erythematosus, and Henoch-Schönlein syndrome may be focally distributed. In addition, focal glomerulonephritis may be found on renal biopsy in patients with asymptomatic proteinuria, asymptomatic hematuria, clinical acute glomerulonephritis, recurrent hematuria, or the nephrotic syndrome. This suggests not a single disease but rather a group of diseases with similar histologic abnormalities.

There are no distinctive laboratory features. Urinary findings vary from massive proteinuria and gross hematuria to minimal abnormalities. Reduction in renal function is usually only moderate, and may be entirely absent. Evidence of preceding streptococcal or other infection is lacking.

Differential diagnosis consists simply in excluding known specific renal disease. In the absence of specific etiology, and with the demonstration histologically of focal renal involvement, the diagnosis of focal glomerulonephritis remains.

Most cases appear to be self-limiting, although since focal glomerulonephritis is a pathologic diagnosis with a variety of clinical presentations, its course also may be extremely variable. Renal failure rarely is reported, although the disease may continue for many years. Treatment is entirely symptomatic unless a specific etiology is determined.

BENIGN RECURRENT HEMATURIA

This condition is characterized by recurrent episodes of gross hematuria, occurring over a period of months or years [17, 50, 140, 158, 285, 308, 343, 468, 500]. The diagnosis of acute glomerulonephritis almost invariably is made with the first episode, when the child presents with the abrupt onset of hematuria and proteinuria, although hypertension, reduced renal function, and edema usually are absent. The recurrent nature of the disease differentiates it subsequently from acute glomerulonephritis. The etiology is unknown.

Recurrent episodes usually begin in association with respiratory infections (usually viral), and a presenting complaint of mild to severe abdominal pain often heralds a new episode. In about half the cases, the urine returns to normal between episodes. In the others, persistent hematuria or proteinuria (or both) can be demonstrated. Function usually remains normal throughout the entire course, although we have seen significant, although temporary, decreases in the glomerular filtration rate during acute episodes.

Since recurrent and especially persistent hematuria and proteinuria usually indicate significant and often serious kidney disease, the diagnosis of benign recurrent hematuria should not be made without thorough examination, including renal biopsy. The initial renal biopsy reveals focal or generalized lesions of proliferative glomerulonephritis. Subsequent biopsies reveal either similar lesions, without progression to scarring or glomerular hyalinization, or complete regression of lesions.

There is no specific treatment. Recovery is the rule, even though the clinical course may continue over many years. Whether or not children with this condition have a higher frequency of kidney disease than adults is not known.

GOODPASTURE'S SYNDROME

In Goodpasture's syndrome severe glomerulonephritis is associated with diffuse pulmonary hemorrhage [192]. Although more than 100 patients with Goodpasture's syndrome have been reported, only a few of these have been children, and in those cases the pathogenesis, clinical features, and course did not appear to be different from those in adults [125, 192, 372, 393, 489]. The prognosis is equally poor at all ages, with most cases ending fatally.

Immunofluorescent staining of renal biopsy

specimens has demonstrated the presence of antiglomerular basement membrane antibodies in all cases [115, 489]. The mechanism of immunization and the source of the immunizing antigen are unknown. Adrenocortical steroid and immunosuppressant therapy has been attempted, with equivocal results.

HENOCH-SCHÖNLEIN SYNDROME

Nephritis associated with anaphylactoid purpura appears to be much more common in children than in adults. However, the disease appears to be much less severe in children, in whom the prognosis usually is good [10, 39, 53, 112, 118, 173, 207, 269, 298, 377, 412, 432, 485].

Most children with the Henoch-Schönlein syndrome have renal involvement, although renal disease is clinically obvious in only one-fourth to one-half the cases. The clinical picture mimics acute poststreptococcal glomerulonephritis, except that the frequency of hypertension may be lower. Normal serum complement activity may provide an important means of differentiating the two conditions.

Renal biopsy early in the course of the disease shows either generalized or focal glomerulonephritis, and recovery is the rule. However, in some 5 to 10 per cent of patients the disease progresses to chronic renal insufficiency. In these cases the histologic picture is indistinguishable from progressive, sclerosing glomerulonephritis [39, 118, 269, 432, 512].

Treatment of the renal complication with adrenal corticosteroids does not appear to be effective although an adequate evaluation has not been done [385]. A few patients with the nephrotic syndrome appear to have benefited from therapy with azathioprine or cyclophosphamide [202, 356, 432, 528].

SYSTEMIC LUPUS ERYTHEMATOSUS

Systemic lupus erythematosus (SLE) is being recognized with increasing frequency in childhood [96, 97, 200, 217, 241, 251, 271, 351, 384, 543]. Approximately 10 per cent of all patients are below the age of 15 years. The same predilection for females is observed in children as in adults, 80 to 90 per cent of cases in children occurring in girls [352, 384, 478].

The onset of disease in childhood is most frequently between 10 and 15 years of age; commonly several years elapse before the correct diagnosis is established. Joint symptoms and rash comprise the most common presenting complaints [97, 251, 351]. Most children have evidence of renal involvement at the time the diagnosis is made, and a significant additional number manifest renal disease during their subsequent clinical course.

Meislin and Rothfield [351] compared a group of 42 children with SLE with a group of 200 adults with the disease. Clinical manifestations were similar except for the more frequent occurrence of hepatosplenomegaly and lymphadenopathy in children. On the basis of their experience, the authors constructed models of survival for adults and children with and without renal involvement. They demonstrated that the presence of renal disease at diagnosis reduced survival among children and adults and that patients whose disease began in childhood without renal disease had a poorer survival rate than adult patients with renal disease. Survival data reported by these authors are in general agreement with other large series in children: 70 per cent survival five years after diagnosis in children without renal disease, 45 per cent in children with renal disease. At 10 years, these figures fall to 55 and 20 per cent, respectively, and by 20 years to 30 and 5 per cent.

Considerable evidence has been accumulated that patients with lupus nephritis are benefited by administration of large doses of adrenocortical steroids and by other immunosuppressant agents. In a retrospective study, Hagge et al. [212] reviewed all the children with SLE seen at the Mayo clinic over a period of 20 years. Survival was longer in patients who had received high doses of steroids than in those receiving no or low doses. Similar favorable experience with adrenocortical steroids and other immunosuppressant and cytotoxic agents has been reported by several authors [4, 97, 98, 202, 212, 356, 389, 476, 520].

Currently we recommend that patients be treated initially with steroids alone, which in nontoxic doses is frequently effective in controlling the disease, as judged by examination of the urine and serum factors. If this goal is not achieved, azathioprine or cyclophosphamide is added to the regimen.

HEREDITARY NEPHRITIS

Hereditary nephritis is the classic example of glomerulonephritis beginning in the child and progressing insidiously to death from renal failure in the adult [11, 22, 81, 83, 92, 172, 169, 188, 191, 208, 234, 270, 314, 348, 374, 403, 423, 424, 438, 447, 449, 516, 517, 529]. This disease (or diseases) is discussed in detail in Chapters 34 and 37. Only a few points will be emphasized here.

The clinical features of hereditary glomerulonephritis may be indistinguishable from typical poststreptococcal acute glomerulonephritis. We have established hereditary nephritis as the correct diagnosis in two children who initially were considered on the basis of clinical and histologic criteria as having mild acute glomerulonephritis. When the children's urine failed to return to normal after six months, further investigation uncovered familial disease. It should be noted in this regard that failure to establish the correct diagnosis of familial nephritis would have suggested that these patients had progressed from acute glomerulonephritis to subacute and chronic disease — a course, as indicated earlier, which we do not believe occurs in children following streptococcal infection.

Wasserman and his colleagues [517] have suggested that serum complement levels, which are normal in hereditary nephritis, may help to distinguish these patients from children with acute poststreptococcal glomerulonephritis.

In a review of 476 members of seven families with hereditary renal disease and deafness, Cassady et al. [81] "uncovered the syndrome successfully mimicking acute and chronic nephritis and pyelonephritis in university hospitals and schools for the deaf." They suggested that familial nephritis might account for a high proportion of cases of childhood "chronic nephritis."

Although the predilection in most reported families has been for males, we have had experience with two families in which only female members were involved. Our experience in children is similar to that reported by others — that is, that corticosteroid and immunosuppressant therapy appears to be of no value, although further evaluation of these agents is needed.

SICKLE CELL DISEASE

Patients with sickle cell (SS) disease have functional and morphologic abnormalities involving many organ systems [41, 42, 46, 86, 159, 452]. Renal manifestations include a concentrating defect [222, 264, 280, 297, 382, 451, 530, 541], hematuria [2, 193, 219, 319, 321, 364, 387, 464, 507], and a peculiar type of progressive nephropathy, at times presenting as the nephrotic syndrome [46], which may lead to renal insufficiency [41, 42, 46, 86, 452, 494].

The prevalence of sickle hemoglobin in American Negroes has been estimated to be 8 per cent; 2 to 3 per cent of these have sickle cell disease. The proportion demonstrating renal involvement is unknown, but the concentrating defect and hematuria are seen in patients with SA and SC hemoglobin as well as in patients with sickle disease. Progressive nephropathy apparently is limited to the latter group.

Clinical and Laboratory Features. During

the first few years of life glomerular filtration rate (GFR) and renal blood flow (RBF) in patients with sickle cell disease tend to be normal or elevated for age [69], similar to the findings in patients with other types of chronic anemia. These functions subsequently decrease, however, so that characteristically they are reduced below normal by early adult life [159].

Studies in adults have suggested that as high as one-third of affected patients may have hematuria, which may be unilateral or bilateral [2, 193, 219, 319, 321, 364, 387, 464, 507]. This abnormality is not rare in children, but precise figures for its frequency are not available. In a survey of 16 asymptomatic children with sickle cell disease we discovered no hematuria, although all subjects demonstrated a concentrating defect.

The concentrating defect is not present early in life, but it is almost constant after two or three years of age [222, 264, 280, 297, 382, 451, 530]. Initially, this abnormality may be reversible since concentrating ability can be restored by blood transfusions [264], but by adolescence it appears to be a permanent defect. In our series of 16 patients, ranging in age from 3½ to 14 years, maximum urinary concentration after water deprivation ranged from 235 to 564 mOsm per kilogram, except for one child of 7 years in whom it reached a level of 1102 mOsm per kilogram. No trend with advancing age was discernible.

Reports of the nephrotic syndrome associated with sickle cell disease are rare [491], but it is probably not an uncommon disorder since we have seen several instances in the past few years. This form of the nephrotic syndrome apparently is totally resistant to steroid therapy, which we believe should not be given since we have had one patient in whom severe sickle crisis appeared to be induced by administration of prednisone.

Chronic renal insufficiency and uremia secondary to sickle cell disease has also been reported, though rarely. It has all the clinical and laboratory manifestations of chronic glomerulonephritis [41, 42, 46, 86, 452, 494]. We have treated four children with this condition and have found evidence of early insufficiency in a number of others. This experience suggests that generalized renal damage secondary to sickle cell disease may be more common in children than generally realized.

Pathologic Changes. Pathologic study of young patients shows certain abnormalities that may be correlated with the known alterations of renal function [41, 46, 86, 364, 494, 541]. The renal medullae are the site of edema, telangiectasia, cicatrization, and tubular obliteration. These changes appear to be sequelae of ischemic necrosis, and by virtue of their predominant location in the papillae, they may be responsible for permanent inability to concentrate urine during water deprivation. The glomeruli in older children are strikingly enlarged and congested, a finding that may be related to increased filtration rate. However, increased vascularity gives way to progressive ischemia, focal disruption, and focal fibrosis. This process progresses to glomerular obliteration in some patients, leading to chronic renal insufficiency. Less severe changes may provide the pathogenesis of declining filtration rate in older patients.

Pathophysiology. The cause of hematuria in the patient without generalized renal damage and chronic renal insufficiency is probably related to papillary congestion and necrosis secondary to red cell sickling, stasis, and hypoxia [219, 364]. Similarly, the concentrating defect appears best explained by sickling of erythrocytes in the vasa recta during descent into the hypertonic relatively hypoxic renal medulla. Vascular stasis may exaggerate the normal degree of hypoxia and thus interfere with medullary sodium transport in the loop of Henle or impair countercurrent-exchange mechanisms of the vasa recta [297, 382, 451]. Osmotic diuresis, with its associated increase in medullary blood flow, might be expected to reverse intravascular sickling in the kidney, by lessening medullary hypoxia and decreasing medullary hypertonicity. Thus, it is of interest that the maximal rate of reabsorption of free water during osmotic diuresis in patients with sickle cell anemia is normal or close to normal, supporting the hypothesis that the concentrating defect is caused by intravascular sickling. Further evidence relating disturbed function specifically to the sickling phenomenon is correction of the concentrating defect in young subjects by administration of multiple blood transfusions [264].

Treatment. No treatment of the various renal abnormalities in patients with sickle hemoglobin is available. Chronic transfusion therapy with suppression of erythropoiesis and elimination of sickle cells from the circulation might prevent progression of renal disease, but it would result in all the complications associated with repeated blood transfusions.

Patients with hematuria secondary to papillary changes require no specific therapy. Gross hematuria rarely is of sufficient magnitude to be significant with regard to blood loss. Hematuria usually subsides spontaneously after several days of rest. Nephrectomy for unilateral hematuria has been carried out in a number of patients, but it is contraindicated in a disease which subsequently may very likely affect the other kidney.

HEMOLYTIC-UREMIC SYNDROME

The association of hemolytic anemia with acute renal disease has been recognized for many decades and given a variety of names [174]. It is a disease seen predominantly in young infants and only rarely after the age of two years [24, 144, 174, 181, 183, 209, 302, 349, 350, 386, 433, 455, 466]. It has no sex predilection. It is a rare condition, but apparent epidemics have been described [183, 349]. A similar condition appears to exist among adults, particularly in women in the postpartum period.

The cause is unknown, but probably there are multiple etiologic factors. The appearance of the disease in epidemic form has suggested a viral agent, but attempts to isolate a virus have been unsuccessful [144, 183]. The report by Mettler [355] of isolation of a microtatobiote from two children with the hemolytic-uremic syndrome and from one adult with thrombotic thrombocytopenic purpura provides further evidence for an infectious etiology.

Many features of the disease suggest an immunologic process, but the Coombs test is invariably negative, serum complement levels are not depressed, and immunoglobulins have not been demonstrated in the kidney. Nevertheless, the changes in the kidney resemble those observed in the Shwartzman phenomenon. There is now evidence that a hypercoagulable state leading to fibrin deposition in the glomerular capillaries and the small vessels of the kidney plays a major role in the pathogenesis of the hemolytic-uremic syndrome [286, 505].

The course of the disease is quite characteristic. Following several days of acute gastroenteritis, an infant or young child, previously well, develops the clinical features of acute glomerulonephritis. In addition, a severe hemolytic anemia is present from the onset or develops within a few days. Thrombocytopenia and its complications may also be present. The course is one of prolonged renal failure with repeated hemolytic episodes. Mild to severe neurologic signs, including irritability, ataxia, convulsions, and coma, may be seen. The disease may either progress to death or gradually abate over a period of several weeks. Both neurologic and renal sequelae are seen, the frequency relating apparently to the severity of the initial process.

Gianantonio reported on a group of 123 patients seen with the hemolytic-uremic syndrome [181, 183]. Twenty per cent died in the acute stage. Follow-up data were obtained on 76 of the survivors [181]. Of these, 33 had recovered clinically at the end of one year, with normal renal function and urinalysis. In a second group of 36 children, renal function remained low or slowly increased to normal, and the urinary sediment usually revealed abnormalities. In the final seven children, GFR remained very low and urinary abnormalities persisted; three of these died in chronic renal failure, and the others had persistent renal insufficiency.

A close correlation was observed between the severity of the acute stage of disease and the ultimate outcome. Thirteen of the 21 patients whose disease was considered mild initially (oliguria for less than seven days) went on to complete recovery; the other eight either recovered slowly or demonstrated progression. Of the 33 patients whose disease was considered moderate during the acute stages (oliguria for 7 to 21 days) the late prognosis was worse. Only three of the 22 patients whose disease was initially considered severe (oliguria for more than 21 days) recovered completely after several years.

Renal lesions in this syndrome fall into two overlapping categories. The cases described originally by Gasser and his colleagues had cortical necrosis [174]; those reported by Royer and his associates [433] had a form of severe glomerulitis, termed thrombotic microangiopathy. Fibrinoid necrosis and thrombosis of arteries and glomeruli are seen in both. The glomeruli in the latter are the site of striking endothelial and mesangial swelling and hyperplasia, and the cells contain extremely large vesicular nuclei. Focal or partial glomerular necrosis is often observed, suggesting a transition stage to cortical necrosis. Renal biopsies in survivors may show chronic progressive glomerulonephritis.

There is no established treatment other than the symptomatic management of acute renal failure and of hemolytic anemia. Adrenocorticosteroids have not been evaluated adequately, but they do not appear to be of benefit. Anticoagulation with heparin has been utilized on the theory that intravascular coagulation and thrombotic obstruction of renal cortical arteries might underly the disease process. The results of this form of therapy are, at best, uncertain.

THE NEPHROTIC SYNDROME (NEPHROSIS)

The nephrotic syndrome is a clinical entity characterized classically by proteinuria, hypoproteinemia, lipidemia, and edema [129]. It is now recognized, however, that in children as in adults the important feature is massive proteinuria and that the secondary features of the syndrome may be present to a variable extent. We agree, therefore, with the definition proposed by Schreiner (page 503) that "the nephrotic syndrome is a clinical entity . . . characterized by . . . massive proteinuria [with] . . . a variable tendency toward edema, hypoproteinemia, and hyperlipemia." In contrast with experience in adults, the nephrotic syndrome in children usually occurs in the absence of recognizable systemic or preexisting renal disease. It may occur, however, as a complication of various systemic diseases (lupus erythematosus, Henoch-Schönlein syndrome, multiple myeloma, sickle cell anemia, malaria, typhus, tuberculosis, syphilis), following renal vein thrombosis, as a result of drug toxicity (trimethadione, mercurials, bismuth, gold salts), or following bee stings or contact with poison oak. It may occur also during the course of chronic glomerulonephritis which was preceded by what appeared to be acute glomerulonephritis, although this sequence is uncommon in adults and extremely rare, if it occurs at all, in children.

The great majority of children in whom the nephrotic syndrome develops have neither recognizable associated disease nor evidence of exposure to known toxic agents [28, 33, 129, 237, 272, 291, 345, 409, 510]. A significant number of such children will have, in addition to the characteristics of the nephrotic syndrome, one or more nephritic manifestations, such as hematuria, reduced kidney function, or hypertension, a fact which has led some observers to consider that all instances of the nephrotic syndrome not associated with recognizable causes represent a state of glomerulonephritis, the initial episode of which may have been missed. However, data obtained from percutaneous renal biopsies have substantiated the view of most pediatricians that the nephrotic syndrome as seen in children is unrelated to acute glomerulonephritis and is distinct from the nephrotic stage of chronic nephritis as seen in adults.

Frequency. The frequency of the nephrotic syndrome in children in the United States has been estimated variously to be 1.9 [486], 2.3 [426], and 2.8 [450] cases per 100,000 white children under 10 years of age. Schlesinger et al. [450] reported a frequency of 1.9 cases per 100,000 white children and 2.8 cases per 100,000 nonwhite children under 16 years of age. These authors found the number of active cases to be 15.7 per 100,000 children below the age of 16. An analysis of the nephrotic syndrome in 425 patients 12 years old or younger showed the age at onset to peak between two and three years, with two-thirds of the cases between one and four and three-quarters less than five years of age [28]. There is a higher prevalence of the disease in boys, the distribution in one series being 291 boys and 175 girls [28].

Etiology. The cause of the nephrotic syndrome is unknown. Even when it occurs in association with some systemic disorder or following toxic exposure, the pathogenetic relationship is not clear and the association is not a consistent one. At one time the nephrotic syndrome in children was considered a disease of hypersensitivity, related to a poorly understood antigen-antibody reaction involving the kidneys [231, 232, 283]. Evidence in favor of this formulation included:

1. The apparent increased incidence of allergic disease in the patients and their families.
2. Reports of low concentrations of serum complement activity during the active stage of the disease.
3. Demonstration of deposits of gamma globulin on glomerular basement membranes.
4. The favorable effects of adrenocortical steroids and other immunosuppressant drugs.
5. Production of the disease in laboratory animals using a variety of immunologic technics.

It has now been shown, however, that in the great majority of children with the nephrotic syndrome the concentration of β_1C globulin in serum is normal [198], and immune deposits are not present on glomerular basement membranes [124]. Finally, the mechanism of action of steroids and other so-called immunosuppressant agents is entirely unknown. At present, therefore, it appears that an immunologic mechanism underlies the disease process in at most a small portion of the children with the nephrotic syndrome. In the remainder, the disease remains truly idiopathic.

Familial Forms of the Nephrotic Syndrome. The occurrence of the nephrotic syndrome in siblings or in consecutive generations of the same family is infrequent [28, 33]. Congenital or infantile nephrosis, which is clearly familial (page 1381), differs from idiopathic childhood nephrosis by its appearance before three months of age and often at or shortly after birth, its lack of responsiveness to steroid therapy, and its poor prognosis. There have been rare instances of the nephrotic syndrome in siblings, with an onset after infancy. In these children the clinical picture and pathologic findings simulate sporadic childhood nephrosis. The possibility that it is a heritable disorder cannot be excluded. Although the frequency of multiple cases of what appears to be idiopathic nephrotic syndrome in the same family cannot be estimated, it appears to be so low that it is justifiable to reassure parents of a child with the disease that there is almost no chance of a second child being affected [33].

Clinical and Laboratory Features. The major clinical and laboratory features of the nephrotic syndrome in children are the same as those in adults [28, 33, 129, 186, 187, 237,

272, 291, 345, 409, 510]. However, the occurrence of this chronic illness in a young child does pose special problems.

Malnutrition and growth failure are common in children in whom the active stage of the disease is prolonged. Poor appetite and the altered metabolism of protein [186, 187] and perhaps of calcium and other nutrients are probably all involved. Malnutrition tends to be obscured by the edema, although changes in the quality of the hair may reveal it. There are striking changes in the cartilage of the ear. Despite the poor nutrition, which with present treatment rarely persists for many months, there is apparently no residual growth impairment if recovery from the disease occurs. Prolonged high-dosage steroid therapy exaggerates the growth retardation, but this effect also appears to be reversible.

A second problem concerns the psychologic reaction of the patient and his family [272]. Although such a reaction is prominent in both children and adults, it is different in children. These psychologic problems are discussed under *Treatment*.

Proteinuria during the active stage of the disease exceeds 1 gm. per square meter of body surface area per 24 hours. About one-fifth of children have hematuria; gross hematuria is exceptional and usually is associated on biopsy with the finding of lobular or proliferative disease. Changes in serum proteins and lipid are the same as in adults [233].

In the great majority of children, serum β_1C globulin is normal [198]. Some investigators believe that hypocomplementemia augurs steroid resistance and a poor prognosis [527]. Although there appears to be such a correlation, we have had experience with one patient who was steroid responsive despite a markedly decreased level of $beta_{1C}$. In this patient the β_1C level returned to normal under treatment, suggesting, therefore, that the significant feature may be the persistence of hypocomplementemia. Tests of urinary protein selectivity have been found in some series to correlate well with steroid response [75, 77, 325]. In our recent experience with 174 children studied at the onset of disease, a similar correlation was found. However, a number of patients with poor selectivity were steroid responsive, and others with highly selective proteinuria were nonresponsive.

In the majority of children tests of renal function are normal, although they may be depressed during severe exacerbations. In occasional children values of urea clearance are significantly above normal.

Differential Diagnosis. The combination of edema, proteinuria, hypoproteinemia, and hyperlipemia defines the nephrotic syndrome; differential diagnosis concerns the underlying diseases with which it may be associated. In only exceptional children can a specific diagnosis be made, such as lupus erythematosus, Henoch-Schönlein syndrome, or drug toxicity. In the great majority of children with the nephrotic syndrome, no underlying systemic or renal disease can be identified. In most of these, light microscopic examination of the renal biopsy reveals a normal or near-normal histologic picture. There is no satisfactory name for this group of patients although the terms *pure lipoid nephrosis* or *minimal change idiopathic nephrotic syndrome* have been proposed. In 10 to 15 per cent of the group without identifiable disease, renal biopsy reveals various types of diffuse or focal glomerulonephritis, including membranous and proliferative lesions. Since the clinical course differs markedly depending upon the associated renal histology, diagnostic investigation should include histologic examination of tissue obtained by percutaneous renal biopsy to permit morphologic as well as clinical classification [45, 124, 510, 521].

Course and Prognosis. The clinical course of the nephrotic syndrome in children tends to follow one of three general patterns: (1) active clinical disease followed by partial or complete remission, the duration of the active stage being as short as a few weeks, but usually one to four or more years; (2) active clinical disease progressing to death due to renal insufficiency during the active stage; and (3) active disease of many years' duration, followed by chronic renal insufficiency. It is difficult even to estimate the proportion of children with the nephrotic syndrome who might be expected to follow each type of course.

In considering prognosis, however, the various types of idiopathic nephrotic syndrome observed in children must be considered separately [480]. Children in the largest group, designated pure nephrosis or minimal change idiopathic nephrotic syndrome, are almost invariably responsive to steroid therapy and appear to have an excellent prognosis. Certain of these patients have frequent relapses and, therefore, are candidates for the development of steroid toxicity. Nevertheless renal biopsies in these children after 10 or more years of active disease usually continue to reveal normal histologic patterns. Infreqently, a progressive type of hyalinization is observed which over the course of years may lead to significant nephron loss and renal insufficiency. At present we are unable to identify these children at the onset of their disease.

Children with the idiopathic nephrotic syndrome whose biopsies reveal some type of glomerulopathy have a poor prognosis [124]. Usually they are unresponsive to steroid therapy. Clinical and histologic examination documents a progressive course, with a fatal outcome in a high proportion at the end of five years. Although there are reports of favorable responses to immunosuppressant drug therapy in this group of patients, there is no convincing evidence that the ultimate outcome is altered by this form of treatment.

The course and prognosis in children with identifiable disease depends upon the particular disease in question. Thus children with nephrotic syndrome secondary to lupus erythematosus, Henoch-Schönlein syndrome, or sickle cell disease have, in general, a poor prognosis. The nephrotic syndrome secondary to certain drugs, such as trimethadione, is usually reversible following withdrawal of the drug, and the prognosis is generally but not uniformly good.

With the improved understanding obtained from studies of renal biopsy tissue from patients with the various types of disease that may underly the nephrotic syndrome, certain clinical features which have been considered to have prognostic value can be better understood. The presence of nephritic manifestations at the time of first observation — leading to the term *nephritis-nephrosis* — has been thought to indicate a poor prognosis. In a recent survey of 72 children [45] one-fourth had a nephritic onset. All patients in the non-nephritic group histologically fell into the classification "minimal change," were responsive to steroids, and were considered to have a good prognosis. This was true also of 7 of the 17 classified as nephritic. The other 10, however, had various types of glomerulopathy, including proliferative, membranous, and lobular disease. Most were unresponsive to steroids, and it was considered that the group carried a very poor prognosis. It appears, therefore, that the presence or absence of a "nephritic" onset is of some prognostic value in that it helps to identify children who may not fall into the minimal change, idiopathic group.

Age of onset does not appear to affect the prognosis up to the age of 10 years; at older ages, however, there is evidence that the case fatality rate increases slowly but progressively [28]. This may be due to the increased incidence with advancing age of other than minimal change, idiopathic disease, rather than a difference in the response with increasing age to the same disease.

The most favorable prognostic feature at the onset of disease remains the initial response to adrenocortical steroid therapy. Complete cessation of proteinuria following treatment indicates a favorable prognosis, with the rare exception of the patient who responds well clinically despite serious progressive glomerulopathy. Incomplete or absent response to adrenocortical steroid therapy is usually associated with a grave prognosis.

Treatment. Nephrosis is a trying disease for the patient, the family, and the physician. Treatment must include measures directed toward control of the outstanding clinical feature, edema, and more importantly, toward attempts to modify favorably the course of the disease and its ultimate prognosis. In addition, because of the chronicity of the disease and the uncertainty of the outcome, the child with nephrosis and his parents need more than the usual amount of psychologic support from the physician.

Since the time of Richard Bright, only two major advances, both in the past 25 years, have been made in the treatment of children with the nephrotic syndrome: (1) the development of antibacterial agents, which have almost eliminated the severe infections that were the principal cause of death in these children, and (2) the development of the therapeutic use of adrenocortical steroids, which in most instances permits complete control of the edema and in children, at least, does appear to modify favorably the underlying disease and the ultimate outcome.

GENERAL MEASURES. The diet of the nephrotic child is that suitable for the normal child. Salt needs to be restricted only during periods of edema, when foods are not salted during cooking, a shaker is not provided, and excessively salty foods are avoided. The protein content of the diet is not altered. No restrictions are placed on the *activity* of the child beyond those which he himself may impose during periods of edema. It is important to maintain associations with other children, but because exacerbations of proteinuria and edema may follow common *upper-respiratory-tract infections,* some limitations are advisable. For example, when contacts with other children during visits or playtimes are planned, more than the usual amount of attention is paid to the possibility of infection in the other children. Although exposure to large groups is best avoided, patients are allowed to attend kindergarten and regular school classes.

Serious intercurrent infections are a real hazard for the nephrotic child. Although continuous prophylaxis with antibiotics is not recommended, it is advisable to administer antibiotics after definite exposure to bacterial infection and to use these agents in therapeutic doses promptly and more liberally for therapy of possible bacterial infection, particularly during periods of edema. In the past, most serious infections were due to the *Pneumococcus,* but at present they are caused more frequently by other organisms, particularly gram-negative bacilli and staphylococci. Until the infecting organisms can be identified, a broad-spectrum antibiotic is indicated.

ADRENOCORTICAL STEROID THERAPY. Although recommendations for specific adrenocortical steroids and dosage schedules vary considerably, the basic aim of all regimens is to maintain the patient free from proteinuria* with the minimal dosage of adrenocortical steroids [15, 16, 62, 70, 99, 283, 368, 410, 426, 479]. We are not convinced that any one of the suggested therapeutic regimens for adrenocortical steroids has any clear advantage over the others, including the following plan which we have used for the past several years. This plan is relatively easy to follow, it utilizes one of the less expensive drugs, and it involves oral medication exclusively.

INITIAL TREATMENT. Adrenocortical steroid therapy is started as soon as the diagnosis is established, prednisone being given orally for 28 days in a dosage of approximately 60 mg. per square meter of body surface area per day, in three or four divided doses; for older chil-

* Daily determination of urinary protein concentration is performed at home by the parents on the first urine specimen in the morning using Albustix or 10% sulfosalicylic acid. These tests constitute the simplest assessment of the most important manifestation of disease activity. They have been extremely valuable in regulating treatment.

dren, usually a daily dosage of 80 mg. is not exceeded. With this regimen, diuresis will occur in the majority of patients within 7 to 21 days and the urine will become free from protein (less than 5 to 10 mg. per 12-hour night specimen). In these cases, after the first 28 days, the dosage of prednisone is reduced to 40 mg. per square meter per day and is given for three consecutive days of each week for an additional four weeks.

TREATMENT OF REFRACTORY PATIENTS. Our experience has been that, with rare exceptions, patients who do not respond to an initial treatment of four weeks of daily therapy and four weeks of intermittent therapy do not respond to continuing steroid therapy alone, even when given in higher dosage. Our recommendation, therefore, is that treatment of such patients with an immunosuppressant drug be considered at this time.

TREATMENT OF RECURRENCES. Patients showing recurrences of proteinuria lasting more than two or three days are begun again on their initial dosage of prednisone, which is continued until the urine is free from protein for three days. Therapy is then changed to the lower dosage, given on an intermittent basis for an additional four weeks, as during the initial course of therapy. If recurrences are frequent (more than every three or four months), daily treatment is followed by several months of intermittent therapy. If this fails to prevent frequent recurrences, patients are considered for combined therapy with an immunosuppressant agent.

Alternate-day steroid therapy, in which a single dose, equivalent to twice the usual daily dose, is given once every 48 hours, has not been successful in our experience, although good results have been reported by others [3, 220, 479, 481, 492, 499]. Until the therapeutic efficacy and the supposed freedom from steroid toxicity of this dosage schedule has been tested against other dosage schedules in a properly designed clinical trial, we do not recommend that it be used.

In addition to hypothalamic-pituitary-adrenocortical suppression, the many and varied side effects of adrenocortical steroid therapy are frequently seen in children with the nephrotic syndrome who are treated with relatively high dosages over prolonged periods [189, 194, 303, 309, 368, 496]. Extensive experience indicates, however, that with proper precautions, serious side effects, such as vertebral compression fractures, arrested growth, or severe Cushing's syndrome, are not seen more frequently in children with the nephrotic syndrome than in children receiving steroids for other reasons.

An occasional child is encountered in whom tapering of steroids after many months of therapy at high dosage is associated with symptoms of headache, lethargy, weakness, anorexia, and vomiting. Treatment is accomplished by providing the minimal dosage of steroid which is adequate to alleviate the symptoms. After a period of two or three months, therapy is stopped. If symptoms reappear, treatment is given for another period of two or three months. In rare instances, supportive therapy may be required for as long as a year before treatment can be discontinued completely.

IMMUNOSUPPRESSANT THERAPY. The use of immunosuppressant drugs, including nitrogen mustard, cyclophosphamide, methotrexate, 6-thioguanine, and azathioprine, has been advocated in the treatment of patients refractory to other forms of therapy [123, 141, 151, 202, 281, 356, 361, 378, 522, 528]. The value of these agents in such patients has not been established, and recommendations regarding their use are under constant revision. Treatment of steroid-responsive children with 6-thioguanine, cyclophosphamide, or azothioprine, either alone or in combination with low-dosage prednisone, has been successful in inducing and maintaining remissions, permitting avoidance or gradual resolution, if present, of steroidal side effects.

Since the use of the newer immunosuppressant drugs must still be considered experimental, patients considered candidates for such treatment should be managed by or in consultation with investigators actively engaged in studying the effect of these drugs in patients with the nephrotic syndrome.

DIURETIC THERAPY. Sodium restriction is capable of slowing accumulation of edema during an exacerbation of the nephrotic syndrome; however, it is usually not successful in eliminating edema. Numerous diuretic agents are available which, combined with moderate sodium restriction, contribute significantly to control of edema.

Since the majority of patients have a satisfactory diuresis within 10 to 14 days after beginning adrenocortical steroid therapy, diuretic agents are not given initially. However, in refractory patients or before diuresis has occurred in very edematous patients who become more edematous during treatment, diuretics may provide symptomatic relief.

Hydrochlorothiazide, 2 to 4 mg. per kilogram per day, is the agent used initially. The thiazide drugs are relatively nontoxic. Hypokalemia is usually not seen if a child is eating a normal diet; it can be avoided under other circumstances by giving potassium supplements. The serum uric acid concentration is frequently elevated. Other side effects, including thrombocytopenia, skin rashes, jaundice, pancreatitis, and hyperglycemia, are either extremely rare or have not been reported in children.

Often thiazides are not effective, and a more potent diuretic must be employed. We have had uniformly good results with the use of furosemide, given either intravenously in a dose of 0.5 mg. per kilogram or by mouth in a dose of 1 to 2 mg. per kilogram, and repeated as needed.

PLASMA EXPANDERS. The principal physiologic stimulus to sodium retention in patients with the nephrotic syndrome is the contracted vascular volume that results from protein depletion [353, 354]. However, efforts directed toward expansion of plasma volume with albumin or other plasma expanders have generally not been effective in inducing a diuresis. At present we use albumin in conjunction with furosemide for the hypoalbuminemic patient with resistant edema who requires vigorous diuretic therapy. In such patients, salt-poor albumin may be given in a dose of 10 to 25 gm. per day followed by intravenously administered furosemide. Attempts should not be made to increase the albumin concentration to the normal range by frequent infusions of albumin. The refractory patient with only a moderate degree of edema is *not* given plasma albumin since the primary goal in treatment is reversal of glomerular lesions, and temporary alleviation of edema through indirect means offers little in the overall management of the patient. Other plasma expanders such as dextran have been abandoned.

THE NEPHROTIC SYNDROME AS PART OF OTHER RECOGNIZABLE DISEASES. The rare instance of the nephrotic syndrome associated with *renal vein thrombosis* or *constrictive pericarditis* can be treated only by alleviation of the underlying condition.

The nephrotic syndrome related etiologically to certain *drugs,* such as trimethadione (Tridione), usually resolves after discontinuation of the offending agent. If not, it is questionable whether or not adrenocortical steroids should be used. At present, we tend not to give them until several weeks or even months after the drug has been stopped. Drugs implicated in producing the nephrotic syndrome should be withheld permanently since their repeated administration may subsequently result in irreversible disease.

The nephrotic syndrome as a manifestation of the renal disease associated with *disseminated lupus erythematosus* and *sickle cell disease* in children is discussed under those headings.

PSYCHOLOGICAL ASPECTS OF THE NEPHROTIC SYNDROME. In considering some of the effects of the nephrotic syndrome in a child, on the child himself, the family, and the physician, it has been stated that:

> An awareness of the psychological reactions and needs of the parents of sick children and the developmental and emotional needs of the young child with nephrosis enables the physician to make a significant continuing contribution to the welfare and comfort of patient and family. The parents need to feel that they can trust the physician to make the best medical decisions for them and their child, and that his decisions are based on expert general medical knowledge tempered with specific, up-to-date information about child development and interest in their individual situation. They also need to feel that the physician trusts them as parents to help him to provide the best care for their child. They need his guidance in providing optimal conditions for development and adjustment of their sick child at home, from a medical, as well as psychological, point of view. They need the physician's support and reassurance in dealing with their own anxieties and mixed feelings, so that they can be as supportive and reassuring as possible in their relationship to the sick child whose attitudes about his illness, his treatment, and himself as a person will largely reflect the attitudes of his parents [272].

Finally, *criteria of recovery* must be considered in formulating therapy and must be included as an important aspect of discussions with the family. Recovery from the nephrotic syndrome must be defined as permanent subsidence of all the manifestations of the disease. Although one can never be absolutely certain that proteinuria may not recur at some future date, and recurrences after 5 or 10 years or more of apparent recovery have occurred, if a year or two has elapsed on a steroid-free regimen without recurrence of proteinuria, permanent recovery is almost virtually assured.

CONGENITAL NEPHROSIS

The nephrotic syndrome occurs infrequently during the first year and particularly during the first three months of life; when it does, it presents certain characteristic features: a high familial incidence, almost complete resistance to therapy, and a fatal outcome [145, 159, 184, 201, 203, 213, 214, 216, 273, 274, 279, 284, 287, 369, 375, 380, 509, 515, 536]. Many of these cases have occurred in newborn and premature infants [145, 203, 279].

Hallman et al. [214] pointed out features of the disease which indicate an onset during intrauterine life: (1) almost without exception the placenta is very large; (2) the birth weight is low due partly, at least, to prematurity; (3) proteinuria and characteristic changes in serum proteins are seen immediately after birth in a great majority of cases; (4) the cranial sutures are wide at birth, indicating that the ossification process is delayed already in utero; and (5) polycythemia and especially the advanced erythroblastosis occasionally seen in newborn infants with congenital nephrosis probably derive from impaired function of the large edematous placenta.

At least 112 families with congenital nephrosis have been described, the great majority occurring either in Finland or in families of Finnish origin [214]. From a genetic study of 57 Finnish families Norio [369] concluded that the disease is transmitted as an autosomal recessive.

The clinical picture and laboratory findings in congenital nephrosis do not differ from the nephrotic syndrome in older children, except for the age of the patients. Although the serum cholesterol is usually elevated in these infants, as in children and adults with the nephrotic syndrome, the distribution of values is shifted to the left due to the developmentally lower values in young infants.

Pathologic findings have varied from glomerular hypercellularity and basement membrane thickening to glomerular sclerosis and hyalinization. Marked dilatation of the cortical tubules, which has been shown by microdissection to be segmental, has led to the term microcystic disease of the kidney, implying some form of primary congenital renal tubular dysplasia [375]. It is more likely, however, that the tubular abnormalities are secondary reactions in immature kidneys to the primary glomerular disease.

Lange and his associates [284] demonstrated the presence of gamma globulin and complement in the glomeruli of an infant with congenital nephrotic syndrome and suggested that the disease might have an immunologic basis. Kouvalainen and his co-workers [274] transplanted skin from infants born with congenital nephrosis to the mother and obtained an accelerated rejection, suggesting previous sensitization of the mother to the fetus.

Total resistance to adrenocortical steroid therapy has been observed consistently, most patients dying of infection or renal failure within the first few months of disease. Survival for many months has been reported exceptionally, with one patient living to the age of three years and 10 months. Successful therapy with a combination of immunosuppressive drugs has not been reported, but further experience with this form of treatment is needed. If the disease is in fact primarily renal, these infants should be considered as candidates for renal homotransplantation.

CHRONIC GLOMERULONEPHRITIS

Chronic glomerulonephritis in children, as in adults, represents a syndrome rather than a single entity. It is characterized by bilateral, nonsuppurative disease of the kidneys, with continued loss of nephrons, progressive reduction in renal function, and ultimately renal insufficiency.

Chronic glomerulonephritis may develop in the absence of any manifestations of previous kidney disease, it may begin with the nephrotic syndrome, or it may follow what appears to be acute glomerulonephritis [19, 60, 65, 93, 135, 344, 411, 510, 522, 523, 526]. Other causes of chronic nephritis in children include anaphylactoid purpura, hereditary nephritis, and "collagen diseases" such as lupus erythematosus and periarteritis nodosa. In certain parts of the world, the hemolytic-uremic syndrome has been recognized as a common cause of renal failure. It was recently pointed out by McCrory [344] that this condition may become "A New Cause for an Old Disease — Chronic Nephritis."

It has been suggested that a common cause of chronic nephritis in adolescents and adults is acute poststreptococcal glomerulonephritis in childhood, usually unrecognized. However, as discussed in detail elsewhere (page 1367), there is no convincing evidence for the progression, following a prolonged latent phase, of acute to chronic glomerulonephritis either in children or, in our opinion, in adults [135]. The recent study by Bacani and his co-workers [19] of rapidly progressive glomerulonephritis in adults, a catastrophic disease that is encountered also in children, suggests that this condition also is unrelated to streptococcal disease.

All histologic patterns are observed on renal biopsy, including membranous nephropathy and the various types of diffuse and focal proliferative glomerulonephritis [60, 411, 510, 523].

The clinical and laboratory manifestations of chronic nephritis in children are the same as those observed in adults, with the additional feature of growth failure. Recovery does not occur once a child has passed into the hypertensive, uremic phase of the disease. However, before the diagnosis of chronic glomerulonephritis is made, a careful search must be made for specific diseases, particularly treatable ones, including pyelonephritis, primary hypertensive disease, and obstructive uropathy.

There is still no form of therapy that appears to alter the course of nonspecific chronic nephritis. However, during much of the course, and often over a period of many months and years, symptomatic treatment can be of great importance. Prolonged restriction of activity is not recommended unless demanded by the symptomatic state of the patient. The child should be encouraged to attend school and to participate in other activities within his limitations. No special changes in diet are needed early in the course of chronic nephritis, and needless restrictions should be avoided.

The evidence to date of favorable effects from treatment with adrenocortical steroids or immunosuppressant therapy is not conclusive. There are reports suggesting, however, that in some patients the process of progressive nephron destruction may be slowed or even halted by such therapy [4, 98, 123, 141–143, 202, 356, 490, 520, 522, 526–528].

FAMILIAL JUVENILE NEPHRONOPHTHISIS

This unusual condition, first described by Fanconi and his associates in 1951 [152], combines a severe renal concentrating defect, anemia, and early development of uremia. In early life children generally are entirely free from symptoms or any evidence of disease, which first appears usually between two and five years of age. Even then the urine may contain neither protein nor formed elements, despite the presence of hyposthenuria, growth retardation, and severe anemia. Subsequently, the disease is invariably progressive, leading finally to renal failure and death in uremia, usually before 15 years of age [59, 152, 195, 205, 206, 210, 211, 229, 236, 249, 268, 311, 326, 360, 429, 461, 474, 488, 514].

Genetic studies suggest that the disease is transmitted as an autosomal recessive, although sporadic cases do occur. Both Strauss and Sommers [488] and Mongeau and Worthen [360] have suggested that familial nephronophthisis, a disease of children, is identical with medullary cystic disease of the kidney, reported first by Smith and Graham [474] and described primarily in adults.

Diagnosis usually is not difficult in the patient presenting with anemia, a concentrating defect which is out of proportion to the degree of uremia, and little or no urinary abnormalities. Hypertension characteristically is absent until the terminal stages of disease. Salt-wasting may be prominent. Differential diagnosis includes nephrogenic diabetes insipidus, congenital urologic malformations, and chronic pyelonephritis; these conditions usually are excluded without difficulty.

The kidneys are reduced in size, demonstrate diffuse atrophy, and contain a variable number of cysts in the medulla and cortex. There are extensive tubular changes consisting primarily of cystic dilatation and interstitial infiltration and fibrosis. Early the glomeruli are normal; later there is periglomerular fibrosis and hyalinization. The histologic picture may be difficult to distinguish from chronic pyelonephritis and chronic interstitial nephritis.

There is no specific treatment. Symptomatic therapy follows the principles and practices described in the sections on chronic renal failure.

POSTURAL PROTEINURIA

Isolated proteinuria of abnormal degree, present only when the subject is in the upright position, has been recognized since the beginning of this century [64]. However, its pathophysiologic and clinical significance still are not clear. An increase in the rate of protein excretion in the urine has been noted in orthostasis in normal subjects and in patients with clear-cut renal disease, as well as in those with so-called "orthostatic proteinuria" [266, 267, 289, 416]. Thus, individuals in the last category differ from normal subjects in that their rate of proteinuria in orthostasis is greater, and they differ from patients with renal disease in that they have no other evidence of any underlying renal abnormality.

The pathophysiology is not fully understood. Increased glomerular filtration of protein has been suggested, although diminished tubular reabsorption cannot be excluded

[470]. Elevated blood pressure in the inferior vena cava has been observed concomitant with orthostatic protein excretion [267], but artificial elevation of the pressure in recumbency fails to reproduce this effect. Proteinuria has also been induced in susceptible individuals by the application of tourniquets to the legs and by norepinephrine administration [288]. Conversely, it has been suggested that the protein may be derived from renal papillary lymph [317], although other studies strongly suggest a vascular derivation.

Much has been written about the benign nature of the disease, which is said to occur in 2 to 5 per cent of adolescents and to be transient in nature. However, a number of lines of evidence now suggest that, at least in certain subjects, postural proteinuria may not be simply a physiologic variant of normal but may represent significant renal disease. In the survey of Randolph and Greenfield [399] of almost 4000 children ranging in age from three weeks to 16 years who had been screened for urinary tract disease, proteinuria was observed on at least one occasion in more than one-third. However, reexamination of the children with one positive test revealed no persistent, intermittent, or postural proteinuria in the entire group. It appears from this study, therefore, that postural proteinuria rarely occurs in the healthy child.

King [265] reported that of 191 apparently healthy young males with postural proteinuria, one-third had developed constant proteinuria when examined five to eight years later. Robinson and his co-workers, in a study of army recruits with what they termed fixed and reproducible orthostatic proteinuria, demonstrated significant abnormalities on renal biopsy in one-half [293, 417].

Ruckley et al. [444] reported light and electron microscopic studies of renal biopsies from seven patients with orthostatic proteinuria. Light microscopy revealed no significant abnormality, a finding similar to our own experience in four children. Focal abnormalities were seen in all glomeruli on electron microscopy.

We have observed the following sequence in many children either recovering from acute glomerulonephritis or going from relapse into remission of the nephrotic syndrome. Initially, proteinuria is constant, although increased during ambulation. Subsequently, abnormal proteinuria is absent when the child is supine, but it is easily demonstrable when the child is in the lordotic position. Finally, proteinuria is absent in both the supine and the erect position. These observations could be interpreted as indirect evidence that postural proteinuria is a minimal expression of true renal disease.

Rowe and Soothill [427] and Ruckley et al. [444] reported nonselectivity in patients with orthostatic proteinuria. The slight proteinuria present in normal subjects has been found by MacLean and Robson [324] also to be nonselective. However, the technical difficulties in determining selectivity with slight degrees of proteinuria and the possibility of nonrenal sources of protein make interpretation of these results extremely difficult. Therefore, it is not possible to state on the basis of the selectivity index whether the nonselective nature of orthostatic proteinuria reflects an exaggeration of normal or is evidence of true renal disease.

Herdman et al. [230] reported five patients with postural proteinuria, only one of whom had other findings of renal disease. All four patients with idiopathic postural proteinuria responded to prednisone therapy with cessation or diminution of proteinuria. The significance of these observations is unknown, although the authors interpreted their results as indicating that the lesion of postural proteinuria may be similar to that underlying the nephrotic syndrome. Of interest is their suggestion that a diagnostic trial of steroid therapy in postural proteinuria might distinguish patients with benign disease from those with a poorer prognosis.

The diagnosis of postural proteinuria is

easily established by comparison between rates of excretion of protein in a timed overnight specimen and in a specimen obtained in the erect and, preferably, lordotic position. Although the prognosis in patients with minimal proteinuria and no other evidence of renal disease generally has been considered good, in the absence of careful long-term follow-up studies of many patients, it must be concluded that the true significance of postural proteinuria is still not known. If postural proteinuria is found, patients should have appropriate investigation to discover specific etiology and pathology. In the absence of demonstrable abnormality, patients should be followed for subsequent development of overt renal disease.

Disorders of Renal Tubular Function

Renal tubular disorders may be defined as conditions in which there is selective impairment of one or more specific tubular functions, in the absence of evidence of a generalized decrease in renal function or depression of glomerular filtration rate. In infants and children it is especially important to emphasize that this definition applies to the early stages of the disease since secondary glomerular damage, which in some conditions is preventable, may appear later. For example, early recognition and proper treatment of distal renal tubular acidosis can prevent the development of nephrocalcinosis and secondary pyelonephritis. In the Fanconi syndrome with cystinosis, on the other hand, progressive renal insufficiency cannot be prevented with presently available treatment.

Defects of tubular function may be single or multiple. Analysis of the disorder may be complicated by the fact that a defect may not represent a primary, specific abnormality, but rather a secondary, functional one. For example, a concentrating defect may be due to potassium deficiency; hyperkaliuria may be caused by secondary hyperaldosteronism; hypercalciuria may result from acidosis; and increased phosphate clearance may be caused by hyperparathyroidism. The reversibility of the abnormality when the primary cause is corrected establishes the defect as functional, but such a clear distinction between functional and specific defects is not always possible.

The cause of many renal tubular disorders is unknown. They may be either acquired or hereditary; in the latter, manifestations may appear at or shortly after birth or be delayed for months or years. Genetic disorders may modify renal function in two ways: (1) through a primary abnormality in a specific tubular function, as in primary renal glycosuria, or (2) by the toxic effect on the renal tubule of accumulated metabolites consequent to an extrarenal metabolic block, as in galactosemia. Both primary and secondary causes may present with identical symptoms and be indistinguishable on the basis of functional and urinary findings. For this reason, a descriptive rather than an etiologic classification is followed in this section.

RENAL GLYCOSURIA

Primary renal glycosuria is a classic, specific, hereditary renal tubular dysfunction in which variable amounts of glucose are excreted in the urine at normal levels of blood glucose [276, 328, 359, 402]. Renal glycosuria occurs also in several generalized disorders of tubular function, such as the Fanconi syndrome, and occasionally in far-advanced renal failure. The pathophysiology of the two types of primary renal glycosuria is discussed in Chapter 30. This condition is undoubtedly present at birth, but its discovery may be delayed until adult life. It is a benign condition, and patients are generally asymptomatic.

The presence of glucose in the urine concurrent with normal blood levels establishes the diagnosis. In the obvious case glucosuria is constant, even during fasting, but in some cases it can be detected only postprandially.

In the few patients with renal glucosuria who have had renal biopsies, the kidney histologically has been normal. However, Monasterio et al. [359] have recently reported alterations in the structure of proximal tubular cells when observed by the electron microscope.

The differentiation of renal glucosuria from diabetes mellitus is essential to avoid dangerous therapeutic errors. In renal glucosuria the fasting blood sugar characteristically is normal and the glucose tolerance test frequently is flattened. The glucose oxidase test will differentiate other types of mellituria.

Therapy is not indicated. The amount of glucose in the urine is independent of the carbohydrate intake, and no dietary restrictions are needed.

AMINOACIDURIAS

The amino acids present in glomerular filtrate are normally almost completely reabsorbed in the proximal tubule. Urine normally contains mainly glycine, taurine, histidine, and glutamine, which are the only ones detected when urine is analyzed by paper chromatography. However, it can be demonstrated by ion-exchange chromatography that most of the plasma amino acids are present in urine, although in very small amounts.

The rate of excretion of amino acids is comparatively greater in infants and children than in adults. Healthy children excrete alpha-amino nitrogen at a rate of approximately 2.5 mg. and infants as much as 8.5 mg. per kilogram of body weight per day. The pattern of urinary excretion of amino acids in children is similar to that in adults, but it may differ markedly in small infants, especially premature neonates, who excrete predominantly serine, alanine, lysine, phenylalanine, tyrosine, cystine, proline, and hydroxyproline. The difference is due primarily to decreased renal tubular reabsorption. Healthy children excrete about 1 per cent of the filtered amino acids, and infants excrete as much as several per cent [61].

Although knowledge of mechanisms involved in tubular transport of amino acids is very limited, it is known that there are three groups of amino acids which compete for tubular reabsorption: The first group includes arginine and lysine; the second, leucine, isoleucine, and histidine; and the third, glycine alone. The absorption of amino acids at the level of the jejunal mucosa appears to involve similar mechanisms in that identical competition for amino acid absorption has been shown. Moreover, in specific defects of amino acid transport, such as cystinuria and Hartnup disease, both tubular reabsorption and intestinal absorption are defective.

Increased urinary excretion of amino acids is due to one of two mechanisms: (1) *overflow aminoaciduria*—i.e., saturation of tubular transport due to an increased filtered load, the plasma level of the amino acid or amino acids involved being elevated; or (2) *renal aminoaciduria,* due either to a specific defect in the reabsorption of one group of amino acids or to nonspecific dysfunction of the proximal tubule resulting in a generalized aminoaciduria, plasma levels characteristically being normal. Only the renal aminoacidurias are considered in this section [87, 180, 370].

Cystinuria. The importance of this defect is that patients are prone to urolithiasis [52, 395]. Tubular reabsorption of cystine, ornithine, arginine, and lysine is abnormal. There is increasing evidence that penicillamine may be useful in the treatment of cystine stones. This disorder is discussed in detail on page 1076.

Hartnup Disease. This is a disorder in which there is abnormal tubular transport of a number of amino acids, particularly tryptophan [357, 458]. A peculiar rash is present, and there are central nervous system manifestations. The disease is described in detail on page 1083.

Hereditary Glycinuria. This condition has been described by DeVries and his co-workers in only one family [113]. It is transmitted as an autosomal dominant and was present in three consecutive generations. The only clinical manifestations were associated with recurrent nephrolithiasis. Urinary excretion of glycine was markedly elevated, whereas the plasma level was normal. Chemical analysis of one calculus revealed primarily calcium oxalate, but 0.5 per cent of free glycine was found. Jejunal transport of glycine was not investigated.

Glucoglycinuria. This condition was described by Käser and his associates in 14 members of a single family [263]. Renal glycosuria was present in association with a marked excretion of glycine. The patients were asymptomatic except for the propositus, who had cystic fibrosis.

Late Vitamin D-Resistant Rickets with Hyperglycinuria. This entity is similar to the more common *familial hypophosphatemia* (page 1108) except for its late onset in adolescence and early adulthood and excessive urinary excretion of glycine [266]. In a patient reported by Scriver et al. glycinuria and hyperphosphaturia were associated with renal glucosuria and abnormal excretion of glycylproline [459].

The relationship, if any, between the various entities and abnormal glycinuria is unknown. Differentiation from *idiopathic hyperglycinemia* in which the hyperglycinuria depends on an overflow mechanism, is important.

Beta-Aminoisobutyric Aciduria. Beta-aminoisobutyric aciduria has no clinical significance. However, the urinary excretion of the metabolite is of interest as a genetic marker.

Nonspecific Defects of Amino Acid Transport. The presence of generalized aminoaciduria is indicative of nonspecific tubular damage and generally is associated with other tubular abnormalities. This type of aminoaciduria usually is not characteristic, most of the plasma amino acids being present in the urine in excessive amounts. However, some differences in the pattern of aminoaciduria may be found depending on the etiology of the tubular dysfunction. Thus cystine is characteristically increased in Wilson's disease, proline in cystinosis, and lysine and tyrosine in Lowe's syndrome.

Generalized aminoaciduria is characteristically present in vitamin D-deficient rickets [88] and may be found as an isolated tubular abnormality in cases of congenital lactose intolerance, hereditary intolerance to fructose, galactosemia, Wilson's disease, heavy-metal poisoning, and malnutrition.

XANTHINURIA

Xanthinuria is an extremely rare cause of urolithiasis in children [111, 518, 537]. Not everyone with xanthinuria has stones, which apparently form only when the urinary concentration exceeds 30 to 40 mg. per 100 ml. Little is known about the pathophysiology which probably involves a specific tubular defect in the transport of xanthine, hypoxanthine, and uric acid.

Xanthine stones should be suspected when radiolucent urolithiasis is detected, since all stones except those formed of xanthine and uric acid are radiopaque.

DISORDERS OF PHOSPHATE TRANSPORT

Familial Vitamin D-Resistant Rickets. This is a form of hypophosphatemic rickets in which the primary abnormality is believed to be an isolated defect in phosphate transport [439, 504, 532]. However, this view is not accepted by many authors, who believe the primary abnormality is intestinal malabsorption of calcium and phosphorus with secondary hyperparathyroidism. The pathogenesis of this condition is described in Chapter 6. Hypophosphatemic rickets generally is transmitted as a sex-linked dominant trait, although other modes of inheritance have been described, suggesting that the term may include more than a single disease.

Onset of symptoms ranges from infancy to several years of age, with clinical evidence of rickets, poor growth, and bone pain. Laboratory features in children do not differ from those in adults, with severe hypophosphatemia being the most striking finding.

Treatment consists of administration of large amounts of vitamin D, 50,000 to 100,000 units or more per day, with an attempt to find an effective dose which does not produce vitamin D toxicity. Serial measurements of blood and urinary calcium should be done to ensure that hypercalcemia is not induced and that the rate of calciuria does not exceed 2 mg. per kilogram of body weight per day. In determining the optimal dosage of vitamin D, the dosage should not be changed more often than every two weeks. Toxicity may require withdrawal of therapy for several weeks. Favorable results have been reported with oral administration of large amounts of phosphate, 1.5 to 2.0 gm. daily added to the ordinary diet.

Sporadic Hypophosphatemic Rickets. Royer [428] has described four cases of sporadic hypophosphatemic rickets of a very severe form. The clinical and biochemical features resemble closely hereditary hypophosphatemia, but renal tubular reabsorption of phosphate is not restored to normal by intravenous infusion of calcium. Treatment is the same as for the familial form of the disease.

Pseudohypoparathyroidism. In this condition, which mimics true hypoparathyroidism, the parathyroid glands anatomically are normal, with no deficiency in parathyroid secretion [315]. The associated skeletal disturbances, retardation of skeletal growth and brachydactyly, are not present in hypoparathyroidism, and are unexplained. Mental retardation has been reported in several patients, and metastatic calcification is common.

Biochemical features are identical to those in hypoparathyroidism, except for the failure of response to parathormone (Ellsworth-Howard test). Treatment consists of administration of large amounts of vitamin D in starting doses of 10,000 units in infants and 25,000 to 50,000 units in older children. In an individual patient, the optimal dose, which avoids both symptoms of the disease and also vitamin D toxicity, must be determined as described above, by frequent monitoring of blood and urinary calcium. Therapy must be continued indefinitely.

MULTIPLE DYSFUNCTION OF THE PROXIMAL RENAL TUBULE (FANCONI SYNDROME)

The name Fanconi syndrome or De Toni-Debré-Fanconi syndrome is given to a disorder involving multiple functional disturbances of the proximal tubule, including prominent defects in the reabsorption of glucose, amino acids, and phosphate [153]. Tubular proteinuria, acidosis, inadequate renal conservation of sodium and potassium, and a defect in maximum concentrating ability may all be present. The term Fanconi syndrome was originally given to the idiopathic form of the disorder. However, cystinosis was soon found to be the most common cause of the "primary" form in children, and many other causes or entities with an associated Fanconi syndrome have been disclosed. In current terminology, the designation Fanconi syndrome is given to any nonspecific, complex, proximal tubular dysfunction, complete or partial, regardless of etiology.

The pathophysiology, and clinical and laboratory features are discussed in detail in Chapter 30.

The clinical picture varies depending on the degree of tubular dysfunction and the etiology. However, characteristic symptoms are common to all forms with complete dysfunction of long-standing duration. Failure to thrive and growth retardation are constant. Bone lesions of rickets, osteoporosis, or both are frequent, despite adequate intake of vitamin D, and may dominate the clinical picture. Polyuria is found occasionally and in the early months of life may cause unexplained fever, dehydration, and constipation. Muscular weakness and paralysis caused by potassium deficiency may also be present.

Serum analysis reveals hypophosphatemia and normal or low levels of calcium. Alkaline phosphatase is increased if there are active osteomalacic lesions. Hyperchloremic acidosis and hypokalemia are frequently present. Rarely, a patient may present with metabolic alkalosis due to chronic renal loss of sodium, chloride, and potassium. Serum levels of amino acids are normal.

The urine contains glucose, and there is a generalized aminoaciduria of the "renal" type. Rate of excretion of phosphate in urine may be normal, but an increased phosphate clearance or decreased coefficient of phosphate reabsorption (TRP) is found. Proteinuria frequently is present.

The urine pH is 6.0 or higher, and the rates of excretion of titratable acid and ammonium are low. However, most patients are able to elaborate an acid urine and to excrete adequate hydrogen ion when stimulated by the administration of an acid load, indicating that the acidosis is of the proximal type — that is, caused by a defect in bicarbonate reabsorption (page 1093). Both the plasma threshold and Tm of reabsorption of bicarbonate have been found low in cases of Fanconi syndrome of varied etiologies [245].

Hypercalciuria is usually found, but in contrast with distal renal tubular acidosis, nephrocalcinosis and lithiasis are exceptional [422]. A defect in maximum concentrating ability may be present; it probably results from the potassium deficiency and hypercalciuria rather than from a specific tubular defect.

The course, prognosis, and specific treatment of the Fanconi syndrome depend on the cause. Secondary dysfunctions will, in general, disappear after withdrawal of the offending cause or treatment of the primary disease. Some general therapeutic measures, applicable to all types of the disease, are considered here.

The bone lesions of rickets and osteomalacia are resistant to vitamin D, and require doses in excess of 25,000 international units (I.U.) per day. Some children require as much as 400,000 I.U. per day, and often remineralization cannot be achieved even with these large doses. Careful monitoring of the calcium concentration in the blood and its rate of excretion in urine is necessary to avoid vitamin D toxicity. Correction of the acidosis is an important measure, but, in contrast with distal renal tubular acidosis, rachitic lesions will not heal until vitamin D is given. The amount of sodium and potassium citrate or bicarbonate necessary to control the acidosis is generally much larger than the dose required in distal renal tubular acidosis. It should be given every 2 to 4 hours, day and night, in a dose sufficient to keep the blood pH and total carbon dioxide within the normal range. As much as 10 mEq. of citrate or bicarbonate per kilogram per day may be required. The administration of potassium is mandatory if hypokalemia is present. When polyuria is present, water requirements should be evaluated carefully, especially during infancy. In spite of all these measures, growth and development often remain poor.

Primary Fanconi Syndromes. CYSTINOSIS. This disease, an inborn error of metabolism, was first recognized at autopsy by Abdehalden in 1903 and established as a clinical entity by Lignac in 1924. It is also known under the names of Lignac-Fanconi syndrome or cystine storage disease. The disorder is characterized by the existence of the Fanconi syndrome in association with deposits of cystine crystals in many tissues of the body. The tubular dysfunction probably represents a secondary abnormality, but it generally appears as a "primary" condition, the cystine storage being undetected [47, 154, 535].

The frequency of cystinosis is estimated to be between 1:20,000 and 1:40,000 of the general population. In one-third of reported cases there is a familial distribution, the disorder being inherited as an autosomal recessive. No abnormality has been detected in heterozygotes.

The defect of cystine metabolism responsible for the accumulation of cystine in the cells of the cornea, reticuloendothelial system, and proximal renal tubular and renal interstitial tissue is unknown. A lack or inactivity of cystine reductase has been suggested but not confirmed. The pathogenesis of the tubular dysfunction is unknown. It is believed to represent a toxic effect of cystine on sulfhydryl-containing enzymes. However, cystine crystals are found mainly in the interstitial tissue and not in the interior of the tubular cells, and some authors believe that the basic cause of the renal disturbances lies in a metabolic or enzymatic deficiency of the tubular cell, the cystine deposits being secondary and noncausative.

The clinical picture arises from involvement of kidney, intestine, eyes, liver, spleen, and lymph nodes. In most cases, however, the picture is dominated by symptoms related to the renal tubular defects, with progressive glomerular insufficiency and death in uremia. The clinical onset occurs in the first months of life, but in rare cases it may be delayed until late childhood. The earliest abnormality, when normal siblings of affected children are studied, is the appearance of aminoaciduria. Soon thirst, vomiting, constipation, chronic dehydration, unexplained fever, and failure to thrive become evident. Growth retardation becomes increasingly severe during the first years of life, and signs of rickets may become predominant. When renal function is studied during this early stage, the glomerular filtration rate is normal, but multiple tubular dysfunctions are usually found. Sometimes, only isolated abnormalities are present: glycosuria, aminoaciduria, or hyperchloremic acidosis. Death may occur during this stage from acute hypokalemia, acidosis, or overwhelming infection. Hepatomegaly, lymphadenopathy, and rarely splenomegaly may appear. Photophobia, if noted, should suggest strongly the diagnosis of cystinosis.

After a variable period, glomerular insufficiency becomes evident and tubular symptoms improve or disappear. This amelioration is only apparent and is due to the progressive destruction of nephrons. After a number of years the glomerular insufficiency becomes so severe that the symptoms are dominated by the uremic syndrome. Death occurs usually before puberty.

Cystine crystals are rectangular or hexagonal, and they are easily seen under polarized light in smears from a bone marrow aspiration, peripheral leukocytes, liver, spleen, or lymph nodes. In about 80 per cent of the cases they can be seen by slit-lamp examination of the cornea. Cystine is soluble in aqueous solution and in formalin; therefore, an alcoholic fixative should be chosen for histologic studies. The absence of cystine crystals in a single bone marrow aspiration does not exclude the condition, and repeated trials over a period of several years may be necessary.

Treatment is symptomatic. The use of penicillamine has been recommended recently, but its usefulness is still undetermined. The possible beneficial effect of a diet poor in cystine and methionine is also unclear.

IDIOPATHIC FANCONI SYNDROME. This entity is most often seen in adults, but it occurs occasionally in children, about 20 cases having been reported in the pediatric age group[48, 94, 153, 245, 248, 292, 422, 534]. Inheritance occurs as an autosomal recessive. The onset is often between the first and second year of life, and the clinical picture is that of the Fanconi syndrome. In contrast with cystinosis, glomerular function is not affected during its evolution, and patients may attain adult life, although severely retarded in growth. Exclusion of cystinosis is obligatory in any isolated Fanconi syndrome appearing in childhood since the finding of cystine crystals indicates a fatal prognosis. Only after a repeatedly negative search for cystine may the syndrome be labeled idiopathic.

LUDER AND SHELDON SYNDROME. Luder and Sheldon found a glucoaminoaciduria in three generations of the same family [320, 465]. Over the course of many years the three affected members of the last generation developed vitamin D-resistant rickets and tubular acidosis.

CEREBRO-OCULORENAL DYSTROPHY (LOWE'S SYNDROME). This entity was described in 1952 by Lowe et al. [316, 404, 436]. It associates the Fanconi syndrome with mental retardation and severe congenital ocular abnormalities. It is a hereditary condition, transmitted by a sex-linked recessive gene, all the affected members being males. Cataracts may develop in female carriers. The cause of the condition is unknown. Chromosomal analyses have been normal, and no specific metabolic block has been detected. Abnormalities of amino acid excretion during ornithine administration have been reported, but their significance is unknown.

The age of onset is variable from early months to late childhood. The presence of cataracts is almost constant, and they frequently coexist with congenital glaucoma (hydrophthalmos). Nystagmus is common and is probably secondary to the blindness. The involvement of the nervous system is very characteristic and combines severe mental retardation with marked muscular hypotonia and tendinous areflexia. Paralyses are never found. Patients may emit a continuous, distressing cry.

A peculiar type of Fanconi syndrome is seen: glycosuria is rare, aminoaciduria is only moderate, a concentrating defect is exceptional, and hypokalemia has never been found. Proximal renal tubular acidosis has been demonstrated. Lowe and his co-workers reported a characteristic organic aciduria. However, this finding has not been confirmed. Osteoporosis is the most frequent bone lesion, but rickets may be present. Retardation in growth and development soon becomes evident. Development of glomerular insufficiency does not occur, but nevertheless the prognosis remains poor due to severe mental retardation and poor vision.

The differential diagnosis includes other conditions in which there is an association of cerebral, ocular, and renal abnormalities. A frequent error is the indiscriminate diagnosis of Lowe's syndrome in a severely retarded child with rickets, aminoaciduria, and ocular anomalies. In many such cases rickets is due to deficiency of vitamin D from inadequate nutrition and lack of sunlight.

There is no specific therapy, but adequate measures to control bone lesions and acidosis should be undertaken.

Secondary Fanconi Syndromes. CONGENITAL CIRRHOSIS WITH FANCONI SYNDROME AND TYROSINURIA ("TYROSINEMIA"). This entity, first reported by Baber in 1956 [18], consists of congenital cirrhosis of the liver and multiple tubular dysfunctions. Tyrosine is present in abnormal amounts in blood and urine, and the term "tyrosinemia" has been suggested [178]. A high degree of consanguinity has been reported. The disease appears to be inherited as a recessive. Gentz and his associates [178] suggest that the condition is an inborn error of tyrosine metabolism associated with lack of p-hydroxyphenylpyruvic acid oxidase; p-hydroxyphenylpyruvic acid is increased in the urine, suggesting an identity with the condition "tyrosinosis" described by Medes. However, on both clinical and biochemical grounds the conditions are probably different.

In cases with very early onset the clinical picture is dominated by liver involvement and is similar to galactosemia. In less severe cases, the Fanconi syndrome is the predominant feature. Hepatomegaly is constant. Death may occur during the early months of life from hepatic insufficiency or be delayed several years, in which case the development of a malignant hepatoma has been reported. The finding of tyrosinemia and tyrosinuria are diagnostic.

The course of the disease is invariably fatal. The effect of a diet low in phenylalanine and tyrosine is still under evaluation. In the only reported cases, improvement was found in renal tubular but not in hepatic function.

GALACTOSEMIA. Galactosemia is an inborn error of galactose metabolism caused by an absence of galactose 1-phosphate uridyl transferase. The accumulation of galactose 1-phosphate has toxic effects in many body tissues, especially liver, brain, cornea, and kidney. The renal toxic effect is primarily an isolated aminoaciduria, but proteinuria, true glycosuria, and tubular acidosis may also be present. The tubular abnormalities disappear quickly when a diet without lactose and galactose is instituted [102].

GLYCOGEN STORAGE DISEASE. One patient has been described by Fanconi and Bickel [154] with a glucoaminophosphaturia. Tubular dysfunction was probably dependent on accumulation of glycogen in the renal proximal tubular cells.

WILSON'S DISEASE. The most frequent renal abnormality is aminoaciduria [503]. Glycosuria, increased phosphate and urate clearances, and hyperchloremic acidosis may also be found. Hypercalciuria is very frequent and urinary lithiasis has been reported in adult cases. The tubular abnormalities probably depend on a toxic accumulation of copper. Treatment of the disease by D-penicillamine will improve the hepatic and neurologic symptoms, but the effect on tubular dysfunction is less evident.

HEREDITARY INTOLERANCE TO FRUCTOSE. Aminoaciduria and hyperchloremic acidosis may be present in this disease. A defect in bicarbonate reabsorption has been documented by Morris [362]. The toxic substance is probably fructose 1-phosphate.

NEPHROTIC SYNDROME. The presence of tubular abnormalities during the evolution of the idiopathic nephrotic syndrome is exceptional [437]. Only 13 cases of a complete Fanconi syndrome have been described in children. It is not known if these patients represent a specific entity or a particular evolution of a noncharacteristic idiopathic nephrotic syndrome.

The clinical picture is rather uniform. During the initial period the nephrotic syndrome is typical, and normal renal histology and function are present. Later, tubular function becomes progressively affected with marked hypokalemia and tetany. In a later stage, glomerular insufficiency is severe, and in all reported cases the patients have died in uremia. The administration of steroids has been ineffective.

EXOGENOUS TOXINS. Proximal tubular damage may follow the exposure to many toxic substances. Heavy metals are especially notorious. Aminoaciduria and glycosuria have been reported in association with lead [89], cadmium, uranium, and mercury intoxication. Chisolm and Leahy [89] found that aminoaciduria and glycosuria were almost constant in lead poisoning in children, and they reported a case with associated increased phosphate clearance and rickets. Other potentially toxic substances include Lysol and some antibiotics, including tetracycline and amphotericin B. The tubular abnormality disappears after discontinuation of the toxic substance, although complete reversal may take weeks or months.

RENAL TUBULAR ACIDOSIS

Two mechanisms are involved in renal excretion of acid: (1) reabsorption of filtered bicarbonate, which is primarily a proximal function; and (2) excretion of hydrogen ion in the form of titratable acid and ammonium, which is primarily a distal function. Abnormalities of these mechanisms are associated, therefore, with loss of bicarbonate into urine due to a defect in bicarbonate reabsorption, termed proximal renal tubular acidosis; impaired excretion of hydrogen ion as titratable acid or ammonium or both, termed distal renal tubular acidosis; or a combination of these mechanisms.

Although the term *renal tubular acidosis* (RTA) is used conventionally to indicate a specific heritable entity characterized by an inability to acidify the urine, a complete classification now requires separation into proximal and distal tubular acidosis, which is used here [419].

Proximal Renal Tubular Acidosis. In this condition hyperchloremic acidosis results from incomplete reabsorption of bicarbonate in the proximal renal tubule [419–421]. The capacity of the distal tubule to reabsorb bicarbonate is exceeded and an acid urine cannot be formed. During metabolic acidosis, with a smaller load of filtered bicarbonate to reabsorb, these patients are able to elaborate urine with a pH of 5.0 or below and demonstrate normal rates of excretion of titratable acid and ammonium. Thus, in contrast to normal children whose renal bicarbonate plasma threshold is 24 to 26 mmoles per liter (21.5 to 22.5 mmoles per liter in infants), these patients excrete bicarbonate in the urine until blood concentrations fall to acidotic levels. If attempts are made to correct the acidosis by administration of bicarbonate, large and frequent doses are required since the bicarbonate is excreted rapidly in the urine once the abnormally low plasma threshold is exceeded.

In these patients the maximal rate of reabsorption of bicarbonate is also low, indicating a defect in rate of production or secretion of hydrogen ion in the proximal segment. As judged by response to administration of acetazolamide, carbonic anhydrase activity is normal.

In the patients described in our original report of the primary form of this disorder, glomerular and other tubular functions were normal, except for one patient who had renal glycosuria as well. Histologically the kidneys revealed no abnormalities [420]. Bone lesions and nephrocalcinosis were absent, the major clinical manifestation being retarded growth. High-dosage bicarbonate or citrate therapy was necessary to assure adequate growth.

All the patients we have studied with primary proximal renal tubular acidosis have been males. The secondary complications frequently observed in distal renal tubular acidosis (see below) have been absent. Several patients apparently have recovered.

Secondary forms of proximal renal tubular acidosis have been demonstrated in association with other tubular dysfunctions in patients with idiopathic Fanconi syndrome (page 1390), cystinosis (page 1389), Lowe's syndrome (page 1391), and hereditary intolerance to fructose [363].

Distal Renal Tubular Acidosis. The net excretion of hydrogen ion is regulated by the distal tubule, and, in consequence, abnormalities in its function may be responsible for tubular acidosis. Abnormalities in distal tubular handling of hydrogen ion theoretically might result in primary defects in acidification of the urine (i.e., establishment of low urinary pH), excretion of titratable acid, or excretion of ammonium. However, the only abnormality that has been documented is an inability to establish an adequate gradient of pH between blood and urine, with secondary impairment in formation of titratable acid and ammonium [6, 419, 462]. A primary defect in excretion of titratable acid has been suspected in some adults with low phosphate excretion; an isolated defect in ammonium excretion has not yet been demonstrated.

PRIMARY DISTAL RENAL TUBULAR ACIDOSIS. The *persistent or adult form* (*Butler-Albright syndrome*) is usually referred to simply as renal tubular acidosis and results from the inability of the distal tubular cell to establish an adequate pH gradient between blood and urine [6, 67]. The majority of cases reported are sporadic, but there are several examples of an increased family incidence, suggesting an autosomal dominant transmission.

The disorder occurs predominantly in females (about 70 per cent of cases) and tends to appear after the age of 2 years, and frequently not until adult life. However, several cases unquestionably have begun in infancy, with vomiting, constipation, anorexia, polyuria, dehydration, and failure to thrive. Growth retardation is most evident beyond infancy and may represent the only clinical abnormality. Bone lesions are frequent, and rickets and osteomalacia are present during childhood and adolescence. Nephrocalcinosis is an almost constant finding and may be demonstrated by x-ray examination. Urolithiasis also is common, but occurs less frequently in children than in adults.

Serum analysis reveals a low pH and bicarbonate concentration with elevation of the chloride. Moderate hyponatremia and hypokalemia are present. The concentration of phosphate in blood is low, with normal or even high levels of calcium. The alkaline phosphatase may be elevated if active osteomalacic lesions are present. The glomerular filtration rate is normal in the young child if adequately hydrated, although variable degrees of glomerular insufficiency are present in adult patients.

Urine pH is usually above 6.0, with low rates of excretion of titratable acid and ammonium, despite concurrent acidemia. Polyuria is marked; it is due to a concentration defect. In the early stages, the hyposthenuria may be corrected by adequate control of the acidosis and potassium deficiency, but subsequent to nephrocalcinosis and tubular damage, it becomes fixed.

The phosphate clearance is increased, as a manifestation of secondary hyperparathyroidism. Hypercalciuria is a constant feature when acidosis is present, and reverts completely to normal after adequate alkali therapy. Hyperkaliuria results not only from a preferential excretion of potassium instead of hydrogen ion, at the level of the distal tubule, but also from secondary hyperaldosteronism triggered by sodium depletion. A low excretion of citrate is characteristic and is probably secondary to the intratubular acidosis and potassium deficiency. Normal urinary levels of citrate can be obtained only after persistent administration of alkali and potassium [439]. The hypercalciuria, hypocitraturia, and alkaline urine are important factors in the development of nephrocalcinosis.

The prognosis in primary distal RTA is good if the diagnosis is established early enough to prevent the development of nephrocalcinosis with secondary pyelonephritis and tubular damage. Treatment consists of correcting the acidosis, following which the bone lesions heal without large amounts of vitamin D, and the growth rate accelerates, patients often regaining their earlier normal growth pattern. Calcium excretion reverts to normal, and further calcium deposits may be prevented. Potassium needs to be given regardless of the serum potassium value; in instances of severe hypokalemia, potassium should be given prior to correction of acidemia.

The *transient or infantile form* (*Lightwood syndrome*) was first recognized by Lightwood et al. in infants with anorexia, vomiting, constipation, failure to thrive, polyuria, and hypotonia [305]. Rickets and nephrocalcinosis were not demonstrated radiologically. The response to alkali therapy was dramatic, and the patients were said to recover spontaneously around 2 years of age. When some patients were studied at an older age, they were reported to have a normal response to ammonium chloride administration. At least 90 cases were documented in England between 1947 and 1953, and a temporary immaturity of the renal tubule was suspected as a possible cause.

The pathogenesis of the acidosis is unclear.

A neutral or alkaline urine was present despite the hyperchloremic acidosis, but no precise studies of hydrogen excretion were performed. Latner and Burnard [290] suspected a bicarbonate reabsorption defect in six infants, and it is possible that a *proximal,* rather than a *distal,* defect was present. Moreover, it appears likely now that this infantile or transient form did not represent a single etiologic entity. Probably most of the cases reported in England were a manifestation of vitamin D toxicity. The peak incidence of the disease coincided with that of idiopathic hypercalcemia. When the vitamin content of foods was decreased, both diseases became rare [304]. Toxicity due to sulfonamides and mercury was also suspected.

SECONDARY DISTAL RENAL TUBULAR ACIDOSIS. Tubular acidosis may be associated with a number of systemic and renal conditions. In many of these the pathogenesis is unclear, and both proximal and distal types may be represented. In most instances, however, an inability to acidify the urine has been reported, indicating the possibility of a deficient distal mechanism [419, 462]. Hyperchloremic acidosis has been documented in cases of primary hyperparathyroidism, hyperthyroidism, vitamin D deficiency (nutritional or secondary to steatorrhea), vitamin D intoxication, idiopathic hypercalcemia, various types of hyperglobulinemia, mercury intoxication, and in the recovery phase of acute tubular necrosis and infantile dehydration. The hyperchloremic acidosis associated with pyelonephritis and obstructive uropathy is accompanied by a urine of maximum acidity and is probably secondary to nonspecific generalized tubular damage.

IDIOPATHIC HYPERCALCIURIA

Idiopathic hypercalciuria is a frequent cause of recurrent lithiasis in adults. It occurs less frequently in children, however, and few cases have been described [38, 152, 430, 440, 543]. The most frequent presenting symptom is growth retardation in association with renal abnormalities such as proteinuria and decreased concentrating capacity. Clinical manifestations also include urolithiasis, nephrocalcinosis, and vitamin D-resistant rickets.

Calcium excretion exceeds 5 mg. per kilogram of body weight per day. Acidosis is not present, and the hypercalciuria does not decrease after administration of sodium bicarbonate. Serum calcium is normal, and serum phosphorus may be normal or low. Renal histology is normal or shows variable degrees of interstitial nephritis. In the cases studied, intestinal absorption of calcium was normal, pointing to a renal tubular abnormality as the cause of the hypercalciuria.

The rate of excretion of calcium can be decreased by administration of diuretic agents or restriction of dietary sodium. Both measures increase proximal reabsorption of sodium and, presumably, calcium as well.

SALT-LOSING DISORDERS

Pseudohypoaldosteronism. This entity, first described by Cheek and Perry in 1958 [84], is believed to represent a failure of the renal tubule to respond to aldosterone, with secondary excessive loss of sodium in the urine, hyponatremia, and hyperkalemia [84, 119, 431, 434]. The five cases reported were all males, but a genetic transmission is unproved.

Affected infants are normal at birth, but after one or two weeks exhibit vomiting, anorexia, failure to thrive, and if treatment is delayed, severe marasmus, with delayed skeletal and psychomotor development, appears. During episodes of dehydration, often triggered by intercurrent infection, patients may have marked vascular collapse or even coma.

The serum sodium concentration is low, and moderate hyperkalemia is present. Despite dehydration and hyponatremia a high rate of excretion of urinary sodium continues. The excretion of 17-ketosteroids and 17-hydroxysteroids is normal, but the excretion of aldosterone is abnormally high, up to 900 micrograms per 24 hours. The administration of DOCA or aldosterone fails to modify the urinary excretion of sodium.

Differentiation from the salt-losing forms of congenital adrenal hyperplasia and adrenal insufficiency is difficult clinically and depends upon appropriate investigation of steroid metabolism. Hypertrophic pyloric stenosis, cystic fibrosis, inappropriate ADH secretion, and other salt-losing nephropathies should also be considered.

The administration of supplementary sodium chloride is the treatment of choice. A dose of about 5 gm. per day is required, following which there is usually dramatic improvement in vomiting, weight gain, and skeletal and psychomotor development. There is some evidence that after some months or years, the need for supplementary sodium chloride decreases, but sufficient data from long-term follow-up studies are not yet available.

Salt-Losing Nephropathies. Excessive urinary loss of sodium occurs together with other tubular abnormalities in the Fanconi syndrome, in distal renal tubular acidosis, and in other tubulopathies; it is found also in association with some forms of generalized renal disease [497]. Limitation of renal capacity to conserve sodium is common in most cases of uremia, but usually a balance between input and output is maintained, urinary wastage becoming evident only under conditions of salt deprivation. However, in exceptional cases, termed *salt-losing nephritis,* the urinary loss of sodium is so marked during periods of normal intake that the patients appear to have Addison's disease. This syndrome has usually been associated with chronic pyelonephritis, medullary cystic disease, and hereditary polycystic disease.

This condition apparently is rare in children, the youngest patient reported being an adolescent. Urinary sodium loss of lesser degree is seen, however, in children with bilateral renal hypoplasia or dysplasia, obstructive uropathy, juvenile nephronophthisis, and interstitial nephritis.

It is important to realize that the salt-losing defect associated with tubular and generalized renal disorders is often unrecognized. Dehydration may be minimal, and the serum sodium may be normal due to compensatory contraction of the extracellular space. However, even in such patients, giving extra sodium is followed by improved well-being, weight gain, and increases in rates of glomerular filtration and renal plasma flow.

POTASSIUM-LOSING DISORDERS

Pseudohyperaldosteronism (Liddle's Syndrome). In 1964 Liddle et al. [300] described this hereditary condition, probably transmitted as an autosomal dominant, in six siblings with hypertension, hypokalemic alkalosis, and negligible aldosterone secretion. The disorder seems to be caused by an unusual tendency of the kidney to reabsorb sodium and excrete potassium even in the virtual absence of mineralocorticoids. These patients differ from normal subjects and from patients with primary aldosteronism in that their electrolyte excretion is unaffected by giving either an inhibitor of aldosterone synthesis or an aldosterone antagonist. Giving both an inhibitor of tubular sodium transport (triamterene) and supplementary potassium chloride serves to return the blood pressure to normal and to correct the hypokalemia.

Hyperplasia of the Juxtaglomerular Apparatus with Hyperaldosteronism and Hypokalemic Alkalosis (Bartter's Syndrome). About 20 patients with this condition are reported in the literature, under such varied names as renal tubular alkalosis, congenital hyperaldosteronism, chronic idiopathic hypokalemia, and congenital hypokalemia [36, 63, 73, 85, 435, 469]. Bartter et al. [36] reported two cases in 1962 and defined the pathophysiology. Several familial cases are documented; it is probably inherited as an autosomal recessive.

Symptoms first occur during infancy, but the diagnosis may be delayed for many years. The earliest symptoms are polyuria, polydipsia, a tendency toward dehydration, constipation, vomiting, and anorexia. Growth retardation is constant, becoming more marked as the child gets older. Muscular weakness is frequent, and very often recurrent tetany is present. The blood pressure characteristically is normal. The outstanding biochemical feature is the marked hypokalemia, often accompanied by hyponatremia, hypochloremia, and metabolic alkalosis. Hypercalcemia and hyperlipemia may also be found. The urine is dilute, with no response to exogenous vasopressin, and contains abundant amounts of sodium, potassium, and chloride, despite the simultaneous hypoelectrolytemia. Glomerular and tubular functions generally are normal. In all cases in which the aldosterone secretion rate has been studied, it has been markedly elevated. The urinary excretion of aldosterone, however, may be normal or even low, if potassium deficiency has not been corrected. The excretion of 17-ketosteroids and 17-hydroxysteroids is normal, and the plasma levels of renin and angiotensin are elevated.

Renal pathologic findings are characteristic. The glomeruli reveal marked hypertrophy of the juxtaglomerular apparatus, and a variable degree of hyalinization. The tubular lesions of potassium deficiency may be present. The zona glomerulosa of the adrenal gland is hypertrophic, with marked lipid infiltration.

The pathophysiology of this disorder is still under study. Bartter believes the primary defect is insensitivity of the arterial and arteriolar muscles to angiotensin. The consequent increase in angiotensin stimulates aldosterone secretion, and potassium loss results. This hypothesis explains the normotension and the decreased response to administration of angiotensin.

Differential diagnosis includes primary aldosteronism, due either to adenoma or to adrenal hyperplasia. The absence of hypertension, sodium retention, and hypernatremia, and the very high levels of renin and angiotensin in Bartter's syndrome differentiate the two conditions. Patients with secondary hyperaldosteronism due to renovascular or malignant hypertension or associated with edematous states should be differentiated easily. Other potassium-losing disorders such as Fanconi syndrome, distal renal tubular acidosis, Liddle's syndrome and some types of pyelonephritis must also be considered.

The prognosis is poor and death may occur suddenly, due to acute electrolyte imbalance or intercurrent infection. There is some evidence that progressive glomerular insufficiency may appear over the course of years.

Therapeutic administration of potassium is mandatory, but if given alone, it is quickly lost in the urine without correction of the hypokalemia. The best results are obtained by the simultaneous administration of spironolactone (Aldactone) with sodium and potassium supplements. Dosage must be adjusted to obtain an equilibrium between intake and excretion. Partial adrenalectomy is without effect and should not be done.

NEPHROGENIC DIABETES INSIPIDUS

Nephrogenic diabetes insipidus (NDI) is a hereditary disorder characterized by insensitivity of the renal tubule to vasopressin [79, 146, 171, 176, 177, 238, 260, 262, 295, 379, 453, 524]. Most of the affected patients are male, suggesting a sex-linked transmission [166, 415]. Heterozygous females may exhibit some degree of polyuria with limitation of concentrating ability. This type of inheritance contrasts with vasopressin-deficient diabetes insipidus which, when genetically determined, is transmitted as an autosomal dominant.

NDI appears shortly after birth. Polyuria and polydipsia generally are not appreciated, and the infant presents with a nonspecific picture of vomiting, anorexia, constipation, unexplained fever, recurrent dehydration, and failure to thrive. In some of these infants thirst is virtually absent ("occult diabetes insipidus") [176]. A marked retardation in psychomotor development is often present; it has been attributed both to the chronic hyperelectrolytemia and to the lack of environmental stimulation, most of the infant's time being spent in drinking and sleeping [446]. In older children, beyond three or four years of age, polyuria, polydipsia, and retarded growth persist, but a more normal balance between intake and output is possible and secondary complications generally are absent.

Examination of the serum, especially in infants, reveals increased concentrations of sodium, chloride, and urea secondary to the negative water balance. Despite dehydration and hemoconcentration, urine is dilute, with a specific gravity between 1.001 and 1.005 (40 to 200 mOsm per kilogram of water). During severe dehydration, with decreased glomerular filtration rate, urinary osmolality may increase, but rarely to even slightly hypertonic levels. Administration of vasopressin changes neither the volume nor concentration of the urine. A water deprivation test to assess maximum urinary concentrating ability is not necessary for diagnosis; it is hazardous and should be avoided.

Insensitivity to vasopressin is the only primary tubular abnormality in NDI, but during dehydration proteinuria and aminoaciduria may be present. The glomerular filtration rate is normal if hydration is adequate.

In most cases the intravenous pyelogram is normal. Although in some reports marked bladder distention and hydronephrosis has been attributed to voluntary retention of large amounts of urine, such findings should suggest the diagnosis of obstructive uropathy with secondary diabetes inspidus, and adequate urologic studies must be done.

The exact pathogenesis of NDI is unknown. Antidiuretic hormone is present in blood and urine, and neurohypophyseal lesions are not found [240]. Increased concentration of electrolytes in sweat has been demonstrated [313]. The precise defect responsible for tubular insensitivity to antidiuretic hormone has not yet been determined. Histologically the kidney is normal, although a shortened proximal segment has been demonstrated by microdissection.

Differential diagnosis includes the hereditary form of diabetes insipidus due to lack of ADH, which also may start very early in life. The response to vasopressin serves to separate these conditions. Several renal disorders may present with a syndrome of vasopressin-resistant diabetes insipidus: obstructive uropathies, renal hypoplasia, hypercalciuria with or without renal tubular acidosis, potassium-losing disorders, and especially familial nephronophthisis.

The prognosis is favorable if the diagnosis is made early in life and adequate therapy is instituted. However, between 5 and 10 per cent of patients die in infancy, and in some cases both mental and physical growth is irreversibly retarded.

Therapy consists in giving water in amount and frequency necessary to compensate for the obligatory urinary loss [101]. In older children this aim is easily attained, but great difficulties may be encountered in infancy, especially when thirst is absent. Administration of solute-poor milk reduces urinary water requirements and helps to maintain an adequate water balance.

The discovery that thiazide diuretics decrease urinary output has facilitated enormously the management of these patients, especially during infancy [126, 454]. The decrease in urine volume observed following administration of the diuretic is accompanied by an increased urinary solute concentration and decreased free water clearance. It has been shown that the effect is mediated through sodium depletion, with increased proximal reabsorption of sodium and water and decreased delivery of fluid to the distal tubule. Giving sodium chloride interferes with the antidiuretic effect which is maximal on a low sodium intake. Furthermore, it can be produced by any diuretic and is not an exclusive property of the thiazides.

References

1. Aas, K. The cellular excretion in the urine of normal newborn infants. *Acta Paediat. Scand.* 50:361, 1961.
2. Abel, M. S., and Brown, C. R. Sickle cell disease with severe hematuria simulating renal neoplasm. *J.A.M.A.* 137:624, 1948.
3. Ackerman, G. L., and Nolan, C. M. Adrenocortical responsiveness after alternate-day corticosteroid therapy. *New Eng. J. Med.* 278:405, 1968.
4. Adams, D. A., Gordon, A., and Maxwell, M. H. Azathioprine treatment of immunological renal disease. *J.A.M.A.* 199: 459, 1967.
5. Albert, M. S., Leeming, J. M., and Scaglione, P. R. Acute glomerulonephritis without abnormality of the urine. *J. Pediat.* 68:525, 1966.
6. Albright, F., Burnett, C. H., Parson, W., Reifenstein, E. C., Jr., and Roos, A. Osteomalacia and late rickets: The various etiologies met in the United States with emphasis on that resulting from a special form of renal acidosis; the therapeutic indications for each etiological subgroup, and the relationship between osteomalacia and Milkman's syndrome. *Medicine* (Balt.) 25: 399, 1946.
7. Alexander, D. P., and Nixon, D. A. Plasma clearance of p-aminohippuric acid by the kidneys of foetal, neonatal, and adult sheep. *Nature* (London) 194:483, 1962.
8. Alexander, D. P., Nixon, D. A., Widdas, W. F., and Wohlzogen, F. X. Gestational variations in the composition of the foetal fluids and foetal urine in the sheep. *J. Physiol.* (London) 140:1, 1958.
9. Alexander, D. P., Nixon, D. A., Widdas, W. F., and Wohlzogen, F. X. Renal function in the sheep foetus. *J. Physiol.* (London) 140:14, 1958.
10. Allen, D. M., Diamond, L. K., and Howell, D. A. Anaphylactoid purpura in children (Schoenlein-Henoch syndrome). *A.M.A. Amer. J. Dis. Child.* 99:833, 1960.
11. Alport, A. C. Hereditary familial congenital hemorrhagic nephritis. *Brit. Med. J.* 1:504, 1927.
12. Ames, R. G. Urinary water excretion and neurohypophysial function in full term and premature infants shortly after birth. *Pediatrics* 12:272, 1953.
13. Anderson, J., Lee, H. A., and Stroud, C. E. Haemodialysis in infants and small children. *Brit. Med. J.* 1:1405, 1965.
14. Aoki, A. Development of the human renal glomerulus: I. Differentiation of the filtering membrane. *Anat. Rec.* 155:339, 1966.
15. Arneil, G. C. Management of the nephrotic syndrome. *Arch. Dis. Child.* 43:257, 1968.
16. Arneil, G. C., and Lam, N. C. Long-term assessment of steroid therapy in childhood nephrosis. *Lancet* 2:819, 1966.
17. Ayoub, E. M., and Vernier, R. L. Benign recurrent hematuria. *Amer. J. Dis. Child.* 109:217, 1965.
18. Baber, M. D. A case of congenital cirrhosis of the liver with renal tubular defects akin to those in the Fanconi syndrome. *Arch. Dis. Child.* 31:335, 1956.
19. Bacani, R. A., Velasquez, F., Kanter, A., Pirani, C. L., and Pollak, V. E. Rapidly progressive (nonstreptococcal) glomerulonephritis. *Ann. Intern. Med.* 69:463, 1968.
20. Bain, A. D., Beath, M. M., and Flint, W. F. Sirenomelia and monomelia with renal

agenesis and amnion nodosium. *Arch. Dis. Child.* 35:250, 1960.

21. Bain, A. D., and Schott, J. S. Renal agenesis and severe urinary tract dysplasias. *Brit. Med. J.* 1:841, 1960.
22. Barber, H. Chronic interstitial nephritis in children; a brother and sister affected. *Brit. Med. J.* 2:1204, 1913.
23. Barger, A. C. Personal communication, 1966.
24. Barnard, P. J., and Kibel, M. Hemolytic-uremic syndrome of infancy and childhood: Report of 11 cases. *Cent. Afr. J. Med.* 11:4, 1965.
25. Barnett, H. L. Renal physiology in infants and children: I. Method for estimation of glomerular filtration rate. *Proc. Soc. Exp. Biol. Med.* 44:654, 1940.
26. Barnett, H. L. Kidney function in young infants. *Pediatrics* 5:171, 1950.
27. Barnett, H. L. Paediatric nephrology: The scientific study of kidneys and their diseases in infants and children. *Arch. Dis. Child.* 41:229, 1966.
28. Barnett, H. L., Forman, C. W., and Lauson, H. D. The nephrotic syndrome in children. *Advances Pediat.* 5:53, 1952.
29. Barnett, H. L., Hare, W. K., McNamara, H., and Hare, R. S. Influence of postnatal age on kidney function of premature infants. *Proc. Soc. Exp. Biol. Med.* 69:55, 1948.
30. Barnett, H. L., Hare, W. K., McNamara, H., and Hare, R. S. Measurement of glomerular filtration rate in premature infants. *J. Clin. Invest.* 27:691, 1948.
31. Barnett, H. L., McNamara, H., Hare, R. S., and Hare, K. Inulin, urea, mannitol, and PAH clearance ratios in premature infants. *Fed. Proc.* 7:5, 1948.
32. Barnett, H. L., and Sereni, F. Kidney function tests in infants and children. *Pediat. Clin. N. Amer.* 2:191, 1955.
33. Barnett, H. L., and Shibuya, M. Nephrosis in children. *Postgrad. Med.* 15:362, 1954.
34. Barnett, H. L., and Vesterdal, J. The physiologic and clinical significance of immaturity of kidney function in young infants. *J. Pediat.* 42:399, 1953.
35. Barnett, H. L., Vesterdal, J., McNamara, H., and Lauson, H. D. Renal water excretion in premature infants. *J. Clin. Invest.* 31:1069, 1952.
36. Bartter, F. C., Pronove, P., Gill, J. R., and MacCardle, R. C. Hyperplasia of the juxtaglomerular complex with hyperaldosteronism and hypokalemic alkalosis: A new syndrome. *Amer. J. Med.* 33:811, 1962.
37. Bearn, J. G. The association of sirenomelia with Potter's syndrome. *Arch. Dis. Child.* 35:254, 1960.
38. Beilin, L. J., and Clayton, B. E. Idiopathic hypercalciuria in a child. *Arch. Dis. Child.* 39:409, 1964.
39. Bergstrand, A., Bergstrand, C. G., and Bucht, H. Kidney lesions associated with anaphylactoid purpura in children. *Acta Paediat. Scand.* 49:57, 1960.
40. Berlyne, G. M., Shaw, A. B., and Nilwarangkur, S. Dietary treatment of chronic renal failure: Experiences with a modified Giovannetti diet. *Nephron* 2:129, 1965.
41. Berman, L. B., and Schreiner, G. E. Clinical and histologic spectrum of the nephrotic syndrome. *Amer. J. Med.* 24:249, 1958.
42. Berman, L. B., and Tublin, I. The nephropathies of sickle cell disease. *A.M.A. Arch. Intern. Med.* 103:602, 1959.
43. Bernstein, J. Developmental Abnormalities of the Renal Parenchyma — Renal Hypoplasia and Dysplasia. In Sommers, S. C. (Ed.), *Pathology Annual 1968.* New York: Appleton-Century-Crofts, 1968. P. 213.
44. Bernstein, J., and Ruben, M. Congenital abnormalities of urinary system: II. Renal cortical and medullary necrosis. *J. Pediat.* 59:657, 1961.
45. Bernstein, J., Spitzer, A., Moore, E., Edelmann, C. M., Jr., and White, R. H. R. Pathologic significance of a "nephritic" onset in childhood nephrotic syndrome. *Amer. J. Path.* 52:47A, 1968.
46. Bernstein, J., and Whitten, C. F. A histologic appraisal of the kidney in sickle cell anemia. *Arch. Path.* (Chicago) 70:407, 1960.

47. Bickel, H., et al. Cystine storage disease with aminoaciduria and dwarfism (Lignac-Fanconi disease). *Acta Paediat. Scand.* 42: (Suppl. 90)1, 1952.
48. Bickel, H., and Thursby-Pelham, D. C. Hyperaminoaciduria in Lignac-Fanconi disease, in galactosemia and in obscure syndrome. *Arch. Dis. Child.* 29:224, 1954.
49. Blumberg, R. W., and Feldman, D. B. Observations on acute glomerulonephritis associated with impetigo. *J. Pediat.* 60:677, 1962.
50. Bodian, M., Black, J. A., Kobayashi, N., Lake, B. D., and Shuler, S. E. Recurrent hematuria in childhood. *Quart. J. Med.* 34: 359, 1965.
51. Boehm, J. J., and Haynes, J. L. Bacteriology of "midstream catch" urines: Studies in newborn infants. *Amer. J. Dis. Child.* 111:366, 1966.
52. Boström, H., and Hambraeus, L. Cystinuria in Sweden: VII. Clinical, histopathological, and medico-social aspects of the disease. *Acta Med. Scand.* 175 (Suppl. 411):7, 1964.
53. Bouissou, H., Dupont, H. G., and Régnier, Cl. L'atteinte rénale au cours du syndrome de Schönlein-Henoch. *Arch. Franc. Pediat.* 16:7, 1959.
54. Boylan, J. W., Colbourn, E. P., and McCance, R. A. Renal function in the foetal and newborn guinea pig. *J. Physiol.* (London) 141:323, 1958.
55. Brescia, M. J., Cimino, J. E., Appel, K., and Hurwich, B. J. Chronic hemodialysis using venipuncture and a surgically created arteriovenous fistula. *New Eng. J. Med.* 275:1089, 1966.
56. Brèt, A. J., Dubois, J. P., and Demay, C. Cortical necrosis and renal thrombosis in the newborn. *Arch. Franc. Pediat.* 21:101, 1964.
57. Bricker, N. S. The control of sodium excretion with normal and reduced nephron populations. *Amer. J. Med.* 43:313, 1967.
58. Bricker, N. S., Klahr, S., Lubowitz, H., and Rieselbach, R. E. Renal function in chronic renal disease. *Medicine* (Balt.) 44: 263, 1965.
59. Broberger, O., Winberg, J., and Zetterström, R. Juvenile nephronophthisis: 1. A genetically determined nephropathy with hypotonic polyuria and azotaemia. *Acta Paediat. Scand.* 49:470, 1960.
60. Brod, J., and Benesova, D. A comparative study of functional and morphological renal changes in glomerulonephritis. *Acta Med. Scand.* 157:23, 1957.
61. Brodehl, J., and Gellissen, K. Endogenous renal transport of free amino acids in infancy and childhood. *Pediatrics* 42:395, 1968.
62. Browth, R. B., Burke, E. C., and Stickler, G. B. Studies in nephrotic syndrome: 1. Survival of 135 children with nephrotic syndrome treated with adrenal steroids. *Mayo Clin. Proc.* 40:384, 1965.
63. Bryan, G. T., MacCardle, R. C., and Bartter, F. C. Hyperaldosteronism, hyperplasia of the juxtaglomerular complex, normal blood pressure and dwarfism: Report of a case. *Pediatrics* 37:43, 1966.
64. Bull, G. M. Postural proteinuria. *Clin. Sci.* 7:77, 1948.
65. Burke, E. C. Chronic nephritis in children: A diagnostic enigma. *Mayo Clin. Proc.* 34:591, 1959.
66. Burke, E. C., and Titus, J. L. Poststreptococcal acute glomerulonephritis in children. *Med. Clin. N. Amer.* 50:1141, 1966.
67. Butler, A. M., Wilson, J. F., and Farber, S. J. Dehydration and acidosis with calcification of renal tubules. *J. Pediat.* 8:489, 1936.
68. Calcagno, P. L., and Lowe, C. U. Substrate-induced renal tubular maturation. *J. Pediat.* 63:851, 1963.
69. Calcagno, P. L., McLavy, J., and Kelley, T. Glomerular filtration rate in children with sickle cell disease. *Pediatrics* 5:127, 1950.
70. Calcagno, P. L., and Rubin, M. I. Physiologic considerations concerning corticosteroid therapy and complications in the nephrotic syndrome. *J. Pediat.* 58:585, 1961.
71. Calcagno, P. L., and Rubin, M. I. Renal excretion of para-aminohippurate in infants and children. *J. Clin. Invest.* 42:1632, 1963.
72. Calcagno, P. L., Rubin, M. I., and Weintraub, D. H. Studies on the renal concentrating and diluting mechanisms in the

premature infant. *J. Clin. Invest.* 33:91, 1954.
73. Camacho, A. M., and Blizzard, R. M. Congenital hypokalemia of probable renal origin. *Amer. J. Dis. Child.* 103:535, 1962.
74. Cameron, G., and Chambers, R. Direct evidence of function in kidney of an early human fetus. *Amer. J. Physiol.* 123:482, 1938.
75. Cameron, J. S., and Blandford, G. The simple assessment of selectivity in heavy proteinuria. *Lancet* 2:242, 1966.
76. Cameron, J. S., and Miller-Jones, C. M. H. Renal function and renal failure in badly burned children. *Brit. J. Surg.* 54:132, 1967.
77. Cameron, J. S., and White, R. H. R. Selectivity of proteinuria in children with the nephrotic syndrome. *Lancet* 1:463, 1965.
78. Campbell, A. C. P., and Henderson, J. L. Symmetrical cortical necrosis of the kidneys in infancy and childhood. *Arch. Dis. Child.* 24:269, 1949.
79. Carré, I. J., and McCoy, J. E. Hereditary Pitressin-resistant diabetes insipidus. *Acta Paediat. Scand.* 48:223, 1959.
80. Carré, I. J., and Squire, J. R. Anuria ascribed to acute tubular necrosis in infancy and early childhood. *Arch. Dis. Child.* 31:512, 1956.
81. Cassady, G., Brown, K., Cohen, M., and DeMaria, W. Hereditary renal dysfunction and deafness. *Pediatrics* 35:967, 1965.
82. Chamberlain, M. J., Shackman, R., Smith, E. K. M., and Wrong, O. M. Haemodialysis in young children. *Brit. Med. J.* 1:1610, 1965.
83. Chappell, J. A., and Kelsey, W. M. Hereditary nephritis. *A.M.A. Amer. J. Dis. Child.* 99:401, 1960.
84. Cheek, D. B., and Perry, J. W. A salt-wasting syndrome in infancy. *Arch. Dis. Child.* 33:252, 1958.
85. Cheek, D. B., Robinson, M. J., and Collins, F. D. The investigation of a patient with hyperlipemia, hypokalemia and tetany. *J. Pediat.* 59:200, 1961.
86. Ching, R. F. The pathology of sickle cell anemia. *Southern Med. J.* 27:839, 1934.
87. Chisolm, J. J., Jr., and Harrison, H. E. Aminoaciduria. *Pediat. Clin. N. Amer.* 7:333, 1960.
88. Chisolm, J. J., Jr., and Harrison, H. E. Aminoaciduria in vitamin D deficiency states in premature infants and older infants with rickets. *J. Pediat.* 60:206, 1962.
89. Chisolm, J. J., Jr., and Leahy, N. B. Aminoaciduria as a manifestation of renal tubular injury in lead intoxication and a comparison with patterns of aminoaciduria seen in other diseases. *J. Pediat.* 60:1, 1962.
90. Clapp, W. M., Holmes, J., and O'Brien, D. Extracorporeal hemodialysis in children. *Amer. J. Dis. Child.* 104:45, 1962.
91. Clara, M. Vergleichende Histobiologie des Nierenglomerulus und der Lungenalveole. *Z. Mikr. Anat. Forsch.* 40:147, 1936.
92. Clark, N. S. Familial renal insufficiency. *Arch. Dis. Child.* 26:251, 1951.
93. Clark, N. S. Nephritis in childhood: A clinical assessment of the Ellis classification. *Arch. Dis. Child.* 31:12, 1956.
94. Clay, R. D., Darmady, E. M., and Hawkins, M. The nature of the renal lesion in the Fanconi syndrome. *J. Path. Bact.* 65:551, 1953.
95. Cohen, J. A., and Levitt, M. F. Acute glomerulonephritis with few urinary abnormalities: Report of two cases proved by renal biopsy. *New Eng. J. Med.* 268:749, 1963.
96. Comerford, F. R., and Cohen, A. S. The nephropathy of systemic lupus erythematosus: An assessment of clinical, light, and electron microscopic criteria. *Medicine* (Balt.) 46:425, 1967.
97. Cook, C. D., Wedgwood, R. J. P., Craig, J. M., Hartmann, J. R., and Janeway, C. A. Systemic lupus erythematosus: Description of 37 cases in children and a discussion of endocrine therapy in 32 of the cases. *Pediatrics* 26:570, 1960.
98. Corley, C. C., Jr., Lessner, H. E., and Larsen, W. E. Azathioprine therapy of "autoimmune diseases." *Amer. J. Med.* 41:404, 1966.
99. Cornfield, D., and Schwartz, M. W. Nephrosis: A long-term study of children treated with corticosteroids. *J. Pediat.* 68:507, 1966.

100. Cort, J. H., and McCance, R. A. The renal response of puppies to an acidosis. *J. Physiol.* (London) 124:358, 1954.

101. Crawford, J. D., and Kennedy, G. C. Chlorothiazide in diabetes insipidus. *Nature* (London) 183:891, 1959.

102. Darling, S., and Mortensen, O. Aminoaciduria in galactosemia. *Acta Paediat. Scand.* 43:337, 1954.

103. Darmady, E. M., Offer, J., Prince, J., and Stranack, F. The proximal convoluted tubule in the renal handling of water. *Lancet* 2:1254, 1964.

104. Davis, J. H., and Faber, H. K. Prognosis in acute glomerulonephritis in children. *J. Pediat.* 27:453, 1945.

105. Dean, R. F. A., and McCance, R. A. Inulin, diodone, creatinine, and urea clearances in newborn infants. *J. Physiol.* (London) 106:431, 1947.

106. Dean, R. F. A., and McCance, R. A. Response of newborn children to hypertonic solutions of sodium chloride and of urea. *Nature* (London) 160:904, 1947.

107. Dean, R. F. A., and McCance, R. A. Phosphate clearances in infants and adults. *J. Physiol.* (London) 107:182, 1948.

108. Dean, R. F. A., and McCance, R. A. The renal responses of infants and adults to the administration of hypertonic solutions of sodium chloride and urea. *J. Physiol.* (London) 109:81, 1949.

109. DeDeuxchaisnes, C. N. M. D., Krane, S. M. The treatment of adult phosphate diabetes and Fanconi syndrome with neutral sodium phosphate. *Amer. J. Med.* 43: 508, 1967.

110. Dent, C. E., and Harris, H. Hereditary forms of rickets and osteomalacia. *J. Bone Joint Surg.* [Brit.] 38:204, 1956.

111. Dent, C. E., and Philpot, G. R. Xanthinuria, inborn error (or deviation) of metabolism. *Lancet* 1:182, 1954.

112. Derham, R. J., and Rogerson, M. M. The Schönlein-Henoch syndrome with particular reference to renal sequelae. *Arch. Dis. Child.* 31:364, 1956.

113. DeVries, A., Kochwa, S., Lazebnik, J., Frank, M., and Djaldetti, M. Glycinuria, a hereditary disorder associated with nephrolithiasis. *Amer. J. Med.* 23:408, 1957.

114. Dickers, S. E., and Tyler, C. Estimation of the antidiuretic, vasopressor, and oxytocic hormones in the pituitary gland of dogs and puppies. *J. Physiol.* (London) 120:141, 1953.

115. Dixon, F. J. The pathogenesis of glomerulonephritis. (Editorial.) *Amer. J. Med.* 44:493, 1968.

116. Dodge, W. F., Daeschner, C. W., Jr., Brennan, J. C., Rosenberg, H. S., Travis, L. B., and Hopps, H. C. Percutaneous renal biopsy in children: II. Acute glomerulonephritis, chronic glomerulonephritis, and nephritis of anaphylactoid purpura. *Pediatrics* 30:297, 1962.

117. Dodge, W. F., Spargo, B. H., Bass, J. A., and Travis, L. B. The relationship between the clinical and pathologic features of poststreptococcal glomerulonephritis: A study of the early natural history. *Medicine* (Balt.) 47:227, 1968.

118. Dodge, W. F., Travis, L. B., and Daeschner, C. W. Anaphylactoid purpura, polyarteritis nodosa and purpura fulminans. *Pediat. Clin. N. Amer.* 10:879, 1963.

119. Donnell, G. N., Litman, N., and Roldan, M. Pseudohypoadrenal corticism: Renal sodium loss, hyponatremia and hyperkalemia due to a renal tubular insensitivity to mineralocorticoid. *A.M.A. Amer. J. Dis. Child.* 97:813, 159.

120. Doxiadis, S. A. Azotaemia in infancy. *Arch. Dis. Child.* 23:50, 1948.

121. Doxiadis, S. A., Goldfinch, M. K., and Cole, N. "Proteinuria" in the newborn. *Lancet* 2:1242, 1952.

122. Drescher, A. N., Barnett, H. L., and Troupkou, V. Water balance in infants during water deprivation: The effects of the protein content of the diet on renal water requirements. *Amer. J. Dis. Child.* 104:366, 1962.

123. Drummond, K. N., Hillman, D. A., Marchessault, V. J. H., and Feldman, W. Cyclophosphamide in the nephrotic syndrome of childhood. *Canad. Med. Ass. J.* 98:524, 1968.

124. Drummond, K. N., Michael, A. F., Good,

R. A., and Vernier, R. L. Nephrotic syndrome of childhood: Immunologic, clinical and pathologic correlations. *J. Clin. Invest.* 45:620, 1966.

125. Duncan, D. A., Drummond, K. N., Michael, A. F., and Vernier, R. L. Pulmonary hemorrhage and glomerulonephritis. *Ann. Intern. Med.* 62:920, 1965.

126. Earley, L. E., and Orloff, J. The mechanism of antidiuresis associated with the administration of hydrochlorothiazide to patients with vasopressin-resistant diabetes insipidus. *J. Clin. Invest.* 41:1988, 1962.

127. Edelmann, C. M., Jr. Unpublished observations, 1959.

128. Edelmann, C. M., Jr., and Barnett, H. L. Role of the kidney in water metabolism in young infants: Physiologic and clinical considerations. *J. Pediat.* 56:154, 1960.

129. Edelmann, C. M., Jr., and Barnett, H. L. Nephrotic Syndrome. In Conn, H. F., and Conn, R. B., Jr. (Eds.), *Current Diagnosis II*. Philadelphia: Saunders, 1968. P. 607.

130. Edelmann, C. M., Jr., Barnett, H. L., and Stark, H. Effect of urea on concentration of nonurea solute in premature infants. *J. Appl. Physiol.* 21:1021, 1966.

131. Edelmann, C. M., Jr., Barnett, H. L., Stark, H., Boichis, H., and Rodriguez-Soriano, J. A standardized test of renal concentrating capacity in infants and children. *Amer. J. Dis. Child.* 114:639, 1967.

132. Edelmann, C. M., Jr., Barnett, H. L., and Troupkou, V. Renal concentrating mechanisms in newborn infants. Effect of dietary protein and water content, role of urea, and responsiveness to antidiuretic hormone. *J. Clin. Invest.* 39:1062, 1960.

133. Edelmann, C. M., Jr., Boichis, H., Rodriguez-Soriano, J., and Stark, H. The renal response of children to acute ammonium chloride acidosis. *Pediat. Res.* 1:452, 1967.

134. Edelmann, C. M., Jr., and Greifer, I. A modified technique for percutaneous needle biopsy of the kidney in infants and children. *J. Pediat.* 70:81, 1967.

135. Edelmann, C. M., Jr., Greifer, I., and Barnett, H. L. The nature of kidney disease in children who fail to recover from apparent acute glomerulonephritis. *J. Pediat.* 64:879, 1964.

136. Edelmann, C. M., Jr., Gruskin, A. B., Oetliker, O., Spitzer, A., and Wolfish, N. The response of piglets to intravenous infusions of water, mannitol, and saline. In preparation.

137. Edelmann, C. M., Jr., Rodriguez-Soriano, J., Boichis, H., Gruskin, A. B., and Acosta, M. Renal bicarbonate reabsorption and hydrogen ion excretion in infants. *J. Clin. Invest.* 46:1309, 1967.

138. Edelmann, C. M., Jr., and Spitzer, A. The maturing kidney. A modern view of well-balanced infants with imbalanced nephrons. *J. Pediat.* 75:509, 1969.

139. Edelmann, C. M., Jr., and Wolfish, N. M. Dietary influence on renal maturation in premature infants. *Pediat. Res.* 2:421, 1968.

140. Editorial. Recurrent haematuria and focal nephritis. *Lancet* 1:413, 1966.

141. Editorial. Treatment of steroid-resistant nephrotic syndrome. *Lancet* 1:644, 1966.

142. Editorial. Immunosuppressive or anti-inflammatory. *Brit. Med. J.* 1:650, 1967.

143. Editorial. Immunosuppressive drugs and chronic renal disease. *Lancet* 1:1093, 1967.

144. Editorial. Haemolytic-uraemic syndrome. *Lancet* 2:271, 1968.

145. Eiben, R. M., Kleinerman, J., and Cline, J. C. Nephrotic syndrome in a neonatal premature infant: Report of a case. *J. Pediat.* 44:195, 1954.

146. Ellborg, A., and Forssman, H. Nephrogenic diabetes insipidus in children. *Acta Paediat. Scand.* 44:209, 1955.

147. Eskeland, G., and Skogrand, A. Bilateral cortical necrosis of the kidneys in infancy. *Acta Paediat. Scand.* 48:278, 1959.

148. Esperanca, M. J., and Collins, D. L. Peritoneal dialysis efficiency in relation to body weight. *J. Pediat. Surg.* 1:162, 1966.

149. Etteldorf, J. N., Dobbins, W. T., Sweeney, M. J., Smith, J. D., Whittington, G. L., Sheffield, J. A., and Meadows, R. W. Intermittent peritoneal dialysis in the management of acute renal failure in children. *J. Pediat.* 60:327, 1962.

150. Etteldorf, J. N., Smith, J. D., Tuttle, A. H.,

and Diggs, L. W. Renal hemodynamic studies in adults with sickle cell anemia. *Amer. J. Med.* 18:243, 1955.

151. Etteldorf, J. N., Shane, R., III, Summitt, R. L., Sweeney, M. J., Wall, H. P., and Burton, W. M. Cyclophosphamide in the treatment of idiopathic lipoid nephrosis. *J. Pediat.* 70:758, 1967.
152. Fanconi, A. Idiopatische Hypercalciurie im Kindesalter. *Helv. Paediat. Acta* 18: 306, 1963.
153. Fanconi, G. Der Frühinfantile nephrotisch-glykosurische Zwergwuchs mit hypophosphatämischer Rachitis. *Jb. Kinderheilk.* 147:299, 1936.
154. Fanconi, G., and Bickel, H. Die chronische Aminoacidurie (aminosaure-diabetes oder nephrotischglukosurischer Zwergwuchs) bei der Glykogenose und der Cystin krankheit. *Helv. Paediat. Acta* 4:359, 1949.
155. Fanconi, V. G., Hanhart, E., Albertini, A. Von, Ühlinger, E., Dolivo, G., and Prader, A. Die familiäre Juvenile nephronophthise (Die idiopathische parenchymatöse Schrumpfnier). *Helv. Paediat. Acta* 6:1, 1951.
156. Feldman, W. Intermittent peritoneal dialysis in the management of chronic renal failure in children. *Amer. J. Dis. Child.* 116:30, 1968.
157. Feldman, W., Baliah, T., and Drummond, K. N. Intermittent peritoneal dialysis in the management of chronic renal failure in children. *Amer. J. Dis. Child.* 116:30, 1968.
158. Ferris, T. F., Gorden, P., Kashgarian, M., and Epstein, F. H. Recurrent hematuria and focal nephritis. *New Eng. J. Med.* 276: 770, 1967.
159. Fetterman, G. H., and Feldman, J. D. Congenital anomalies of renal tubules in a case of "infantile nephrosis." *Amer. J. Dis. Child.* 100:319, 1960.
160. Fetterman, G. H., Shuplock, N. A., Philipp, F. J., and Gregg, H. S. The growth and maturation of human glomeruli and proximal convolutions from term to adulthood: Studies by microdissection. *Pediatrics* 35: 601, 1965.
161. Fine, R. N., DePalma, J. R., Lieberman, E., Donnell, G. N., Gordon, A., and Maxwell, M. H. Extended hemodialysis in children with chronic renal failure. *J. Pediat.* 73: 706, 1968.
162. Fine, R. N., Korsch, B. M., Grushkin, C. M., and Lieberman, E. Hemodialysis in children. *Amer. J. Dis. Child.* 119:498, 1970.
163. Fleisher, D. S., Voci, G., Garfunkel, J., Purugganan, H., Kirkpatrick, J., Jr., Wells, C. R., and McElfresh, A. E. Hemodynamic findings in acute glomerulonephritis. *J. Pediat.* 69:1054, 1966.
164. Fomon, S. J., Harris, D. M., and Jensen, R. L. Acidification of the urine by infants fed human milk and whole cow's milk. *Pediatrics* 23:113, 1959.
165. Forbes, G. B. Methods for determining composition of the human body: With a note on the effect of diet on body composition. *Pediatrics* 29:477, 1962.
166. Forssman, H. On hereditary diabetes insipidus with special regard to a sex-linked form. *Acta Med. Scand.* (Suppl. 159):1, 1945.
167. Freedman, L. R., Phair, J. P., Masafumi, S., Hamilton, H. B., and Nefzger, M. D. The epidemiology of urinary tract infections in Hiroshima. *Yale J. Biol. Med.* 37:262, 1965.
168. Friis-Hansen, B. Body water compartments in children: Changes during growth and related changes in body composition. *Pediatrics* 28:169, 1961.
169. Friis-Hansen, B., Skadhauge, E., and Zetterström, R. Fluid and electrolyte metabolism in nephrogenic diabetes insipidus. *Acta Paed. Scand.* (Suppl. 146):57, 1963.
170. Frölich, T. Zwei Falle von hereditärer, familiärer, kongenitäler Nephritis. *Jb. Kinderheilk.* 64:244, 1906.
171. Fuhrmann, W. Ein erbliches Nierenleiden mit dem Leitsymptom der Hämaturie. *Z. Kinderheilk.* 82:514, 1959.
172. Gachet, F. S. Course and prognosis of hemorrhagic nephritis in children. *Amer. J. Dis. Child.* 61:1175, 1941.
173. Gairdner, D. Schönlein-Henoch syndrome (anaphylactoid purpura). *Quart. J. Med.* 17:95, 1948.
174. Gasser, C., Gautier, E., Steck, A., Siebenmann, R. E., and Oechslin, R. Hämoly-

tisch-urämische Syndrome. *Schweiz. Med. Wschr.* 85:905, 1955.

175. Gauer, O. H. Osmo control versus volume control. *Fed. Proc.* 27:1132, 1968.
176. Gautier, P. E., and Prader, A. Un cas de diabète insipide néphrogène chez un nourrisson avec absence initiale de soif (diabète insipide occulte). *Helv. Paediat. Acta* 11: 45, 1956.
177. Gautier, P. E., and Simpkiss, M. The management of nephrogenic diabetes insipidus in early life. *Acta Paediat. Scand.* 46:354, 1957.
178. Gentz, J., Jagenburg, R., and Zetterström, R. Tyrosinemia. *J. Pediat.* 66:670, 1965.
179. Gessner, I., Krovetz, L. J., Benson, R. W., Prystowsky, H., Stenger, V., and Eitzman, D. V. Hemodynamic adaptations in the newborn infant. *Pediatrics* 36:752, 1965.
180. Ghadimi, H., and Schwachman, H. Evaluation of aminoaciduria in infancy and childhood. *A.M.A. Amer. J. Dis. Child.* 99:457, 1960.
181. Gianantonio, C. A., Vitacco, M., Mendilaharzu, F., and Gallo, G. The hemolytic-uremic syndrome: Renal status of 76 patients at long-term follow-up. *J. Pediat.* 72: 757, 1968.
182. Gianantonio, C. A., Vitacco, M., Mendilaharzu, J., Mendilaharzu, F., and Rutty, A. Acute renal failure in infancy and childhood. *J. Pediat.* 61:660, 1962.
183. Gianantonio, C. A., Vitacco, M., Mendilaharzu, F., Rutty, A., and Mendilaharzu, J. The hemolytic-uremic syndrome. *J. Pediat.* 64:478, 1964.
184. Giles, H. McC., Pugh, R. C. B., Darmady, E. M., Stranack, F., and Woolf, L. I. The nephrotic syndrome in early infancy: A report of 3 cases. *Arch. Dis. Child.* 32:167, 1957.
185. Giovanetti, S., and Maggiore, Q. A low nitrogen diet with proteins of high biological value for severe chronic uraemia. *Lancet* 1:1000, 1964.
186. Gitlin, D., Cornwall, D. G., Nakasato, D., Oncley, J. L., Hughes, W. L., Jr., and Janeway, C. A. Studies on the metabolism of plasma proteins in the nephrotic syndrome: II. The lipoproteins. *J. Clin. Invest.* 37:172, 1958.
187. Gitlin, D., Janeway, C. A., and Farr, L. E. Studies on the metabolism of plasma proteins in the nephrotic syndrome: I. Albumin, gammaglobulin and iron-binding globulin. *J. Clin. Invest.* 35:44, 1956.
188. Goldbloom, R. B., Fraser, F. C., Waugh, D., Aronovitch, M., and Wiglesworth, F. W. Hereditary renal disease associated with nerve deafness and ocular lesions. *Pediatrics* 20:241, 1957.
189. Goldbloom, R. B., Hillman, D. A., and Santulli, T. V. Arterial thrombosis following femoral venipuncture in edematous nephrotic children. *Pediatrics* 40:450, 1967.
190. Goldman, H. I., Karelitz, S., Acs, H., and Seifter, E. The relationship of sodium, potassium, and chloride concentration of the feeding to the weight gain of premature infants. *Pediatrics* 30:909, 1962.
191. Goldman, R., and Haberfelde, G. C. Hereditary nephritis; report of a kindred. *New Eng. J. Med.* 261:734, 1959.
192. Goodpasture, E. W. The significance of certain pulmonary lesions in relation to the etiology of influences. *Amer. J. Med. Sci.* 158:863, 1919.
193. Goodwin, W. E., Alston, E. F., and Simons, H. J. Haematuria and sickle-cell disease. *J. Urol.* 63:79, 1950.
194. Gootman, N., Gross, J., and Mensch, A. Pulmonary artery thrombosis. *Pediatrics* 34:861, 1964.
195. Gordillo, G., Alvarez, R. G., and Bessudo, J. Nefronoptisis juvenil familiar, nefropatia tubulo-intersticial cronica idiopatica, o enfermedad quistica medular. *Bol. Med. Hosp. Infantil* (Mexico) 24:533, 1967.
196. Gordon, H. H., McNamara, H., and Benjamin, H. R. The response of young infants to ingestion of ammonium chloride. *Pediatrics* 2:290, 1948.
197. Goss, R. J. The Functional Demand Theory of Growth Regulation. In Goss, R. J. (Ed.), *Adaptive Growth*. New York: Academic, 1964. P. 259.
198. Gotoff, S. P., Fellers, F. X., Vawter, G. F., Janeway, C. A., and Rosen, F. S. The

beta-1-C globulin in childhood nephrotic syndrome. *New Eng. J. Med.* 273:524, 1965.

199. Greifer, I. Clinicopathology and Natural History of Acute Glomerulonephritis in Children. In Metcoff, J. (Ed.), *Acute Glomerulonephritis, Proceedings Seventeenth Annual Conference on the Kidney*. Boston: Little, Brown, 1967. P. 165.
200. Gribetz, D., and Henley, W. Systemic lupus erythematosus in childhood. *J. Mount Sinai Hosp. N.Y.* 26:289, 1959.
201. Grupe, W. E., Cuppage, F. E., and Heymann, W. Congenital nephrotic syndrome with interstitial nephritis. *Amer. J. Dis. Child.* 111:482, 1966.
202. Grupe, W. E., and Heymann, W. Cytotoxic drugs in steroid-resistant renal disease. *Amer. J. Dis. Child.* 112:448, 1966.
203. Gruskay, F. L., and Turano, A. Nephrosis in the newborn infant: A syndrome difficult to explain by existing theories of etiology. *A.M.A. Amer. J. Dis. Child.* 94: 117, 1957.
204. Gruskin, A. B., Edelmann, C. M., Jr., and Yuan, S. Maturational changes in renal blood flow in piglets. *Pediat. Res.* 4:13, 1970.
205. Grüttner, R., and Lenz, W. Zur Kenntnis und zur Differential diagnose der familiären Nephronophthise im Kindesalter. *Arch. Kinderheilk.* 155:271, 1957.
206. Grüttner, R., Lenz, W., and Seifert, K. Ein weiterer Beitrag zur Nephronophthise des Kindesalters. *Arch. Kinderheilk.* 164: 12, 1961.
207. Guazzelli, C. L'interessamento renale nella syndrome d'Schönlein-Henoch. *Riv. Clin. Pediat.* 72:439, 1963.
208. Guthrie, L. G. Idiopathic or congenital hereditary and family hematuria. *Lancet* 1:1243, 1902.
209. Habib, R., Mathieu, H., and Royer, P. Le syndrome hémolytique et urémique de l'enfant. *Nephron* 4:139, 1967.
210. Hackzell, G. Fall av familiär juvenil nephronophthis hos en 7-arig flicka. *Nord. Med.* 48:179, 1952.
211. Hackzell, G., and Lundmark, C. Familial juvenile nephronophthisis. *Acta Paediat. Scand.* 47:428, 1958.
212. Hagge, W. W., Burke, E. C., and Stickler, G. B. Treatment of systemic lupus erythematosus complicated by nephritis in children. *Pediatrics* 40:822, 1967.
213. Hallman, N., and Hjelt, L. Congenital nephrotic syndrome. *J. Pediat.* 55:152, 1959.
214. Hallman, N., Norio, R., and Kouvalainen, K. Main features of the congenital nephrotic syndrome. *Acta Paediat. Scand.* Suppl. 172:75, 1967.
215. Hansen, J. D. L., and Smith, C. A. Effects of withholding fluid in the immediate postnatal period. *Pediatrics* 12:99, 1953.
216. Hansen, M. F., and Coye, R. D. Congenital nephrosis with renal arteriolar hypertrophy. *Amer. J. Dis. Child.* 102:28, 1961.
217. Hanson, V., and Kornreich, H. Systemic rheumatic disorders in childhood. *Bull. Rheum. Dis.* 17:435, 1967.
218. Harrison, H. E., and Harrison, H. C. Hereditary metabolic bone diseases. *Clin. Orthop.* 33:147, 1964.
219. Harrow, B. R., Sloane, J. A., and Liebnam, N. C. Roentgenologic demonstration of renal capillary necrosis in sickle-cell trait. *New Eng. J. Med.* 268:969, 1963.
220. Harter, J. G., Reddy, W. J., and Thorn, G. W. Studies on an intermittent corticosteroid dosage regimen. *New Eng. J. Med.* 269:591, 1963.
221. Hatemi, N., and McCance, R. A. Renal aspects of acid base control in the newly born: III. Response to acidifying drugs. *Acta Paediat. Scand.* 50:603, 1961.
222. Heinemann, H. O., and Cheung, M. W. Renal concentrating mechanism in sickle cell anemia. *J. Lab. Clin. Med.* 49:923, 1957.
223. Heller, H. Antidiuretic hormone in pituitary glands of newborn rats. *J. Physiol.* (London) 106:28, 1947.
224. Heller, H., and Lederis, K. Maturation of the hypothalamoneurohypophysial system. *J. Physiol.* (London) 147:299, 1959.
225. Heller, H., and Zaimis, E. J. The antidiuretic and oxytocic hormones in the posterior pituitary glands of newborn infants and adults. *J. Physiol.* (London) 109:141, 1953.
226. Henneman, P. H., Dempsey, E. F., Carroll,

E. L., and Henneman, D. H. Acquired vitamin D-resistant osteomalacia: A new variety characterized by hypercalcemia, low serum bicarbonate and hyperglycinuria. *Metabolism* 11:103, 1962.

227. Heptinstall, R. H., and Joekes, A. M. Focal glomerulonephritis: A study based on renal biopsies. *Quart. J. Med.* 28:329, 1959.

228. Herbert, H. J. Acute glomerulonephritis in childhood; a study of the late prognosis of twenty-seven cases. *J. Pediat.* 40:549, 1952.

229. Herdman, R. C., Good, R. A., and Vernier, R. L. Medullary cystic disease in two siblings. *Amer. J. Med.* 43:335, 1967.

230. Herdman, R. C., Michael, A. F., and Good, R. A. Postural proteinuria: Response to corticosteroid therapy. *Ann. Intern. Med.* 65:286, 1966.

231. Heymann, W. Pathogenesis of the nephrotic syndrome: Considerations based on clinical and experimental studies. *J. Pediat.* 58:609, 1961.

232. Heymann, W., and Lund, H. Z. Nephrotic syndrome in rats. *Pediatrics* 7:691, 1951.

233. Heymann, W., Nash, G., Gilkey, C., and Lewis, M. Studies on the casual role of hypoalbuminemia in experimental nephrotic hyperlipemia. *J. Clin. Invest.* 37:808, 1958.

234. Hobolth, N. Hereditary nephropathy with haematuria. *Acta Paediat. Scand.* 52:581, 1963.

235. Hodgman, J. E., Schwartz, A., and Thrupp, L. D. Bacteriuria in the premature infant. *Pediat. Res.* 1:303, 1967.

236. Hooft, C., Roels, H., and Herpol, J. A case of Fanconi's familial juvenile nephronophthisis. *Helv. Paediat. Acta* 14:217, 1959.

237. Hooft, C., and van Acker, K. J. The natural history of the idiopathic nephrotic syndrome in childhood. *Ann. Paediat.* (Basel) 207:1, 1966.

238. Holliday, M. A. The distal nephron and disorders of its function. *J. Pediat.* 57:23, 1960.

239. Holliday, M. A. Diagnosis and treatment: Acute renal failure. *Pediatrics* 35:478, 1965.

240. Holliday, M. A., Burstin, C., and Hurrah, J. Evidence that the antidiuretic substance in the plasma of children with nephrogenic diabetes insipidus is antidiuretic hormone. *Pediatrics* 32:384, 1963.

241. Holman, H. Systemic lupus erythematosus: A review of certain recent developments in the study of this disease. *J. Pediat.* 56:109, 1960.

242. Holten, C. The dependence of the normal kidney function on the size of the body. *Acta Paediat.* 12:251, 1931.

243. Houston, I. B. Urinary white cell excretion in childhood. *Arch. Dis. Child.* 40:313, 1965.

244. Houston, I. B. Personal communication, 1967.

245. Houston, I. B., Boichis, H., and Edelmann, C. M., Jr. Fanconi syndrome with renal sodium wasting and metabolic alkalosis. *Amer. J. Med.* 44:638, 1968.

246. Hoyer, J. R., Michael, A. F., Fish, A. J., and Good, R. A. Acute poststreptococcal glomerulonephritis presenting as hypertensive encephalopathy with minimal urinary abnormalities. *Pediatrics* 39:412, 1967.

247. Hutchings, R. H., Hickman, R., and Scribner, B. H. Chronic hemodialysis in a preadolescent. *Pediatrics* 37:68, 1966.

248. Illig, R., and Prader, A. Primäre Tubulopathien: II. Ein Fall von idiopathischem Gluko-Amino-Phosphat-Diabetes (De Toni-Debré-Fanconi-Syndrom). *Helv. Paediat. Acta* 16:622, 1961.

249. Ivemark, B. I., Ljungqvist, A., and Barry, A. Juvenile nephronophthisis: II. A histologic and microangiographic study. *Acta Paediat. Scand.* 49:480, 1960.

250. Jackson, C. M., and Shiels, M. Compensatory hypertrophy of the kidney during various periods after unilateral nephrectomy in very young albino rats. *Anat. Rec.* 36:221, 1927.

251. Jacobs, J. C. Systemic lupus erythematosus in childhood: Report of 35 cases. *Pediatrics* 32:257, 1963.

252. Janovský, M., Martínek, J., and Stanincová, V. Antidiuretic activity in the plasma of

human infants after a load of sodium chloride. *Acta Paediat. Scand.* 54:543, 1965.

253. Janovský, M., Martínek, J., and Stanincová, V. The distribution of sodium, chloride, and fluid in the body of young infants with increased intake of NaCl. *Biol. Neonat.* 11:261, 1967.
254. Jäykkä, S. The problem of dormant fetal organs: The kidneys, lungs and the gut. *Biol. Neonat.* 3:343, 1961.
255. Joseph, M. C., and Polani, P. E. The effect of bed rest on acute hemorrhagic nephritis in children. *Guy. Hosp. Rep.* 107: 500, 1958.
256. Kagan, B. M., Felix, N., Molander, C. W., Busser, R. J., and Kalman, D. Body water changes in relation to nutrition in premature infants. *Ann. N.Y. Acad. Sci.* 110:830, 1963.
257. Kallen, R. J. A method for approximating the efficacy of peritoneal dialysis for uremia. *Amer. J. Dis. Child.* 111:156, 1966.
258. Kallen, R. J., Zaltzman, S., Coe, F. L., and Metcoff, J. Hemodialysis in children: Technique, kinetic aspects related to varying body size, and application to salicylate intoxication, acute renal failure and some other disorders. *Medicine* (Balt.) 45:1, 1966.
259. Kandall, S., Edelmann, C. M., Jr., and Bernstein, J. Acute poststreptococcal glomerulonephritis: A case with minimal urinary abnormalities. *Amer. J. Dis. Child.* 118:426, 1969.
260. Kao, M. Yun-Chen, and Steiner, M. M. Diabetes insipidus in infancy resistant to Pitressin. *Pediatrics* 12:400, 1953.
261. Kaplan, S. A., Strauss, J., and Yuceoglu, A. M. Conservative management of acute renal failure. *Pediatrics* 25:409, 1960.
262. Kaplan, S. A., Yuceoglu, A. M., and Strauss, J. Vasopressin-resistant diabetes insipidus. *A.M.A. Amer. J. Dis. Child.* 97:308, 1959.
263. Käser, H., Cottier, P., and Antener, I. Glucoglycinuria, a new familial syndrome. *J. Pediat.* 61:386, 1962.
264. Keitel, H. G., Thompson, D., and Itano, H. A. Hyposthenuria in sickle cell anemia: A reversible renal defect. *J. Clin. Invest.* 35:998, 1956.
265. King, S. E. Postural adjustments and protein excretion by the kidney in renal disease. *Ann. Intern. Med.* 46:360, 1957.
266. King, S. E. Albuminuria (proteinuria) in renal diseases: II. Preliminary observations on the clinical course of patients with orthostatic albuminuria. *New York J. Med.* 59:825, 1959.
267. King, S. E., and Baldwin, D. S. Renal hemodynamics during erect lordosis in normal man and subjects with orthostatic proteinuria. *Proc. Soc. Exp. Biol. Med.* 86:634, 1954.
268. Kobayashi, A., Imai, M., Murata, H., and Sata, H. Familial juvenile nephronophthisis: Report of two cases in two siblings. *Acta Paediat. Jap.* 9:1, 1967.
269. Kobayashi, O., Wada, H., Kanasawa, M., and Kamiyama, T. The anaphylactoid purpura-nephritis in childhood. *Acta Med. Biol.* (Niigata) 13:181, 1965.
270. Kopelman, H., Asatoor, A. M., and Milne, M. D. Hyperprolinemia and hereditary nephritis. *Lancet* 2:1075, 1964.
271. Kornreich, H. K., Drexler, E., and Hanson, V. Antinuclear factors in childhood rheumatic disease. *J. Pediat.* 69:1039, 1966.
272. Korsch, B., and Barnett, H. L. The physician, the family, and the child with nephrosis. *J. Pediat.* 58:707, 1961.
273. Kouvalainen, K. Immunological features in the congenital nephrotic syndrome: A clinical and experimental study. *Ann. Paediat.* (Fenn.) 9 (Suppl. 22):1, 1963.
274. Kouvalainen, K., Vaino, T., Hjelt, L., and Hallman, N. Behavior of skin grafted from infants to mother in congenital nephrosis families. *Ann. Paediat.* (Fenn.) 8: 173, 1962.
275. Krakower, C. A., and Heino, H. E. Relationship of growth and nutrition to cardiorenal changes induced in birds by a high salt intake. *Arch. Path.* 44:143, 1947.
276. Krane, S. M. Renal Glycosuria. In Stanbury, J. B., Wyngaarden, J. B., and Fredrickson, D. S. (Eds.), *The Metabolic Basis of Inherited Disease* (2d ed.). New York: Blakiston Div., McGraw-Hill, 1966. P. 1221.
277. Kunin, C. M., Deutscher, R., and Paquin, A. J., Jr. Urinary tract infection in school

children: An epidemiologic, clinical and laboratory study. *Medicine* (Balt.) 43:91, 1964.

278. Kunin, C. M., Zacha, E., and Paquin, A. J., Jr. Urinary tract infections in school children: I. Prevalence of bacteriuria and associated urologic findings. *New Eng. J. Med.* 266:1287, 1962.
279. Kunstadter, R. H., and Rosenblum, L. Neonatal glomerulonephritis and nephrotic syndrome in a 1,320 gm prematurely born infant. *A.M.A. Amer. J. Dis. Child.* 88: 611, 1954.
280. Kunz, H. W., Mellin, G. W., Cheung, M. W., and Pratt, E. L. Impairment of urinary concentration in sickle cell anemia. *A.M.A. Amer. J. Dis. Child.* 86:512, 1953.
281. Lagru, G., Bariéty, J., Canlorbe, P., Vassal, J., and Milliez, P. La chimiothérapie dite immunodépressive dans les syndromes néphrotiques primitifs de l'enfant. *Presse Med.* 75:1773, 1967.
282. Lamy, M., Royer, P., and Frézal, J. *Maladies Héréditaires du Métabolisme Chez l'Enfant.* Paris: Masson, 1959. Vol. 1, p. 259.
283. Lange, K., Slobody, L., and Strang, R. Prolonged intermittent ACTH and cortisone therapy in the nephrotic syndrome; immunologic basis and results. *Pediatrics* 15:156, 1955.
284. Lange, K., Wachstein, M., Wasserman, E., Alptekin, F., and Slobody, L. B. The congenital nephrotic syndrome. *Amer. J. Dis. Child.* 105:338, 1963.
285. Lannigan, R., and Insley, J. Light and electron microscope appearances in renal biopsy material from cases of recurrent haematuria in children. *J. Clin. Path.* 18: 178, 1965.
286. Lanzkowsky, P., and McCrory, W. W. Disseminated intravascular coagulation as a possible factor in the pathogenesis of thrombotic microangiopathy (hemolytic-uremic syndrome). *J. Pediat.* 70:460, 1967.
287. Laron, Z., et al. Infantile nephrosis in two siblings: Case report. *Ann. Paediat.* (Basel) 195:337, 1960.
288. Lathem, W. Renal circulatory dynamics and urinary protein excretion during infusions of 1-norepinephrine and 1-epinephrine in patients with renal disease. *J. Clin. Invest.* 35:1277, 1956.
289. Lathem, W., Roof, B. S., Nickel, S. F., and Bradley, S. E. Urinary protein excretion and renal hemodynamic adjustments during orthostasis in patients with acute and chronic renal disease. *J. Clin. Invest.* 33: 1457, 1954.
290. Latner, A. L., and Burnard, E. D. Idiopathic hyperchloraemic renal acidosis of infants: Observations on site and nature of lesion. *Quart. J. Med.* 19:285, 1950.
291. Lawson, D., Moncrief, A., and Payne, W. W. Forty years of nephrosis in childhood. *Arch. Dis. Child.* 35:115, 1960.
292. Leaf, A. The Syndrome of Osteomalacia, Renal Glycosuria, Aminoaciduria, and Hyperphosphaturia (The Fanconi Syndrome). In Stanbury, J. B., Wyngaarden, J. B., and Fredrickson, D. S. (Eds.), *The Metabolic Basis of Inherited Disease* (2d ed). New York: McGraw-Hill, 1960. P. 1222.
293. Lecocq, F. R., McPhaul, J. J., and Robinson, R. R. Fixed and reproducible orthostatic proteinuria: V. Results of a 5-year follow-up evaluation. *Ann. Intern. Med.* 64:557, 1966.
294. Lee, H. A., and Sharpstone, P. Haemodialysis in paediatrics. *Acta Paediat. Scand.* 55: 529, 1966.
295. Lestradet, H. Le Diabète insipide néphrogénique idiopathique héréditaire. In Hottinger, A. and Berger, H. (Eds.), *Problèmes Actuels de Pédiatrie.* Basel; Karger, 1960. Vol. 6, p. 376.
296. Lestradet, H., Correa, C. E. C., and Broyer, M. L'exploration de la fonction d'acidification du tubule rénal par une epreuve courte utilisant une surcharge intraveineuse du chlorydrate de L-Arginine. *Rev. Franc. Etud. Clin. Biol.* 9:885, 1964.
297. Levitt, M. F., Hauser, A. D., Levy, M. S., and Polimeros, D. The renal concentrating defect in sickle cell disease. *Amer. J. Med.* 29:611, 1960.
298. Lewis, I. A. The Schönlein-Henoch syndrome (anaphylactoid purpura) compared with certain features of nephritis and rheumatism. *Arch. Dis. Child.* 30:212, 1955.

299. Lewy, J. E., Salinas-Madrigal, L., Pirani, C., and Metcoff, J. Clinical and morphological correlates in acute glomerulonephritis. *Pediat. Res.* 2:318, 1968.
300. Liddle, G. W., Bledsoe, T., and Coppage, W. S., Jr. A Familial Renal Disorder Simulating Primary Aldosteronism but with Negligible Aldosterone Secretion. In Baulieu, E. E., and Robel, P. (Eds.), *Aldosterone.* Oxford, Eng.: Blackwell Scientific Publications, 1963. P. 353.
301. Lieberman, E., and Donnell, G. N. Recovery of children with acute glomerulonephritis. *Amer. J. Dis. Child.* 109:398, 1965.
302. Lieberman, E., Heuser, E., Donnell, G. N., Landing, B. H., and Hammond, G. D. Hemolytic-uremic syndrome: Clinical and pathological considerations. *New Eng. J. Med.* 275:227, 1966.
303. Lieberman, E., Heuser, E., Gilchrist, G. S., Donnell, G. N., and Landing, B. H. Thrombosis, nephrosis, and corticosteroid therapy. *J. Pediat.* 73:320, 1968.
304. Lightwood, R., and Butler, N. Decline in primary infantile renal acidosis: Aetiological implications. *Brit. Med. J.* 1:855, 1963.
305. Lightwood, R., Payne, W. W., and Black, J. A. Infantile renal acidosis. *Pediatrics* 12:628, 1953.
306. Lincoln, K., and Winberg, J. Studies of urinary tract infections in infancy and childhood: II. Quantitative estimation of bacteriuria in unselected neonates with special reference to the occurrence of asymptomatic infections. *Acta Paediat. Scand.* 53:307, 1964.
307. Lincoln, K., and Winberg, J. Studies of urinary tract infection in infancy and childhood: III. Quantitative estimation of cellular excretion in unselected neonates. *Acta Paediat. Scand.* 53:447, 1964.
308. Livaditis, A., and Ericsson, N. O. Essential hematuria in children — Prognostic aspects. *Acta Paediat. Scand.* 51:630, 1962.
309. Livanou, T., Ferriman, D., and James, V. H. T. Recovery of hypothalamo-pituitary-adrenal function after corticosteroid therapy. *Lancet* 2:856, 1967.
310. Ljungqvist, A. Fetal and postnatal development of the intrarenal arterial pattern in man: A micro-angiographic and histologic study. *Acta Paediat. Scand.* 52:443, 1963.
311. Ljungqvist, A., Victorin, L., and Winberg, J. Atypical nephronophthisis: A clinicopathologic study of juvenile patients without hypotonic polyuria. *Acta Paediat. Scand.* 56:164, 1967.
312. Lloyd-Still, J. D., and Atwell, J. D. Renal failure in infancy with special reference to the use of peritoneal dialysis. *J. Pediat. Surg.* 1:466, 1966.
313. Lobeck, C. C., Barta, R. A., and Mangos, J. A. Study of sweat in Pitressin-resistant diabetes insipidus. *J. Pediat.* 62:868, 1963.
314. Løken, A. C., Hanssen, O., Halvorsen, S., and Jølster, N. J. Hereditary renal dysplasia and blindness. *Acta Paediat. Scand.* 50:177, 1961.
315. Lowe, C. U., Ellinger, A. J., Wright, W. S., and Stauffer, H. M. Pseudohypoparathyroidism (the Seabright bantam syndrome). *J. Pediat.* 36:1, 1950.
316. Lowe, C. U., Terrey, M., and MacLachlan, E. A. Organic-aciduria, decreased renal ammonia production, hydrophthalmos and mental retardation. *A.M.A. Amer. J. Dis. Child.* 83:164, 1952.
317. Löwgren, E. Studies on benign proteinuria with special reference to the renal lymphatic system. *Acta Med. Scand.* Suppl. 300:52, 1955.
318. Lubowitz, H., Slatapolsky, E., Shankel, S., Rieselbach, R. E., and Bricker, N. S. Glomerular filtration rate: Determination in patients with chronic renal disease. *J.A.M.A.* 199:252, 1967.
319. Lucas, W. M., and Bullock, W. H. Hematuria in sickle cell disease. *J. Urol.* 83:733, 1960.
320. Luder, J., and Sheldon, W. A familial tubular absorption defect of glucose and amino-acids. *Arch. Dis. Child.* 30:160, 1955.
321. Lund, H. G., Cordonnier, J. J., and Forbes, K. A. Gross hematuria in sickle cell disease. *J. Urol.* 71:151, 1954.
322. Lyttle, J. D. The Addis sediment count in normal children. *J. Clin. Invest.* 12:87, 1933.

323. MacKay, E. M., MacKay, L. L., and Addis, T. The degree of compensatory renal hypertrophy following unilateral nephrectomy. *J. Exp. Med.* 56:255, 1932.
324. MacLean, P. R., and Robson, J. S. Unselective proteinuria in acute ischemic renal failure. *Clin. Sci.* 30:91, 1966.
325. MacLean, P. R., and Robson, J. S. A simple method for determining selectivity of proteinuria. *Lancet* 1:539, 1967.
326. Mangos, J. A., Opitz, J. M., Lobeck, C. C., and Cookson, D. U. Familial juvenile nephronophthisis: An unrecognized renal disease in the United States. *Pediatrics* 34:337, 1964.
327. Manley, G. L., and Gollipp, P. J. Renal failure in the newborn: Treatment with peritoneal dialysis. *Amer. J. Dis. Child.* 115:107, 1968.
328. Marble, A. Renal glycosuria. *Amer. J. Med. Sci.* 183:811, 1932.
329. Martínek, J., Janovský, M., Stanincová, V., and Slechtová, R. The effect of vasopressin on the water diuresis and excretion of Na, Cl, K, and urea in infants. *Nephron* 1:322, 1964.
330. McCance, R. A. The maintenance of stability in the newly born: 1. Chemical exchange. *Arch. Dis. Child.* 34:361, 1959.
331. McCance, R. A. The maintenance of stability in the newly born: 2. Thermal balance. *Arch. Dis. Child.* 34:459, 1959.
332. McCance, R. A. The Bearing of Age Upon the Maintenance of Electrolyte Stability. In Stewart, C. P., and Stenger, Th. (Eds.), *Water and Electrolyte Metabolism.* Amsterdam: Elsevier, 1960. P. 23.
333. McCance, R. A. Age and Renal Function. In Black, D. A. K. (Ed.), *Renal Disease.* Philadelphia: Davis, 1962. P. 157.
334. McCance, R. A., Naylor, N. J. B., and Widdowson, E. M. The response of infants to a large dose of water. *Arch. Dis. Child.* 29:104, 1954.
335. McCance, R. A., and von Finck, M. A. The titratable acidity, pH, ammonia and phosphates in the urines of very young infants. *Arch. Dis. Child.* 22:200, 1947.
336. McCance, R. A., and Widdowson, E. M. Renal function before birth. *Proc. Roy. Soc.* [Biol.] 141:488, 1953.
337. McCance, R. A., and Widdowson, E. M. Hypertonic expansion of the extracellular fluids. *Acta Paediat. Scand.* 46:337, 1957.
338. McCance, R. A., and Widdowson, E. M. The response of the newborn puppy to water, salt, and food. *J. Physiol.* (London) 141:81, 1958.
339. McCance, R. A., and Widdowson, E. M. Renal aspects of acid base control in the newly born: 1. Natural development. *Acta Paediat. Scand.* 49:409, 1960.
340. McCance, R. A., and Widdowson, E. M. Mineral metabolism of the foetus and newborn animal. *Brit. Med. Bull.* 17:132, 1961.
341. McCance, R. A., and Young, W. F. The secretion of urine by newborn infants. *J. Physiol.* (London) 99:265, 1941.
342. McCarthy, J. M., and Pryles, C. V. Clean voided and catheter neonatal urine specimens. *Amer. J. Dis. Child.* 106:473, 1963.
343. McConville, J. M., West, C. D., and McAdams, A. J. Familial and nonfamilial benign hematuria. *J. Pediat.* 69:207, 1966.
344. McCrory, W. W. A new cause for an old disease — chronic nephritis. *J. Pediat.* 72:912, 1968.
345. McCrory, W. W., and Fleisher, D. S. The Nephrotic Syndrome. In Gairdner, D. M. T. (Ed.), *Recent Advances in Pediatrics* (2d ed.). Boston: Little, Brown, 1958. Chap. 9, p. 227.
346. McCrory, W. W., Fleisher, D. S., and Sohn, W. B. Effects of early ambulation on the course of nephritis in children. *Pediatrics* 24:395, 1959.
347. McCrory, W. W., Forman, C. W., McNamara, H., and Barnett, H. L. Renal excretion of phosphate in newborn infants. *J. Clin. Invest.* 31:357, 1952.
348. McCrory, W. W., Shibuya, M., and Worthen, H. G. Hereditary renal glomerular disease in infancy and childhood. *Advances Pediat.* 14:253, 1966.
349. McLean, M. M., Jones, C. H., and Sutherland, D. A. Hemolytic-uremic syndrome: A report of an outbreak. *Arch. Dis. Child.* 41:76, 1966.
350. McQuiggan, M. C., Oliver, W. J., Littler,

540. Yunibhand, P., and Held, U. Der Einflusz der zunehmenden Hydropenie auf Nierenmark, Serum und Urin be Albinoratten. *Helv. Physiol. Pharmacol. Acta* 23:139, 1965.

541. Zarafonetis, C. J. D., Steiger, W. A., Molthan, L., McMaster, J., and Colville, V. F. Renal defect associated with sickle cell trait and sickle cell disease. *J. Lab. Clin. Med.* 44:959, 1954.

542. Zetterström, R. Idiopathic Hypercalcemia and Hypercalcuria. In *Mod. Probl. Paediat.* 3:478, 1957.

543. Zetterström, R., and Berglund, G. Systemic lupus erythematosus in childhood: A clinical study. *Acta Paediat. Scand.* 45: 189, 1956.

43

Immunologic and Genetic Aspects of Kidney Transplantation

D. Bernard Amos

Transplantation of kidneys is becoming an accepted treatment for end-stage renal disease. While excellent results are being obtained with ever-increasing frequency, it must be remembered that the procedure is still experimental and that the results often fall considerably short of the optimum. In cases in which there is a pronounced incompatibility between the donor and the recipient, graft rejection is frequently so severe as to be uncontrollable by current therapeutic procedures. Even if a severe immunologic rejection is controlled, the kidney may be permanently damaged, leaving the patient with hypertension, proteinuria, and a kidney that functions poorly.

The contrast between a successful and a mediocre transplant is so great that the high overall survival rate of kidney grafts must not be accepted as the only criterion. With our presently available knowledge it is possible to increase the rate of success. With additional research the proportion of completely successful transplants should rise still further.

The acceptance of any graft is dependent upon its failure to provoke an effective immune response on the part of the recipient. This may be achieved in many ways. The recognition system of the recipient may be blunted, specifically as in the induction of tolerance or nonspecifically by the use of immunosuppressive agents such as antilymphocyte serum. The effector system may be impaired by drugs, by lymphocyte depletion, by complement depletion, and probably by stabilization of the lysosomes of the host cell. The graft may be feebly antigenic, as in the case of bone, or may be placed in a "favored site" as in the case of a corneal transplant. Finally, the antigenic patterns of donor and recipient may be alike as in grafts between monozygotic twins, or differences may be minimal as in grafts between certain siblings. Most or all of these procedures are used in avoiding transplant rejection.

Some of these factors are discussed in this chapter; in particular, I shall review information relating to the transplantation antigens, discuss what "compatible" and "incompatible" relationships may involve, describe the immunogenic criteria for donor selection, and discuss some aspects of the immunologic process. For general information on the history and development of transplantation the reader is referred to the monographs by Starzl [44] and by Calne [13]. The early literature has been comprehensively reviewed by Woodruff [54]. The trend of the results of transplantation can be followed by comparing the successive reports of the Kidney Transplant Registry [23, 34–37, 40]. Several monographs have appeared on organ and tissue transplantation [18, 42], and three committee reports deal with the overall problems of transplantation.

Transplantation Antigens

The antigens relevant to kidney graft rejection are obviously substances found on the vascular endothelium and in the tubule, glomeruli, and interstitial tissue of the kidney itself. It is difficult to obtain information about these antigens per se. It is believed that certain factors are found only in the kidney, but these appear to have little relevance to graft rejection since they are shared by all kidneys. These antigens may be relevant to the recurrence of disease but are proper to a study of autoimmunity rather than of transplantation immunity.

The important transplantation antigens in all species so far studied are widely distributed among the tissues including the white cells. In certain species, such as rat and mouse, they are also found on the red cells. They are known as isoantigens or alloantigens and differ from individual to individual. Some of them also function as xenoantigens and as such are recognized by other species. Other xenoantigens are common to all members of a species and are known as species-specific antigens. These antigens have relevance to transplantation between members of different species or genera but are not involved in grafts within a species.

Since the transplantation or histocompatibility alloantigens are present on the white cell, it is most convenient to test for their presence by such means as leukoagglutination, lymphocyte cytotoxicity, or complement fixation.

Transplantation was first shown to be a practicable therapeutic procedure for the relief of chronic renal disease through a series of grafts from monozygotic twin donors [31]. Two-year survival rates were approximately 90 per cent, and excellent renal function was obtained. Recurrence of the original disease in the transplanted kidney later became a problem. Even this appears to have been minimized by recipient nephrectomy before transplantation, by the continuous use of antibiotics, and, in some instances, by the administration of immunosuppressive drugs.

Early attempts at the transplantation of kidneys from cadavers were only moderately successful. Most of the kidneys failed to function or failed early. One exceptional kidney functioned well for over five months [24].

The operative technics developed were adequate, but the problem of transplant rejection was, and to a lesser extent still is, difficult to solve. A major impetus to transplantation practice was provided by the discovery in several laboratories that drugs used as cancer chemotherapeutic agents were effective in suppressing certain types of immunologic response [41, 47]. These drugs, such as methotrexate and 6-mercaptopurine, were most effective in preventing the development of immunity to relatively weak antigenic factors in skin or tumor homografts in laboratory animals, but had relatively little effect on an established, strong immune response.

Similar findings are emerging from clinical results. Drug therapy proved to be effective in controlling the rejection of about half the kidneys taken from close relatives, and about 20 per cent of kidneys from cadavers. Immunologic reactivity remained a problem in that the function of many of the surviving kidneys was less than optimal. While a few of the earliest transplanted kidneys are still surviving, the majority have now ceased to function.

One of the factors contributing to the death of the patient was depression of bone marrow function or toxicity to the liver through overtreatment with drugs. This tendency was possibly exaggerated by the introduction of corticosteroids and other agents such as actinomycin to aid in the control of rejection.

Improvements in patient management and in the use and handling of new drugs have resulted in a progressive improvement in survival rates as reported in the Kidney Transplant Registry [40]. Interestingly enough, several classes of living donors used in the early attempts — that is, distant relatives and nonrelatives — are now rarely utilized. Figures for these categories are not significantly better than those for cadaveric donors; in fact, the survival of kidneys from live unrelated donors is slightly inferior to that of cadaveric kidneys [37].

The extent of the immunologic barrier is still apparent from a consideration of the difference in survival between kidneys from close relatives as compared to those from cadavers. As will be discussed later, about one-fourth of all sibling donors would be expected to be highly compatible with their recipient. Parent-child, child-parent, and half of the sibling-sibling combinations will, on the average, be more compatible than unrelated donors.

The survival curve is the mean result obtained from two populations. The most highly compatible grafts behave, under only moderate immunosuppression, like grafts from monozygotic twins. The least compatible elicit an almost overwhelming immunologic response that can be controlled only with great difficulty if at all.

Not apparent from the survival curve is another effect of incompatibility — that is, impairment of function. While patients with the most successful transplants have high creatinine clearances, normal blood pressures, and low plasma creatinine and urea levels, many recipients, especially those receiving cadaveric grafts, suffer from some degree of hypertension or proteinuria and have other evidences of impairment of renal function.

It is the task of the immunologist and of the immunogeneticist to find means whereby the most compatible kidneys can be selected, and to seek methods of preventing or overcoming the immunologic response when some degree of incompatibility is unavoidable. Information about the transplantation antigens was gained when, in 1958, Dausset [17] tested similar agglutinins for white cells in the serum of several multitransfused patients. Van Loghem et al. [29] and Miescher [32] also found leukoagglutinating antibodies. Dausset's antigen is noteworthy in that on later investigation it was shown to be associated with skin graft rejection. Factors described by other investigators were not further studied, and their specificities are unknown. Van Rood and van Leeuwen [49] and Payne and her colleagues [38] described an ever-increasing number of leukoagglutinins; while Walford et al. [52], Terasaki and McClelland [45], and others began to define an increasingly wide variety of antigens detected by a cytolytic method. Shulman and his co-workers [43] carried out similar studies using complement-fixation procedures, as did van der Weerdt and Columbani and their colleagues [16, 48].

By 1965 the result was an accumulation of information about a relatively large number of factors described by symbols which varied from laboratory to laboratory. Following a series of comparative studies on cells from the same donor panel at a practical workshop in Leiden, it was learned that many laboratories had produced sera that detected the same factors [10]. Van Rood et al. [51], Amos [1], and Payne et al. [38] recognized some constant genetic association between their various factors. Dausset and the Ivanyis [19], basing their extrapolation on data collected from typing unrelated subjects, suggested that all the well-defined antigens they could detect belonged to a single system. Bach and Amos, separately and in collaboration, soon confirmed this by skin graft experiments combined with leukocyte typing and mixed leukocyte culture reactions on a number of closely related subjects [2, 7, 8]. These investigators also showed that the antigens of this system were the major histocompatibility factors in man [3, 7].

The locus, or rather the gene complex, soon came to be called HL-A, and a committee was organized by the World Health Organization to designate the antigenic factors controlled by it. In September, 1968, the first six factors were named and a model system for defining new factors was established.

Relatively few of the specificities have received official recognition as yet. This will change rapidly, but the complexity of the system is so great that it will be many years before the definitive table can be drawn. Even at this time, the identity of some of the designated antigens has not been fully determined.

There exists then a large number of antigenic factors controlled by a single genetic unit. It is probable that a considerable length of chromosome is involved. This is implied by the ability of chemists to separate out molecules having distinctive antigenic properties. The molecular weight of these products is about 50,000 [26]. It is not known whether the antigenic specificities are an integral part of the protein molecule, whether each molecule determines one or many specificities, or whether the actual determinant is a side chain attached to the protein. The antigens appear to contain little or no lipid, but could contain up to 10 per cent of carbohydrate. Yields of purified product are so small that less than 1 mg. is obtained from 50 gm. of spleen.

Separation of the antigenic material into at least five fractions by column chromatography suggests that several molecules are produced simultaneously [9]. Since each might require the activation of 250 nucleotide triplets, the length of chromosome involved must be considerable. Several reports of possible examples of recombination within the HL-A genetic units have already appeared, but none as yet fully satisfies the criteria suggested for proof of recombination within this system [53].

As might be expected by this degree of genetic complexity, the number of different alleles or haplotypes is enormous. Ceppellini and his colleagues analyzed 44 HL-A units from 22 subjects tested at the Turin workshop and found them all to be different [15]. Amos et al. [4] analyzed 140 additional allelic units and found that including the Italian series there were at least 170 different configurations. Since each individual carried two HL-A genetic units, the probability of finding unrelated individuals who share the same two alleles is less than 1 per 100,000. It is important to keep in mind the distinction between family members and unrelated subjects. Within a single family only four alleles can be present. Despite the complexity of each allele, the characteristics are inherited as a single unit, just as the various Rh alleles are inherited as single units [2]. In both Rh and HL-A genotyping, at least 25 per cent of siblings must share the same two alleles. Between families and between individuals, the differences between HL-A serotypes may be extreme. An example of the antigenic representation of four typical alleles from one family is given in Table 43-1.

Compatibility in a Functional Sense

It has been established then that HL-A is a complex genetic unit which controls an un-

Table 43-1. Antigenic Representation of Four Typical Alleles from Family 0102

Genotype	Father AB	Mother CD	Ma AC	Ja AC	Sa BC	Ri AD	Antisera Detecting Factors Controlled by Allele
Haplotype							
A	+	0	+	+	0	+	Ca8, Ril 7/65, RA 1/67/BeB, RA P-1, RA 1/67, Joc 11/66, GW 7/65, Cutten 2701
B	+	0	0	0	+	0	RB P-1, RB 1/67/JM, RB 1/67/AB, SD P-3, BHP-1/RA, BM 5/66
A + B	+	0	+	+	+	+	DAL 2/67/KS, DAL P-1, RB 1/67, BM 12/66
C	0	+	+	+	+	0	AJ 5/67, McM 9/65, SHO 9/65, Ma9
D	0	+	0	0	0	+	None
C + D	0	+	+	+	+	+	JPO 11/66
B + C	+	+	+	+	+	0	Pig 1/67, NW 11/65
A + D	+	+	+	+	0	+	None
B + D	+	+	0	0	+	+	None
A + C + others	+	+	+	+	+	+	DK 9/66/SD, DK 9/66/ROD, DK 9/66, BHP-1, DAL 2/67, FS 1/67, NW 3/65, CAR 2/66, JT P-1, KH 1/67, KH 1/67/FL, Anderson
O	0	0	0	0	0	0	PAY 2/66, ENN 12/65, WB P-1, SA 9/66, SA 4/65, FS P-1, NW 3/65/NH, RA; HF P-1, ROY 6/65, P. Bu 3/66, L. Bu 11/66, L. Bu 7/65, MH P-1, Cou 3/65, JD 6/65, MJ 9/67, Sc30, Harris, Thompson, Willett

known number of antigenic specificities and that perhaps as many as 100,000 unrelated donors would have to be tested in order to find one who was antigenically identical to a given recipient. To find an exactly identical donor for each recipient is manifestly impracticable, and from experience in renal transplantation we know that approximately one out of 10 cadaveric kidneys behaves as if it came from an HL-A identical donor. One of our own recipients with a perfectly functioning kidney and who receives only low doses of immunosuppression could be distinguished from his donor by the reactions of no less than 6 antisera out of the 46 used in the comparison. Obviously complete identity between donor and recipient is not needed any more than it is needed in blood transfusion.

Good analogies can be drawn from animal experimentation and from knowledge of the Rh system. Hildemann et al. [22] studied skin graft rejection between mice differing at a single locus. In one direction involving a difference at the H-1 locus, a graft might be rejected in a few days, while the reciprocal graft would persist for weeks or even months. The first graft is functionally incompatible, while the reciprocal, although it involves incompatibility at the same locus, is functionally compatible. In blood transfusion practice the only Rh antigen commonly considered is D. Transfusion from a phenotypically CDe donor to a cDE recipient would be unlikely to give rise to serious sensitization, whereas transfusion from a cDe donor to a cde recipient should be avoided. The first transfusion would be functionally compatible but antigenically incompatible, while the second would be functionally and antigenically incompatible.

It seems unlikely that all HL-A antigens are equally strong, but there is no clear information concerning this. It may be inferred that those factors that frequently elicit circulating antibodies are more likely to be potent than those that do not — thus, 4a, HLA-2, and HLA-7 could perhaps be taken as possible strong antigens — but other factors such as gene frequency and the difference between the induction of delayed and of immediate type hypersensitivity may be very important. A further complication is that certain combinations of antigens may be highly immunogenetic, while the same factors in different combinations are feebly so. For example, HLA-2 in combination with HLA-12 might be more effective than HLA-2 in combination with HLA-7. It is probable that some of these complex problems will take years to resolve.

It is essential to gain further information if the immunogeneticist is to advise on donor selection. Two experimental models have been explored. The first has been used by van Rood and his associates [51] and by Dausset and his colleagues [20]. A panel of subjects was typed with a battery of antisera and the reactions obtained were compared. The selected donor possessed the antigen to be studied — for example, HLA-2 — whereas the recipient did not. From several such donors possessing the HLA-2 antigen, the one who otherwise resembled the recipient most closely was selected. The recipient was then immunized against him and given grafts from three donors possessing HLA-2 and from three negative donors. Grafts from the antigen-positive donors were rejected in an accelerated fashion; grafts from the negative (control) donors were not.

Under similar experimental circumstances five of the antigenic factors were shown to have transplantation activity. The method is rather cumbersome and subject to considerable error, however, and it appears to have been dropped in favor of an indirect analysis in which the success of a transplant is correlated with the number and nature of the incompatibility involved. This has been the approach of Terasaki and his co-workers [46] and van Rood and his colleagues [50], who prospectively or retrospectively typed kidney donors and recipients; and of Ceppellini, Dausset and Amos who carried out similar studies with skin graft donor recipient pairs. While there is an overall correlation between incompatibility and the survival or function of grafts exchanged between unrelated individuals, it is difficult to make a prediction on an individual basis.

An account of one of our earlier experiments may serve as an illustration of the difficulties faced. Cells from some 30 volunteer subjects were tested with the 30 or so antisera available to us. The reaction patterns were compared and eight pairs who were relatively compatible were identified. These 16 subjects were arranged in groups of four so that each group included two "compatible" pairs. There were, of course, numerous incompatibilities between pairs. Skin grafts were exchanged so that each subject received a graft from a "compatible" and an "incompatible" donor. The experiment took many weeks of preparation, each typing being repeated several times. The outcome, which had been awaited with pleasant anticipation, was disastrous. Although a few grafts followed the expected pattern, overall there was no correlation and many of the "incompatible" grafts outlasted the "compatible" ones. Obviously our assumption of what constituted "compatibility" was wrong, and we had failed to detect a number of potent antigens. We therefore immunized many of the subjects who rejected their grafts rapidly with lymphocytes from their "compatible" donor and obtained a series of antibodies which ipso facto detected new specificities. The experiment was repeated with somewhat better, but still far from perfect, results. Similar results have been obtained by many other investigators [14, 50], who obtained a mean difference in survival between "compatible" and "incompatible" grafts of about two days. One of the immediate tasks is to obtain additional reagents which will identify the missing specificities.

The problem is simplified when close relatives are used in skin or organ grafting. Apart from ABH blood-group factors, only antigens of the HL-A system appear to function as strong antigens.

A representation of inheritance of the HL-A factors is given in Figure 43-1. The parents each possess homologous chromosomes that bear the HL-A genetic units. Each child inherits one of these units from each of his parents. For convenience, the paternal units are designated A and B, the maternal units C and D. A child will inherit A or B from the father, C or D from the mother, so only the combinations AC, AD, BC, or BD are possible. Suppose a patient having several siblings had inherited the A and C determinants or alleles, the first sibling to be considered as donor could be AC, AD, BC, or BD with equal probability. The chances are one in four that he too would be AC. In this event both donor and recipient would have inherited the

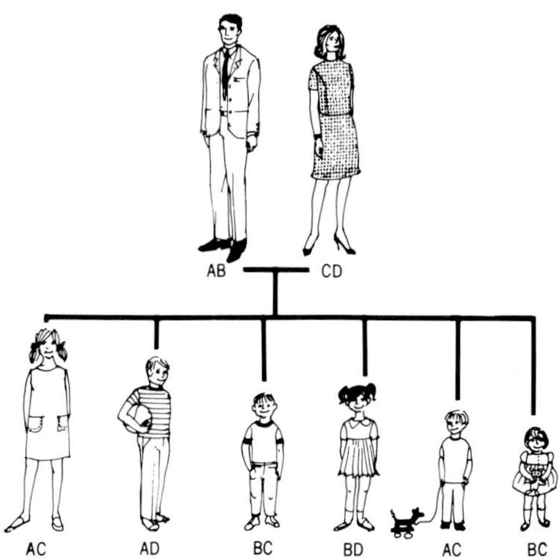

Figure 43-1. Representation of the inheritance of chromosomal determinants of the HL-A system. "A + B" are carried by the paternal gametes, "C + D" by the maternal gametes. Only four genotypes can occur within a family. The HL-A alleles differ greatly from family to family.

same two factors and would be identical with respect to the HL-A antigens. It therefore does not matter that the HL-A system is extremely complex or that the A, B, C, and D alleles differ from family to family. Within a family there is a 1 in 4 chance that a given donor will be HL-A identical with respect to the patient.

This is the ideal transplant situation. Skin grafts last from 15 to 41 days (mean, 23 days), and kidney grafts function well with only minimal immunosuppressive therapy. Similarly, the worst transplant situation occurs when donor and recipient differ at both alleles. The resemblance between them may be no better than that found between two unrelated subjects. In practice, skin graft survival is approximately the same as that found between unrelated subjects.

There is a one in two chance that a given sibling will share one allele with the patient, and each parent, of course, shares one allele. This is the most interesting experimental situation since donor and recipient differ only with respect to the products of a single allele. This then is the relationship in which it is easiest to examine the correlation between differences for individual antigenic specificities and graft rejection. As might be expected, skin graft rejection times vary widely (from 7 to 33 days), and the mean survival time lies between the 11-day survival for grafts differing at two alleles, or unrelated grafts, and the 23 days for zero difference. We are at present attempting to correlate incompatibility for the various antigenic factors and rejection time [5]. Despite this simplification, the problem of deciding which are the most potent antigens is by no means resolved. Frequently two alleles differ with respect to a large number of antigens, and there is no evidence that all the antigens can yet be identified. The problem of identifying the missing factors is compounded by variability in the individual immune response. An example of the variability between subjects was given by an analysis of Duke family 0099 [53]. Grafts from five related donors were placed on two siblings who were HL-A identical. The mean rejection time of all the grafts by one recipient was 20.6 days, whereas that of grafts from the same five donors to the other recipient was 27.8 days. At present the existence of variability in the immune response between different recipients is not exploited in clinical practice, but as will be suggested later, it should be, for it may provide an explanation for the prolonged survival of many incompatible kidney grafts.

To summarize, there does not now appear to be any simple method of defining the functional antigenic strength of the antigens or of the alleles. Bach and his colleagues are attempting to equate the degree of stimulation observed in mixed lymphocyte cultures with the intensity of skin graft rejection. Other tests, such as the irradiated hamster test of Ramseier et al., may prove to be useful, but the major effort is being put into a comparison of serotype and graft survival, a very cumbersome and time-consuming type of bioassay, fraught with many difficulties.

The Reaction Against the Incompatible Graft

As soon as the blood supply becomes established, antigen leaves the kidney via the renal vein and presumably gets trapped by phagocytic cells in the lungs, liver, spleen, and lymph nodes. In the absence of immunosuppression, the release of antigen induces the production of antibody and results in the appearance of specifically reactive lymphoid cells in the circulation. These two factors can act synergistically or antagonistically with each other. One of the possible ways in which some of the immunosuppressive agents can act is to alter the phase of the components of the response. For example, antibody from a late-phase (hyperimmune) animal can block the early phase of lymphoid responsiveness. Lymphoid cells are soon seen cuffing the small vessels and later crowding into the interstitial spaces. It is thought that these cells can exert their effect independently of antibody and in the absence of complement. A good case has been made for this in isolated systems or by the transfer of lymphoid cells in inbred animals. The role of antibody is less securely established and has tended to be overlooked because free antibody can rarely be detected in the animal or patient bearing a renal homograft. Milgrom et al. [33] have shown that this is because the kidney acts as a very efficient sponge and soaks up antibody directed against it. After removal of the kidney, high titers of cytotoxic antibody are found in the serum. A second kidney transplanted at a time when antibodies are present in high titer will be immediately rejected if it contains antigens which cross-react with those of the first kidney.

A direct demonstration of the effects of antibody has recently been reported. A kidney from a unilaterally nephrectomized dog was transplanted to a normal recipient. After four days, the recipient was irradiated and the second kidney from the original donor was transplanted to the lymphocyte-depleted animal. After four hours, the second kidney was replaced in the original donor where it was immediately rejected [21]. It is, of course, impossible to say that no lymphoid cells were trapped during these four hours, but the cellular depletion of the recipient through x-ray and the speed and manner of rejection suggest that an Arthus-like response is involved.

Donor Selection

It may be helpful to give a brief account of the screening process employed by our transplantation group in screening out incompatible donors.

Medically and psychologically suitable recipients are asked if there are other family members. The family is contacted separately and members are asked if they will donate. The whole family is invited to the laboratory, and blood for leukocyte typing and blood grouping is drawn. The cells are tested against a battery of some 60 sera defining a variety of different specificities. The investigation is repeated on the following day. By including all family members, including those who are obviously unable to donate, it is possible to follow the inheritance of the four alleles. Immunologically the ideal donor (class 1) is one who shares the same two HL-A alleles and who is ABO compatible. If no such donor is available, a sibling or parent sharing one allele is sought. Suppose the patient is designated AC, the choice would be between the A*B* or the C*D* parent, or between a parent and an A*D* or a *B*C sibling — that is, the donor will be incompatible for B or D. An HL-A identical sibling who is not available as a donor can be used as a substitute for the recipient in a model graft experiment. Grafts from the B or D incompatible donors are followed. If a graft survives for more than 15 days, the donor is categorized as class 2a; if for less than 14 days, as a class 2b.

Even if no HL-A identical test donor is available, graft survival can be tested. A BC graft to the mother or a graft from the father to an AD sibling both test some attributes of incompatibility for the B allele, and grafts to the father or from the mother can test the D allele. In all, there are six relationships involving the same one-allele incompatibility. Note that (1) they do not all necessarily measure the same antigens and that (2) variability in the immunologic status of the test subject can influence the result.

When skin grafting is impracticable or impossible, recourse may be had to the degree of stimulation in mixed lymphocyte culture or the phenotypic similarity on serotyping. These two tests are regarded by us as only a rough guide, and donors selected in this way are put into class 3. Some of our class 3 relationships would be regarded as class A matches by other laboratories, but it is emphasized that at present we regard phenotyping or MLC results between non-HL-A identical siblings as a very rough guide only to histocompatibility. As typing improves, the guide will improve in its reliability, but until all the transplantation antigens are known, phenotyping can present grave errors in interpretation. We do regard it as highly advisable in the selection of cadaver donors, but prefer to avoid using live donors selected on this basis.

Immunosuppression

Without the use of immunosuppressive drugs there would be very few transplants. With the exception of the thalidomide drugs which are largely untried except in baboons, the only impressive agent is antilymphocyte serum (ALS) [55]. The serum is produced in one species (often the horse) against thymus or other lymphoid cells of another species (e.g., man). It is interesting that although this material has been made sporadically and its lympholytic effect known for very many years, only recently has it been used to suppress the immune response. Its effects in laboratory animals, especially when coupled with thymectomy, are dramatic. It not only will suppress the homograft response, but also facilitate the production of immunologic unresponsiveness in the adult and permit the survival of grafts across wide species barriers [30]. Its full potential in man has not been realized, largely because it has been used in a completely uncontrolled manner and with little regard to standardization.

In the laboratory, as in the clinic, ALS is the focus of frenzied activity. We know fairly well what it is not, and what it does not do, but what it is and what it does are unknown. It is not simply an antibody directed against lymphocytes, since preparations having immunosuppressive activity can be made by immunization against fibroblasts, tumors, and other nonlymphoid sources [28]. Gamma globulins are active both in vivo and in vitro, whereas a highly lymphocytolytic 19S macroglobulin can destroy lymphocytes without causing effective immunosuppression [25]. A highly purified preparation can be absorbed out from an antilymphocyte serum and then eluted from lymphoid cells. By analogy with studies on the induction of immunologic unresponsiveness with enhancing antibodies, it is possible that ALS has an effect on the antigens of the donor instead of, or in addition to, those of the host, but this is purely speculative. Other suggestions proposed are that the antiserum "blinds" the recognition system of the lymphocytes, that it acts by lymphoid depletion, or that it destroys certain cells of thymic origin.

Even in its present crude state, antilymphocyte serum does appear to have immediate clinical value, although it also introduces additional risks such as those of anaphylaxis and nephritis. It is usually used synergistically with other forms of therapy including azathioprine and corticosteroids.

Other methods of immunosuppression which at one time appeared to be of value have generally been abandoned as being ineffective or hazardous. These include generalized or local irradiation, thymectomy, splenectomy, and thoracic duct drainage.

The Immunologic Cripple

The immunologic cripple was thought of as a rarity until quite recently. Patients with Hodgkin's disease, leukemia, or aggammaglobulinemia were obvious exceptions. Now it is realized that many children who suffer from recurrent infections during childhood, some going on to die with bronchiectasis or other complications, have rather subtle forms of immunologic deficiencies. R. H. Buckley et al. [12] have described normal immunoglobulin levels in childhood and have identified a series of abnormalities involving the three major immunoglobulins associated with a predilection toward disease.

The reduced immunocompetence of patients with nephritis has been known for years, and it was generally concluded that their immunologic depression was due either to their uremia or to their impaired protein uptake. Patients treated adequately with hemodialysis are no longer uremic but retain their depressed immune state; some patients with nutritional problems are not necessarily handicapped immunologically.

C. E. Buckley [11] has recently conducted a study of the immunoglobulin levels of patients with intractable renal disease and found a variety of abnormalities. We have been struck with the alarmingly high frequency of hypertension or of frank renal disease in the siblings of our transplant subjects and have begun to wonder to what extent the two conditions, immunologic incompetence and renal disease, coexist — just as autoimmune diseases and impaired immunologic reactivity coexist in hybrids of certain mouse strains.

Considerably more work on this point is needed, but it seems a distinct possibility that the most relevant determination to make in a transplant recipient is his degree of immunocompetence. If immunologic reactivity is really impaired, the patient will require less immunosuppression and will accept a more histo-incompatible graft than will a normal recipient.

From the studies of Kirkpatrick et al. it appeared that transplant recipients rapidly regained their ability to respond to a variety of delayed allergens [27]. While this may be true of delayed hypersensitivity, it seems possible that they do not regain full immunologic competence. Buckley [11] finds their immunoglobulin levels remain upset even when they receive a well-functioning kidney maintained on very low doses of drug. Bach found that the lymphocytes of some patients in the Denver series failed to respond to any cell in mixed culture; others failed to respond to their donor [3, 6]. This seemed to be particularly true of the incompatible patients who had survived for over two years. In all three studies the patients were receiving immunosuppressive drugs, and "control" studies on patients receiving a transplant for reasons other than glomerular disease are essential.

Even in normal subjects, the ability to respond to microbial antigens, to injections of lymphocytes, or to skin grafts varies widely from person to person. The effect of certain viruses in reducing immunologic reactivity is being established, just as other microbial products are known to exaggerate the immune response. These factors all merit attention.

To summarize, the immunologic responsiveness of the transplant recipient has been almost totally ignored; yet it may be the most critical factor in determining whether or not he will accept a graft and whether or not he will develop a recurrence of his original disease.

Overall Considerations

Transplantation is becoming accepted as a way of treating end-stage kidney disease. It is both more and less than this. Transplantation is not an end in itself; the ideal approach is through prevention, not treatment. Even when immunosuppression, tissue typing, and tolerance are understood and intelligently applied, transplantation will remain an expensive, painful, and somewhat hazardous expedient. Transplantation does, however, offer a unique way of studying renal disease: for short-term studies of renal function, transplants to a nonabdominal site may serve to harvest antibodies and immune cells in a concentrated form; from an analysis of recurrence of disease in the transplant, the etiology of the disease and its pathogenesis may be studied.

There has been an avalanche of articles on kidney transplantation and the student is referred to such monographs as the Proceedings of the Second International Congress of the Transplantation Society [39], Advance in Transplantation [18], and to the texts on kidney transplantation by Calne [13] and by Starzl [44].

Since this chapter was completed there have been a number of significant advances. Most investigators now believe that the antigens exist as members of two segregant series. Each series is determined by a specific genetic determinant. According to this concept, each individual possesses only four HL-A antigens, two of the first series and two of the second. At least fourteen first series and nineteen second series antigens have been proposed. Since gene frequencies vary greatly between different allelic forms and some combinations occur more frequently than would be expected by chance, the probability of finding donor and recipient possessing the same four antigens also varies greatly. Cross reactivities between antigens are recognized and it appears probable that the chance of a strong rejection crisis is diminished when donor and recipient, although differing in their antigenic profile, differ only by cross-reacting antigens. An example of cross reactivity would be HLA-3 and HLA-11. A recipient who carried HLA-3 would be expected to react less strongly against tissues from a cross-reacting HLA-11 donor than from a non-cross-reacting HLA-9 donor. The cross reactivities have been only partially explored. The existence of cross reactivity can explain why apparently mismatched donors may, not infrequently, provide quite acceptable kidneys. To what extent serologic cross reactivity will coincide with immunogenic cross reactivity is not yet known, but it is known from the work of several investigators using hapten-carrier complexes that cross reactivity in cellular and humoral terms is not always coincidental.

It is also being recognized that we cannot always demonstrate some of the apparently well defined antigens. Dr. Yunis encountered an antibody produced in a multiparous woman that reacted strongly with all cells carrying HLA-12 except those from her husband and children. However, cells from these family members would absorb her antibody. We called the cytotoxicity-negative immunization-positive phenomenon CNIP, and the more common cytotoxicity-negative absorption-positive situation CNAP. A second example of CNIP has been encountered at Duke where an individual, immunized against a donor whose cells were consistently negative when tested with anti-HLA-2 sera, produced an anti-2. The donors' cells were subsequently found to absorb all 2-positive sera available, but still would not react directly. Presumably, an artifact due to inadequate fixation of complement is responsible for both CNIP and CNAP.

Certain generalizations made in this chapter as first written still hold. It is clear from many reports that grafts from genotypically HL-A identical siblings are almost invariably accepted and that skin grafting to other family members provides a fairly accurate estimate of the immunogenicity of the alleles carried in that family. There is a correlation between phenotypic similarity and graft survival among unrelated pairs, but this is most clearly seen at the extremes of phenotypic identity for, or divergence at, the four HL-A antigens. There is little indication that any particular HL-A specificity is more immunogenic than another. The mixed-lymphocyte reaction is often of help in assessing HL-A identity in families in which serotyping is ambiguous. Pairs differing at both alleles generally stimulate more than pairs differing only by one allele. Unfortunately, in our own series we have found the correlation between individual MLC (mixed lymphocyte culture) results and skin-graft survival between individuals differing at one allele to be low.

In summary, April 1971, the results of kidney grafting are becoming ever more encouraging. Survival rates continue to improve, our knowledge of enhancement is increasing rapidly, and a number of organs have now been transplanted successfully in animals using only alloantiserum for immunosuppression. Even with our presently imperfect knowledge of so many facets of organ transplantation, there can be no disputing that thousands of patients who would have died from chronic renal failure are now leading productive lives.

Acknowledgments

Supported in part by grants (5 KO6 A118399, and GM 12535) from the U.S. Public Health Service.

References

1. Amos, D. B. Some Results on the Cytotoxicity Test. In Balner, H., Cleton, F. J., and Eernisse, J. G. (Eds.), *Histocompatibility Testing, 1965*. Copenhagen: Munksgaard, 1966. P. 151.
2. Amos, D. B. The inheritance of leukocyte antigens. *Transplantation* 5:1015, 1967.
3. Amos, D. B., and Bach, F. H. Phenotypic expressions of the major histocompatibility locus in man (HL-A): Leukocyte antigens and mixed leukocyte culture reactivity. *J. Exp. Med.* 128:623, 1968.
4. Amos, D. B., Ward, F. E., and MacQueen, J. M. Analysis of the Haplotypes (Alleles) of the Turin Workshop Families. In Rose, N. R., and Milgrom, M. (Eds.), *Proceedings*

of the International Convocation on Immunology. Basel: Karger, 1969.

5. Amos, D. B., Ward, F. E., Zmijewski, C. M., Hattler, B. G., and Seigler, H. F. Graft donor selection based upon single locus (haplotype) analysis within families. *Transplantation* 6:524, 1968.
6. Bach, F. Personal communication.
7. Bach, F. H., and Amos, D. B. Hu-1: Major histocompatibility locus in man. *Science* 156:1506, 1967.
8. Bach, F. H., and Kisken, W. A. Predictive value of results of mixed leukocyte cultures for skin allograft survival in man. *Transplantation* 5:1046, 1967.
9. Boyle, W. Soluble HLA iso-antigen preparations. *Transplant. Proc.* 1:491, 1969.
10. Bruning, J. W., van Leeuwen, A., and van Rood, J. J. Leucocyte Antigens. In *Histocompatibility Testing, 1965*. Copenhagen: Munksgaard, 1966. P. 275.
11. Buckley, C. E. In Soklik, W. J. (Ed.), *Zinsser Microbiology* (15th ed.), New York: Appleton-Century-Crofts, 1972.
12. Buckley, R. H., Dees, S. C., and O'Fallon, M. Serum immunoglobulins: I. Levels in normal children and in uncomplicated childhood allergy. *Pediatrics* 41:600, 1968.
13. Calne, R. Y. *Renal Transplantation* (2d ed.). Baltimore: Williams & Wilkins, 1966.
14. Ceppellini, R., Mattiuz, P. L., Scudeller, G., and Visetti, M. Experimental allotransplantation in man. I. *Transplant. Proc.* 1: 385, 1969.
15. Ceppellini, R. A Preliminary Report on the Third International Workshop on Histocompatibility Testing. In *Advance in Transplantation*. Copenhagen: Munksgaard, 1968. P. 195.
16. Colombani, J., Colombani, M., and Dausset, J. Indirect Antiglobulin Consumption Test for the Detection of Human Antibodies Against Skin Cells, Leukocytes, and Platelets. In Balner, H., Cleton, J. F., and Eernisse, J. G. (Eds.), *Histocompatibility Testing*. Washington, D.C.: Nat. Acad. Sci.-Nat. Res. Council, pub. 1229, 1965. P. 163.
17. Dausset, J. Iso-leuco-anticorps. *Acta Haemat.* (Basel) 20:156, 1958.
18. Dausset, J., Hamburger, J., and Mathé, G. *Advance in Transplantation, Proceedings of the First International Congress of the Transplantation Society*. Copenhagen: Munksgaard, 1968.
19. Dausset, J., Ivanyi, P., and Ivanyi, D. Tissue Alloantigens in Humans. In Balner, H., Cleton, F. J., and Eernisse, J. G. (Eds.), *Histocompatibility Testing, 1965*. Copenhagen: Munksgaard, 1966. P. 51.
20. Dausset, J., Rapaport, F. T., Ivanyi, P., and Colombani, J. Tissue Alloantigens and Transplantation. In *Histocompatibility Testing, 1965*. Copenhagen: Munksgaard, 1966. P. 63.
21. Foker, J., Clark, D., Pickering, R., Good, R., and Varco, R. Studies on the mechanism of canine renal allograft rejection. *Transplant. Proc.* 1:296, 1969.
22. Hildemann, W. H., Morgan, M., and Frautnick, L. Immunogenetic components of weaker histoincompatibility systems in mice. *Transplant. Proc.* 2:24, 1970.
23. Human Kidney Transplant Conference. Summary of proceedings. *Transplantation* 2:147, 1964.
24. Hume, E. M., Merrill, J. P., Miller, D. F., and Thorn, G. W. Experiences with renal homotransplantation in the human: Report on nine cases. *J. Clin. Invest.* 34:327, 1955.
25. James, K., and Medawar, P. B. Characterization of antilymphocyte serum. *Nature* (London) 214:1052, 1967.
26. Kahan, B. D., Reisfeld, R. A., Epstein, L. B., and Southworth, J. G. Biological Activities of a Soluble Transplantation Antigen. In Curtoni, E. S., Mattiuz, P. L., and Tosi, R. M. (Eds.), *Histocompatibility Testing, 1967*. Copenhagen: Munksgaard, 1967. P. 295.
27. Kirkpatrick, C. H., Wilson, W. E. C., and Talmadge, D. W. Immunologic studies in human organ transplantation. *J. Exp. Med.* 119: 727, 1964.
28. Levy, R., and Medawar, P. B. Nature and mode of action of antilymphocyte antiserum. *Proc. Natl. Acad. Sci. U.S.A.* 56:1130, 1966.
29. Loghem, J. J. van, van der Hart, M., and Borstel, H. The occurrence of complete and incomplete white cell antibodies. *Vox Sang.* 2:257, 1957.
30. Medawar, P. B. Biological Effects of Heter-

ologous Antilymphocyte Sera. In Rapaport, F. T., and Dausset, J. (Eds.), *Human Transplantation.* New York: Grune & Stratton, 1968. P. 501.

31. Merrill, J. P., Murray, J. E., Harrison, J. H., and Guild, W. R. Successful homotransplantation of the human kidney between identical twins. *J.A.M.A.* 160:277, 1956.
32. Miescher, P. Leucopénie chronique par "auto anticorps." *Acta Haemat.* 11:157, 1954.
33. Milgrom, F., Litvak, B. I., Kand, K., and Witebsky, E. Humoral antibodies in renal homograft. *J.A.M.A.* 198:226, 1966.
34. Murray, J. E., Gleason, R., and Bartholomay, A. Second report of the Human Kidney Transplant Registry. *Transplantation* 2:660, 1964.
35. Murray, J. E., Gleason, R., and Bartholomay, A. Third report of the Human Kidney Transplant Registry. *Transplantation* 3:294, 1965.
36. Murray, J. E., Gleason, R., and Bartholomay, A. Fourth Report of the Human Kidney Transplant Registry. *Transplantation* 3:684, 1965.
37. Murray, J. E., Barnes, B. A., and Atkinson, J. Fifth report of the Human Kidney Transplant Registry. *Transplantation* 5:752, 1967.
38. Payne, R., Tripp, M., Weigle, J., Bodmer, W., and Bodmer, J. A new leukocyte isoantigenic system in man. *Cold Spr. Harb. Symp. Quant. Biol.* 29:285, 1964.
39. Proceedings of the Second International Congress of the Transplantation Society. *Transplant. Proc.* 1:1, 1969.
40. Registry Advisory Committee eighth report of the Human Kidney Transplant Registry. *Transplantation* 11:328, 1971.
41. Schwartz, R. and Dameshek, W. The effects of 6-mercaptopurine on homograft reactions. *J. Clin. Invest.* 39:952, 1960.
42. Seventh International Transplantation Conference. *Ann. N.Y. Acad. Sci.* 129:1, 1966.
43. Shulman, N. R., Aster, R. H., Leitner, A., and Miller, M. C. Immunoreactions involving platelets: V. Post-transfusion purpura due to a complement-fixing antibody against a genetically controlled platelet antigen. *J. Clin. Invest.* 40:1597, 1961.
44. Starzl, T. E. *Experience in Renal Transplantation* Philadelphia: Saunders, 1964.
45. Terasaki, P. I., and McClelland, J. D. Microdroplet assay of human serum cytotoxins. *Nature* (London) 204:998, 1964.
46. Terasaki, P., Mickey, M., Mittal, K., Singal, D., and Patel, R. A review of histocompatibility testing of 400 kidney transplants. *Transplant. Proc.* 1:372, 1969.
47. Uphoff, D. E. Alteration of the homograft reaction by A-methopterin in lethally irradiated mice treated with homologous marrow. *Proc. Soc. Exp. Biol. Med.* 99:651, 1958.
48. van der Weerdt, C. M., van de Wiel-Dorfmeyer, H., Engelfriet, C. P., and van Loghem, J. J. A New Platelet Antigen. In *Proceedings of the Eighth Congress of the European Society of Haematology.* Basel: Karger, AG, 1961. P. 379.
49. van Rood, J. J., and van Leeuwen, A. Leukocyte grouping: A method and its application. *J. Clin. Invest.* 42:1382, 1963.
50. van Rood, J. J., and van Leeuwen, A. Leukocyte typing of unrelated donor-recipient pairs. *Transplant. Proc.* 1:372, 1969.
51. van Rood, J. J., van Leeuwen, A., Schippers, A. M. J., Vooys, W. H., Frederiks, E., Balner, H., and Eernisse, J. G. Leukocyte Groups, the Normal Lymphocyte Transfer Test and Homograft Sensitivity. In Balner, H., Cleton, F. J., and Eernisse, J. G. (Eds.), *Histocompatibility Testing, 1965.* Copenhagen: Munksgaard, 1966. P. 37.
52. Walford, R. L., Gallagher, R., and Sjaarda, J. R. Serologic typing of human lymphocytes with immune serum obtained after homografting. *Science* 144:868, 1964.
53. Ward, F. E., Southworth, J. G., and Amos, D. B. Recombination and other chromosomal aberrations within the HL-A locus. *Transplant. Proc.* 1:352, 1969.
54. Woodruff, M. F. A. *The Transplantation of Tissues and Organs.* Springfield, Ill.: Thomas, 1960.
55. Woodruff, M. F. A., and Anderson, N. A. The effect of lymphocyte depletion by thoracic duct fistula and administration of antilymphocyte serum on the survival of skin homografts in rats. *Ann. N.Y. Acad. Sci.* 120:119, 1964.

44

Kidney Transplantation

J. A. Mannick and R. H. Egdahl

While one may argue whether or not kidney transplantation in man has a sufficiently high rate of success to make it an acceptable method of therapy for the majority of patients with terminal renal failure, it nevertheless is clear that renal transplantation is being performed more and more frequently in an increasing number of medical centers in the United States and Europe. As of this writing nearly 1200 human kidney transplants have been reported to the Kidney Transplant Registry in Boston [72], and there are unquestionably an additional significant number of which the registry has no specific knowledge. Thus it seems appropriate to review the present status of kidney transplantation as therapy for uremic patients and to consider briefly some of the possibilities for improving the safety and increasing the applicability of this technic.

Historical

While there had been a number of prior attempts at renal transplantation in man, it was not until 1952 that this procedure was studied in a systematic way by Hume and his co-workers [41, 42]. In a series of cadaver kidney transplants in uremic patients Hume demonstrated that the transplanted kidneys could function for short periods and could, while functioning, effect a considerable improvement in the uremic state. As animal experimentation had suggested, no truly long-term function of these transplants was obtained.

Shortly thereafter, in 1955, Merrill and Murray and their associates [64, 76] reported the first successful kidney transplants between identical twins. Since, in this case, there was no antigenic difference between the donor and the recipient of the transplanted organ, normal renal function resulted and has persisted in some recipients of twin kidneys for many years [73]. However, the rejection of the transplanted organ by the immune system of the new host appeared to present an insurmountable obstacle to the application of kidney transplantation in uremic patients, other than identical twins, if significant survival of the transplanted organ were to be achieved.

Following the demonstration in the laboratory that blood-cell chimerism and permanent or semipermanent tolerance of allografts could be obtained following lethal total-body irradiation and allogenic (from another individual of the same species) bone marrow transplantation in a number of animal species [55, 56], a few attempts at applying this technic to patients in terminal uremia were made in the late 1950's. Unfortunately, these patients all died of the effects of the irradiation [75].

The first successful human kidney allograft (a graft of tissue from an allogenic donor) was performed by Merrill and his associates in 1959 [63]. The kidney in this case was exchanged between a pair of nonidentical twins. The immune response of the recipient was suppressed, but not destroyed, by sublethal total-body irradiation, and subsequent mild rejection attempts on the part of the new host were treated with steroids as well as supplemental irradiation. However, the modern era of kidney allografting in man clearly begins with the observation by Schwartz and his coworkers in 1959 [90] that the antimetabolite 6-mercaptopurine (6-MP) would inhibit the immune response in mammals. Thus with 6-mercaptopurine, or more recently with its analogue azathioprine, the clinical investigator had a chemical tool which would permit protracted survival of at least some kidney allografts in patients who would otherwise have succumbed to uremia. This new era was ushered in by Hamburger and his colleagues [32], who combined 6-mercaptopurine treatment with sublethal total-body irradiation in an initial series of human renal allografts; long-term success was obtained in several patients.

Present Status of Renal Transplantation in Man

SELECTION OF ORGAN RECIPIENTS AND DONORS

It is generally agreed that recipients of renal allografts should be terminally uremic and no longer manageable by conservative means. Whether or not such patients should, at this point, be considered for renal transplantation or chronic hemodialysis is not always clear. It seems certain, however, that for uremic patients who cannot obtain a place in a chronic dialysis program or who are already in such a program and are doing badly, renal transplantation offers the only alternative to death. Since kidney transplantation and the associated immune suppressive therapy cannot be considered innocuous procedures, it seems logical at present to restrict attempts at renal allografting to reasonably young patients who, except for uremia, are potentially healthy and free of other life-threatening disorders. These patients should have a normal lower urinary tract, no evidence of serious infection, and, because of the uncertainty of the outcome of transplantation at present, should be possessed of emotional stability and reliability.

Ethically the most acceptable kidney donor is obviously a cadaver since the donor in this case cannot be injured by removal of the kidney. It is now generally agreed that the major blood group of the kidney donor should be compatible with that of the recipient [39, 40, 94, 97]. Thus a type O cadaver becomes the universal donor, as in the case of blood transfusion, and the type AB cadaver can donate only to a type AB recipient. Whether or not an attempt should be made to match antigens on nucleated cells, particularly nucleated white blood cells, between donor and recipient prior to transplantation, is currently under extensive investigation [4, 15, 81, 95, 101]. At present, however, the majority of cadaver transplants (whether or not any form of matching or typing is carried out) are performed without regard to the results of leukocyte typing procedures.

It is generally agreed that the cadaver donor should be age 60 or younger and have normal renal function at the time of death. If possible the cadaver donor should be free of systemic infection and preferably should not have had a prolonged period of hypotension and inadequate renal perfusion prior to death. Since there have been a number of instances of transplantation of malignant tumors along with a cadaver kidney [59, 61], it is now the opinion of most transplantation groups that cadavers with malignancies other than primary brain tumors should not be utilized as kidney donors.

It goes without saying that obtaining a cadaver as soon after death as possible is desirable as far as the function of the transplanted organ is concerned. The death of the kidney donor must be anticipated by enough time to permit the transplant team to prepare to remove the kidneys when natural death occurs. Kidneys from persons who die suddenly and unexpectedly are seldom obtained sufficiently promptly to be suitable donor organs.

The kidneys are removed under sterile conditions. The left kidney is ordinarily removed first because of the lesser likelihood of duplication of the renal artery on that side and because the renal vein is longer. However, both kidneys are commonly used for transplantation if two suitable recipients are available. The kidneys are ordinarily cooled by perfusion with cold electrolyte solution usually containing colloid and heparin [19, 22]. After they have been cooled to 2 to 4° C., the kidneys can be stored successfully for from 2 to 6 hours without unacceptable deterioration in potential renal function. It is now clear that the time the kidneys spend at normal body temperature following cessation of normal heart action and prior to their removal and cold perfusion, the so-called "warm time," determines to a large extent the degree of ischemic damage that takes place and the degree to which complete functional recovery will occur after transplantation. Needless to say, acute tubular necrosis of greater or lesser degree is common in cadaver renal transplants in the immediate post-transplant period [22, 39, 40, 69, 73, 74, 100]. Many transplant groups now believe that a warm time after death of more than one hour makes cadaver kidneys unacceptable for transplantation. Quick and easily applied biochemical tests may soon permit an objective answer to be obtained at the time the kidneys are removed as to whether or not there has been sufficient ischemic damage to make transplantation undesirable [87].

In the case of living kidney donors consideration for the welfare of the donor becomes paramount. While it is now generally considered that success of kidneys transplanted from nonrelated living donors is not sufficiently high to warrant the potential risk to the organ donor [39, 72], most groups seem convinced that if the potential donor is a parent or sibling of the proposed recipient, the one- or two-year success rate is sufficiently high to justify kidney donation [72]. The immediate and long-term risk to the donor appears slight if he is in good health and has normal renal function. The tendency to consider kidney donation by parents or siblings of the intended recipient as ethically justifiable has recently been reinforced by evidence that typing and matching technics are quite effective within a family group in predicting whether or not a donor or recipient will be relatively compatible or incompatible [4, 6, 7, 39, 81, 95]. Thus if the proposed related donor appears to be compatible with the recipient by leukocyte matching, the chances of success of the transplant appear very good.

TECHNICS OF TRANSPLANTATION

Figure 44-1 shows the usual technic of human kidney transplantation. The kidney is placed in the recipient pelvis. It has been customary to position the kidney so that the ureter is anterior — that is, the left kidney is placed in the right pelvis and the right kidney in the left pelvis. The renal artery is ordinarily sutured end to end to the hypogastric artery of the recipient and the renal vein end to side to the external iliac vein. An end-to-side anastomosis between the renal artery and the common or external iliac artery of the recipient is frequently used as an alternate procedure. Several methods of reestablishing the continuity of the urinary tract are currently in vogue. The most

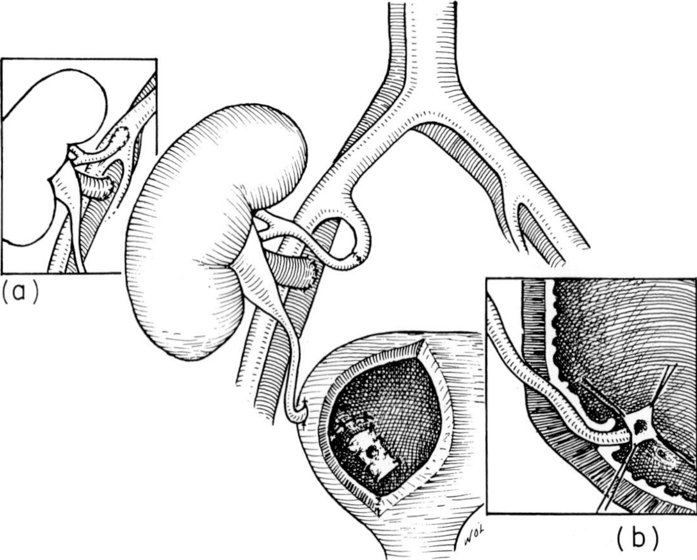

Figure 44-1. Customary technic of kidney transplantation. Renal artery is sutured end to end to hypogastric artery of recipient and renal vein end to side to recipient's external iliac vein. In alternative procedure (*a*) renal artery may be sutured end to side to recipient's common or external iliac artery. Ureter is implanted into bladder after traversing a submucosal tunnel (b).

commonly utilized technic is ureteroneocystostomy, with implantation of the donor ureter into the bladder. However, some groups prefer ureteropyelostomy, utilizing the recipient ureter and suturing it end to end to the pelvis of the transplanted kidney [52]. Other groups now prefer an end-to-end ureteroureterostomy [2]. The entire operation in the recipient is carried out retroperitoneally through an oblique lower-quadrant abdominal incision. The customary position of a renal transplant is illustrated by the intravenous pyelogram shown in Figure 44-2.

IMMUNOSUPPRESSIVE THERAPY

Granted a technically successful transplantation and a viable donor kidney, the success of renal transplantation clearly hinges upon the adequacy and safety of the immunosuppressive therapy given to the organ recipient. It is also clear that suppression of the transplantation immune response is much less difficult when the donor and recipient are highly compatible than when the incompatibility between the two is great. Nevertheless, since information concerning compatibility is often of questionable reliability at present, and is commonly not known at the time of transplantation, relatively standard immunosuppressive practices are found throughout the United States and Europe.

The basic immunosuppressive drug in almost all transplant programs is azathioprine, which is administered just before or at the time of transplantation in doses of 3 to 4 mg. per kilogram of body weight daily [39, 94]. Azathioprine is maintained at the highest dose compatible with preservation of a normal white blood cell count in the recipient and is continued indefinitely. The maintenance dose is usually 2 to 3 mg. per kilogram. It has been found that the patient must have adequate renal function to tolerate azathioprine at these dosages [39, 40]. If there is a preliminary period of renal shutdown, as is often the case with cadaver kidney transplants, the azathioprine dosage must be promptly and drastically reduced. Otherwise severe toxicity to the bone marrow and leukopenia will ensue.

Glucocorticoids, usually in the form of prednisone, are administered to the transplant recipient as adjunctive immunosuppressive therapy. Two general approaches to glucocorticoid administration are now used: (1) ad-

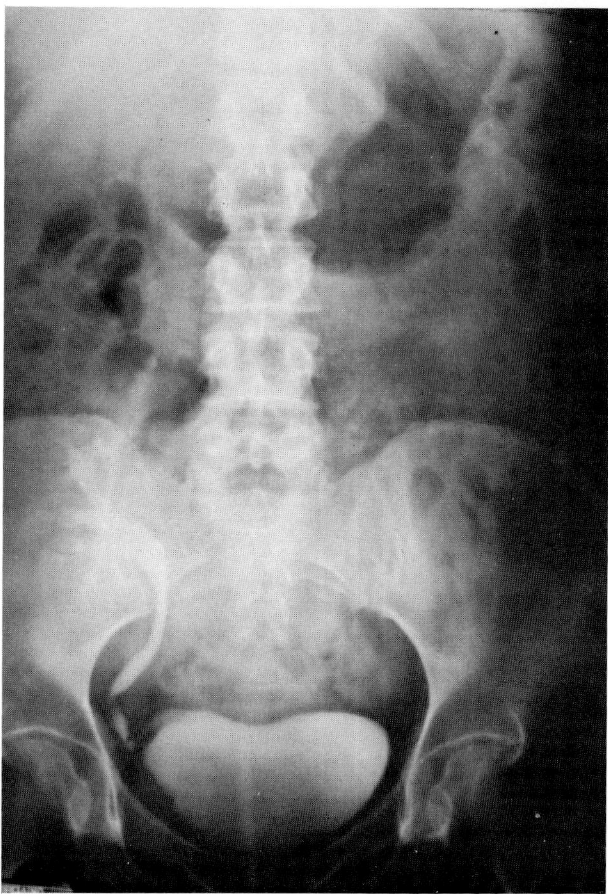

Figure 44-2. Intravenous pyelogram performed 6 weeks after bilateral nephrectomy and renal allografting in one of the authors' patients.

minister corticosteroids in high doses initially at the time of transplantation and then reduce the dose gradually thereafter until a rejection episode supervenes or until the patient has reached a low maintenance dose of 5 or 10 mg. of prednisone a day [40, 69, 100]; or (2) reserve corticosteroid therapy until a rejection crisis appears in the post-transplant period and then institute steroid therapy at high dosages [33, 94]. In any event it is the custom in almost every transplant group to increase corticosteroid dosage at the time of an attempted rejection of the transplanted kidney.

The diagnosis of attempted transplant rejection, called a "rejection crisis" [94], is ordinarily made apparent by deteriorating renal function, falling urine output, an active urinary sediment, fever, leukocytosis, increase in size of the transplant by palpation or x-ray, and local tenderness of the tissues surrounding the transplant [39]. In some cases, many features of a rejection crisis are mimicked by nonimmunologic events such as ureteral obstruction or leakage, or by vascular obstruction. Thus there have been a number of reports describing further methods of distinguishing an acute rejection crisis by the appearance of lymphocytes in the urine [47, 50], by changes in the excretion of certain enzymes [50, 77, 82], by increased amounts of immunoglobulin light chains in the urine [25], by changes in the level of serum complement or its components [17, 28], and by increased levels of circulating alpha globulins [83] among others. In most

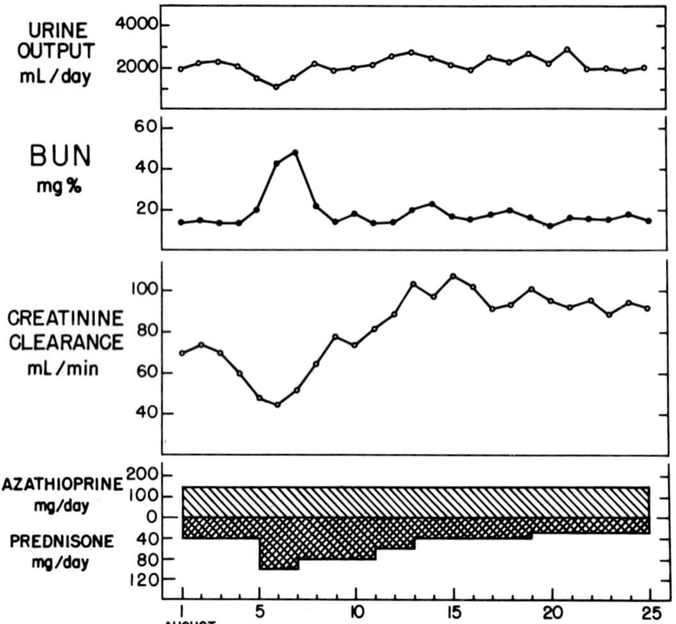

Figure 44-3. Clinical course of one of the authors' patients who received a cadaver renal allograft 3 weeks earlier. The mild rejection episode, evidenced by falling urine output and creatinine clearance and by rising blood urea nitrogen (BUN), was promptly reversed by increasing the dose of prednisone temporarily.

instances, however, examination of the patient and a few simple laboratory tests are sufficient to establish the diagnosis of attempted rejection, and treatment may be promptly begun. A rejection crisis in one of the authors' patients successfully aborted by increasing the dose of steroids is illustrated in Figure 44-3.

Formerly actinomycin C and presently actinomycin D are utilized by some transplant groups in repeated intravenous doses at the time of attempted transplant rejection as additional antirejection therapy [40, 74, 94]. Because of their toxicity, actinomycins are ordinarily not used as maintenance therapy.

Local irradiation to the kidney transplant itself is widely utilized in dosages of 100 to 150 R given on alternate days at the time of rejection crisis [40, 94, 100], or in some instances as initial antirejection therapy at the time of transplantation and for several days subsequently [39, 40]. The efficacy of treating a systemic response — transplant rejection — by local irradiation of the transplanted organ, has only recently been established experimentally. However, animal studies show quite clearly that local irradiation does inhibit the rejection of transplanted kidneys, possibly both by interfering with the carrying of antigen from the transplant by host leukocytes and by destruction of leukocytes currently engaged in attacking the transplanted organ [48, 49]. The total dose of irradiation administered to the kidney is, of course, limited because of the dangers of radiation nephritis [54].

Total-body irradiation of the recipient in sublethal doses has been abandoned in most centers because of the difficulty of management of the postradiation period of marrow aplasia. However, total-body irradiation is still utilized as the initial immunosuppressive maneuver by Hamburger and his associates [33].

COMPLICATIONS OF RENAL TRANSPLANTATION

The complications of renal transplantation fall into two groups, technical complications and complications related to transplant rejection and immunosuppressive therapy. While there are, of course, occasional technical disasters with regard to the vascular anastomoses, the greatest source of technical difficulty with kidney transplants has been in the reconstruction of the urinary tract. There has been a surprising amount of difficulty with bladder closure following ureteroneocystostomy [2, 39]. This is perhaps related to poor tissue healing properties associated with chronic uremia, and the administration of large doses of steroids. Then, too, the donor ureter may be partially devascularized in the proximal portion ordinarily utilized for the ureteric anastomosis, and this problem, occasionally aggravated by the involvement of the ureter in attempted rejection [31], can result in disruption of the distal portion of the donor ureter with ureteral leakage.

In order to avoid these problems some groups have preferred to utilize an anastomosis between the very proximal donor ureter and distal recipient ureter [2], or pyeloureterostomy utilizing the pelvis of the donor kidney and the ureter of the recipient [52]. However, both procedures have resulted in a significant number of urinary leaks as well [2, 39]. While many of the urologic complications are fully amenable to surgical correction and may resolve spontaneously with proper drainage, these complications can unfortunately result in local sepsis which may spread, in a patient treated with immunosuppressive agents, and cause the death of the recipient.

However, the chief clinical problems following renal transplantation are related to the immune attack of the recipient upon the transplanted organ and the attempts to prevent this rejection with immunosuppressive therapy. Certainly the most common cause of death of kidney transplant recipients is a combination of relentless rejection of the transplanted organ coupled with overwhelming infection, which in turn is directly related to intensive antirejection therapy with immunosuppressive drugs [39, 94, 100]. Figure 44-4, a photomicrograph of a kidney allograft removed at autopsy from a patient who died of this combination of acute rejection and infection, illustrates the pathology of acute rejection. Note the massive in-

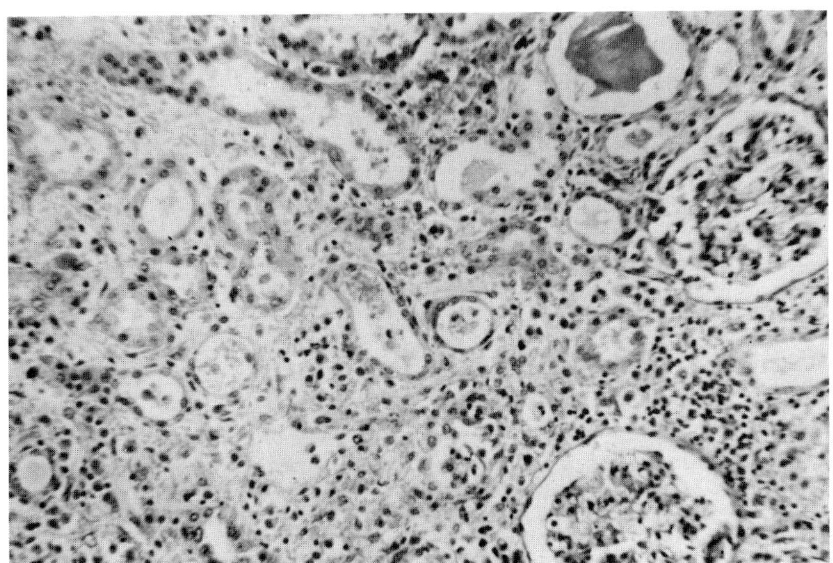

Figure 44-4. Photomicrograph of kidney transplant removed at autopsy from a patient who died of a combination of rejection of the transplant and pulmonary infection 8 weeks after transplantation. Intense round cell infiltration of the renal parenchyma and tubular destruction are evident. Hematoxylin and eosin. × 10.

filtration of the renal parenchyma with host round cells and the tubular destruction.

In addition to abrogating the host defenses against environmental pathogens, the immunosuppressive agents currently utilized have other toxic manifestations as well. Azathioprine and other similar compounds are directly toxic to the bone marrow and must be carefully controlled in order to prevent severe marrow aplasia and leukopenia. This problem, of course, complicates the already weakened resistance to infection. There is also evidence that azathioprine is hepatotoxic in some individuals and therefore must be used with extreme caution in patients with any evidence of liver disease [39].

Most transplant patients receive long-term corticosteroid therapy and are thus subject to all complications of continued steroid usage [39, 94], including in some instances fat embolism [77]. Finally, attempted withdrawal of corticosteroids may lead to arthralgia, joint effusions, fever, and malaise as noted in other conditions when steroids are withdrawn after a period of prolonged administration [39, 94]. In addition, in some transplantation patients steroid withdrawal is accompanied by a peculiar syndrome termed "transplant lung" [39, 40, 92]. This condition is manifested by evidence of alveolar-capillary block and diffuse mottling of the lung fields by chest x-ray. It may occur during a period of steroid withdrawal following kidney transplantation or may be associated with evidence of attempted rejection of the kidney transplant on the part of the new host. While it has been suggested that this condition may represent an infectious complication of immunosuppressive therapy, there is fairly convincing evidence that it is fundamentally an immunologic phenomenon and may ordinarily be reversed by increasing steroid dosage again.

RESULTS OF HUMAN TRANSPLANTATION

The results of kidney transplantation in man utilizing currently available immunosuppressive technics are known with considerable accuracy because of the work of the Kidney Transplant Registry under the supervision of Dr. Joseph Murray. The available evidence indicates that a kidney transplanted from a close relative of the recipient has approximately an 80 per cent chance of surviving for one year following transplantation. A kidney transplanted from an unrelated cadaver donor has approximately a 40 per cent chance of surviving for one year [72]. The survival rate at two years is not greatly different from that at one year. Patient survival is probably somewhat better than kidney transplant survival by 10 or slightly more percentage points [39]. While these results clearly demonstrate that there is considerable room for improvement with respect to both the safety and the efficacy of kidney transplantation, it is also apparent that many individuals have been offered one or more years of relatively normal existence who otherwise would almost certainly have died of renal failure [78]. It is also likely that while kidney transplant survival may not have increased dramatically over the past two or three years a real increase in patient survival has taken place. This probably results from the increasing experience of most transplant groups in utilizing immunosuppressive therapy and the willingness of most groups to accept rejection of the kidney when this appears inevitable rather than pressing immunosuppressive therapy to the point of threatening the patient's life. Indeed, a considerable number of patients have received a second, and even a third, kidney transplant following the failure of the first [39, 40, 72]. The survival of the second and third kidney allografts has not been notably poorer on the average than that of first allografts.

It is of interest to compare the success rate of kidney transplantation and that achieved by chronic hemodialysis in expert hands. One-year patient survival in chronic dialysis programs is now said to approach 90 per cent

[12]. While patient survival following kidney transplantation at one year is not quite this high, it is not greatly different when one considers patients who have had donation of a kidney by a close relative. The one-year survival of patients receiving cadaver kidneys is of course significantly less than that achieved by chronic dialysis. On the other hand, it is generally agreed that most patients who have a successfully functioning kidney transplant feel quite normal and well, whereas only a minority of the patients on chronic dialysis fail to note some continuing disability from their chronic absence of renal function [12].

Now that kidneys have been transplanted between individuals other than identical twins in considerable numbers for a period of five years, it has recently become evident that the continued function of even highly successful renal allografts may be seriously jeopardized in many instances by the problem of "late rejection." This process, recently described by several groups engaged in clinical transplantation [34, 35, 39, 81, 98, 99], appears to result from a subtle but relentless immunologic attack of the new host upon the graft tissue which is different in character and intensity from the acute rejection crises that often occur in the early post-transplant period. These late rejection changes include subintimal hyperplasia of the small arteries and arterioles in the renal parenchyma and glomerular changes, resembling those seen in lupus nephritis, which may be accompanied by the nephrotic syndrome [35].

It has been suggested that while early acute rejection episodes are primarily mediated through immune-competent cells of the host, these late changes may be the result of deposition of humoral antibody [34, 39, 81]. In any event an increasing number of patients have been reported with late rejection of renal allografts occurring from two to five years following transplantation [35], and the progressive changes of late rejection in these cases have ordinarily taken place despite the continued administration of immunosuppressive agents in the form of azathioprine and steroids [34, 35, 81]. These findings suggest, therefore, that the survival of many kidney allografts must be considered self-limited by uncontrolled immunologic rejection, even though a number of years of useful renal function may be obtained for the recipients.

Recent Developments and Prospects for the Future

TYPING

The evidence that kidney transplants from related donors are more likely to succeed than those from unrelated individuals [39, 72, 99], and that even among the latter some have done remarkably well [39, 72], strongly suggests that presently available immunosuppressive therapy is much more effective when the incompatibility between the donor and the recipient of the kidney transplant is small enough. It seems likely, therefore, that if methods can be found to match the genetically determined transplant antigens present on the somatic cells of the donor and the recipient of an organ graft, the chances of survival of the graft will be markedly enhanced.

A number of methods of attempting to match kidney donors and recipients with respect to transplantation antigens have been suggested. Three methods — the normal lymphocyte transfer test, the mixed lymphocyte culture test, and serologic typing of leukocytes — have received or are currently receiving extensive evaluation both clinically and experimentally.

Lymphocyte Transfer Test. The normal lymphocyte transfer test, described by Brent and Medawar [14] in laboratory animals, consists of the intradermal injection of normal peripheral blood lymphocytes from the proposed transplant recipient into each of a panel of prospective transplant donors. The intensity of the reaction (in all likelihood an immunologic reaction of the injected lymphocytes against the transplant antigens of the prospective donor) is thought to be an indication of the antigenic disparity between the donor and the recipient. The impressions of various investigators as to the potential usefulness of this test in man have been mixed [5, 15, 18, 27]. While the evidence is still incomplete, it seems clear that the normal lymphocyte transfer test will not prove to be a sensitive index of incompatibility, but it may have a role to play in confirming the compatibility of a potential donor selected by other means. The test has the drawback of requiring injection of human cells and plasma into a healthy individual with the attendant risk of transfer of disease.

Mixed Lymphocyte Culture Test. The mixed lymphocyte culture test, originally described by Bain et al. [8] and by Bach and Hirschhorn [7], is performed by placing peripheral blood lymphocytes obtained from the proposed donor and recipient of a kidney transplant into tissue culture together. Experimental evidence indicates that the degree to which the two populations of lymphocytes stimulate one another to proliferate and to undergo transformation to blast cells may be correlated with the degree of genetic disparity between the individuals who have donated the lymphocytes [3, 6]. Additional evidence suggests that the results of the mixed lymphocyte culture test correlate well with the rejection times of skin allografts in monkeys [71] and within family groups in man [6]. Some recent observations indicate that the results of this test may be related to the acceptance or rejection of kidney transplants in man [84].

From the extensive evaluation performed by Bach [6] and by Amos [3] it seems likely that positive stimulation in the mixed lymphocyte culture test is obtained only when individuals differ genetically with respect to one or more alleles of a strong histocompatibility locus termed HL-A by most investigators. Lesser degrees of incompatibility are not detected by this technic. This in itself probably does not seriously affect the test's usefulness. Available evidence suggests that the chance of finding two individuals compatible at the HL-A locus in the population at large is less than one in 1000 [3, 6]. Thus the mixed lymphocyte culture test appears most likely to be of use in determining which members of a sibling or family group are compatible at the HL-A locus where the chances of compatibility within a more closely related population are far greater. Figure 44-5 shows the clinical course of one of the author's patients who received a renal allograft from a sibling, apparently compatible at HL-A as determined by mixed lymphocyte culture. Excellent function of the transplant has been maintained on minimal immunosuppressive therapy.

The mixed lymphocyte culture test has the disadvantage that a considerable period of time is required before the results are known — a minimum of five days in tissue culture plus whatever time is necessary to read the result either in terms of per cent of cell transformation or in the degree of cell division as indicated by the uptake of radioactive precursors into DNA. Thus the test appears to have little hope of providing information quickly as to the compatibility or incompatibility of a prospective cadaver donor.

Serologic Typing of Leukocytes. Matching of the donor and recipient of a kidney transplant by the results of serologically typing blood leukocytes is based upon the premise that circulating antileukocyte antibodies, found in patients who have received multiple blood transfusions or in females after multiple pregnancies, are directed against transplantation antigens on the surface of these cells [86, 101]. That this is indeed the case is suggested by recent attempts to compare the results of serologic typing of lymphocytes by leukoagglutination or cytotoxic methods with the fate of tissue allografts transplanted between the lymphocyte donors [4, 81, 95, 98]. Certainly in one sizable series the results of lymphocyte

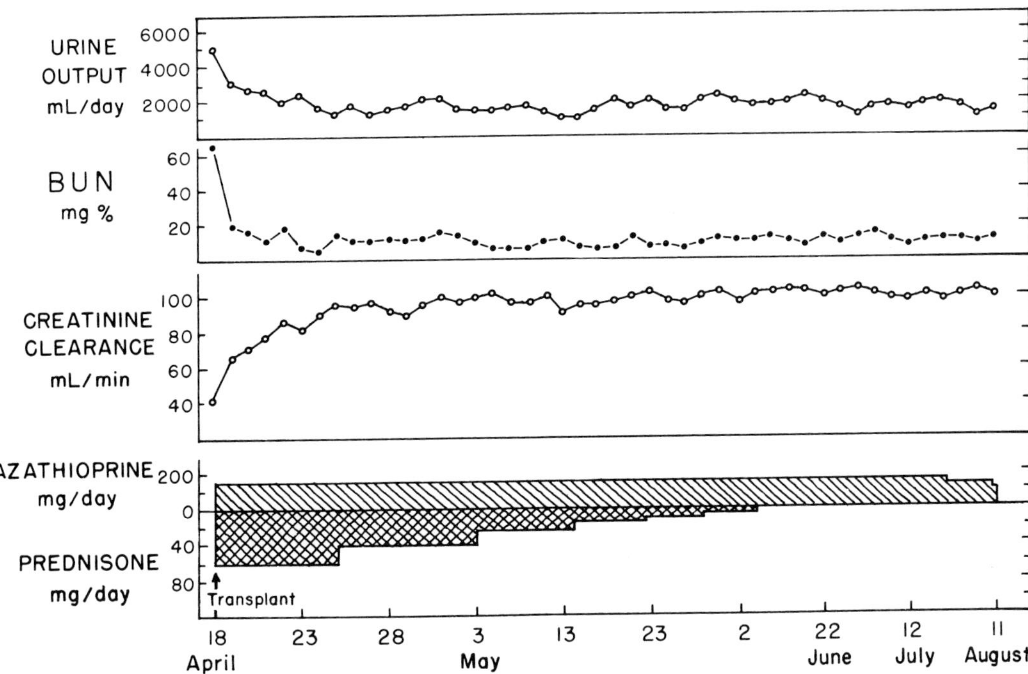

Figure 44-5. Clinical course of one of the authors' patients who received a kidney transplant from a sibling donor apparently HL-A identical as indicated by the mixed lymphocyte culture technic. No rejection crises were noted, and steroids could be discontinued. Azathioprine therapy has been continued until the present. She remains well 5 years after transplantation.

typing appear to have correlated well with the survival of human kidney allografts [95, 98].

When further correlations have been made among the various lymphocyte groups, detected by the vast number of available antisera, and the apparent strength of the transplantation antigens they define within the human population, serologic leukocyte typing may very well prove to be of major importance in predicting the likelihood of success of an organ transplant in man. However, as in the case of the other methods of matching donor and recipient, the precise degree to which this technic will be able to detect all significant antigenic differences between individuals remains to be determined. At the present stage of its development it seems clear that serologic typing of lymphocytes will predict with considerable accuracy the compatibility of members of the same family group [4]. However, the correlation of the results of this form of typing with transplant success between unrelated individuals has been less good [39].

Unfortunately under ordinary circumstances the practical usefulness of any method of typing, no matter how effective, is seriously limited by the lack of a large number of available kidney donors. In the case of living donors the choice, if it exists at all is ordinarily between two or three members of a family group. The use of typing to select the best donor under these circumstances may be of moderate value. In the case of cadaver donors there is ordinarily only one donor available at any given time and the decision to be made is simply whether or not incompatibility is so extreme as to preclude kidney survival even with optimum immunosuppressive management.

One possible solution to the problem of a

limited supply of donor organs consists of having a large group of potential recipients maintained on chronic hemodialysis. Under these circumstances each available cadaver donor would be matched with all the potential recipients, and the most suitable recipient would receive the kidney. Even if this were universally possible, however, it would not represent full utilization of the information available from typing and matching methods even at their current state of development. What is clearly needed is a breakthrough in the field of organ preservation. Unfortunately, it still remains beyond the capabilities of any known method to preserve a kidney in vitro for periods longer than a day or two even under optimum circumstances [9, 51, 57]. Thus the availability of a large bank of suitably typed cadaver organs for transplantation remains a dream for the future.

IMPROVED IMMUNOSUPPRESSIVE THERAPY

Antilymphocyte Serum. Clearly the most interesting and publicized innovation in the field of kidney transplantation is the utilization of antilymphocyte serum in the treatment of patients with renal allografts. As the name suggests, antilymphocyte serum (ALS) is an antiserum raised in a foreign species against the lymphocytes of the species to be treated. Such antisera have proved in the laboratory to be the most powerful immunosuppressive agents so far encountered with respect to transplantation immune responses [26, 53, 67]. Antisera raised in the rabbit against various rodent species have produced prolongation of skin allograft survival across strong antigenic barriers which has been truly spectacular [53, 67, 104]. Antisera raised in the horse against dog lymphocytes have produced clear-cut prolongation of canine renal allografts, but the potency of ALS in dogs has been somewhat less than that noted in smaller animals [37, 43, 65, 66, 79]. Antisera raised in the horse against human lymphocytes have been administered to a considerable number of human recipients of kidney transplants [95]. The potency of the material in man is open to question, although the currently available evidence suggests that it is useful in augmenting previously available immunosuppressive drugs in the prevention of transplant rejection. Unfortunately, because clinical administration of ALS alone to human patients has been very rare, interpretation of the effects of ALS has been clouded by the concomitant administration of azathioprine and corticosteroids [39, 95].

One of the difficulties in evaluating ALS, particularly different preparations of ALS, with regard to its immunosuppressive potency has been the poor correlation of the effects of ALS in vivo with any in vitro test. Thus the leukoagglutination and leukocytotoxicity titers obtained in the test tube with ALS appear not to correspond with the ability of the serum to suppress the transplantation immune response in laboratory animals [44, 53]. Similarly the immunosuppressive effect of ALS is not correlated with its ability to reduce the circulating lymphocyte counts in animals to which it is administered [44]. The mechanism of action of ALS, therefore, remains to be delineated. In addition, the problem is confused because while ALS clearly reacts with circulating lymphoid cells, it is not specific for these cells and reacts with most other nucleated cells from the same animal species [53, 85].

The advantages of ALS as an immunosuppressive agent include its clearly demonstrated potency in laboratory animals, its presumed lack of bone marrow toxicity (that it is not completely innocuous in this regard has recently been demonstrated [23]), and the absence of serious interference with resistance to infection in laboratory animals given ALS in dosages that produce marked inhibition of the transplantation immune response [53, 66].

The disadvantages inherent in the use of ALS stem from its being a foreign protein (and therefore antigenic in the new host) and an antibody with cross-reactivity for many other tissues as well as lymphoid tissue. There is little doubt that in most instances the administration of ALS or immunoglobulins extracted from this serum is accompanied by humoral antibody formation in the recipient animal against the ALS protein [26, 43, 85]. With persistent administration, this immune reaction of the host against the antiserum may result in greater or lesser degrees of serum sickness. In the case of kidney transplant recipients any such reaction is of course accompanied by the danger of immune complex nephritis. It appears likely that the administration of the 7S gamma globulin extracted from ALS, which contains in most preparations the major portion of the immunosuppressive activity [85], may reduce the incidence of serum sickness. Certainly there is evidence that the danger of immune complex nephritis is reduced as the size of the complexes is diminished [20]. Thus the 7S gamma globulin would be expected to have less potential for inducing this untoward complication than whole serum or 19S gamma globulin. It is also possible that the combined administration of antilymphocyte globulin (ALG) with an immunosuppressive drug such as azathioprine may reduce the incidence of immune reactions to foreign protein and thus may increase the safety of ALG administration [95, 102]. In any case the clinical use of modest doses of ALS or ALG for short periods in patients with renal allografts so far has not resulted in serious disability or evidence of glomerular damage in the transplanted kidneys [95].

A second danger in the use of ALS or ALG is the possibility that this material may induce direct nephrotoxic nephritis. There is good evidence that in animals antilymphocyte globulin cross-reacts strongly with kidney antigens [30, 46, 85]. This potential hazard appears to argue against the chronic use of antilymphocyte antisera in kidney transplant recipients.

In summary it appears likely that ALG may prove very useful in the initial treatment of patients with kidney allografts. Experimental evidence suggests that the combined use of ALG and azathioprine [102] will be a potent therapy in the prevention of early graft rejection and may contribute considerably to the safety of kidney transplantation by decreasing or eliminating the need for large doses of steroids [95]. It does not appear likely, however, that ALS or ALG will prove to be the solution to the problem of late allograft rejection since chronic use of antilymphocyte antisera is not likely to prove feasible in the near future because of the dangers of serum sickness and direct nephrotoxicity.

Thoracic Duct Drainage. Woodruff and Anderson [104] have demonstrated in laboratory animals that lymphocyte depletion by thoracic duct drainage is associated with protracted survival of skin allografts. That this is also true in man has been shown by the work of Tunner and his colleagues [89]. Whether or not this adjunctive maneuver will enhance the effectiveness of presently available immune suppressive therapy in patients with kidney allografts is not entirely clear [24]. There have been encouraging reports from one series of clinical trials [88].

Other Approaches. With the demonstration that some episodes of acute renal allograft rejection are associated with intrarenal alterations in the coagulation mechanism [13, 16, 96], several centers now have under way a cautious clinical trial of anticoagulants as supplementary antirejection therapy [13, 16, 96].

Other apparently safe approaches to the problem of immunosuppressive therapy include the finding of Mowbray [68, 70] that an alpha globulin fraction obtained from normal mammalian serum has potent immunosuppressive properties without noticeable toxicity. This work has been confirmed and expanded in the author's laboratory [21, 58]. There is current interest as well in the use of mitogens such as phytohemagglutinin in the suppression of the immune response in vivo. A considerable immunosuppressive effect has been reported for some mitogens without evidence of significant systemic toxicity [80, 93]. However, neither of these two potentially useful new classes of immunosuppressive agents has been studied sufficiently in the laboratory to warrant a clinical trial.

THE POSSIBILITY OF IMMUNOLOGIC TOLERANCE

In 1953 Billingham et al. [11] and, independently, Hasek [36] succeeded in inducing specific unresponsiveness to subsequent tissue allografts by the administration of living lymphoid cells from the prospective donor to animals still in utero. This phenomenon, called "specific immunologic tolerance," was thought to result from exposure of the mammalian host to foreign antigens while still immunologically immature and incapable of mounting an immune response. It was postulated that these foreign antigens were subsequently recognized by the maturing immune system as self rather than nonself and specific unresponsiveness toward these antigens resulted through a "central" failure of the immune system of the tolerant host. Immunologic reactivity to other foreign antigens remained normal. It was subsequently determined that such tolerant animals were chimeras in that they contained lymphoid cells of both donor and host type [10].

It was assumed for a number of years that the ability to acquire specific immunologic tolerance was an exclusive property of the immature mammal. However, Shapiro and his co-workers [91] and others [29] have more recently demonstrated that in adult mice massive and repeated intravenous and intraperitoneal doses of lymphoid cells from members of an inbred donor strain result in the induction of specific unresponsiveness in a single allogenic recipient to subsequent tissue grafts from the donor strain. This specific unresponsiveness induced by massive quantities of foreign antigen is termed *immunoparalysis* by some investigators. However, it is currently impossible to distinguish this state from immunologic tolerance induced in immature animals [60].

Specific immunologic tolerance appears to be the ideal solution to the problem of graft rejection in clinical organ transplantation since by definition tolerance implies specific unresponsiveness to the graft in question with maintenance of normal immune responsiveness against other foreign antigens. There are, however, pitfalls in attempting to induce tolerance in man. In the first place, it has been almost universally true that induction of tolerance has been successfully achieved only by means of the injection of lymphoid tissue. Thus any attempt at inducing tolerance is plagued with the possibility of graft-versus-host disease. This pathologic process results from an immunologic reaction of the foreign lymphoid cells against the new host when these cells are introduced into an immunologically incompetent individual or one specifically tolerant of these cells [10, 103, 105]. Secondly, the quantities of foreign tissue required for the induction of tolerance in adult animals are very large [29, 91]. Thus, in successful experiments multiple genetically identical donors are required to induce tolerance in a single recipient.

One possible solution to the problem of graft-versus-host disease in the attempted induction of tolerance has been afforded by the work of Martinez et al. [60]. These workers have shown that subcellular antigenic material extracted from lymphoid cells may, if administered in sufficiently large quantities over a sufficiently long period, induce a significant degree of immunologic tolerance to subsequent skin allografts in mice even when the donor and recipient are dissimilar with respect to strong histocompatibility antigens.

The acquisition of sufficiently large quantities of transplantation antigen from the lymphoid tissue of any one donor, however, still remains a problem to be solved before attempting to utilize such technics in the field of clinical transplantation. However, some hope that such utilization of subcellular antigenic material for induction of tolerance might be possible clinically has come from the work of Medawar [62] and of Hoehn [38], who have shown that the concomitant administration of immunosuppressive agents with the infusion of transplantation antigenic material considerably increases the tolerance-producing potential of the antigens infused. Thus it is conceivable that with utilization of the proper immunosuppressive agents the quantities of antigen necessary to induce significant tolerance clinically might not be prohibitively large.

The possibility still exists, however, that the achievement of permanent tolerance in adult humans may require the infusion of living lymphoid cells and the maintenance of a chimeric state. If true, this may preclude at least for the foreseeable future any widespread attempts at inducing tolerance in man because of the fear of graft-versus-host disease. Utilization of antilymphocyte globulin or other immunosuppressive agents, however, may permit the safe induction of chimerism by inhibiting graft-versus-host disease as well as the reaction of the host against the engrafted cells. Whether or not this is possible has yet to be demonstrated decisively.

Nevertheless, it appears logical to continue to work toward the goal of inducing specific immunologic tolerance to kidney grafts in man. It seems likely that only the attainment of this ideal will permit consistently successful transplantation of vitally needed tissues and organs while at the same time enabling the recipient to protect himself against environmental pathogens by eliminating the need for long-term suppression of normal immune responsiveness.

References

1. Abaza, M. H., Noland, B., Watt, G. J., and Woodruff, M. F. A. Effect of antilymphocytic serum on the survival of renal homotransplants in dogs. *Transplantation* 4:618, 1966.
2. Al-Askari, S. Urologic Aspects of Renal Transplantation. In Rapaport, F. T., and Dausset, J. (Eds.), *Human Transplantation*. New York: Grune & Stratton, 1968.
3. Amos, D. B. HU-1 major histocompatibility locus in man. *Science* 156:1506, 1967.
4. Amos, D. B., Hattler, B. G., Hutchins, P., McCloskey, R., and Zmijewski, C. M. Skin donor selection by leucocyte typing. *Lancet* 1:300, 1966.
5. Amos, D. B., Nicks, P. J., Peacocke, N., and Sieker, H. O. An evaluation of the normal lymphocyte transfer test in man. *J. Clin. Invest.* 44:219, 1965.
6. Bach, F. H. Transplantation: Problems of histocompatibility testing. *Science* 159: 1196, 1968.
7. Bach, F. H., and Hirschhorn, K. Lymphocyte interaction: Potential histocompatibility test *in vitro*. *Science* 143:813, 1964.
8. Bain, B., Vos, M. R., and Lowenstein, L. Development of large immature mononuclear cells in mixed leukocyte cultures. *Blood* 23:108, 1964.
9. Belzer, F. O., Ashby, B. S., Gulyassy, P. F., and Powell, M. Successful seventeen-hour preservation and transplantation of human-cadaver kidney. *New Eng. J. Med.* 278:608, 1968.
10. Billingham, R. E., and Brent, L. Acquired tolerance of foreign cells in newborn animals. *Proc. Roy. Soc.* (*Biol.*) 146:78, 1957.
11. Billingham, R. E., Brent, L., and Medawar, R. B. Actively acquired tolerance to foreign cells. *Nature* (London) 172:603, 1953.
12. Bluemle, L. W., Jr. Current status of chronic hemodialysis. *Amer. J. Med.* 44: 749, 1968.
13. Braun, W. E., and Merrill, J. P. Urine fibrinogen fragments in human renal allografts. *New Eng. J. Med.* 278:1366, 1968.

14. Brent, L., and Medawar, P. B. Tissue transplantation: New approach to "typing" problem. *Brit. Med. J.* 2:269, 1963.
15. Bridges, J. M., Nelson, S. D., and McGeown, M. G. Evaluation of lymphocyte transfer test in normal and uremic subjects. *Lancet* 1:481, 1964.
16. Calne, R. Y., White, H. J. O., Hebertson, B. M., Millard, P. R., Davis, D. R., Salaman, J. R., and Samuel, J. R. Heparin in delayed transplant function. *Lancet* 1:1178, 1968.
17. Carpenter, C. B., Gill, T. J., Merrill, J. P., and Dammin, G. J. Alterations in human serum β_1C-globulin (C′) in renal transplantation. *Amer. J. Med.* 43:854, 1967.
18. Carpenter, C. B., Glassock, R. J., Gleason, J. M., Corson, M., and Merrill, J. P. The application of the normal lymphocyte transfer reaction to histocompatibility testing in man. *J. Clin. Invest.* 45:1452, 1966.
19. Cleveland, R. J., Lee, H. M., Prout, G. R., Jr., and Hume, D. M. Preservation of the cadaver kidney for renal homotransplantation in man. *Surg. Gynec. Obstet.* 119:991, 1964.
20. Cochrane, C. G., and Hawkins, D. Studies on circulating immune complexes: III. Factors governing the ability of circulating complexes to localize in blood vessels. *J. Exp. Med.* 127:137, 1968.
21. Cooperband, S. R., Bondevik, H., Schmid, K., and Mannick, J. A. Transformation of human lymphocytes: Inhibition by homologous alpha globulin. *Science* 159:1243, 1968.
22. Couch, N. P., Curran, W. J., and Moore, F. D. The use of cadaver tissues in transplantation. *New Eng. J. Med.* 271:691, 1964.
23. DeMeester, T. R., Anderson, N. D., and Shaffer, C. F. The effect of heterologous antilymphocyte serum on mouse hemopoietic stem cells. *J. Exp. Med.* 127:731, 1968.
24. Ellis, F. Renal homograft response following thymectomy and thoracic duct drainage in goats. *Transplantation* 5:21, 1967.
25. Epstein, W. V., Gulyassy, P. F., Tan, M., and Rae, A. I. Effect of renal homotransplantation on the metabolism of the light chains of immunoglobulins. *Ann. Intern. Med.* 68:48, 1968.
26. Gray, J. G., Monaco, A. P., Wood, M. L., and Russell, P. S. Studies on heterologous antilymphocyte serum in mice. *J. Immun.* 96:217, 1966.
27. Gray, J. G., and Russell, P. S. Donor selection in human organ transplantation; possible screening test. *Lancet* 2:863, 1963.
28. Guiney, E. J., Austen, K. F., and Russell, P. S. Measurement of serum complement during homograft rejection in man and rat. *Proc. Soc. Exp. Biol. Med.* 115:1113, 1964.
29. Guttmann, T. D., and Aust, J. B. Acquired tolerance to homografts produced by homologous spleen cell injection in adult mice. *Nature* (London) 192:564, 1961.
30. Guttmann, T. D., Carpenter, C. B., Lindquist, R. R., and Merrill, J. P. Renal transplantation in the inbred rat: III. A study of heterologous anti-thymocyte seras. *J. Exp. Med.* 126:1099, 1967.
31. Haber, M. H., and Putong, P. B. Ureteral vascular rejection in human renal transplants. *J.A.M.A.* 192:157, 1965.
32. Hamburger, J. A., Vayasse, J., Crosnier, J., Auvert, J., Lalanne, C. M., and Hopper, J. Renal homotransplantation in man after radiation of the recipient: Experience with six patients since 1959. *Amer. J. Med.* 32: 854, 1962.
33. Hamburger, J. A. Experience with 45 renal homotransplantations in man. *Lancet* 1:985, 1965.
34. Hamburger, J. A. A reappraisal of the concept of organ "rejection" based on the study of homotransplanted kidneys. *Transplantation* 5:870, 1968.
35. Harland, W. R., Holden, K. R., Williams, G. M., and Hume, D. M. Proteinuria and nephrotic syndrome in rejection of kidney transplants. *New Eng. J. Med.* 277:769, 1967.
36. Hasek, M. Vetetativine hybridisace zivocichu spojenim krenich obehu v embryonalnim vyvojhi. (Vegetative hybridization of animals by parabiosis during embryonic development.) *Cesk. Biol.* 2:265, 1953.

37. Hinchey, E. J., and Bliss, J. Q. The prolongation of canine renal homograft survival by heterologous serum. *Canad. Med. Ass. J.* 95:1169, 1966.
38. Hoehn, R. J. Induction of tolerance to mouse tail skin homografts by combining paired immunosuppressive agents and cellular antigens. *Transplantation* 3:131, 1965.
39. Hume, D. M. Kidney Transplantation. In Rapaport, F. T., and Dausett, J. (Eds.), *Human Transplantation.* New York: Grune & Stratton, 1968. P. 110.
40. Hume, D. M., Lee, H. M., Williams, G. M., Wolf, J. S., Prout, G. R., Slapak, M., Kauffman, H. M., Jr., and Cleveland, R. J. The comparative results of cadaver and related donor renal homotransplants in man, and the immunologic implications of the outcome of second and paired transplants. *Ann. Surg.* 164:253, 1966.
41. Hume, D. M., Merrill, J. P., and Miller, B. F. Homologous transplantation of the human kidney. *J. Clin. Invest.* 31:640, 1952.
42. Hume, D. M., Merrill, J. P., Miller, B. F., and Thorn, G. W. Experiences with renal homotransplantation in the human: Report of nine cases. *J. Clin. Invest.* 34:327, 1955.
43. Iwasaki, Y., Porter, K. A., Amend, J. R., Marchioro, T. L., Zuhlke, V., and Starzl, T. E. The preparation and testing of horse antidog and antihuman antilymphoid plasma or serum and its protein fractions. *Surg. Gynec. Obstet.* 124:1, 1967.
44. Jeejeebhoy, J. F., and Vela-Martinez, J. M. Studies on the mode of action of heterologous antilymphocyte plasma. *Transplantation* 6:149, 1968.
45. Jones, J. P., Engleman, E. P., and Najarian, J. Systemic fat embolism after renal homotransplantation and treatment with corticosteroids. *New Eng. J. Med.* 273:1453, 1965.
46. Katz, D. H., Unahue, E. R., and Dixon, F. J. Nephritogenic properties of cross-reacting kidney-fixing antibodies to heart, spleen and muscle. *J. Immun.* 98:260, 1967.
47. Kauffman, H. M., Clark, R. F., Magee, J. H., Rittenbury, M. S., Goldsmith, C. M., Prout, G. R., Jr., and Hume, D. M. Lymphocytes in urine as an aid in the early detection of renal homograft rejection. *Surg. Gynec. Obstet.* 119:25, 1964.
48. Kauffman, H. M., Cleveland, R. J., Dwyer, J. J., Lee, H. M., and Hume, D. M. Prolongation of renal homograft function by local graft radiation. *Surg. Gynec. Obstet.* 120:49, 1965.
49. Kauffman, H. M., Cleveland, R. J., Robertshaw, G. E., Graham, W. H., and Hume, D. M. Inhibition of the afferent arc of the immune response to renal homografts by local graft radiation. *Surg. Gynec. Obstet.* 123:1052, 1966.
50. Koo, G. C. G., Monagham, E. D., Gault, M. H., and MacLean, L. D. Comparative value of lymphocyturia serum and urinary enzymes in the diagnosis of renal homograft rejection. *Surg. Forum* 16:256, 1965.
51. Ladaga, L. G., Nabseth, D. C., Besznyak, I., Hendry, W. F., McLeod, G., and Deterling, R. A. Preservation of canine kidneys by hypothermia and hyperbaric oxygen: Long-term survival of autografts following 24-hour storage. *Ann. Surg.* 163:553, 1966.
52. Leadbetter, G. W., Monaco, A. P., and Russell, P. S. A technique for reconstruction of the urinary tract in renal transplantation. *Surg. Gynec. Obstet.* 123:839, 1966.
53. Levey, R. H., and Medawar, P. B. Nature and mode of action of antilymphocytic antiserum. *Proc. Nat. Acad. Sci. U.S.A.* 56:1130, 1966.
54. Liu, C. T., and Overman, R. R. Effects of whole-body irradiation in renal function and renal hemodynamics in the dog. *Radiat. Res.* 25:552, 1965.
55. Lorenz, E., Uphoff, D., Reid, T. R., and Shelton, E. Modification of irradiation injury in mice and guinea pigs by bone marrow injections. *J. Nat. Cancer Inst.* 12:197, 1951.
56. Main, J. M., and Prehn, R. T. Successful skin homografts after the administration of high dosage x-irradiation and homologous bone marrow. *J. Nat. Cancer Inst.* 14:1023, 1955.
57. Manax, W. G., Bloch, J. H., Longerbeam, J. K., and Lillehei, R. C. Successful 24 hour *in vitro* preservation of canine kidneys by the combined use of hyperbaric oxygena-

tion and hypothermia. *Surgery* 56:275, 1964.

58. Mannick, J. A., and Schmid, K. Prolongation of allograft survival by an alpha globulin isolated from normal blood. *Transplantation* 5:1231, 1967.
59. Martin, D. C., Rubini, M., and Rose, V. J. Cadaveric renal homotransplantation with inadvertent transplantation of carcinoma. *J.A.M.A.* 192:82, 1965.
60. Martinez, C., Smith, J. M., Blaese, M., and Good, R. A. Production of immunological tolerance in mice after repeated injections of disrupted spleen cells. *J. Exp. Med.* 118:743, 1963.
61. McIntosh, D. A., McPhaul, J. J., Jr., Peterson, E. W., Harvin, J. S., Smith, J. R., Cook, F. E., Jr., and Humphreys, J. W., Jr. Homotransplantation of a cadaver neoplasm and a renal homograft. *J.A.M.A.* 192:1171, 1965.
62. Medawar, P. B. Use of antigenic tissue extracts to weaken immunological reaction against skin homografts in mice. *Transplantation* 1:21, 1963.
63. Merrill, J. P., Murray, J. E., Harrison, J. H., Griedman, E. A., Bealy, J. B., and Dammin, G. J. Successful homotransplantation of the kidney between nonidentical twins. *New Eng. J. Med.* 262:1251, 1960.
64. Merrill, J. P., Murray, J. E., Harrison, J. H., and Guild, W. R. Successful homotransplantation of human kidney between identical twins. *J.A.M.A.* 160:277, 1956.
65. Mitchell, R. M., Sheil, A. G. R., Slafsy, S. F., and Murray, J. E. The effect of heterologous immune serum on canine renal homografts. *Transplantation* 4:323, 1966.
66. Monaco, A. P., Abbott, W. M., Othersen, H. B., Simmons, R. L., Wood, M. D., Flaz, M. H., and Russell, P. S. Antiserum to lymphocytes: Prolonged survival of canine renal allografts. *Science* 153:1264, 1966.
67. Monaco, A. P., Wood, M. L., Gray, J. G., and Russell, P. S. Studies on heterologous antilymphocyte serum in mice: II. Effect on the immune response. *J. Immun.* 96:229, 1966.
68. Mowbray, J. F. Effect of large doses of an α_2-glycoprotein fraction on the survival of rat skin homografts. *Transplantation* 1:15, 1963.
69. Mowbray, J. F., Cohen, S. L., Doak, P. B., Kenyon, J. R., Owen, K., Percival, A., Porter, K. A., and Peart, W. S. Human cadaveric renal transplantation; report of twenty cases. *Brit. Med. J.* 2:1387, 1965.
70. Mowbray, J. F., and Hargrave, D. C. Further studies on the preparation of the immunosuppressive alpha$_2$ protein fraction from serum and its assay in mice. *Immunology* 11:413, 1966.
71. Moynihan, P. C., Jackson, J. F., and Hardy, J. D. Lymphocyte transformation as an *in vitro* histocompatibility test. *Lancet* 1:453, 1965.
72. Murray, J. E., and Barnes, B. A. The World-Wide Status of Kidney Transplantation. In Rapaport, F. T., and Dausett, J. (Eds.), *Human Transplantation.* New York: Grune & Stratton, 1968.
73. Murray, J. E., and Harrison, H. J. Management of 50 patients with kidney transplants including 18 pairs of twins. *Amer. J. Surg.* 105:205, 1963.
74. Murray, J. E., Merrill, J. P., Dammin, G. J., Dealy, J. B., Alexandre, G. W., and Harrison, H. J. Kidney transplantation in modified recipients. *Ann. Surg.* 156:337, 1962.
75. Murray, J. E., Merrill, J. P., Dammin, G. J., Dealy, J. B., Walter, C. W., Brooke, M. S., and Wilson, R. E. Study on transplantation immunity after total-body irradiation: Clinical and experimental investigation. *Surgery* 48:272, 1960.
76. Murray, J. E., Merrill, J. P., and Harrison, J. H. Renal homotransplantation in identical twins. *Surg. Forum* 6:432, 1955.
77. Noble, R. E., Najarian, J. S., and Brainard, H. D. Urine and serum lysozyme measurement in renal homotransplantation. *Proc. Soc. Exp. Biol. Med.* 120:737, 1965.
78. Ogden, D. A., Porter, K. A., Terasaki, P. I., Marchioro, T. L., Holmes, J. H., and Starzl, T. E. Chronic renal homograft function. *Amer. J. Med.* 43:837, 1967.
79. Pichlmayr, R., Brendel, W., and Zenker, R. Production and effect of heterologous anticanine lymphocyte serum. *Surgery* 61:774, 1967.

80. Pierre, R. L., Younger, J. B., and Zmijewski, C. M. Effect of phytohemagglutinin on skin allograft survival in mice. *Proc. Soc. Exp. Biol. Med.* 126:687, 1967.
81. Porter, K. A., Dossetor, J. B., Marchioro, T. L., Peart, W. S., Rendall, J. M., Starzl, T. E., and Terasaki, P. I. Human renal transplants. *Lab. Invest.* 16:153, 1967.
82. Prout, G. R., Jr., Macalalag, E. V., and Hume, D. M. Serum and urinary lactic dehydrogenase in patients with renal homotransplantation. *Surgery* 56:283, 1964.
83. Riggio, R. R., Schwartz, G. H., Stenzel, K. H., and Rubin, A. L. Alpha-2-hyperglobulinemia as a humoral indicator of the homograft reaction. *Lancet* 1:1218, 1968.
84. Rubin, A. L., Stenzel, K. H., Hirschhorn, K., and Bach, F. Histocompatibility and immunologic competence in renal homotransplantation. *Science* 143:815, 1964.
85. Russell, P. S., and Monaco, A. P. Heterologous antilymphocyte sera and some of their effects. *Transplantation* 5:1086, 1967.
86. Terasaki, P. I., and McClelland, J. D. Microdroplet assay of human serum cytotoxins. *Nature* (London) 204:998, 1964.
87. Terasaki, P. I., Martin, R. C., and Smith, R. B. A rapid metabolism test to screen cadaver kidneys for transplantation. *Transplantation* 5:76, 1967.
88. Tilney, N. L., and Murray, J. E. The thoracic duct fistula as an adjunct to immunosuppression in human renal transplantation. *Transplantation* 5:1024, 1967.
89. Tunner, W. S., Carbone, P. P., Blaylock, W. K., and Irvin, G. L. Effect of thoracic duct lymph drainage on the immune response in man. *Surg. Gynec. Obstet.* 121:334, 1965.
90. Schwartz, R., Eisner, A., and Dameshek, W. The effect of 6-mercaptopurine on primary and secondary immune responses. *J. Clin. Invest.* 38:1394, 1959.
91. Shapiro, F., Martinez, G., Smith, J. M., and Good, R. A. Tolerance of skin homografts induced in adult mice by multiple injections of homologous spleen cells. *Proc. Soc. Exp. Biol. Med.* 106:472, 1961.
92. Slapak, M., Lee, H. M., and Hume, D. M. Transplant lung — a new syndrome. *Brit. Med. J.* 1:80, 1968.
93. Spreafico, F., and Lerner, E. M. Suppression of the primary and secondary immune response of the mouse by phytohemagglutinin. *J. Immun.* 98:407, 1967.
94. Starzl, T. E. *Experience in Renal Transplantation*. Philadelphia: Saunders, 1964.
95. Starzl, T. E., Groth, C. G., Terasaki, P. I., Putnam, C. W., Brettschneider, L., and Marchioro, T. L. Heterologous antilymphocyte globulin, histoincompatibility matching and human renal homotransplantation. *Surg. Gynec. Obstet.* 126:1023, 1968.
96. Starzl, T. E., Lerner, R. A., Dixon, F. J., Groth, C. G., Brettschneider, L., and Terasaki, P. I. Shwartzman reaction after human renal homotransplantation. *New Eng. J. Med.* 278:642, 1968.
97. Starzl, T. E., Marchioro, T. L., Holmes, J. H., Hermann, G., Brittain, R. S., Stonington, O. H., Talmage, D. W., and Waddell, W. R. Renal homografts in patients with major donor-recipient blood group incompatibilities. *Surgery* 55:195, 1964.
98. Starzl, T. E., Marchioro, T. L., Porter, K. A., Moore, C. A., Rifkind, D., and Waddell, W. R. Renal homotransplantation: Late function and complications. *Ann. Intern. Med.* 61:470, 1964.
99. Starzl, T. E., Marchioro, T. L., Terasaki, P. I., Porter, K. A., Faris, T. D., Herrmann, T. J., Vredevoe, D. L., Hutt, P. P., Ogden, D. A., and Waddell, W. R. Chronic survival after human renal homotransplantation. *Ann. Surg.* 162:749, 1965.
100. Straffon, R. A., Hewitt, C. B., Kiser, W. S., Stewart, B. H., Nakamoto, S., and Kolff, W. J. Clinical experience with the use of 79 kidneys from cadavers for transplantation. *Surg. Gynec. Obstet.* 123:483, 1966.
101. Walford, R. L., Gallagher, R., and Troup, G. M. Human lymphocyte typing with isologous antisera: Technical considerations and a preliminary study of the cytotoxic reaction system. *Transplantation* 3:387, 1965.
102. Weil, R., and Simmons, R. L. Combined immunosuppression for canine renal allograft prolongation: Antilymphocyte serum

plus prednisolone or azathioprine. *Ann. Surg.* 167:239, 1968.

103. Woodruff, M. F. A. Can tolerance to homologous skin be induced in the human infant at birth? *Transplant. Bull.* 4:26, 1957.

104. Woodruff, M. F. A., and Anderson, N. A. Effect of lymphocyte depletion by thoracic duct fistula and administration of antilymphocytic serum on survival of skin homografts in rats. *Nature* (London) 200: 702, 1963.

105. Woodruff, M. F. A., and Sparrow, M. Further observations on the induction of tolerance of skin homografts in rats. *Transplant. Bull.* 4:157, 1957.

Index

Index

This Index covers both volumes. Volume I contains pages 1–734; Volume II contains pages 735–1456.

A DEATH ON THE OCEAN WAVE

By the same author

Fiction

Unbecoming Habits
Blue Blood Will Out
Deadline
Let Sleeping Dogs Die
Just Desserts
Murder at Moose Jaw
Caroline R
Masterstroke
Class Distinctions
Red Herrings
Brought to Book
The Rigby File (ed)
Business Unusual
A Classic English Crime (ed)
A Classic Christmas Crime (ed)
Stop Press
Death and the Visiting Fellow
Death and the D'Urbervilles

Non-fiction

It's a Dog's Life
John Steed – the Authorised Biography
HRH The Man Who Would Be King (with Mayo Mohs)
Networks (Who we know and how we use them)
The Character of Cricket
The Newest London Spy (ed)
By Appointment – 150 years of the Royal Warrant and its Holders
My Lord's (ed)
The Duke – a Portrait of Prince Philip
Honourable Estates – the English and their country houses
A Life of Love – the Biography of Barbara Cartland
Denis – the Authorised Biography of the Incomparable Compton
Brian Johnston – the Authorised Biography
Beating Retreat – Hong Kong Under the Last Governor
A Peerage for Trade – a History of the Royal Warrant
Village Cricket
Princess Margaret – A Life Unravelled

A Death on the Ocean Wave

Tim Heald

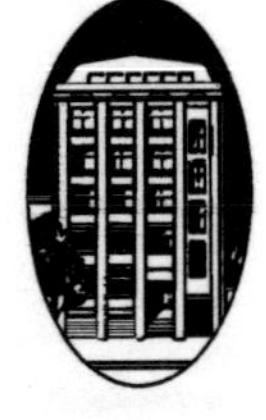

ROBERT HALE · LONDON

First published in Great Britain 2007

ISBN 978-0-7090-8326-9

Robert Hale Limited
Clerkenwell House
Clerkenwell Green
London EC1R 0HT

2 4 6 8 10 9 7 5 3 1

Typeset in 11/15pt Sabon
by Derek Doyle & Associates, Shaw Heath
Printed and bound in Great Britain
by Biddles Limited, King's Lynn

CHAPTER ONE

The *Duchess* didn't look like a cruise ship. She had two funnels, round port holes, scrubbed wooden decks and a jaunty air of sea-worthiness which suggested a bygone era in which passengers travelled by sea because that was the best and possibly the only way of getting from A to B. The *Duchess* was all brass, teak and jolly Jack tar. She was the pride and joy of Riviera Shipping, the smartest, most eclectic and most expensive shipping line of the twenty-first century. No bingo and balcony, no chrome and casino: this was P.O.S.H.

Doctor Tudor Cornwall stood on the Budmouth Quayside and sighed. Middle age was making him conservative and old-fashioned. He who had once been an awkward, progressive maverick, castigated by his opponents as a dangerous leftie was now reduced to celebrating the traditional lines of a ship that looked like a ship.

'Nice, eh?' he said to the gamine figure at his side.

Elizabeth Burney smiled. 'Yeah,' she said. 'Sort of thing I used to have in my bath when I was a kid.'

They could have been father and daughter. He, grizzled, tweedy, beetle-browed, overcoated, feeling the cold of a bright, sharp October morning; she, booted, be-jeaned, cotton-shirted, cashmere-sweatered, unbothered by the chill;

he, fifty-something; she, twenty-something. But not father, not daughter – guest lecturer; research assistant.

He was looking forward to the assignment. Some people didn't enjoy transatlantics. They were bored by day after day of featureless ocean. The rise and fall of the dangerous deep made them sick and alarmed; consequently they couldn't eat; conversely they drank too much. Tudor, on the other hand, relished the unaccustomed isolation; he liked getting no signal on his mobile; he enjoyed caviar and cold, dry château-bottled Muscadet. Applause was gratifying as well. Likewise recognition. As Reader in Criminal Studies at the University of Wessex, head of an increasingly well-regarded department, author, expert, broadcaster, aspiring television personality, Dr Tudor Cornwall was on the verge of celebrity. Actually, in his own worlds of Wessex and criminal studies he was a celebrity, albeit a minor one. 'Minor' celebrity, he reflected, was a bit like 'minor' poet or 'minor' public school. It was almost a pejorative. Never mind, on the good ship *Duchess* he was a guest lecturer and therefore *ipso facto* a celebrity grade one, alpha male. He was not a vain man but the notion gave a keen edge to his anticipation.

The girl, on the other hand, was just beginning. She was a blank page, the beginning of a book, could go anywhere, could become anything. Not that she was unformed. Far from it. She was a precociously developed personality, smart and streetwise way beyond her years. Tasmanian by birth and upbringing she was as far from home as it was possible to be. An uprooted orphan, she never spoke of family or friends down under. It was as if she had drawn a line under her past, wiped the slate clean, moved on. She herself would never have used such clichés for she was naturally original and inventive. But she seemed to have no past. It was as if she had been beamed in from outer space – which, in a sense, she had.

They had met when Tudor was on a Visiting Fellowship in that far-off land. Even then she had an ambiguous, shady reputation. She was the protégé of Tudor's oldest but false friend, Ashley Carpenter. Probably his mistress, though that was too old-fashioned a word to describe their relationship. She was also alleged to be the college thief, though this, too, was an assumption without serious substance. She had been foisted on Tudor in what, at the time, had seemed like a final act of revenge by Carpenter. Subsequent events had cast doubts on this. Tudor still thought of her as some sort of Trojan horse, but he no longer regarded her as hostile. She seemed well disposed, affectionate even, and she was awfully bright. Although he couldn't admit it, even to himself, he was more than a little in love with her. She, on the other hand, didn't appear to be in love with anyone. She never mentioned Ashley Carpenter.

'Well, star pupil,' said the Reader in Criminal Studies, grasping the handle of his battered leather suitcase, 'shall we go on board?'

She smiled up at him.

'Why not?' she said. 'She's home for a week.'

'Not quite a week,' he said. 'We dock in New York in six days' time.'

She hefted her rucksack on to her shoulders.

'That's hair splitting,' she said. 'I think of it as a week. Call it a nautical week. Like a knot. Chronological equivalent of a sea-mile.'

Her teacher sucked his teeth. 'A week is a week. Six days is six days. You can't have it both ways.'

'I like having it both ways,' she said. 'Suits my temperament. If I say six days is a week then a week is six days. That's the meaning of meaning.'

'Oh shut up,' he said. 'Stop being tiresome and precocious.'

There were procedures to be gone through. There were, reflected both Tudor and Elizabeth, always procedures to be gone through. This was what so much of life had become: a procedure to be gone through. Tudor's professional life should have been divided into teaching and researching and writing. Instead it was dominated by form-filling and pen-pushing and answering to a faceless, humourless, gormless bureaucracy. Elizabeth's particular bugbear were the immigration authorities who seemed to have an antipathy to Australians in general and her in particular. These were particular procedural problems, but both of them were confronted with the increasing regimentation and regulation of modern life. For free spirits such as them the experience was hobbling. For professional crime-studiers who believed that everything they did should be individual, intuitive, quirky and idiosyncratic the constant drive to make them conform to a grim post-Stalinist pattern of behaviour was a constant reproach. Crime didn't stick to rules. That was the whole point.

The pre-boarding procedures took place in a large corrugated-iron shed cursorily tricked out with tired bunting and frayed red carpet. As formalities went these were agreeably perfunctory. Luggage went through an X-ray screening machine and was then whisked off to their cabins. It was a listless examination as was the body search, performed by bored men and women out-sourced from some private agency and abetted by hand-held metal detectors. Tudor and the girl knew that it was all a charade, a sop to the terror instilled in so many westerners by the destruction of the World Trade Centre. It meant nothing but it made people feel good, or at any rate less bad. It created the illusion that the President of the United States was doing something. Likewise the British Prime Minister. Tudor knew perfectly well, and his talks with his friends and contacts in the Intelligence Services confirmed, that if any terrorist organization worth its salt wanted to do something horrible to a cruise liner it was a doddle.

Nevertheless the two of them submitted to the more or less pointless formalities with a good grace before striding purposefully up the gangplank and submitting their shiny new ID cards to the beaming Filipino purserette at the vessel's entrance.

'Welcome aboard,' she said. The badge attached to her crisp, starched white shirt, said 'Cherry.'

Tudor and Elizabeth smiled back.

Cherry consulted a chart on the baize-covered table in front of her, then turned to a gallery of hooks behind her and picked off two old-fashioned keys with heavy wooden tags.

'Two floors up,' she said. 'Boat deck, aft. Adjacent cabins.'

She smiled with what might have been innuendo but might just have been friendliness.

Tudor and Elizabeth smiled back in a blank semi-expressionless way that ignored any suggestion of suggestiveness, accepted their keys and moved off in the direction of the stairways which were carpeted in blue and lined with photographs and portraits of assorted aristocrats and royals from Britain and beyond. Two decks up they turned left along the *Duchess*'s starboard corridor until at the very end they found their cabins.

'I'd like to be on deck when we sail out,' said Tudor. 'Why don't I see you by the Lido Bar in half an hours' time?'

'Where's the Lido Bar?' she asked, wide-eyed, innocent.

'You'll find it,' said Tudor. 'She's a small ship. If in doubt ask a uniform.' Tudor had guest-lectured on the *Duchess* before. He knew his way around. So, metaphorically at least, did Elizabeth even though this was her first time on board.

The cabin, like the ship, was old-fashioned. After all, the *Duchess* had been built in Gdansk some twenty years earlier when Lech Walesa was strutting his stuff. Poles were fine shipbuilders but, like the Pope and Walesa, they were essentially traditionalist. Thus Tudor's cabin had sturdy mahogany furnishings and a serviceable *en-suite* bathroom but no gold taps and no balcony. Indeed it didn't even have a window but a couple of large, brass-surrounded port holes. Port holes on a modern cruise-ship. Good-selling point, he reckoned.

His cases would come in good time and be stored in the walk-in fitted cupboard. He eyed the half-bottle of champagne on the coffee table and decided to broach it later, then picked up the heavy vanilla envelope with 'Doctor Tudor Cornwall, Guest Lecturer, Cabin BD77' written in inky loops on the outside, and opened it with his fingers, thinking, slightly pompously, that a line of Riviera's pretensions really ought to provide paper-knives in its boat deck cabins.

There was a stiffy inside bidding him to a Captain's Cocktail Party in the ballroom that evening after they had set sail. He noticed that the Captain – though 'Master' was the preferred moniker – was still Sam Hardy. He had sailed with Sam before. Several times. He must be getting on for retirement age. Not that Sam had much to do with sailing the ship. He was a Captain Birds Eye sort of captain, all jovial bonhomie and silver whiskers, more at home waltzing round the dance floor with elderly widows or telling noon-time jokes over the Tannoy from the bridge. The actual work was done by his officers. Well, that was unfair, conceded Tudor. Being mine host and master of ceremonies on a ship like the *Duchess* was a twenty-four hour permanent smile, constant charm, never-a-cross-word sort of job, and in a way far harder work than actually making sure the old ship got safely from one side of the Atlantic to the other. Tudor wouldn't have liked being master of the *Duchess* but it suited old Sam Hardy. The ladies liked him and that was all that mattered.

There was another envelope, similarly addressed though this time in typewriting.

Tudor smiled. He knew what this was and he smiled as he read it.

'Hi Tudor!' it ran. 'Good to have you aboard again. I really look forward to more of your criminal experiences and I know the lucky passengers are in for a real treat as usual. We'll be having a short briefing in the cinema at 9.00 p.m. this evening for guest lecturers, gentlemen hosts and other entertainers. And I'd be delighted if you and your companion could join me and the rest of the team for dinner in the Chatsworth Room at 7.30 for 8.00. Look forward to catching up. Best, Mandy xx.' 'Mandy' and the kisses were handwritten and underneath were the words 'Mandy Goldslinger. Cruise director.' He liked Mandy. They, too, had worked together in the past. She was of a certain age and uncertain antecedents: Coral Gables by way of Budapest. She could, up to a point, have been one of the Gabor sisters if life had panned out differently. Her virtues of brash street-wise American pzazz perfectly complimented the stolid all-British joviality of Skipper Sam.

Tudor put the two missives back on the table and contemplated the bowl of fruit: apple, banana, two kiwi fruit, red and white grapes. Standard issue for Guest Lecturer Grade One. He wondered who his colleagues would be, what the passengers would be like. The lumpen passenger list was always pretty much the same. Likewise the lecturers. But voyages such as this invariably threw up the odd surprise.

He was sure this would be no exception.

Thinking which, he picked up his key and set off in the direction of the Lido Bar, whistling a happy tune.

•

CHAPTER TWO

Tudor was not a sailor in the practical sense of knowing a quarter deck from a poop or being able to tie a sheepshank or a bowline but he took a real pleasure in things nautical. It was a vicarious spectator's pleasure but none the less genuine for that. Watching the *Duchess* cast off her chains before being tug-nudged gently out to sea was always mesmerizing. He had little real understanding of what was happening, but he derived an expert's enjoyment from watching other experts at work. You didn't have to be C.S. Forester or Patrick O'Brien to do that.

The ship's orchestra, all seven of them, were playing 'When the Saints Go Marching In' from a balcony on the deck above and white-clothed trestle-tables were laid out with canapés and bottles of sparkling white Spanish wine.

Tudor took a glass of Cava and a miniature chipolata on a toothpick, walked to the rail and contemplated.

The members of the band seemed even older than the passengers. They had a slightly louche, left-over air that Tudor associated with a certain sort of seaside resort or spa. People who he'd assumed were long dead turned up in resorts such as Budmouth, or ships such as the *Duchess*, all wrinkles and hip-replacements. Many of them were orphaned so that one was likely to encounter Gerry without the Pacemakers (now there was a sick geriatric joke), Wayne Fontana without the Mindbenders or Brian Poole without the Tremeloes. Ancient has-beens strutting their last at the end of the pier. At least the *Duchess*'s orchestra had each other, wearied by age though not yet quite condemned. They played the 'Saints' with a lugubrious panache, their moustaches improbably dyed, their paunches straining against the buttons of striped pseudo-Edwardian waistcoats, wispy hair lapping discoloured collars. They might, reflected Tudor, have known better days, they might have been drowning but they were still playing on. Dying but not dead, bloodied but unbowed. In a moment they'd do 'Land of Hope and Glory'. At least the ship's orchestra was maintaining a pretence and doing so with conviction.

This was not always the case with the passengers who in some cases closely resembled what Tudor imagined were the walking dead. Watching from the rail, drink and sausage in hand, he had a sense that he was the only man alive. This was unfair. He knew it as soon as he thought it. There were some sprightly nonagenarians tripping the light prosaic before his eyes on the lido deck. Men and women were mocking age and infirmity, shaking their zimmers at the Grim Reaper and embarking with stoicism and gritted teeth on what for some was almost certainly the Last Great Cruise.

One or two had already changed for dinner: men in white tuxedos with brightly coloured waistcoats and cummerbunds, buckled shoes, sleek silver hair and gold fillings; women in long ball gown concoctions that would not have shamed Barbara Cartland and beehive hair-do's that suggested a golf-club dinner-dance in Surrey circa Coronation Year. Tudor told himself to stop being ageist and snobby. He himself wasn't that smart nor that young any more. Those still in day clothes had an air of *Carry on Cruising*: male tattoos of a bruiser, sergeant's mess quality Hawaiian shirts, golf shoes; sandals with knee-length socks, pearls, cardigans. Everything said money and middle Britain; Thatcherland; suburban and provincial. 'Shut up,' Tudor said to himself. 'This is your audience. If you want to be a celebrity you've got to make people like this like you.' Even as he said it, half of him at least thought the game not worth the candle.

'Doctor Cornwall,' said a smoky estuarine voice at his elbow, 'nice to see you again. Muriel and I wondered whether you might be on board.' When Tudor too obviously didn't recognize him, he said, 'St Petersburg the year before last. Freddie Grim, ex-Flying Squad. Used to work with Slipper of the Yard.'

'Of course,' said Cornwall, suddenly remembering all too well. Slipper was the man who had developed an obsession with the Great Train Robber, Ronnie Biggs. Freddie Grim had been close to him. If Cornwall's memory was not playing tricks Freddie Grim had accompanied Slipper on the notoriously unsuccessful trip to Brazil where they had so ignominiously failed to secure the robber's extradition.

'Great Train Robbery,' he said hopefully and was relieved when Grim's mouth cracked in a satisfied grin, revealing a set of unnaturally even teeth and letting out a halitosis breeze of stale tobacco and lunchtime beer. He was wearing a blazer with the badge which appeared to be that of the Metropolitan Police Bowls Club and a matching cravat.

'Spot on,' said the former policeman. 'See our Ron's trying to get let out on compassionate.'

Biggs was in Belmarsh prison where he was supposed to have suffered a couple of strokes. His solicitor was having no luck at all in presenting his client as more sinned against than sinning.

'Giving us the *Bounty* again?'

Tudor nearly always did his 'Mutiny on the *Bounty*' talk on board ship. In it he proved beyond reasonable doubt that Captain Bligh was strict but fair and that his survival in a small open boat was due to consummate seamanship. It seemed an appropriate subject for a cruise and invariably proved popular. His audiences tended to sympathize even if they felt Bligh's rules were strictly administered. In fact, *particularly* if strictly administered. Most of them were almost certainly floggers if not hangers. Probably both.

'You remember Muriel,' said Grim, indicating a small, mousy woman at his side, who smiled and seemed embarrassed.

'Of course,' lied Tudor. Muriel was infinitely forgettable and looked as if she knew it. Her husband did not exactly cast a long shadow but it was long enough to render Muriel effectively invisible.

'Hope we don't have a rough crossing,' said Muriel's husband. 'Muriel's not the world's greatest sailor, are you, pet?'

'To be honest,' she said, 'I'd rather be at home with the cats. But Freddie says you're only young once and travel broadens the mind.'

Grim seemed pleased to be credited with such an original thought.

'What do they know of England, I always say,' he said, unexpectedly, 'who only England know?'

Tudor nodded sagely and was rescued by the arrival of Elizabeth Burney who had not changed for dinner and was still showing no sign of feeling the cold. Not even a goose bump.

'Elizabeth is my research assistant,' he said. 'She's doing a criminal studies Ph.D.'

It was disconcerting to see that the Grims didn't believe him. Their hand-shaking and smiling were polite but incredulous. Almost immediately Freddie and Muriel moved away on the pretext of more food and drink. Cruising, even aboard as serious a ship as the *Duchess*, was unhealthily often about more food and drink.

'You want to know who's top of the bill speakerwise?' asked Elizabeth, sipping her wine and gazing appreciatively at the rippling, tattooed muscles of burly stevedores doing serious stuff with crates and ropes.

'I thought *I* was top of the bill speakerwise, as you so charmingly put it,' said Tudor, smiling at her in protective mode.

'Well, I'm afraid Sir Goronwy Watkyn's on board.'

Tudor almost choked on his Cava.

'You're joking,' he said, when he'd done some dramatic coughing and throat clearing, 'Not that fraudulent Welsh goat? And I suppose that means the ghastly Myfanwy's on board, no doubt with her bloody harp.'

Actually the ghastly Myfanwy never brought her own harp but commandeered the instrument belonging to the ship's harpist. This inevitably caused grief and allegations of broken strings. She was a rotten harpist but fancied herself on account, of course, of being Welsh. As for her husband, Tudor loathed him with a passion. He was famous for a series of fantasy-style detective stories set in some Tolkien-like Middle Kingdom full of monsters and wizards and featuring a Grand Bard of the Gorsedd who was the first of the great detectives. In Tudor's estimation they were utter tosh but they had made Goronwy Watkyn millions of pounds and earned him a knighthood for 'Services to Literature.' When he was not writing about his ridiculous bard he wrote a series of gritty contemporary police procedurals set, Tudor thought, in

Aberystwyth, or it might have been Bangor. These featured a detective called Dai Jones and were written under the pseudonym J.P.R. Morgan. It was all complete rubbish. Watkyn liked to use his title, habitually wore canary-yellow ankle socks and an overly neat goatee which waggled ridiculously when he talked – which was incessantly.

'You've just ruined my trip,' said Tudor almost meaning it, 'And who in heaven's name do you imagine the bloke in the white robe is? The one with the harem in attendance. Surely he shouldn't be drinking alcohol? Not in that outfit!'

'He's called Prince Abdullah and beyond that we know practically nothing whatever except that he's paid in full and the money's good.' The speaker was a blue-ish blonde with vivid make-up in a silk kaftan slit oriental style virtually up to the waist. The heels of her shoes were ridiculously high, especially for being on a ship, and she jangled with bangles. Tudor suspected, but didn't know for sure, that the rocks on her rings were real.

'Mandy!' he exclaimed, kissing her on both cheeks. 'Mandy, this is Elizabeth Burney, my star post-graduate pupil at the University of Wessex, who's come along to help out. Elizabeth this is Mandy Goldslinger, the fabulous Cruise Director of the good ship *Duchess*.'

'*Enchanté*,' said Ms Goldslinger extending a hand with astonishingly long almost witch-like fingernails painted in gilt-flecked purple.

'Hi,' said Elizabeth.

Tudor could have been mistaken but the encounter did not somehow suggest love-at-first-sight. Inside his head he heard the all-too-familiar clinking of ice cubes.

'I hope you've run the appropriate security checks,' said Tudor, not joking.

'Oh you crime people!' said Ms Goldslinger, loudly enough

to make some adjoining passengers turn round curiously. 'That's exactly what that cutie, Goronwy Watkyn said. You're all the same. Too too paranoid.'

'You can't be too careful,' said Tudor. 'You know how vulnerable cruise ships are to international terrorism. They could be kamikaze-wives. Has anybody looked under their jellabas?'

'Tudor darling,' said the cruise director, 'Prince Abdullah is a hundred per cent kosher. I personally have checked with my dear friend Eddie Mortimer who does communications for Kofi Anan at the United Nations and he tells me that the Prince has a great humanitarian record and is a prominent member of the Yemeni royal family.'

'The Yemenis don't have a royal family,' said Elizabeth, 'it's a Marxist republic.'

'Oh Yemeni shemeni,' said Mandy. 'The Prince wouldn't hurt a fly. Matter of fact hurting even flies is against his religion. He's a sweetie.'

'You'll be sorry if they've all got bombs in their shoes,' said Tudor. The ship's orchestra had not moved on to 'Land of Hope and Glory' but were playing 'Hearts of Oak'. Tudor reckoned they were in for a good half-hour of songs nautical and marine.

'Who are those two sitting on thrones?' he asked, noticing a man in a safari suit with a much younger blonde wife. They were both smoking and sitting in upholstered chairs. Although not actually behind rope or barbed wire they looked as if they had been cordoned off from the vulgar herd. They had their own table with their own cloth, their own canapés, their own bottle in their own ice bucket.

Mandy frowned.

'Those are the Umlauts,' she said. 'They think they own the ship. Trouble is they more or less do.'

'Expand,' said Tudor. 'I don't understand.'

'Oh shucks,' said Mandy unexpectedly. She took a long swig from her glass and wiped her brow. On the shore and the lower decks, dockers and seamen were doing really serious things with ropes, chains and hawsers. They were cutting the remaining umbilical links between the *Duchess* and Budmouth. Slowly but unmistakably the ship began to move away from the quayside. Her siren sounded. The band was playing 'A Life on the Ocean Wave.' Passengers were leaning over the rails and waving at anyone they could see on shore. Some shorebound onlookers waved back. Others maintained an air of stolid indifference. Tudor felt oddly moved. He was pleased that Elizabeth seemed to share his elation to the extent even of waving at a couple of stout workers on the quayside. They waved back cheerily.

'Umlaut takes the Imperial Suite for at least six months of the year. He treats the ship as his office and home. He makes his own rules. He does deals with Zurich and New York and the City and Tokyo and the Middle East.'

'What sort of deals?' asked Tudor, only half paying attention.

'Money,' said Mandy. 'Money, money, money. Mrs Umlaut, Frau Umlaut, is dripping in diamonds, festooned with fur and treats everyone on board as if they were personal staff. Mr Umlaut, Herr Umlaut, Gottfried to his friends – if he had any – is rude beyond belief, tells the captain what to do, makes the rules as he goes along, believes that money can buy anything and anyone.'

'They don't sound altogether attractive,' said Tudor.

Mandy Goldslinger looked thoughtfully across the broadening band of murky water which now separated the vessel from the United Kingdom.

'I could cheerfully murder the Umlauts,' she said. 'I really could.'

CHAPTER THREE

Entering the ballroom for the welcome party was like coming on to the set of a modern-dress version of HMS *Pinafore*. Tudor half expected the ship's officers lined up in white and blue with gold braid on their wrists and shoulders to launch into a chorus of 'He's hardly ever sick at sea/ so give three cheers and one cheer more/ for the hardy Captain' and so on. The stagey impression of faux-seamanship took its cue from the Master himself who was, naturally, first in line. Captain Sam, universally known, for obvious reasons, as 'Kiss me Hardy' was straight from Central Casting. The skipper had what the Royal Navy refers to as a 'full set,' meaning a moustache and beard. These were white in Santa Claus style. Indeed, if one could imagine Father Christmas in the uniform of a Merchant Navy captain you would have a pretty good idea of what Captain Hardy actually looked like for he was a big, pink-faced fellow who shook like jelly when he laughed which was often. He didn't actually bellow out 'Ho, ho, ho!' or even 'Yo, ho, ho!' but you would not have put it past him.

The Master recognized Tudor and greeted him cordially enough though with less joviality than he managed for complete strangers.

When Tudor introduced Elizabeth Burney, Hardy called her

'Little Lady' which was a big mistake. The Master was excellent with women of advanced years and preferably limited intelligence; the younger and brighter they got the less at ease he seemed. Despite the fact that he exuded a sort of mariner's braggadocio which suggested – was designed to suggest – extreme virility, Tudor had doubts about his true sexuality. Helped out at tea parties, if you asked Tudor. Not that Tudor had the slightest objection to men who helped out at tea parties. Some of his best friends came into just that category. But he was uneasy with pretence, uncomfortable with deceit. After all it was part of his trade and he, as much as the next man, disliked mixing business with pleasure.

The canapés and Cava had been moved from the lido deck to the ballroom with the Riviera Line's customary expedition and lack of fuss. The ship's orchestra had, however, been replaced by a female duet playing 'Greensleeves' on classical guitar and cello. They looked Baltic: high cheekbones, possibly deceptive innocence, elegant but cheap strapless dresses, probably fresh out of the conservatoire in Riga, Tallin or Vilnius.

Tudor and Elizabeth negotiated the line of immaculate, beaming, hand-shaking ship's officers; avoided having their photograph taken, took a gesture of food and drink and headed for a far-off corner of the room from which better to survey the crew and crowd.

'Is it always like this?' the girl asked, looking around wide-eyed yet not innocent. They were out in the English Channel now and there was a breeze. Force Three perhaps. The curtains of the ballroom, tasselled purple, swayed gently and so did some of the passengers. It would be rougher before they reached New York. It always was and despite the ship's sophisticated stabilizers it would keep a lot of paying customers in their cabins. It seemed an expensive way of making yourself sick.

An elderly man in a white tuxedo, a spangled turquoise cummerbund with matching made-up bow tie, and sleek white hair, shimmered over.

'Doctor Cornwall,' he said proffering a much-ringed hand, 'Ambrose Perry.'

'Ah,' said Tudor, medium-term memory working overtime. 'Ambrose Perry, the gentleman host.'

'That am I,' said the over-groomed old gent in a curiously archaic and unconvincing turn of phrase which suited his general demeanour and appearance.

Tudor remembered that Mr Perry had once owned and run a hairdresser's salon in Bromley called, he thought Daphne's. He was a brilliant gentleman host: attentive, unthreatening, with a mean fox-trot and a devilish paso doble. In the afternoons – or *après-midis* as he described them – he called bingo or played bridge. He also picked up gossip like nobody's business. Gentlemen hosts aboard the *Duchess* were privy to more secrets than the barmen.

'Prince Abdullah *and* the Umlauts,' said the host, 'that's a double whammy we've never seen before.'

'Is that a problem?' asked Tudor, all *faux-naïf*.

'Problem?!' exclaimed Mr Perry, 'A "many-pipe problem" as your Sherlock Holmes might have said. Herr Umlaut and the Prince are not exactly bosom companions. And the accommodation question is unanswerable.'

'How do you mean?' asked Elizabeth. She had no idea what he meant.

'I mean,' said Ambrose, a tad stuffily, 'that on most of the *Duchess* voyages either the Herr Doctor or the Prince travel and that invariably they do so without the other. Never the twain shall meet. However, on this occasion they have been, as it were, double-booked. And alas, there is room, accommodationally speaking for but one top banana on board.'

He spoke a very strange English. Both Tudor and Elizabeth independently supposed that he must originally have come from somewhere else.

'Surely you can have as many top bananas as you like?' said Elizabeth.

'There is only one Imperial Suite,' said Ambrose. 'On voyages when the Prince is on board without the Umlauts he is always given the Imperial. So he is used to it. It confers status. Unassaillable status. On those occasions when the Umlauts are on board without the Prince it is they who are installed in the Imperial. They, too, are used to it and they, too, enjoy the status. The Imperial comes complete with a butler whereas the likes of you and I have to make do with bowls of fruit.'

Tudor suspected that gentlemen hosts probably had to share cabins with each other. In the complex hierarchy of life aboard the *Duchess* a guest speaker ranked higher than a gentleman host by several degrees. Guest speakers were among the elite of the non-paying passengers though, Tudor conceded, some guest speakers were more equal than others and he had a horrid feeling that, at least in the eyes of the Master and the shipping line, he was out-ranked by Sir Goronwy Watkyn. He was afraid Watkyn would have the better cabin.

'So you're saying that whoever gets the Imperial Suite is universally acknowledged to be Top Banana.' Elizabeth was catching on fast, as usual. 'And on most voyages there is no contest but that on this occasion someone has to decide who gets it and the verdict went to the Umlauts. . . .' She paused for thought and then said, 'Who decides? They presumably don't just flip a coin?'

'It would be the Master's judgement that decided,' said

Perry, 'Everything on board ship is down to the Master. He is indeed *master of all he surveys*.'

'But surely,' said Tudor, 'that sort of thing is decided by the company? And it depends on how much money changes hands?'

'Maybe,' said Perry, 'maybe not. I think the Captain's word is final. What's more I'm fairly certain that's how the Prince and the Umlauts would see it.' And he shimmered off in the direction of the dance floor whence duty and some very old women were beckoning him to do something appropriate with the last of the remaining light fantastic.

'What an odd bloke!' said Elizabeth when he was out of earshot – not far, as he was obviously acoustically threatened despite being hearing-aid-enhanced. Deaf as a post notwithstanding the pink plastic stuffed into his right ear.

A waiter came past with a tray of drinks and Tudor and Elizabeth both exchanged empty glasses for full.

'You do need to pace yourself on board ship,' said Tudor, in headmasterly mode. 'Sometimes you feel there's nothing to do except eat and drink, especially on transatlantic runs.'

Swilling and browsing seemed pretty pervasive except for the small knot of old people gliding about the dance floor. Cello and classical guitar made an unlikely dance band but some of those on board had the sort of itchy feet which would have bopped to Beethoven or charlestoned to Chopin. These were serious dancers and although in conventional pedestrial mode many of them would have been stiff to the point of virtual paralysis, they seemed when dancing to glide as if on ice. The pair from the University of Wessex watched with admiration and disbelief.

'Och, Dr Cornwall,' said a broad Scottish voice which was almost as much of a stereotypical Scottish voice as the Captain's was a bucolic English one. Actually, thought Tudor,

Scots, even caricature ones like this, never quite said 'Och' but it was a reasonable Sassenach rendition of the noise a Scot makes at the beginning of his first paragraph.

'Angus Donaldson,' said the uniformed figure who boasted a ruddy wind-burned face and a set of whiskers almost as full as the Captain's. His beard and moustache, however, were as black as the Master's were silver. He looked about twenty years younger. 'We sailed on the *Baroness* a few years back. Sardinia and Sicily as I recall. You mounted a spirited defence of Captain Bligh in your talk on the *Bounty*.'

'He'll be doing it again,' said Elizabeth flirtatiously and Tudor introduced her.

'You were Master of the *Baroness*,' said Tudor, tentatively.

'Aye,' said Donaldson. 'She was a grand wee vessel. I was very happy with her, but, as they say, you have to move on, draw a line under things, so here I am on the flagship of the fleet.'

'Forgive me,' said Tudor, squinting at Donaldson's gold braid stripes, 'But what's your title here?'

'You mean, why am I not captaining the ship?' He laughed, though not sounding wildly amused. Then he lowered his voice. 'I'll let you into a secret,' he said, 'when it comes to actually sailing the ship, that's the responsibility of the Staff Captain and the Staff Captain is yours truly. The Staff Captain is by way of what on dry land would be called the Chief Executive or perhaps the Chief Operating Officer. The Master would be the Chairman or the President. He's the senior officer but he doesn't actually *do* a great deal.'

Tudor wondered why he was telling him this, perilously close as it was to insubordination. He hardly knew the man.

Staff Captain Donaldson obviously noticed Tudor's surprise.

'Don't get me wrong, Doctor,' he said, 'Sam Hardy's a fine

man and a grand sailor in his day and in his way. I'm not saying his position is purely cosmetic but, well you know how it is. Being the life and soul of the party and a convincing figurehead is a full-time job of its own. It would be asking too much to expect him to steer and navigate as well.'

'Quite,' said Tudor, bearing in mind the old adage about ceasing to dig when you'd created a deep hole.

They were saved from further embarrassment by Mandy Goldslinger ringing a handbell.

'Hi, ladies and gentlemen, girls and boys,' she shouted. 'Welcome aboard the good ship *Duchess*. I'm your Cruise Director Mandy and we're going to have ourselves a ball together during the next few days. However before we do it's my wonderful job to introduce our wonderful captain so that he can introduce y'all to his wonderful crew. I know some of you have sailed on this great ship before and so you'll know what a truly great captain we're privileged to have at the helm. Those of you who are on board for the first time are privileged to have the opportunity of finding out what true captaincy really is. So without more ado, let me present the finest skipper on the seven seas, the pride and joy of Her Majesty's Merchant Navy, the one and only, irreplaceable, irresistible Captain Samuel Hardy.'

Saying which she set down her bell on the table at her side and clapped her hands in a vigorous invitation to everyone else to do the same. Behind her on stage the ship's orchestra who had reappeared as if by magic played a few jaunty bars of 'Rule Britannia' and the Master, preening his elegant moustaches in a gesture which not even the simplest passenger could have mistaken for modesty, acknowledged the plaudits of the multitude before gesturing for silence, as if the applause was all too much for him.

'Welcome, ladies and gentleman, to the finest ship afloat,'

he began and continued in a spirit of effusive bonhomie for a minute or two before introducing Staff Captain Donaldson, the Chief Engineer, the Purser, the Head Housekeeper, the Executive Chef and others, all of whom smiled and waved and were rewarded by enthusiastic clapping and even the occasional unexpected wolf-whistle.

Finally, when he had done, the Master raised his glass, and said, 'As they say on the other side of the English Channel. *Bon Voyage*! I wish you all a calm passage and a safe arrival in New York City.'

Tudor shrugged at his pretty protégé.

'Tempting fate a bit wouldn't you say?' he asked softly.

'I'd say so,' she replied. 'What do you imagine the captain said to the passengers when the *Titanic* set sail?'

'Much the same, I imagine,' said Tudor.

'You bet,' she said.

CHAPTER FOUR

Elizabeth Burney shivered on the spiral staircase leading to the Chatsworth Restaurant and pulled her Tasmanian Trefusis stole tight about her shoulders.

'I feel like I'm in the cast of an Agatha Christie. *Murder on the Nile* maybe,' she said. 'Is it always like this?'

' "As if", not "like" if you don't mind,' he said pedantically.

'Oh, for f***'s sake,' she said, 'Can you do content not context and answer the question?'

Tudor winced. He knew he had fuddy-duddy tendencies.

'Cruise ships are natural settings for Agatha Christie type mysteries,' he said, in pedagogic mode. 'In some respects you could argue that the modern cruise ship is the conscious equivalent of the twentieth-century house-party. Or at least that's what it aspires to. Equally you could say that ships like the *Duchess* are deliberately trying to ape the great transatlantic passenger liners of the same period. The passengers reflect this. So yes.'

'So yes,' she mimicked, giggling lightly, 'it's like being on stage for a matinée of *The Mousetrap*.'

'Yes,' he said, 'I know what you mean. Cruising's a bit like that.'

She giggled again and was still smiling when they entered

the dining room which was doing its best to live up to its name. Seeing the pastiche oil paintings on the panelled walls Tudor remembered a quip about a Duke of Devonshire at his stately pile selling off old masters to pay for young mistresses. These paintings were ersatz old masters unlike the real duke's paintings in the real Chatsworth and like the room itself they were part of a charade or pantomime. This was part of the essence of cruising. The experience involved a voluntary suspension of disbelief. For the duration of the voyage passengers entered a world of fantasy and make-believe. For most of them this was entirely agreeable. For some, some of the time, it was not.

This was now the case for Dr Tudor Cornwall who found himself obliged to dine at a table for four with Sir Goronwy and Lady Watkyn. This was Tudor's idea of purgatory. Sir Goronwy droned on through the prawn cocktail, droned on through the brownish steak Diane, droned on through the Black Forest gâteau and droned on through the coffee and petits fours. Whenever the drone seemed to stop in order to allow the speaker a pause for breath, Lady Watkyn managed to get in a sycophantic coda which prevented either Tudor or Elizabeth putting an end to what represented the verbal equivalent of a record-breaking marathon snooker break.

In one way or another Watkyn droned on about himself. As a professional Welshman he possessed all the verbosity of the most long-winded Methodist preacher but without the redeeming belief in the Almighty. As far as Sir Goronwy Watkyn was concerned there was only one God and that was Sir Goronwy Watkyn. He would have said that his conversation – he would never have accepted that it was actually a monologue – ranged far and wide. In a sense this was true for, beginning with crime fiction, its origins, its history, its current strengths and weaknesses he rabbited on through politics from his own parish in the Marches just outside Montgomery, to Welsh politics – with special reference to the Plaid – British politics, European politics and global politics. He could do terrorism, cricket, crochet, crosswords. You name it. His knowledge may not have run very deep but it ran impossibly wide. And every topic he covered had an ill-concealed subtext which was, of course, Sir Goronwy Watkyn. You might think that, for instance, he was delivering a detailed and dispassionate account of British military operations in Iraq, but before long he himself would make an entrance. Sometimes he would appear as a name-dropping British Council lecturer, sometimes as a military expert who had done national service in the Royal Welch Fusiliers; sometimes as a young man who had once canoed up the Euphrates, perhaps as an author who had once set a novel in Biblical Babylon. It was, in Tudor's opinion, self-opinionated and self-obsessed tripe. Impressive in its way, rather like a model of the Empire State building made entirely of matchsticks, or the world's biggest Cornish pasty, but tripe nonetheless. The dreaded Myfanwy's breathy little encomia filled the tiny silences like the pitter-patter of confetti. 'So right, darling . . . so very, very right . . . that was the time the Prime Minister phoned to ask . . . Watty's laver bread is the best in the whole of Wales.' And so on.

It was said of him that if he simply dropped God's name then all was normal. Thus when Sir Goronwy confided, 'I was walking down to the club and happened to bump into God. Had a most interesting chat,' that was OK. The time to worry was when he said, 'I was walking down to the club when I bumped into Goronwy Watkyn.' That was when you knew you were in trouble and Goronwy was due for one of his periodic periods in the bin.

After a while Tudor started to play a game of guessing how

many times the old wind-bag would use the words 'I' or 'me' in the next five minutes. The incidence of both was astonishingly high and increased noticeably in proportion to the ingestion of alcohol which was itself significant. Riviera Shipping might have been conservative on the food lines but it was generous with the claret.

Mandy Goldslinger was at a table with two gentlemen hosts and the Baltic classical guitarist. They seemed to be having a much better time than the Cornwall-Watkyn table. There was evidence of four-way conversation, story-telling, jokes and even laughter. The two boys and two girls of the celebrity, all-singing, all-dancing, all-smiling cabaret team of whom no one on board had previously heard, were evidently enjoying an incestuous luv-in. Mandy's deputy, an androgynous wet-behind-the-ears Yorkshire tyke, was hosting a ventriloquist, the water-colour teacher and the computer lecturer. And so on. There were about thirty diners in all.

Just as Tudor was floating into a Goronwy-induced miasma of total inattention and ennui he heard a Watkynism which brought him suddenly back to something approaching life.

'Blah . . . blah . . . Goronwyblah . . . bach . . . hwyl . . . aberblah . . . blahgynolwyn . . . blah . . . watkynblah . . . last voyage of the *Duchess*.'

Tudor reacted like a schnauzer stung by a wasp.

'Last voyage of the *Duchess*?' he repeated, fumbling his way out of half-asleep.

'Last voyage of the *Duchess*, boyo,' said the Welsh knight, taking a long sip of the Australian sticky with which Riviera Shipping had rounded off their largesse. 'The old girl's swan-song. At least the last voyage in these particular colours. Dare say she'll re-emerge as a hospital ship for the Swiss Navy or a nautical knocking shop for the dictator in some banana republic. Or a Central African kingdom. There's a public-school educated emperor with a lot of wives in Equatorial Bongo-Bongo land who might just about fit the bill. In any event' – he sipped again, fleshy lips kissing the glass with an almost lascivious caress – 'it's the last time you and I will tread the boards of these particular decks.'

'Are you sure?' asked Tudor, experiencing a frisson of anticipatory alarm. He was beginning to have a bad feeling about this trip.

'This Oz Auslese is warming to the cockles of my old Celtic heart,' said the theatrical old crime writer. 'Sure? Nothing's sure in life. That's the only certainty about our drab existence wouldn't you say? Dylan Thomas has a memorable passage about madness and sanity, but alas I've forgotten it. Ah Dylan, Dylan. How I miss the dear darling boy. . . .'

'I remember the line perfectly,' said Tudor, sharply, for he was vexed.

Sir Goronwy shot him a threatened look from under beetling white eyebrows. The eyes were unfocused in a fuddled fashion.

'How did you know?' he asked tetchily.

'One does,' said Tudor, matching the older man's bad temper with his own. 'And how come too that you knew that this was the *Duchess*'s last voyage with Riviera?'

Sir Goronwy smiled elliptically.

'As you suggest,' he said, 'there are things that one simply knows as if by osmosis, picked up on the ether, plucked from the wings of gossip, born to one's ears on the silvery threads of ethereal whispers from one knows not where.'

'Someone told you late one night and you've forgotten who,' said Tudor.

The old fraud was not to be easily riled.

'I never reveal my sources save in works of genuine written scholarship,' said Sir Goronwy. 'In verbal communication seldom if ever. Confidences are not to be betrayed but evidence must be acknowledged. My dear old father, the Reverend Ebenezer Watkyn of Abergynolwyn, of whom you may have heard me speak, was a past master of the telling reference, the learned footnote, the bibliophiliac bibliography, in short of knowledge lightly worn yet properly acknowledged.' He paused, breathless at last and waved at a passing waiter for more dessert wine.

'Ebenezer, Goronwy's da, was a fine man,' said Lady Watkyn, quick as a flash, 'And a wonderful preacher. Held his congregations in the palm of his hand he did, just as if they'd been a lump of dough and they about to be baked into a loaf of bread and fed with the fishes, just as the Good Book tells us.'

It was apparent to Tudor and to Elizabeth Burney that Sir Goronwy was not the only Watkyn the worse for wear alcoholically speaking.

Tudor was wondering whether to go through the charade of intelligent conversation when the Cruise Director shimmered across clanking with costume jewellery and gleaming all over.

'Dahling,' she said breathily, 'would you mind playing musical chairs so that I can sit with these gorgeous people?'

Elizabeth Burney regarded this as a virtually divine intervention and did as she was asked with an alacrity which might have been considered impolite even by the stone cold sober. Sir Goronwy and Lady Watkyn however seemed barely to notice but just continued their seamless droning duet. This was, reflected Tudor, as dispassionately as he was able, a remarkable conversational accomplishment – the sort of thing that ought to go into the *Guinness Book of Records* alongside Gyles Brandreth's longest ever after-dinner speech.

'What's all this,' he hissed, ignoring the Welsh, 'about the

Duchess being sold? On her last voyage in Riviera colours I'm reliably informed.'

'Reliable, sweetie?' Mandy Goldslinger smiled a sceptical smile implying that this was not even mere gossip but a positive untruth. She could have been right for there was not much to do with Riviera Shipping that Mandy did not know. Cruise Director was a title that did her far less than justice.

'It came from the horse's mouth,' said Tudor. 'At this very table. Sir Goronwy himself, no less.'

At the mention of his name the Welsh knight came to an unprecedented pause and the slack of his jaw was not, for once, taken up by his harpist harpie wife.

'You're not taking my name in vain I trust. Very verily, all is vanity,' he said theatrically and evidently rather pleased with a joke which only he and his wife seemed to understand.

'Not in the least,' said Tudor pleasantly. 'I was simply confirming with Mandy here what you told me earlier about this being the last voyage of the MV *Duchess*.'

'I always think of the dear thing as the RMS *Duchess* though I suppose she carries no mailbags these days,' said Sir Goronwy. 'The Royal Mail in any case no longer being as regal as it was in the days when the postman rang twice and always came on time. New Labour is little more than republicanism in sheep's clothing though the concept is insulting to sheep, which is as sacred to my nation as the leek or the daffodil.'

Some of Tudor's best friends, Tudor reflected, were Welsh. Indeed as his name suggested he had plenty of Celtic blood himself. He did not, however, wish to claim kinship with the Watkyns.

Mandy Goldslinger cut through this Celtic cackle like a knife through low cholesterol health spread.

'If Riviera are selling,' she said with an air of ill-defined menace, 'then who, I would like to know, is buying? Riviera, as you know, is owned by Atlantic and Pacific, which in turn is owned by Galactic and Global which means, effectively, that there is no one else in the market.'

Sir Goronwy smiled saliverly.

'I'm told that the two most likely purchasers are both on board,' he said, 'and already at daggers drawn. It wouldn't surprise me if we had some dramatic events to entertain us before we arrive in New York.'

He gave a knowing wink and a portentous belch and seeing that his glass was empty rose unsteadily to go in search of a refill.

CHAPTER FIVE

They had a good day in Cork.

Had Tudor been a more flippant, Wodehousian figure, he might have described it as 'an absolute corker' or 'jolly corking run-ashore,' but being the man he was he simply said, that evening when they were back on board nursing a couple of Boris the Barman's lethal but delicious cocktails, 'I rather enjoyed today.'

Elizabeth, who was beginning to read her supervisor as well as he would like to think *he* read *her*, said succinctly, 'Me too.'

Until a few months earlier she had barely been out of Tasmania and then only to the Australian mainland and, just once, to New Zealand on a hiking holiday. Coming to England she had been amazed at how like her own homeland it was, despite being on the other side of the planet. She knew the history and understood how the affinities had arisen but she was nevetheless viscerally amazed at having travelled so many thousands of miles to end up, nearly, exactly where she had begun.

Yet as she settled in she found that the superficial similarities of cricket and culture, custom and convention were exactly that – superficial. There were profound differences of language and idiom; a pervasive defeatism where she had grown up with optimism and the idea of 'can do'. She felt she had grown up in a place which lived outdoors and where anything was possible. Now she was in a country with low horizons where there was nearly always some sort of bureaucratic regulation that prevented you doing anything interesting or unusual.

She loved being in England because of its complexity and its history. Life in Wessex, even at its not particularly good university, had a texture that was missing in the breezy, nonchalant, new land of her youth.

And now Ireland. She had been told that Cork was not the true Ireland but that it was a place apart: *Corcaigh* – she was irritated by the Gaelic sub-title to everything from road-signs to picture postcards especially the curlicued typeface which she thought pretentious and naff. This didn't stop her and her boss buying postcards – views of tiny typical whitewashed cottages with donkeys. They wrote messages on them for folks back home in a dark pub where they drank cold black Guinness and marvelled at the efficacy of the recent smoking ban which seemed to have been obeyed with remarkable un-Irish alacrity. The juke box played fiddle and squeezebox folk songs of vaguely Republican sentiments. Afterwards they moved to a brighter less sepulchral pub and lunched off big meaty mutton chops and colcannon with more Guinness to drink followed, greatly daring, by an Irish coffee heavily impregnated with Tullamore Dew and with the cream correctly unwhipped and poured over the back of a silver spoon so that it sat fat and mildly yellow on top of the Guinness-black coffee. After lunch they visited St Fimbar's Cathedral which seemed like the rest of the city familiar and yet stridently un-English, then took a cab back to the ship, nodding and smiling uncomprehendingly at the driver's travelogue and what sounded like a long, gloomy weather forecast.

It was oddly reassuring to be back on the *Duchess*. Already she had taken on a familiar home-like quality even though she was no more than a floating hotel. It was part of the attraction of cruising that the ship took on an almost protective coccoon-like air so that after the adventures of a day in some foreign port (well, actually as often as not, seen from the synthetic safety of a chaperoned tour bus) one could relax, feel pampered and unthreatened. Travel without danger, holidays without fuss.

Supplies and fuel had been taken on board in the Irish Republic and so too had passengers. Elizabeth got talking to a group of new arrivals in the bar while Tudor toyed in a desultory manner with the *Irish Times* crossword.

Presently she rejoined him.

'They're a press group,' she said. 'Their leader seems to be a PR person called Jeffrey who could be English, but all the others are Irish and seem to have names beginning with F. The blokes are called Finn, Flan, Fergal, Fingal and even Fimbar and the hackettes have names like Fiannula or Fenella or Felicitas.'

'That sounds like a nun,' said Tudor.

'Doesn't look like a nun,' she said. 'The whole lot are straight out of central casting. Boozing and betting people and they talk funny.'

'I can guess,' he said, 'and what are they here for?'

'Classic freebie,' she said. 'They all, more or less seem to have commissions from Irish papers and magazines. Do you really think there's such a thing as the *Tipperary Tatler*? One of the Fiannulas says she's doing a style piece for them.'

'Anywhere can have a *Tatler*,' said Tudor, caustically. 'Most places do. It's a licence to print money. Even in Tipperary they'll pay money to see if Finn and Flan are sharing a quiet joke over a pint of Guinness in the Fiddler's Flea. Or whatever. *Tatlers* are just parish magazines with ball gowns and black ties. Upwardly mobile gossip.'

'Well,' said Elizabeth thoughtfully, 'Fiannula, or one of them, is doing a style piece for the *Tipperary Tatler.* The other Fiannulas are writing the same sort of drivel for the same sort of non-publications. So are the Finns and the Fimbars. All a complete waste of time and money. They're only here for the beer.'

'And the fruit machines,' said Tudor. 'Oh, and all the romance that goes with a life at sea. They'll write bland complimentary pieces and they'll appear in their publications with bland, complimentary photographs and everyone will be happy.'

'Is that the way it is?' she asked.

'That's the way it is,' said Tudor. 'Way of the world. Nothing really what it seems. All make-believe. Pay enough money and you can make anything happen. Or appear to happen.'

'You don't believe that.'

'I believe that's how it would be if it weren't for people like me. Like us. Whistle-blowers. The incorruptible.'

The girl stared moodily into her drink and said nothing.

After a while Tudor sunk the last of his cocktail and said, 'Come outside. I think this should be a rather spectacular departure. It usually is. I did it once in the *QE2.* Breathtaking.'

It took a lot to take Elizabeth's breath away but the Irish leave-taking came close. It was dusk as they sailed down river, past the twinkling lights of Cobh and the fairy-tale silhouette of the cathedral and it was as if the whole of Ireland had turned out to wave them on their way across the Atlantic to what so many Irish people regarded as new Ireland across the water where the Irish could be free from the English yolk and your Kennedys and your Reagans walked tall and inherited the earth.

And the Irish lined the waterfront in their smart French, German and Italian cars and they sounded their horns and they flashed their lights and they cried out in the lowering dark and the passengers on board the *Duchess* waved back and some of them smiled, and some of them called back and some of them wept a little for it was all quite magical in a Gaelic way and they stayed on deck until the last winking shaft of light from the beacon on the ultimate cliff disappeared into the evening fog and the ship was truly on her own, utterly so, without land or escort, destined for thousands of miles of dangerous and desolate ocean before they came to the land of the free.

'Time for dinner,' said Tudor with an Englishman's tin tongue.

'You go,' she said, 'I'll catch up.'

He waited a moment, then saw that she really did want to stay and savour the moment. As he walked towards the door that led indoors, he glanced back and saw that she was leaning on the rail gazing down on the white wake gleaming in the dark below. As the ship gathered speed the foaming fan grew more turbulent stretching out in a giant V astern. A handful of gulls still followed them wheeling and mewing before they turned back to the safety of dry land and left the little vessel to the mercy of the ocean. You could almost be forgiven for thinking anthropomorphically of the *Duchess* as she seemed to lengthen her gait and began to stretch out to the even marathon runner's stride which would, in a few days, God willing bring her safely to port.

She was pitching and rolling now as the sea buffeted her and the more she moved the noisier she became. Tudor could never work out whether the rattling and whining of a ship at sea was protest or pleasure but he found the noise oddly comforting – the regular thump of the engines, the sigh of the wind through wire and rigging, the plangent rasp of rivets and plates. This, after all, was what the ship had been built for and she had made countless voyages such as this. The knowledge was reassuring though the future was, as always uncertain.

It was an oddity of all journeys, he reflected, glancing up at the sky which had cleared to reveal a full moon and a Milky Way, that they were at the same time similar yet unique. Each time he took the train from Casterbridge to Waterloo he passed through the same countryside, the same towns, the same stations. Often he showed his ticket to the same guard, smiled a silent greeting to the same passengers, bought coffee from the same girl in the buffet. Yet all these people like himself were older every time, a step or two nearer death, a page or so nearer the end.

Crossing the Atlantic was more glamorous than travelling from Wessex to London and yet the voyage contained the same elements of routine and surprise. Once on board they would all fall easily into observing the fixed points that each person created – meals being pre-eminent but lectures and film shows and bridge sessions all playing their part so that in a way life on ship was almost dull, particularly if you were seated at a table with the Welsh Watkyns.

And yet no two voyages were ever quite the same. However many times the *Duchess* crossed from Britain to America there were always moments of the unexpected to chip away at monotony. Mostly the deviations were trivial, unnoticeable even. Drama was not something the cruise companies encouraged and on the whole they were successful in lulling their customers into a sybaritic somnolence undisturbed by anything untoward.

Tudor spent several moments hesitating on the deck thinking these thoughts, lost in reflections of self-indulgent banality even though they had to do with such fundamental and universal questions as the meaning of life.

He was so abstracted that the sudden opening of the door took him quite by surprise though he realized as he jumped that it was ridiculous to find oneself discomposed by the sudden opening of a door. That was what doors did after all. They opened and shut. Even on board ship. And he was silly, too, to be surprised by the figures who emerged on to the moonlit deck. He would have expected them to have been safely ensconced in their suite, the three waiting hand and foot on the one.

'Good evening,' said Prince Abdullah politely, as he led his three wives into the bracing night.

Tudor inclined his head and said 'Good evening' back. The Prince spoke the greeting like an old-fashioned Englishman, public-school educated, BBC-modulated. Just the tiniest trace of a foreign inflection. The eyes of his wives looked out at Dr Cornwall, the rest of them concealed in jellabas and yashmaks.

He wondered what they were thinking and continued to do so even as he perused his menu at the dinner table a few moments later and considered the great questions which dominated life on ship: whether to have the pâté or the soup; the duck or the beef, whether to drink white or red.

He didn't even notice that the Watkyns were not with him.

CHAPTER SIX

Tudor was woken by noise in the middle of the night.

For a moment he felt hopelessly, helplessly disoriented as one does when woken suddenly and unexpectedly between alien sheets. It was a klaxon. Deep disorientating noise of an indeterminate character, the sort of thing you'd use on torture victims in Guantánamo or the Lubyanka. Noise so penetrating that it had an almost physical character. It hurt.

Seeing the mahogany panelling, the port hole and his towelling bath robe slung across the end of his bed, feeling the regular sway of his room and hearing the throb and mutter of the vessel's nuts and bolts he quickly remembered where he was. The noise was the blast of the ship's klaxon, usually sounded only as a test or the prelude to the mandatory boat drill.

Seconds later it ceased. A series of metallic clicks followed and then a female voice spoke.

'Good morning ladies and gentlemen,' it said, pleasantly and with a soft Irish lilt which could under other circumstances have seemed quite beguiling. 'We're sorry to have disturbed your sleep and in a moment or two we'll let you resume your slumbers. This is simply to tell you that the ship has now been taken over by the People's Liberation Army of

United Ireland. There will be a further announcement in due course but for the time being we ask everyone to remain calm and to stay in your cabins. As far as we can ascertain there are at present no passengers in public areas of the ship. If there is any passenger away from their cabin we ask them to return there. If anyone is found outside their cabin we cannot be responsible for the consequences. However, if everyone stays in bed and goes back to sleep you may rest assured that you will be perfectly safe. Thank you for your attention.'

There was a click and the Tannoy went dead.. Tudor switched on the bedside light and looked at his watch. 4.30. The chances of any passenger being up and about, even an insomniac fruit machine user, were remote. It was the best possible moment for a take-over. He rubbed his eyes and considered his position. Any ordinary sensible passenger would do as asked and stay put. Going back to sleep might be a tall order but it was certainly the sensible course of action.

He had doubts, however, whether he was an 'ordinary sensible passenger'. As a guest speaker his role was ambiguous. He was not an ordinary passenger, but he was not a member of the crew either. Did that confer obligations? How, he wondered, would Sir Goronwy Watkyn react? And there was the added complication, was there not, that he, like Watkyn, was an expert on crime. If, as it appeared, this was an act of piracy, a maritime hi-jack, then this was as much of a crime as the Mutiny on the *Bounty*, on which, he remembered with a start, he was due to speak later this morning.

He was about to decide that going back to sleep would be a dereliction of duty when his phone rang.

It was Elizabeth. The Irish People's Liberation Army might have performed the revolutionary's text-book first task of commandeering the radio station, but they clearly hadn't disabled the communications system. Passenger was still able to talk unto passenger.

'What did you make of that then?' she asked, obviously excited.

'Shhh,' he said nervously and a touch theatrically. 'You don't want someone to hear.'

'Oh come on,' she said. 'Someone is far too bothered trussing up the captain and officers, making sure the crew don't stage a counter-attack. They're not going to bother with cabin-to-cabin communication. They've got other things to do. I think it's my gang though. The so-called Irish travel hacks. I told you there was no such thing as the *Tipperary Tatler*. That was Fiannula on the loudspeaker system.'

'You sure?'

'Pretty sure,' she said.

'Are you surprised?'

He could almost hear her thinking down the line.

'Surprised but not surprised,' she said.

She was good at ambivalence. Properly expressed it carried academic conviction. Certainty was risky. It was fine if you were right, but mistakes were very bad. Bets, she reckoned were, on the whole, better hedged. On the one hand, on the other hand, might end up as a drawn match but it was better to share the points than earn none.

'So what should we do?' asked Tudor.

'We?' she asked. 'What's this *we*, Kemo Sabe? I see no *we* I'm a mere menial. I do as I'm told.'

This was being economic with the truth but at the moment it suited her and it was true that she was, technically, the led and he the leader. He taught, she learned. She sat at his feet, at least as far as the casual observer was concerned. The reality might be different, but she was not going to let on, at least when it didn't suit her.

'You're the boss,' she said. 'I'm staying in bed till they sound the all-clear.'

'OK,' he said, not feeling remotely OK. 'I'll call you after the all-clear.'

He put the phone down.

She was right. It was disconcerting that she was so often right. She was younger than him. And a girl. On both counts she should have been wrong and yet she wasn't.

He lay back and sighed.

'Am I man or am I a mouse?' he asked himself, not sure whether it was a rhetorical question, whether he had the answer, whether he cared, whether he knew, whether, well, anything really. . . .

'Man or mouse,' he said out loud. 'Discuss.'

It was a question that had bothered him almost all his life and was doing so now with increasing frequency. It disturbed him in the dark and silent small hours when one was particularly prone to doubt and loss of confidence. In youth he had been relatively confident of his manhood but as the years passed that confidence evaporated. He had read in one of the colour magazines only a week or so earlier that a man's testosterone disappeared faster and faster after the age of something like eighteen. Not that testosterone had ever been his sort of thing. If anything he had always cultivated a sort of refined femininity albeit on the uncompromisingly masculine grounds that girls seemed to like that sort of thing. The Morgan motor car was an exception, he supposed, but that had come relatively late in life and was deliberately designed to compensate for the rodent attacks on his virility. Anyway even the Morgan was a subdued symptom of blokeishness. A hardcore *Maxim* reader would have opted for a Harley-Davidson.

He shook himself. Only a mouse, he told himself, would

behave like this. No proper man would conduct such a private conversation at a moment of crisis. It was pusillanimous prevarication. Cometh the hour cometh the man should have been his rallying cry. Not cometh the man cometh the mouse.

He considered his options. Option A was to turn over and go back to sleep. That was the extreme-mouse solution – white mouse tending to albino. The pink-eyed way out. In any case even if he took this cowardly way out it wouldn't work properly becaused he was far too tense and excited to go back to sleep. The nautical motion of the old ship might be soporific, but the apparent terrorist hijack was far too bracing for even a drowse or a day-dream.

Option B was to get up, have a shave and a shower, dress and be prepared for the terrorists' next move. This was more seductive than A if only because it gave him something to do as well as affording him more time to think. He had to admit that it was still pretty mousy behaviour but on the other hand he would present a tougher, more effective proposition if he were scrubbed up. Also it didn't represent a complete campaign, just part of it. A necessary prelude you might say. Option B might be mouse-like but it could quite easily slip into something altogether more manly. He decided to leave the problem as a straight choice between A and B, leaving consideration of C and possibly further letters of the alphabet until later. He had always admired Fabius Cunctator more than Hannibal. There was a difference between bravery and bravado.

The shower was hot and the shave close. He had, as usual brought his own soap, brown Pears in a box, and he applied shaving soap with an old Trumper's brush with genuine bristles removing it with a new Gillette blade in a safety razor. He quite liked the idea of an old-fashioned razor which you sharpened by stropping, but he was anxious not to appear too much of a fogey. Indeed for someone who gave the impression of not caring about his appearance he cared very much indeed. He believed that such deceptive nonchalance had to be worked at.

As he washed and shaved himself he considered his next move. Yet again he shrank from the really serious decision by just considering what he should wear. If he were going to indulge in serious counter-terrorist activity he would need to convey gravitas and authority. That meant a collar and tie. The tie should definitely not be Channel Four Newscaster with its mutton-dressed-as-lamb garishness but something plain and sober. Not club or old-school-striped which would be unacceptably Fogeyish. He had a green number with white polka-dots which would just about do. Also a plain creamy yellow shirt with gold monogrammed cuff-links. Dark-grey worsted trousers and a dark blue jacket more in the style of an Ivy League reefer than a British blazer. Blue socks and a pair of dark-grey loafers he had picked up in a closing-down sale in a small shoe-shop behind the Frari church in Venice.

When he had packed himself into this outfit he contemplated the result with a satisfaction verging on the smug. He was weathering well, he told himself, and he looked as if he was at the very least a head of department, which indeed he was. It was an image which, he reckoned, inspired respect if not exactly awe. Even Irish terrorists would think twice before tackling him. He looked the sort of man policemen might still, even in the early twenty-first century, call 'Sir'.

Wondering whether the bags under his eyes indicated wisdom or fatigue, the crow's feet healthy scepticism or unhealthy late nights, the flecks of grey at the temple seniority or senility, he found the mouse reasserting itself. There was something wrong with the picture in front of him and he knew that it was a question of conviction. He might have fooled other people into thinking that this was a commanding presence but he didn't fool himself. Not for a minute. He knew that the Tussaud-like image really was just a waxwork façade. He longed to be able to snuff out candles with the flicker of an eyelid at forty paces, but he knew deep down that he would melt at the strike of a match.

He sat down heavily on the bed. Option B was now complete. It was too late for Option A. It was time therefore to consider C and any alternatives he could bring to mind. C was confrontation. If he adopted it he would leave his cabin, walk to the bridge and command the hijackers to put down their weapons and submit to his citizen's arrest.

C for crazy. Even if he were a cross between James Bond and Spiderman this was a really bad idea. If the terrorists were even half serious they'd shoot him on sight. Of course they would. That's what terrorists did. It had happened time and again during his lifetime and before. Moreover, having spent a lifetime studying crime in all its aspects he knew this better than most. The ordinary bloke who 'has a go' is a certain suicide. He might make an adulatory obituary in the next day's paper but that was all.

Option D was to sit down and read a book. Another mousy idea but safe and sensible. He could phone a friend. That meant Elizabeth in the cabin next door but what good could that do? For different reasons he couldn't involve her in either his cowardice or his riskiness. The one would be too embarassing and the other, well, ungentlemanly. In a curious old-fashioned way, he rather cared about that.

He was still wrestling feebly with these choices when his phone rang.

He picked it up and realized that the necessity of making a

choice had been removed. The decision was being made for him.

The voice was familiar.

And Irish.

CHAPTER SEVEN

'Doctor Cornwall?'

'This is he,' he said, wishing he wasn't.

'You're wanted on the bridge.'

'By whom?' Tudor was surprised by the bolshiness in his voice. If the person to whom he was speaking was the person he thought it was, asking questions, particularly in that tone of voice, was risky.

'Us,' said the voice with Celtic ambiguity. 'We'll send an escort. They'll be with you presently.'

Tudor shrugged. No question now of his sitting in the cabin and reading a book. He wondered what they wanted from him and whether heroics would be required. If he had been seriously contemplating such a course of action he felt somewhat thwarted. A potential initative had been removed. Had he come bursting on to the bridge unannounced he would have held the upper hand. Surprise was a key element in conflict of any kind. All the manuals said so.

Presently there was a sharp knock on the door. The knock had an unpleasantly peremptory quality. It was not a question expecting the answer 'no' nor even entertaining the idea. More of an affirmation of authority.

'Come,' said Tudor, using the expression and the tone of voice he assumed at home in the university when one of his students came calling.

The door was unlocked despite the advice to bolt it while asleep. Tudor had an aversion to locked doors even though it made him vulnerable. It was now flung open with abrupt violence and a stocky figure in a balaclava helmet and combat fatigues stood in the doorway, beckoning. The knocker's left hand held what looked like some sort of pistol. Although firearms came within Tudor's area of knowledge, they were not a speciality. Whatever the man held it gave off an air of metallic menace. The person had not spoken but it exuded male body-language and, more potently and convincingly, male body odour. Strong pong of beer, tobacco and unwashed armpit.

It said nothing but jerked its right hand in an uncouth beckoning fashion while the left pointed the gun barrel at Cornwall's midriff. Compliance seemed desirable even if mousy. In any case Tudor was curious. He had never been involved in a nautical hi-jack before. It would prove an invaluable teaching tool as well as a terrific subject for future cruise lectures. Reasoning thus he did as he was gestured. He was good at rationalizing weakness.

The hijacker shoved him roughly to one side, shut the door and prodded him in the small of the back with what Tudor took to be his gun barrel. Activated in this crude manner he walked.

They went as far as the elevators, ascended three decks to bridge level, exited, walked to a door marked with a red skull and crossbones and words 'Danger. Crew only!' translated into French, Spanish and some script which could, to Tudor, have been Japanese, Chinese or any language from east of Suez. Passing through was the nautical equivalent of going through the green baize door in a stately home which separated upstairs from downstairs, ladies and gentlemen from maids and players. The contrast between passenger accommodation and crew quarters was almost total. Carpet became lino; chandelier, neon strip; polished mahogany, raw steel. In a single second one went from pampered indolence to forced labour. Tudor tried, vainly, to remember the lunar astronaut's oracular words about the instantaneous step for man and mankind but only found himself wondering whether the crew slept in hammocks. It would be difficult to find such anachronistic class distinctions on dry land.

Tudor was thinking of all this in a dreamy academic sort of way when he suddenly realized that he and his demon prodder had emerged on to the bridge. 'Bridge', like so many words on board ship, was misleading for in no way did the area in which Tudor now found himself resemble a structure traversing a road, railway or river. Much less a game of cards. This dimly lit room with its flickering screens and panoramic, wrap-round view of the moon-lit ocean deep was a nerve-centre or control-room but in no recognizable way a 'bridge'. It took him a blinking second or so to accustom himself to the dim half-light and even then he saw only through a glass darkly.

There were five officers on watch. At least that was what he assumed the ghostly white figures to be. He could not make out their features, or their badges of office but their white uniforms glowed in the gloom. Each one of them was being shadowed – literally – by a darker person whom Tudor took to be one of the terrorist team from the Emerald Isle. This was all the hijackers had had to do – break on to or in to the Bridge, commandeer the *Duchess*'s public address system – the maritime equivalent of a banana republic's national broadcasting centre and post office – and Bob's your uncle, the revolution's triumphed and the regime is toppled.

The gorilla-guerilla escort prodded him towards a diminutive shadow which looked female and in charge. These were difficult things to assess in the crepuscular light but Tudor guessed that it was Fiannula or Ffion or whoever the girl from the fictitious *Tipperary Tatler* was and that she was the ring-leader and also the voice who had spoken to everyone over the ship's public address system.

'Doctor Cornwall,' she said in a voice that confirmed that she was a girl and also the voice on the Tannoy. Her air of authority was sufficiently obvious for him to think that his intuition about being the boss was also correct.

'*Tipperary Tatler*,' he said, hoping to fit the last piece into this little jigsaw. It sounded the sort of name Ian Fleming might have given a Bond girl.

'Very astute, Dr Cornwall,' she said, in a brogue so husky and Gaelic that he felt sure it must have been fake. No real Irishwoman would speak like that. It was like something from *Father Ted*, 'I know you're a professional,' she said, 'it's why we asked you to step up here. We're keen to have a plausible mouthpiece.'

'What exactly are you playing at?' he asked, feeling like the mouse that roared, a frisson of daring translating into courage. Yet the remark didn't, he felt, require real courage because, he sensed intuitively, that this was just a game. These people weren't real.

'We're not playing at anything,' said *Tipperary*, lilting. 'This is no game. You'd better believe it.'

'Listen,' said Cornwall, 'it's easy to do what you've done so far because that's the way civilized societies are. We don't live in a police state. Not in Ireland. Not in the UK. Not in the United States. And most certainly not on board an ocean liner such as this. Everything is based on tolerance and trust which means no obtrusive security devices, no armed goons patrolling everywhere, no CCTVs, nothing to make people scared or tense. If you go on holiday you don't expect to end up in Guantánamo. And the only way one can prevent people like you doing what you've just done is by creating a world that is simply not acceptable. Being civilized opens the way for the uncivilized.'

'I agree. Western society is soft, vulnerable. We've just demonstrated that.' She sounded, thought Tudor, more than slightly mad. But you'd have to be more than slightly mad to do what they'd just done.

'You do realize,' said Tudor, 'that what you've done is easy because those in charge have no choice but to make it easy. The reason it doesn't happen more often is that real professionals understand that the only part of an operation such as this which is viable is phase one. The deterrent lies in the certainty of effective response.'

'You're the expert,' said the girl. 'That's why you're here.'

'You could have commandeered Sir Goronwy Watkyn,' said Tudor, playing for time.

'He's fiction,' she said, 'we deal in fact. We also think he's yesterday's story. And a windbag. We know your stuff, Dr Cornwall. You'll do. You suit our purposes perfectly well.'

'Thank you,' said Tudor, 'I'm flattered.'

He was too, up to a point and in a manner of speaking. It was always good to score points over his old crime writer rival even in dodgy circumstances such as this and the circumstances couldn't get much dodgier. Here he was, ivory-tower man, effectively the hostage of a gang of fanatical Irish terrorists on the bridge of a hijacked cruise liner in the middle of the Atlantic Ocean.

In theory he should have known exactly how to behave but, he had to concede, theory was what he knew about and this, disturbingly and threateningly, was the real thing. It was 'Who wants to be a Millionaire?' syndrome. Any fool could answer

Chris Tarrant's patsy questions when they were sitting in an armchair in the comfort of their own home, preferably with a hot milky drink and a packet of chocolate digestives or Jaffa cakes to hand. Plonk them down on one of those uncomfortable stools in the studio under the full glare of the studio lights and the deceptively amiable quiz-master himself and all was utterly different. The mind went blank. One no longer knew what two and two equalled, let alone what the capital of French Equatorial Africa was or who invented the kitchen scales.

'You're not meant to be flattered,' she said. 'Like I said, we deal in facts. You're our man, Dr Cornwall. You're part of the deal. We didn't pick our ship or our cruise at random. We wanted the *Duchess* and we wanted you. An expert on crime. Academic. Cutting edge. The sort of guy Jeremy Paxman would invoke in a crisis. Larry King even. Someone who will play well on the airwaves. Also help us in other ways. You play ball with us; we'll play ball with you.'

Tudor found himself levitating. It had happened to him once or twice before on the rare occasions when he had found himself in an unaccustomed or threatening session. There had been one such moment when he was summoned to 10 Downing Street for what sounded like a routine consultation with a Whitehall committee of jobsworth bureaucrats only to find himself alone on a sofa with Tony Blair. And another when he agreed to address a meeting of Animal Rights Activists and found himself not, as he had expected, a neutral imparter of inside information, but a target, an enemy alien, a subject of verbal abuse which threatened to teeter over a brink into something more physical. It didn't quite, but he was glad to escape unscathed. On another occasion he had fallen out of a boat off the Cornish coast and had five minutes of thinking he was about to drown.

All three times he had enjoyed what he could only describe as an 'out-of-body-experience'. It was if his soul or brain, (call it what you like depending on the state of your beliefs and he being cheerfully agnostic simply wasn't sure) had left his body and settled at a point a few feet above his head. From this vantage point the thinking part of his being was able to make a far more rational assessment of the situation than if it had remained at head level. The one common factor was that the disembodied regarded base camp with a mixture of disdain and hilarity. From six feet above his head Dr Tudor Cornwall looked, regrettably, a trifle absurd.

It was the same now except that in this case the other principal figure cut little more of a dash than Cornwall. It seemed from on high that the girl was all mouth and no knickers as they say on Tyneside. She was bluffing.

It was all very well knowing this in theory, quite another to act on it. Spaceship Cornwall beamed the message down to base but it was quite another matter for base to act on it.

Cornwall found himself running through his internal 'man or mouse' routine once more. 'Man' would have called the bluff; 'mouse' would have played safe and gone along with the implausible manner and the gun-barrel pointing at the small of his back from an unnervingly close distance. He had a choice and very little time to make it.

'The weapon,' he said, in a voice which was far firmer than he felt, 'which your friend is pointing at me in such a threatening and, if I may say so, melodramatic and superfluous a fashion, intrigues me. I don't think I recognize it. Not, I think, a Mauser or a Walther and certainly not a Smith & Wesson. I doubt it's Czech or Russian. Beretta I somehow doubt. Chinese perhaps. I don't think I've seen anything quite like it before.'

He was bluffing himself. He knew next to nothing about

firearms. In theory maybe, but certainly not in practice. Motivation was his forte not the crude business of execution. He was not a Ludlumite as in Robert of that ilk who devoted whole pages to the minutiae of small-arms.

'How should I know?' asked the girl. 'I leave that sort of thing to others. I do brain not brawn.'

'The truth,' said Cornwall, 'is that you haven't a clue, because' – and here he surprised himself as much as everyone else in the room, by spinning round deftly and grabbing hold of the menacing barrel – 'it isn't a real gun at all.'

CHAPTER EIGHT

He was right. It wasn't a Smith & Wesson. Or a Beretta. Or a Walther or Mauser. In fact it wasn't any sort of gun, just a crude piece of make-believe, a piece of black metal piping taped to a roughly hewn wooden butt. It was enough to deceive a startled innocent on a dark night, especially if the owner was wearing a balaclava helmet and combat fatigues. As a blunt instrument wielded with force and precision it might have maimed or even killed but as deployed here on board the *Duchess* it was just a piece of play-acting.

For a moment there was silence.

It was the girl who broke it.

'We didn't want anyone to get hurt,' she said. The words sounded lame.

Tudor turned back to her.

'Oh really,' he said. 'Can't you do better than that?'

A further silence followed. A mid-Atlantic stand-off. Tudor couldn't help feeling rather pleased with himself, but at the same time horrified at what might have been. His alter-ego, that disembodied part of him which had been hovering above his head but which now seemed, mysteriously to have returned to base, had given the correct advice but it was reckless and dangerous counsel. How could it have known? Did it know? Had he acted on a certainty or a desperate hunch. Should he be dead? Was he really a man? Or was he just a mouse in man's clothing? These worries pounded away at him as he tried to concentrate on the immediate issue and maintain his imitation of Action Man, Bond, the cutting edge rather than his preferred mode of cerebral onlooker.

Eventually he said, 'I think you and I had better sit down and have a little chat.'

To his gratification and, once more, surprise, she agreed at once.

There was a room off the bridge, a curious sort of R and R place with a couple of beds, a coffee-maker, some armchairs and a general slightly desperate air of getting-away-from-it all-but-only-just. It was somewhere for those on watch to take forty winks when the situation allowed. A halfway house.

They sat down in two chairs facing each other and said nothing. It was thought-gathering time before the match or the duel or whatever sort of competition this was going to be. Chess? Poker? Tennis? Fencing? Pistols at dawn? Tudor ran through the metaphors and remained unsure. All he knew was that this was adversarial and tricky. They didn't know who was going to lead the first card, make the first serve, take strike. He almost felt like tossing a coin.

'You going to keep that balaclava on? I know what you look like. There's no need to hide.'

She seemed to think about it, then removed the woolly disguise and flicked her head like a dog after a swim. Thick auburn hair bounced down to her shoulders. She was freckled, high cheek-boned, would have been attractive but for an off-putting set of the jaw, an air of fanaticism bordering on madness. Or was Tudor fantasizing? Maybe she just looked a bit silly.

She still said nothing, waiting for him to play a second card.

'So what on earth is this all about?' he said, trying to sound grown-up without being pompous, and not sure he was succeeding, 'What are your demands?'

'It's not as simple as that,' she said, scornfully. 'You know that.'

'Maybe,' said Tudor, 'but if we're going to negotiate, we need to have some sort of agenda. We can't negotiate nothing.'

'What did you have in mind?' she asked, sounding almost as if she meant it.

'Oh come on.' Tudor's exasperation was genuine. 'You're the one who's hijacked the ship. Terrorists have causes. That means reasons, demands. You've effectively taken us all hostage so you have to come up with terms. You release us in return for...well, in return for whatever it is that you want.'

'Who says so?'

'It's the convention.'

'We don't believe in convention. That's why we're here.' She flicked her head back, thrust out her jaw and challenged him to argue. 'Suicide bombers don't make demands,' she continued. 'The 9/11 guys didn't ask for anything. They just killed people, destroyed an American icon, panicked Dubya and his cronies into an idiot reaction. But they didn't fly into the twin towers waving a piece of paper with an agenda on it.'

'You haven't killed anyone,' said Tudor evenly, 'or destroyed anything. You're not suicide bombers. Even your guns are fake.'

'We've taken the ship,' she said, 'we can do what we like. If we want to kill people, we'll kill people. If we want to blow things up, we'll do that too.'

'You don't understand, do you?' Tudor wasn't bluffing. He didn't think she did.

'Understand what?'

'That the way Western democracies work is by appearing as unlike dictatorships as possible. In a dictatorship authority is always visible. Dictatorships rule on the basis of fear and coercion whereas democracies operate by consent. Dictators use iron fists; elected leaders hide them in velvet gloves. That doesn't mean they're not there.'

'I really don't need a lesson in political theory,' she said, disdainfully, 'Particularly one for twelve year olds.'

'Well excuse me but I think you do,' said Tudor, condescendingly. 'You seem to think that you and your friends have won something, that you've proved a point. That's not the case.'

'We control the ship,' she said. 'I want you as a mouthpiece. You're hostage number one and you'll come to no harm provided you do as you're told.'

She was blustering. Tudor told her so, angrily now.

'It's like the Falklands,' he said. 'Britain as a mature democracy had a relaxed attitude to the islands and didn't maintain a serious military garrison. That seemed to make them vulnerable to a rapacious dictatorship. So the Argentinians did what you've done. They took the islands and they were able to do so because they were not obviously defended. They were part of the free world and we treated them like that. However the Argentine Government were hopelessly naïve and in due course, and with a distressing and unnecessary loss of life, they were expelled and the government of General Galtieri was overthrown. It's the same here. The nature of the *Duchess* is that she appears vulnerable. In fact she has to appear vulnerable if she is to perform her essential function. No one wants to take a holiday on a floating fortress. However there are detailed and sophisticated plans for dealing with situations such as this and people like you.'

'Malvinas,' she said, 'they were the Malvinas. And that's a

grotesque Enid Blyton version of what actually happened and it has nothing, absolutely nothing to do with what's happening here and now.'

She was still blustering.

He told her so, angry now, 'and if you don't listen to me you'll end up dead. Your friends, too. Any time now the Master-at-Arms will press the button, put the relevant plan into action and you lot will be finished.'

She smiled the truculent smile of the super-confident or the impossibly naïve. Both, actually, thought Tudor.

'We could throw you overboard right now,' she said. 'You don't seem to realize. We're in charge. We are the masters now. We control the ship.'

Tudor shrugged.

'If you say so,' he said. In a sense, he supposed, she was right. His Falklands analogy was actually quite accurate, but the period between the coup or invasion or hijack or whatever and the arrival of the cavalry was a dodgy one. His own position like that of the officers on the bridge was undeniably fraught. For the time being at least.

'So. All right. What do you want?'

She appeared to relax.

'That's more like it,' she said. 'We'll make a little video. You'll have a list of our demands to read out but you'll frame it with a sympathetic and expert explanation of what's going on and why we're right.'

'And what *are* your demands?' he asked.

She smiled, apparently feeling that she'd regained an initiative. 'That's for me to decide and for you to find out. So are you going to co-operate?'

'I don't seem to have any alternative,' he said. 'But I wish you'd listen to what I have to say.'

'There'll be plenty of time for that,' she said. 'You and I are going to be spending quite a time with each other. I shall be interested in hearing some of your theories. And you may learn a thing or two by seeing what terrorism and hijacking are like in real life.'

Somewhere out on the crepuscular bridge a phone rang. After a few shrill tintinnabulations they ceased and an Irish voice spoke in surly monosyllables. Then a combat-geared figure appeared in the doorway.

'It's the girl,' said the goon. 'She wants to speak to the professor.'

Tipperary Tatler considered the request for a moment, then shrugged and said, 'I don't see why not. Give him the phone.'

Which he did. The woman's acquiescence seemed, to Tudor, further evidence of amateurism. In a similar situation he wouldn't have let himself talk to anyone except under strict supervision.

'Tell her,' said the Irish leaderene, 'that we'll be sending down a video shortly.'

'I'm to tell you that they'll be sending down a video.'

'Oh.' Elizabeth Burney sounded pertly amused.

'And we expect to see it broadcast on the ship's closed circuit TV within the half-hour,' said Tudor's captor, and he duly and obediently repeated the expectation, which was greeted with a sharp disbelieving laugh.

'I'm with the Master-at-arms,' said Elizabeth. 'He's an ex-SAS major with a karate platinum belt and a very old-fashioned moustache. He seems unnervingly anxious to kill people. Dishy but disturbing. I think you should warn your new friends that they have real trouble pending. Meanwhile there's just one thing he needs to know.'

'I'll pass the message on,' said Tudor.

'The major wants to know if they're armed.'

'Absolutely not,' he said. 'I'm fine. And being treated very nicely thank you.'

The goon and the girl looked at him, irritated, as if they were having second thoughts about allowing this conversation, as well they might.

'Just tell your friend that we'll be sending out the video shortly and meanwhile not to do anything stupid. And that goes for everyone else on board.'

Tudor smiled. 'I'm to tell you not to do anything stupid and that goes for everyone else on board,' he parroted.

'I'm sure Major Timbers will be trembling at the knees,' she said. 'Meanwhile we'll look forward to the film show. Take care. Over and out.'

There was a click, a buzz of static, then a dialling tone.

He handed the set back.

'Right,' he said, 'if we have a film to make I think I ought to have a look at the script.'

'I'm glad you're seeing sense,' she said.

'Sense is emphatically not what I'm seeing,' he said. 'Far from it. I've told you that I think you've got yourself in to a mess and it's going to become more of a mess and much much worse for you the longer you persevere with this silly charade. My playing along with what you want doesn't imply surrender or acquiescence or anything at all except, well . . . "playing along with you". I'll do just that but it doesn't mean you're out of trouble.'

She smirked in a way that seemed mildly deranged, then took a piece of paper from some hidden fold in her garment and handed it to Tudor.

'Demands,' she said. 'I'd like you to read them to camera but I don't want it to look as if you're being coerced in any way. So no script. Just a few cue-words and phrases. The whole thing should look like a nice cosy interview on daytime "Judy". Definitely Richard and Judy rather than Paxman or Humphries. Think David Frost. It's a conversation not an interrogation.'

'Anything you say,' he said, frowning over the green child-like handwriting. 'George Bush and Tony Blair to apologize profusely and in person at United Nations for invasion of Iraq. President Putin to withdraw all Russian troops from Chechnya.' He glanced up. 'You don't think perhaps you're being just a tiny bit optimistic?' he asked. She looked back just as scornfully and he glanced down again. 'Religious schools to be abolished,' he read. 'Hunting with hounds to be universally outlawed.'

'Are you going to make eating meat an offence?' he asked, not altogether good-naturedly.

She scowled.

'I know you think we're being naïve,' she said, 'but the fact is that most people around the world agree with us. But they're too oppressed and frightened to say so.'

Tudor nodded, all too aware that the way he did it made the gesture seem patronizing.

'Just let me rough out some notes,' he said, yawning. He suddenly felt extraordinarily tired, light-headed even. A combination of age and stress, he supposed.

Seconds later he realized he was passing out.

Only a nano-second later, he actually did so.

CHAPTER NINE

He felt as if he were coming out from under an anaesthetic. His throat was dry and sore at the back. His chest ached and his vision was blurred. He was aware of concerned, smiling, female, almost beatific faces looking down on him and wishing him well. The feeling was impotent but agreeable.

'Er . . .' he said.

'No need to say anything,' said an Australian voice which he recognized as Elizabeth Burney's. 'You've been through a little bit of an ordeal. Done well. We're all impressed. Even me.'

He tried to speak again and failed once more.

'Don't worry,' she said, 'Major Timbers says it usually takes about twenty minutes to get your voice back. After that you'll be talking quite normally. So I've got a magical little window of opportunity into which I can get a word. A rare treat.' She giggled. Tudor had an uneasy feeling that her head had been turned by the galloping major with the moustache and exotic belt.

'So sshhh!,' She put a finger to her mouth. 'You've been gassed as I imagine you know. Rupert won't be too specific about it. Just describes it as "standard-issue kit" – whatever that means.'

Rupert eh? So the major had a first name already.

'He's the Master-at-Arms,' she said, wide-eyed, 'but I expect you knew that. Most people on board call him "the Jaunty" or "the Jonty". You learn something new every day. Every ship has one. Well, every ship except Filipino rust-buckets or Taiwanese fishing smacks. Our friends, the Irish, never had a prayer against a top-class Jonty with a crack team. Major Rupert has a crack team. They double up as everything you can imagine. One of the gentleman hosts is a genius with a jemmy; his explosives expert is a drummer in the jazz band; two of the wine-waiters are snipers with medals from Bisley. You wouldn't want to mess with them even if you were serious al-Qaeda suicide-squaddies. And these guys certainly aren't.'

She smiled encouragingly.

'They're in the brig. They'll be interrogated properly. Rupert supervises that with the two ballroom dancing instructors. He does nasty and the wife does nice. It's all rather wonderful.'

He wanted to ask more about the gas and she seemed to guess as much.

'Rupert's keeping pretty shtumm about some aspects of the operation,' she said. 'He won't say exactly what the gas was and he won't say how it was introduced. He was actually rather keen to storm the bridge with stun-grenades and stuff. He seemed a bit depressed that we all wanted something stealthier and unmessy. He said storming the bridge would be good training for his "boys" but I think the real reason was that he wanted to hurt someone, maybe kill them. I get the impression that, provided it can be justified, he's slightly into killing people. Anyway whatever sent you all to beddy-byes was presumably pumped in through the air-conditioning or maybe the sprinkler system.'

The other smiling female mopped Tudor's brow with some sort of dampish cloth. It smelt of disinfectant and cheap scent, like the sort of face-towel flight attendants give out on airlines. He seemed to be back in his cabin rather than the ship's sick-bay.

'We retrieved the list of demands which was babyish, frankly, but I dare say you found time to read it before the gas hit.'

She sighed.

'We'll leave you now,' she said. 'Try and get some sleep. I'll come back in an hour or so. You may have forgotten but it's Sunday. I thought we might go to church service. They're doing matins at eleven which is just over an hour's time. You can say thank you to God for your safe deliverance.'

The girls left. Their absence rendered him oddly deflated.

He couldn't sleep so stayed supine, staring at the ceiling and thought. He was alive but could easily have been dead. At least he thought he was alive. Limbo or purgatory, if not heaven or hell, could perfectly well have been a cabin on the *Duchess* being ministered to by a couple of pretty girls. On balance, however, he was reasonably convinced that he was alive and moderately well on the high seas. He had, though, behaved recklessly and must try not to do so again. Had the Irish hijackers been even moderately professional he would almost certainly not have been spared. On the other hand he had got away with it and would, with reasonable luck, be regarded as some sort of hero. Cool in a crisis and an expert at this sort of thing; not just an armchair expert. In any event he would certainly have put one over on Sir Goronwy Watkyn. Not to mention Chief Inspector Emeritus Freddy Grim.

But what on earth had that gang been playing at? It was almost as if they were students pulling off a stunt during rag week. He wondered what would happen now. The ship was beyond territorial waters and therefore beyond any one country's jurisdiction. International law of the sea would apply although this was, he confessed to himself, not one of his major areas of expertise. Maritime Law he knew was based on the Laws of Oleron which had been codified by Eleanor of Aquitaine. In the event of mutiny on board a Royal Naval ship the mutineers were tried by courts martial and if found guilty hanged from the yard arm in front of the assembled crew. This was what happened to the guilty *Bounty* men. At the Spithead Mutiny of 1797 it was judged that their demands were legitimate, therefore no one was strung up. At the Mutiny of the Nore which followed shortly it was judged that the legitimate demands had all been satisfied after Spithead so the ring-leaders were executed, as was traditional when every man-jack took part of the insurrection and mass execution of all hands would have been impractical.

On merchant ships mutineers were tried by civil courts. However, if he were honest he couldn't be certain what was done to passengers who rose up against the ship's legitimate authority. It wasn't a frequent occurrence. Bearing in mind the so-called war on terrorism which had been carried on since the destruction of the New York World Trade Centre on 9/11 anyone attempting to hijack a cruise-ship could reasonably expect to be shot out of hand. The US Marine Corps didn't take prisoners.

He sighed.

It was all quite mystifying. And the 'demands' had been grotesquely naïve. It was almost as if the gang had gone into operation demanding the answer no, determined to fail. But what would be the point of that? Perhaps they had been hired by Riviera so that the shipping line could be made to look good. There was a horrid plausibility about that in the modern world. On the other hand the ragtag band of brothers and sisters he had encountered on the bridge didn't feel like actors from Central Casting. Tudor was not, by nature, a conspiracy theorist belonging firmly in the cock-up camp. He found it inconceivable that even in the age of spin a cruise company would stage an act of high-seas piracy in order to demonstrate the reliability of their own security procedures and systems.

This afternoon he was scheduled to deliver his 'Mutiny on the *Bounty*' talk. This seemed at one and the same time both more and yet less significant. The incident this morning gave him first-hand experiences on which to draw and yet a contemporary brush with disaster made a history lecture seem pretty irrelevant. Why care about mid-Pacific mid-eighteenth century when you'd experienced a state-of-the-art, man-of-the-moment equivalent in the here-and-now? Tudor would have his work cut out to demonstrate the reason for talking about the *Bounty* when what everyone wanted to know about was the *Duchess*. Heigh-ho!

He dozed. Images flickered across his subconscious like scenes from an old movie. He saw lifeboats from *Titanic* overturning; Trevor Howard as Captain Bligh berating Marlon Brando as Fletcher Christian – were they actually in the same movie?; Jack Hawkins in *The Cruel Sea*; Humphrey Bogart as Captain Queeg rolling dice in the Herman Wouk classic whose name eluded him. *The Caine Mutiny* that was it. Mutiny seemed the operative word and yet what had happened this morning was not a mutiny in the accepted sense.

His mind was wandering. Bloody nerve gas. Bound to have a disorientating effect. Wouldn't be a nerve gas if it didn't. It would wear off presumably. Timbers and Co must be aware of its properties. He'd be right as rain in a minute or so. Church parade would sort him out. Hand of God and all that. Thinking of Timbers and his lot though gave one pause for thought, didn't it? It was obviously essential in the post-9/11, Iraq-invasion world for ships such as the *Duchess* to carry discreet private armies as protection against terrorism in any shape or form, but private armies were, almost by definition, susceptible to bribes and blandishments. That was, after all, the definition of a mercenary.

What God abandoned, these defended,
And saved the sum of things for pay.

Housman. It was a cynical trade. You made yourself available to the highest bidder. Patriotism, loyalty, belief, fanaticism, call it what you like...these buttered no parsnips with men like Major Timbers. Both the Umlauts and the Prince of Araby could match any bids made by, well, anyone. On the other hand, Tudor guessed, selling out to the highest bidder would, if it meant changing sides in mid-stream, be ultimately bad for business. Trust might be too cosy a word for terrorism and its counterpart, but there would have to be honour among thieves. If you got a reputation for breaking contracts you wouldn't last long even in that murky world.

He must have dozed off again for when he was next aware of anything it was of a hand on his shoulder and the radiant and intelligent eyes of Elizabeth Burney staring into his.

'Church parade,' she said, half-mocking, half-affectionate, not even marginally respectful. 'If you're not feeling a whole lot better already you will be after a hymn or two and some robust words from our glorious captain. I had a quick look at the menu and they're doing "Eternal Father Strong to Save"; the Old Testament lesson is Genesis Seven.'

'There went in two and two unto Noah into the ark . . . the

male and the female,' intoned Tudor wearily. 'That's a bit corny.'

'Attaboy,' said Elizabeth clapping her hands together. 'No permanent ill-effects from nerve gas. Just like Shiver-my-Timbers said.'

'Shiver-my?' repeated Tudor.

'Someone called Major Timbers simply has to have a nick-name,' she said. 'And I don't, under the circumstances, see how it could conceivably be anything else.'

'And I suppose the second lesson is Matthew, Chapter Twenty-four, verse Thirty-eight.'

' "For as in the days that were before the flood they were eating and drinking, marrying and giving in marriage, until the day that Noe entered into the ark, and knew not until the flood came and took them all away." '

'How did you know that?' asked the girl, impressed.

'They always do a double-Noah on the first Sunday after embarcation,' he said. 'It's a bit obvious, but passengers seem to like it. The idea of being descended in some curious way from Mr and Mrs Noah rather appeals to them though I don't think the ark would have satisfied modern safety regs and I don't suppose the catering would been any great shakes.'

'No rum punch in the captain's bar,' said Elizabeth. 'I always imagine the ark must have been incredibly smelly.'

'Probably,' said Tudor. He was beginning to feel a lot better. Heroic even. He stood up and went into the bathroom where he splashed his face liberally with cold water.

'Five minutes before kick off,' she said, chirpily, opening the cabin door and hustling him outside.

They walked briskly and in silence along the corridors and up to the doors of the cinema which doubled up, on these occasions, as morning chapel, ecumenical. It was slightly unconvincing, tasteless even, but not as unconvincing or even, in a manner of speaking, tasteless as the figure standing at the entrance clutching a Bible and prayer book and wearing a cassock and a sanctimonious expression.

It was Freddie Grim, but to Tudor's amazement, no longer retired Detective Chief Inspector Grim, but the Reverend Grim. Policeman Fred appeared to have taken to Holy Orders.

CHAPTER TEN

Grim's was a bizarre sermon. ' "Water, water everywhere and not a drop to drink",' he began, in a nasal sing-song voice which reminded Tudor of Jonathan Miller's vicar in 'Beyond the Fringe.' ' "My brother Esau is an hairy man, but I am a smooth man".' Grim's words made about as much sense. His theme was H_2O but he was drowned by it, engulfed. No ark for Grim.

In a perverse way Tudor quite enjoyed trying to work out what exactly it was that the newly ordained preacher was trying to say. He was certainly moving in a mysterious way but it was difficult if not impossible to work out what lay behind the mystery and if there was any method at all in the apparent madness. Tudor wouldn't have given him a licence.

Meanwhile the *Duchess* was heading into a storm. The curtain behind the makeshift altar was waving mesmerizingly and metronomically at the beginning of the service but by the time they reached the second hymn it had moved from the gentle sleepy seduction of Force Five to the dangerous billowing of Eight or Nine. Preacher Grim had to brace his sea legs and hold fast to the lectern. One or two of the congregation wove an uneasy path out of the cinema.

'The animals went in two by two,' said Reverend Grim. 'Two by two. Not individually one by one; not even in threesomes where one of them would have been what later generations call a gooseberry; not in a herd, nor a flock, nor a crowd, nor a group, nor a team, but two by two.'

Here he paused and glared round the auditorium as the curtain flapped behind him and the floor rose and fell.

'Two by two,' he repeated, 'two by two.'

'The animals are going out two by two,' whispered Elizabeth behind her hand as another queasy couple made for the exit.

Grim now seemed lost for words, his attention distracted by the gathering storm and the diminishing congregation. Then, with an obvious effort, he pulled himself together and relaunched himself. 'When,' he said, 'in a previous life I was often confronted by sin and its wages I found myself deliberating on the subject long and hard. Long and hard.' And here, he stared around the cinema with the demonic gaze of an Old Testament prophet or a Methodist preacher in the Wesleyan tradition.

'Why's he repeating everything?' asked Elizabeth in another whisper.

'Because he can't think what to say next,' said Tudor unkindly. 'Or,' he added even less kindly, 'because it's something they taught him in preaching college. Trick of the trade.'

'What I learned in a life surrounded by criminals and immersed in crime was that actually the most serious crime of all, that of murder, the taking of human life, which is not only a crime against humanity but a sin against God, murder is very rarely a criminal crime. That is to say that in my experience – in my very varied and lengthy experience – I very rarely came across criminals who killed.

'Murder was much more frequently . . . very much more frequently...committed by those who, like the animals who went into the ark, lived their lives two by two. For as the wife said of her husband, or it could just as well have been the husband saying of the wife, when asked, if during their long marriage, he, or she, had ever considered divorce, replied, "Divorce never, murder frequently." He stared at the now thin congregation, eyes revolving unnervingly and was rewarded with a mild titter.

'Lady Longford,' said Tudor under his breath, 'speaking of the noble Earl.'

'It's a very old joke,' whispered Elizabeth, 'and almost certainly apocryphal.'

God alone knew where Freddie Grim went from here. He seemed to be talking about the perils yet sanctity of marriage and to be pegging his remarks to the notion that many of those cruising aboard the Good Ship *Duchess* were celebrating significant wedding anniversaries. For couples such as this read animals two by two; for the *Duchess* read the ark; and presumably for Noah read the Master of the *Duchess*, Sam Hardy.

It was odd, thought Tudor, that the Master was not present. Perhaps, aware of the impending storm, he had decided that his place was on the bridge. Yet that seemed unlikely for Sam Hardy only ever thought of the bridge as the place to be when he was showing passengers around it. He would normally be here with a big black prayer book leading matins the way ship captains were popularly supposed to.

'So you see,' said the preacher, 'nothing could seem cosier or more companionable, or safer than a voyage at sea in the company of one's beloved partner. The ark represented sanctuary and safety. She was a refuge from a naughty world. Indeed in that particularly disastrous moment in the world's history she represented the only place in which one could live. Everybody else perished.

'And yet' – and here he wagged a finger at his now seriously depleted audience – 'and yet, the safety of the closed room which is another way of looking at a modern cruise liner or an ancient ark is a deception and a delusion. There is no safety at sea, no safety in an enclosed space but, above all, my brothers and sisters there is no safety with those you consider your nearest and dearest. It was Jean Paul Sartre, no Christian he, who told us that hell is other people. *Huis Clos*.'

He paused and gazed round again. Tudor had a distinct impression that either he or the preacher were going mad. 'It was right for Noah,' said Grim. 'Noah was six hundred years old when he built the Ark and when he disembarked he lived on for another three hundred and fifty. And it was all right for those who sailed with him. But it wasn't all right for those that were left behind. Remember what happened? ' "Every living substance was destroyed which was upon the face of the ground, both man and cattle, and the creeping things, and the fowl of the heaven, and they were destroyed from the earth: and Noah only remained alive, and they that were with him in the ark".'

'What's he trying to say?' muttered Elizabeth.

'I think he's telling us that he knows his Bible inside out,' said Tudor, 'otherwise I just don't get it.'

'So what, in the end, did God mean by this?' asked Grim. 'What is the underlying message in the story of Noah and the ark and the animals that went in two by two and all those creeping things and the clean and the unclean? What possible relevance can it have for the rest of us?'

And now he looked around with a baleful air of triumph as if he had come to the end of a difficult task but had prevailed in the end.

'Our Master on board this ship will not live to be nine hundred and fifty years old as Noah did,' he said. 'But at the same time we would do well to ponder the words with which our Lord ended the dreadful story of the flooding of the earth and the saving of the human race on board ship. He said, ' "I will not again curse the ground any more for man's sake; for the imagination of man's heart is evil from his youth; neither will I again smite any more every thing living, as I have done".'

And here the retired policeman smiled a huge grin of baleful self-satisfaction, crossed himself and said, 'And so in the name of God the Father, God the Son and God the Holy Ghost, Amen.' After which in a voice subtly changed from that of inspirational preacher to official factotum, he announced that the final hymn was to be "Eternal Father strong to save whose hand hath bound the restless wave" and during it a collection would be taken in aid of the Royal National Lifeboat Association.

Tudor sang lustily and gave generously; Elizabeth remained stumm and gave nothing. At the end of the hymn they all bowed their heads while Grim pronounced a blessing and told them to go in peace. This they duly did.

'Fascinating sermon,' said Tudor, outside in the lobby. 'Fascinating' was one of the most useful words in his semantic armoury, suggesting huge enthusiasm while actually doing no such thing. He suspected, from Grim's sickly grin of acknowledgement that the policeman/priest recognized the device for what it was.

'I'm glad you enjoyed it,' he said.

It was on the tip of Tudor's tongue to point out that he hadn't broached the matter of enjoyment, but instead he said, guardedly, 'Plenty of food for thought,' he said.

'Drink for thought,' said Elizabeth accurately but unhelpfully. 'One of the most liquid addresses I've ever heard.'

Grim turned his rheumy eyes on her as if noticing her for the first time.

'Thank you my dear,' he said, clearly not meaning it.

He then reverted to Tudor and said, 'Certain amount of excitement this morning, I understand.'

It was a question masquerading as a statement.

' "Exciting" is a bit strong,' said Tudor wearily and warily. 'All in a day's work for people such as you and I. There was an incident of sorts but it was all easily resolved. No harm done. A handful of silly people handcuffed together in the brig but nothing that couldn't be resolved by a mixture of intellectual rigour and a straight bat.'

'How very British,' said Grim. 'I look forward to hearing more in due course.'

Saying which he turned to other members of the congregation who were still filtering out into the Sunday morning.

'I fancy a walk round the deck,' he said to Elizabeth Burney. 'Coming?'

She said she thought that sounded like a half decent idea and would probably do him good so they went up a flight of stairs to the promenade deck, shoved open one of the heavy doors and were beaten back by the wind which was rising in strength.

'OK?' asked Tudor.

'Yup,' she said, looking frail and vulnerable but no longer fooling her mentor.

They leaned into the wind and walked.

Seconds later they bumped into Mandy Goldslinger. She was wearing a designer track-suit and walking in the wrong direction.

'*Dottore*!' she screeched above the gathering storm. 'You're dead. It's official. How's it feel?'

She was clutching a piece of paper. It turned out to be the hard copy of an e-mail from the obituaries department of the *Daily Telegraph* in London. The author was David Twiston-Davies, the paper's chief obituarist and he was researching a eulogy of the distinguished Criminal Student Dr Tudor Cornwall who, he was reliably informed, had just perished at sea under distressing and violent circumstances.

'Good, eh?' cackled La Goldslinger mirthlessly. 'Never believe anything you read in the newspapers. Had you on the right ship though. Or off it, eh!' and she shoved him in the shoulder almost knocking him over.

'Ah,' said Tudor, making the obvious connection with the sinister amateurs with whom he had been grappling earlier in the day. 'Not *Tipperary*?'

'I thought that might interest you,' she said. 'You might want to run it past the prisoners in the bilges. But that's not all.'

A larger than usual wave rocked the boat causing all three to stagger and clutch on to the nearest railings. The next revelation from Mandy Goldslinger also made Tudor and Elizabeth stagger though not as literally as the wave.

'I called Twiston-Davies,' she said, 'to tell him that you were still very much alive. He sounded halfway between relieved and irritated. Said he'd put a lot of work in on the piece and was I quite sure as they were rather hoping to make you their lead – it being a slow death day. He also said his informant was absolutely adamant about your having passed away. He was an old friend of yours as well, apparently. The Visiting Professor at the IISWP.'

'Don't tell me,' said Tudor, 'I think I can guess.'

But Elizabeth Burney did the guesswork for him.

'Ashley Carpenter,' she said. 'It has to be Ashley.'

Ms Goldslinger arched immaculately painted eyebrows and glanced from one to the other.

'How did you know?' she asked.

Tudor and Elizabeth glanced at each other and shrugged.

'He had to crop up sooner or later,' said Tudor.

Elizabeth simply frowned.

'Greatly exaggerated,' he said, 'rumours of my death.'

' 'Course you're not dead, darling,' said the cruise director. 'I know a stiff when I see one. Had enough in my day. Hardly a cruise goes by when a gentleman host or his client doesn't topple off the perch and end up in the refrigerator between the lobster and the Aberdeen Angus rib-eye.'

Elizabeth Burney looked incredulous and seemed on the verge of speech but Tudor quelled her with a vividly alive-looking glare.

'So the Twister thinks I'm dead,' he said. 'How so? Who's his source?'

'Well,' said Mandy with a lascivious leer, 'the story seems to have come out of the International Institute for the Study of World Republicanism.'

'Which must be somewhere in North Carolina,' said Tudor.

'Or Bulgaria,' said Elizabeth.

'Close but no cigar,' said Mandy. 'You're on track. It's not really international, it doesn't really study anything, it . . . oh well, shit, it's a Mickey Mouse sort of a place but they seem to have stacks of money and nothing much to do but make trouble and stuff.'

The stormy winds did blow and the trio braced their legs as the Arabian wives marched past in close formation and billowing burnooses, eyes firmly straight ahead and undeviating.

'So the International Institute for the Study of World Republicanism told the *Daily Telegraph* I was dead. Where are they when they are at home if not Bulgaria or North Carolina? Don't tell me. Bolivia. They're big in La Paz.'

' 'Fraid not,' said the cruise director. 'Irish outfit. The postal address is Limerick.'

CHAPTER ELEVEN

Ashley Carpenter was Moriarty to Tudor's Sherlock Holmes.

It wasn't as simple as that. How could it be? Fact was, in his experience, always more complicated and far-fetched than fiction. He and Carpenter had an edgy, complex reality that the melodramatic Victorian cut-outs of Holmes and Moriarty necessarily lacked.

Carpenter had been satisfactorily absent from Tudor's life for a while now, to such an extent that Tudor almost believed he had vanished for good, perished in some unobserved disaster at his own Reichenbach Falls perhaps, or vanished into Mexican gunsmoke like Ambrose Bierce. Yet so far, Ashley had never quite gone away, and he always cropped up unexpectedly just when Tudor had almost forgotten him.

Not that he could ever entirely forget, not as long as the precocious Elizabeth Burney remained under his wing. Elizabeth was Carpenter's legacy, a farewell gift after that Visiting-Fellowship which made Tudor wince whenever he thought of it.

The two of them had been best of friends at university – or so Tudor believed. Only years later when Ashley invited his former fellow-student to spend a semester in his hometown 'uni' did Tudor come to believe otherwise. Ashley had asked him down under and then done a bunk and set Tudor up on a murder rap. It sort of hadn't worked out and in some curious and still unexplained act of final revenge Carpenter had bequeathed him Elizabeth, his own former mistress. Or so Tudor believed. It was not something he and Elizabeth ever discussed. Indeed until now the words Ashley Carpenter had scarcely passed their lips. Theirs was an unusual relationship, founded largely on evasion and unspoken words.

They had in the phrase of the day, 'moved on.' In another piece of bromide vernacular they had drawn a line under what had gone before. And yet as they both knew neither option was really available. Life and lives were not like that. They were all of a piece. You could not simply create a new identity for yourself and repudiate all that had gone before. Your past was part of your present and would inevitably inform your future. And Ashley Carpenter was part of Tudor's past and Elizabeth's as well. Try as they might they could not eradicate him and pretend he had never been. Now here he was, back with a vengeance.

'So,' said Tudor, as the ship tossed and they turned back down the starboard promenade deck, buffeted by the gale-force wind, 'did you know anything about this?'

'Of course not.' The girl looked put out. 'Ashley's history.' she said. 'You know that.'

Cornwall leaned against the rail and looked out over the swirling whitecaps, feeling the salt on his face. 'Maybe you're Ashley's sleeper. You've been put in place, lulled me into a false sense of well-being and acceptance and then just when I least expect it you explode. An emotional suicide bomber, programmed to go off at the most lethal moment.'

She snorted. 'Clever analogy,' she said, 'but insulting. I'm shocked. Anyone would think you didn't trust me.'

'Let's go in,' he said abruptly. 'I need a strong coffee and a straight think.'

It was a relief to escape the raw wind and spume and to find oneself rocking comparatively gently at the bar while Boris's espresso machine fizzed and fumed.

'Did you like Ashley?' he asked the girl.

She wrinkled her nose. 'That's sort of the wrong question,' she said thoughtfully. 'Liking or not liking was never part of the equation with Ashley. He was a sort of Svengali figure and I was mesmerized. You don't like or dislike people in situations like that. I was in thrall. *Thrall*. There's a word. I'm not even exactly sure what it means but that's what I was in. Bad place to be. Much better off out of it.'

Their coffees came. The ship rocked.

'Maybe I was in thrall to Ashley once upon a time too,' said Tudor. He felt comfortable suddenly. The insecurity of the abortive hijacking and the threat of the storm outside seemed to have abated. Disconcertingly he found himself thinking of modern shipwrecks. *Titanic*, of course, but more recently the car ferry *Estonia* which capsized in the Baltic in 1994 killing more than 800. Tudor's own opinion regarding the disaster was that it was an accident brought about by faulty design, shoddy maintenance – greed, indiscipline and a furious storm. There was however, a conspiracy theory led by a former TV reporter called Jutta Rabe. Tudor had read her book and talked to many of those concerned. Jutta Rabe had made a film of the tragedy starring Greta Scacchi as an intrepid German TV reporter. Tudor had thought it ridiculous. However he could not completely discount the theory that the ship's bows had been blown off by explosive charges planted by former KGB agents who escaped in a lifeboat and were never found. The notion seemed fanciful and melodramatic, but then conspiracy theories nearly always did and sometimes they were correct.

More to the point, in a way, was the sense of complete security which preceded the capsize. Hundreds of people were drinking in the bars; many others were in their cabins, tucked up, asleep, lulled there by the seductively soporific motion of the ship. Much as now, moving to and fro on a bar stool, contemplating a serious double espresso in five star comfort alongside a pretty person with dangerous legs and lips. What could be safer?

It reminded him of that remark in Conan Doyle about the smiling English countryside actually being a much more dangerous place than the snarling English city. Boris' Bar on the *Duchess* had an almost womb-like quality with its serried ranks of single malts and insect-riddled tequilas. Boris himself shimmered about shaking cocktails smoothly and exuding a reassuring charm. The carpets were thick. The sepia prints of ancient ships and seafarers spoke of history and tried and tested values. There was a scent of expensive cigar and Chanel.

Yet . . . it would be stretching a point to say that they were sitting in a floating death-trap but this place was nowhere as safe as it seemed. Like life itself. One of the obvious discoveries he had made in the course of his academic career was that the only way most people got through life was because they believed that life would always continue in a placid almost somnolent almost entirely predictable fashion. If you could see the horrors around the corner you'd give up immediately, slash your wrists or throw yourself somewhere from a great height.

This was an obvious fact but academics devoted their lives to stating the obvious in a mildly obfuscatory manner designed to impress the laity. It was almost a definition of his role: to spend a long time and much research in order to demonstrate a proposition which most people thought too obvious to be worth discussing. You took some corny old adage such as 'Pride comes before a fall' and conducted a number of case-studies, got a market research company to issue questionnaires to demonstrate that in 51 per cent of all known cases pride did indeed come before a fall, but that notwithstanding this, the chances of it doing so were significantly greater if you were a low earning smoker from the Scottish borders than if you were an affluent retired non-smoker in the Home Counties.

The proposition he now considered was how the time to really worry about some unexpected disaster was when you were feeling most secure. That was when these things struck. That was what happened on the *Estonia* and the *Titanic*. Those on board, believed, against all the evidence that the vessels were unsinkable. 'Blow, blow thou winter wind/ Thou art not so unkind/ As man's ingratitude.' Shakespeare. *As you Like it*. But had Shakespeare ever really been in a tempest? Were his storms truly convincing? Did he, like J.M.W. Turner, lash himself to the mast of a struggling ship in order to experience the reality of a storm at sea. Did it really matter? What price imagination?

'Penny for them,' said Elizabeth, at his elbow.

'I was just thinking how good the coffee was and how much I needed it. Also that I'm speaking this afternoon and I'm not sure how much enthusiasm I can really muster for the *Bounty* and Bligh.'

'I don't believe a word of it,' she said. 'You were thinking about Ashley. Trying to get inside his head.'

'Why ask if you know the answers?' he said, 'Little Miss Know All.'

She was right of course. If she had been wrong he wouldn't have been so unreasonably irritated. Getting inside the head of your opponent, the criminal, was one of the first essentials of good detection. It was the most obvious reason for the

West's inability to cope with al-Qaeda. Very few westerners, especially those in the security services, had the knowledge and sophistication to get inside the heads of Islamic preachers or disaffected Asian youths. He, Tudor, probably didn't have what it took to get inside the head of Ashley Carpenter. Nevertheless he knew that that was where the answers lay. Psychological understanding.

It was why the old-fashioned custom whereby coppers hung out with villains, drank in their dens, flirted with their molls and were, shamefully, often as bent as the criminals they were supposed to be chasing, was in some ways more effective than the modern ivory tower methods involving DNA and the internet. Same went for crime reporting. The old-fashioned ways may have seemed primitive or politically incorrect but they were often effective.

'You're away with the fairies,' she said. The ship lurched suddenly and their coffee cups slid in unison down the bar counter spilling as they went.

'I suppose,' he admitted. Then, in self-vindication, said, 'I was only thinking. There's a lot to think about.'

'Fancy sharing some of them?'

He looked at her, wondering, not for the first time, what was going on inside that pretty little head of hers and then cursing himself for being so patronizing even though he was keeping these male-chauvinist thoughts to himself.

'The more I know about crime,' he said, 'the more I understand how little I know. That's life, but even so. I mean, I think Ashley is obsessional about me for some reason I don't properly understand. I always liked him. Or thought I did. He seems to hate me. I don't understand why. And if I don't fully understand why I'll never be able to predict what he'll do next. Which is true of nearly all criminal activity.'

'Ashley is beyond understanding,' she said, with feeling.

'He's almost certainly criminally insane which means that someone who is sane and law-abiding is in serious trouble when it comes to comprehending what makes Ashley tick. I don't think anyone who isn't barmy can ever properly come to terms with someone who is – despite what shrinks say. But, hey, I thought this cruise was supposed to be a rest?'

Tudor retrieved his coffee and sipped.

'That's the theory,' he said. 'Sometimes they are. Just as often they're so stressful you need a holiday when you get home.'

He suddenly felt a need to unburden himself and slip into confessional mode. However, he was saved by the bell – literally. The bell was electronic and amplified and signified twelve noon. When it had finished sounding a voice came over the Tannoy. It was Scottish.

'Hi, ladies and gentlemen, boys and girls,' it began unpromisingly. 'This is your Staff Captain, Angus Donaldson, speaking from the bridge. It is twelve noon and we are approximately three hundred miles west of Ireland steaming at a speed of approximately fifteen knots through winds of around Force Seven. And the first thing I should say, apart from wishing all and every one of you a very good day, is to apologize on behalf of the Master of the *Duchess*, Captain Sam Hardy. Unfortunately, Captain Sam became unwell in the night and is suffering from laryngitis.

'I am happy to tell you that he is not actually suffering. Indeed he ate a hearty breakfast and he would be here with us talking to you today were it not for the fact that due to the illness from which he is suffering he has lost his voice completely.'

Captain Donaldson had clearly not lost his. One after another not particularly funny Scottish jokes, followed each other in a staccato stand-upspeakery of one-liners.

Interspersed among these there were one or two more or less pertinent facts about the ship's position and prospects. Donaldson did not, at any stage, allude to the dramatic incident involving the *Tipperary Tatler* girl and her friends. After about five minutes of wittering he signed off with an old chestnut about an Englishman, a Welshman and a Scotsman and what people wore under their kilts.

Tudor looked at his pupil and she gazed back at him.

'What do you make of that?' he asked. 'Old Captain Birds Eye seemed his usual implausible self last night.'

'That's what I thought,' she said.

'So?'

'Fishy,' she said, arching her eyebrows. 'Captain overboard perhaps? A bridge too far?'

Tudor frowned but said nothing.

CHAPTER TWELVE

They lunched off caviar in the Dowager's Diner and sat at a table next to Prince Abdullah. Tudor always lunched off caviar when guest-lecturing. It was an extravagance he could otherwise not afford and it was relatively slimming despite the soured cream and the blinis. The restaurant, despite its kitsch name, was extravagantly elegant and reserved for the use of those in suites or the most expensive staterooms. Tudor and Elizabeth Burney somehow just made the cut largely thanks to the good offices of Mandy Goldslinger. Only Sir Goronwy and Lady Watkyn of the other guest speakers were similarly honoured. Little Freddie Grim was a class or two below in the Baroness Brasserie and gentlemen hosts such as Ambrose Perry were way beneath the salt and, almost, the water-line in the Butler's Pantry.

The Prince ate mulligatawny soup, steak and kidney pudding, and jam roly poly. In between courses he smoked untipped Passing Cloud cigarettes. Tudor and Elizabeth watched out of the corners of their eyes with an almost awed fascination.

Eventually when all three were drinking coffee and the Prince was smoking yet another cigarette, he spoke.

'I do hope,' he said, in a nasal parody of an Oxford-BBC-

Wodehousian accent, 'that my smoking does not cause offence.'

Tudor and Elizabeth, both of whom would have much preferred a non-smoking dining-room, shook their heads and murmured polite nothings.

Evidently encouraged by this the Prince unbent.

'Smoking at mealtimes is customary in my country,' he said, smiling. 'Just as it used to be in yours. However, the use of nicotine appears to have become unfashionable. In fact' – and here he leaned towards them in a conspiratorial way – 'in fact, I am sorry to say that as the result of pressure from certain non-smoking passengers, the owners of the *Duchess* went so far as to propose a shipboard ban on the practice. Happily they have now desisted.'

The Prince was clearly eager to impart a confidence so Tudor encouraged him to do so.

'What made them do that?' he asked innocently.

'Aha,' said the Prince, stubbing out a cigarette and immediately lighting another. 'Money. As you say it speaks louder than words.'

Neither Tudor nor the girl were sure how to respond to this truism so they said nothing. However they both smiled in an encouraging way designed to make the Prince confide further.

'Between you and I,' he said conspiratorially, 'it was that fellow Umlaut. He is not a good man, Herr Umlaut. Not one of us.'

Tudor was tempted to say '*Ach so*!' or 'Don't mention the war'. Instead he merely muttered something inane about some of his best friends being German. He didn't much like the look of the Umlauts either, but it had nothing to do with xenophobia. He just didn't like the look of them. It was as simple as that. Or as complex. The half-empty, half-full argument.

'In any event,' said the Prince, 'he was easily defeated. I simply told the shipping company that if the *Duchess* was declared a no-smoking zone I should like my money back. With interest. And as I have booked the two largest and most expensive suites for the best part of the next ten years this represented a substantial amount of spondulicks, at least as far as a not particularly well-managed medium-sized commercial company is concerned.

'My grandfather made a fortune trading with river steamers on the Euphrates. He also built the world's largest yacht. You have probably heard of her. *The Ethel Selina* named after my grandmother who was English and came from Letchworth. My beloved Granny Ethel.' The Prince smiled and blew a blue smoke ring at the ceiling watching it wistfully as it dissolved above him.

'Owning your own yacht, however, is, as you would put it, a mug's game. Which is why I prefer to make my home aboard the *Duchess*.'

This was not an option available to either Tudor or Elizabeth but they nevertheless nodded in dutiful agreement as if they too were in the Forbes' Magazine top hundred richest people in the world list. Then for a moment the three of them contemplated the coincidence which had thrown together in such weird incongruity. Tudor was about to break the gathering ice with a hastily put-together platitude when the ship's klaxon sounded.

It was the daily message from the bridge but, contrary to usual practice, it was not the captain.

Tudor took a sip of wine and frowned.

'The captain seemed in good voice yesterday evening,' he said.

'Stentorian,' agreed Elizabeth.

'Like the proverbial foghorn,' said Prince Abdullah as the

staff captain chuntered on with longitudes, latitudes, gale warnings and ancient jokes.

None of the three could be bothered listening. It was perfectly obvious that they were sailing through stormy weather but that they were more or less on schedule. This was the Atlantic Ocean after all and the sturdy old *Duchess* was designed to cope with her. She might toss about a bit but she would emerge unscathed and on time. After all she had been doing so for the best part of thirty years.

'I sense some form of rodent assailing the nostrils,' said the Prince. Tudor wondered what sort of language school had taught him to maul the English tongue in such a peculiarly archaic manner. Actually it probably wasn't a language school but some sort of mad tutor hired through some hopeless rival of Gabbitas and Thring, the educational employment agency.

'The Master's vocal chords appeared to be functioning with their usual stentorian efficiency,' said the Prince. 'Would you care to join me in a sticky?'

Tudor and Elizabeth looked at each other warily. It had been a hard and unusual day so far and Tudor had a lecture to deliver. Even so, both felt that they were on the verge of an interesting break-through. They were not exactly making a new friend but they seemed on the verge of crashing a hitherto forbidding barrier. In an unexpectedly threatening little world they could use any ally they could find. It would be good to have Prince Abdullah on side, however precariously.

They settled for a Calvados apiece.

'You come here often?' asked Tudor, disingenuously, as the Staff Captain finally signed off with yet another ghastly joke.

The Prince sighed. It seemed to Tudor that the sigh was both weary and wary – a sign of fatigue and caution.

'I feel at home here,' he said, 'but perhaps not as at home as I once did.'

Tudor and Elizabeth hung on his words, smiling encouragingly, saying nothing.

'They tried to stop smoking,' said the Prince, 'until I persuaded them that it was an abuse of civil liberties. Dashed impertinence. Like this hand-washing rigmarole. I don't hold with it.'

Because of something called the Norovirus, previously known as the Norwalk Virus, passengers were required to go through a ritual hand cleansing when boarding the ship or entering any of the restaurants. All passengers were given a piece of paper which contained the admonition: *we would like to remind you that the simplest preventative measure you can take to help maintain our healthy environment is to wash your hands frequently and thoroughly with soap for at least twenty seconds and rinse them well under running water. We strongly recommend that you follow this procedure each time you use the toilet, after coughing or sneezing, and before eating, drinking or smoking. Avoid touching your mouth.*

'Bloody cheek,' said the Prince, blowing blue smoke at the ceiling. 'If I want to wash my hands before smoking I'll decide for myself, thank you. I haven't been spoken to like that since I was eight years old and that was by matron at my boarding prep.'

The Prince seemed angry.

'I have been sailing on the *Duchess* for many years and I would like to sail on the *Duchess* for many years to come,' he said. 'I have paid the company massive quantities of spondulicks, much of it on account and in advance. In return I expect service and deference. Part of which' – and here his voice went up an octave or so – 'involves having a captain who is capable of being on the bridge and speaking to the ship's passengers on a daily basis. Laryngitis, shlaryngitis, as my Jewish friends would say. Nelson would never have succumbed to such a thing. Horatio would have remained on the bridge at all times and spoken with the voice of an Englishman.'

Tudor felt that the Prince was in danger of muddling his Horatios but he said nothing, just nodded sympathetically and sipped his apple brandy.

'I'm speaking this afternoon,' he said, feeling that it was probably time to change the subject and wondering how much alcohol the Prince had consumed and whether this might prove to be a problem. He had always understood that Islam, to which presumably the Prince subscribed, involved an abstinence from alcoholic beverages, but he had seen enough of a certain sort of privileged adherent of any number of supposedly puritan creeds to realize that there were always some who considered themselves to be above the law, even if that law was God's.

'Ah. Break a leg!' said the Prince unexpectedly. 'I make it a practice never to attend lectures but I shall catch a little of what you have to say on the closed circuit television in my stateroom. On what are you holding forth?'

'I'm doing the Mutiny on the *Bounty*,' said Tudor.

'How apposite,' said the Prince. 'Or perhaps not. I trust that our gallant captain is faring better than Captain Bligh at the hands of Fletcher Christian and his fellow desperadoes even if his voice has escaped him. Do you have anything new to tell us?'

'Well . . .' Tudor thought for a moment. 'Not new exactly but my interpretation differs fundamentally from the view that Bligh was some sort of tyrannical bully who got his just deserts.'

'Ah,' said the Prince, 'a revisionist view.'

'You could say so,' said Tudor.

'I'm not sure that I share your charitable view of ships'

captains,' said the Prince. 'Certainly in modern times I believe that they should subscribe to the view that the passenger is always right. Particularly when the passenger is myself.'

Saying which he rose unsteadily to his feet, smiled over enthusiastically, waved a hand in farewell and made for the exit, banging in to one or two tables as he did so.

CHAPTER THIRTEEN

His talk went well. The *Bounty* was an obvious subject. Even if everyone hadn't seen one or other of the movies and got a fix on Charles Laughton or Marlon Brando they still had a good idea of the basic story. Tudor was a Bligh man, believing that the captain of the ship was a maligned figure and a great seaman and that Fletcher Christian was unfairly romanticized. He had a good academic grasp of the subject and had even, once, visited Pitcairn Island and talked to the descendants of Fletcher Christian and his accomplices. On this occasion, however, he didn't think it appropriate to be too academically rigorous. The sort of audience you got in the ballroom of the *Duchess* was unlikely to want anything too demanding, especially after lunch.

What went down well, as always, with a cruise-ship audience was to try to evoke a picture of the ship as an island entire unto itself, a little self-contained community far from the reach of outside civilization. This was, of course, far more true in the relatively empty and unsophisticated world of the eighteenth century. Today on oceans teeming with merchant ships and under constant surveillance by satellite and other electronic devices, one was never as isolated as the vulnerable little HMS *Bounty*. Nevertheless, as the morning's events had so dramatically demonstrated a ship at sea was, well, a ship at sea.

'No e-mails; no mobile; not even the most primitive ship's radio,' he said, theatrically. 'Nowadays the Tahitian authorities would have sent a helicopter or a gunboat and the mutineers would have been subdued with stun-guns and taken away to face the international law of the sea. Even in the middle of the Atlantic or Pacific oceans the odds are that there is another vessel within an hour or so even if it's only a Liberian registered container ship or a Taiwanese oil tanker. But back then you were well and truly on your own. And, incidentally, despite everything that has happened in the last century or so this is still a very lonely and vulnerable place to be.'

At this point he always stared around the audience hoping to instil a moment of fear and awe but knowing only too well that the swaying curtain behind him and the memories of a gargantuan alcohol-fuelled lunch behind them and of a similarly proportioned tea in prospect would be enough to lull his listeners into a sense of security however false. Besides, many of them, if not actually asleep, were certainly not paying proper attention.

At home in his lecture room at the University of Wessex on the Casterbridge campus he would have allowed himself the luxury of a snide sarcasm, but here in front of an audience of paying punters he was not as much in charge as he would have wished. He was not exactly a member of the crew but he certainly wasn't a professor addressing a bunch of students. This audience was composed of paying customers and since they paid the piper they called the tune. At home he would have been seriously rude at the expense of a sleeping student; on board ship he was compelled to allow the sleepers to snore on.

After forty minutes or so he stopped and invited questions. This was a risky enterprise. Sometimes the ship's bore moved in and droned on for minutes on end, not asking a question but simply enjoying the sound of his own voice. It was usually *his* but sometimes *hers*. In his experience there was no sexual discrimination when it came to narcolepsy. On marginally less boring occasions an 'expert' of some kind stepped up and contradicted something Tudor had said. Sometimes these people were ignorant cranks with bees in their bonnets; on other sometimes embarrassing occasions they knew more than he did. Best, under those circumstances, to put your hands up and surrender.

This time it was little Umlaut. Tudor hadn't noticed him, sitting there at the back unobtrusively, in the classic position of the man who doesn't want to be recognized, identified, called upon to speak. He was in the aisle seat of the person who wishes to escape without being called upon to do anything. Anonymity seeped from every pore. Yet the diffidence was oddly unnatural. Tudor had seldom met a man who was so obviously confident in himself.

'This morning,' said Umlaut, with assumed diffidence, '*Heute morgen*. Something happened. Very mysterious. Quite alarming. May you please tell us what precisely took place?'

'I'm terribly sorry,' said Tudor, surprised and a little discomfited, 'but I'm really here to talk about the Mutiny on the *Bounty*. I'm afraid today's events just aren't within my remit.'

'Forgive me, but were today's events not a little reminiscent of the events concerning Captain Bligh and Mr Christian?'

He had a funny way of talking, thought Tudor. It was a little like listening to dialogue written by a thriller writer whose first language was not actually English. Tudor had someone in mind but could not for the moment remember who it was. He knew several thriller writers like that.

'I really can't comment,' said Tudor. 'But you seem to know something that the rest of us do not and perhaps you would care to share that information. In what sense were today's events reminiscent of the Mutiny on the *Bounty*, Doctor Umlaut? I think we should be told.'

The little doctor looked shifty and Tudor realized that he hadn't expected his name to be known, much less called out in public.

'Private information,' he said, unconvincingly. 'I have private information that as we are outside national waters and therefore subject to no national jurisdiction but only the law of the sea, you were called in to advise on the legality of a complicated and delicate situation. No?'

'No,' said Tudor, 'or rather no comment. However on the matter of legality and jurisdiction I believe that you're mistaken. When a criminal matter arises in international waters it is treated as if the case had arisen in the country in which the vessel concerned is registered. As you know many ships today are registered, as a matter of convenience, in countries such as Liberia or Panama where justice and the law is administered with, how shall I put it, a somewhat lighter touch than some of us are used to. Luckily, however, the ship on which we have the good fortune to sail is registered in Southampton. Therefore, any misdemeanours that occur on board will be treated as if they had taken place in Great Britain itself. Malefactors will be dealt with according to Her Majesty's law. This applied, of course, to HMS *Bounty* herself. When finally apprehended those mutineers who did not evade the long hand of Brtish justice were brought back to Blighty, tried in properly constituted courts martial and, for the most part, hanged from the yard arms of His Majesty's ships at Spithead. We take a more enlightened view these days, I'm happy to say, but now if you'll excuse me I'm afraid we're completely out of time and in fairness to the macramé class, which is scheduled to begin in only five minutes, I must wind up. Thank you for coming and I look forward to seeing you at my next lecture.'

'Sod!' he said to himself, as he acknowledged the slightly half-hearted clapping. 'Try not to sound so pompous.' He knew it was a failing. When rattled, he succumbed to verbal diaorrhea, used long words where short ones would do and generally banged on. He knew instinctively that he should shut up and sit down but something in his nature made him long-winded and patronizing. He did himself no favours.

'Alpha until the questions,' said a voice at his elbow.

It was Elizabeth, grinning with the insubordinate affection he found so beguiling.

'To be honest,' he said, 'I wasn't expecting questions. Brits are usually too embarrassed. It's an American thing, running up to the microphone as soon as the speaker's finished and telling him he knows nothing.'

'Australians do it,' she said. 'We're not shy either. It's a completely British thing that false modesty. I find it rather unattractive. As you know.'

'Yes, I know,' he said, 'but Doctor Umlaut is German.'

The audience had vanished as if by magic and they were alone on stage. The only person in sight but not earshot was the sound technician in his box of tricks at the far end of the auditorium.

'German extraction,' she said. 'He hasn't lived in Germany since he was a child. He's from Leipzig. His family came out soon after the Russians moved in. He owns an island or two, but if he lives anywhere he seems to live on board ship. Useful tax dodge I imagine, and the communications are presumably excellent.'

'What exactly does he do?' Tudor wanted to know, His young protégée seemed to know practically everything there was to know about the German-sounding doctor.

She shrugged. 'Arms, property, drugs, second-hand cars, prostitution.' She sighed. 'That's what I suspect. In other words nothing nice. But it won't show up anywhere. All the paperwork will prove that he is a perfectly above-board banker of some kind. Assets, acquisitions . . . legalized gambling with other people's money. Making squillions out of ordinary people's life savings. Shunting money around so that it breeds. You know my opinion of men like Umlaut.'

'It's called capitalism,' said Tudor, mildly irritated, because once upon a time he too had had scruples and ideals and now he feared they had just become jealousy and suppressed rage. He didn't see why, in a just society, good university lecturers such as himself shouldn't inherit the earth. But somehow they didn't and it was all left to shysters like Umlaut. Never mind, he would never be able to pass through a needle and attain the Kingdom of God.

Elizabeth jabbed him playfully in the ribs.

'You know you don't believe that for a moment. You think it's theft just the same as I do.'

'No matter,' he said. 'It doesn't much matter what we think of him, nor how he makes his money. What was he getting at when he asked those strange questions? Why did he ask them in front of everyone else? Does he know something we don't?'

'You mean, is he in on the plot?'

Tudor thought for a moment. 'I suppose I do,' he said. 'I mean there are two ways of looking at this morning's fiasco. Either it was just a lot of scatterbrained Irish students indulging in an elaborate sort of rag-week stunt, or it was something altogether more significant and sinister which simply misfired.'

'We don't know that it's misfired,' said Elizabeth.

'What do you mean by that?'

'The voyage isn't over yet,' she said. 'We have three or four days before we hit New York. We're only halfway through the mystery.'

'But they're locked up,' he protested.

'That's only a key-turn. Just as easy to unlock as to lock.'

'That's silly,' he said.

'I wish I shared your certainty,' she said. 'I think there's more to this than meets the eye. I didn't care for Umlaut's questioning whatever the subtext is. I'm not happy about the captain's laryngitis. I'm deeply suspicious of half the passengers. I think we're all at risk and frankly I'd rather be safe back home in the good old U of W.'

Tudor smiled at her.

'There's absolutely nothing to worry about,' he said, wishing he felt as certain as he sounded. 'As long as I'm here representing law'n'order and intellectual rigour we have nothing to fear.'

He glanced up at the ceiling and cocked an ear for noises off.

'You know,' he said, 'unless I'm much mistaken the storm has abated and the tempest past. All sounds calm. The worst is behind us. Why don't we go outside and take another turn on deck and see if the waters are as placid as I sense?'

She stared at him as if he were deranged. Which she sometimes thought he was.

'All right,' she said, at last, 'why not?'

CHAPTER FOURTEEN

The water had become placid as the proverbial mill pond. Extraordinary, mused Tudor, how the sea could move in moments from gurly and growly to butter-wouldn't-melt-in-my-mouth. One moment the depths were all menace, the next they were stroke-your-brow-and-hold-my-hand. The wind had dropped and there were no whitecaps. All was quiet and calm. You could have sculled across this ocean in a skiff.

'Sail ho!' exclaimed a breathy voice just behind them.

Tudor and Elizabeth turned abruptly and saw Mandy Goldslinger in a Florida female approximation of a sailor suit. She wore white trousers and a white jacket, with much gold braid, buttons, epaulettes and a blue belt tightly buckled. She looked like the runner up in the best first mate competition, senior section. She smelt vaguely as if she had been drinking margaritas, swayed slightly despite the new calm but was tipsy rather than drunk.

'Sail ho!' she repeated loudly and liltingly in what she must have thought was a good imitation of a cry from the crow's nest. As she called out she gesticulated in the direction of a distant horizon and when Tudor and Elizabeth followed her outstretched hand with their eyes they were surprised to see a shape. It was not merely a ship shape but also, as the cruise director suggested, a ship under sail. A lot of it. Billowing in the prescribed manner.

'A ship,' said Cornwall fatuously.

'Not any old ship, darling,' said Mandy, 'a barquentine no less. Four masts, the tallest little short of two hundred and thirty feet; the most forward square-rigged and the three behind rigged fore and aft. I'd judge that she carries the best part of, oh I'd say around thirty-six thousand square feet of sail, and she's something over two thousand tons and about three hundred and sixty feet long. Modern, very. Judging from the way she sails I'd say she was built in Belgium possibly in the Langerbrugge Yard in Ghent. But I'd say she was registered in Luxembourg, though Swedish owned. Can't be much more than ten years old. Ask me another.'

She smiled in triumph.

'You're making it up,' said Elizabeth, visibly impressed.

'*Au contraire*,' said Mandy. 'But I'll admit we've had the bins on her from the bridge. And that wondrous display of sail doesn't entirely account for the speed she's making. That's from her twelve cylinder diesel engine which generates thirteen hundred and fifty horsepower with seven to one reduction gear operating a four-blade variable-pitch aluminium/bronze propeller that gives a speed of twelve knots—'

'Stop, stop!' said Tudor. 'My ears are bleeding.'

Ms Goldslinger laughed, a husky tinkling sound much practised and rehearsed.

'You didn't know my alter ego was Jane of *Jane's Ships*, did you? Don't worry. She's an old friend; *Star Clipper*. Klaus or Jurgen is at the wheel. They're twins so can't tell them apart. And my friend Jeffrey Rayner's on board. He says they have a surprise for us and when Jeffrey says 'surprise' he means *surprise*.'

'Like what?' Tudor wanted to know.

'He wouldn't say. Surprisingly shtumm. I thought we'd pay a visit in one of the Zodiacs. Want to come?'

Tudor glanced at the girl with a raised interrogative eyebrow and she nodded back.

'We'll give you life jackets, but I'd wear something waterproof. Warm too. It may look calm and not very far but mid-Atlantic in an open boat gets kinda choppy and chilly.' Mandy smiled a wintry smile at Elizabeth. If looks could kill this wouldn't quite have done the job but it would certainly have maimed. Or frozen. It was the coolness rather than the ferocity that was marked. Elizabeth smiled back but her eyes were almost as glacial as the cruise director's.

Five minutes later the two guests were back in yellow woolly hats decorated, slightly improbably, with the logo of the University of Wessex. They also wore anoraks. Mandy Goldslinger in a figure-hugging *Duchess* weatherproof catsuit looked superior and ushered them slinkily to a rope ladder suspended from a door several decks down. At the bottom a black inflatable bobbed dangerously alongside with three crew members lounging nonchalantly in charge. Just as they were about to set off they were joined by two thirty-something men in black wet suits. Neither Tudor nor Elizabeth recognized them. They nodded curtly. Presumably, thought Tudor, they were security officers of some sort or another. He wondered who exactly was in charge. He vaguely assumed it was Mandy Goldslinger though he wasn't entirely sure.

It was a bumpy ride. The boat's rubber bottom slapped the water as the skipper revved the show-off outboards in a display of nautical muscle-flexing. From high up on the *Duchess* the ocean looked oily and placid; down here it felt rough as stubble. As the *Duchess* receded so she began to look more and more like a stylized child's toy safely at anchor in a bath tub. Conversely, as the four-masted barquentine got closer and closer she looked more and more like the real thing. She gleamed like a well-trained thoroughbred in the paddock and if you hadn't known that she was a creature of the twentieth century with the gear to match you would have suspected her of being a close blood relation of the *Cutty Sark* bringing home tea from China at a rate of wind-blown knots.

A flight of wooden steps had been lowered over the side of the ship and two blond able-bodied seamen were standing at the bottom ready to assist the passengers' landing. Mandy Goldslinger and Elizabeth went first, armed expertly from taut rubber to polished teak and followed closely by Tudor and the two wet-suits. At the head of this collapsible staircase stood an epauletted, white-haired skipper in tropical drill and a dapper figure in white canvas trousers, espadrilles and a striped Breton jerkin whom Tudor supposed to be Mandy's friend Jeffrey Rayner. As she kissed him full on the lips Tudor felt his suspicions confirmed.

As he stepped gingerly on to the wooden deck Mandy introduced him to Rayner and the Captain who apparently had a German name that Tudor did not quite catch.

'Jeffrey and the captain have one of our boats,' said Mandy.

'I didn't know that one of our boats was missing,' said Tudor.

The wet-suits had vanished.

'No reason why you should,' said Mandy. 'Boat overboard!' She honked a brassy laugh and stopped abruptly when no one else joined in. 'Well,' she said, 'that's not a usual cry on board ship. On the other hand, our boat must have gone overboard and you'd think someone would have seen it and raised an alarm.'

There was a longish silence.

'Seems to me,' said Elizabeth, 'that almost anything could

disappear overboard on a big ship like ours without anyone noticing.'

Mandy Goldslinger went quickly into PR mode, assisted by the obvious fact that she disliked Elizabeth Burney very much, 'The crew on the *Duchess* is highly trained to detect and report the slightest irregularity at all times and in all places,' she said.

'Oh come on, Mandy,' said Tudor, 'you know that isn't true. It can't be. It's half a mile at least just to walk round the Promenade Deck. And at night when it's dark and there are virtually no outside lights, you simply couldn't see an object go over the side. And in anything more than a slight breeze you wouldn't hear it either.'

'Just a little plop as it hit the surface,' said Elizabeth. 'Plop. Then vanish never to be seen again. Easy peasy.'

'Yes,' said Mandy, 'well.' And she took out a cigarette and lit it. The captain asked her to put it out. She did, but looked furious.

'So what exactly happened?' asked Tudor. 'I mean you were just sailing along and suddenly you saw one of our lifeboats in the middle of the Atlantic.'

'Well no.' Rayner looked bothered. He and the captain had decided it was unwise to say too much on open insecure lines but now they were all together in, as it were, private, they felt secure enough to reveal that there was another ship involved. The barquentine had spotted this before they were aware of the *Duchess* lifeboat. Indeed had it not been for the presence of the larger vessel they might not have seen the lifeboat at all. She was an elderly rust-bucket of the sort that seemed to sink periodically and usually east of Suez and, thought Tudor, nearly always full of pilgrims *en route* to the Haj. But hush, that was prejudice. Rayner and the captain reckoned she was a retired cross-channel steamer of some description. She was flying an Irish flag and bore the name *Michael Collins* on her bows and stern as well as the unlikely claim to be registered in the landlocked African republic of Chad.

All attempts to establish contact with the ship failed totally. The *Michael Collins* did not respond to shouts on the loud-hailer, flags sending semaphore signals, an Aldis lamp flickering Morse Code and, least of all, to anything to do with electronics. Jeffrey Rayner had tapped her name into Google on one of the barquentine's computers and had discovered that she was some sort of floating university campus.

'Based in Limerick,' said the Captain.

'Some sort of self-proclaimed Institution for the Study of—'

'World Republicanism,' chipped in Tudor and Elizabeth, speaking in unison.

Mandy Goldslinger looked long-suffering but unsurprised. The captain and Jeffrey Rayner exchanged glances. They had never previously heard of such a thing and it obviously sounded as bogus to them as it had previously done to Tudor and Elizabeth.

'Ashley Carpenter strikes again,' said Tudor. 'Originally I assumed this was cock-up, but I'm beginning to wonder if it might not be conspiracy after all. Mind if I have a look at the boat?'

No one objected. The lifeboat had been taken on board and was sitting on the after-deck alongside the swimming-pool and looking like some sort of beached fish. It was out of its element and far from home.

Tudor clambered in. There was a brownish stain on the port side just where there was a hole in the side presumably for a rowlock, though the lifeboat had a moderately powerful inboard engine. The *Duchess* lifeboats were carefully maintained so there should have been no need to row.

'Blood?' asked Tudor, staring hard at the stain.

'We assumed so,' said the captain.

'What exactly happened?' asked Tudor, frowning knowledgeably at the supposed bloodstain.

It wasn't entirely clear what 'exactly' happened because the whole incident was so murky. *Star Clipper* had been bowling along, minding her own business and doing her inimitable greyhound-of-the-sea act when they had stumbled, as it were, on the SS *Michael Collins*, doing something furtive with the *Duchess*'s lifeboat which appeared to be tied up alongside. As soon as the *Michael Collins* realized that the sailing ship was keen to establish what was going on, the old Afro-Irish ship turned tail and scuttled off.

Tudor listened attentively to what the two men had to say and, at the same time, paced up and down the wooden lifeboat not entirely sure what he was looking for, not at all sure what exactly was going on, but uneasily aware that he himself was a part of what was happening.

The boat was essentially open and undecked, designed to take between thirty and forty survivors who would have been packed tightly on the plank-like seats. She may have been a seaworthy craft but she was primitive. There were two lockers in the bows, one on which side, secured only by doors with only rudimentary latches such as you might find in any old country cottage. Without knowing quite why he was doing so Tudor opened one of these doors and felt inside. His hand encountered something squared off and brick-like. He grasped it and lifted it out. It was cold and metallic and, as he stared at it thoughtfully, he heard Elizabeth cry out, 'That's gold. You've struck gold!'

And after he had handed it to her and knelt down to look inside the locker he realized that he had indeed struck gold, for there, packed neatly in the compartment where he had expected to find life-jackets or torches or iron rations, were a great many ingots, stacked neatly as logs in a fire-basket.

'Finders keepers,' he said, softly and facetiously.

It was a veritable treasure trove.

On inspecting a sample ingot Tudor was pleased to find that, as he suspected, the letters GR were stamped on the base. To the uninitiated this might have suggested 'George Rex' and indicated an English king called George. Tudor knew, however, that it merely indicated that the gold had been supplied by his old sparring partner Guy Roberts, now knighted and therefore 'Sir' Guy but better known as 'Golden Balls', 'Mr Goldbar', 'Goldilocks' or any one of a number of similar sobriquets involving the precious metal.

Guy was an Eton and Oxford-educated smoothie who had unexpectedly gone into the world of gold-trading which was traditionally dominated by Essex-boy traders in leather jackets. Guy had taken this world by storm to such an extent that within a decade he was the world's leading expert on the subject.

One of his stocks-in-trade was supplying gold bars to the mega-rich as an insurance against fluctuations in markets of all kinds. He gave billionaires the chance of the plutocratic equivalent of hiding used fivers under the mattress or the stair carpet. His clients were men such as Umlaut or Prince Abdullah and he offered them a rainy-day safety net. The Umlauts and Abdullahs of this world avoided tax by having their offices and headquarters in a floating tax haven. The naïve pirates from the Emerald Isle had come up with the luck of the Irish. Stumbling on this sort of treasure trove was a brilliant fluke. But being flukey didn't make it less brilliant.

CHAPTER FIFTEEN

The lifeboat and the gold ingots returned to the *Duchess* whence, presumably, they had come. No one aboard the *Star Clipper* seemed distressed by their departure; indeed they seemed relieved to be rid of them.

'So what do you make of that?' asked Elizabeth, as they clambered back on board the cruise ship. Turning back on the promenade deck they leaned against the rail and watched the barquentine let out sails and gather speed on her passage towards the Mediterranean. Music of some kind came wafting across the waves. It could have been Van Gelis or something more classical. Distance lent the melody charm and ambiguity.

There was no one else in earshot.

'I've heard of returning to the gold standard,' said Tudor, 'but I never thought I'd see it in practice. How much do you imagine that gold's worth?'

'Ask me another,' said Elizabeth. 'Stocks and shares may break my bones but gold . . .' She shrugged. 'I simply don't know. But that's a lot of gold. A hundred ingots, do you think? And whatever else gold keeps its price. Safer than houses. Maybe not as spectacular as a shrewd property investment or Princess Margaret's jewellery but as safe as, well, houses.'

'Safer than bricks and mortar, wouldn't you say?'

Tudor frowned into the gathering gloom.

'I'd say they were kilo bars. And if you're talking about two hundred pounds an ounce, which I guess you are, then each bar is worth about seven grand, I would have thought we were looking at at least five hundred bars which would add up to around three and a half million quid. Not a lot these days but a useful stand-by for moments of need. Better than a piggy bank.' This was unexpected.

'You what?' He was taken by surprise. One minute she professed complete ignorance and the next she came up with some arcane remark which indicated exactly the reverse. Maddening woman.

'I'd say that the gold bars in that lifeboat add up to about three and a half million quid.'

The information hung in the salty air like a corpse waiting for dissection. A skilful forensic wielding of the scalpel should carve out some missing secrets. In clumsy hands, however, the knife might reveal nothing at all.

'So,' said Tudor thoughtfully, 'you're telling me that one of the *Duchess*'s lifeboats went AWOL in the middle of the night with three and a half million pounds of gold ingots on board. It fetches up against an unlikely floating college of an equally improbable Irish university which is surprised by our elegant flying greyhound of the sea. The Irish rustbucket does a bunk and the boat fetches up with Jeffrey and his pals with the loot intact but no human occupant and a sinister-looking bloodstain on board.'

'*Presumed* bloodstain,' said Elizabeth sharply. 'We don't know it was blood and we've no way of proving it one way or the other. Not until we reach New York.'

'I don't want to wait till New York; I want to solve this at sea. As you say – one way or another. I don't trust any police force to get this one right. Least of all the Americans.'

Like many Englishmen he was sceptical about American expertise while actually having very little real first-hand experience of it. He was prejudiced and convinced of his own skills. Sometimes this self-confidence was justified and sometimes not. On this occasion he did not have to compete with any form of official police force but on the other hand he had some experienced opposition from among his fellow passengers. He was almost forgetting Sir Goronwy Watkyn and the former CID inspector, Freddie Grim. No doubt also senior members of the *Duchess*'s crew would also want their pennyworth. He would have to move fast for all sorts of reasons. In a sense, too, he already had an excess of evidence and a surfeit of information: idiotic Irish terrorists in the brig, gold ingots in an abandoned lifeboat, a mysterious bloodstain and a missing captain. It was almost too much.

He was less and less inclined to believe the story of laryngitis explaining the captain's disappearance. A throat infection was too much to swallow in more ways than one. As far as he was concerned the captain was missing. It was not just his voice that was lost.

'You could just wash your hands of the whole thing. Leave it till we dock in New York and let the professionals handle it.'

'I *am* the professional,' he said coldly. 'As you perfectly well know I have a professional reputation to maintain. If we reach the United States with these mysteries unsolved the name of the University of Wessex will be mud.'

Elizabeth did not say what she was thinking which was that sometimes her boss could seem a little absurd. She admired him much of the time and there was no doubting his knowledge and abilities. Sometimes, however, he over-reached himself and she was beginning to wonder whether this might not be one of those occasions.

'Penny for them,' she said, wrinkling her nose and looking quizzical, 'What are your thoughts, oh Mighty One?'

She had the rare knack of being able to send him up without his being irritated. Or, she sometimes thought, even noticing.

'There are only two people on board ship who strike me as being rich enough to have that sort of loot on board. Likewise the same two people are just the sort of oddball, fly-by-night characters who might want to have ready cash in a reliable but disposable form. Your average Goldman Sachs wunderkind wouldn't be on the Gold Standard.'

'But Umlaut or Prince Abdullah might be?'

'What made you think of those two?' Tudor asked, irritably.

'I'm not stupid,' she said. 'Or hadn't you noticed?'

He smiled.

'So whoever was in the lifeboat nicked Umlaut or the Prince's pocket money and was about to transfer it to the Irish university rustbucket when they were surprised by the *Flying Dutchman*.'

'So the thief,' she said, pursing her lips in thought, 'went aboard the floating Irish ivory tower but left the gold on the lifeboat because he was a guilty thing surprised.'

'Something like that,' agreed Tudor.

'He couldn't have boarded the sailing ship. Jeffrey would have told us. I've known Jeffrey for years. He wouldn't connive in a crime like that. Not any sort of crime actually. Straight as a die, Jeffrey.'

'And there's a connection between the abortive hijacking and the theft of the gold bars and the disappearance of the captain,' said Tudor. 'Besides which our mutual friend Ashley Carpenter is involved.'

'So it seems,' she agreed.

'Don't you think we should talk to Umlaut and Abdullah and find out which of them owns the gold?'

This obvious next move was deferred by the sudden arrival of Sir Goronwy Watkyn looking majestic but bothered in a sort of Celtic Merlin mode. His mane of white hair was awry and a black cape fastened with a brass chain at the neck flapped theatrically in the breeze.

'Crime at sea, I understand,' said the old knight. 'Never fear there is no such thing as a perfect crime, especially when Sir Goronwy Watkyn is at hand. Do we have a body?'

'Everything is under control,' said Tudor.

'Not what I hear, dear boy,' said Sir Goronwy patting Tudor's shoulder in a gesture that managed to be both avuncular and threatening, 'Never fear though. Uncle Goronwy will sort everything out.'

'Thank you,' said Tudor, 'but everything is under control and there's no need for anyone else to be bothered.'

'No bother. No bother at all.' The old Celt tossed his head and gazed out at the horizon. 'It's a rare privilege to be able to do in practice what I have spent a lifetime perfecting in theory.'

'It's all right,' said Tudor. 'I've been in communication with all concerned and, as I say, it's under control. There's no need for you to be involved in any way. Just act normally and carry on with the lecturing.'

'What I say now.' The old man lowered his voice so that his listeners had to strain to catch what he was saying over the sibilant sighing of the sea, 'What I always say is *Cherchez le pied*.' He beamed with self-satisfaction.

'You sure you don't mean *cherchez la femme*,' said Elizabeth, a little obviously.

'Certainly not!' he said with asperity, '*Cherchez* chiropody, if one is being alliterative. The answer lies in the feet. People tell palms or look for character in a person's face but I tell you now that the solutions to practically everything may be found below the ankle. Just mark my words. I concede that this is a discovery I have made late in life but it is none the less valid for being belated.'

He inclined his head in an old-fashioned thespian manner and seemed on the verge of clicking his heels and kissing Elizabeth's hand. At the last moment however he seemed to think better of it and simply turned and disappeared indoors.

'Silly old phoney!' said Tudor.

'I suppose so,' said Elizabeth. She frowned. 'And talking of feet I'm afraid PC Plod is heading our way.'

It was indeed Grim, the unlikely lay-reader, formerly of the Metropolitan Police who was heading their way. His appearance lived up to his surname. He looked serious and forbidding in a curmudgeonly disobliging sort of way. Not at all the expression you'd expect to find on the face of a lay preacher on a Sunday after matins.

'I've had words with the First Officer, Cornwall,' said Freddie, 'And I take an exceedingly dim view. It seems to my good self that you have abrogated an entirely inappropriate level of responsibility in the matter of what appears to be prima facie an act of piracy on the High Seas. What have you got to say for yourself?'

'I have nothing to say for myself,' said Tudor, 'I simply don't know what you're talking about. And when you say 'First Officer' to whom are you referring?'

'Angus Donaldson, of course. As well you know.'

'Forgive me, Freddie,' said Tudor in a friendly familiar fashion which was calculated to infuriate, 'but Donaldson's actual title is Staff Captain and he's not in charge. The boss is Captain Hardy, the Master.'

'The Master is, as you well know, indisposed. Not even I

have been able to make contact with him. In view of this, er, indisposition Angus Donaldson is in charge whether he is First Officer or Staff Captain. Captain Donaldson has told me something of what appears to have taken place and was much relieved when I explained details of my former life and qualifications. From now on I am in charge and you can cease whatever activities you have been indulging in. From what I am able to glean from Captain Donaldson this is a case for the professionals.'

'I'm not actually entirely certain about that,' said Tudor. 'With the greatest possible respect to your former life and all that I rather had the impression that you had retired and moved on to what might aptly describe as higher things.'

'This is no time for facetiousness,' said Grim, who never had time for facetiousness of any kind. 'An attempt has been made to hijack this ship in the middle of the ocean and I understand there has also been an attempt at theft or robbery involving a stolen lifeboat and a mysterious vessel now vanished.'

'The lifeboat I can assure you is safely recovered and back on board together with its cargo or whatever it was.'

'Whatever it was indeed,' said the former inspector, pouncing on the phrase as if it was a fugitive from justice that he was about to apprehend with a snap of his official handcuffs. 'Whatever was it?'

'I would have thought Captain Donaldson would have told you whatever it was if he had indeed entrusted the enquiry to you. I mean, I hate to pull rank and all that, but (a) the Captain who, as we all know is Sam Hardy, Master of the *Duchess* is in charge, and (b) I am already involved in this affair *faute de mieux*.'

'Don't try and bamboozle me with fancy frog phrases,' said Grim. 'I may not be a professor but that doesn't make me stupid.'

But before this conversation could degenerate further they were interrupted. It was Mandy Goldslinger looking alarmed and dishevelled.

'Gentlemen, gentlemen,' she said breathlessly, 'I need your help. Something's happened.'

CHAPTER SIXTEEN

'What do you mean "something's happened"?'

Tudor took Mandy Goldslinger by the elbow and pulled her out of earshot. He did not want Grim to overhear. Elizabeth was doing a good job of blocking the former policeman while attempting merely to seem flirty and ingratiating.

'It's your ring-leaderene,' shouted Mandy, in a stage-shriek designed to rise above the wail of the waves and the sigh of the sea. 'She's escaped. Vanished. Done a bunk. She's at large. Somewhere on board ship. Dangerous. Maybe armed.'

'What?' asked Tudor semi-rhetorically. '*Tipperary Tatler*? How so? Who let her out?'

La Goldslinger sighed. 'Classic cock-up,' she said. 'Your Irish captives asked for refreshment. The infinitely civilised British acquiesced. Jeez, you Brits. Cup of tea, Mr Bin Laden? Absolutely. Earl Grey or Lapsang Souchong? No problem. Milk? Sugar? So that's what happened. Little stewardess is sent in to the prisoners with a tray of tea and cucumber sandwiches. I speak metaphorically but only just. She is hit on head. Again, I speak metaphorically. Your friend the flame-haired temptress from Tipperary takes her outfit and exits left with a load of empties. Hey fucking presto she's part of the crew. Every girl who carries a tray on board this ship is bog-Irish or fake Filipino. No one knows who they are. Your girl is just part of the herd.'

'You're telling me that the leader of a gang of international pirates has been captured and locked up only to be allowed to walk free without any let or hindrance?'

'Seems about the size of it,' said Mandy.

'You mentioned tea,' said Tudor glancing at his watch. 'I could do with a cup. Maybe a cucumber sandwich.' He glanced back at Grim. 'In private.'

'OK,' she said. 'Butler's Pantry in ten minutes. I'll make sure we have a quiet table to ourselves.'

She left, presumably to arrange tea and Tudor returned to his long-suffering sidekick and the aggrieved Grim.

'Look, Freddie,' he said, laying an ingratiating hand on the ex-copper's shoulder, 'There really isn't any need for you to be involved, not least because there's nothing to be involved, as it were *in*.' He laughed, aware that he was sounding donnish. 'Naturally if there *is* anything to be involved in you'll be the first person to be, well, involved. But right now there's nothing whatever to worry about. I've been thinking about your sermon too. Very thought provoking if I may say so.'

'The Lord moves in mysterious ways,' said Grim. 'Me, too. You'll never know where I'll turn up next or in what guise. Just like our Lord. He is everywhere and nowhere. Now you see Him; now you don't. You would be well advised not to sup with the Devil even using a long spoon. Best, by far, to stay alongside your old pal Freddie.'

Tudor had never noticed quite how yellow Freddie's teeth were when he smiled. Nor how bad his breath. Perhaps the mouth had deteriorated since leaving the force.

'I'll think about it Freddie,' he said, 'but really, there's no need for concern. Sam Hardy runs a tight ship. None of us will come to any harm while he's in charge.'

'Tight,' said Freddie, 'is the operative word. Sam Hardy is a drunk, as well you know. Ho, ho and a bottle of rum is not just a figure of speech in his case. Speaking as one who hasn't touched a drop of the hard stuff since I went on the wagon many years ago I know of what I speak.'

'Well . . .' began Tudor, but Grim silenced him with a finger to his mouth. 'Say no more,' he said. 'You know where to find me if you need professional help.'

It was on the tip of Tudor's tongue to say something clever and superior but he thought better of it and said nothing, simply stared out to sea for a moment, then said to the precocious Elizabeth, 'Why don't you ferret around while I have a cucumber sandwich and a cup of Earl Grey with la Goldslinger? I'll see you in a cabin later.'

'OK,' she said, grinning. 'We don't have ferrets in Tasmania but I think I know what you're saying. I'll sniff around.'

'Unobtrusively,' he said.

She smirked back at him. 'Obtrusive? *Moi*? I'll be discreet as the day is long. I'll be virtually invisible. No one will have the first idea of what I'm doing.'

'Not just a pretty face, are you?'

'On the contrary,' She was still smirking. 'That's exactly what I'll be. Just a pretty face. Plus pert breasts, fine cheekbones, a neat bum, long legs and an almost tiny waist. Combine all those and everyone will think I'm here for ornament only. That's the way of the world. I shall pass without notice.'

'That'll be the day,' Tudor spoke with feeling.

They both went indoors, she, on a predatory prowl; he for a cuppa in the Butler's Pantry.

When he arrived he wondered, not for the first time, who

was fooling who and why. What was the thinking behind a scene like this? Who had originally thought of the idea of taking the Ritz to sea? Whose bright idea was it to recreate the Palm Court complete with tinkling tea-cups and crustless egg sandwiches and crustless cucumber sandwiches and crustless smoked salmon sandwiches, scones and strawberry jam and cream, miniature swiss rolls and miniature sausage rolls and miniature jam tarts and Dundee Cake. 'Dundee Cake.' He seemed to remember Cary Grant rolling the words off his tongue in some old Hitchcock movie just before biting into a slice of said cake and rolling that round his tongue instead of words. Come to that why wasn't Cary Grant sitting at a table being charming to some old duck who was spending her late husband's legacy? Or more likely yet, why wasn't Cary Grant out on the dance floor schmoozing round with another elderly widow with money to spend on afternoon tea in the Butler's Pantry? What was that story about Cary Grant? The one about the newspaper reporter who cabled the film star in connection with a feature he was writing and simply sent a message saying 'How old Cary Grant?' to which Grant replied, quick as a flash, 'Old Cary Grant fine. How you?' Palms. They even had palm trees weaving gently in the wind to the sounds of Strauss, or was it Offenbach being scratched out by the trio of young Latvians or Lithuanians from the conservatoire on some Baltic beach. And talking of Cary Grant, he recognized the fellow in the off-white linen suit shuffling round the dance floor and shouting into the hearing-aid of his blue-rinsed partner as he executed a nimble 'one-two-three, one-two-three, one-two-three' which would have more than passed muster at any *thé dansant* in any palais from Shanghai to Shoreham. It was Ambrose Perry, the gentleman host. There should have been 'Let them eat cake,' he muttered to himself: Battenburg, Pontefract, simnel, Victoria sponge,

Dundee dammit. He could murder an eclair or what they used to call soap cakes at school in cricket matches when the headmaster's wife did the honours with the huge chipped urn and the huge chipped tea-pots and. . . .

'Are you all right, sir? May I be of any assistance?' It was a waiter in striped trousers and black jacket doing a passable imitation of a landlubber maitre d' at the Ritz.

'All right?' said Tudor, aware that Mandy Goldslinger was waving at him from a far corner of the pantry where she had secured an isolated table for two in a secluded corner. It wasn't quite screened off, but Ms Goldslinger's haughty demeanour and icy stare was more than enough to repel boarders.

'You looked, if I may say so, sir,' said the waiter doing a plausible Jeeves imitation, 'a little under the weather.'

It was increasingly rare to find a genuine waiter on a cruise ship these days. Even the gentlemen hosts were more host-like than gentlemanly. Only the officer class were British. The other ranks were mostly all foreign. Tudor heard his inner voice saying these things and was horrified. He sounded like his father.

'No, I'm fine, thank you,' said Tudor.

'You still look a little green,' said the waiter, 'and feverish. I think you may be running a temperature. Perspiration on the brow. I hope we're not about to be struck by one of those bugs. The *Duchess* has been bug-free for as long as I've been on board but, as you say, there's always a first time.'

'Thank you. Thank you,' said Tudor. 'Not to worry. Really.'

'You kept repeating something about Dundee cake,' said the waiter. 'It's not a standard item, but as you're with Miss Goldslinger I'm sure some can be arranged. May I fetch you Dundee cake?'

'Thank you, no,' said Tudor. 'But water would be good. A

glass of water.'

'Certainly, sir. Sparkling or still? Ice? Lemon or lime?'

'Just water, thanks. And, er . . . thanks.'

He looked at the man suspiciously. He was too good to be true.

'You all right?' Mandy Goldslinger had changed into a curious tea-drinking outfit – a sort of black lamé cat-suit with a high collar. More Vegas than vicarage.

'I'm fine. I wish people would stop suggesting otherwise.'

'You don't look fine. You look ill. Would you like brandy?'

'The man's bringing me water.'

'The man's Shane. Been with the ship for years. Queen of the Butler's Pantry. He's from Toowoomba in Queensland. Cute,eh? Surprised you hadn't noticed him already.'

'Must have been on shore leave whenever I've been on before,' said Tudor.

She poured Earl Grey from a silvery teapot.

'This'll put the hair back on your chest,' she said. 'Twining's best. We had Sam Twining himself on board once, showing us how to do a proper brew. A lot depends on the water. We have special tea water just for the Pantry. Malvern I believe. Just like Her Majesty. Did you know that your Queen Elizabeth takes bottles of Malvern Water wherever she goes? Especially for brewing afternoon tea. We have royal authors on board regularly. That's one thing they all agree on.'

Tudor felt very tired. He put a hand to his head.

'You don't have to do a sales pitch for me, Mandy,' he said, 'I've read the brochure. I've heard Sam Hardy doing his spiel.'

Her mood changed.

'I need to talk to you about Sam,' she said, sounding serious and almost human.

'Yes,' he said.

Shane of Toowoomba shimmered over with the glass of

water which he deposited deftly on the table in text-book manner with the non-carrying hand crooked behind his back. He smiled synthetically. All very Butler's Pantry, thought Tudor, still wondering at the incongruity of it all. The ship bumped, reminding him that they were still at sea.

'I'm worried about Sam.'

'Yes,' said Tudor. He was not in the mood to be helpful.

'You see,' she said, 'Sam and me.' She now sounded coy, almost girlish. Tudor wondered if this was an act like everything else about her.

'The truth is,' she continued, 'that Sam and me – Sam and I that is – we, the two us, are an item. We're an item. That is we, if you see what I mean. Sam and I are, like, together. We're an item. Except that the company has a rule about members of crew you know, well, we have to pretend. When we're on board together. Everyone's been, well, you know, very British about us, but if the company found out one of us would have to go.'

'I see,' said Tudor, not really seeing. He would have been surprised by this revelation if he had been particularly interested but he wasn't. He didn't care about Mandy's private life. Nor the Captain's. He wasn't really into private lives, he thought ruefully. Perhaps that was his problem.

'So why are you worried?' he asked, sipping his water.

'Because I can't find him. And I can't get into his cabin. The lock's been changed so my key doesn't work.'

CHAPTER SEVENTEEN

The Baltic strings were playing a polka. Tudor could imagine lads and lasses in some northern Tivoli strutting their stuff under the larches in summer dusk while an orchestra on a wooden nineteenth century bandstand oompahed out a number such as this. Ambrose Perry and his colleagues and partners did not, however, strut or trip the light fantastic. Instead they swayed gently and shuffled around the floor making sure their lady-passengers remained upright and followed them more or less in time to the music. It was, in its way, an impressive performance. Tudor thought of flying buttresses holding up an ancient abbey and was impressed enough by the metaphor to make a mental note to use it in a paper for a learned journal at some future date.

'An item,' he said. 'You and Sam Hardy. The two of you.'

Like royalty, he often, when nonplussed, repeated the remark just vouchsafed, if necessary more than once. It gave him valuable thinking time.

'Yes,' said Ms Goldslinger, dabbing at her mascara with a frilly handkerchief. 'Sam and me. The two of us. An item.'

Royal-speak was catching.

On the far side of the dance floor Tudor could see Prince Abdullah and his harem. The Prince was not smoking as the Butler's Pantry was a smoke-free zone. Instead he was glowering around a cucumber sandwich. The wives poured him tea, fed him food and generally fawned. Tudor wondered idly how many there were and whether they had particular duties or rosters – toenail cutting wife, a nostril hair-removing wife, a Scotch-pouring wife. Their eyes sparkled from their almost-all concealing Muslim headdresses and their bodies shimmered seductively under their supposedly chaste robes. He'd be prepared to bet they owed more to Dior or St Laurent than a cut-price couturier in the soukh back home.

'So you've been having it off with the captain.'

Tudor was aware he sounded indelicate.

Mandy Goldslinger blushed to the roots of her hair – which did not exactly match the unsplit ends. Time for a visit to the ship's coiffeuse he thought to himself.

'The physical side of things between Sam and myself is only part of the chemistry between us. We think of ourselves as human beings not like, you know, "sex toys".'

'I'm sorry,' he said, 'I didn't mean to imply anything else. But let's, as you say, cut to the chase. You haven't seen Sam Hardy for a while and you can't get into his cabin because it's locked and the locks have been changed.'

'Yup,' she said.

'So who's in charge?' he asked her, expecting her to answer 'Angus Donaldson' which, gratifyingly, she did.

'So did he change the locks?'

'Not personally, no. Angus isn't a DIY person.'

'That's not what I meant. Did he order the locks changed? Is he responsible for Sam's disappearance?'

'I honestly don't know,' she said, looking disturbingly weepy. 'In Sam's absence Angus is the boss.'

'Some people say that Angus is the boss whether Sam is around or not.' Tudor tried not to sound uncharitable. 'Sam is brilliant PR; great Captain Birds Eye. Passengers adore him.

He could read tide tables or Lloyd's Log and they'd hang on his every word, but when it comes to actually sailing the ship one isn't quite so sure. In a seafaring sense there are those who think old Sam is past his sell-by date.'

'That's not fair,' said Mandy indignantly. 'He's one of the great sailors as you know perfectly well. He still keeps a Troy on the Fowey River and he sails it himself whenever he can get down to Cornwall.'

'Which isn't often.'

'He's kept very busy. The *Duchess* isn't the *Duchess* without him.'

'Which is now.'

'I don't know,' she said, 'I simply don't know.' She took a mouthful of thin China tea. 'This isn't like him. He's never gone AWOL on a voyage before. Never in all the years I've known him.'

Tudor looked out across the Butler's Pantry like an ancient mariner on the qui-vive for icebergs or albatrosses. Prince Abdullah was still glowering and when Tudor followed his gaze he saw that he was glowering at his arch-enemy Doctor Umlaut who was sitting with his wife at a corner table which had Umlaut all over it. You sensed that this was table Umlauts-for-the-use-of-only and that should any common or garden ordinary passenger try to usurp it they would get short shrift from Shane the maitre d' from Toowoomba. What made Tudor frown almost as menacingly as Prince Abdullah was that there were three at the Umlaut table and the third party was none other than his precocious side-kick and Ph.D. student, Elizabeth Burney. She seemed relaxed, at ease – as indeed did the Umlauts. It was if they had known each other for years. Tudor was no lip-reader, but from the shapes their mouths were making he would have said they were not speaking English.

Mandy was talking. Tudor wrenched his gaze away from the tableau before him and paid attention to her. She was agitated.

'I've been on the *Duchess* for longer than I care to remember,' she said, 'and every other voyage I've been on has been almost totally without incident. Ocean flat as duckpond; passengers friendly and appreciative; crew efficient and courteous; no serious illness; no more than occasional fatalities and then always from natural causes on account of advanced years and chronic long term illness. The *Duchess* has never had what other ships had: no mystery bugs; no sewage in the staterooms; no bloody pirates. Just cruisy-cruisy. All quiet on the Western Approaches. No man, woman or child overboard. Just what the doctor ordered. Everything always passed off without incident. But this voyage is just one long incident after another. I think there's a Jonah on board.' She narrowed her eyes. 'You're not a Jonah, are you?'

The three girls were now playing the Radetsky March which presumably called for a military two-step. Ambrose Perry and his colleagues and their charges went on shuffling gently just the same. It would take more than a change of tempo from the orchestra to make them break sweat. Besides, if they did there would have been fatalities among the old ladies. Not that there was any sign of stumbling among the dancers. The swell of the ocean beneath was insufficient to cause more than the occasional gentle shift of the goalposts and their pace was so stately that there was no danger of falling.

'I'm a guest speaker in good standing, as well you know,' said Tudor, 'and for all his faults the same is true of Sir Goronwy. I don't think you can be a regular cruiser and Jonah too. So that rules out Prince Abdullah and Doctor Umlaut as well. They're recidivists.'

'I'm not superstitious,' said Mandy, 'but I *am* bothered. This voyage is becoming a nightmare. First we have that mad Irish hijack which is nipped in the bud, but then the ring leader gets sprung. Meanwhile a mysterious Flying Irishman turns up and does a bunk, but not before one of our lifeboats comes alongside her with a cargo of gold bars. And then they're surprised in mid ocean by this bloody great sailing ship. So we get the lifeboat and the gold back but the captain is missing. Or seems to be. Or might be or might not. And whoever was in charge of the lifeboat has vanished. Along with the captain.'

'Unless the person who was in charge of the lifeboat was the captain himself.'

'But why in God's name would Sam make off in a lifeboat with several millions worth of gold bars and then vanish, presumably either overboard or into the bowels of the mad Irish university ship? Which may or may not have your would-be obituarist Professor Ashley Carpenter on board.'

'Hmmm,' said Tudor. 'Put like that I concede it does sound pretty odd. You weren't selling this as a mystery cruise, were you? Or a celebrity whodunit?'

'It's not funny, dammit.'

She noticed that Tudor had suddenly stopped even pretending to pay attention to what she was saying but was focused uncompromisingly on the dance floor. The three-piece orchestra had switched to something Argentinian and tango-like. Surprisingly wild and raunchy. Gypsy music. The lead violin tossed her head and bared her teeth. The cellist and the pianist followed suit. Ambrose Perry and the others continued to shuffle, but a new and unexpected couple had taken to the floor and were executing what looked to Tudor's admittedly inexpert and untutored eye like a pretty passable piece of Latin-American exhibitionism. It was Dr Umlaut and Elizabeth Burney. Frau Umlaut did not look pleased.

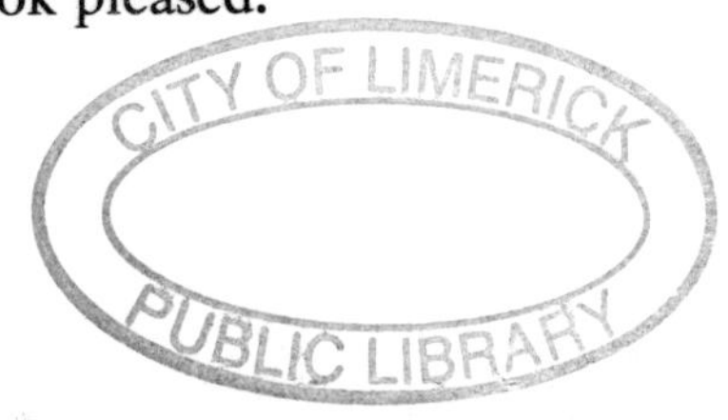

'Good grief!' exclaimed Tudor. Little Miss Burney never ceased to surprise him. She was unrecognizable, all hips and slinkiness and as if she had a rose or carnation clutched between her canines. Something clenched between the buttocks too, he thought, and then checked himself. Little Umlaut wasn't bad either in a predictably mechanical parade-ground manner. He did the samba-rumba-tango or whatever, not like a Latin but in the manner of the Prussian Guard, as if taught by some Teutonic drill sergeant. The whole cabaret was a revelation. People noticed, even Ambrose Perry. Beside him Mandy Goldslinger gaped.

'Is that your little girl with that Kraut?'

'Elizabeth dancing with Dr Umlaut. Looks like it, yes.'

'If you call that dancing. Jeez. We don't get that kind of thing on the *Duchess* on the average cruise.'

Tudor gazed at the elderly stick-insects and mountainous jellies all around the pyrotechnical little German and his precocious Tasmanian sidekick and could see only too well that this must be true.

'We have to find Captain Sam,' said Tudor, bringing them both back to earth.

'Too right,' said Mandy.

'But it's sort of difficult to find someone if the powers-that-be deny that he's missing.'

'Can't we overrule Donaldson?'

'Not without Sam. Sam's the only man on board who out-ranks him. Sam can order him to do anything he likes but no one else can. Without Sam he is Sam, if you follow me.'

Tudor took a long draught of water and as if by magical osmosis Shane appeared with a chilly replacement. Tudor nodded gratefully and the maitre d' bared his fangs in acknowledgement.

'What you mean,' said Tudor, 'is that if Donaldson won't

admit there's a problem we can't solve it.'

'You could put it like that.'

'Suppose I insist on seeing Sam.'

'You can insist as much as you like,' she said. 'I've tried that. He just says that Sam isn't well enough to see anyone, that he's sedated, that he can't speak because of the laryngitis and he specifically asked not to see anyone.'

'How could he do that if he's incapable of speech?'

'I imagine he wrote it down on a piece of paper. Sign language maybe. It doesn't matter. Angus Donaldson's word is law unless Sam is able to overrule him. And, what's more, can be seen to be able to overrule him.'

The three girls stopped playing their sexy foot-stamping number and acknowledged the applause of the tea-dancers and tea-drinkers. Some of the applause appeared to be aimed at Elizabeth and Dr Umlaut. Tea was now officially over. Drinking up time. Nothing to eat between now and olives and nuts in the happy hour which would begin in less than half an hour's time. There were plenty of passengers on board who browsed and sluiced on a non-stop basis. That's what they paid for.

Tudor pursed his lips.

'You're right,' he said, eventually, 'we've a lot of mysteries for just one little cruise. I'm not sure if they're connected or just coincidental. And I can't work out whether Captain Sam constitutes a mystery or just a straightforward medical indisposition.'

'The change of locks is a clincher, wouldn't you say?'

'I've only got your word for that,' he said.

'Are you calling me a liar?'

'Of course not. But. Well, there may be another explanation. A perfectly respectable one.'

'Nobody else knows about Sam and me,' she said.

'Don't be silly,' he said. 'I may not know this ship particularly well but one thing I do understand about closed societies such as this: you can't keep secrets. Everybody knows what everyone else is doing.'

'No one knows where Sam is. Or who changed the locks. Or why. Or about the gold. Or the lifeboat. Or the mysterious ships in mid-ocean. Life is suddenly nothing but secrets.'

'Not for long,' he said with certainty. 'I simply don't believe you can keep secrets on the *Duchess*. Not for any length of time.'

He looked up. Elizabeth was standing breathing heavily and perspiring gently. A bead of sweat stood out on her upper lip.

'Did I hear the word secret?' she said. 'I think you're right. Secrets will out. People can't keep them. Particularly during a *thé dansant* and revisiting the time of their life.'

Her two elders regarded her with a mixture of suspicion and admiration.

'Time to change for the next round,' she said. 'Dinner soon. Black tie evening.'

CHAPTER EIGHTEEN

Tudor turned on the television in his cabin and was surprised to find a man talking about the Mutiny on the *Bounty*. He seemed quite articulate and to know about what he was talking. He did not look well, however, and was, pale if not exactly green about the gills. His tie was loosely tied, exposing the top button of his shirt. Occasionally he paused to take a sip of water from a glass on the table at his elbow.

It was a moment or two before Tudor realized that he was watching himself. He had been on the verge of saying that the lecturer was not nearly as good as *he* was. In fact, he was about to disagree with him about the 'inward happiness and peculiar pleasure' experienced by Captain Bligh when he was cast off the *Bounty* in the ship's boat. Would whoever was lowered over the side of the *Duchess* in the lifeboat have experienced similar emotions? 'Inward happiness and peculiar pleasure' were indeed the words that Bligh had written at the time in his running log. Whoever went off in the *Duchess*'s boat had kept no log. Or if he had, it hadn't turned up.

He turned himself off. It was disconcerting to see himself in that way but at least the image was controllable. Good PR as well. He wondered how many others on board ship were dressing for dinner and watching his earlier performance.

Freddie Grim? The Goronwy Watkyns? Prince Abdullah and his wives? The Umlauts? The Master? The Staff Captain? Mandy Goldslinger? Ambrose Perry and the gentlemen hosts? Who knew? He was tempted to ask 'Who cared?' But he knew that although he would never admit it to the world at large there was a part of him, probably a dominant part, that cared quite a lot. He craved an audience. Pity that he didn't come across better on TV.

There was a knock at the door and he abandoned his half-tied bow tie and went to open it. It was Elizabeth dressed to kill and for dinner. She was wearing the classic little black dress. It began late and finished early which, at *her* age and with *her* figure, was allowable. In a few years she'd have to start dressing a little more like mutton but for the time being she could do lamb and get away with it.

'Hi!' he said, non-committal as ever, and then, rather out of character, added, 'You're looking particularly nice.'

'Thanks,' she said, giving him a peck on the cheek. 'And you look a bit the worse for wear. Do you want me to tie your tie? Why don't you have a clip-on? Particularly when you so obviously can't tie your own. So how was La Goldslinger? What was so important?'

'I saw you with Umlaut. Dancing.'

'Of course.' She smelt nice as well as looking nice. Especially standing close behind him as she deftly fixed the tie around his neck. But she was about the same age as his daughter would have been if he had one. 'Nifty little mover our Walter.' She pronounced the name in an un-English way. 'Vultur'.

'Vultur,' he repeated, sounding idiotic.

'My new friend,' she said, pulling the black silk ends tight and straightening the tie in the glass. 'There,' she said, 'perfecto. Good enough to be fake. Yes, Dr Umlaut is Vultur and his wife is Irmgarde. They asked me to dinner in their suite. They have their own butler. I declined.'

'And Irmgarde doesn't mind you dancing with Vultur?'

'Not at all,' she smiled. 'It's good for him. He needs the exercise. He was the young foxtrot champion of Basel in his youth. She has a funny leg so she can't dance any more. They used to be very good she says. So no. No objections.'

'Charming,' said Tudor, feeling his teeth gritting. 'So Basel. Swiss not Kraut?'

'*Schwitzer-kraut*,' she said. 'Pharmaceuticals. Umlaut, Umlaut and Umlaut. Or something like that. His great grandfather invented the oral contraceptive. At least I think that's what he meant. He was a bit coy about it. So what's your news? What did La Goldslinger want? Don't tell me, it was a proposition: she wants to get you into bed.'

He turned round and took his jacket off its hanger. He was wearing braces, plain dark-blue ones with gold-coloured clips; his shoes had toe-caps and laces and were highly polished. He was that sort of man. Dull, he thought to himself. When all was said and done he was dull. He so very much wished not to be and made every effort to be interesting. But deep down he knew that he wasn't. Elizabeth on the other hand was. It was annoying. Very.

'No Madam Goldslinger did not make a pass.' He shrugged into his dinner jacket and patted non-existent dandruff off the shoulders.

'Snap then,' she said. 'Vultur didn't make a pass at me either. Though I wouldn't put it past them at dinner. I have a feeling they're a kinky couple. I suspect she likes to watch. Only guessing but there's something about them that's kind of fishy. In a sexual way. Know what I mean? Anyway, tell me: what *did* la Goldslinger want?'

He patted his pockets to make sure he had keys, wallet and

a handkerchief.

'She's been having an affair with the Captain. With Sam Hardy.'

'Yes,' she said. 'I thought you knew that.'

He looked at her sharply. 'Did you know?'

'Everybody knew.'

'Mandy thought it was a secret.'

'Oh,' she shrugged, 'people who are having illicit affairs always assume they've managed to keep their guilty secret when they've failed to do so. You know that.'

'I suppose.' It was years since Tudor had enjoyed an illicit affair or even harboured a guilty secret. His professional studies told him that what the girl said was true but he knew it only in a professional academic sense. Vicarious, not visceral. It was at moments like this that he wondered if his copper friends such as Chief Inspector Trythall back home at the Wessex Constabulary didn't have a point. Trythall's approach to crime was sharp-end stuff. His was ivory-tower. It was a point Trythall enjoyed making. He himself countered by arguing that a certain dispassionate, cool academic examination was more valuable than gut reactions. But, privately, he had doubts. At moments such as this he wondered if he were too thin-blooded.

'People like Mandy Goldslinger never seem to understand how visible they are. She's a celebrity on board ship. Likewise old Popeye Sam Hardy. She can't sneeze without the passengers and crew catching a cold. Nor he.'

She sat down on Tudor's bed and yawned.

'Been quite a day,' she said, 'I hadn't imagined cruising would be so exciting. So Mandy let you into a secret that the rest of them have been sharing for as long as the relationship's been going on. Then what? I got something useful out of Vultur so you'd better have something other than *l'affaire*

Hardy-Goldslinger. Sounds like a new ship's cocktail – a local take on the Harvey Wallbanger.'

'The Harvey Wallbanger was invented by Duke Antone in the 1950s,' said Tudor. 'A local surfer called Harvey had a bad day on the beach and consoled himself in the Blackwatch Bar run by Antone with rather too many of the Duke's special Screwdrivers which were vodka and orange with a dash of Galliano. When he got up to go he couldn't find the door and kept bumping into walls. Hence Harvey Wallbanger.'

'I'm impressed,' said Elizabeth stifling a second yawn, 'so what else did Mandy tell you?'

'That she's lost her lover. She can't find Sam any more than anyone else. But what's really sinister is that they've changed the locks on his cabin door. Mandy had a set of keys but now she can't get in.'

'So who's "they"?'

'I don't know. Angus Donaldson's in charge if Sam's not with us. He gives the orders, has the authority. If someone else changed the locks Angus would have the right to overrule them.'

'So why would Donaldson change the locks?'

'So that people like Mandy couldn't get into the captain's cabin.'

'And why would he want to do that?'

'Because the cabin contains something that he doesn't want Mandy to find.'

She frowned. 'Or nothing,' she said.

'How do you mean?'

'It's like the dog in the night,' she said. 'Not the barking but the lack of barking. The conceit is that Captain Sam is lying in his own bed speechless on account of his laryngitis. But suppose he's been bumped off and tipped overboard, then there's no one in the Captain's cabin and the emptiness has to be concealed from prying eyes.'

'So,' said Tudor, aware that he was not functioning at the top of his range, 'Angus Donaldson is responsible for the murder of Captain Sam and is covering up by having the locks changed, shutting the cabin up and keeping the keys.'

'It's a theory,' said Elizabeth. 'Perfectly plausible. Except that in a few days we'll be docking and the NYPD will be all over the *Duchess* like marauding ants.'

'So he's got till then to work out a final solution.'

'Yup,' said the girl, tossing her head. 'I guess you're right. Nothing else you have to tell me?'

'No,' he said, sitting down heavily in one of his two status-conferring armchairs, 'Your turn now. Go ahead. Shoot.'

'Well,' she said, giving the impression of a story-teller who is anxious to make the most of a good, if tall tale, 'you've noticed that the Umlauts and Prince Abdullah aren't exactly the best of pals.'

'It hadn't escaped my notice,' said Tudor drily. 'But you wouldn't expect it? They both behave as if they owned the ship. Naturally they can't stand the sight of each other. It's alpha-male stuff. Testosterone. Everything is part of the game. Take the wives. Parading them around the ship is the sheikh's way of putting two fingers up at Walter. Poor old Walter's only got Irmgarde. Or did, until you came along and inveigled him on to the dance floor.'

She turned mildly pink.

'It's one way to get the little man to spill beans,' she said. 'Anyway who said Prince Abdullah was a sheikh?'

'You know what I mean,' said Tudor. 'Personally I have a feeling he's a phoney so it doesn't much matter whether he's a fake-sheikh or a fake-prince. It's the fakery that's significant, not the title to which he's pretending.'

'Hmmm,' said Elizabeth. 'I don't know about Middle-

Eastern titles but I think the money's real. He's loaded. So is Herr Doktor Umlaut.'

'OK,' said Tudor, 'they're both rich as Croesus and Umlaut's ancestor made a fortune out of oral contraceptives. What else did he tell you?'

'Guess,' she said.

'Oh, for heaven's sake. I'm not in the mood. He's challenging Prince Abdullah to a duel. Pistols at dawn.'

'Many a true word,' she said. 'It's not a duel in that sense but it is a kind of *mano-a-mano* deal. Kids in the playground stuff. Umlaut wants to buy the ship.'

'And so does the Prince.'

'Right on,' she said. 'They both want it and the board is split. There's an Umlaut faction and a Prince Abdullah faction. What's more, the split extends beyond the boardroom. Sam Hardy is the on-board rep of one of the factions and Angus Donaldson of the other. Umlaut is a Donaldson man; the Prince is a Sam supporter. Neither of them will stop at anything.'

'So.' Tudor looked at his watch and wondered if they should venture back into what for the moment passed as the outside world and prepare themselves for the next round of gourmandizing. 'Both these shady plutocrats want to buy the ship. Whichever one succeeds will effectively bar the vanquished one from ever setting foot on board again.'

'*Ja-wohl* as Vultur would say.'

'And are you telling me that your little Basel billionaire might have bumped off Captain Sam?'

She looked thoughtful. 'I'm not saying he did,' she said eventually, 'and I'm not saying he didn't. But he had at least half a motive and he's more than unscrupulous enough. It's a chance.'

'Interesting,' he said. 'It hadn't occurred to me that the

rivalry was quite so intense.'

'No,' she agreed, 'me neither. Whose side are you on?'

'We don't take sides,' he said. 'You know that.'

CHAPTER NINETEEN

The bar outside the entrance to the Chatsworth restaurant was called the Mitford, a little act of homage to one of the best known Devonshire Duchesses – Debo, youngest of the famous Mitford sisters. A portrait of her hung in a prominent position alongside photographs of herself and her sisters, including Nancy, the novelist, Diana, the wife of Sir Oswald Moseley, Unity, the friend of the Führer who shot herself in a park in Munich, and the radical Jessica who settled in the United States and wrote a best-seller about American funeral customs.

Riviera Shipping's design department had done a sparky job on the bar which exuded exactly the sort of brittle period charm Tudor associated with the Mitford girls. It was almost decadent but in a chintzy chocolate box way that saved it from being dangerous. Just right for a cruise liner. No threat.

All tables were taken so Tudor and Elizabeth sat on bar stools and picked abstractedly at olives, Twiglets and tiny cheese biscuits presented in small silvery bowls of the sort you might expect a Mitford girl to encounter in a Grand Hotel. Sitting on bar stools made one susceptible to interruption and so it proved. The interloper, in a white tuxedo of the sort one would expect to see at a sub-standard award ceremony involving C-list celebrities, was Ambrose Perry, gentleman host. He was, briefly, unattached.

'Formidable tango,' he said, easing himself on to the stool next to Elizabeth, 'Where did you learn?'

'Tasmania,' said Elizabeth. 'I did a dance minor at uni. We had an exiled Chilean poet who'd been a senior diplomat under Allende. Should have seen his fandango. Cool.'

'I thought you were remarkable. I myself have earned a modest crust from ballroom exertions of one sort or another and I know enough to recognize quality. Accept, please, my felicitations.'

'Will you have a drink?' asked Tudor, who had already ordered a couple of Harvey Wallbangers in acknowledgement of their earlier conversation. Perry said he wouldn't mind if he did and his was a white wine spritzer.

'Enjoying your cruise?' he asked conversationally and, apparently, innocently.

'Yes,' said Elizabeth. 'She's a great ship. Food and drink's excellent. Company ditto. What more could a girl want?'

'You should have seen the *France*,' said Ambrose. 'She was the ultimate. The acme. Never been a ship like her.'

Elizabeth nibbled a pretzel.

'She must have been amazing,' she said. 'But I like the *Duchess*. She's cute.'

'The *France* was never cute,' said Perry. He had a face like a lizard. All wrinkle. The eyes were slits and you half-expected a forked tongue to flick out from behind the pursed lips and spear an olive from the silver bowl. Or maybe an errant insect if one should fly within range. He could be any age but even if he wasn't he seemed ancient. 'I'm not sure the *Duchess* is cute either, but the *France* had a touch of class. More than a touch. She was class through and through.'

He sipped at his spritzer and patted his mouth with a linen

napkin immediately afterwards, removing the salty aftermath of a peanut. He was fastidious – fussily so.

'I'm glad you're enjoying the trip,' said Elizabeth, unconvincingly.

'I didn't say I was enjoying it,' said the host. His fastidiousness clearly extended to speech and judgement as well as dress and manners. 'Gentlemanly hosting is a job. Enjoyment would be an inappropriate response. Satisfaction maybe, but enjoyment, no. It would be like having fun. My job is to enable others to have fun not for me to have fun myself.'

'Oh,' said Elizabeth feeling, rightly, that she had been put in her place.

'And are your old ladies enjoying themselves?' asked Tudor, sensing that this was the question Ambrose Perry was waiting for.

'I believe so,' he said, appearing to think quite hard about what was the correct answer, 'The ship-board activities are exemplary as they always are. The little girls from Latvia play prettily and, as you know, with *brio* when it is appropriate. The bingo is well called. The bridge is popular and the pairs well-matched. Few play chess but boards and pieces are there as always and one or two of us if not in quite the Grandmaster class are always ready to oblige. The jigsaws are stimulating. The library well stocked. Fruit machines are not to my taste nor to that of the majority of my ladies. The food and drink throughout are delicious. With all this I find no fault.'

Both Tudor and Elizabeth could sense a big 'but' looming.

Elizabeth anticipated it.

'But,' she said helpfully.

Ambrose did not look like a man who wanted help. Particularly from a woman. At least not from a young woman. It occurred to both Elizabeth and Tudor that when it came to women Ambrose was like a conservative oenophile. He liked only old vintages. Anything *spritzig* made him nervous. Beaujolais Nouveau upset him. Younger elements would say that he only liked women when they were past their sell-by date. It was not that he didn't like women. He would not have been doing the job that he did if he didn't. But he only really liked old ducks. He was a sexually inverted snob – unimpressed by nubility.

'But nothing,' he said, sipping another sip of spritzer and nibbling a nut. 'However, there is, how shall I put this? There is a *mood*.' He pronounced the word as if it were the noise a cow might make, giving it an extra syllable or two, as if building an extra section into its middle.

'A mood,' repeated Tudor. 'How do you mean, "mood"? Bad mood, good mood, foul mood, moody mood.' Drink and fatigue were making him facetious. Elizabeth dug a pointy toe into his shin.

'I'm not entirely sure I'd qualify the mood one way or another,' said Ambrose, 'but I definitely detect one. You could call it an atmosphere if you preferred. It might perhaps be one of anticipation. Or merely heightened awareness. It may, of course, pass. But' – and he speared an olive and regarded it thoughtfully before popping it between his overly regular dentures – 'there again, it may not.'

Tudor and Elizabeth were not entirely sure what he was talking about but judged it better not to admit it. Better to say nothing. Thus encouraged he might expand and become more intelligible. They both therefore had another sip and another olive.

Presently, Perry said, 'Mrs Potts, for example. Olive. With whom I was sharing the floor earlier. She senses a mood too.'

'Can you be more specific?' asked Tudor, not sure whether Olive Potts' analysis of mood or atmosphere was worth knowing. Or that of Ambrose Perry come to that. Still, it was better, surely, to know what people were talking about than to be left stumbling through a fog of ambiguity.

'This morning's business,' said Perry, 'is a case in point. One minute, confusion, strange voices on the public address system, clear indications of something amiss. Then suddenly and for no apparent reason, all is suddenly well again. The ship continues on its way as if nothing has happened. In Olive Potts' eyes that creates uncertainty. An unsettled atmosphere. A bad mood.'

'I thought,' said Tudor, deliberately disingenuously, 'that this morning's stuff was some sort of anti-terrorist exercise. I'm afraid I didn't take it terribly seriously. I assumed it was a sort of Bush-Blair inspired equivalent of lifeboat drill. If it isn't Health and Safety Regulations it's the War on Terror. Even on board ship.'

'That's what you were lecturing on, surely,' said Perry. 'Captain Bligh and the *Bounty* was the eighteenth-century equivalent of what we're experiencing today. Fletcher Christian was the contemporary equivalent of a suicide bomber. Captain Bligh was in charge of Neighorurhood Watch.'

'I didn't see you at the talk,' said Tudor supiciously.

'No,' said Perry, 'I watched you on TV when I was preparing for dinner. Very good if I may say so, but not necessarily conducive to improving the mood. A little like showing the film *Titanic* as a matinée on board.'

'Well,' said Tudor, 'I wouldn't go as far as that. You wouldn't get the Mutiny on the *Bounty* happening in this day and age. We've become far too sophisticated.'

Ambrose Perry rolled a nut round his mouth and seemed on the verge of spitting it out but evidently thought better of it and chewed and swallowed instead.

'I'm delighted to hear you say so,' he said. 'But I have to say that the Master's laryngitis is disturbing some of my elderly friends. Mrs Dolly Mather-Jenkins from New Jersey for instance. She is of a naturally nervous disposition, but she is concerned at the Master's silence. Even if he can't speak one might hope that he would come among us if only to be hail fellow and well met in silence.'

'I understand he's not at all well,' said Elizabeth. 'Doctor says he must get some rest.'

Tudor glanced at her and wondered if he should kick her shins too. Why were they both telling porkies?

'I'm sorry to hear it,' said Ambrose. 'I've always had a softish spot for Master Sam whereas there is something not entirely to my taste when it comes to the Scottish Staff Captain. My ladies, I have to report, are of a similar mind.'

'I'm sorry to hear it,' said Tudor. 'But I hope you'll allay their fears. I'm sure you will. I can't think of more capable hands for them to be in.'

He drained his glass and smiled at Elizabeth.

'I think it's time we went in, don't you?'

'I'm really not terribly hungry,' she said. 'I think I'll just stick to a couple of ounces of Beluga and a lightly seared *filet*. Or maybe a tuna steak.'

Tudor got off his stool and stood aside.

'*A bientôt*,' he said pleasantly to the gentleman host who smiled not altogether agreeably and raised his glass at their retreating forms.

'Rum cove,' said Tudor, as they paused to wash their hands in the new regulation sani-fluid at the door of the Chatsworth restaurant.

'Rum's the word,' said Elizabeth, raising her eyebrows.

It was too. There was rum everywhere. Or a mixture of rum and brandy and Grand Marnier depending on whether one was having babas or crêpes Suzettes or steak Dianes or dinde Duchesse or choufleur Chatsworth or moules Mitfords. Rum or not, strong spirits were everywhere leaping towards the low ceiling as men in striped trousers and jet black jackets set fire to food of every description after smothering it in alcohol. The room was like a veritable Hell's Kitchen – Hieronymus Bosch meets the *Sunday Times* Colour Supplement: Delia with Danger.

The two of them threaded their way gingerly past the various table-side conflagrations nodding in a correctly friendly way to the Umlauts, Prince Abdullah and wives, the Grims, the Goronwy Watkyns and various other old or new acquaintances.

Their stewardess, Helga, brought iced water and menus to their now familiar table.

'Neither of us is terribly hungry, I'm afraid,' said Tudor. They both smiled ingratiatingly.

'How about a little Beluga, followed by a rare steak with spinach?' asked Helga in flawless English. She had been here before. 'And shall I send Igor?'

Igor was the sommelier with a superior jacket and a tastevin suspended from his neck. He'd know that because Tudor was paying for the wine he would have a cheap bottle. That meant he would not rate special glasses, or indeed, much in the way of special attention either.

Tudor gazed around the Chatsworth and smiled.

'You wouldn't get away with this on dry land,' he said. 'In fact I'm quite surprised they get away with it in mid-Atlantic. There must be international safety regulations which tell you how high flames are allowed to go in the dining-room. I'm surprised they're allowed flames at all. Read, mark etcetera etcetera for you will not see the like again. At least not anywhere with an ounce of political correctness.'

The two of them gazed around this anachronistic temple of

1950s cooking at the table.

'Restaurants were like this once,' said Tudor, 'before you were born. In the days when Sir Bernard and Lady Docker were the stuff of the William Hickey Column in the *Daily Express* and all was right with the world. That was before huge salaries for footballers and commodity brokers, when the workers wore clogs and the Trades Unions—'

He didn't finish the sentence for a few tables away there was an uncontrolled explosion, a whoosh of flame greater even than that which was usual for the Chatsworth room and a plume of smoke which suggested that one of the penguin-outfitted maitre d's had made a dreadful mistake.

'Bomb,' said Elizabeth. 'Bombe Surprise!'

CHAPTER TWENTY

She was right. It was a big bang.

Tudor swore.

'That wasn't a gastro-explosion,' he said, 'that was the real thing. An Ambrose Perry. His old ladies are going to be in a serious mood now.'

The way in which the Chatsworth staff transformed themselves from food and drink flunkeys to para-medics was impressive. Tudor was reminded of military bandsmen who, in time of war, doubled up as stretcher-bearers.

In fact stretchers were called to the table in a far corner of the room though from what Tudor and Elizabeth could see there was no great need for them. The people who were being stretchered off were walking wounded. They must have been shocked and they would surely have suffered a degree of burning, but they were not dead and they did not appear to have been seriously injured. It looked from a distance as if there were two guests on the casualty list and perhaps a couple of members of staff. The silence which had descended upon the room lifted as abruptly as it had fallen. It was replaced by a buzz of conversation several decibels higher than the muted level of what had gone before.

Suddenly waiters emerged through the swing doors to the

galley carrying trays on which there were enough filled brandy balloons to provide each diner with a glass. Classic treatment for shock. Nothing was said. It was all done crisply, efficiently and with a uniformly stiff upper lip.

'Well,' said Elizabeth, accepting the proffered medicine, 'quite a day. And I thought cruising was an escape and a relaxation. Silly me!'

'Oh, I think appearances are deceptive,' said Tudor. 'It's like effortless superiority. The more effortless it appears the more effort has actually gone into it. Same on board ship. The smoother and more relaxed everything seems to be the more blood, sweat and tears it has actually cost.'

'You reckon?'

'I reckon,' he said. 'I also have a sense that whatever it was may have been aimed at your new friends Herr Doctor and Frau Umlaut. Weren't they sitting over there?'

They both peered in the direction of the pall of smoke which hung blue and acrid over what little remained of the dining table in the far corner. Someone had moved swiftly with a fire extinguisher so there was a lot of foam about. Also charred table and cloth. Essentially, however, it seemed that damage was minimal. The shock was considerable; the explosion spectacular; the consequences depressing but the short-term effects nothing much.

And so to caviar and steak and a Chilean Merlot. The sang-froid was so thick you could have cut it with a standard-issue butter knife let alone one of the sabre-toothed specialist jobs which came with the *filet*. But this was a British ship and although her Britishness had been diluted her *esprit* was undimmed. Rule Britannia and all that. Britons never ever would be slaves. And all that as well.

'A murder attempt that failed?' asked Tudor, 'Or a signally successful warning? It's one or the other.'

'Conspiracy or cock-up,' said Elizabeth. She ordered her caviar straight without egg, onions or sour cream. Ever the purist.

'If the victims were the Umlauts, the greatest enemy they have on board is Prince Abdullah. Do you think he's trying to kill them?'

'It's so easy,' she said, 'someone just has to drop some paraffin on to the steak Diane or whatever, just before the waiter lights his match and *pouf!* you've singed the King of Spain's beard. In a manner of speaking. If you see what I mean.'

'And anyone can have done it?'

She shrugged. 'If that's what it was. After all, you can apparently blow up a Boeing with a mixture of Vodka, lemonade and toothpaste so it really wouldn't be too difficult to lethalize a flambéed steak or crêpe. Simplicity itself. Do you imagine the powers-that-be will slap a ban on table-side cooking? I would. Remember your friend *Tipperary Tatler* is on the loose. Perhaps it's her doing.'

They both stared ruminatively into space and wondered how long it would be before an element of panic was introduced to the ship. Once that happened it would spread as rapidly and inexorably as germs in the air-conditioning or a dreaded lurgy in the galley.

'Gosh,' said Tudor, snapping out of his reverie. 'What's this?' Between his knife and fork there now rested a piece of stiff creamy card with the ship's crest on it and his name printed in crude black ink capital letters. DOCTOR TUDOR CORNWALL. He stared at it suspiciously and then turned it over. On the other side was a message.

'MYOB,' he read. 'Or you're next. And you'll be all fire and no smoke.'

'MYOB?' queried Elizabeth.

'An acronym for Mind Your Own Business,' said Tudor. 'Haven't heard that since, oh, university I suppose. It was a catch-phrase of Ashley Carpenter as a matter of fact.'

'I never heard him use it.' Elizabeth had been Carpenter's pupil in the not-so-distant bad old days. Her relationship had been more than academic so she should have known about his own business.

'You came after that time,' said Tudor. 'He would have adopted a new range of acronyms and acrostics by your day. Or abandoned them altogether. Always up with the latest fashion was our Ashley.'

'Do you think' – Elizabeth looked implausibly ingenuous – 'that MYOB is a signal that he's on board and pulling strings? Seems a strange message otherwise.'

Caviar came. The helpings seemed larger even than usual. If it were true that an army marched on its stomach it was even more true, thought Tudor, of a cruise liner full of paying passengers. Give the punters too much to eat and they'll be lulled into a false sense of security before you can say knife.

'There's no way that Ashley Carpenter can be on board the *Duchess*,' said Tudor. 'I mean, we'd know.'

'Not necessarily,' said Elizabeth. 'He's a terrible tease.'

'He didn't get on in the UK,' said Tudor, 'and I'm pretty sure he didn't embark in Cobh.'

'Maybe,' said Elizabeth, 'he came in the other night. Off the Irish lectureboat. Swapped places with the Captain.'

Tudor rubbed his chin and ate a mother-of-pearl spoonful of Beluga. They did things properly in the Chatsworth.

'Why would he do that?'

'No telling with Ashley,' she said. 'He hates you, that's obvious, and he's keen to get back at me for some reason. Also he has increasing tendencies to megalomania. I don't see any reason for not thinking that he's up to his ears with this gang of hijackers wherever they come from and whoever they are. He's quite doolally.'

'First of all the Irish press party or whoever they are stage a ham-fisted attempt to hijack the ship,' he said. 'They fail but *Tipperary Tatler* escapes and is still at large.'

'Possibly attempting to incinerate the Umlauts.'

'Precisely,' said Tudor, 'and, for the sake of an alternative theory, warning me off with anonymous notes.'

'OK.' The girl shovelled Beluga into her mouth. She clearly found the dainty spoon too mimsy. Caviar wasn't meant to be nibbled, not where she came from.

'Do we think that Ashley and *Tipperary Tatler* are in cahoots?'

'I don't know,' said Elizabeth. 'Ashley was always attracted to dangerous Bohemian redheads. And I think because he sees himself as a failure in conventional terms he wants to remedy the situation with the most radical solution he can find. In other words, violence. He wants to shoot his way into *Who's Who*. The only way he can even manage a footnote in history is by bombing his way in. He's the John Wilkes Booth of our times. He can't be a great man himself so he'll kill one to secure a vicarious destiny. Greatness by proxy. What do you think? You were his contemporary.'

This was true. Tudor and Ashley had competed for the same girl; argued at the same tutorials; got drunk together; played squash against each other; rowed briefly in the same eight; drank beer and sometimes Scotch in each other's company; lied on each other's behalf. Been friends. Now, for reasons that Tudor still found difficult to clearly comprehend they had become the best of enemies. It was something to do with jealousy, though quite what he was not entirely sure. Ashley seemed to him, as he always had done, at least as much a suitable subject for envy himself.

He had no inkling of this enmity until Ashley had invited him down under as a visiting fellow and plotted against him in a cunning and almost lethal way. One legacy of that bizarre encounter was Elizabeth Burney who had once been Ashley's own star pupil and also much much more. Now she was his though only in an academic and never in a million years a carnal one. He had hoped that Ashley would vanish but like the proverbial bad penny he kept turning up when least expected or wanted. The girl and he had privately christened him a latter day Moriarty to Tudor's Holmes. Now here he was once more. Apparently. Perhaps.

Now Mandy Goldslinger also turned up, breathing heavily, flushed, flustered and wearing a little black dress which, as is the way with little black dresses, particularly when worn by ladies of a certain age and a particular disposition began too early and finished too late. Or something like that. It certainly seemed to Tudor that there was not enough of it.

La Goldslinger's impressive breast was heaving with a combination of over-exertion and over-emotion. She appeared to have been running in a literal and metaphorical top gear. And quite possibly been at the brandy.

'There's someone in the Captain's cabin,' she said, breathlessly.

'Someone?' Tudor was intrigued. 'You mean someone other than a skipper stricken by laryngitis?'

'If it's Sam he wouldn't submit to house arrest. I don't think Sam's on board, wherever he is. I think there's someone else in there.'

Elizabeth and Tudor looked at each other meaningfully. They were both thinking Ashley Carpenter. Neither said anything. Professor Carpenter was unlikely to mean anything to Mandy Goldslinger.

'How do you know?' asked Elizabeth.

'A tray,' said the Cruise Director. 'I saw someone with a tray with dinner on it. They knocked on the door and it was opened from inside. The girl went in.'

'Girl?'

'Yes. A stewardess. In *Duchess* uniform.'

'Did you notice anything about her particularly?' Tudor wanted to know but he could tell from her expression that Mandy couldn't tell one member of crew from another. Or didn't. They were like servants to a feudal aristocrat. They all looked the same and were, basically, beneath notice. They merely fetched and carried. A bartender on board mixed cocktails. Why would one know his name or face?

'She was just one of those girls.'

'*Tipperary Tatler*,' said Elizabeth in a 'Eureka! I've got it' tone of voice which owed more to intuition than forensics. There was no reason on earth for thinking that the captain's cabin girl was the Irish terrorist. Elizabeth was playing a hunch. She was good at it, but Chief Inspector Trythall would not have approved. No method, he would have said – typical girl. He, like any good copper, marched inexorably through the alphabet taking in every letter as he went. Not for him these sudden inspired leaps from A to Z.

Mandy Goldslinger looked at her as if she were mad.

'The Irish terrorist girl who escaped,' said Tudor helpfully. 'She originally claimed to work for this fictitious magazine so we've named her after it. Sorry!'

La Goldslinger gave the lady Cruise Director's equivalent of a snort, managing with a gesture and something between a sniff and a sneeze, that she just hated having to deal on equal terms with delinquent children.

'I don't see that the identity of the serving girl is relevant,' she said, sounding like Queen Elizabeth I reprimanding an over-familiar courtier, 'the point is, surely, that the Captain's cabin is occupied.'

'And you previously thought it was empty?'

'Well, yes. Maybe. What do you think's happened to Sam? Has he been murdered?'

'You could take things at face value,' said Tudor, not believing himself or even convinced that he was saying what he heard, 'that poor old Sam's got laryngitis, doesn't want to be disturbed and has lost his voice.'

'The day old Sam loses his voice,' boomed a familiar Celtic foghorn, 'is the day I have it off with the Pope. My view is that old Sam's finally done a runner. Jumped ship and taken the crown jewels with him. He always was a shifty old bugger.'

Mandy Goldslinger began to cry.

CHAPTER TWENTY-ONE

It was indeed Walter and Irmgarde Umlaut who had suffered incendiary indignity in the Chatsworth that night. Their wounds were, however, more cosmetic than damaging. What's more the Umlauts were very cross. Vultur, in particular, was incandescent.

You had to hand it to them, thought Tudor, they were back in the Chatsworth in time for a brace of champagne sorbets and a couple of double espressos. Regular undaunted Prussian Guards, they didn't frighten easily. Blackened but unbowed.

Sir Goronwy and Lady Watkyn passed unsteadily by their table and paused. 'I'm giving them the Porthole Murder tomorrow,' said the bardic Watkyn portentously. 'Steady the Buffs and all that. Not too near the bone, I hope.'

'You mean Gay Gibson, James Camb, the *Durban Castle*, Khaki Roberts and all that?'

'I didn't know it was a speciality of yours,' said the Welshman.

'It isn't,' said Tudor. 'I've read Herbstein's book that's all.'

'Ah.' Sir Goronwy's eyes were rheumy and his expression sceptical, 'Port holes, missing persons, illicit sex...recurring perils of life at sea.'

Mandy Goldslinger sniffed tearfully.

'I have great faith in the Celtic tendency,' said Sir Goronwy. 'The Welsh and the Scots will see us through.'

'But not, I think, the Irish,' said Tudor meaningfully.

'Perhaps not,' said Watkyn. 'On which note I'll bid you *adieu*.'

'Pompous git,' said Elizabeth.

'What was all that about the Port hole case?' asked Mandy, still lachrymose.

'A stewardess on a ship called the *Durban Castle* vanished one night. She was pushed through a port hole by a man called Camb who got off on a technicality. Well, wasn't hanged. He did a long stretch in Dartmoor. Sex that went wrong is what it looks like. Happens quite often on ocean liners. They seem to be havens of innocence and safety but in reality they're hotbeds of lust, crime and sudden death. Like the benign, smiling English countryside. Like the *Duchess*.'

A sombre silence ensued.

'We have a missing captain which may have a perfectly innocent explanation,' said Elizabeth, 'and an attempted hijack which may have been a silly student prank. And a lifeboat loaded with gold ingots which was returned intact. So, *ipso facto*, no provable crime has been committed.'

'That's one interpretation,' said Tudor, 'but the other is that we have a murder or abduction, attempted theft on an extremely ambitious scale and a thwarted act of piracy on the high seas.'

'None of which you can prove.'

Caviar plates were cleared. Steak came.

'You don't like Donaldson,' said Tudor, addressing Mandy Goldslinger.

'Of course not,' she said. 'Why should I? He's been after Sam's job for years but he's not up to it. And he disapproves of the relationship between the two of us.'

'So he knows.'

'He's never said anything outright but he knows. Or at least suspects. He and Sam work in the same office. If you see what I mean. And Angus isn't stupid.'

'But straight.'

'No reason to think otherwise,' she said. 'Like I said, I don't care for him, but I can't pin a dishonesty rap on him. He's always acted by the book.'

'And where does he fit in the present scheme?' asked Tudor. 'Sam is out of it. Whether it's just laryngitis or something more serious is irrelevant. I hate to seem insensitive but that's the way it is. Angus is the man we have to deal with whether we like it or not.'

Mandy sighed. 'Angus sails the ship,' she said. 'That's his job. That's his expertise. Sam is front of house. Sam is the image. He's what the punters enjoy; what they trust; why they sign up for the *Duchess*; why they love Riviera Shipping.'

'But Sam's the boss,' said Elizabeth. 'Angus has to defer if they disagree.'

'They don't disagree,' said Mandy, 'not openly. They can't. Their duties just don't overlap. It's like Sam's front of house and Angus is the chef.'

'That's the theory,' said Tudor. 'What about the reality?'

'What you see is what you get.' The Cruise Director seemed surprised. A lifetime of selling illusion might have robbed her of the ability to distinguish between fact and fiction, thought Tudor. She couldn't do her job if, to an extent, she didn't believe her own publicity. That made her an unreliable witness. On the other hand she was the only member of staff in whom he could really trust. Or could he? So many grey areas. It made life unsettling but it was the nature of the job. Criminal affairs did not concern certainties. Post-mortems reflected the mortems themselves: grey, shadowy, murky, always open to doubt and debate. It was part of what made crime so fascinating.

'You're telling me that Angus and Sam were – are – peas in a pod?' asked Tudor.

'Of course not,' said Mandy Goldslinger, with something approaching asperity. Except that Cruise Directors didn't do asperity. They did schmooze and spin.

'You mean they told one story and lived another,' said Tudor.

'No.' She was irritated now, even though she knew that Tudor was a necessary ally. 'They lived the same story and told the same story. They were both reading from the same hymn sheet. There's no argument. They were a team – whatever they may have felt privately.'

Silence ensued. The atmosphere in the Chatsworth was edgy. It would have been extraordinary if it had been anything else. Atmospheres were elusive concepts. Tudor and Trythall argued about them incessantly. Trythall and other police procedurals denied their existence and believed that even if they did exist they were irrelevant to what actually happened. The presence of the seriously singed Umlauts didn't help any more than the obvious truculence of those at Prince Abdullah's table, leering across the room. There was an atmosphere and you could cut it with the proverbial knife.

'I don't like it,' said Elizabeth. 'I'm getting bad vibes.'

'Relax,' said Mandy Goldslinger, 'everything's under control.' She wasn't convincing, didn't sound as if she meant it. The little tub in the middle of the vasty deep suddenly seemed a terribly vulnerable place to be.

'I need to talk to Donaldson,' said Tudor. 'He's in charge whether we like it or not.'

'You,' said Elizabeth, 'have no standing in any of this. Goronwy Watkyn and Freddie Grim are just as well qualified.

In any case, Angus Donaldson simply has to take us to our destination and the American authorities will sort everything out. So relax. Go with the flow.'

'I disagree,' said Tudor. 'I don't think the American authorities *will* sort it out. My sense is that they still have a blind spot when it comes to Irish republicans, and Irish republicans are one of the threads we're contending with here. I think the American process is even more susceptible to hot-shot lawyers than the British one. I think they'll be out of sympathy and kilter with what is still, despite the Prince and the Umlauts, a British-owned shipping line. So actually my view is that American so-called justice will screw up and we'd be much better solving the whole thing at sea before we dock.'

'You sound like a crusty old xenophobe,' Elizabeth laughed scornfully. 'I thought you were better than that.'

'Tudor may be right,' said Mandy Goldslinger unexpectedly. 'I'm not too happy about the idea of the NYPD followed by the course of American justice. I can see our poor little ship being impounded for months if not years while nothing much happens at vast expense.'

'And Mandy's American,' said Tudor with a self-satisfaction bordering on triumphalism.

'If you're determined to try to solve it single-handed without benefit of due legal and forensic process then I think you have to see Angus Donaldson and have a serious discussion with him.' Elizabeth was being uncharacteristically sensible, even pedantic. 'In Sam's absence Donaldson's in charge. You simply have to get his clearance. As we've said there's already a sort of official ship's system for sorting out misdemeanours at sea even if it's only a semi-competent Master-at-Arms and his minions. You've also got Freddie Grim and Goronwy Watkyn, both of whom think their credentials are as good as yours. Or better.'

She was right. They all knew it.

'No time like the present,' he said, smiling at Mandy. 'Can you fix?'

'Sure,' she said. 'Angus and I have very correct and cordial relations. There'll be no problems.'

She stood and left. Tudor sighed and gazed round the emptying restaurant. Staff were stacking, polishing glasses, laying tables for next morning's breakfast. Passengers had mostly left heading for the cinema or the ballroom where the evening entertainment of crooner, crooneuse, stand-up comedian and the ship's dancers, mainly classically trained Romanians would have to be introduced in just under ten minutes. A job for La Goldslinger though she might have delegated it to one of her two assistants in view of the pressing matter of pinning down the Staff Captain.

The ship lunged lightly, reminding them, as she did from time to time, that she was a ship and not a grand hotel. It was such a strange phenomenon, this salty escape which was in its way a self-imposed imprisonment. Hell was gentlemen hosts, he mused. Or other passengers. Or nothing to do but eat and drink and be fried lobster-pink by sun, sea and wind. After a day or so it took him ten minutes to decide whether to have a gin and tonic or a Tom Collins.

'May we join you?'

It was Vultur and Irmgarde, fresh from bonfire night.

They were both clutching coffee cups and liqueur glasses and looking blackened but unbowed.

'I apologize,' said Doctor Umlaut, 'for the earlier diversion. It must have been upsetting for everybody.'

'Not as much as for you,' said Tudor politely.

'It is nothing,' he said, as they sat down heavily. Tudor and Elizabeth's table was a four, laid for two, but with a quartet of chairs, 'but whether a mistake or something more sinister, well . . .' He grinned. 'Occasionally I feel times at sea are in need of a little enlivening. Storm perhaps. An outbreak of stomach sickness. A man overboard. Don't you agree?'

'Up to a point,' said Tudor. 'But on the whole people come on the *Duchess* to get away from that sort of unpleasantness. It's like country-house weekends. People didn't go away expecting to find a body in the library, a suspicious butler, an adulterous hostess and Miss Marple or Monsieur Poirot asking a lot of impertinent questions and coming up with some embarrassing answers. They just wanted to play billiards and croquet, drink champagne and flirt. Same with being on board the *Duchess*. Passengers come for a quiet life – eat, drink, be quietly merry, tango with a gentleman host or a beautiful passenger and generally escape unpleasant reality.'

'My turn to say "up to a point",' said Doctor Umlaut, smiling, 'and to observe that life isn't like that. A truism verging on a cliché. There is a sense that a great ship is a microcosm of the greater life in the world outside. Not unlike the country-house you describe. And if reality should rear its ugly head it is much more difficult to escape its clutches on board ship than on dry land. Perhaps that is a paradox too.'

He's trying to tell me something, thought Tudor, but he's being so elliptical that I'm not sure what he means. He wasn't altogether sure that Umlaut himself knew.

'What I mean to say,' said the little man, seeming to sense the lack of comprehension and the ambiguity that had caused it, 'is that nothing is ever what it seems and never more so than in an isolated, hot-house atmosphere such as this, from which, for a while at least, there is no escape. But you will know this from your academic studies. Forgive me. I am presuming too much, encroaching on an area of expertise which is foreign to me just as it is familiar to you.'

Tudor nodded his head but said nothing.

'And,' Doctor Umlaut abruptly changed the subject, 'talking of academic interests. I thought your talk on HMS *Bounty* most interesting. What is your next subject please?'

'Piracy,' said Tudor. 'Tomorrow at eleven.'

Doctor Umlaut inclined his head. 'I have often wondered,' he said, 'about the exact distinction between privateers, buccaneers and pirates.'

'It can be a perilously thin line,' said Tudor, 'but in essence an act of piracy is when a ship is seized out of control of her legal master and crew by those who have boarded the vessel in disguise as passengers. When captured they were hanged in chains on prominent headlands as a warning to others. Or staked to the ground at Execution Dock in Wapping to be drowned by the rising tide.'

Mrs Umlaut let out a little yelp of disgust but her husband seemed quite amused.

'The last pirate was executed in England in 1840,' added Tudor, 'but the United States executed one in 1862.'

Doctor Umlaut shook his charred head and smiled.

Tudor half-expected him to say '*Ach so*!' which was almost exactly what he did, adding the single line, 'History is so often an act of repetition, don't you think? Even at sea there is nothing new under the sun.'

CHAPTER TWENTY-TWO

Angus Donaldson's cabin shook, trembled and rattled causing Tudor to quite involuntarily do much the same.

'We seem to be making good speed,' said Tudor.

'Aye,' said Donaldson, who was a man of few words save when cracking ancient jokes over the Tannoy. He hailed from the Kingdom of Fife and was loose-limbed and bearded. His family were all fisher-folk and his brother and nephews still manned a small herring trawler in the town of Anstruther. Angus had come south and been with Riviera Shipping most of his adult life.

'Should be in New York on schedule if not before,' said Tudor conversationally.

'Happen,' said Donaldson.

They were both standing and Donaldson suddenly and awkwardly motioned his guest to sit. They both did so. The Staff Captain's cabin had two armchairs, upright and not particularly comfortable. Donaldson did not offer his guest any refreshment. Instead he said, 'I'd like to extend the company's thanks in the matter of apprehending the ruffians who attempted to hijack the vessel.'

He was not only a man of few words, he had a funny way with them.

There was a black and white masked ball in the Great Hall that evening and Tudor was already wearing his black tie and dinner jacket which seemed a marginal cop-out but could hardly be more black and white. His bog-standard black mask, purchased in the ship's boutique was in his pocket. For the time being he was instantly recognizable.

'That's very kind of you,' said Tudor. 'Thank you.'

The Staff Captain flashed an official smile of acknowledgement and then said, a touch ominously, 'But.'

The monosyllable hung in the air between them for what seemed like a long time. Then Donaldson repeated it making it seem even worse second time round.

'That will be all. It was Ms Goldslinger's initiative to embroil you in the unpleasantness that occurred earlier and I'm afraid she exceeded her authority. No harm done fortunately, but from now on the proprieties will be observed and Riviera Shipping will take care of things in the normal way.'

'You can't behave "in the normal way",' protested Tudor, 'when events just aren't normal.'

The Staff Captain shrugged. 'Riviera Shipping is prepared for every eventuality,' he said, as if reciting from an instruction manual.

Tudor shrugged back but could think of no immediately sensible riposte. It was abundantly clear that the company was not prepared for every eventuality. The Irish had taken it by surprise: Tudor had saved its bacon. Now the captain was off sick believed missing, and the ring-leader of the pirates had escaped. A key passenger had almost been incinerated. An empty lifeboat had been recovered with hundreds of thousands of pounds-worth of gold ingots and possibly a bloodstain. Ashley Carpenter had planted an obituary notice of his good self. There was nothing normal in any of this and, as far as he could see, the official response had been non-existent.

No wonder Donaldson shrugged. A collective shrug seemed to be the official reaction. Not good enough in his estimation.

'Anyway,' said Donaldson, 'while thanking you for your valuable assistance I must point out, again on behalf of the company, that you are engaged solely as a guest speaker so that while we appreciate your continued efforts in that capacity we must ask that you in no way exceed or deviate from the terms of your contract.'

'Say again,' said Tudor, in the vernacular he had picked up from the crew's communication. No one in the navy seemed ever to use the word 'repeat'.

'I say again,' said Donaldson, 'stick to what you've been hired to do. Lecture the passengers. Understood?'

He made it sound very like a threat and Tudor finally took the hint, made only the flimsiest pretext of an excuse, and left.

The masked or was it 'masqued' ball that followed was as surreal an affair as he had expected and feared. He and Elizabeth had bought the most basic Venetian-style masks from Ye Shoppe situated aft on the boat deck. Ye Shoppe had obviously bought a job lot of such things from a manufacturer with an obscurely Middle Eastern sounding name in Skegness. The masks were heavily sequinned and came in two kinds. One was a sort of permanent business of the type airlines provided to shut out light when attempting to sleep and came with elastic bands which fitted over the ears. These not only left your hands free for dancing, or whatever, and would have been useful for gentleman hosts attempting to prevent their leaning partners from toppling over. They also ensured that the disguise did not slip. The other kind came on sticks like sartorial lollipops. They were cheaper, meant that at least one hand had to be kept clutching it and were imperfect at hiding one's identity. In other words these masks slipped.

Music was provided by the ship's resident band, the Dukes of Dixie, an elderly gaggle of jazz musicians who had originally played together in the far-off days of Radio Luxemburg. Transferring to the later pirate radio ship, *Caroline*, moored for a while in the middle of the North Sea the Dukes had rather taken to the ocean wave so that when she was launched the *Duchess* was, in every way, made for them. Once svelte, lean and darkly handsome, the Dukes had become grey, tubby and mildly seedy, but they could still hold a tune and belt it out satisfactorily. Their lead singer who called himself Hiram G. Billy, but whose real name was something quite different, could have rasped a bronchial rap with George Melly who must have been much the same age.

The dancers seemed, on the whole, to have some difficulty keeping up with the Dukes but that didn't really matter much. Meanwhile, waiters shimmered about the ballroom with sparkling drinks of uncertain provenance and the ship rolled.

'If Mom and Dad could see me now,' muttered Elizabeth, as she led Tudor round the floor and peeked over the top of her hand-held mask.

'I know what you mean,' said her partner, perspiring. It seemed awfully hot to him though not, apparently, to everyone else.

From time to time passing dancers waved, bowed or in other ways made themselves known to Tudor and Elizabeth. This was polite but tantalizing since without exception they appeared to have masks which worked and which in many cases seemed to have come from more exotic and expensive places than Ye Shoppe or Skegness.

Much of this dress was decidedly fancy so that Tudor in his regulation dinner jacket and Elizabeth in her almost equally regulation little black dress felt ill-prepared and out-of-place. They were not real cruisers in the sense that the majority of the *Duchess*'s passengers clearly were. They lacked the wardrobe and they grew restless with too much indolence and pleasure. Most of the disguised dancers, however, were having a ball.

'Who *are* all these people?' asked Elizabeth, as they shuffled round the small and undulating floor. 'I mean have we, like, been introduced?'

The Dukes seemed to accelerate their syncopations as if to emphasize their difference from the paying passengers. Quick, quick, slow seemed to become fast, fast, quick but it made little apparent difference to the gentlemen hosts, their partners and those who followed. They stuck to their own time and beat which was, of course, a great deal more leisurely than the Dukes' geriatric frenzy. Sticking to their own time and beat was, Tudor reflected, what passengers did best. The *Duchess* had guidelines which needed to be adhered to but within these confines her clientele did pretty much as they pleased in their own distinctive fashions. It was, up to a point, the purpose of cruising.

From time to time fellow-revellers bumped into Tudor and Elizabeth or they into them. Because, however, they were masked neither Tudor nor his partners knew who they were. This, Tudor supposed, was another of cruising's golden rules. One was always bumping into people. You were seldom sure who they were and the odds were that you would never see them again. This didn't matter for they were ships that pass in the night. Or to be precise, they were *on* ships that pass in the night. Or to be even more precise, they were *like* ships that pass in the night.

'Ouch!' exclaimed Elizabeth. 'You just trod on my toe.'

'Sorry,' he said. 'I wasn't thinking.'

'Yes, you were,' she riposted. 'Thinking too much. You may not be the niftiest dancer ever known but you're not a foottreader. Penny for them.'

'What?'

'The thoughts.'

The band was playing something Tudor thought dimly was by Gershwin though one Dukes' melody sounded pretty much like another. They were that sort of band and made that sort of noise. Syncopated muzak. Rentabilk.

'I don't know,' he said, 'I was all over the place.'

'Including my feet,' said Elizabeth with feeling, though less feeling than a few moments earlier when Tudor had first stepped on them.

One of Prince Abdullah's wives cannoned off them and bounced away at around forty-five degrees giggling coquettishly. She was, surprisingly, locked in a stiff embrace with an obvious gentleman host in a vaguely Mexican-eagle head-dress and mask. The Aztec eagle had the hallmarks – tottering dexterity, louche innocence – of Ambrose Perry but then so many of the gentlemen hosts were similar walking oxymorons. The girl might not have been one of Abdullah's brides but she wore a jellaba – which obviated the need for a mask – and Tudor was so influenced by the clichés of ship-board life that he had begun jumping to conclusions he would never have reached on shore. Whatever, the girl had dancing eyes and seemed familiar. Tudor had an odd sense that the Prince's harem was increasing every knot. It was as if they were multiplying by some strange osmotic reproductive process. This could have been an illusion.

The band seemed to be playing 'The Eton Boating Song' souped up. Presumably a Humphrey Lyttleton adaptation created perhaps for a Beaulieu jazz festival of the 1950s. It was like all the other noises made by the band but somewhere in among the farty-brassy stridences you could just about make out the plangent notes of the old rowing number with its references to jollity and togetherness which seemed apt and to 'feathering' which didn't.

Mandy Goldslinger slunk past, facially disguised but instantly recognizable on account of her constricted and cantilevered carcass entubed in sequins and lamé and doing something mildly South American with a black-masked figure in the uniform of a ship's doctor. She waved a touch too gaily. The game Doctor and Frau Umlaut, recognizable by their singes, limped past forlornly. Prince Abdullah sat on a sofa surveying the hordes, smoking implacably.

'Mass murderers,' said Tudor. 'Looking around here I'd say they might all have done it.'

'That's silly,' said Elizabeth.

'Maybe,' said Tudor. 'But it's life and death as well. Nearly everyone prancing around this room is capable of murder.'

'So what?' Elizabeth had to shout in to his ear as they shuffled round the Great Hall, 'We're all *capable* of murder. Ashley taught me that and you say the same. But as you also say, the fact that we're *capable* of murder doesn't make us all murderers. We could all commit all sorts of crimes but that doesn't turn us into criminals. Civilization is about the suppression of instinct. If we all did what we could and, more importantly, if we all did what we'd really like then life would be impossible. We'd all be killing each other, nicking each other's possessions, having sex with each other's partners and Christ knows what.'

The band had moved on to 'Amazing Grace'. Strange how they managed to make the same noise all the time and yet underlay it with a just recognizable tune.

'I still think the room is full of potential killers,' said Tudor, as they cannoned off a couple who had the ample paunch and posterior of the Goronwy Watkyns. Whoever they were they made no acknowledgement of acquaintance but waddled off, wiggling, more or less in time to the music.

'That's silly too,' said Elizabeth. 'I think you've overdone it. I think you should go to bed.'

'I do feel tired,' said Tudor. 'It's been a rough old day. But I still think there's more murder and more crime at sea than most people admit. Which means that there are plenty of criminals afloat. And plenty right here all round us, thinly disguised or not.'

'Bed,' she said, 'definitely time for bed.'

And for a fleeting moment Tudor thought he caught a whiff of double-entendre.

CHAPTER TWENTY-THREE

Once more he slept fitfully. This actually meant that he tossed and turned and had trouble breathing when on his back and even more when he turned over and tried lying on his stomach. The ship was noisy and the ride bumpy but neither of these was the problem. He slept well on ships, even in storms and this wasn't a storm in the accepted sense. He was dog-tired as well so sleep should have come easily, but somehow it didn't. Once or twice he got up and peered out of the port hole, awed as usual, by the vast expanse of white capped nothingness of the mid-Atlantic.

Donaldson's words bothered him. In a sense they were not new. He had been living with the strictures of hard-bitten professionals for the whole of his working life. Back home, his old mucker Trythall was permanently on his shoulder, a copper's copper now holding the exalted rank of Detective Chief Inspector in the local constabulary. Trythall had always taken an avuncular view: OK sonny, abstract theories are all very well in your ivory tower, but when it comes to real life you should leave it to real men like me – people who've actually been out on the beat, felt a few collars, witnessed nature red in tooth and claw, been there and done that. You stick to your books and papers, your lectures and tutorials. You're fiction: we're fact.

He sighed up at the ceiling. Dawn was breaking through the night outside and forcing lightness through the porthole. Newer ships had square windows and balconies. The *Duchess* belonged to a different generation when seaworthiness was the first consideration in ship-building. She was almost defiantly old-fashioned and seaworthy. A professional to her fingertips.

Which brought him back to his sleep-disturbing unease. Was he a genuine professional? Of course he was. He ran a fine department in an adequate university. It was, in fact, a flagship outfit – an alpha institution in an otherwise beta organization. He personally enjoyed international respect among his peers. He had a job and he was good at it. His alumni prospered. Likewise his papers and pamphlets. He teetered on the brink of celebrity, was already world-famous in Wessex. And yet, deep down in his heart of hearts, he feared that men like Trythall and Donaldson were right. He was an amateur and they were professionals; he was a Gentleman and they were Players.

He got up again and went to the porthole. Away in the distance he could make out a huge container ship buffeting through the waves. He was reminded of John Masefield's catchy little poem 'Cargoes' which he had learned by heart as a child. They hadn't had container ships in Masefield's day, just chunky little tramp steamers with cargoes of pig-iron. That wasn't quite right. Pig-lead. He closed his eyes.

Funny, he could have sworn it was 'pig-iron' not 'pig-lead' and a 'Tramp steamer' not a 'coaster.' Just showed how fallible memory was and yet memory was a cornerstone of conventional British justice. Evidence in court was memory-based, almost by definition. Yet memory was almost always flawed. Tramp steamers, he thought, squinting at the ugly container vessel on the horizon, had been consigned to history along with bobbies on bicycles. Somehow everything seemed to bring him back to police procedure. He supposed he must have learned the Masefield at about the time that he was first getting to know Sherlock Holmes and Lord Peter Wimsey. Privately he still stuck to the belief that these two were the best detectives ever with Holmes right out in front of Wimsey, and the rest limping along in their wake. As for real-life detectives they were nothing compared to the giants of fiction. Whisper it not to the likes of Donaldson and Trythall but they were mere pygmies in the police pantheon.

Day really was beginning to dawn now. He realized as he watched fingers of pink illuminating the ocean that it had been a while since they had seen the sun or even a hint of blue sky. They had been sailing under and over steel grey. A metaphor for life, he thought gloomily. His existence was seldom punctuated even by shafts of crepuscular pink but was almost uniformly monotone. No, that was an exaggeration. There were a number of highs in his life of lows but in the still small hours it never seemed like that, particularly after a dressing down from a man such as Angus Donaldson. He knew he should rise above such sermons but he was absurdly thin-skinned besides which there was more than a shadow of doubt about the worth of what he was doing. In his heart of hearts he doubted even whether Wessex should have a university of its own and whether, anyway, the University of Wessex was worthy of the name. His department was degree-giving. You could graduate with a Bachelor of Arts in Criminal Studies or even, God help him, a Ph.D. in Criminal Studies complete with tasselled mortar board and a banana and orange hood to your rook-like black gown. Was it all a farce? The Vice-Chancellor had even tried to foist Lord Archer of Weston-super-Mare on him as one of a batch of celebrity honorary ordinands but at least Tudor had been able to resist that one. No honorary degree from Wessex for Jeffrey. Not even over his dead body.

He sat down heavily on the bed. Now there was a success. Lord Archer of Weston-super-Mare. He was a real pro. But here Tudor really did tell himself to take a grip. There were crimes to consider, disappearances to be explained and he really could not afford the luxury of contemplating Jeffrey Archer.

He supposed he should do as he was commanded by Donaldson. After all the man was in charge of the ship and had a right to be obeyed without question. That was the way they did things in the Merchant Marine. You did as you were told without demur. If there was to be a debate you had to wait until after the event. Quite unlike civvy street and in particular to a man such as Tudor Cornwall whose natural instinct honed by years of practice was to subject everything to relentless, forensic examination.

Someone knocked on the door and he glanced at his watch. 6.30. Far too early for room service even if he had ordered such a thing. He presumed it was a human knock and not a ship's rodent scratching. If it were human it could be an enemy, dangerous. *Tipperary Tatler* perhaps still dangerously at large. Or someone suspicious like Freddie Grim or Prince Abdullah or . . . well, as he had observed on the dance floor of the Great Hall the previous night, almost everyone was more or less suspicious. He simply couldn't afford to be paranoid and terrified of every early morning knock on the door. Nevertheless caution was advisable.

'Who is it?' he asked in a stage whisper.

'It's me,' said a strong, female Antipodean voice, 'Elizabeth.'

'Oh,' he replied, apprehensive though not for quite the same fearful reasons as a few seconds earlier. 'What is it?'

'I wanted to see you. Let me in. The door's locked.'

He put on a *Duchess* towelling bath robe with the ship's logo of anchor and tiara over the breast pocket, unlocked the door and admitted a windblown waif in tight jeans and a turquoise tank top. She was blue lips, tousled hair and damp, salty spray.

'Brill sunrise,' she said. 'I've been up on the foredeck or whatever you call it. You know, just under the bridge. I was the only person there. It was just miraculous. One minute it's so dark you can still see the stars and that container ship away on the left was still lit up—'

'Port,' said Tudor pedantically.

'You what?'

'Port,' he said. 'On board ship left is port and right is starboard.'

'That's just affectation,' she said. 'Any case you no more know your port from your starboard than your arse from your elbow. You're even more of a landlubber than I am.'

'It's not an affectation actually,' said Tudor, uncomfortably aware that he was sounding even more pompous. 'If you say "right" or "left" there's room for ambiguity. If you're facing the stern it could be your left or the ship's left. If it's port or starboard it's always the same. See what I mean? Did you say you were watching the sunrise over the bows. You sure you don't mean the stern?'

'Unlike you,' she said, 'I do know my arse from my elbow, my port from my starboard and, above all and most certainly, my bows from my stern and my front from your back.'

'And you saw the sun come up while you were standing forrard.'

'Amazing. First of all you just have a sort of general pink haze and then this amazing sort of red cricket ball emerges and pops up. It's like a beachball being squeezed out of a swimming pool. You know? Now you see it, now you don't. Or rather, the other way around. Now you don't see it, then you do. Exciting. It almost fizzed. First real sun I've seen all trip.'

'You sure you were in the bows?'

'Don't be silly. Look on the TV.'

The TV set had no fewer than eighteen channels. Half a dozen were dedicated to movies; three to a loop of in-house lecturing, including Tudor himself – to his chagrin; others were devoted to sales of various *Duchess*-related products including shore excursions where appropriate. Channel Three was 'The View from the Bridge' with classical music. Tudor turned it on and was rewarded by Handel and a magnificent view of the sharp end of the *Duchess* ploughing towards a gloriously rising sun. 'Thine be the Glory' Judas Maccabeus. Epic stuff.

'See,' said Elizabeth. 'Stern indeed. Did we have a bet on it?'

'Not that I can remember. You can have a second boiled egg for breakfast.'

'Big bloody deal,' she grinned. 'I slept like a log till six. How about you?'

' 'Fraid not,' he said. 'Donaldson's slightly got to me. I have a feeling we should pull back; leave things to sort themselves out; let Donaldson and his security team take care of it all.'

'Security team!?' Elizabeth looked sexily angry. 'Those goons! You must be joking.'

'To be honest I hadn't given them much thought. But my strong impression is that Donaldson is concerned to try to keep a lid on the situation; prevent things getting out of hand; hand it over to competent authorities as soon as possible.'

'And you feel like letting him?'

Tudor shrugged. 'If I'm asked to help – as I was by Mandy

Goldslinger – then I'll do what I can. But if I'm expressly told not to interfere I don't feel I have much alternative.'

'That's a bit weedy.'

'It's life,' he said. 'When the chips are down I have to admit that I have no authority. Also my skills are essentially theoretical. You could be the regius professor of law at Oxford or whatever but that doesn't mean that you'd be competent to lead for the prosecution or defence at a big case at the Old Bailey.'

'On the contrary,' said Elizabeth, 'you'd be a damned sight better than most barristers. You always say so and I believe you. I think you're right. I also think you'd make a better first of conducting a criminal investigation. Probably better than the average senior cop back in the UK and most certainly than some jumped up security guard on board ship.'

'I don't know,' he said, 'we're all prone to self-doubt. I'm all very well on paper, lecturing, sitting in my ivory tower. But sometimes I feel I should stay there and leave real life to the people who deal with real life. I just do theory and I should stick to it.'

'Well, maybe,' she said, 'but I think you have a duty to be involved. 'We have every reason to believe that Sam Hardy, the legitimately appointed Master of the *Duchess* has been removed from his position against his will and possibly even murdered. I think you have a perfect right – duty even – to insist on his being released or produced. And until and unless that's done you should investigate like fury.'

'It's not as simple as that,' he said, glancing at his watch. 'They'll be serving breakfast in a moment and I'm feeling peckish. I'm going to have a shave and a shower then I'll see you up there. If you're there ahead of me I'll have porridge and a couple of boiled eggs with brown toast and black coffee.'

'And mine's mixed berries, low fat yoghurt and camomile tea,' she said, letting herself out. 'I guess you could poison us with any of that, though my money's on the dispenser which "sanitizes" your hands. That's a murder weapon if ever I saw one. Sir Goronwy Watkyn in the Chatsworth with the hand-sanitizer. Beats Colonel Mustard in the conservatory with the lead piping any day.'

And she laughed.

CHAPTER TWENTY-FOUR

Breakfast aboard the *Duchess* was always a muted, even subdued, affair. The morning after the masked ball it was, inevitably, even quieter and more sparsely populated than usual.

The meal was served between 7 and 9.30 but that was ship's time which by now was in a little warp all of its own. In the middle – or thereabouts – of its voyage to the United States, the *Duchess* was chronologically behind home but ahead of her destination. She lost an hour a day throughout the voyage, so that by the time she arrived in New York, she was five miles behind her base in the United Kingdom and existing at the same time as the millions of Americans living along the Eastern Seaboard. In mid-Atlantic she was as isolated in time terms as she was geographically. This compounded her sense of loneliness, isolation and vulnerability. In terms of the ideal setting for a closed-room classic Agatha Christie murder she knocked a snow-bound country house into any number of cocked hats.

In a real terrestrial stately home, of course, there would have been a hotplate on a sideboard with silver topped dishes of kidneys and kedgeree from which silent guests would have helped themselves. The *Duchess* was more grand hotel than grande dame with what the trade called 'silver service' from waiters and waitresses with names such as Waclav and Natalia, all immaculate in starched jackets and with manners and skills that their United Kingdom counterparts simply couldn't have deployed. Tudor found this mildly depressing though not sufficiently to put him off his boiled eggs which came just as he preferred with firm whites, gungy yolks and crisp brown soldiers. Elizabeth dabbed at a light moustache of low-fat yoghurt and eyed him disapprovingly.

The crew to passenger ratio on board the ship was amazingly high. There were almost as many people driving the ship and attending to the clients' needs as there were paying punters. Given that the passengers were for the most part elderly and infirm and the crew fit and youthful it would have been a doddle for a mutiny to have succeeded. Overpowering resistance, should the masses behind the green baize door have risen up in rebellion, would have been ridiculously easy. Over the years Tudor had witnessed some ugly moments when passengers took against crew or, less obviously, vice versa. But none had ended in tears.

'That's a heart attack on a plate,' said Elizabeth virtuously.

'Nonsense,' said Tudor. 'Two *not* hard boiled eggs represent a mild palpitation at worst. Fay Weldon as much as said so. "Go to work on an egg".'

'That was an advertising campaign on behalf of the Egg Marketing Board if I'm correctly informed,' she said. 'But for a man of your age and in your condition they're a bad idea in anything other than moderation.'

'I can't help my age,' said Tudor, 'but there is nothing at all wrong with my condition. I'm in perfectly good nick. And certainly in good enough nick not to be damaged by a couple of boiled eggs for breakfast.'

She seemed unimpressed.

'Boiled eggs are bad for you,' she said. 'End of story. But more to the point, "Are you a detective or not?" People like Trythall and Donaldson are right in a way. You're all fur coat and no knickers. Most of the time, operating in the UK the way you do you're in the same position as a critic to an author or a concert. Power possibly, but no responsibility. Now here, for once, you're outside police jurisdiction, away from the rule of law, you have a serious possibility of showing the world that you're not just a load of hot air but a real power to be reckoned with. This is a serious chance to prove yourself. Take it, run with it, come first past the post and you're made for life – fail and everyone's criticism is justified.'

'That's pretty harsh.'

'It's life,' she said, smiling.

'A defining moment?'

'You could say that.'

'If I cop out I remain a peripheral figure, properly despised by those at the sharp end like Detective Chief Superintendent Trythall and Captain Donaldson.'

'You said it.' She spooned low-fat yoghurt on to her berries, blue, black, straw, rasp. Waclav poured her more camomile tea. Natalia poured him more black coffee.

Away in the distance the Umlauts, still charred, were breakfasting off cured herring, pumpernickel and Darjeeling tea with lemon. They seemed agitated and presently Walter placed his napkin carefully to the left of his place, pushed back his chair and walked slowly to Tudor and Elizabeth's table where he asked if he might sit. They naturally acquiesced.

'You understand, naturally,' he began, 'that the man Abdullah and I are not the best of friends.'

No one said anything.

'Enemies, in fact.'

Tudor and Elizabeth both nodded.

'He is not, of course, a prince.'

There seemed nothing they could say and they didn't, though Elizabeth smiled encouragingly.

'And his wives are not wives.'

'Really!' said Tudor. 'I've had my suspicions about the so-called wives ever since we set sail.'

Elizabeth shot him a glance which was half amused, half exasperated. It seemed to say 'Men!'

'And they have been multiplying,' said Dr Umlaut. Waclav asked if he'd like something to drink and he said he'd like to continue with Darjeeling and a slice of lemon.

'Multiplying?' asked Tudor.

'There are now more than there were when we embarked,' he said. 'I can't say for certain how many more but there has been a definite increase. You know that Abdullah is attempting to acquire the ship and make it his own. With compulsory smoking everywhere.'

'I understood as much,' said Tudor, 'but I understand that you too aspire to taking over the ship.'

'Only in order to prevent this horrible person,' said the Doctor, 'My position is entirely, as you would have it, reactive. If this so-called "Prince" were not in the frame I would be more than content to let the status quo maintain itself.'

'Well that's by the by,' said Tudor. 'The fact is that you and Prince Abdullah, Prince or not, are in the middle of what is, in effect a boardroom war. From a seat in the grandstand it's quite difficult to call the shots. As an impartial observer I...well let's just say I find it very difficult to become partial. I'm not sure I should take sides.'

'But there is good,' said Umlaut, 'which is me. And there is bad, which is that man.'

'With respect,' said Tudor, meaning as always when those

words are uttered, nothing of the sort, 'we only have your word for that.'

'My word is my bond,' said the little man, bristling in a burnt-out way.

'That too. This wouldn't stand up in court. You need proof, corroborative evidence.'

'That's what we look to *you* for. You are our resident expert. You run a department of criminal affairs at a university. You are the expert. Much better than police. They have no brain.'

'It's very kind of you to say so,' said Tudor, 'but I'm afraid I'm off the case. The captain has ordered me to back off.'

'But we have no captain. The captain is missing. This is the heart of the mystery. This is why you are essential. It is you who must discover the body. Or the living person. We rely on you. The whole ship relies on you.' He sounded quite distraught.

'The drill is that the senior officer aboard is the man in charge. The official line is that the Master himself is indisposed due to laryngitis. Because he can't speak the captaincy automatically devolves on to his number two, Angus Donaldson. That means that Donaldson is in charge. And Donaldson has ordered me off the case. Whatever you or I think about that it really leaves me with no options. Sorry.'

Waclav brought a pot of Darjeeling and some lemon slices. The three of them sat in silence while he poured.

When he had retreated, Umlaut said, 'I also am sorry.'

'I'm not sure I agree with your sit rep,' said Elizabeth. 'If you have good reason to believe that the right and proper captain of the ship, namely Sam Hardy, has been abducted, maybe even murdered, and that Angus Donaldson might conceivably have been involved in the crime, then surely you're duty bound to solve the mystery no matter what. If

Donaldson's position as *de facto*, substitute boss has been wrongfully obtained then all bets are off. I'm not convinced Donaldson has the right to tell you what to do.'

'Mind if I join you?' It was Mandy Goldslinger looking as if she had slept as fitfully as Tudor. She had rings under her eyes, her hands shook and her voice sounded husky.

'Tomato juice, Waclav,' she said, 'heavy on the Tabasco and Worcester. Very black coffee.' She sat down without waiting for a say-so.

'Couldn't help hearing that,' she said, 'and I agree and then again I don't. If it's any consolation I've had a shot across the bows from Donaldson just like Tudor has. And according to the rules he has authority on his side. I mean he's the number two and there's no number one and therefore in the absence of the said number one the number two takes the top spot. Do I make myself clear?'

'Not entirely,' said Tudor, 'but I think we call get your drift.'

'On the other hand,' continued the Cruise Director, 'if the number two has only got into pole position on account of nefarious behaviour towards his superior officer and captain then all bets are off and it's permissible to investigate. Not just permissible but imperative.'

'May an old man pull up a chair?'

It was Sir Goronwy Watkyn looking as if he had enjoyed a better night's sleep than anyone.

'It appears,' he said, extracting an empty a chair from an adjacent table, 'that willy-nilly we find ourselves as players in the sort of puzzle in which I and the good Doctor here' – he nodded almost conspiratorially in the direction of Tudor Cornwall – 'specialize – though usually as arbiters rather than participants.'

'We are together here whether we like it or not,' said

Umlaut. 'It is inescapable. We are in on the act. We are on stage. We cannot just be in the audience.'

'Our friend has a certain logic on his side,' said Sir Goronwy portentous as ever. 'In life on land an inspector calls. In a situation such as this, one dials nine nine nine and policemen arrive, lawyers are retained and the whole apparatus of detection, apprehension, trial and sentence is gone through in the traditional manner. Out here however we are in, as it were, a nautical jungle. There are no policemen, no lawyers, no trials, no juries. On this occasion, quite fortuitously, we have a number of experts of whom I have the honour to be one. This expertise should be utilized. We would be failing in our duty if we were to do otherwise and particularly if we were to stand idly by.'

'But,' protested Tudor, 'we have absolutely no legal authority. Besides, in a day or so the ship will be docking and the whole matter can be handed over to the legitimate authorities.'

'But those authorities will be American,' said Umlaut, 'and the ship is registered in the United Kingdom. This presents the first of many dilemmas. The pirates are, I believe, Irish. American justice is, as you say, notoriously one-eyed with regard to the Emerald Isle. The Abdullah man comes from I know not where. So where does this leave us? In a state of much confusion. I certainly am in such a state.'

'Seems to me,' said Elizabeth, 'that Donaldson is, on the one hand a prime suspect, and on the other, judge and jury. That's not right.'

They all thought about this while the staff replenished their drinks.

'I don't trust Donaldson,' said Mandy Goldslinger, 'and I fear for Sam.' She seemed tearful.

Tudor pushed his chair back. 'I'm sorry,' he said. 'I'm sure you'll forgive me but I have a lecture to deliver at eleven and I need to prepare. Also I have a letter to write.'

He smiled around at the little group which seemed dissatisfied if not exactly open-mouthed. He glanced out of the window – a big square job at this more exalted level than his stateroom. Outside the day had turned sullen gun-metal grey and the sky was quite without features.

CHAPTER TWENTY-FIVE

His talk on pirates seemed to go reasonably well. He had done it many times before and was able to speak for forty-five minutes or so without notes. The producer in the box at the back of the theatre was an old acquaintance now and trusted him not to do anything ridiculous, to keep his voice level consistent, speak slowly, and perhaps above all not to attempt anything too ambitious on the joke front. There were between 100 and 150 in the audience which was marginally more than for his 'Mutiny on the *Bounty*' lecture. He decided on a blazer with an open-necked shirt which seemed to him to combine informality and gravitas to more or less the right degree. He used a hand-held mike and walked about on the stage, pausing occasionally to sit but not, as some speakers, did, venturing down into the actual auditorium. That, he considered, was too Billy Graham.

One or two of his listeners went to sleep or at least closed their eyes and opened their mouths which might, or might not, have been the same. He spotted Freddie Grim and his wife; Ambrose Perry and at least one Abdullah 'wife' though not the Prince himself. No Umlaut, no Goldslinger, no Watkyns and no Elizabeth. They could have been continuing their post-breakfast discussions or merely skipped his talk.

Elizabeth, at least, had heard it several times before.

Mid-morning was prime time for speaking because on the whole the passengers had not yet had recourse to the bottle. Any time after lunch was bad, though evenings were worst. Mercifully this was not a lecture time zone and the après-dinner slots were all filled by stand-up comics and dancers who reported whole rows of passengers sleeping off the evening meal in preparation for the midnight buffet. In the middle of the morning audiences were inclined to be, relatively speaking, wide awake.

When he finished there was a ripple of polite applause and he took two or three questions. He always dreaded questions on the grounds that they would either be wince-makers such as 'Do you write under your own name?' or even, most shaming of all 'What did you say your name was?' or, arguably worse, would come from someone who knew more about pirates than he did or even, God save him, was a pirate or retired pirate him or herself. 'Thus when I boarded a cargo ship called *Polaris* in the Malacca Strait . . .' or 'Out of two hundred and thirty-seven reported incidents of piracy in the Indian Ocean last year how many would you say . . .'

Mercifully on this occasion the questions were all placid half-volleys along the lines of 'Why Blue Beard and not some other colour?' and 'Is there a future for piracy?' These were easily swatted away and when he had finished he received another round of applause warmer than the first.

As the audience filed out for early cocktails one of them headed for the stage and as he came down the steps into the body of the hall came up very close and whispered in a breathy almost stage-Irish, 'Great talk, Dr Cornwall. Now just smile at me bravely and make a show of saying something sensible. But don't try anything silly or you're dead meat.'

It was an Abdullah wife, but masquerading under the

anonymity-conferring robes was none other than the missing girl herself, *Tipperary Tatler*.

She prodded him in the ribs with something metallic feeling. 'This is loaded,' she said, 'and I shan't hesitate to use it.'

'You wouldn't dare,' he said.

They were alone in the theatre now. The lights were dim. The sound box and projectionist's room were empty too. It was just the two of them. If she were to carry out her threat and shoot him dead she would have no difficulty in getting away and vanishing back into the safety of the Prince's harem. The threat was real. Tudor thought of calling the bluff but decided that it would be the silly side of valour. He had no wish to end his life shot dead in the theatre of the *Duchess* after one of his talks. People would say it was a more than usually disappointed member of his audience expressing disgust. That would taint the obituaries. Seriously, he told himself, there was no point in taking unnecessary risks. Besides he had sent his letter which was the nearest he could think of to an SOS for Eddie Trythall. He wondered if it would get through.

'Try me,' said the woman. 'I'm perfectly happy to pull the trigger and I'm quite confident I'd get clean away. If not then *tant pis*. The Americans will be thoroughly understanding. Unlike the Brits. They like us. Now just walk normally and naturally out the door and turn left. I'll keep guiding you.'

Tudor shrugged and did as he was told. On balance he didn't think he had a serious alternative. Outside the library they almost bumped into Freddie Grim who smiled and gave him an odd look but said nothing. *Tipperary* obviously sensed trouble for she gave him a snarling jab with the gun – always supposing it was a gun. It could have been anything, but Tudor still reckoned it was not a bluff worth calling. Besides he was curious. Once the ship lurched unexpectedly and

Tudor stumbled. The woman jabbed him again and hissed an obscenity. They took the stairs upwards and then walked forward along the boat deck before cutting inside.

Finally they reached what was clearly their destination.The door said 'Captain. Private'. Tudor arched an eyebrow as the woman took a key from her pocket, opened the door, gave Tudor a shove in the back which propelled him inside, closed the door behind him and disappeared. Tudor was not at all sure what or whom to expect but it was lax of him not to expect the disarmingly but unconvincingly friendly figure he found in front of him sitting at the captain's desk scribbling something on a notepad.

'Tudor,' said the man, tall, lean, fifty something, in corduroy trousers and a tweed jacket with a roll-neck sweater. He looked what he was: a provincial academic. But what he really was, was Tudor's nemesis; his Moriarty, the blast from the past who was not at all what he had seemed and had come back to haunt him on what now seemed to be a regular basis.

'Ashley,' he said, trying to appear unfazed as if encountering his former undergraduate contemporary and friend was the most natural thing in all the world. Maybe it was. Ashley had become the bad penny in his life. He was always turning up when least expected and least wanted. Why not now?

The basic facts about Ashley were simple enough. He and Tudor had been contemporaries at Oxford University many years ago and had both entered academic life as young dons in criminal affairs departments on opposite sides of the world: Ashley in Australia whence he came; Tudor in the UK. From time to time their paths had crossed, mainly at academic conferences in different parts of the globe but inevitably they drifted apart. Then, suddenly, out of the blue, Ashley had invited Tudor to be Visiting Fellow in his faculty at university in Tasmania. Tudor accepted but when he arrived Ashley had vanished without explanation. He reappeared but not before a woman had been murdered by a form of remote control and Tudor was suspected of the crime. Only then did Ashley return, determined, apparently, to have his old 'friend' convicted. He failed. Tudor returned to the University of Wessex but found that he had acquired a formidably bright Ph.D. student in Elizabeth Burney, former protégée and erstwhile mistress of Ashley himself. Elizabeth seemed to have changed sides and had been loyal and clever ever since the transition. But there was always the possibility, embedded deep and immovably in Tudor's sub-conscious – that she was some form of sleeper. One day perhaps she would be 'activated' by Ashley and used against him.

Quite what had motivated this late flowering lust for revenge was quite beyond Tudor. It was too simple and unrigorous to simply shrug and say that he must have gone mad. But there was a deep, smouldering resentment that was not going to go away and which threatened to haunt the pair of them for the rest of their lives. Now, just when he thought that his false friend had gone into permanent hibernation he erupted again. And here he was. It was all simplicity itself yet complex beyond belief.

'Sit down, do,' said Carpenter. 'Make yourself at home. Can I get you anything?'

'Thank you, no,' said Tudor.

'You're looking well. I enjoyed your drone on Pirates. Picked it up on closed circuit TV. For various reasons I'm not leaving the cabin or I'd have come and attended in person.Very professional. Like the way you wander about. And good work with the hand-mike. Very practised.'

'Thank you very much.' Tudor inclined his head. 'So to what do we owe this unexpected pleasure?'

Ashley smiled a smug superior smile.

'Well,' he said, 'it's a long story, but it all arose out of my visiting fellowship at this really quite bizarre university. It's not like any other academic institution I've been associated with. Very liberating. Not conventional at all. We teach traditional subjects and disciplines but in a non-traditional way. For example, the old-fashioned notion that the teachers are in some way "in charge" of the students – that's out of the window. It's a true democracy. Like I say, very liberating.'

'So you thought you'd do some liberating beyond the college walls?'

Ashley laughed though he didn't seem to find the remark particularly funny.

'I have to admit that knowing that you and Elizabeth were on board gave the idea an extra piquancy, but liberating the *Duchess* seemed a perfect idea. She's both marvellously high-profile and incredibly vulnerable. The easiest possible target but also the most headline-grabbing.'

'But plan A didn't work?'

'Evidently not,' said Ashley, 'though there was always an element of fantasy in that, don't you think? It was always unlikely that our gallant little band would actually take the ship over and I'm delighted that you were able to call their bluff. It should prove a thoroughly educational experience for the children. I trust they'll learn from it. But I always thought Plan B was more likely to be successful. As indeed appears to be the case.'

He did look intolerably smug, thought Tudor. He had never seemed smug at Oxford. Rather the reverse. Perhaps, however, that apparent callowness had really been an inferiority complex that he and others had been too insensitive to recognize. Maybe the English of that generation had seemed insufferable. Maybe they had inflicted humiliations without quite knowing that they were doing so. He had not consciously felt arrogant at the time but perhaps that was how he had looked.

It was all immaterial anyway. The harm was done and he was now, in mid-life, lumbered with a stalker of alarming ingenuity and determination.

'What about Sam Hardy?'

'Sam?' repeated Carpenter in an absurdly conversational way as if they were making tea-time small talk and Tudor had just asked about one of the neighbours.

'Sam's fine,' he said.

'Then where is he? He's not here. He's supposed to have laryngitis.'

'Alas poor Sam!' murmured Ashley, pressing the ends of his fingers together and closing his eyes as if in deep contemplation. 'So very greedy when it came down to it. They say everyone has his price but even so.'

'Is he OK?' Tudor did not wish the Master dead.

'He's fine, like I said. A distinguished guest on our floating campus somewhere over there on the ocean deep. Doesn't have his gold, of course, though there was never any question of his being allowed to keep that.'

'And you,' said Tudor. 'What about you? I don't get it. I just don't understand.'

'You never did,' said Ashley abruptly. 'I'm another story altogether.' He glanced at his watch. 'We have plenty of time so I'll tell you some of it. Not all, mind. We need to retain a few surprises up our sleeve, don't you agree?'

CHAPTER TWENTY-SIX

'Once upon a time,' said Ashley, 'or should I ask if you're sitting comfortably? Or are both those gambits too patronizing for you?'

'Just get on with it,' said Tudor. He disliked being played with and if this was a cat and mouse situation he didn't honestly see that Ashley was entitled to the cat position. He himself had at least as many shots left in his locker, didn't he?

'Actually I think I'll start at the end and work backwards,' said Ashley. 'You could say that the early history is water under the bridge, or that we've drawn a line under it – except, of course, that I don't suppose I ever shall. But let us for the time being concern ourselves with the here and now.'

'Let's,' said Tudor sharply. The cabin creaked.

'Sam Hardy first then. Sam is, as you know, something of a joke. However passengers seem to love him and he does the Jolly Jack Tar bit to the manner born. He remains, as far as Riviera are concerned, an asset even though everyone, most of all Sam, knows that the asset is dwindling. He is a certain age; he is a little too fond of pink gins – made always, as you know with Plymouth full strength, the angostura left in and just a splash of still Malvern. No ice. Definitely no ice. Sam's pension arrangements are dodgy to non-existent and when offered the opportunity of jumping ship with several million pounds worth of gold ingots I'm afraid he needed distressingly little persuasion.

'I – we – were able to offer him the bolt hole he needed and which otherwise he would never have secured. Who knows, he might even have been able to hang onto the gold if your friend Mr Rayner hadn't so disobligingly and unexpectedly heaved into view aboard his wretched *Clipper*.'

'That was bad luck.'

'Yes,' agreed Ashley, 'very. But by then Sam was safely on board our vessel and I had swapped places and was ensconced in his very comfortable quarters aboard the *Duchess*.'

'So,' said Tudor, 'things weren't going to plan.'

'Not to plan A perhaps,' agreed Ashley, 'but I was still happy that we were more or less adhering to plan B. Maureen, the *soi-disant* editor of the *Tipperary Tatler* whom you now know quite well had mercifully broken out from the brig and was a valuable aide, disguised in one of my friend Abdullah's wives' voluminous robes. And we were only a few days out from New York where we could, indeed can, be guaranteed an enthusiastic welcome from the likes of Senator Kennedy and his followers. You simply can't underestimate the strength of the Irish lobby in the States and when a certain sort of feisty Irish band cocks a snook at the former Imperial power then you're on to a certain winner. It might have been better to have managed the take-over of the *Duchess* in mid-Atlantic but there would have been complications – after all what were we to do with several hundred elderly Brits in corsets and on zimmers? In New York they can simply be wheeled ashore while we enjoy day upon day of singular propaganda scoop.'

'But you'll be arrested by the American authorities. There'll be a trial. You haven't a hope.'

'Don't worry your tiny head on that subject,' said Ashley. 'The ground has been well prepared. In any case what exactly would we be tried for?'

'Hang on,' said Tudor, 'let's go back to Sam for a second. What's his part in all this?'

'Sam's what you might call a stool-pigeon or a stalking horse. I'm not sure. Your command of arcane idiom was always so much greater than mine. Just one reason I hated you so much. Sam, a victim of his own blind greed, is now as it were a visiting fellow aboard our hall-of-residence at sea. As such you could say that he is a sort of hostage. Were anyone to attempt anything desperate with relation to the *Duchess* then Sam might suffer. Riviera Shipping might not mind that, but they'd hate the publicity. Why would anyone want to put their trust and their life's savings at the disposal of a company which allowed their most illustrious sea captain to be abducted on the high seas and then, as it were, be thrown to the sharks, walk the plank, or whatever? Again, you're the one with the idiom. Write your own metaphor.'

'So Sam is being held against his will? He's effectively been kidnapped.'

Ashley smiled.

'It's a nice point isn't it? Sam left the *Duchess* quite voluntarily with several million pounds in gold. He boarded our vessel entirely of his own accord and without any coercion because he believed that we could guarantee him and his loot a safe haven. So in that sense and up to that point I plead innocence. It is conceivable that now Sam, having lost his ill-gotten gains, may be having second thoughts. Difficult to say and even more difficult to prove. Eventually, I dare say, he'll be put ashore to face whatever music lies in store. For the time being, however, he remains afloat where he may conceivably be of use to me and mine as a sort of bargaining tool, guarantee, call him what you will.'

'Hostage,' ventured Tudor.

'I'd rather not use that word. It carries mildly pejorative undertones. Not appropriate.'

'So that's Sam Hardy.'

'Yes,' said Ashley, 'that's Sam Hardy. I'm sorry about Mandy Goldslinger. She's distraught, I understand, and the truth may prove even more unpalatable. Sam has rather let her down She won't like it. Woman scorned and all that. I wouldn't want to get the wrong side of La Goldslinger.'

'No,' Tudor agreed. 'And the others?'

'Watkyn's working for MI6 and Grim for 5. But, of course you knew that.'

'Of course,' Tudor lied. The information actually came as rather a shock. He had put both men down as ineffectual independents. All, piss and wind. Maybe they still were but it sounded as if they had official backing which made them more of a force to be reckoned with. Though perhaps 'force' was the wrong word.

'Watkyn's Six and Grim's Five,' said Tudor. 'Are you sure that's right?'

'Five, Six, who cares?' asked Ashley rhetorically. 'Both as useless as each other. The umbrella description is "security services" or something like that, but whatever you call them they're no bloody good. Loada wankers.'

'You're telling me that Watkyn and Grim work for the British security services?'

Ashley shrugged and smiled. 'Same way Goldslinger works for the CIA. *Work* is pitching it a bit high. Security is clearly a misnomer. Nevertheless and up to a point, well, yes. Though I'm never sure whether Watkyn works for Six and Grim for Five or vice versa. Six is the flaky upmarket FCO one and five the working class nitty-gritty Home Office equivalent so I think I'm right. Could be wrong. The name of the game, after all, is bluff, counter bluff, triple bluff and bluff *ad infinitum*. Ask John le Carré – he worked for both. Then invented his own. He was right. It's a never-never land that one makes up as one goes along. You know that as well as I do.'

'Yes,' said Tudor, bridling. 'Well.'

'And, of course, Mandy Goldslinger is CIA.'

'Now you are fantasizing,' said Tudor irritably. 'she'll be upset about Sam but if she's a CIA agent then the Pope's the King of Swaziland.'

'You don't know that,' said Ashley, 'about Goldslinger. I buy what you say about the Pope and His Majesty the King of Swaziland, but now I've sown a seed about Goldslinger you'll never be absolutely a hundred per cent sure about her. That's the wonderful thing about sowing seeds. No smoke without fire. I'm not suggesting that your friend Mandy is a very important cog in the American Intelligence wheel but I most certainly think she's not above an expensive meal with some chap from the Grosvenor Square Embassy and that she's quite happy to betray little confidences for a couple of dry martinis and a *filet mignon*. Way of the world. Wouldn't you agree?'

In a sense and up to a fashion Tudor did. Uncertainty and innuendo were oxygen in the world of espionage, and espionage certainly came within the ambit of his department. Why else would he be lobbying so hard for an Honorary Doctorate for John le Carré?

'You're mad,' he said, sensing that attack was the best form of defence, if not always at least where Ashley Carpenter was concerned.

'Oddly enough,' said Ashley, 'you're by no means the first person to say that. Little Elizabeth used to say it often. It's a question of definition I suppose but, mad certainly isn't the word I'd use. Obsessed or obsessive might be nearer the mark and possibly even something I'd admit to. Mad is very loose. Byron mad? I don't think so; "bad and dangerous to know" rather more plausible. I think mad is too often just a loose term of abuse. That's the way you're using it. You're just calling me mad because I'm on your back and you can't shake me off. Furthermore you don't understand what's going on so you're flailing around and seeking to explain things by branding me mad. I'm profoundly unconvinced.'

And he made a pyramid of his palms and rested his chin on the fingertips.

'Smug bastard,' thought Tudor, but also mad as the proverbial hatter.

Out loud he said, 'I don't think any court of law would find you completely sane. And you're certainly not rational.'

'Oh Tudor, Tudor,' said Ashley acting exasperated. 'You're so conventional and English. Who in their right mind would wish to be found sane by a court of law? The very idea.'

He laughed. Tudor thought the laugh manic but, as he conceded ruefully, he would, wouldn't he?

'OK,' said Tudor, 'let's cut out the verbiage and introspection. What happens now?'

Ashley appeared to contemplate for a while, as if he was thinking about his plans for the first time. Then he said, 'What would you do in my position? And what would you *like* me to do?'

'Never answer a question with a question,' said Tudor repeating a mantra he had learned at his first boarding-school or even perhaps, though he would never dare mention it, from a nanny or governess. More cause for resentment.

'Masterly inactivity,' said Ashley. 'There has been too much action for one transatlantic crossing so for the remainder of the voyage we shall do as little as possible.'

'And when we dock. . . ?'

'Ah,' said Ashley complacently, 'then activity will resume. We shall disembark most but not all the passengers. Most of the crew will remain on board. I shall tell the authorities that you and your accomplice, well, maybe we should extend the focus of our accusation to include more than just little Miss Burney, and include one or two other players such as the Umlauts perhaps, or even your friend Mandy Goldslinger, that you and yours have been involved.'

'Have been *what*?' Tudor was incredulous. 'You *are* mad. No one is going to believe you.'

'On the contrary, dear boy. In today's "war on terrorism" people will believe what they want to believe. I have friends in the requisite high places, including the press and television. The basic tale will be that, together with my trusty band of free spirits, I have foiled a plot, fiendishly conjured up by your good self, to commandeer one of the most famous ships in the world and use her for your own nefarious ends.'

'But that's crazy,' said Tudor, 'that's what *you* were attempting. Not me. You're standing reality on its head.'

'In a manner of speaking,' conceded Ashley, 'but mirror images are what so much of life is about, don't you think? You have made yourself believe that I am the fruitcake determined on a desperate bid to hijack the *Duchess*, hold the Master to ransom and so on and so forth. But why not you, pray? Why should you be presumed innocent? I should add, incidentally, that I have been busy sowing seeds. The American authorities and my friends in high places are prepared for something much like this. There has been a whispering campaign. Tip-offs. As soon as we reach New York they will be ready and waiting. You will be surprised at the extent of documentary evidence. Convincing stuff, if I say so myself.'

He sat back and smirked.

Tudor was unnerved and would have been more so had he not known, or at least suspected, that he was privy to information which Ashley was not. Even so he felt chilled.

CHAPTER TWENTY-SEVEN

Sea and sky were grey and sullen and would have seemed threatening and filled with menace were it not such a relief to escape his enemy's presence.

Elizabeth was leaning over the rail on the helicopter deck gazing out at the two widening white lines of wash behind them. She seemed pensive.

'The Master is on the *Michael Collins*,' he said, 'somewhere out there.' And he gestured at the huge anonymity of the sea.

'Are you sure?' she asked, not unreasonably. 'How do you know? Where have you been? People have been looking for you.'

'That's what I'm about to tell you,' he said. 'Sam Hardy and Mr X have done a swap. The mystery guest is in Sam's cabin waiting to pounce. Guess who?'

'I hate silly games,' she said. 'Tell me.'

He told her.

'That's so surprising it's not surprising,' she said. 'I was half expecting him.'

'You didn't know anything?'

'Of course not.' She seemed mildly irritated. 'Ashley's past history as far as I'm concerned. Not you though. Not by the sound of it. Why's he here? Just to make trouble for you?'

'That, and I don't know . . . I think he's flipped. I mean this bogus sounding so-called Irish university and their floating campus. I think they've gone to his head, infected his brain. I actually think he sees himself as some sort of latter day Che Guevara. I'm not joking. He believes his own publicity, thinks he can change the world. There are people like that.'

'Mostly writing columns for the *Daily Mail*,' said Elizabeth sharply. 'I'm not convinced academics and others should try too much real world stuff. I've just been having a chat with Major Timbers.'

'Oh him,' said Tudor, 'I'd forgotten about him.'

This was true. Tudor found the Major instantly forgettable. This was true of most majors.

'I think he's quite fanciable, if you like that sort of thing.'

'And do you?'

'I might.' There was a glint in her eye. She was only doing it to tease.

'The Major is a great one for men and boys, chaps staying out of the kitchen if they can't stand the heat, leave it all to the professionals, *sang-froid*, gung-ho, stiff upper-lip, straight bat and when the chips are down the Brits do this sort of thing supremely well.'

'And you believe him?'

'Not really,' she smiled. 'On the other hand I was hoping this would be a quiet crossing and we could all relax. That's what he said: "Just relax and go with the flow".'

'He said that?'

'His very words.'

'He thinks he has everything under control?'

'That's what he said.'

'That sort of person always says that sort of thing,' said Tudor. 'They said it before the Fall of Singapore. You know, "Don't worry our men are supremely well prepared and the

Japanese can't see in the dark".'

'And "don't like it up 'em, Captain Mainwaring".'

'Precisely,' said Tudor. 'False optimism; whistling in the dark, a Dickensian "something will turn up" characteristic of the British middle-classes. Something always does turn up in my experience, but seldom what you expect.'

'It was men like Major Timbers who won the war,' said Elizabeth. 'They made Britain great. My father always told me so. All phlegm, grit and stoicism.'

'All moustache and no chin,' said Tudor, 'they're what makes Britain mediocre.'

'You should know,' said Elizabeth. The remark seemed meaningless since Tudor was clean-shaven and had a jaw which did not exactly jut but was a jaw nonetheless, but it was intended to be hurtful. Tudor was duly hurt. He felt vulnerable and unwanted.

'I think people like the Major are a menace,' he said with feeling. 'They're second-rate to the core, but they get away with murder because in some unexplained way they are able to pass themselves off as "Players" whereas they're "Gentlemen". I grant you that there used to be a caricature of brilliant amateur detectives and plodding professional policemen which was unfair to the police but the pendulum has swung too far the other way. You won't find brilliance or intuition among the boys in blue and sometimes you find pedestrianism and downright incompetence. If the shenanigans on board ship were left to plodders like the Major nothing would ever be solved.'

As if to add credence to this judgement the bardic figure of Sir Goronwy Watkyn came into view walking with exaggeratedly bowed legs as if to tell the rest of those on board that he was, among many other things, a salty old sea-dog of great experience. He shook his shaggy locks in Tudor's direction and said, 'Been warned off by the acting skipper. Little Grim likewise. A diabolical liberty. Crime occurs and you have real experts on hand with none of the concomitant obstruction of the local constabulary and you don't just ignore what we have to offer – you positively shackle it. Outrageous.'

With his low opinion of Watkyn and Grim, Tudor was inclined to side with Angus Donaldson, but at the same time he recognized that a strike against them was part of a strike against himself as well.

'And another thing.' The old Welshman looked as if he had a long list of 'other things' about which to complain. 'Bloody Donaldson seems to have stopped talking to the ship from the bridge. No noon message. What's more the chart showing the ship's progress hasn't been updated. According to what's on it we haven't moved at all for at least forty-eight hours.' He peered out into the murky gloom. 'We could be absolutely any bloody where. I shall complain to my agent when we get home.'

Tudor thought privately that this was a threat unlikely to alarm Riviera Shipping. He also noted that if the old boy was correct about the captain's non-speak regarding the ship's position it served to confirm his innermost suspicions and make his letter to Donaldson all the more worthwhile.

'He must be under a lot of strain with the Master's laryngitis and everything.'

'Laryngitis, my arse,' said Sir Goronwy. 'Believe that and you'll believe Wales have a half-decent football team. Sam Hardy's no more got laryngitis than I have. The day he loses his voice will be the day I lose mine.'

The thought of Goronwy Watkyn losing his voice was indeed preposterous. Some sort of plastic container floated into the wake and bobbed about for a while reminding them all of man's threat to the world. There was no sign of fish nor fowl, just the *Duchess* and hundreds of humans.

'We could be anywhere,' said Watkyn gloomily, 'and I'm not at all convinced Donaldson and his people know what they're about. That Major Wood is all piss and wind. I'm not happy about the Abdullah cove nor the Umlaut dwarfs. Neither up to any good. And someone must have dropped a firecracker in the Krauts' crêpes Suzettes last night. One of the Prince's wives if you ask me. I noticed one stroll past just before the conflagration. And what's happened to the Irish press party? Haven't had sight nor sound for days now. All passed out down below somewhere, I suppose. And the other morning we seemed to have some sort of emergency and then we don't have an emergency.'

'It was a drill,' lied Tudor, 'not a real emergency. A fake.'

'Huh!' Sir Goronwy cleared his throat emphysematically. 'I shall be glad to be back in the Land of My Fathers. I usually enjoy these trips but present company excepted this has been a bit of a downer. Haven't even sold many books. And there's something badly wrong somewhere. I feel it in my water. Talking of which would anyone care for a snifter. The drink of the day's negroni.'

The trio tottered off to the Rum Locker a small sepulchral bar which had somehow missed out on the usual stately home nomenclature and had passable negronis mixed by Klaus, a middle-aged, strawberry-nosed bartender from Dresden who had been with the ship since her maiden voyage. Nothing significant was said over this drink which presently blurred into a second and was followed by food and more drink and by more drink and more food and by a little bit of lying down and a little bit of walking around the promenade deck and a snooze in the cinema and tea and sandwiches and a look in on the bingo and a rehearsal of the dance troupe and an abortive shop, not knowing whether or not to invest in some duty-free which would probably be cheaper in Tesco in Casterbridge, and a bit of a lie-down and a shower and another stroll and a perusal of the evening's menu and a spin through the old movies on the stateroom TV and an attempt at reading an H.R.F. Keating 'Inspector Ghote' mystery spoiled with the sudden realization that it had been read already and one knew whodunit and a nodding off while lying down and a changing for dinner and, in short, all the little procrastinations and indulgences of a day at sea aboard the *Duchess*.

Yet for Tudor it was not just a typical day at sea for he was all too aware of his *bête noire*'s presence, usurper of the Captain's cabin, determined apparently to destroy his life but slowly, stealthily, twisting the knife gently. Carpenter was not interested in a quick kill. Tudor guessed that Ashley would like him arrested, maybe even tried, but would prefer to have him released so that he could resume the slow torture.

And yet was the whole elaborate scheme really just another piece of slowly savoured revenge? Sam Hardy must have been a willing thief motivated, surely, by greed, not any feelings towards Tudor. Relations between the two men had always been cordial.Or had they? And the Prince and his harem. And the Umlauts. Little Grim. Ambrose Perry the gentleman host. Mandy Goldslinger. Donaldson. He knew he was being paranoid and yet when did justified suspicion shade into neurosis?

Whenever he almost lost himself in food, drink, slumber, ambling or some spectator sport Tudor found himself shaken back into suspicion and fear. He should, by now, be relaxed and euphoric but instead he was a seething mess of worry and nerves. Every time he saw a woman in concealing robes he found himself shivering with apprehension. He flinched whenever there was a gastronomic combustion in the Chatsworth Restaurant. He searched for a hidden meaning whenever anyone addressed him, even if it was Waclav or

Natalia asking if he would like the prawn cocktail or the chicken liver parfait. The pop of a champagne cork made him jump. He saw stalkers in the shadows on deck.

In bed, he slept but did not sleep. He tried reading and failed. He counted sheep and failed at that too. He played tic-tac-toe with Elizabeth but found it impossible to concentrate. He reviewed his life and his achievements, decided that he was an abject failure, that every crucial decision had been a wrong one, that he should never have been an academic, should never have specialized in Criminal Affairs and, perhaps most particularly, he should never have met Ashley Carpenter much less befriended him.

Not for the first time in the last few years and, he feared, not for the last, he cudgelled his mind for memories of Carpenter. Was it a girl? Was it something to do with rowing? Or their studies? Had something happened in a tutorial? Or was it life after university? Did this enmity hinge on later life? What was it? What possible slight or injustice could have triggered such an obsessive hatred? Or was he imagining the entire feud?

At last, alone, he turned out the light and saw that the sky had cleared and a full moon shone pale on an ink-black sea. There were no whitecaps – only a gentle roll and swell which made the old ship creak and sway. The rhythms and sounds usually soothed him to sleep, but tonight every movement and every noise triggered a nervy response, a sudden sitting-up in bed, a pad to the lavatory, a sip of water, a mop of brow, another fruitless attempt at memory.

Try as he might he slept only in fits and starts, woken even by his own soft snoring. He was a wreck.

CHAPTER TWENTY-EIGHT

He must have dozed off though he would later deny it. At first he thought his snoring had woken him again, but then he realized that the noise came from outside. Even though his waking wooziness he recognized it immediately: helicopter. He hurried to the porthole and stared out. The night was clear and away on the horizon he could see flickering lights which must have been on the shore. His stateroom was on the port-side. That could mean only one thing. He was right. Close to the ship the bulbous shape of a big whirly-bird hovered alongside. She looked like a Puma but in all honesty he knew very little about helicopters. He suspected she came from Culdrose near Helston in Cornwall, the biggest helicopter station in Europe. That was if his supposition was correct. In any event, if he was right, it was one of ours.

He glanced at his watch. It said 4 a.m. though they had been through so many time changes announced and unannounced that the information might have meant anything. The point was that it was still dark though there was just a hint of light at the edges of the picture before him.

Behind him the bedside phone shrilled. He picked it up and heard a clipped English voice say, 'Dr Cornwall, sir. Captain Donaldson presents his compliments and would be pleased if you could present yourself as soon as possible at the helicopter landing pad on Boat Deck.'

It was on the tip of his tongue to reply 'Aye, aye, sir', but it was not in Tudor's nature to be flippant, particularly at times like this which was not just the middle of the night but crucial in the unfolding of the convoluted drama of the past few days. Or so he assumed. The phone sounded again. This time it was Elizabeth.

'Is that a helicopter?' she asked fatuously. Tudor excused her on the grounds of her obvious sleepiness.

'Landing imminent he said,' he said. 'Donaldson has been kind enough to invite me to help greet her despite his warning me off. I suggest you join us if you want a bit of excitement or interest at least.'

'Is it American?' she asked, not unreasonably.

'I'd be very surprised,' he said, 'but I'll see you up there and explain then.' Saying which he replaced the receiver, pulled on a woollen rollneck, corduroy trousers and a pair of desert boots, ran a comb through his hair, grimaced at his pouchy eyes and designer stubble, put his room card key in his pocket and hurried out almost colliding with a be-jeaned and fleece-topped Elizabeth in the corridor outside.

'I don't understand,' she said.

'If I'm right,' he said, as they waited for the elevator in the foyer by one of the endless gift shoppes on board, 'we're in British territorial waters and Detective Chief Superintendent Eddie Trythall of the Wessex Constabulary is about to take over the investigation.'

The lift-doors slid open, they got in and Tudor pressed the Boat Deck button.

'But,' she protested, 'we should be taking on the New York pilot somewhere around the Nantucket light.'

'*Should* doesn't come into it,' he said. 'If I'm right

Donaldson and his crew turned the ship round and hardly anyone noticed.'

'Huh?' she said, still drowsy. This information was clearly too much to assimilate.

'In a few hours' time, if I'm right, we'll be tying up alongside the quay at Budmouth,' he said, as the doors slid open on to the Boat Deck foyer.

'What makes you think that?' she asked, rubbing sleep from her eyes and yawning.

'The sun rises in the east and sets in the west, yes?'

'I suppose,' she said. 'Geography was never my strong point. Or is it astrology. Red sky in the morning, shepherd's warning; red sky at night, shepherd's delight. That's about as much as I can do on dawns and dusks.'

'Trust me,' said Tudor. 'So when you came back down and said you'd just seen the most exquisite sunrise over the bows I put two and two together.'

They pushed through a heavy door out on to the open deck and heard the thudding metallic clatter of the chopper low overhead. The blades were creating a heavy down-draught like a mechanical whirlwind. A little knot of officers standing on the edge of the helipad was literally holding on to its collective hat. Donaldson was among them and seeing Tudor and the girl managed something almost resembling a smile.

'Got your letter, Doctor,' he shouted, over the wind and rattle of the helicopter, 'and passed it on to my Board. They seem to take a more, shall we say, lateral view of procedures than I sometimes do myself. If I'm not much mistaken your man is on board.'

'Good. Thank you,' said Tudor, 'and congratulations. It was clever to turn her round with no one noticing.'

'Aye,' said Donaldson, looking momentarily pleased with himself in a monosyllabic Fife fashion, 'the weather was on our side. So overcast and grey you couldn't make out any features at all. Could have been anywhere.'

'Except for one dawn.'

'Didn't last long,' said the acting Captain.

'Long enough.'

'Happen.'

'She's coming down, sir,' said one of the younger officers whom Tudor had never seen before. He noticed Major Timbers in a dark-blue track suit. He looked muscular and menacing in the gloom. Tudor doubted his mental capacity but not his combat skills. He looked as if could kill with his bare hands – not something to which Tudor aspired.

The onlookers backed against the wall of what, in agreeable weather, did service as a Lido Bar, called, since this was, after all, the good ship *Duchess*, the Croquet Lawn. It did a good line in Pimms of various otherwise forgotten varieties. There was even an Imperial one using brandy and champagne. It seemed a long way away as the helicopter throbbed slowly deckward, swayed once or twice and then hit the surface, bounced almost imperceptibly and came to a halt. The pilot cut the engine and the blades turned slower and slower before eventually coming to a full stop. There was a short pause, then a door slid open and a burly figure in a belted trench coat and tweed cap stepped with surprising agility on to the deck of the *Duchess*. Eddie Trythall of the Wessex Constabulary.

Donaldson went forward to greet him. 'Chief Superintendent Trythall I presume,' he said, and the two shook hands perfunctorily. Then, almost at once, the policeman spotted and recognized the academic, his lifelong sparring partner. The two had known each other almost as long as Ashley and Tudor. Their mutual respect might have been grudging but it was at least genuine. As was their affection.

'Doctor!' said Trythall. 'Got your message. Let me deploy

these men – with the permission and assistance of the Master, of course,' he added, recognizing that proprieties had to be observed even though there was no technical need and even though he wanted to listen to what Tudor had to say far more than he wanted to have his ear bent by a Merchant Navy captain from Anstruther, no matter how seamanlike he might be.

For a few moments he and Donaldson engaged in an earnest confabulation. Then Major Timbers was summoned and evidently co-opted into some sort of liaison role involving Trythall's policemen who, Tudor was impressed to see, appeared to be heavily armed, to be wearing flak jackets and to be accompanied by two enormous German Shepherd dogs. He almost felt sorry for the girl called *Tipperary Tatler*, for Professor Carpenter, the Prince and his harem, and anyone else who looked like getting in the way of the forces of conventional law and order.

Presently this conference was over; men were deployed; and the police gave every indication of behaving with their customary efficiency. It was not a pretty sight, nor marked by the sort of intellectual rigour Dr Cornwall prided himself on displaying on campus. Despite this – perhaps because of it – the effect was scary. You wouldn't want to get on the wrong side of this lot.

'Now,' said Eddie, rubbing his hands and blowing into the cold night air. 'Time for a nice hot cup of tea and a quiet chat.' He stared meaningfully at Major Timbers, at Elizabeth, at Angus Donaldson, and added with quiet menace. 'With my old friend Dr Cornwall. In private.' There was a pause which might properly have been described as pregnant and even ugly but which flattened out into an almost deferential acquiescence. Donaldson instructed a Filipino steward to take the policeman and the detective don to the wardroom while everyone else peeled off.

This officers' day-room which, thankfully, paid not even lip-service to the prevailing theme of 'dead *Duchess* upstairs' but was dominated by a large photograph of a youngish Queen Elizabeth II and several dozen shields presented by other ships from around the world as well as ports where the *Duchess* had at one time or another been made welcome. Inside, the Chief Superintendent removed his cap and coat, sat down heavily on a leatherette sofa and said, laughing, 'Well this is a turn-up for the book, old son.'

'You could say that,' agreed Tudor. 'It's good to see you. They wouldn't pay much attention to me even though I think I've got the whole thing more or less wrapped up. If there are any uncrossed "t's" or undotted "i's" I'm sure that between us we can do the necessary.'

Tea, hot, sweet, rough Indian and quite unlike the refined stuff served in the passenger areas, arrived in short order together with digestive biscuits. Trythall dunked one in his mug and said, 'One stroke of luck was that we had a frigate in mid-Atlantic. HMS *Truro*. She happened to be passing when we had a mildly alarming message from our friend Rayner aboard the *Star Clipper*. As a result I'm happy to say that the not-so-good-ship *Michael Collins* was boarded by a party from the Special Boat Service and Captain Sam Hardy was discovered tied up and indubitably being held against his will. He was not a happy bunny. I have to say that the ship shows every sign of failing every known regulation regarding health and safety at sea. She's being escorted to Falmouth by the *Truro*. Against all the rules, of course, but frankly there's bugger all anyone can do about it.'

'Captain Sam went aboard of his own accord,' said Tudor. 'He was hoping to make off with several million pounds worth of gold ingots.'

The Chief Superintendent dunked more biscuit.

'I have a feeling that might complicate our case,' he said. 'I see no very good reason why Captain Sam shouldn't have been abducted against his will by these obvious terrorists. It's in everyone's interests for him to look like a really good guy, wouldn't you say?'

'Certainly simpler,' said Tudor.

'Yes, well. That's my news. What's yours?'

So Tudor told him about the Irish take-over bid; how it was foiled; how Ashley Carpenter had come on board; how the *Tipperary Tatler* girl had disguised herself as one of the Prince's brides and incinerated the Umlauts; how the Prince and the Umlauts were at daggers drawn in their ambitions to gain control of the ship albeit, as far as he could judge, by more or less legal boardroom means; how that old windbag Goronwy Watkyn had tried to get in on the act and that slimy little creep Freddie Grim, whom they both remembered from his days in the Met. And how he had serious reservations about a gentleman's host called Ambrose Perry but suspected that he was guilty of nothing much worse than battening on elderly ladies who liked to believe that they were doing the rhumba with him. And how he had a soft spot for Mandy Goldslinger even though her infatuation with Captain Sam was remarkably silly. That, of course, didn't make her a criminal. Far from it in fact. She was actually rather gullible and for all her Lauren Bacall affectations a bit of an ingénue.

Detective Chief Superintendent Trythall listened to this baroque tale with a half-smile playing around his tea-wettened, biscuit-crumbed lips and eventually said, 'It looks as if your old mate Professor Carpenter has given himself enough rope to hang himself with. I don't know what the rest of his gang will get. Time off for gullibility, I should think. But the case against Carpenter strikes me as cast-iron, watertight.

We should be able to get him off your back for a good many years.'

'You reckon?' Tudor was dubious, 'He'll get the best possible defence lawyers if he doesn't conduct his own case. Which would probably help us. He's brilliant at wriggling out of impossible situations. He's done it before and I have a horrible feeling he'll do it again.'

'Don't see how he can manage it this time,' said Trythall. 'And if we go easy on everyone else we should be able to find plenty of witnesses to testify against him.'

He paused and drank some sweet tea.

'Even so,' he said, 'I don't fully understand this obsession. How come he hates you so much? It's not rational.'

'No,' said Tudor, shaking his head with disbelief. 'He used to be my best friend. At least I thought he was.'

'That's the problem then,' said Eddie. 'Like the marriage partner who thinks they've been wronged; you must have been too close.'

'I suppose,' said Tudor. 'I hope we can have him sent down for a long spell in clink but I have an unpleasant feeling he'll be back. He's a man obsessed. A little thing like prison won't put him off.'

With which thought they sat and contemplated the remains of their tea. Outside the wind started to sigh and the old ship pitched and rolled as if in one final dismissive nautical V-sign before reaching the haven of her home port.

A day after docking, Elizabeth and Tudor shared a bottle of vintage Bitschwiller in Henchards wine bar and conducted a desultory post-mortem.

Donaldson's role bothered him.

On the face of it he was dour, unimaginative and honest as the day was long. Tudor doubted whether he had the wit to